# HANDBOOK OF PERSONALITY DISORDERS

## Also Available

*Integrated Treatment for Personality Disorder:
A Modular Approach*
Edited by W. John Livesley, Giancarlo Dimaggio,
and John F. Clarkin

*Practical Management of Personality Disorder*
W. John Livesley

# Handbook of Personality Disorders

## Theory, Research, and Treatment

SECOND EDITION

Edited by
W. John Livesley
Roseann Larstone

THE GUILFORD PRESS
New York   London

Copyright © 2018 The Guilford Press
A Division of Guilford Publications, Inc.
370 Seventh Avenue, Suite 1200, New York, NY 10001
www.guilford.com

Paperback edition 2020

All rights reserved

No part of this book may be reproduced, translated, stored in a retrieval system,
or transmitted, in any form or by any means, electronic, mechanical, photocopying,
microfilming, recording, or otherwise, without written permission from the publisher.

Printed in the United States of America

This book is printed on acid-free paper.

Last digit is print number:  9  8  7  6  5  4  3  2

The authors have checked with sources believed to be reliable in their efforts to provide
information that is complete and generally in accord with the standards of practice that are
accepted at the time of publication. However, in view of the possibility of human error or
changes in behavioral, mental health, or medical sciences, neither the authors, nor the editors
and publisher, nor any other party who has been involved in the preparation or publication
of this work warrants that the information contained herein is in every respect accurate or
complete, and they are not responsible for any errors or omissions or the results obtained
from the use of such information. Readers are encouraged to confirm the information
contained in this book with other sources.

**Library of Congress Cataloging-in-Publication Data**

Names: Livesley, W. John, editor. | Larstone, Roseann, editor.
Title: Handbook of personality disorders : theory, research, and treatment /
    edited by W. John Livesley, Roseann Larstone.
Description: Second edition. | New York : The Guilford Press, [2018] |
    Includes bibliographical references and index.
Identifiers: LCCN 2017023842 | ISBN 9781462533114 (hardback) |
    ISBN 9781462545926 (paperback)
Subjects: LCSH: Personality disorders—Handbooks, manuals, etc. | BISAC:
    PSYCHOLOGY / Personality. | MEDICAL / Psychiatry / General. | SOCIAL
    SCIENCE / Social Work. | PSYCHOLOGY / Clinical Psychology.
Classification: LCC RC554 .H36 2018 | DDC 616.85/81—dc23
LC record available at *https://lccn.loc.gov/2017023842*

# About the Editors

**W. John Livesley, MD, PhD,** is Professor Emeritus in the Department of Psychiatry at the University of British Columbia, Canada. His research focuses on the structure, classification, and origins of personality disorder, and on constructing an integrated framework for describing and conceptualizing personality pathology. His clinical interests are directed toward developing a unified approach to treatment. Dr. Livesley is a Fellow of the Royal Society of Canada. He is a past editor of the *Journal of Personality Disorders*.

**Roseann Larstone, PhD,** is Research Associate in the Northern Medical Program at the University of Northern British Columbia, Canada. She holds an adjunct appointment in the Faculty of Medicine at the University of British Columbia. Her research has focused on personality and psychopathology, adolescent social–emotional development, and adolescent mental health. Dr. Larstone is currently involved in community-based research and program evaluation in the area of health promotion for mental health service recipients. She is a past assistant editor and current editorial board member of the *Journal of Personality Disorders*.

# Contributors

**Timothy A. Allen, MA,** Institute of Child Development, University of Minnesota, Minneapolis, Minnesota

**Emily Ansell, PhD,** Department of Psychology, Syracuse University, Syracuse, New York

**Arnoud Arntz, PhD,** Department of Clinical Psychology, University of Amsterdam, Amsterdam, The Netherlands

**Anthony W. Bateman, MD,** Anna Freud National Centre for Children and Families, London, United Kingdom

**Lorna Smith Benjamin, PhD, ABPP,** Department of Psychology, University of Utah, Salt Lake City, Utah

**David P. Bernstein, PhD,** Department of Clinical Psychological Science, Maastrict University, Maastricht, The Netherlands

**Donald W. Black, MD,** Department of Psychiatry, Roy J. and Lucille A. Carver College of Medicine, University of Iowa, Iowa City, Iowa

**Nancee Blum, MSW,** Department of Psychiatry, Roy J. and Lucille A. Carver College of Medicine, University of Iowa, Iowa City, Iowa

**Sarah J. Brislin, MS,** Department of Psychology, Florida State University, Tallahassee, Florida

**Nicole Cain, PhD,** Department of Psychology, Long Island University, Brooklyn, New York

**Chloe Campbell, PhD,** Research Department of Clinical, Educational and Health Psychology, University College London, London, United Kingdom

**Andrew M. Chanen, PhD,** Orygen, The National Centre of Excellence in Youth Mental Health, Melbourne, Australia; Centre for Youth Mental Health, University of Melbourne, Melbourne, Australia

**Lee Anna Clark, PhD,** Department of Psychology, University of Notre Dame, Notre Dame, Indiana

**John F. Clarkin, PhD,** Department of Psychiatry, Weill Cornell Medical College, New York, New York

**Maartje Clercx, MSc,** Faculty of Psychology and Neurosciences, Maastricht University, Maastricht, The Netherlands

**Emil F. Coccaro, MD,** Department of Psychiatry and Behavioral Science, Pritzker School of Medicine, University of Chicago, Chicago, Illinois

**Stephanie G. Craig, PhD,** Department of Psychology, Simon Fraser University, Burnaby, British Columbia, Canada

**Kenneth L. Critchfield, PhD,** Department of Psychology, James Madison University, Harrisonburg, Virginia

**Elizabeth Daly, PhD,** Department of Psychology, University of Notre Dame, Notre Dame, Indiana

**Kate M. Davidson, PhD,** Institute of Health and Wellbeing, University of Glasgow, Glasgow, United Kingdom

**Roger D. Davis, PhD,** Department of Psychology, Ateneo de Manila University, Port Charlotte, Florida

**Jennifer R. Fanning, PhD,** Department of Psychiatry and Behavioral Science, Pritzker School of Medicine, University of Chicago, Chicago, Illinois

**Peter Fonagy, PhD,** Research Department of Clinical, Educational and Health Psychology, University College London, London, United Kingdom

**John G. Gunderson, MD,** Department of Psychiatry, Harvard Medical School, Boston, Massachusetts

**Michael N. Hallquist, PhD,** Department of Psychology, The Pennsylvania State University, University Park, Pennsylvania

**Julie Harrison, PhD,** Harrison Psychological Consultations, Indianapolis, Indiana

**André M. Ivanoff, PhD,** School of Social Work, Columbia University, New York, New York

**Kerry L. Jang, PhD,** Department of Psychiatry, University of British Columbia, Vancouver, British Columbia, Canada

**Carsten René Jørgensen, PhD,** Department of Psychology, Aarhus University, Aarhus, Denmark

**Christie Pugh Karpiak, PhD,** Department of Psychology, University of Scranton, Scranton, Pennsylvania

**Stephen Kellett, PhD,** Centre for Psychological Services Research, University of Sheffield, Sheffield, United Kingdom

**Robert F. Krueger, PhD,** Department of Psychology, University of Minnesota, Minneapolis, Minnesota

**Roseann M. Larstone, PhD,** Northern Medical Program, University of Northern British Columbia, Prince George, British Columbia, Canada

**Mark F. Lenzenweger, PhD,** Department of Psychology, State University of New York at Binghamton, Binghamton, New York; Department of Psychiatry, Weill Cornell Medical College, New York, New York

**Kenneth N. Levy, PhD,** Department of Psychology, The Pennsylvania State University, University Park, Pennsylvania

**Marsha M. Linehan, PhD, ABPP,** Department of Psychology, University of Washington, Seattle, Washington

**W. John Livesley, MD, PhD,** Department of Psychiatry, University of British Columbia, Vancouver, British Columbia, Canada

**Jill Lobbestael, PhD,** Department of Clinical Psychological Science, Maastricht University, Maastricht, The Netherlands

**Patrick Luyten, PhD,** Faculty of Psychology and Educational Sciences, University of Leuven, Leuven, Belgium; Research Department of Clinical, Educational and Health Psychology, University College London, London, United Kingdom

**Paul Markovitz, MD, PhD,** Interventional Psychiatric Associates, Santa Barbara, California

**Birgit Bork Mathiesen, PhD,** Department of Psychology, University of Copenhagen, Copenhagen, Denmark

**Kevin B. Meehan, PhD,** Department of Psychology, Long Island University, Brooklyn, New York

**Robert Mestel, PhD,** Helios Clinics, Berlin, Germany

**Theodore Millon, PhD** (deceased), Institute for Advanced Studies in Personology and Psychopathology, Port Jervis, New York

**Marlene M. Moretti, PhD,** Department of Psychology, Simon Fraser University, Burnaby, British Columbia, Canada

**Leslie Morey, PhD,** Department of Psychology, Texas A&M University, College Station, Texas

**Theresa A. Morgan, PhD,** Department of Psychiatry and Human Behavior, Alpert Medical School, Brown University, Providence, Rhode Island

**Roger T. Mulder, MD, PhD,** Department of Psychological Medicine, University of Otago, Christchurch, New Zealand

**Morgan R. Negrón, MA,** Department of Psychology, University of Notre Dame, Notre Dame, Indiana

**Shani Ofrat, PhD,** Department of Psychology, University of Minnesota, Minneapolis, Minnesota

**Lacy A. Olson-Ayala, PhD,** VA Greater Los Angeles Healthcare System, Los Angeles, California

**Joel Paris, MD,** Department of Psychiatry, McGill University and Jewish General Hospital, Montreal, Quebec, Canada

**Christopher J. Patrick, PhD,** Department of Psychology, Florida State University, Tallahassee, Florida

**Anthony Pinto, PhD,** Department of Psychiatry, Donald and Barbara Zucker School of Medicine at Hofstra/Northwell and Zucker Hillside Hospital, Glen Oaks, New York

**Maria Elena Ridolfi, MD,** Fano Department of Mental Health, Fano, Italy

**Clive J. Robins, PhD, ABPP, ACT,** Department of Psychiatry and Behavioral Sciences, Duke University, Durham, North Carolina

**Anthony C. Ruocco, PhD,** Department of Psychology, University of Toronto, Toronto, Ontario, Canada

**Anthony Ryle, DM, FRCPsych** (deceased), St. Thomas' Hospital, London, United Kingdom

**Maria Cristina Samaco-Zamora, PhD,** Department of Psychology, University of San Francisco, San Francisco, California

**Jaime L. Shapiro, MA,** Department of Psychology, University of Notre Dame, Notre Dame, Indiana

**Rebecca L. Shiner, PhD,** Department of Psychology, Colgate University, Hamilton, New York

**Merav H. Silverman, MA,** Department of Psychology, University of Minnesota, Minneapolis, Minnesota

**Erik Simonsen, MD,** Institute of Clinical Medicine, Faculty of Health and Medical Sciences, University of Copenhagen, Copenhagen, Denmark

**Andrew E. Skodol, MD,** Department of Psychiatry, College of Medicine, University of Arizona, Tucson, Arizona

**Tracey Leone Smith, PhD,** Center for Innovations in Quality and Effectiveness and Safety, Michael E. DeBakey Veterans Affairs Medical Center, Houston, Texas

**Paul H. Soloff, MD,** Department of Psychiatry, University of Pittsburgh School of Medicine, Pittsburgh, Pennsylvania

**Don St. John, MA, PA-C,** Department of Psychiatry, Roy J. and Lucille A. Carver College of Medicine, University of Iowa, Iowa City, Iowa

**Jennifer L. Tackett, PhD,** Department of Psychology, Northwestern University, Evanston, Illinois

**Katherine N. Thompson, PhD,** Orygen, the National Centre of Excellence in Youth Mental Health, Melbourne, Australia; Centre for Youth Mental Health, University of Melbourne, Melbourne, Australia

**Marianne Skovgaard Thomsen, PhD,** Department of Psychology, University of Copenhagen, Copenhagen, Denmark

**Emily N. Vanderbleek, MA,** Department of Psychology, University of Notre Dame, Notre Dame, Indiana

**Philip A. Vernon, PhD,** Department of Psychology, Western University, London, Ontario, Canada

**Michael G. Wheaton, PhD,** Department of Psychology, Barnard College, New York, New York

**Thomas A. Widiger, PhD,** Department of Psychology, University of Kentucky, Lexington, Kentucky

**Stephen C. P. Wong, PhD,** Department of Psychology, University of Saskatchewan, Saskatoon, Saskatchewan, Canada

**Aidan G. C. Wright, PhD,** Department of Psychology, University of Pittsburgh, Pittsburgh, Pennsylvania

**Noga Zerubavel, PhD,** Department of Psychiatry and Behavioral Sciences, Duke University, Durham, North Carolina

**Mark Zimmerman, MD,** Department of Psychiatry and Human Behavior, Alpert Medical School, Brown University, Providence, Rhode Island

# Preface

Since the first edition of the Handbook was published nearly 20 years ago, much has changed in the study and treatment of personality disorder (PD). Most importantly, the emergence of PD from relative obscurity to become the important area of clinical practice and research noted in the first edition has been consolidated perhaps more than could have been envisioned at the time. Research has increased substantially in quantity and scope. New areas of inquiry have opened up, and old ones have been extended in new ways. Topics that were previously largely domains of theoretical speculation are now active areas of empirical inquiry. It is not just that empirical research has been consolidated and extended; similar changes have occurred in clinical practice. New therapies have been developed, adding richness and depth to our therapeutic armamentarium and, more importantly, a substantial increase in outcome studies is beginning to form a solid foundation for evidence-based treatment. These developments continue to challenge traditional ideas and are opening up new perspectives on the essential nature of PD, its causes and development, and more effective treatments.

Given progress on so many fronts, it seemed timely to consider a second edition of the *Handbook* to document these changes, to comment on the current state of knowledge, and perhaps even to consider potential new directions. However, the progress being made and the increased data about PD, along with the current state of knowledge, presented something of a challenge in planning and organizing the volume. Although we wanted to produce a text that is comprehensive and represents the overall scope of the current study of PD, it was clear that we could not include all developments. Even with the first edition, we needed to be selective about what to include and how to approach the concept of PD. The progress of the last two decades added to the challenge. One of the difficulties that we faced is that the growth in empirical research that has so enriched the PD database has also added to the fragmentation of the field, and we wanted to find ways to foster the idea of integration or at least begin to connect different areas of scholarship.

As with the first edition, our intent to emphasize empirical findings led to us continue to organize the volume around major themes such as conceptual and theoretical issues, psychopathology, etiology and development, epidemiology and course, assessment, and treatment rather than specific diagnoses, because we continue to be concerned about the validity of categorical or typal diagnoses whether described in terms of criteria sets or trait constellations. However, we have softened our stance a little on this matter by including a few chapters on specific diagnoses. The reason is not that we think evidence on the validity of categorical diagnoses has changed: to the contrary, the evidence against categorical diagnoses has strengthened substantially in the intervening years. Rather, clinical knowledge about PD is largely organized around specific diagnoses, and recent interesting developments have occurred in our understanding of the psychopathology associated with some putative disorders that we thought should be discussed. Consequently, we have included chapters on diagnoses that show some resemblance to empirically derived structures, namely, antisocial/psychopathic, obsessive–compulsive, and borderline PDs. Our assumption is that these patterns of psychopathology have some degree of validity and will ultimately be represented in some way in any future evidence-based taxonomy. In contrast to our softened position on specific diagnoses, we have been more rigorous in the section on treatment in our emphasis on evidence-based approaches. We only invited chapters on specific therapies that were supported by at least one randomized controlled trial and on approaches that were evidence-based.

In editing this volume, we also wanted to promote a greater interest in two issues that seem important for the continued development of the field and the construction of more effective treatment methods: greater attention to theoretical and conceptual issues, and a broader interest in the psychopathology of PD. The most pressing problems confronting the study of PD seem to us to be conceptual rather than empirical. The value of collecting ever more data is compromised by the lack of conceptual and theoretical frameworks needed to organize and systematize these data into a coherent account of PD. However, conceptual progress since the publication of the first edition has been limited. Also, our emphasis on empirical findings means that we decided not to include chapters describing general theories of either PD or specific diagnoses unless they are based on empirical evidence. We consider this approach to be reasonable, because the field seems to be moving away from interest in grand theories that seek to explain all aspects of a given disorder or even PDs as a whole. Unfortunately, these theories have not been replaced by more specific conceptual developments focusing on specific issues such as the structure and nature of the disorder and etiology and development. We have tried to address this issue by including chapters that draw attention to the problem by discussing the importance of theoretical and conceptual development and the challenges of developing more integrative frameworks in an attempt to promote discussion of how to begin connecting and even integrating different approaches. We have also tried to foster attention to the need to think in a more integrative way by providing brief introductions to each section that discuss the key themes illustrated by the chapters in the section, and, in some instances, we propose tentative links between the ideas discussed in the different contributions.

We also wanted to promote greater interest in the subtleties, nuances, and complexities of clinical presentations. An unfortunate consequence of the DSM preoccupation with reliability and hence with diagnostic criteria sets is that clinical interest has increasingly focused on the simplest and most overt aspects of personality pathology, leading to an almost total neglect of personality processes and functioning, and the complex interaction between different domains of personality pathology. It has even led to a tendency to neglect trying to understand the person manifesting the diagnostic criteria under consideration. The result is an impoverished understanding of the descriptive richness of these disorders. Unfortunately, we found it difficult to address this problem to the degree we think necessary, although a few chapters do address some aspects of the problem.

The idea for the first edition of the *Handbook* came from Seymour Weingarten, Editor-in-Chief at The Guilford Press, and we are very grateful to him for his continued help and support. We also appreciate the support we have received from others at Guilford, including Jim Nageotte and Jane Keislar. We also want to acknowledge the help of our authors for both their support and advice and their tolerance and patience. Finally, we especially want to thank our respective spouses, Ann and Chris, for their continuous support and encouragement and also for the remarkable tolerance they have shown in the final months of this project as we struggled to bring to a conclusion what at times seemed an interminable project.

As with the first edition, our hope is that this volume will not only help to disseminate current knowledge about PD but also encourage readers to become even more aware of the complexities of PD and to question some of the fundamental assumptions that continue to dominate and limit the field. We would also like to think that this handbook will contribute to a better and more enlightened understanding of a disorder that is so painful and misunderstood.

# Contents

## I. CONCEPTUAL AND TAXONOMIC ISSUES     1

1. Conceptual Issues     3
   W. John Livesley

2. Theoretical versus Inductive Approaches to Contemporary Personality Pathology     25
   Roger D. Davis, Maria Cristina Samaco-Zamora, and Theodore Millon

3. Official Classification Systems     47
   Thomas A. Widiger

4. Dimensional Approaches to Personality Disorder Classification     72
   Shani Ofrat, Robert F. Krueger, and Lee Anna Clark

5. Cultural Aspects of Personality Disorder     88
   Roger T. Mulder

## II. PSYCHOPATHOLOGY     101

6. Identity     107
   Carsten René Jørgensen

7. Attachment, Mentalizing, and the Self     123
   Peter Fonagy and Patrick Luyten

8. Cognitive Structures and Processes in Personality Disorders     141
   Arnoud Arntz and Jill Lobbestael

9. Taking Stock of Relationships among Personality Disorders and Other Forms of Psychopathology     155
   Merav H. Silverman and Robert F. Krueger

## III. EPIDEMIOLOGY, COURSE, AND ONSET — 169

10. Epidemiology of Personality Disorders — 173
    *Theresa A. Morgan and Mark Zimmerman*

11. Understanding Stability and Change in the Personality Disorders: Methodological and Substantive Issues Underpinning Interpretive Challenges and the Road Ahead — 197
    *Mark F. Lenzenweger, Michael N. Hallquist, and Aidan G. C. Wright*

12. Personality Pathology and Disorder in Children and Youth — 215
    *Andrew M. Chanen, Jennifer L. Tackett, and Katherine N. Thompson*

## IV. ETIOLOGY AND DEVELOPMENT — 229

13. Genetics — 235
    *Kerry L. Jang and Philip A. Vernon*

14. Neurotransmitter Function in Personality Disorder — 251
    *Jennifer R. Fanning and Emil F. Coccaro*

15. Emotional Regulation and Emotional Processing — 271
    *Paul H. Soloff*

16. Neuropsychological Perspectives — 283
    *Marianne Skovgaard Thomsen, Anthony C. Ruocco, Birgit Bork Mathiesen, and Erik Simonsen*

17. Childhood Adversities and Personality Disorders — 301
    *Joel Paris*

18. Developmental Psychopathology — 309
    *Rebecca L. Shiner and Timothy A. Allen*

19. An Attachment Perspective on Callous and Unemotional Characteristics across Development — 324
    *Roseann M. Larstone, Stephanie G. Craig, and Marlene M. Moretti*

## V. DIAGNOSIS AND ASSESSMENT — 337

20. Empirically Validated Diagnostic and Assessment Methods — 341
    *Lee Anna Clark, Jaime L. Shapiro, Elizabeth Daly, Emily N. Vanderbleek, Morgan R. Negrón, and Julie Harrison*

21. Clinical Assessment — 367
    *John F. Clarkin, W. John Livesley, and Kevin B. Meehan*

22. Using Interpersonal Reconstructive Therapy to Select Effective Interventions for Comorbid, Treatment-Resistant, Personality-Disordered Individuals — 394
    *Lorna Smith Benjamin, Kenneth L. Critchfield, Christie Pugh Karpiak, Tracey Leone Smith, and Robert Mestel*

## VI. SPECIFIC PATTERNS — 417

### 23. Clinical Features of Borderline Personality Disorder — 419
Joel Paris

### 24. Theoretical Perspectives on Psychopathy and Antisocial Personality Disorder — 426
Christopher J. Patrick and Sarah J. Brislin

### 25. Clinical Aspects of Antisocial Personality Disorder and Psychopathy — 444
Lacy A. Olson-Ayala and Christopher J. Patrick

### 26. Obsessive–Compulsive Personality Disorder and Component Personality Traits — 459
Anthony Pinto, Emily Ansell, Michael G. Wheaton, Robert F. Krueger, Leslie Morey, Andrew E. Skodol, and Lee Anna Clark

## VII. EMPIRICALLY BASED TREATMENTS — 481

### 27. Cognitive Analytic Therapy — 489
Anthony Ryle and Stephen Kellett

### 28. Cognitive-Behavioral Therapy — 512
Kate M. Davidson

### 29. Dialectical Behavior Therapy — 527
Clive J. Robins, Noga Zerubavel, André M. Ivanoff, and Marsha M. Linehan

### 30. Mentalization-Based Treatment — 541
Anthony W. Bateman, Peter Fonagy, and Chloe Campbell

### 31. Schema Therapy — 555
David P. Bernstein and Maartje Clercx

### 32. Transference-Focused Psychotherapy — 571
John F. Clarkin, Nicole Cain, Mark F. Lenzenweger, and Kenneth N. Levy

### 33. Systems Training for Emotional Predictability and Problem Solving — 586
Nancee Blum, Donald W. Black, and Don St. John

### 34. Psychoeducation for Patients with Borderline Personality Disorder — 600
Maria Elena Ridolfi and John G. Gunderson

### 35. Pharmacotherapy — 611
Paul Markovitz

### 36. A Treatment Framework for Violent Offenders with Psychopathic Traits — 629
Stephen C. P. Wong

### 37. Integrated Modular Treatment — 645
W. John Livesley

Author Index — 676

Subject Index — 694

# PART I
# CONCEPTUAL AND TAXONOMIC ISSUES

# CHAPTER 1

# Conceptual Issues

W. John Livesley

It is difficult to characterize the current state of the study of personality disorder (PD). The field is obviously vigorous and productive. Extensive empirical data are being collected about an increasingly wide range of topics. In important areas, conclusions based on empirical findings are replacing traditional ideas that were more speculative in nature. However, the field is hampered by the lack of a coherent conceptual framework to guide research and systematize findings, resulting in a mass of information that often seems to lack coherence. This makes it difficult to evaluate the extent to which progress is being made because science is organized knowledge (Medawar, 1984): It involves facts and findings that have internal coherence because they are held together by general principles and laws. Current theories of PD do not offer a solution to this problem: Most are conceptual positions rather than actual theories and are insufficiently developed to bring coherence to the field (Lenzenweger & Clarkin, 2005).

This situation reflects the early state of the field's development. All sciences begin this way, amassing vast amounts of relatively unrelated observations. This is how biology started as natural history. Viewing the situation from the perspective of Kuhn's (1962) description of the nature of scientific change, the current situation may be viewed as either characteristic of the preparadigmatic phase in the development of a science or as a period that Kuhn referred to as "extraordinary science." In the preparadigmatic phase, data collection dominates, but there is uncertainty about the value and significance of these data. As a result, scholars practice science, but the results of their efforts do not constitute a science. Kuhn also noted that the phase is marked by multiple schools of thought and intense debates about legitimate methods, problems, and standards of evidence that serve more to define the different schools than to produce agreement. In some ways, this seems an apt commentary on contemporary study of PD. Extensive data are being collected. Multiple schools and perspectives exist, such as cognitive therapy, psychoanalysis, trait psychology, neurobiology, interpersonal theory, behavioral theory and therapy, traditional phenomenology, and so on, each with its own focus of interest, methodology, and mode of explanation. Since communication between schools is limited, knowledge tends to get stovepiped. From time to time, there is talk of integration, but it never occurs.

However, it may also be argued that the study of PD does have a paradigm and has for much of its recent history: the paradigm of the medical model than underpins contemporary psychiatry. The model has structured the field and informs most aspects of practice and research. However, recently, concerns have been raised about the model and its relevance to mental disorders, raising additional concerns about the conceptual foundations of the study of PDs.

Although the medical model is usually assumed to be a unitary framework, there are several versions (Bolton, 2008). The version implicitly adopted by psychiatry is a somewhat simplified form of the traditional disease-as-entity model of modern medicine (Sabbarton-Leary, Bortolitti, & Broome, 2015). With this model, symptoms are organized into discrete syndromes that are explained by an underlying impairment that is generally assumed to be biological. The model's appeal to psychiatry is understandable given its success in general medicine, and its assumed relevance was undoubtedly bolstered by its success at the beginning of the 20th century with the discovery that general paresis, a relatively common form of psychosis at the time, was a form of tertiary syphilis due to the spirochete *Treponema pallidum*. This created the expectation that major causes of other mental disorders would also be identified (Pearce, 2012). Despite the fact that a century later this early success has not been repeated, the idea that "big causes" will be identified for mental disorders lingers on, with infectious agents being replaced with causes such as genes, with major effects and specific impairments in neural mechanisms.

This version of the medical model was adopted by the neo-Kraepelinian movement (Klerman, 1978), which sought to reaffirm the medical foundations of psychiatry. Since the neo-Kraepelinian perspective formed the conceptual foundation for DSM-III and subsequent editions, this version of the model underpins much of the contemporary study of PD. Recently, however, several authors have noted that the disease-as-entity version of the model is not applicable to many disorders in general medicine, let alone mental disorders (Bolton, 2008; Kendler, 2012b). The model does not work for disorders with a complex, multifaceted etiology. Since most mental disorders, and certainly most PDs, have this feature, the models' relevance to the study of PD requires reconsideration.

Kuhn referred to periods in the evolution of a science when an established paradigm is no longer viable as periods of extraordinary science. Current problems with the medical model and problems arising from the neo-Kraepelinian paradigm, most notably the failure to identify discrete diagnostic categories and the extensive patterns of diagnostic co-occurrence among all forms of mental disorder, may be considered to create within psychiatry, and hence within PD, a situation resembling Kuhn's ideas of extraordinary science (Aragona, 2009). In such periods, progress is fragmented, there is widespread disagreement about appropriate methods and procedures, extreme and speculative concepts emerge, and there is usually an increased interest in the philosophical assumptions of the field. The latter point is interesting given the recent spate of texts and articles on the philosophy of psychiatry.

Whether the current situation represents the preparadigmatic or extraordinary science periods in the emergence of a science of PD is a matter for philosophers of psychiatry to explore. However, both perspectives have similar consequences: Either way, the field needs an agreed paradigm and conceptual framework to guide the acquisition and interpretation of empirical findings. However, such developments need not involve a sudden change. The Kuhnian model of scientific progress is one of revolutionary change, with the creation of a new paradigm that leads off a period that he called normal science, in which progress is incremental until another paradigm crisis. Other views of scientific progress consider change to occur for a variety of reasons and to involve a more gradual process. This seems more appropriate to PD. This chapter explores these issues. In the first section, I begin by briefly tracing the history of the field prior to the publication of DSM-III in 1980 because current conceptions of PD have tangled roots that continue to exert an influence. The second section deals with what is referred to as the "DSM era," dating from the publication of DSM-III to the publication of DSM-5. DSM-III was a landmark event that helped establish systematic empirical research on PD and the assumptions underlying DSM-III continue to shape and dominate the contemporary study of PD. Although authors of successive revisions of DSM often emphasize the distinctiveness of their revision, continuity across editions is extensive compared to the differences between them (Aragona, 2015). The section focuses particularly on the impact and relevance of the medical model and the problem of diagnostic validity. The third section examines principles that may contribute to a new conceptual framework for a science of PDs, including an alternative version of the medical model. In the final section I briefly consider how these principles might contribute to a more coherent nosology.

### Early Conceptions of PD

Although interest in personality patterns that are similar to modern PD diagnoses date to antiquity, Berrios (1993) argued that the contemporary concept of PD only truly emerged with the work of Schneider (1923/1950). Nevertheless, several developments during the 19th century helped to structure current ideas. The term "character" was widely used during that time to describe the stable and unchangeable features of a person's behavior. Writings on the topic also used the concept of "type," and Berrios noted that "character" became the preferred term to refer to psychological types. Although the term "type" was used in the contemporary sense to describe discrete patterns of behavior, the term "personality" was used largely to refer to the mode of appearance of the person (Berrios, 1993), a usage derived from the Greek term for "mask." Gradually, the term took on a more psychological meaning when used to refer to the subjective aspects of the self. Hence, 19th-century writings about the disorders of personality referred to mechanisms of self-awareness and disorders of consciousness, and not to the behavior patterns that we now recognize as PD. It was only in the early 20th century that the term "personality" began to be used in its present sense. However, it is interesting to note the recent resurgence of interest in self-awareness as a core impairment of PD.

The evolution of the concept of PD during the 19th century was influenced by studies of moral insanity by Pritchard (1835) and others. Although "moral insanity" is often considered the predecessor of psychopathy, Pritchard's description shows little resemblance to Cleckley's (1941/1976) concept of psychopathy or DSM antisocial personality disorder (ASPD; Whitlock, 1967, 1982). Rather, Pritchard used the term to describe forms of insanity that did not include delusions. The predominant understanding of the time was that delusions were an inherent component of insanity, an idea developed by John Locke. The term "moral insanity" described diverse conditions, including mood disorders that had in common the absence of delusions. Berrios (1993) suggested that Pritchard encouraged the development of a descriptive psychopathology of mood disorders that promoted the differentiation of these disorders from related conditions and the differentiation of personality from other disorders by distinguishing more transient symptomatic states from more enduring characteristics. This important development promoted the emergence of PDs as a separate diagnostic group. Interest in moral insanity continued throughout the 19th century. Maudsley (1874) extended Pritchard's concept with the observation that some individuals seemed to lack a moral sense, thereby differentiating what was to become the concept of psychopathy in the more modern sense. Toward the end of the 19th century, German psychiatrist Julius Koch proposed the term "psychopathic" as an alternative to moral insanity. At about the same time, the concept of degeneration, taken from French psychiatry, was introduced to explain this behavior.

The significance of these developments was that the idea of psychopathy as distinct from other mental disorders gained acceptance, which set the stage for Schneider's concept of psychopathic personalities as a distinct nosological group. Before this occurred, however, Kraepelin (1907) introduced a different perspective by suggesting that personality disturbances were attenuated forms (*formes frustes*) of the major psychoses. Kraepelin's seminal contributions to nosology with the distinction between dementia praecox and manic–depressive illness are generally considered to firmly establish the medical model as the basis for conceptualizing and classifying mental disorders. Subsequently, Kretschmer (1925) took the idea of PDs as attenuated forms of mental state disorders further by positing a continuum from schizothyme through schizoid to schizophrenia—an idea that anticipated current thinking about schizophrenia spectrum disorders. The notion that PDs such as borderline personality disorder (BPD) are on a continuum with some major mental state disorders rather than distinct nosological entities, and hence that PDs are not a distinct nosological grouping, continues to be raised intermittently despite extensive conceptual and empirical evidence to the contrary.

Nonetheless, the overriding assumption of psychiatric classification for much of the last century has been that mental state disorders and PDs are distinct, although the nature of this distinction has differed across conceptual frameworks. Jaspers (1923/1963) offered a cogent theoretical rationale for the distinction by differentiating personality developments from disease processes. The idea had little impact on American psychiatry, although it is probably worth revisiting. Personality developments are assumed to result in changes that are understandable in terms of the individual's previous personality, whereas the changes associated with disease processes are not predictable from the individual's premorbid status. Jaspers suggested that these different forms of psychopathology require different methods of classification, with conditions arising from disease processes being conceptualized as either present or absent and hence classified as discrete categories, whereas PDs (and neuroses) should be classified as ideal types. This issue is still unresolved and contributed to much of the confusion associated with the DSM-5 classification of PD.

Schneider's volume *Psychopathic Personalities* published in 1923 was a landmark event that largely established the contemporary approach to PDs. Berrios (1993) suggested that by adopting the term "personality," Schneider made concepts such as temperament and character redundant. There is much to be said for this position, although, unfortunately, this clarity has not been widely accepted (for further discussion, see Chanen, Tackett, & Thompson, Chapter 12, this volume). Schneider also made the important conceptual distinction between abnormal and disordered personality, an issue of current significance given the demonstrated continuity between PDs and normal personality. Schneider defined abnormal personality as "deviating from the average." Thus, abnormal personality merely represents the extremes of normal personality variation. However, Schneider also recognized that this was not an adequate definition of pathology because extreme variation does not necessarily imply dysfunction or disability. He referred to the subgroup of abnormal personalities that are dysfunctional in a clinical sense as psychopathic personalities, which were defined as "abnormal personalities who either suffer personally because of their abnormality or make a community suffer because of it" (p. 3). Schneider did not discuss abnormal personality in detail but concentrated instead on describing 10 varieties of psychopathic personality: hyperthymic, depressive, insecure (sensitives and anankasts), fanatical, attention-seeking, labile, explosive, affectionless, weak-willed, and asthenic. Here the term "psychopathic personality" was used to cover all forms of PD and neurosis. In the preface to the ninth edition, written in 1950, Schneider noted that the term "psychopath" was not well understood and that his work was not the study of asocial or delinquent personality. He added that "some psychopathic personalities may act in an antisocial manner but . . . this is secondary to the psychopathy" (p. x). Thus, he avoided the tautology inherent in conceptions of ASPD that are defined in term of social deviance, whereupon the diagnosis is then used to explain deviant behavior.

Although psychopathic personalities were portrayed as types, it is important to note that Jaspers's (1963) and Schneider's (1923/1950) concept of ideal type was not that of a simple diagnostic category, as is the case with DSM-III to DSM-5. Ideal types are patterns of being rather than diagnoses. According to Jaspers, an ideal typology consists of polar opposites such as dependency and independence or introversion and extraversion. Diagnosis does not involve ascribing a typal diagnosis. Instead, individuals are compared to contrasting poles of the type to illuminate clinically important aspects of their behavior and personality. Thus, the typology is essentially a framework for conducting clinical assessment and formulating individual cases. Moreover, ideal types are not stable in the sense that DSM diagnoses were originally assumed to be stable. Instead, some are episodic and reactive. Thus, Schneider's (1923/1950) system represents a more complex understanding of types and the relationship between normal and disordered personality than that of DSM-III to DSM-5. Although he used the term "type," his conceptualization implicitly acknowledges continuity with normal personality. In addition, Schneider's "types" are not discrete categories; rather, they refer to individuals at the extremes of a continuum, much as Eysenck used the term later to refer to those as the poles of the continuum introversion–extraversion. In this sense, Schneider anticipated current ideas derived from trait models that PDs represent extremes of normal variation, although he added criteria to differentiate pathological from nonpathological variation. Schneider also disagreed with Kraepelin's idea that PDs are systematically related to the major psychoses, although he assumed that personality affected the form that a psychosis takes. Schneider's position is not without problems, particularly in regard to the definition of suffering. Nevertheless, he introduced into the classification of PD a conceptual clarity that has rarely been matched.

Within British and American psychiatry, the concepts of psychopathy and psychopathic personality were defined more narrowly to describe what we now call ASPD, although the two are not synonymous. Descriptions of psychopathy and, later, descriptions of PDs, were largely based on clinical observation. Theoretical factors that influenced Jaspers (1963) and

Schneider (1923/1950) played little part in nosological development, and various definitions emerged as individual clinicians emphasized different facets of these disorders and different aspects of the overall class.

Parallel to these developments, psychoanalytic concepts also contributed to classification and enriched ideas about personality pathology, but in the process they increased diagnostic and descriptive confusion. Although Freud was not primarily interested in PD, his theory of psychosexual development led to descriptions of character types associated with each stage (Abraham, 1921/1927) that became the basis for dependent, obsessive–compulsive, and hysterical (changed to histrionic in DSM-III) PDs. This development shifted assumptions about etiology away from the biological mechanisms stressed by the medical model toward psychosocial factors. Subsequently, the concept of character was formulated more clearly by Reich (1933/1949), who proposed that psychosexual conflicts lead to relatively fixed patterns that he referred to as "character armor." Reich also influenced diagnostic concepts of PD because his interest in treating characterological conditions with psychoanalysis led to the description of individuals who were neither psychotic nor neurotic, which ultimately led to concept of BPD, also considered largely psychosocial in nature. The phenomenological tradition was also interested in borderline conditions, although these were understood differently. The "border" in which these phenomenologists were interested was between normality and psychosis stemming from observations that patient's family members often showed unusual features, a conception that was more rooted in the medical model. Hence prior to DSM-III, the term "borderline" referred to a variety of syndromes derived from diverse positions (Stone, 1980) and hence conceptualized and described differently: Those derived from phenomenological psychiatry were largely descriptive concepts, whereas those based on psychoanalysis were described in terms of inner mental structures and processes. Later, psychoanalytic concepts of PD were further extended with the formulation of narcissistic conditions by Kohut (1971) and others. This period from approximately the 1930s to the 1970s was associated with strong reactions against the medical model by many psychoanalysts and to a substantial decrease in interest in classification, although much more so in America than in Europe.

The 1960s and 1970s saw the first empirical investigations with pioneering work of Grinker, Werble, and Drye (1968), followed quickly in the United Kingdom with studies by Presly and Walton (1973) and Tyrer and Alexander (1979). However, the pre-DSM-III era was dominated by clinical description by the classical European phenomenologists and clinical constructs formulated by psychoanalytic thinkers.

Thus, DSM-III was developed in the context of a rich but confusing array of conceptions of PD (see Rutter, 1987). These included PD as (1) a *forme fruste* of major mental state disorders as proposed by Kraepelin (1907) and Kretschmer (1925); (2) the failure to develop important components of personality, as illustrated by Cleckley's (1941/1976) concept of psychopathy as the failure to learn from experience and to show remorse; (3) a particular form of personality structure or organization as illustrated by Kernberg's (1984) concept of borderline personality organization defined in terms of identity diffusion, primitive defenses, and reality testing; and (4) social deviance as illustrated by Robins's (1966) concept of sociopathic personality as the failure of socialization. In the background there also lurked the idea of abnormal personality in the statistical sense, as represented by conceptions of PD derived from normal personality structure. These different conceptions also placed different emphases on the medical model as the basis for conceptualizing PDs.

### The DSM Era

The DSM-III classification and the relatively minor revisions in DSM-III-R, DSM-IV, and DSM-5 (except for parts of the alternative models listed in Section III) have dominated research and treatment. Despite frequent revisions, continuities across editions far outweigh specific changes (Aragona, 2015), and these continuities have profoundly influenced all aspects of the field. The DSM-III decisions to place PDs on a separate axis, and to diagnose them using the diagnostic criteria approach used with other disorders, stimulated clinical interest and empirical research. It is perhaps ironic that these innovations have had such a lasting impact because neither has stood the test of time. Multiaxial classification was abandoned for DSM-5, and the assumption of discrete categories is inconsistent with empirical findings. Nevertheless, the development of diagnostic criteria for PDs was an important step: It encouraged construction of semistructured interviews during the 1980s that in turn facilitated empirical research. Although these measures are unlikely to make a strong contribution to future research, they established the importance of psychometrically sound measures.

To appreciate the impact of DSM-III, it is useful to recall the context in which it was developed. In the decades preceding its publication, psychiatry was under attack from many directions (Blashfield, 1984). First, psychiatry's credibility was challenged by concern about diagnostic reliability and marked international differences in diagnostic practices. Second, concerns were voiced from multiple sources, including humanistic psychology, psychoanalysis, and the antipsychiatry movement, about the emphasis placed on the medical model and its relevance to psychiatry. Third, criticism also arose from sociology and labeling theory that the diagnostic labels psychiatrists used became self-fulfilling prophecies that strongly affected the person being labeled. This criticism was reinforced by Rosenhan's (1973) study showing that mental health professionals could not differentiate severely mentally ill from healthy individuals. The study involved eight healthy individuals seeking admission to 12 different inpatient units. They reported accurate information about themselves except their names (to preserve their privacy) and having heard a voice saying a single word such as "thud" or "hollow." All were admitted for an average of about 22 days, and in 11 instances, participants were diagnosed as having schizophrenia; the other participant was diagnosed as having mania. In all cases, the discharge diagnosis was schizophrenia in remission.

These criticisms led to the formation of the neo-Kraepelinian movement (Blashfield, 1984) that reaffirmed psychiatry as a branch of medicine and the medical model as the foundation for conceptualizing and treating mental disorders. The neo-Kraepelinian credo, as summarized by Klerman (1978), consisted of nine propositions that strongly influenced DSM-III. The propositions with most impact on the classification of PD included the following: psychiatry is a branch of medicine; there is a boundary between the normal and the sick; there are discrete mental illnesses; diagnostic criteria should be codified; and research should be directed at improving the diagnostic reliability and validity. In the rest of this section I critically examine the DSM classification in terms the medical model and the problem of validity. The intent is not to provide an in-depth review of DSM-III–DSM-5 but rather to highlight issues that are critical to improving the conceptualization and diagnostic classification of PD. A more detailed review of official classifications is provided by Thomas Widiger (Chapter 3, this volume).

## The Medical Model

The medical model was the foundation for understanding mental disorders and hence for classification for much of the early 20th century. Subsequently, its role was diluted by the impact of psychoanalysis, and its relevance was challenged by the various critiques of psychiatry discussed earlier. The neo-Kraepelinians sought to change this situation. As a result of their influence on DSM-III, their version of the medical model exerted an enormous impact both directly through an emphasis on discrete syndromes and the search for a major causes and specific pathologies for given diagnoses, and indirectly through the neglect of possible contributions of other perspectives, most notably normal personality research. The neo-Kraepelinan understanding of the medical model more than anything else accounts for the way the study of PD has evolved over the last 30 years and for the failure of the DSM to show evidence of consistent improvement across revisions. This section explores the relevance of this model to PD and its impact on the field.

### Relevance to PD

The medical model adopted by psychiatry works best for disorders with a specific etiology and pathogenesis. It does not work well when disorders have complex etiology involving multiple interacting mechanisms (see Kendler, 2012a, 2012b). This circumstance clearly applies to PDs: A wide range of psychosocial and biological risk factors has been identified in the last two decades. Psychosocial factors are extremely variable, ranging from attachment problems to cultural influences (see Paris, Chapter 17, this volume). Each factor seems to exert a small effect, and none is necessary or sufficient to cause disorder. Biological influences have a similar structure. Although PDs are heritable, multiple genes contribute to the predisposition toward PDs, each having a small effect, so that the absence of a given gene probably has little effect. More importantly, PD does not appear to be explained by a specific genetic mechanism (Turkheimer, 2015). This situation also appears to apply to other biological risk factors. Although there is in PDs an underlying biology in the general sense that any psychological process must be accompanied by some kind of neural event, major biological cause has not been identified. Here, the term "major biological cause" is used in Meehl's (1972) sense of a biological factor that is found in all individuals with the disorder but not in individuals without the disorder. The failure to find major biological cause is not specific to PDs but has proved elusive for most mental disorders (Turkheimer, 2015). This does not mean that the effort to unravel the biological mechanisms associated with PDs is unimportant. To the contrary, such research can only add to our understanding of these conditions and enhance treatment options. It does, however, mean that these mechanisms need to be understood as part of a complex etiology, and that they are unlikely to be very helpful in resolving taxonomic problems.

The etiology of PD also incorporates a complexity not observed with most medical conditions: The diverse etiological factors contributing to a given clinical picture often influence different components of psychopathology. For example, with the DSM diagnostic construct of BPD, trauma and abuse may primarily affect emotional reactivity and stress responsivity, whereas consistent invalidation may primarily affect self pathology through the development of self-invalidating thinking. This is a very different circumstance from that occurring with many medical conditions in which the primary causal factor is implicated in most symptoms.

Recently, other concerns about the relevance of the medical model to psychiatry have emerged that go beyond matters of etiology by raising questions about the very nature of mental disorders that have prompted the suggestion that psychiatry has a unique status among medical specialties (see Gadamar, 1996). One such conceptual challenge relates to the fact that psychiatry addresses a far wider range of "symptoms" than other medical disciplines (Varga, 2015). Whereas most general medical disorders are diagnosed through relatively straightforward symptoms consisting primarily of sensations, perceptions, and motility anomalies, mental disorders are diagnosed on the basis of more complex, less readily observed features, including actions, emotions, beliefs, meaning systems, interpretations, motivations, thoughts, and cognitive processes. With PDs, the situation is even more complex. Other mental disorders bear some similarity to general medical disorders in that they may also be represented by symptoms and signs, as are the disorders of general medicine, albeit with more complex symptoms. However, PDs are also diagnosed on the basis of attitudes and traits (Foulds, 1965, 1976), and current diagnostic conceptions also include identity problems, self pathology, relationship issues, and narratives. This introduces a different order of complexity, one that is difficult to capture fully using the disease-as-entity version of the medical model espoused by psychiatric nosology.

A second problem is that features used to diagnose PDs are not necessarily indicative of disorder, a circumstance that applies to other mental disorders. This contrasts with the symptoms of general medicine. Pain, for example, always indicates a change for the normal state, even if the pain is transient and without lasting diagnostic significance. However, it is hard to find a feature of PD that invariably indicates disorder. In fact, it is hard to find any feature that does not occur in healthy individuals. Thus, the significance of a diagnostic item cannot be determined in isolation: It always needs to be evaluated within the context of the person's total personality and life experience.

The problems created for the medical model approach to classification and diagnosis are compounded by the diverse psychopathology of PD and by the way pathology extends to all parts of the personality system. As a result, many psychopathological features are common to multiple putatively distinct diagnoses, and few features are specific to a given condition. Discrete and nonoverlapping clusters of symptoms so characteristic of general medical disorders do not occur with PD. This fact that this has often been downplayed and even ignored by DSM in order to create distinct types has sometimes been distorted the way PD is represented. A good example is the decision to exclude quasi-psychotic features and transient psychotic states from BPD criteria in DSM-III in an attempt to ensure a clear distinction from schizotypal personality disorder, a decision later reversed in DSM-IV.

The rich and diverse pathology observed in all cases creates the additional problem of how to decide what features to focus on for diagnostic purposes. With most disorders in general medicine, symptoms are obvious, few in number, easily identified, and closely related to tissue pathology. PDs are palpably different in this respect in that they represent differences in kind. As a result, rules or guidelines are needed to establish what is and what is not pertinent to diagnosis. Currently such guidelines are poorly developed. With DSM, diagnostic features were selected through a committee process presumably guided by traditional clinical opinion. As a result, most sets of criteria are a mixture of items that include general behaviors, specific behaviors, traits, interpersonal matters, self-problems, and self-attitudes, and the constructs used vary widely across diagnoses. The case could be made that some medical conditions are symptomatically more diverse than has been suggested. However, this merely strengthens the case against applying the diseases-as-entity model to PDs. Such disorders tend to have a complex etiology, and these are the disorders that have prompted the observation that the medical model is not even applicable to some disorders of general medicine (Bolton, 2008; Kendler, 2012b).

The contemporary study of PDs has either largely neglected these problems or reframed them in terms of the medical model. Thus, diagnostic criteria are commonly referred to as "symptoms" of PD even though they are highly inferential in nature and radically different in content and form from the symptoms of general medicine. The traditional medical practice of defining symptoms as features of illness that patients complain about is neglected in what often seems to be an attempt to medicalize PDs. Similarly, diagnostic overlap due to the absence of discrete boundaries between putatively distinct disorders and the failure to conceptualize distinct entities is referred to as "comorbidity," although the term was originally developed to refer to the co-occurrence of distinct conditions. This casual use of "medical" creates that impression of continuity between psychiatry and general medicine when there are important differences and imply the relevance of the medical model when this is not the case. The rigid application of such a narrow version of the medical model to PDs has led to the continued use of a mode of diagnostic assessment ill-suited to either understanding and treating the heterogeneity and individuality of clinical presentations or providing the foundation for a science of PD.

## Consequences of the Medical Model

The version the medical model applied to psychiatry and PD has hindered progress by focusing attention on the identification of discrete types, decreasing interest in alternative models, and inadvertently leading to a neglect of psychopathology.

### Assumption of Discrete Categorical Diagnoses

A brief examination of recent articles in key journals or conference presentations reveals the extent to which research and treatment are dominated by the assumption that disorders distinct from each other and from normal personality variation exist. We only need to look at how DSM performs in practice to see that the system is fatally flawed. The rampant patterns of diagnostic co-occurrence refute the neo-Kraepelinian assumption of discrete disorders on which DSM-III to DSM-5 rest, and the problem is compounded by the prevalence of *personality disorder not otherwise specified* (Verheul & Widiger, 2004). There is no need to look beyond DSM to realize that it fails to meet its design criteria. However, if we turn to research designed to evaluate the system, the magnitude of the problem is even more apparent. We have known for nearly a quarter of a century that the features of PD are continuously distributed (see early reviews by Livesley, Schroeder, Jackson, & Jang, 1994; Widiger, 1993), conclusions confirmed by the failure of more recent studies to identify replicable personality types (Eaton, Krueger, South, Simms, & Clark, 2011; Leising & Zimmermann, 2011; Widiger, Livesley, & Clark, 2009). However, the dominance of the medical model is such that the field is impervious to empirical evidence on this point. Perhaps the most blatant example of disregard for evidence is provided by DSM-5: Although the Personality and Personality Disorders Work Group concluded that "personality features and psychopathological tendencies do not tend to delineate categories of persons in nature" (Krueger et al., 2011, pp. 170–171), categorical diagnoses were retained and the work group even opted to retain typal diagnoses in the alternative model presented in Section III of DSM-5.

The consequences of the persistence reliance on categorical diagnoses are not trivial. Considerable research effort is devoted to studying problems such as diagnostic overlap, which are largely artifacts of the assumption of discrete disorders, and to identifying the most effective way to diagnose each type. However, the effects of pursuing pseudoproblems are modest compared to the extent to which the category assumption distorts research by influencing the problems studied, the research questions asked, and the methods used. It also promotes the assumption that there is a limited array of PDs as opposed to multiple ways in which personality can be disordered, an alternative clinical conception that I explore later.

*Inattention to Psychopathology*

An unintended consequence of the DSM's adherence to medical model and attendant emphasis on reliability is the comparative neglect of the broader psychopathology of PDs. There is a tendency to assume that DSM is the ultimate authority on a disorder and its psychopathology leading to a preoccupation with whether patients "meet criteria" for a given condition (Andreasen, 2006). There is also a tendency to equate diagnostic criteria with the diagnostic construct rather than to recognize criteria as a few of many possible indicators of an underlying condition. The authority placed in sets of DSM criteria also had an ossifying effect that has discouraged exploration of alternative conceptual frameworks. Some authors also see see this stance as contributing to a growing disconnect between advances in the neurosciences and psychiatry (Hyman, 2010). However, more concerning in the case of PDs is how heightened concern with reliability has led to an impoverished understanding of psychopathology. Diagnostic criteria are essentially lists of relatively superficial features selected from a wide range of possibilities rather than definitive definitions as is so often assumed. Each criterion also tends to be seen as a distinct "self-contained" entity that can be assessed independently of the personality and the individual's other qualities and life experiences. The result, as Andreasen (2006) noted, is that DSM inadvertently led to a neglect of descriptive psychopathology and to a dehumanizing effect on clinical practice. Although Andreasen was referring to the general impact of DSM, her comments seem especially pertinent to PDs. The syndrome-based descriptive categories of DSM seem remarkably crude when viewed against the rich psychopathology of individual cases. They are simply lists of common features divorced from any coherent understanding of the disorder and the complex processes critical to understanding the psychopathology involved.

*Neglect of Normal Personality Science*

Another indirect consequence of the medical model is the failure to draw on normal personality research in the search for better conceptual and taxonomic models. This neglect is curiously inconsistent with the medical model that the field seeks to emulate. Disorder is a normative concept that can only be understood with reference to some kind of norm. Within medicine, the norm is the normal structure and function of a given system (Bolton, 2008). This suggests that the norm for understanding PD is normal personality. However, conceptions of normal personality were largely neglected in formulating classifications including DSM-5. This neglect is somewhat understandable, since normal personality research is at an early stage compared to the biological sciences underlying general medicine. Nevertheless, personality science is substantially more advanced than the study of PD and it has the potential to enrich ideas about classification and treatment.

## The Problem of Validity

DSM-III was primarily concerned with improving diagnostic reliability to address attacks on psychiatry's credibility, with the assumption that once this problem was solved, attention would subsequently focus on validity (Klerman, 1986). This progression has not occurred. As a result, it is difficult to find evidence that DSM-IV/5 is more valid than DSM-III, or indeed that it is more valid than the taxonomy Schneider proposed nearly a century ago. Nevertheless, proponents of DSM commonly proclaim the validity of both the system and specific diagnoses. Such claims often reflect different understandings of the meaning of diagnostic validity. As Kendell and Jablensky (2003) noted, validity is often confused with clinical utility—the issue of whether a diagnosis is clinically informative. One could argue that DSM PDs have clinical utility because clinicians find them useful, but evidence of validity is lacking.

Confusion also occurs because validity is often approached from the different perspectives of clinical medicine and academic psychology. Although these perspectives are sometimes intertwined, they tend to be pursued independently and they originated from different concerns. Within medicine, the issue of validity is less prominent, probably because most syndromes are relatively clear cut. Instead, the primary concern is to validate disease status (Zachar & Jablensky, 2015), which is largely a matter of establishing that a person had a given disease. Psychology, from the outset of psychological assessment and test construction, was concerned with reliability (i.e., with whether an attribute is being measured in a consistent way) and validity (i.e., with whether an attribute is being measured accurately). The major development in validity was the elaboration of construct validity by Cronbach and Meehl (1955). Psychological tests are primarily concerned with assessing attributes that are hypothetical constructs, such as intelligence or neuroticism. Construct validation is concerned with demonstrating that a measure actually assesses the construct in question. This is largely a matter of providing evidence to support inferences drawn from the measurement of the construct (Cronbach, 1971). Prior to Cronbach and Meehl, there had been dissatisfaction with the way validity was conceptualized and evaluated. Subsequently, the psychological literature referred to content, criterion, and construct validity.

The differences between medical and psychological approaches to validity became somewhat blurred in psychiatry. The classical contribution to validity in psychiatry was Robins and Guze's (1970) article on establishing the diagnostic validity of specific diagnoses such as schizophrenia. They proposed five phases of validation—clinical description, laboratory studies, differentiation from other disorders, studies of outcome, and family studies—that provide a standard that a psychiatric diagnosis should meet (Zachar & Jablensky, 2015). Application of this approach to PDs reveals major deficiencies. Clinical description is inadequate: Many patients, in some studies, the majority, do not meet criteria for any specific diagnosis and hence the prevalence of the PD not otherwise specified category. Differentiation from other disorders is also poor, with most patients meeting criteria for multiple disorders. However, the important issue for validating PDs is that Robins and Guze's approach shows the same concern with validating indicators of a diagnostic construct focus as the construct validation approach. Also, the proposed phases of validation incorporated elements of content, criterion, and construct validity (Cloninger, 1989), although construct validity is represented only by delimitation from other disorders. Despite these similarities, Robins and Guze's framework differs substantially from the construct validation model because it strongly reflects the medical model espoused by the neo-Kaepelinian movement that they helped to found by emphasizing the kinds of external validators that are appropriate for confirming a diagnosis in general medicine. The problem is that such validators are not readily available for many mental disorders including PDs. This suggests the need to consider alternative strategies such as those used to validation psychological instruments, most notably Loevinger's (1957) seminal integration of different forms of validity within an overarching framework for conceptualizing and establishing the construct validity of assessment instruments. Although Loevinger was primarily concerned with improving test structure, her approach is relevant to developing and evaluating psychiatric classifications (Skinner, 1981) and offers a model for constructing and validating classifications of PD (Blashfield & Livesley, 1991; Livesley & Jackson, 1991; see also Jacobs & Krueger, 2015).

As conceptualized by Loevinger (1957), construct validity has three components: substantive, structural, and external components. With PDs, "substantive validity" is largely a matter of developing precise definitions of diagnostic constructs based on theoretical considerations and selecting diagnostic items that conform to this definition. This important step establishes a theoretical taxonomy that is then evaluated empirically. DSM-III may be said to represent such a theoretical classification except that it was not constructed to meet the requirements of substantive validity as outlined by Loevinger. Internal or "structural validity" refers to the extent to which the relationships among components of the theoretical classification are supported by empirical evidence. This step establishes an iterative process in which evaluation leads directly to changes in the theoretical classification that are subsequently reevaluated. Over time, the process progressively enhances validity. "External validity" refers to the extent to which the classification and specific diagnoses predict clinical outcomes, have descriptive validity (i.e., differentiate among postulated disorders), and whether the classification is generalizable across different populations. Loevinger argued that construct validity "is the whole of validity from a scientific point of view" (p. 636) and that the three components "are mutually exclusive, exhaustive of the possible lines of evidence for construct validity, and mandatory" (p. 636).

This framework profoundly influenced test construction. Subsequently, Skinner (1981) showed how it could usefully be applied to psychiatric classification. In contrast to Loevinger's profound impact on psychological assessment, Skinner's innovative proposal was largely ignored because psychiatric nosologists have not been interested in the detailed steps needed to establish a classification that possesses construct validity (Blashfield & Livesley, 1991). Nevertheless, the construct validation framework is especially pertinent to classifying PD due to the lack of external validators that could serve as a "gold standard" against which to validate diagnostic constructs (Jacobs & Krueger, 2015) and the need for an iterative process that systematically enhances the system (Livesley & Jackson, 1991, 1992). It is also relevant because the complexity of personality pathology and the diverse ways personality pathology may be organized for diagnostic purposes mean that greater attention needs to be given to structural validity.

## Substantive Validity

Construction of a carefully defined theoretical classification resembles Robins and Guze's (1970) phase of clinical description. This is crucial step because definitions have a pivotal role in concept formation in science (Hempel, 1961). For this reason, the theoretical classification should include a comprehensive set of diagnostic constructs that encompass all aspects of personality pathology, and each construct should be specified by a set of exemplars (diagnostic criteria or items) that systematically samples all facets of the construct. Failure to meet these requirements incurs the risk of limited coverage of the overall domain of PD and inadequate or biased representation of a constructs.

The attention given to substantive validity in personality assessment contrasts markedly with the almost casual way classifications of PD are constructed. Whereas test construction pays careful attention to construct definition and systematic item development, successive editions of DSM have been produced without systematic definitions of diagnoses or concern with ensuring criteria sets that comprehensively assess all facets of the diagnosis. This has led to serious and repeated concerns about whether all manifestations of PD are adequately represented and to a tendency to equate criteria sets with the construct, as noted earlier. It has also led to the failure to incorporate important features in the criteria for some diagnoses and excessive diagnostic co-occurrence. For example, with BPD, the conflict between neediness and desire for closeness and fear of abandonment and rejection that is generally considered a core feature of the disorder, is poorly represented. Similarly, the impulsivity criterion fails to recognize the multidimensional nature of impulsivity. As a result, the tendency to experience a sense of urgency observed in these patients is not represented. More problematically, this behavior is assumed to be identical to the impulsivity associated with ASPD, leading to inappropriate overlap with this condition. With careful attention to definition and explicit criteria for establishing and validating diagnostic constructs, issues about of what diagnoses should be included or excluded from a classification become little more than political jousts between different factions, as occurred with DSM-5.

## Structural Validity

Structural validity is a necessary feature of classifications (Jacobs & Krueger, 2015). It refers to the extent that diagnostic criteria for a given disorder observed in samples of individuals with the disorder converge with the organization proposed by the theoretical classification. In DSM terms, structural validity requires evidence that diagnostic criteria for a given diagnosis are internally consistent and sort into the diagnostic entities proposed. With DSM PDs, problems with substantive validity pale in comparison to fundamental problems with structural validity. The failure to find evidence that PDs form discrete categories is a challenge to the classification's basic tenet. Also, structural analyses of DSM personality criteria and PD traits have consistently failed to find structures resembling DSM diagnoses (see early reviews by Livesley et al., 1994; Widiger, 1993). Instead, multiple studies show that four broad factors or dimensions underlie PDs (for a review, see Widiger & Simonsen, 2005). These factors represent emotional dysregulation and associated interpersonal problems centered on attachment insecurity and dependency, dissocial behavior, social avoidance, and compulsivity. The four-factor structure, one of the more robust findings in the field, is stable across measures, samples (clinical and nonclinical), and cultures. Since these factors cut across DSM-IV disorders, they explain much of the overlap among diagnoses. Unfortunately, these dimensions show limited resemblance to traditional diagnoses: None match DSM diagnoses closely, although similarities exist between these factors and clinical concepts of borderline, schizoid/avoidant, antisocial/psychopathic, and obsessive–compulsive personalities.

### External Validity

External validity is based on evidence that the classification shows meaningful relationships with external variables, especially etiological factors and clinical outcomes such as prognosis and response to treatment. As noted previously, external validators are difficult to identify for PD. Even the use of clinical outcomes is a problem because most treatments are relatively nonspecific, with similar effects across different disorders. Nevertheless, concerns have arisen about the external validity of DSM diagnoses. Thus, doubts have been voiced about the value of DSM diagnoses for treatment planning (Sanderson & Clarkin, 2002), and studies suggest that severity of personality pathology is a better predictor of outcome than specific diagnoses (Crawford, Koldobsky, Mulder, & Tyrer, 2011). Also, for reasons discussed earlier, etiology, which was so useful in establishing diagnoses of general medicine, is not helpful with PD. Nevertheless, as Jacobs and Krueger (2015) noted, psychiatric nosology has placed considerable emphasis on external validation, which is often tautological, because common validators such as external variables linked to impairment, disability, and dysfunction are not necessary independent of the diagnoses but rather are incorporated in it. The challenges of external validation are strong reasons for concentrating substantive and structural validity. Systematic application of Loevinger's construct validation framework to PD would eliminate many of the problems with current classifications (Jacobs & Krueger, 2015).

## The Persistent Influence of Clinical Tradition and the Medical Model

As the previous discussion documents, we have known for more than a quarter of a century that although the DSM PD classification lacks structural validity, the field largely functions as if this were not a problem. To move beyond this situation, we need to understand why evidence is neglected and why the field clings to a version of the medical model that does not even apply to some areas of general medicine. Two issues stand out. First, psychiatry is strongly influenced by the philosophical notion of essentialism: the idea that disorders have an underlying nature or pathology (Zachar & Kendler, 2007). Second, cognitive heuristics have a considerable impact on clinical thinking.

### Essentialism and the Medical Model

Psychiatry's identification with essentialism is understandable. Psychiatrists' formative experiences with medical disorders seem to have an "essence" in the form of a defined pathophysiology and specific etiology. Not surprisingly, these assumptions were transferred to mental disorders leading to the reification of diagnostic constructs. Although Robins and Guze's (1970) discussion of diagnostic validity had a considerable impact, the field has never really adopted the broader concept of construct validity or shed the primary concern of medicine with confirming diagnoses. Consequently, psychiatric nosology has primarily been concerned with establishing the best way to diagnose conditions whose validity is never seriously questioned. This was clearly illustrated by the way the DSM-5 PDs work group functioned. The validity of diagnoses that have received the most empirical attention was taken for granted; hence, the focus was on how best to diagnose them.

The impact of essentialism is illustrated by Richard Dawkins (2009), the evolutionist, who suggested that essentialism is the reason why it took until the mid-19th century and Darwin to formulate the idea of evolution through natural selection, when the fossil record had been understood for centuries. Essentialism, which led to the idea that each species has an immutable essence or basic nature that cannot be changed, made it difficult to accept the idea that a species can gradually change, until it eventually becomes a new species. Although Dawkins's views have been challenged, his argument illustrates how rigid adherence of essentialism can seriously hinder scientific progress. Essentialism pervades ideas about PD and the field functions as if there is an essence to conditions such as BPD and psychopathy. However, as Kendler

(2012b) subsequently noted, an "approach which assumes that (mental) diseases have single clear essences, is probably inappropriate for psychiatry (and for much of chronic disease medicine). Rather, our disorders can be more realistically defined in terms of complex, mutually reinforcing networks of causal mechanisms" (p. 17). Nevertheless, nosological endeavors continue to assume that the task is to capture the essence of current diagnostic constructs with appropriate diagnostic criteria. Thus, if one set of criteria does not work well, the assumption is that it should be modified, not that the concept should be questioned.

## The Impact of Cognitive Heuristics

The assumption of discrete diagnoses also persists because it is consistent with everyday cognitive strategies and heuristics used to organize information into categories. Our cognitive system seems to have evolved to organize information into categories and force exemplars that struggle several categories into a single specific category. As several authors have noted, PD diagnoses are essentially prototypical categories organized around classical cases that function as heuristics for organizing clinical information (Hyman, 2010). Despite the emphasis placed on diagnostic criteria, most clinicians make a diagnosis by matching patients to their conception of a given disorder. Prototypes seem "real" and intuitively convincing because they are organized around classical cases that are easily recalled; hence, they seem to validate the prototype. In contrast, less prototypical cases are less accessible and more difficult to remember despite that fact that they constitute the majority of cases. It is interesting to note as an aside that DSM-5 seriously considered using prototypes as the basis for classification and diagnosis, and even developed a draft proposal to this effect. Such is the impact of cognitive heuristics on clinical decisions.

Confusion about the value of prototype diagnosis seems to arise because prototypical thinking, like other cognitive heuristics, is effective under some circumstances. These mechanisms permit rapid decisions in situations in which it is better to make a wrong decision if it leads to cautious behavior than to make a slow decision. For example, in the environment in which these mechanisms evolved, it was better to identify a possible predator quickly when there was not a predator than to fail to identify and respond quickly to an actual predator. However, this does not mean that the conclusion or product of prototypical categorization is invariably correct or that it is useful when making considered decisions. Heuristics are useful because they introduce considerable economy into cognitive functions by organizing information so as to make it readily accessible. However, this economy is achieved at a cost—the process is subject to biases that introduce error into decision making (Kahneman, Slovic, & Tversky, 1982). These biases affect not only thinking in everyday situations but also decision making in professional situations ranging from finance and investing (Ferguson, 2008) to medical practice. These biases consolidate the clinician's conviction that there are discrete categories of disorder. Given this conviction and its consistent reinforcement in clinical practice, empirical findings are unconvincing. Also, the considerable discrepancy between empirical findings and traditional clinical concepts seems to foster both heuristic thinking and the philosophical assumptions of essentialism that become mutually reinforcing.

## Summary and Concluding Comments

Three broad arguments advanced in this section challenge some of the fundamental assumptions underlying the contemporary current study of PD. First, the applicability of the disorder-as-entity syndromic version of the medical model espoused by psychiatric nosology has been questioned given the etiological complexity of these conditions and their diverse and wide-ranging psychopathology, including the absence of pathognomonic features. Second, the DSM categorical classification has been shown to lack structural validity. Third, it has been argued that the construct validation framework is the most appropriate methodology for constructing and evaluating a classification of PDs given the psychopathology of PDs and the limited opportunities for external validation.

## Charting a New Course

The conclusions drawn in the previous section point to the need to chart a new course. There seems little point in repeatedly doing the same thing, as occurs with the regular revisions to our main classifications, in the hope of a different outcome. A new conceptual framework is needed to guide research and treatment that also captures the complexity of PD. In a sense, the conclusions drawn in the previous section are alarming: They appear to challenge the very identity of psychiatry and create uncertainty about how to proceed. However, they may also be liberating conclusions that free the study of PD from the procrustean bed of the syndromic version of the medical model with its discrete syndromes based on concepts derived from diverse and often incompatible sources. Also, there are obvious and potentially fruitful ways to proceed.

Alternative versions of the medical model might be examined for their relevance to understanding mental disorders, including PDs, and the study of PD could do what medicine has always done: Turn to its basic sciences and fundamental disciplines to form a new and more broadly based conceptual framework. However, it seems important to not only turn to the biological sciences but also look further afield and add psychology and philosophy to this list. Drawing on these disciplines, three principles are proposed to establish the metatheoretical underpinnings that could contribute to an alternative conceptual foundation of a science of PD: (1) The normative framework for conceptualizing PD is normal personality; (2) the most appropriate metastructure for describing and explaining normal and disordered personality is evolution; and (3) a comprehensive account of PD requires multiple levels of description and explanation, and a plurality of perspectives. I discuss these principles in the following section and revisit the medical model before briefly considering how such conceptual framework would impact classification.

### Normal Personality

The first strut of a conceptual framework was introduced earlier when I noted that the exclusive focus on the medical model leads to neglect of normal personality science as a source of concepts that might contribute to a valid classification. The principle establishes normal personality as the normative framework for diagnosing PDs and conceptualizes these disorders as pervasive impairments to the structure and functions of normal personality. Although this principle seems obvious—what other frame of reference is possible?—its adoption would lead to a different understanding of PD.

First, implementation of this principle requires that concepts and classifications of PD be consistent with the findings of normal personality research. This requires the field to relinquish typal concepts of PD, since these were abandoned by normal personality study nearly a century ago and to instead adopt a taxonomy that recognizes that personality pathology is continuous with normal personality variation. Second, the principle implies a more comprehensive view of personality pathology. Normal personality is broadly conceived to be a loosely organized system with multiple structures and processes forming a complex dynamic system. Disorder in such a system invariably encompasses all aspects of the system, leading to multiple forms of impairment rather than to circumscribed patterns. Such a perspective would be clinically useful because it focuses on all aspects of personality, not merely those included in criteria sets including strengths and assets. It also draws attention to assessing broad domains of personality dysfunction such as symptoms, impaired regulatory and modulatory mechanisms, interpersonal impairments, and self pathology (Livesley & Clarkin, 2015; see Clarkin, Livesley, & Meehan, Chapter 21, this volume).

Third, the study of normal personality has traditionally been concerned with not only the contents of personality (traits, motives, expectations, etc.) but also the organization and coherence of personality functioning. Although this aspect of personality has not be a prominent feature of DSM criteria, it provides the basis for developing a systematic definition of PD. Since some form of personality dysfunction is common—most people have some kind of personality quirk—it is important to differentiate dysfunction from disorder. Disorder is more pervasive and involves extensive disorganization of the personality system. Potential markers of such disorganization are the failure to develop a coherent self-structure and chronic interpersonal dysfunction (Livesley et al., 1994). This proposal creates a distinction between the core or defining features of PD and characteristics, such as traits, that delineate individual differences in the way disorder is manifested.

Finally, normal personality study would be useful in defining the scope of a conceptual model of PD. Over half a century ago, Kluckhohn and Murray (1953) made the often cited proposal that personality needs to account for how every person is like all other persons, like some other persons, and like no other person. The idea suggests that an integrative framework for PD needs to account for (1) features common to all individuals with PDs; (2) features common to some individuals with PDs, that is, individual differences in PD; and (3) features unique to the individual. Kluckhohm and Murray's statement captures a dilemma that has troubled personality science since its inception—the quandary between the nomothetic approach, with its search for broad and preferably universal laws, and the idiographic concern with uniqueness. Researchers are rightly concerned with the nomothetic nature of science, but clinicians cannot afford to ignore the substantial impact of the individuality and uniqueness of individual cases on treatment. For the last 40 years, common and unique features have been neglected in the search for discrete categories of individual differences. However, if a conceptual model is to have clinical utility, it needs to explain both clinically important individual differences and the universal and idiographic features of PD. Unfortunately, this requires an approach to diagnostic classification that is at odds with that of the DSM.

## Evolution

As McAdams and Pals (2006) noted, "Personality psychology begins with human nature, and from the standpoint of the biological sciences, human nature is best couched in terms of human evolution" (p. 206). Millon (1990) made a similar point abut PD (see Davis, Samaco-Zamora, & Millon, Chapter 2, this volume). The notion that personality structures and processes evolved because they enhanced the reproductive success of our remote ancestors provides a broad conceptual framework for understanding normal and disordered personality. The idea anchors personality constructs to adaptive biological mechanisms and forces a consideration of what personality structures and processes are designed to do. Such a perspective brings structure to the complexity of personality phenotypes and focuses attention of the functions of personality mechanisms and how they are impaired in PD.

However, evolutionary psychiatry has not gained much attention, largely because most proposals have sought to offer evolutionary explanations for established diagnoses. Since many diagnoses are simply heuristics, the resulting explanations look contrived (Troisi, 2008). Some formulations also assume that disorder results from a mismatch between the ancestral and contemporary environment—an idea that is not very tenable (Dupré, 2015). However, the framework being proposed does not adopt either approach. Instead, evolution is used as part of a metatheoretical context for conceptualizing normal personality. Since evolution works through the formation of mechanisms that evolved to solve problems occurring in the ancestral environment, an evolutionary perspective implies that *personality structures and processes are either based on, or are the products of, adaptive mechanisms.* These mechanisms form the basic architecture of personality. Since adaptive mechanisms, evolved to solve specific adaptational problems, they are relatively specific in nature (Tooby & Cosmides, 1990). PD is assumed to involve impairments to these mechanisms. Hence, evolution is proposed as a way to conceptualize and thereby clarify the structure that PD takes rather than to explain its occurrence.

Nevertheless, an evolutionary perspective would substantially influence how PD is conceptualized and studied. First, it implies that normal and disordered personality are shaped by an adaptive architecture that places constraints on personality development. However, this does not imply genetic determinism. Adaptive personality mechanisms, such as those underlying personality traits, are influenced by a large number of alleles, each having a small effect. Each allele is probably best considered as increasing the probability of the individual behaving in a given way. Also, the mechanisms linked to personality appear to be highly plastic. During development, they undergo substantial developmental elaboration that gives rise to a variety of phenotypes. The polygenic nature of genetic influences means that we are unlikely to find "genes for personality disorder" or to explain the disorder in terms of a specific genetic mechanism (Turkheimer, 2015), although we are likely to find genes with small effect linked to specific personality characteristics.

Second, the idea that personality phenotypes are based on specific genetically based adaptive mechanisms anchors personality constructs to biological mechanisms and makes the identification and elucidation of these mechanisms a primary research focus. This proposal is consistent with contemporary emphases of mechanisms, as illustrated by the Research Domain Criteria (RDoc) initiative of the National Institute of Mental Health, that seeks to base diagnosis and research on basic biological mechanisms. However, as I argue shortly, it involves a broad conception of mechanisms as neuropsychological structures that need to be studied using an array neurobiological and psychological methodologies.

Third, since adaptive mechanisms evolved to solve a specific problems (Tooby & Cosmides, 1990), the mechanisms underlying personality are context specific—evolution leads to mechanisms designed to have a specific function not general purpose mechanisms. Hence, the adaptive architecture of personality and PD is complex and highly specific, a proposal that is consistent with the specificity of genetic influences on personality (Livesley, Jang, & Vernon, 2003). This means that the basic constructs used to conceptualize PD need to be relatively narrow in their conception rather than broad like constructs used by current models and classifications.

Fourth, an evolutionary perspective also draws attention to the significance of the interpersonal aspects of personality. In a discussion of the origins of the human mental apparatus, Alexander (1989) argued that a powerful factor in the rapid elaboration of the mental apparatus, including personality, is the need to adapt to the pressures of living in social groups. The threats facing our remote ancestors during the period when the human genome evolved did not emanate from competition from other species because these threats had been largely overcome, but primarily from competition with other individuals from the same species. Successful competition under these circumstances required the evolution of mechanisms that enabled individuals to cooperate effectively with members of their own group. This required a host of adaptations involving language, cognition, and interpersonal behavior. Thus significant aspects of personality have social origins. Finally, it should be noted that an evolutionary perspective means that any account of the etiology of PD should include an understanding of both the distal factors that shaped personality mechanisms in our remote ancestors and proximal factors that constitute risk factors for PD.

### Levels of Explanation and Pluralism

A full account for the different aspects of disordered personality requires an understanding of biological, psychological, and cultural factors. These factors break down into multiple levels of description and explanation: (1) genetic (molecular and aggregated); (2) neurobiological (molecular and systems); (3) neuropsychological mechanisms; (4) psychological mechanisms; (5) personality constructs and dispositions; (6) personal narratives; and (7) sociocultural processes. Note that the term "level" is used in this context in a general way to refer to differences in abstractness and generalization. Hence, it is being used in the way that the term "strata" is used in geology. Although some levels or strata were laid down before others, none is intrinsically more important than the rest.

The different levels of explanation fall into roughly into two groups. The first two, and possibly three, levels are concerned with publically observable phenomena in the form of neurobiology and overt behavior. The remaining levels deal with epistemologically private activities of mind—cognitions, intentions, meaning systems, and so on, that are largely inferred (Kendler, 2012b). This dichotomy causes a tendency to assume that the more observable levels are in some way more important or essential that than more inferential levels. However, PD is primarily a psychological disorder in the sense that its manifestations and treatment are primarily psychological. Also, in the sense that the matter of whether a given phenomenon is indicative of disorder or not is a normative question that can only be decided by reference to psychological functioning. This does not mean that the biological levels are unimportant or less essential, just that they are simply facets of a comprehensive understanding of the disorder.

Since the subject matter of each level is distinct and not reducible to that of other levels, the study of PD needs to avoid what Daniel Dennett (1995) called "greedy reductionism" and Panksepp and Northoff (2009) called "ruthless reductionism." Within a multilevel explanatory framework, all levels are necessary for a comprehensive account of PD, and no single level is more important or fundamental than the rest. This is an important point because a significant feature of the current *zeitgeist,* especially in American psychiatry, is to view psychiatry as clinical neuroscience. However, this is too limited a perspective for conceptualizing PD, and probably many other mental disorders.

Each level of explanation needs its own language, constructs, and modes of explanation, and the conceptions that emerge at each level are not explicable using the constructs and modes of explanation of the level below. We cannot explain fully higher-level psychological structures such as self and identity even in terms of lower-level psychological mechanisms such as attention and memory, let alone in terms of biological mechanisms, despite the progress being made in understanding the neural mechanisms associated with these phenomena. The distinctiveness of each level and the importance of all levels for a comprehensive account of PD requires the conceptual framework for PD to be based on what has been called "empirically based conceptual pluralism" (Kendler, 2012a; Longino, 2006). "Pluralism" is the general idea that some natural phenomena cannot be fully explained by a single theory or single mode of investigation (Kellert, Longino, & Waters, 2006). Since a comprehensive understanding of the different levels of personality pathology cannot be provided by a single approach but rather requires contributions from multiple disciplines and different fields within a given discipline, pluralism seems to be the most relevant philosophical approach.

With this approach, different models would be constructed to account for the phenomena at each level. For most levels, multiple models are likely to be needed to provide a full account of the phenomena involved. Although each level is in a sense self-contained, the models need to be consistent with empirical findings about other levels, although one-to-one correspondence across levels is unlikely and unnecessary. The models developed for any level are a facet of a comprehensive account of PD. Consequently, the combination of models developed for all levels form a loosely organized descriptive and explanatory structure rather than a defined theory of PD. To use a term coined by Cartwright (1999), this structure forms a "dappled world." And, within this dappled world, any account of PD would be incomplete if any facet or level of explanation were missing.

An implication of a pluralistic perspective is that the constructs used to account for PD, including diagnostic constructs, are constructions, and as such they may be useful for some purposes but not others. This idea is at odds with the disease-as-entity syndromic model and with the essentialist assumptions that Zachar and Kendler (2007) suggested underlie contemporary psychiatry. Both assume that diagnoses are fixed entities and that the task is to find the optimal way to represent them. Pluralism is also at odds with most contemporary theories of PD. Earlier, I suggested that current theories are in an early stage of development; however, from the perspective of pluralism, some also appear to be misconceived since they attempt to offer a comprehensive, unified, and often one-dimensional explanation of PD, although components of some of these theories may undoubtedly contribute to explanation at specific levels.

The syndromic model and the assumptions of some theories also differ from the way philosophy of science is conceptualizing scientific explanation, especially in the biological and psychological sciences, which largely involve models of various kinds (Dupré, 2015). Models are representations of a phenomenon that make the phenomenon more accessible (Bailor-Jones, 2009). They do not provide a total representation of the phenomenon but rather highlight some features and downplay others to facilitate understanding of the critical features of the phenomenon. With PD, models make a phenomenon at a given level of explanation understandable in terms of its important features and functions.

## *The Medical Model Reconsidered*

The medical model adopted by the neo-Kraepelinians and DSM postulates the occurrence of disease entities with distinct and clearly defined boundaries. This is more stringent than the models used by contemporary medicine, which accept that conditions such as some forms of hypertension are extremes of normal variation, a direct equivalent to the idea of PDs as extremes of normal personality variation. Models used by medicine also recognize that some symptoms of a disease such as fever and cough are not due to the disease entity itself but rather are adaptive ways for the body to respond to disease (Bolton, 2008). Again, such responses do not seem so different from the defense mechanisms proposed by psychoanalysis or the coping mechanisms proposed by cognitive therapy to deal with psychological adversity.

It is also clear that the models actually used by medicine accept that some syndromes are defined by a coherent cluster of symptoms that does not arise from a common etiology because they represent the failure of a functional system that may occur for diverse etiological reasons (Nesse & Stein, 2012). Congestive cardiac failure and renal failure are examples. Again, the model is far removed from that of modern psychiatry. However, it does not seem a far stretch to see this formulation as being akin to the idea that some forms of PD may similarly represent dysfunction in a specific personality system due to different combinations of risk factors. This approach seems to work for medicine because it is based on a detailed understanding of the normal anatomy and physiology of these systems that can be used to explain symptoms. Psychiatry and PD cannot draw on a similarly rich understanding of the functioning personality systems. Nevertheless, they provide a more appropriate conceptual framework than the neo-Kraepelinian credo.

Given the complexity and diversity of models in general medicine, it is puzzling why contemporary psychiatry has so uncritically embraced a version of the model so ill-suited to mental disorders. It is as if psychiatry, which in many ways is considered to occupy the bottom of the totem pole of medical specialties, responded to criticisms from the antipsychiatry movement by seeking to be more medical than general medicine by adopting a more extreme version of the medical model than that of medicine itself. Nevertheless, it is clear that the study of PD need not totally discard the medical model; rather, it should adopt a more liberal version that is compatible with the other principles needed to form a coherent conceptual basis for the field.

## Diagnostic Classification

Problems with the neo-Kraepelinian conception of the medical model and the poor structural validity of current classifications point to the need for a new approach that does not require the occurrence of discrete types. The proposal that conceptions of PD be compatible with those of normal personality, along with the notion that PD represents a pervasive disorganization of the personality system, suggests that it may be more productive to think of PD as single diagnostic entity that is expressed in multiple ways rather than a set of discrete types. In previous publications, I have suggested that these ideas imply a two-component structure to a classification of PD: (1) a representation of general PD and (ii) a system for describing clinically important individual differences in the manifestations of PD (Livesley, 1998; Livesley et al., 1994, 2003).

To flesh out this framework requires attention to both the purposes for which classification is used and accommodation of the complex psychopathology of PD. Blashfield and Draguns (1976) noted that psychiatric classifications serve the multiple purpose of providing the nomenclature needed for communication, facilitating information retrieval, providing a set of descriptive constructs, predicting outcomes, and forming the foundation for concept development and theory construction. Besides these functions, classifications also serve a variety of administrative functions. Given these diverse usages, it probably unrealistic to expect a single system to cover all contingencies. If we factor into this mix the complex psychopathology of this disorder that leads to individual cases showing features common to all with the disorder, features shared with some with the disorder, and features unique to the individual, the idea of a single classification looks even less feasible. Classification is one area in which a plurality of concepts and models seems especially useful.

To make the task of exploring an alternative approach more manageable, let us consider only the clinical and research functions of a classification. Clinicians are primarily concerned with establishing a diagnosis in order to predict outcome and plan treatment. Most diagnostic evaluations are conducted either as part of a general clinical evaluation or specifically to plan treatment. Although the traditional assumption is that the same diagnostic scheme may be applied to both situations, the needs of these situations are different. With a general evaluation, the intent is to establish whether the patient has a PD or not. This does not require a detailed evaluation of the nature of the disorder or domains of impairment. What matters is whether the patient has a PD that co-occurs with another mental disorder because it is the presence of general PD, not the nature of the disorder, that has implications for clinical management. Assessment prior to initiating treatment specifically for PD is a different matter. Here, assessment of severity is also important because prognosis is more a function of severity than any specific diagnosis (Crawford et al., 2011). Also, severity is useful in determining treatment intensity and the relative balance of supportive or generic treatment methods versus more specific change-focused interventions (see Clarkin et al., Chapter 21, this volume). Treatment planning also requires information on the major constellations of traits present. The four-factor model of personality traits described earlier is sufficient for this purpose. It is assess the broad constellations of emotional dysregulation (emotional and interpersonal traits), dissocial traits, social avoidance, and compulsivity because these four patterns of disorder are managed somewhat differently (Livesley & Clarkin, 2015). However, a different kind of information is needed to select interventions or modules and tailor treatment to the needs of the individual—information about the specific impairments of individual cases (see Clarkin et al., Chapter 21, this volume). Earlier four domains were described: symptoms, regulation and modulation impairments, maladaptive interpersonal behavior, and self pathology. Assessment of functional impairments associated with these domains makes it possible to tailor treatment to the individual. Since these domains cover a wide range of impairments, a variety of constructs and methods are often required to cover the different levels of explanation involved, and the depth of the assessment of each domain would depend on the nature of the treatment being planned. An additional benefit of incorporating domain assessment into the overall scheme for diagnostic assessment is that it focuses attention on the functional aspects of personality pathology and on specific mechanisms, an important step toward the development of mechanism-based treatment (Livesley, 2017; Schnell & Herpertz, in press).

Diagnosis for research purposes is different. Again, specific DSM diagnoses are not generally helpful because it is difficult to see how data collection organized around diagnoses that lack structural validity can make a substantial contribution to a science of PD. As with clinical practice, different kinds of research have different assessment requirements. For example, with some epidemiological research, a diagnosis of PD and possibly severity may be sufficient because these predict some outcomes better than do specific diagnoses. If more detailed information is required, this assessment could be supplemented with information on the four constellations mentioned earlier.

Many kinds of research, both biological and psychological, however, are not concerned with diagnosing PD but rather with investigating specific mechanisms or constructs. In these cases, a relatively narrow assessment of the construct of interest is needed because adaptive mechanisms have relatively specific functions. This requires the classificatory scheme to include a comprehensive set of specific constructs. Identification of this component of the classification is more challenging, since our understanding of the mechanisms underlying personality pathology is limited. One initial solution would to focus on the specific or facet-level traits identified through structural analyses of PD traits such as emotional intensity, emotional reactivity, attachment insecurity, lack of empathy, low affiliation, and so. A possible refinement of the approach would be to use a combination of methods to define specific constructs as a step toward delineating specific mechanisms. This would involve identifying a specific or facet-level trait based on factor-analytic studies, then refining the construct using behavioral genetic methods, an evolutionary analysis of the adaptive functions of the phenomenon, and any relevant neurobiological information. For example, research on emotional dysregulation may focus on specific components such as anxiousness, emotional intensity, and emotional reactivity. Anxiousness could initially be defined on the basis of factor analyses of normal and disordered personality and behavioral genetic analyses, showing that anxiousness is a homogeneous construct. Evolutionary analyses could then be used to light on the adaptive functions of anxiousness and a possible underlying adaptive mechanism. For example, Gray (1987) suggested that anxiousness is based in the behavioral inhibition system, a mechanism for managing threat. Together these approaches suggest an initial descriptive formulation of anxiousness and associated mechanism that would be used to construct an assessment instrument. The results of subsequent neurobiological and psychological research on the structure and functioning of the mechanism could then be used to revise the construct. Thus, this kind of research requires a diagnostic assessment system that is far more detailed and specific than is currently needed for most clinical purposes. The specific traits listed in Section III of DSM-5 provide a possible source of some primary traits that might be used for this purpose. However, the value of the overall list is seriously compromised by the fact that the original version was heavily influenced by a committee process that potentially introduced bias into the final list.

In summary, I have argued in this chapter that there are serious conceptual problems with contemporary conceptualizations and classifications of PD. The current mishmash of diagnoses compiled from diverse sources and based on inappropriate assumptions derived from the neo-Krepaelinian position is not conducive to building a coherent body of scientific knowledge about PD. For this purpose, we need a more broadly based conceptual framework and a different approach to diagnostic classification that would replace the current focus on specific diagnoses with a multifaceted scheme that combines diagnosis and assessment, and makes it possible to tailor assessment to the purposes for which it will be used.

Diagnostic assessment would begin by establishing a single diagnosis—whether a patient has a PD. This would be sufficient for many general clinical purposes and some research endeavors. The nature and depth of any subsequent assessment would depend on its intended purpose. For many research purposes, subsequent assessment would focus on specific mechanisms. However, diagnostic assessment for treatment requires a different kind of evaluation. In view of what we know about the nature and functions of personality and the complex interrelationships among components of personality pathology, assessment prior to therapy requires a broader and more nuanced understanding of the individual's personality system, problems, and assets. This is needed to construct the kinds of narrative case formulations required to plan a structured treatment strategy and to help patients in turn to construct more meaningful narratives and scripts for managing their problems and organizing their lives. Viewed in this way, it becomes clear why a multiple-component diagnostic assessment is needed and why the study of PD needs to be open to the idea of incorporating a plurality of perspectives.

## REFERENCES

Abraham, K. (1927). *Selected papers on psychoanalysis*. London: Hogarth Press. (Original work published 1921)

Alexander, R. (1989). Evolution of the human psyche. In P. Mellars & C. Stringer (Eds.), *The human revolution: Behavioral and biological perspectives on the origins of modern humans* (pp. 455–513). Edinburgh, UK: Edinburgh University Press.

Andreasen, N. C. (2006). DSM and the death of phenomenology in America: An example of unintended consequences. *Schizophrenia Bulletin, 33*(1), 108–112.

Aragona, M. (2009). The role of comorbidity in the crisis of the current psychiatric classification system. *Philosophy, Psychology, Psychiatry, 16*, 1–11.

Aragona, M. (2015). Rethinking received views on the history of psychiatric nosology: Minor shifts, major continuities. In P. Zachar, D. St. Stoyanov, M. Aragona, & A. Jablensky (Eds.), *Alternative perspectives on psychiatric validation* (pp. 27–46). Oxford, UK: Oxford University Press.

Bailor-Jones, D. M. (2009). *Scientific models in the philosophy of science*. Pittsburgh, PA: University of Pittsburgh Press.

Berrios, G. E. (1993). European views on personality disorders: A conceptual history. *Comprehensive Psychiatry, 34*, 14–30.

Blashfield, R. K. (1984). *The classification of psychopathology*. New York: Plenum Press.

Blashfield, R. K., & Draguns, J. G. (1976). Evaluative criteria for psychiatric classification. *Journal of Abnormal Psychology, 85*, 140–150.

Blashfield, R. K., & Livesley, W. J. (1991). A metaphorical analysis of psychiatric classification as a psychological test. *Journal of Abnormal Psychology, 100*, 262–270.

Bolton, D. (2008). *What is mental disorder?* Oxford, UK: Oxford University Press.

Cartwright, N. (1999). *The dappled world: A study of the boundaries of science*. Cambridge, UK: Cambridge University Press.

Cleckley, H. (1976). *The mask of sanity* (5th ed.). St. Louis, MO: Mosby. (Original work published 1941)

Cloninger, C. R. (1989). Establishment of diagnostic validity in psychiatric illness: Robins and Guze's method revisited. In L. V. Robins & J. E. Barrett (Eds.), *The validity of psychiatric diagnosis* (pp. 9–18). New York: Raven Press.

Crawford, M. J., Koldobsky, N., Mulder, R., & Tyrer, P. (2011). Classifying personality disorder according to severity. *Journal of Personality Disorders, 25*, 321–330.

Cronbach, L. J. (1971). Test validation. In R. L. Thorndike (Ed.), *Educational measurement* (2nd ed., pp. 443–507). Washington, DC: American Council of Education.

Cronbach, L. J., & Meehl, P. E. (1955). Construct validity in psychological testing. *Psychological Bulletin, 52*, 281–302.

Dawkins, R. (2009). *The greatest show on Earth*. New York: Free Press.

Dennett, D. C. (1995). *Darwin's dangerous idea*. New York: Simon & Schuster.

Dupré, J. (2015). What can evolution tell us about the healthy mind? In K. S. Kendler & J. Parnas (Eds.), *Philosophical issues in psychiatry III: The nature and sources of historical change* (pp. 259–271). Oxford, UK: Oxford University Press.

Eaton, N. R., Krueger, R. F., South, S. C., Simms, L. J., & Clark, L. A. (2011). Contrasting prototypes and dimension in the classification of personality pathology: Evidence that dimensions, but not prototypes, are robust. *Psychological Medicine, 41*, 1151–1163.

Ferguson, N. (2008). *The ascent of money: A financial history of the world*. New York: Penguin.

Foulds, G. A. (1965). *Personality and personal illness*. London: Tavistock.

Foulds, G. A. (1976). *The hierarchical nature of personal illness*. London: Academic Press.

Gadamar, H.-G. (1996). *Philosophical hermeneutics* (D. E. Linge, Ed., & Trans). Berkeley and Los Angeles: University of California Press.

Gray, J. A. (1987). *The psychology of fear and stress.* Cambridge, UK: Cambridge University Press.

Grinker, R. R., Werble, B., & Drye, R. C. (1968). *The borderline syndrome.* New York: Basic Books.

Hempel, C. G. (1961). Introduction to the problems of taxonomy. In J. Zubin (Ed.), *Field studies in the mental disorders* (pp. 3–22). New York: Grune & Stratton.

Hyman, S. E. (2010). The diagnosis of mental disorders: The problem of reification. *Annual Review of Clinical Psychology, 6,* 155–179.

Jacobs, K. L., & Krueger, R. F. (2015). The importance of structural validity. In P. Zachar, D. St. Stoyanov, M. Aragona, & A. Jablensky (Eds.), *Alternative perspectives on psychiatric validation* (pp. 189–200). Oxford, UK: Oxford University Press.

Jaspers, K. (1963). *General psychopathology* (J. Hoenig & M. W. Hamilton, Trans.). Baltimore: Johns Hopkins University Press. (Original work published 1923)

Kahneman, D., Slovic, P., & Tversky, A. (1982). *Judgement under uncertainty: Heuristics and biases.* Cambridge, UK: Cambridge University Press.

Kellert, S. H., Longino, H. E., & Waters, C. K. (Eds.). (2006). *Scientific pluralism.* Minneapolis: University of Minnesota Press.

Kendell, R. E., & Jablensky, A. (2003). Distinguishing between validity and utility of psychiatric diagnoses. *American Journal of Psychiatry, 160,* 4–12.

Kendler, K. S. (2012a). The dappled nature of causes of psychiatric illness: Replacing the organic–functional/hardware–software dichotomy with empirically based pluralism. *Molecular Psychiatry, 17,* 377–388.

Kendler, K. S. (2012b). Levels of explanation in psychiatric and substance disorders: Implications for the development of an etiologically based nosology. *Molecular Psychiatry, 17,* 11–21.

Kernberg, O. F. (1984). *Severe personality disorders.* New Haven, CT: Yale University Press.

Klerman, G. L. (1978). The evolution of a scientific nosology. In J. C. Shershow (Ed.), *Schizophrenia: Science and practice* (pp. 99–121). Cambridge, MA: Harvard University Press.

Klerman, G. L. (1986). Historical perspective on psychopathology. In T. Millon & G. L. Klerman (Eds.), *Contemporary directions in psychopathology: Toward DSM-IV* (pp. 3–28). New York: Guilford Press.

Kluckhohn, C., & Murray, H. A. (1953). Personality formation: The determinants. In C. Kluckhohn, H. A. Murray, & D. M. Schneider (Eds.), *Personality in nature, society, and culture* (pp. 53–67). New York: Knopf.

Kohut, H. (1971). *The analysis of the self.* New York: International Universities Press.

Kraepelin, E. (1907). *Clinical psychiatry* (A. R. Dienfendorf, Trans.). New York: Macmillan.

Kretschmer, E. (1925). *Physique and character.* New York: Harcourt Brace.

Krueger, R. F., Eaton, N. R., Clark, L. A., Watson, D., Markon, K. E., Derringer, J., et al. (2011). Deriving an empirical structure of personality pathology for DSM-5. *Journal of Personality Disorders, 25,* 170–191.

Kuhn, T. S. (1962). *The structure of scientific revolutions.* Chicago: University of Chicago Press.

Leising, D., & Zimmermann, J. (2011). An integrative conceptual framework for assessing personality and personality pathology. *Review of General Psychology, 15,* 317–330.

Lenzenweger, M. F., & Clarkin, J. F. (Eds.). (2005). *Major theories of personality disorder* (2nd ed.). New York: Guilford Press.

Livesley, W. J. (1998). Suggestions for a framework for an empirically based classification of personality disorder. *Canadian Journal of Psychiatry, 43,* 137–147.

Livesley, W. J. (2001). Commentary on reconceptualising personality disorder categories using trait dimensions. *Journal of Personality, 69,* 277–286.

Livesley, W. J. (2010). Confusion and incoherence in the classification of personality disorder: Commentary on the preliminary proposals for DSM-5. *Psychological Injury and Law, 3,* 304–313.

Livesley, W. J. (2017). Psychotherapy for personality disorder: Where are we? Where should we go from here? Where do we need to end up? In J. L. Ireland, C. A. Ireland, M. Fisher, & N. Gredecki (Eds.), *International handbook on forensic psychology in secure settings* (pp. 194–216). London: Taylor & Francis.

Livesley, W. J., & Clarkin, J. F. (2015). Diagnosis and assessment. In W. J. Livesley, G. Dimaggio, & J. F. Clarkin (Eds.), *Integrated treatment for personality disorder: A modular approach* (pp. 51–79). New York: Guilford Press.

Livesley, W. J., & Jackson, D. N. (1991). Construct validity and the classification of personality disorders. In J. Oldham (Ed.), *Personality disorders: New perspectives on diagnostic validity* (pp. 3–22). Washington, DC: American Psychiatric Press.

Livesley, W. J., & Jackson, D. N. (1992). Guidelines for developing, evaluating, and revising the classification of personality disorders. *Journal of Nervous and Mental Disease, 180,* 609–618.

Livesley, W. J., Jang, K. L., & Vernon, P. A. (2003). The genetic basis of personality structure. In T. Millon & M. J. Lerner (Eds.), *Handbook of psychology* (Vol. 5, pp. 59–83). New York: Wiley.

Livesley, W. J., Schroeder, M. L., Jackson, D. N., & Jang, K. L. (1994). Categorical distinctions in the study of personality disorder: Implications for classification. *Journal of Abnormal Psychology, 103,* 6–17.

Loevinger, J. (1957). Objective tests as instruments of psychological theory. *Psychological Reports, 3,* 635–694.

Longino, H. E. (2006). Theoretical pluralism and the scientific study of behavior. In S. H. Kellert, H. E. Longino, & C. K. Waters (Eds.), *Scientific pluralism* (pp. 102–131). Minneapolis: University of Minnesota Press.

Maudsley, H. (1874). *Responsibility in mental disease.* London: King.

McAdams, D. P., & Pals, J. L. (2006). A new Big Five: Fundamental principles for an integrative science of personality. *American Psychologist, 61,* 204–217.

Medawar, P. B. (1984). *The limits of science.* New York: Harper & Row.

Meehl, P. E. (1972). A critical afterword. In I. I. Gottesman & J. Shil (Eds.), *Schizophrenia and genetics* (pp. 367–416). New York: Academic Press.

Millon, T. (1990). *Toward a new personology.* New York: Wiley-Interscience.

Nesse, R. M., & Stein, D. J. (2012). Towards a genuinely medical model for psychiatric nosology. *BMC Medicine, 10,* 5.

Panksepp, J., & Northoff, G. (2009). The trans-species core SELF: The emergence of active cultural and neuro-ecological agents through self-related processing with subcortical-cortical midline networks. *Consciousness and Cognition, 18,* 193–215.

Pearce, J. M. S. (2012). Brain disease leading to mental illness: A concept initiated by the discovery of general paralysis of the insane. *European Neurology, 67,* 272–278.

Presly, A. J., & Walton, H. J. (1973). Dimensions of abnormal personality. *British Journal of Psychiatry, 122,* 269–276.

Pritchard, J. C. (1835). *Treatise on insanity.* London: Sherwood, Gilbert & Piper.

Reich, W. (1949). *Character analysis* (3rd ed.) New York: Farrar, Straus, & Giroux. (Original work published 1933)

Robins, E., & Guze, S. B. (1970). Establishment of psychiatric validity in psychiatric illness: It application to schizophrenia. *American Journal of Psychiatry, 126,* 983–986.

Robins, L. (1966). *Deviant children grow up.* Baltimore: Williams & Wilkins.

Rosenhan, D. L. (1973). On being sane in insane places. *Science, 179,* 250–258.

Rutter, M. (1987). Temperament, personality, and personality disorder. *British Journal of Psychiatry, 150,* 443–458.

Sabbarton-Leary, N., Bortolitti, L., & Broome, M. R. (2015). Natural and para-natural kinds in psychiatry. In P. Zachar, D. St. Stoyanov, M. Aragona, & A. Jablensky (Eds.), *Alternative perspectives on psychiatric validation* (pp. 76–83). Oxford, UK: Oxford University Press.

Sanderson, C., & Clarkin, J. F. (2002). Further use of the NEO-PI-R personality dimensions in differential treatment planning. In P. T. Costa, Jr., & T. A. Widiger (Eds.), *Personality disorders and the five-factor model of personality* (2nd ed., pp. 351–375). Washington, DC: American Psychological Association.

Schneider, K. (1950). *Psychopathic personalities* (9th ed., English trans.). London: Cassell. (Original work published 1923)

Schnell, K., & Herpertz, S. C. (in press). Emotion regulation and social cognition as functional targets of mechanism-based psychotherapy in major depression with comorbid personality pathology. *Journal of Personality Disorders.*

Skinner, H. A. (1981). Toward the integration of classification theory and methods. *Journal of Abnormal Psychology, 90,* 68–87.

Stone, M. (1980). *The borderline syndromes.* New York: McGraw-Hill.

Tooby, J., & Cosmides, L. (1990). On the universality of human nature and the uniqueness of the individual: The role of genetic and adaptation. *Journal of Personality, 58,* 17–67.

Troisi, A. (2008). Psychopathology and mental illness. In C. Crawford & D. Krebbs (Eds.), *Foundations of evolutionary psychology* (pp. 453–475). New York: Erlbaum.

Turkheimer, E. (2015). The nature of nature. In K. S. Kendler & J. Parnas (Eds.), *Philosophical issues in psychiatry III: The nature and sources of historical change* (pp. 227–244). Oxford, UK: Oxford University Press.

Tyrer, P., & Alexander, M. S. (1979). Classification of personality disorder. *British Journal of Psychiatry, 135,* 163–167.

Varga, S. (2015). *Naturalism, interpretation, and mental disorder.* Oxford, UK: Oxford University Press.

Verheul, R., & Widiger, T. A. (2004). A meta-analysis of the prevalence and usage of personality disorder not otherwise specified (PDNOS). *Journal of Personality Disorders, 18,* 309–319.

Whitlock, F. A. (1967). Pritchard and the concept of moral insanity. *Australian and New Zealand Journal of Psychiatry, 1,* 72–79.

Whitlock, F. A. (1982). A note on moral insanity and the psychopathic disorders. *Bulletin of the Royal College of Psychiatrists, 6,* 57–59.

Widiger, T. A. (1993). The DSM-III-R categorical personality disorder diagnoses: A critique and alternative. *Psychological Inquiry, 4,* 75–90.

Widiger, T. A., Livesley, W. J., & Clark, L. A. (2009). An integrative dimensional classification of personality disorder. *Psychological Assessment, 21,* 243–255.

Widiger, T., & Simonsen, E. (2005). Alternative dimensional models of personality disorder: Finding a common ground. *Journal of Personality Disorders, 19,* 110–130.

Zachar, P., & Kendler, K. S. (2007). Psychiatric disorders: A conceptual taxonomy. *American Journal of Psychiatry, 164,* 557–565.

Zachar, P., & Jablensky, A. (2015). Introduction: The concept of validation in psychiatry and psychology. In P. Zachar, A. D. S. Stoyanov, M. Aragona, & A. Jablensky (Eds.), *Alternative perspectives on psychiatry validation: DSM, ICD, RDoC, and beyond* (pp. 3–24). Oxford, UK: Oxford University Press.

# CHAPTER 2

# Theoretical versus Inductive Approaches to Contemporary Personality Pathology

Roger D. Davis, Maria Cristina Samaco-Zamora, and Theodore Millon[1]

The ways we can observe, describe, and organize the natural world are infinite. As such, the terms and concepts we create to represent psychological phenomena are often confusing and obscure (Rounsaville et al., 2002). Some terms are narrow, others are broad, and still others are difficult to define. Of course, not all phenomena related to the subject need be attended to at once. Certain elements may be selected from the vast range of possibilities because they seem relevant to the solution of a specific question. To create a degree of reliability or consistency among those interested in a subject, its elements are defined as precisely as possible and classified according to their core similarities and differences (Dougherty, 1978; Tversky, 1977; Zachar & Kendler, 2010). In subjects such as personology and psychopathology, these classes or categories are given specific labels that serve to represent them. This process of definition and classification is indispensable for systematizing observation and knowledge.

Unfortunately, progress in the classification of personality disorders (PDs) has failed to advance with the speed anticipated when DSM-III was launched in 1980. Latent causes are diverse and intertwined, difficult to segregate out from the "background noise" of their interactions. A multitude of genetic and constitutional factors on the one hand, and family and social factors on the other, ensure that each person is to some extent a unique composite that resists understanding, leading to excessive comorbidity and the predominance of PD not otherwise specified (NOS) within the "classical PD categories" of DSM-III through DSM-IV-TR and now DSM-5. This complexity not only challenges the Kraepelinian assumption that disease and health are fundamentally discrete, it challenges the assumption that classification in psychopathology might ever graduate from largely descriptive professional conventions to some gen-

---

[1] In the mid-1990s, I (R. D. D.) was a graduate student, and the late Ted Millon was my mentor. Nearly every weekday morning, Ted and I would have wide-ranging discussions about personality and psychopathology in the study beside his home. In one way or another, most of these discussions had classification issues at their base. Most of the time, it was Ted talking and me listening. Ted had been a major figure in the development of DSM-III. He was a firm believer in the multiaxial model and had therefore been concerned that the DSM represent total individuals, not just their major diagnoses. But how to do that in the best way? Eventually, we began to look at theories of personality as objects to be classified. All theories are representations, and all representations are necessarily flawed. The question then becomes "Can these theories be grouped in some way that reveals shared characteristics, thereby highlighting their strengths and weaknesses?" Looking back on the body of Ted's work, I think it is accurate to say that nearly every problem discussed in the personality disorders was either anticipated or commented on by Ted Millon in some way. This chapter is an outgrowth of those morning discussions that Ted led nearly two decades ago.

uinely scientific system that "carves nature at its joints." Current controversies regarding the PDs are representative: Which content area and its organizing principles—the interpersonal, behavioral, cognitive, existential, biophysical, or psychodynamic—is most fundamental? Or should personality pathology take its lead from dimensions of normal personality, perhaps one of the lexical models, such as the Big Five or Hexaco models? Should the PDs be organized as dimensions, categories, prototypes, circumplices, or as regions in some higher-dimension space? Thus far, the field lacks solid answers to these questions.

Complicating matters further is the recent discovery by 270 scientist collaborators in the Reproducibility Project, who successfully replicated only 39 of 100 studies published in three leading psychology journals in 2008 (Open Science Collaboration, 2012, 2015). Perhaps some of the 61 studies that failed replication are false negatives, but the authors noted that only 47% of the effects sizes found in the original research were contained in the 95% confidence interval of the replication effect size. Such regression toward the mean suggests that failures of replication mostly constitute false positives. If so, this would mean that much of the empirical literature in psychology is the rationalized result of systematic misinformation dressed up as scientific fact. It would further mean that the human ritual of setting out hypotheses, reviewing literature, gathering data, conducting statistical analyses—all the meticulous steps involved in producing "rigorous scientific research" capable of passing peer review in our most prestigious journals—potentially produces mythology as often as it reveals objective reality. As Ioannidis (2005, p. 696) stated in the title of his landmark article, "Most published research findings are false." Contrast the 61% failure rate of the Reproducibility Project with the use of $p < .05$ as the criterion of significance, which is specifically intended to prevent false positives 95% of the time.

What else is there? To what source or authority might we appeal for reassurance if our experimental methods are demonstrably inadequate? Thomas Kuhn (1975) suggested that progress is guided by some prevailing paradigm. Rather than seek to overturn and reject cherished ideas, researchers instead seek to build a body of confirmatory evidence. Only where new findings cannot be assimilated into the structure of existing ideas is there mounting pressure for change. The transition from the categorical disease model—as represented by the "classical PDs" of DSM-III through DSM-IV-TR, now carbon-copied into the main body of DSM-5—to the dimensional model of personality traits—as represented by the Alternative Model given in Section III of DSM-5—constitutes one such example. As shown by the controversies inspired by this transition, much of what actually happens in personality is really just arguing that a certain approach is consonant with the assumptions of a particular paradigm. For the Alternative Model, the assumption is that because personality consists of traits, pathological personality consists of pathological traits. In turn, traits entail dimensionality and continuity, leading to a paradigm shift away from the categorical model based on this assumption. Scientific "progress," then, is as much about argumentation as it is about "hard data."

In fact, the paradigm itself is likely to dictate what are considered to be hard data. In classical psychoanalysis, for example, free association provides evidence of unconscious drives. In cognitive psychology, the purpose is to unearth cognitive schemas that serve to organize perceptions of the self, world, and others. In behaviorism, the focus is on what is observational and measureable, so that only counts and frequencies are important. Paradigms involve assumptions that structure data and dictate what qualifies as data. Each paradigm therefore obtains a means of insulating itself against falsification: Inconsistent findings are typically based on what the paradigm rejects as data. Each paradigm thus builds its own cadre of devotees and acquires a kind of immortality. Scientific revolutions, then, are not so much concerned with replacing old paradigms, but instead involve increasing enthusiasm for new ones. Paradigms tend to accumulate and, like old generals, never really die, they just fade away (Meehl, 1978). They are greatly assisted in this mission by the seeming inability of any single empirical study to reveal objective truths about nature, even at the $p < .05$ threshold, and the tendency of published effect sizes to be reduced by half upon replication.

## Three Epistemic Choices for Structuring Personality Theories

In this chapter, we try to find a way to step outside and understand the structure and evolution of the many theories that are put forward in personality and its pathologies. We organize approaches to abnormal personality in terms of three major epistemic "choice points." In philosophy, epistemology is concerned with the nature of knowledge. Since any representational system is not reality—the map is not the territory—we seek to understand whether these fundamental choices naturally lead us to characteristic advantages, issues, and sets of problems. We further argue that a taxonomy of models exposes their weaknesses, thereby suggesting "standard plans of attack," as well as means of defending against these attacks. These three epistemic choices structure the criticism of current and future personality theory.

Being able to systematically generate the strengths and pathologies of various models is important to personality. It is far better to predict the critiques of various models—both the advantages and the failings—than it is to wait for such criticism to unfold over decades. Let us remember that the journey from the categorical disease model of PDs to the trait dimensions of the Alternative Model took 35 years, almost the length of an entire scientific career. If some method of classifying personality theories could be found that would automatically unfold and expose shortfalls, not only would that save time but it would also suggest a method by which these theories can be more self-consciously considered. Perhaps it could identify holes in the literature and suggest which theories would fill them. Toward these ends, we have identified three fundamental decisions, choice points, or dimensions that seem to describe the criticism of most contemporary theories of abnormal personality.

### Approach: Inductive versus Theoretical

Two broad approaches to the scientific adventure may be identified. In the first, we go to nature in order to understand what nature has in it. Our emphasis is on identifying and describing all the phenomena of the subject domain. We seek to build a comprehensive list of what our science is to be about, then look for relationships between the entities that we have just observed. This approach may be called "inductive" because it is literally created "from the ground up," based on our store of observations. Lest it degenerate into a list or catalog, all inductive taxonomies eventually need a means by which to transform their naive and merely descriptive observational summaries into scientific principles. Making this transit, from observation and description to latent entities whose relationships are explained by scientific principles, is the main problem of induction. Carl Linnaeus, for example, became famous for his *Systema Naturae*, which categorized all life on earth. As encyclopedic as he was, however, Linnaeus could only create categories based on superficial appearances: Things that looked alike were classified together. In early versions of his work, whales were considered fishes, since both swim in the ocean. Truly scientific classifications that sought to elucidate the Tree of Life, based on the work of Charles Darwin and the theory of evolution, would come later. The philosopher of science, Carl Hempel (1965, p. 139–140) framed this progression from a prescientific classification based on naive categories to one based on genuine scientific principles in terms of stages:

> The development of a scientific discipline may often be said to proceed from an initial "natural history" stage . . . to more and more theoretical stages, in which increasing emphasis is placed upon the attainment of comprehensive theoretical accounts of the empirical subject matter under investigation. The vocabulary required in the early stages of this development will be largely observational: It will be chosen so as to permit the description of those aspects of the subject matter which are ascertainable fairly directly by observation. The shift toward systematization is marked by the introduction of new, "theoretical" terms, which refer to various theoretically postulated entities, their characteristics, and the processes in which they are involved; all these are more or less removed from the level of directly observable things and events.

In the second approach to the development of scientific knowledge, an imaginative theorist starts with some set of observations that are difficult to reconcile, perhaps even contradictory, and imagines the underlying structures, mechanisms, or formula that explains them. Here, progress often involves synthesizing previously disparate theories of limited scope in order to create a more comprehensive formulation that both unifies and simplifies heretofore unrelated domains. Physics and mathematics often evolve according to this motive. Cartesian coordinates provided the foundation of analytic geometry, invented by René Descartes in order to graph the results of various algebraic functions. Prior to this, algebra and geometry were considered separate branches of mathematics. Likewise, James Clerk Maxwell unified electricity, magnetism, and light. And of course, Albert Einstein unified matter with energy, and space with time, through general relativity.

Every system of psychopathology must identify its constructs, speculate on their causes, and provide guidance for their treatment. As the evolution of the various DSM editions have shown, however, just agreeing on "what the syndromes of psychopathology are" is fraught with controversy. The fundamental constructs do not leap out at us, each awaiting some systematic description in order to take its rightful place in the DSM as our periodic table of mental disorders. Instead, the problem of personality pathology is that we cannot even agree what the fundamental constructs are. There are too many ways of "slicing the pie." Are the PDs just "out there" in nature waiting to be discovered? Or are they also human constructions, and thus part "kernel of truth" and part distortion? Naturally, then, we turn to theory as a means of "fixing" the number and nature of psychopathologies. The promise of theory is to tell us which disorders are "real" and which are merely symptoms, or perhaps even illusions.

The principle problem of theory is the opposite of induction. The distinction between a good theory and a good fantasy may be exceedingly thin. The problem for the theorist, then, lies in making the transit back from the world of latent variables to the world of observations, in order to demonstrate that these observations accord well with the predictions of the theory. Numerous obstacles stand in the way of this mission, most notably problems with measurement, such as ceiling and floor effects, the sensitivity of variables, false positive and false negatives, method variance, diverse ways of operationalizing constructs, and reliability concerns. These issues prevent psychological theories from being subjected to strong threats of falsification, since we can never be sure whether failures of prediction are due to poor theories or poor measures.

### Scope: A Single Construct versus a Whole Taxonomy

The second decision is concerned with scope: Are we focused intensely on a single construct or an entire taxonomy of constructs? The study of personality needs both. Focusing on a single construct leads to highly detailed treatments that unearth indicators and covariates, while situating the construct relative to, and distinguishing it from, its near neighbors. Any number of books have been written about single PDs, including dependent PD (Bornstein, 1993), borderline PD (BPD; Linehan, 1993), narcissistic PD (Ronningstam, 2005), and histrionic PD (Horowitz, 1991). On the other hand, some authors seek to either invent or characterize an entire taxonomy of personality constructs. Beck's *Cognitive Theory of Personality Disorders* (Beck, Davis, & Freeman, 2014), Benjamin's *Interpersonal Diagnosis and Treatment of Personality Disorders* (1996), McWilliams's *Psychoanalytic Diagnosis: Understanding Personality Structure in the Clinical Process* (2011), and Millon's *Disorders of Personality* (1981, 1996, 2011) are notable exemplars concerned with characterizing an entire constellation of personality constructs, regardless of how these constructs come to exist or may be derived.

### Content: A Single Domain versus Multiple Domains

The third decision is concerned with content: With what domain(s) of variables will our model be concerned? Historically, these domains have been associated with various schools, for example, the psychoanalytic, the interpersonal, the behavioral, the biophysical, and the cognitive schools. The boundary between domains is somewhat arbitrary, so that more circumscribed, but also relevant, domains could be identified, perhaps existential and cultural approaches. In fact, there is no limit to the number of domains in which personality might be described. Historically, the biophysical approach emerged first, followed later by psychoanalysis and behaviorism. The interpersonal school developed largely as a reaction to psychoanalysis. Other domains may emerge as the century progresses. Nothing prevents it. Which of these is personality? They all are. As such, it seems impossible to reduce any particular school to any other. Each domain is concerned with principles that seem to govern its own variables. The variables of other domains are viewed as being constrained by those of the preferred domain, but are not reducible to the preferred domain. For example, a temperamental construct such as irritability might be associated with interpersonal aggression, but not invariably so. Likewise, irrational cognitions might predict existential crises, but not invariably so. Similarly, neurobiological structures might predict certain cognitions, but not invariably so.

Nevertheless, exponents of particular historical schools do attempt to present their own organizing principles as integrative, thus bridging the gap between domains. For example, the object relations school of psychoanalysis is concerned with mental representations. These representations are imprinted early in development and preempt future relational models—their main psychoanalytic feature—but must also be described as interpersonal, because they are models about important persons—most notably attachment figures—as well as cognitive, because they are representations rather than realities. In aspiring to create models, then, some domains must be identified as core (or predictive), whereas others must be identified as peripheral (or predicted or constrained). Will our efforts be narrowed to some single domain? Or will they seek to combine multiple domains?

We now consider combinations of the three epistemic dimensions previously described. Crossing the three dimensions leads to a cubic model. Each corner of the cube is a unique combination. In the interest of brevity, however, we discuss the four corners associated with theory, but only a single model association with induction, which we term the inductive–lexical–factor–trait tradition.

## Theoretical Models of PD

Assuming one's temperament is oriented more toward theoretical explanation rather than inductive description, how might one approach the topic of personality? A circumplex of theoretical models can be generated by crossing considerations of scope (one PD or an entire taxonomy) with considerations of content (one perspective or domain or school vs. many), as shown in Figure 2.1.

### Single PD–Single Perspective

This approach is concerned with developing an explanation of the origins, characteristics, or perpetuating factors of a single PD through a single personality perspective. Examples in-

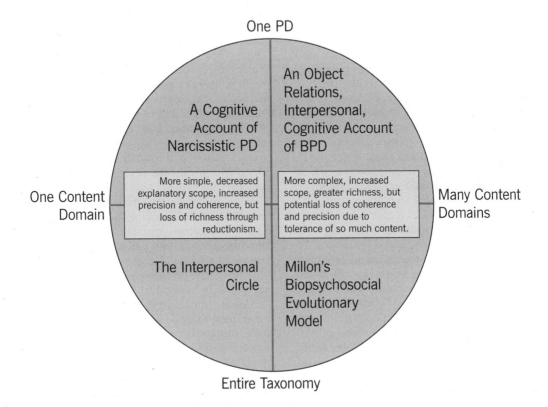

**FIGURE 2.1.** The circumplex model of theoretical species for abnormal personality.

clude a cognitive theory of obsessive–compulsive PD (OCPD), an object relations theory of BPD, an interpersonal theory of dependent PD, and so on. The goal is not to generate the existence of the disorder from the theoretical principles of the content domain, but instead to apply those principles as a means of understanding the disorder from a particular theoretical perspective. Why does the disorder exist? We do not know, but we can try to determine what a particular perspective has to say about it. In this sense, both the disorder and the perspective are prior to the theory. We have only to apply the theory to the disorder in order to obtain the result. The advantage of this model is simplicity. By narrowing attention to a single content domain, practitioners who are comfortable with the theoretical principles of this domain may quickly begin to apply them to the PD. Unfortunately, simplicity is also a vice, since it is usually recognized that a single perspective cannot supply a complete explanation of the PD. For this reason, there may be no claims that, for example, a cognitive theory of paranoid PD represents the "one true theory" of the disorder. Instead, the intent may be to apply the theory in order to understand its limits, or simply to make the disorder accessible to clinicians who subscribe to the theory.

Nevertheless, some such theories are quite imaginative. The classical view of narcissism, for example, contends that it results from developmental arrests or regressions to earlier periods of fixation. As an important elaborator of the narcissism construct, Kohut (1971) does not challenge the content as such, but rather the sequence of libidinal maturation, which, he believed, has its own developmental line and sequence of continuity into adulthood; that is, it does not fade away by becoming transformed into object-libido, as contended by classical theorists, but unfolds into its own set of mature narcissistic processes and structures. Pathology occurs as a consequence of failures to integrate one of the two major spheres of self-maturation, the "grandiose self" and the "idealized parent imago." If disillusioned, rejected, or if one experiences cold and unempathic care at the earliest stages of self-development, serious pathology, such as psychotic or borderline states will occur. Trauma or disappointment at a later phase will have somewhat different repercussions depending on whether the difficulty centered on the development of the grandiose self or on the parental imago. What is notable is that Kohut's theory is a developmental pathway for the self, to the extent that the meaning of the term "narcissism" is significantly changed from that of narcissistic PD. However, it is difficult to see how such developmental accounts could ever give rise to more comprehensive taxonomies, such as Axis II disorders in DSM-IV. Here again, we see the sometimes razor-thin boundary between theory and imagination.

### Single PD–Multiple Perspectives

The desire here is to illuminate a single personality construct by combining principles or variables from various theoretical perspectives. The disorder of interest is given first; its "existence" is assumed. The theorist works backward from there. Cognitive, interpersonal, behavioral, existential, psychoanalytic object relations, temperament—all are considered raw material for understanding the genesis and perpetuation of the specific disorder. If some additional perspective is later discovered, it too can be weaved into the existing account in order to further increase the explanatory scope of the model. For the most part, authors who excel at combining ideas from various perspectives seem to have adopted their PD as a topic on which to build their career, progressively expanding and refining their narrative as time moves forward. Since the PD itself represents their point of departure, they can be agnostic with regard to any particular theoretical school, being free to assimilate content and constructs from whatever sources seem to be most useful. The result is a rich eclectic account that assimilates constructs from a variety of personality content domains, along with lucid case descriptions that illuminate the interplay of these constructs.

Some examples may be helpful. In discussing BPD, Lieb, Zanarini, Schmahl, Linehan, and Bohus (2004) sort the nine DSM-IV diagnostic criteria into affective (inappropriate anger, emptiness, affective instability), cognitive (transient paranoid ideation, identity disturbance), behavioral (recurrent suicide-related behaviors, impulsivity), and interpersonal criteria (efforts to avoid abandonment, unstable relationships). This implicitly presents BPD as an eclectic combination of domains. In reviewing dependent PD, Bornstein (1993, p. 19) considers a related construct, dependency, which he divided into motivational (desire for guidance, approval, and support), cognitive (powerless self, powerful others), affective (anxious about independence), and behavioral (seeking help and reassurance) components. As can be seen, the one PD–multiple perspectives combination is compatible with the medical disease paradigm, wherein each PD is potentially viewed as being an independent disease process or, at least, the label for such a process. Since the focus is on a single PD, it is an empirical question as to whether the vulnerabilities, developmental pathways, mechanisms, and so on, generalize to other disorders. They might or might not. Grouping diagnostic criteria, however, involves the add-on assumption that the outcroppings of abnormal personality afflict the entire matrix of the person. In contrast, the disease model that underlies the DSM makes no assumptions about personality domains.

The weakness of this approach is some lack of precision and theoretical coherence. Different authors may reach somewhat different formulations of the same disorder. When DSM-III was published in 1980, BPD was created to facilitate the research of John Gunderson. By the time DSM-5 arrived, there were many published theories about the genesis of BPD, all of them somewhat similar, yet also somewhat different. Each author seems satisfied to hit the target in a slightly different place. The disorder accumulates a rich literature, as each author has his or her own creative ideas that sound reasonable and require discussion. In turn, this leads to cycles of scholarly comparison and contrast as others attempt to read beyond these overlapping accounts in order to abstract some set of common themes that are believed to be fundamental. Attempts at integration have the following quality: "Among those researchers and theorists who have written extensively about XYZ personality disorder, Researcher A, Theorist B, Researcher C, and Theorist D stand out. Though there are areas of agreement and disagreement, all believe that Principle E, Principle F, Principle G, and Principle H are fundamental, though there are differences of emphasis. . . . These principles are reviewed in relation to core problematic features of personality disorder XYZ as described in the DSM (or ICD)." Assuming that the personality disorder has reached a critical mass of prevalence, it can become the fixation point for many theorists and researchers, and enjoy an enormous output of scholarship as all possible correlates of the disorder are elucidated and weighed for their significance and interrelationships. The disorder accumulates a considerable literature, but there is no guarantee that whatever formulation of the disorder is currently popular represents the final word about its nature. Increasingly sophisticated accounts interweave diverse variables in order to give authors and readers the feeling that real advances are being made. The PDs continued from DSM-IV-TR into the Alternative Model have reached this threshold. When the literature becomes too woolly, new reviews offer tractable condensations that frame existing controversies, and the process starts over.

From a scientific perspective, these theories are satisfying because they tend to be eclectic rather than doctrinaire. Today, it is fashionable to assume that variables across all the previously mentioned domains have genuine predictive power. However, such theories are also not as satisfying as they could be, simply because they do not attempt to explain why the entire constellation of PDs exists as it does. As such, if the PD suddenly disappears—as, for example, sadistic PD appeared in DSM-III-R only to disappear in DSM-IV—then the scientific status of the theory is suddenly imperiled, if only because the disorder is no longer seen as "legitimate." The question "Why do we have these PDs rather than others?" is never addressed. Answering this question requires some deeper set of principles that unify the PDs. This is discussed below in the multiple PDs–multiple perspectives section.

### *Single Perspective–Taxonomically Focused*

In this approach, the theoretical principles of a particular perspective are used to treat an entire taxonomy of PDs. The weaker forms of this epistemic combination apply the principles of a particular school to some set of PDs or constructs, which are already given, not deduced from the theory. An example is Beck's cognitive theory of PDs. This approach gives rise to no PDs from out of its own principles. Instead, it explains the importance of the cognitive domain to all mental disorders, then distinguishes each PD from the others in terms of their characteristic cognitive profiles. If certain taxonomic constructs, such as sadistic PD, are described for one edition of the DSM, only to be deleted later, so be it.

In a deductive theory, the theory describes axes or polarities, and a taxonomy is created directly from the theory as combinations of these. The creation of the taxonomy in turn provides evidence of the surplus meaning and value of the theory. The principles are claimed to be fundamental, so that the taxonomy "carves nature at its joints." This succeeds to the extent that the theory is compelling. In fact, this chapter is an example of this deductive approach, based on the dimensions of one versus many for taxonomic scope, part versus whole for personality content, and inductive versus deductive as the point of departure for the scientific adventure.

The exemplar of this approach is the interpersonal circle. The circumplex first debuted in an article by Freedman, Leary, Ossorio, and Coffey (1951), and was then further developed by Timothy Leary (1957). These theorists crossed two orthogonal dimensions, dominance–submission (the vertical axis) and hostility–affection (the horizontal axis; also called love–hate and communion), creating an interpersonal circle that they further divided into eight segments or themes, each representing a different mix of the two fundamental variables. The dependent, for example, was represented as consisting of approximately equal levels of affection and submission, while the compulsive, which Leary called the "responsible–hypernormal," consisted of approximately equal levels of affection and dominance. The four quadrants of the circumplex, Leary suggested, parallel the temperaments or humors of Hippocrates, while the axes of the circle parallel Freud's two basic drives. Each segment of the circle was further differentiated into a relatively normal region, closer to the center, and a relatively pathological region, closer to the edge. Thus, the circumplex may be used not only to generate a taxonomy of personality traits, but also to represent continuity between normality and pathology. The interpersonal circle also states that interactions obey the principle of complementarity: Love pulls for love, and hate pulls for hate. Dominance pulls for submission, and submission pulls for dominance.

The most radical development of interpersonal theory is Benjamin's (1974, 1996) structural analysis of social behavior (SASB), which integrates interpersonal conduct, object relations, and self psychology in a single geometric model. Benjamin's point of departure lies in the synthesis of Leary's classic interpersonal circle with Earl Schaefer's (1965) circumplex of parental behavior. As every parent knows, there is a fundamental tension between controlling and guiding children, and in allowing them to gradually become masters of their own destiny.

Parents must either let their children grow up to become genuinely mature beings who realize their own intrinsic potentials along a unique developmental path, or else demand submission and deny autonomy, effectively making the child an extension of the parent. Schaefer's model therefore places autonomy-giving at the opposite of control, not submission, as with the Leary circle. The horizontal axis, however, remains the same.

The primary intellectual attraction of the interpersonal circle is its enormous theoretical coherence, which gives rise to a tight coupling of taxonomy, process, and content. For those readers persuaded by interpersonal theory, this will be enough. They are ready to believe that the Leary circle or the SASB carves nature at its joints. And perhaps it does. But this also involves believing that the interpersonal perspective is fundamental to all others, that it provides the core and foundation of human personality, without which the other domains could neither function nor flower. Certainly, there are strong arguments to be made here. Attachment may be seen as the first interpersonal relationship, and attachment theory has been linked to the development of object representations that endure across the lifespan. Likewise, the cognitive domain can be coerced into an interpersonal mold, since thinking is often thinking about someone or about relationships rather than thinking about inanimate objects or abstract ideas. Even thinking about one's job involves thinking about oneself as embedded in the human world. Coordinating other domains to one's favorite taxonomy increases scope but may involve some loss of precision. Benjamin (1986) explored coordinating affective and cognitive descriptors to the circumplices of her SASB model.

Many readers will note that neither the Leary circle nor the SASB produce a comprehensive taxonomy of personality pathology. For these critics, the interpersonal circle becomes an interesting but incomplete theory of personality. The retort—given from a perspective internal to the theory—is that while neither the interpersonal circle nor the SASB model produce the DSM-IV/5 classical personality disorders, these disorders nevertheless have a strong interpersonal component, and some PDs may not stand the test of time anyway. PDs that are likely to be rejected—such as the sadistic and the self-defeating were rejected in DSM-IV and the dependent, schizoid, paranoid, histrionic, depressive, and negativistic in the DSM-5 Alternative Model—cannot provide a strong critique of interpersonal taxonomy.

## Multiple Perspectives–Taxonomically Focused

The primary theoretical task here is to discover a set of theoretical principles that can then be combined to yield a taxonomy deductively, based on the theory. Typically, the theory is based on some related domain in which powerful scientific principles are already well known. If this related domain is believed to be strongly related to personality, then the case can be made that the personality theory derived from this domain carves nature at its joints. As with the interpersonal circle, the taxonomy provides evidence of the surplus meaning and value of the theory. To the extent that the principles can be claimed to be fundamental, the taxonomy can be claimed to "carve nature at its joints." The key defining feature of this approach, however, is that the theoretical principles cut across existing perspectives or schools and provide a way to integrate them. These principles are intended to answer the question "Why this particular set of personality constructs rather than some other?"

Philosophers of science agree that the system of kinds undergirding any domain of inquiry must answer the question that forms the point of departure for the scientific enterprise: Why does nature take this particular form rather than some other? Accordingly, one cannot merely accept any list of kinds or dimensions as given, even if arrived at by committee consensus. Instead, a taxonomic scheme must be justified, and to be justified scientifically, it must be justified theoretically. Taxonomy and theory, then, are intimately linked. Quine (1977) makes a parallel case:

> One's sense of similarity or one's system of kinds develops and changes . . . as one matures. . . . And at length standards of similarity set in which are geared to theoretical science. The development is away from the immediate, subjective, animal sense of similarity to the remoter objectivity of a similarity determined by scientific hypotheses . . . and constructs. Things are similar in the later or theoretical sense to the degree that they are . . . revealed by science. (p. 171)

The deductive approach generates a taxonomy to replace the primitive aggregation of categories or dimensions that preceded it. This generative power is what Hempel (1965) meant by the "systematic import" of a scientific classification. Meehl (1978) has noted that theoretical systems comprise related assertions, shared terms, and coordinated propositions that provide fertile grounds for deducing and deriving new empirical and clinical observations. What is elaborated and refined in theory, then, is understanding, an ability to see relations more clearly, to conceptualize categories more accurately, and to create greater overall coherence in a subject, that is, to integrate its elements in a more logical, consistent, and intelligible fashion. Pretheoretical taxonomic boundaries that were set according to clinical intuition and empirical study can now be affirmed and refined according to their constitution along underlying polarities. These polarities lend the model a holistic, cohesive structure that sharpens the meanings of the taxonomic constructs derived by allowing their comparison and contrast along the axes that constitute the theory.

In contrast to the three epistemic combinations outlined earlier, we might ask whether there is any theory that (1) honors the nature of personality as the patterning of variables across the entire matrix of the person and (2) derives a taxonomy of personality theory deductively. Such a theory is necessary for at least two reasons. First, the natural direction of science is toward theories of increasing scope. In theoretical physics, for example, quantum gravity is an attempt to unify quantum mechanics with the theory of relativity. Second, personality is not exclusively behavioral, cognitive, or interpersonal but rather an integration of all these. But how are we to create a theory that breaks free of the "grand theories of human nature" that are all part of the history of psychology? How do we "rise above" the historical schools—interpersonal, cognitive, psychodynamic, and behavioral—in order to integrate them?

The key lies in finding theoretical principles for personality that fall outside the field of personality proper. Otherwise, we could only repeat the errors of the past by asserting the importance of some new set of variables heretofore not emphasized, building yet another perspective that misses a scientific understanding of the total phenomenon. Herein lies the distinction between the terms "personality" and "personology." Strictly speaking, a science of personality is limited to partial views of the person that may be internally consistent but cannot be total.

In contrast, personology is from the beginning as a science of the total person. In the absence of falsifying experiments, various perspectives on personality tend to develop to high states of internal coherence, becoming "schools" that resist integration and contribute to the fragmentation of psychology as a unified discipline. In so doing, they also create conceptions of personality that intrinsically conflict with the nature of the construct itself. A science of personology ends this long tradition of fractiousness and creates a theoretical basis for a completely unified science of personality and psychopathology.

One attempt to create a comprehensive theoretical model was developed by Millon (1990). For Millon, evolution was the logical choice as a scaffold from which to develop a science of personality. Just as personality is concerned with the total patterning of variables across the entire matrix of the person, it is the total organism that survives and reproduces, carrying forth both its adaptive and maladaptive potentials into subsequent generations. While lethal mutations sometimes occur, the evolutionary success of organisms with "average expectable genetic material" is dependent on the entire configuration of the organisms' characteristics and potentials. Similarly, psychological fitness derives from the relation of the entire configuration of personality characteristics to the environments in which the person functions. Beyond these analogies, the principles of evolution also lie outside personality proper, and thereby form a foundation for the integration of the various historical schools, which escapes the part–whole fallacy of the dogmatic past. A taxonomy of personality styles and disorders based on evolutionary principles faces one central question: How can these processes best be segmented so that their relevance to the individual person may be drawn into the foreground?

The *first* task of any organism is its immediate survival. Organisms that fail to survive have been selected out, so to speak, and fail to contribute their genes and characteristics to subsequent generations. Whether a virus or a human being, every living thing must protect itself against simple entropic decompensation, predatory threat, and homeostatic misadventure. There are literally millions of ways to die. Evolutionary mechanisms related to survival tasks are oriented toward life-enhancement and life-preservation. The former are concerned with improvement in the quality of life, and gear organisms toward behaviors that improve survival chances and, one hopes, lead them to thrive and multiply. The latter are geared toward orienting organisms away from actions or environments that threaten to jeopardize survival. Phenomenologically speaking, such mechanisms form a polarity of Pleasure and Pain.

The *second* universal evolutionary task faced by every organism relates to homeostatic processes employed to sustain survival in open ecosystems. To exist is to exist within an environment, and once an organism exists, it must either adapt to its surroundings or adapt its surroundings to conform to and support its own style of functioning. Whether the environment is intrinsically bountiful or hostile, the choice is essentially between a passive versus an active orientation, that is, a tendency to accommodate to a given ecological niche and accept what the environment offers versus a tendency to modify or intervene in the environment, thereby adapting it to oneself.

The *third* universal evolutionary task faced by every organism pertains to reproductive styles that maximize the diversification and selection of ecologically effective attributes. All organisms must ultimately reproduce to evolve. To keep the chain of the generations going, organisms have developed strategies by which to maximize the survivability of the species. At one extreme is what biologists have referred to as the r-strategy. Here, an organism seeks to reproduce a great number of offspring, which are then left to fend for themselves against the adversities of chance or destiny. At the other extreme is the K-strategy, in which relatively few offspring are produced and given extensive care by parents. Although individual exceptions always exist, these parallel the more male "self-oriented" versus the more female "other-nurturing" strategies of sociobiology. Psychologically, the former strategy is often judged to be egotistic, insensitive, inconsiderate, and uncaring, while the latter is judged to be affiliative, intimate, protective, and solicitous (Gilligan, 1981; Rushton, 1985; Wilson, 1978).

By combining these polarities, the classical DSM personality disorders may be reproduced. For example, the histrionic is said to be active and other-oriented, while the narcissist is passive and self-oriented. The dependent is passive and other-oriented, whereas the antisocial is active and self-oriented. These form the interpersonally imbalanced PDs. The schizoid is passive and detached, whereas the avoidant is active and detached. The compulsive (passive) and negativistic (active) are interpersonally conflicted, not knowing whether to turn to self or others. The sadistic (active) and masochistic PDs (passive) are said to represent a reversal of pain and pleasure. The paranoid, borderline, and schizotypal PDs are severe PDs. The advantage of Millon's model is that it provides a theoretical account for the DSM PD constructs that actively generates these constructs. Moreover, the dimensions that give rise to the PDs are specifically determined by the theory.

Because each traditional perspective on personality represents a partial view of an integrated whole, the PDs can each then be given descriptors within these perspectives. Table 2.1 shows these descriptors for narcissistic PD.

## Inductive–Factor–Trait Models

In the final third of this chapter, we discuss inductive approaches to personality. As with theoretical models, these could be divided in terms of the three epistemic polarities, as shown in Figure 2.2. In the interest of space, however, we focus on factor-analytic approaches, since it is these that attempt to describe entire taxonomies of personality.

As problems with the categorical DSM PDs were being documented in the mid-1990s, a new inductive paradigm was rising in research on normal personality traits (John, Naumann, & Soto, 2008). The strength of the paradigm lay in the comprehensiveness of its claims: that

---

**TABLE 2.1. Domains of the Confident–Narcissistic Personality**

Behavioral level

- Expressively haughty (e.g., acts in an arrogant, supercilious, pompous, and disdainful manner, flouting conventional rules of shared social living, viewing them as naive or inapplicable to self; reveals a careless disregard for personal integrity and a self-important indifference to the rights of others).
- Interpersonally exploitive (e.g., feels entitled, is unempathic and expects special favors without assuming reciprocal responsibilities; shamelessly takes others for granted and uses them to enhance self and indulge desires).

Phenomenological level

- Cognitively expansive (e.g., has an undisciplined imagination and exhibits a preoccupation with immature and self-glorifying fantasies of success, beauty or love; is minimally constrained by objective reality, takes liberties with facts and often lies to redeem self-illusions).
- Admirable self-image (e.g., believes self to be meritorious, special, if not unique, deserving of great admiration, and acting in a grandiose or self-assured manner, often without commensurate achievements; has a sense of high self-worth, despite being seen by others as egotistic, inconsiderate, and arrogant).
- Contrived contents (e.g., internalized representations are composed far more than usual of illusory and changing memories of past relationships; unacceptable drives and conflicts are readily refashioned as the need arises, as are others often simulated and pretentious).

Intrapsychic level

- Rationalization dynamics (e.g., is self-deceptive and facile in devising plausible reasons to justify self-centered and socially inconsiderate behaviors; offers alibis to place oneself in the best possible light, despite evident shortcomings or failures).
- Spurious architecture (e.g., morphological structures underlying coping and defensive strategies tend to be flimsy and transparent, appear more substantial and dynamically orchestrated than they are in fact, regulating impulses only marginally, channeling needs with minimal restraint, and creating an inner world in which conflicts are dismissed, failures are quickly redeemed, and self-pride is effortlessly reasserted).

Biophysical level

- Insouciant mood (e.g., manifests a general air of nonchalance, imperturbability, and feigned tranquility; appears coolly unimpressionable or buoyantly optimistic, except when narcissistic confidence is shaken, at which time either rage, shame, or emptiness is briefly displayed).

*Note.* Adapted from Millon (n.d.).

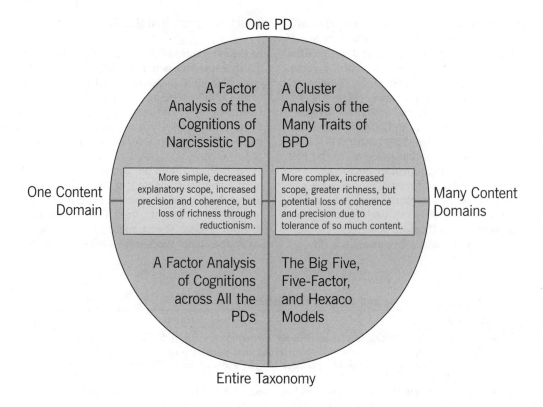

**FIGURE 2.2.** The circumplex model of inductive species for abnormal personality.

it could provide an overarching framework by which to organize and understand personality traits. We refer to this as the "inductive–lexical–factor–trait" tradition. The quadruple dashes are intended to indicate that the parts cohere together strongly, so strongly that they combine a philosophy of science, a data source, a methodology, and a unit of analysis, in that order.

Interestingly enough, the new paradigm has its foundations in the 19th century. A polymath and half-cousin to Charles Darwin, Sir Francis Galton (1822–1911), helped lay the foundations for many sciences. He developed the weather map for meteorology and pioneered the forensic use of fingerprints in criminology. Galton (1884) was also the first to describe the lexical hypothesis, the notion that all the important dimensions of individual differences have already become encoded in the language. Put simply, if a trait is important enough, then there is a single word for it. And conversely, if an aspect of personality cannot be described in a single word, it cannot be that important. Turning to the dictionary as a resource for such dimensions, Galton "estimated that it contained fully one thousand words expressive of character, each of which has a separate shade of meaning, while each shares a large part of its meaning with some of the rest" (p. 181). Galton therefore became a figure of seminal importance in the history of personality. He also described the properties of the normal distribution and invented the concept of correlation, later mathematically formalized by his student Karl Pearson. In turn, correlation led to the invention of factor analysis, a means of extracting latent variables from a correlation matrix.

With factor analysis and the lexical hypothesis in place, the foundation was laid for the new paradigm. The methodology was simple enough: If the most important dimensions of personality are encoded in the language, then those traits are already in the dictionary. So go to the dictionary, find them, and catalogue them. Winnow the traits down to some manageable number, say 500, then administer questionnaires of these traits to hundreds of subjects, enough to meet the sample size requirements for a reliable factor analysis. Position the resulting broadband factors as "supertraits" in a hierarchical model in which the original traits constitute lower-order dimensions or "facets." Argue that your methodology has identified the most important universals in human nature. Write items necessary to transform some of the underlying traits into scales, thereby producing a hierarchically structured inventory. Compare other inventories to your new invention. Show how your factors organize and clarify the scales of any competing inventory, and argue that any holes in their content—content found in your factor model but not found in the competing inventory—make assessment with the competing inventory incomplete.

The previous paragraph puts the history and agenda of the "inductive–lexical–trait perspective" into a tidy package. The reasons for its momentum seem sound: With induction, we go to the world to see what the world has in it. Observation comes first. The subject domain is sampled broadly, thereby establishing a claim that the resulting model is complete, for if we do not sample broadly, others will, thereby possibly deriving additional dimensions and supplanting our work. Next, some methodology organizes and structures our observations into a taxonomy, perhaps categories (e.g., cluster analysis), hierarchical dimensions (e.g., factor analysis), or circumplices (e.g., factor analysis, structural equation modeling, multidimensional scaling). Finally, the subject domain is reconsidered through the resulting classification system, which now is presumed to "carve nature at its joints," if only because the sampling is comprehensive and the methodology so ostensibly rigorous. With the inductive–lexical–trait tradition, the lexical approach provides justification for selecting the traits, factor analysis provides the inductive methodology that derives the dimensions, and the dictionary provides a claim to comprehensiveness.

## History of the Five-Factor Model

A long list of researchers has made contributions to the emergence of the inductive–lexical–trait tradition. In 1936, Gordon Allport, then at Harvard University, and his graduate student, Henry S. Odbert, undertook a large-scale lexical study, surveying some 400,000 terms from *Webster's New International Dictionary*. Over 18,000 "personality descriptive" terms were identified. These were further classified into (1) stable dispositions; (2) states, attitudes, emotions, and moods; (3) social evaluations; and (4) miscellaneous, which included terms related to physical characteristics, talents, and abilities. Norman (1963) used the 1961 edition of *Webster's International Dictionary* to follow up on the Allport and Odbert study. He deleted terms that were obscure, obsolete, evaluative, or physical, ending with nearly 2,800 terms deemed to represent stable personality traits. Norman used a peer nomination strategy, whereby each subject was required to rate multiple other group members, thus achieving high reliabilities for the ratings. In reporting his findings, Norman (p. 574) stated that "analyses yielded clear and consistent evidence for the existence of five relatively orthogonal, easily interpreted personality factors."

The contributions of Lewis Goldberg (1993) represent one high-water mark. Over 20 years ago, Goldberg (1993) chronicled the saga of the Big Five, including his own contributions. Goldberg stated

> during the decade roughly from 1975 to 1985, I was continuously carrying out analyses of these various data sets in an effort to discover a scientifically compelling taxonomic structure. It was as if I were looking through a glass darkly: In each analysis, I would discover some variant of the Big-Five factors, no two analyses exactly the same, no analysis so different that I couldn't recognize the hazy outlines of the five domains. For nearly a decade I wondered as if in a fog, never certain how to reconcile the differences obtained from analysis to analysis. (p. 29)

Another precedent was set with Costa and McCrae's (1992) publication of the five-factor model (FFM). These authors (1978, 1980) began with cluster analyses derived from Cattell's (Cattell, Eber, & Tatsuoka, 1970) condensation of Allport and Odbert's (1936) some 4,500 stable dispositions, thereby recovering Extraversion and Neuroticism. Also emerging from these analyses was the Openness factor, which combined traits such as "imaginative" and "experimenting" based on Cattell. From these broad factors, Costa and McCrae developed their NEO Personality Inventory (1985). The Revised NEO Personality Inventory (NEO PI-R) was published in 1992, and is now the NEO-PI-3 (McCrae, Costa, & Martin, 2005). Each major factor is measured as a combination of six facets, chosen on the basis of their historical importance to personality theorists. The authors have argued strongly for replacing the traditional PDs with the FFM (Costa & McCrae, 1992).

## Effects of the FFM on the PD Area

Induction naturally appeals to our instincts as scientists. Methodologically driven models resist making a priori theoretical commitments and therefore appear to be pure science. The FFM has had a number of salutary effects on abnormal personality. First, factor models assume there is no sharp division between normality and pathology, only a smooth unbroken gradation. In contrast, the DSM classification has been criticized as being archaically categorical (e.g., Widiger, 1993). Second, a factor model is almost always sufficient, which means that it accounts for most of the variation in the dataset from which it was developed. Third, where the factors are extracted to be uncorrelated, cognitive economy is further maximized, since the majority of traits are linked to only one factor. Fourth, factor models are parsimonious, extracting between three and seven factors, regardless of the variables factored (Block, 1995). Fifth, based on parsimony and sufficiency, we can speculate that a factor model might serve as a dimensional taxonomy to which all of personality psychology can be anchored. This challenges other models. Sixth, since factor models are explicitly constructed to telescope almost all of the variance in a particular domain into a handful of dimensions, they necessarily maximize the possibility of finding statistically significant relationships between some measure of the resulting factors and criterion variables in adjacent domains of study. In contrast, DSM-IV and DSM-5 PD constructs exist only within the realm of pathology, with no official endorsement of more normal variants that might encourage their application within related fields. Seventh, lexical factor models systematically force PD content experts to consider the breadth of personality. Because each factor constitutes a significant domain of content, it can be argued that PD prototypes need to be sketched against the canvas of the FFM (or some other inductive factor model) in order to ensure that essential content is not inadvertently excluded. For example, Widiger and his associates (Widiger & Mullins-Sweatt, 2009) have translated the PD prototypes into FFM traits. Each PD prototype is thereby anchored to what is (at first glance) universal and cross-cultural in human nature. Eighth, factor models support the term "personality pathology" over "personality disorder" as the name for our field. By failing to formally recognize specific pathological traits, the content of DSM-IV-TR PD-NOS was largely void and undescribed, despite its excessive prevalence. Ninth, factor models are explicitly mathematical and provide some assurance that the fuzzy domain of the social sciences can be quantified like the harder sciences of chemistry and physics. And tenth, there is little doubt that the FFM has provided important impetus to the study of abnormal personality, which had become a largely stagnant area controlled from the top down by DSM Work Groups. A certain level of controversy is necessary for an area to progress, and the hegemonic claims of the FFM have produced that healthy controversy and increased interest in the area.

Most of this chapter section is concerned with the FFM, as it represents the most persuasive exemplar of the inductive–lexical–factor–trait tradition. The FFM enjoys these benefits because it combines a philosophy of science, a data source, a methodology, and a dimensional representation of its constructs. Technically, the Big Five is lexically derived, while the FFM is lexically inspired—the facet traits were chosen by its authors to represent constructs of widespread interests to psychologists—but the criticisms of the two models are—from the perspective of this chapter—very similar, since both emphasize induction.

## Lack of "Stopping Rules"

In this chapter, we argue that both the advantages and disadvantages of any particular personality model are largely built into the model in advance, depending on the epistemic choices made. The strengths of any particular model are also its weaknesses. This suggests strategic lines of attack against any model, and also ways of defending against those attacks. We now apply this assertion to the FFM. Factor analysis is intended to telescope an existing set of variables into some smaller set. By factor-analyzing lexical trait terms, a much smaller set of variables is produced. The case can then be made—as it is by the FFM, the Big Five, and other lexical models of personality—that these constructs are fundamental.

Recall, however, that the main problem of any inductive model lies in making the transition from constructs that function merely as descriptive summaries to constructs that encode a scientific theory. As such, it is not clear that the FFM dimensions are fundamental or that they are the "best dimensions." And it may never be clear. The primary task of any science is to unify the phenomena of its subject domain, not merely catalogue them. By generating a taxonomy directly from some set of dimensions, a deductive theory explains why these particular disorders exist rather than others. The interpersonal circle thus argues that the transactions of any dyad can be explained in terms of the two dimensions of control and affiliation. What is fundamental is the space described by the dimensions. In Millon's (1990) evolutionary model, the theory justifies the existence of the taxonomy and promises that the taxonomy "carves nature" at the joints determined by the theory. If someone asks why these particular disorders are to be preferred, the answer is found in the underlying theory.

Why, then, are there five factors? What is special about the number five? According to McCrae and John (1998), the existence of five factors, rather than four or six, is simply a historical accident. Five major dimensions of personality are simply an enduring feature of our psychological world, just as seven continents are an enduring feature of our physical world. The contingent processes of evolution have produced five factors. Obviously, this suggests that the number of factors could change over evolutionary time. Perhaps it also suggests that the variance allocated between factors could change. As such, the question "Why are there five factors?" is not meaningful—at least, not meaningful if you are a proponent of the FFM. We are asked simply to accept the dimensions yielded by the methodology: There are five dimensions because five are what is found, and no deeper reason. From this perspective, factor analysis functions somewhat like the Hubble Space Telescope: Just as the larger and larger telescopes identify fainter and fainter objects, factor analysis can be seen as an empirical method of identifying smaller and smaller dimensions of human nature. Factor analysis becomes a systematic method for making distinctions. Essentially, it tells us the next distinction worth making. When the next distinction to be made is less significant than the facts at hand—when the eigenvalue of the next factor falls below 1.0, for example—extraction stops. The major features of the subject domain have been identified.

In practice, however, drawing the line at five or six factors, or seven factors, has proven to be somewhat arbitrary. This is a primary weakness of induction: There is always more that could be described. Someone always finds a way of justifying an additional factor. Ironically, an enormously rigorous methodology is employed in order to obtain a rigorous and empirically unassailable solution, yet as the distinctions become progressively finer—as the factors become slimmer—it gradually becomes apparent that there is no real solution to the number of factors problem. Yes, there is the eigenvalue greater than 1 criterion, the scree test (Cattell, 1966), parallel analysis (e.g., Fabrigar, Wegener, MacCallum, & Strahan, 1999) and perhaps other methods for choosing the number of factors. But there is no method of solving unequivocally the number of factors problem derived exclusively from within the data. Essentially, the variance accounted for by each successive factor progressively trails off. From the perspective of a deductive theoretical model—such as the interpersonal circle or Millon's model—factor analysis is likely to mistake small distinctions (small factors) as significant, and thereby extract too many dimensions. From a deductive theoretical perspective, it is the theory that dictates the number and nature of the dimensions.

Many important criticisms of the FFM derive from lack of "stopping rules" internal to the data. Famous among these is the content and name of the fifth factor. Terms noted by Goldberg (1993) in a Big Five context include Intellect and Intellectance (Hogan, 1986) and Culture (Norman, 1963). In the FFM, the fifth factor, Openness to Experience, is a pervasive motivation to examine and re-examine one's experiences (McCrae, 1994). We do not cover this debate again, except to note that PDs probably make more sense when discussed from a Big Five-like interpretation of Culture as the fifth factor. Culture is the product of advanced experiences with socialization, and to be uncultured is to lack such experiences. Synonyms of the term "uncultured" include "coarse," "ignorant," "crude," and "vulgar." All of these suggest a developmental failure of socialization. Early developmental pathology is an important feature generic to personality pathology. Someone whose personality is coarse, crude, and vulgar currently has no home in the FFM. The antagonism pole of the Agreeableness factor provides one possibility, but such a person—the "smiling buffoon" or "town fool"—need not be disagreeable. A broader interpretation of the fifth factor is therefore necessary. Perhaps for this reason, Openness is not generally recognized as being related to the personality categories of DSM-IV/5 (Schroeder, Wormworth, &

Livesley, 1992). Does this mean that only four dimensions are responsible for personality pathology? Does it mean that the DSM-IV/5 PD categories are lacking essential content related to intellect? Does it mean that the fifth factor of the FFM should be revised to better accord with the Big Five? These questions are hard to answer.

The Hexaco model provides another important example of the issues that inductive factor models have with stopping rules. Apparently, one man's noise is another man signal. In the Hexaco model, six factors are recognized instead of five. The sixth factor is named Honesty–Humility, which has dishonesty and arrogance as opposites. Lee and Ashton (2005) argue that the sixth factor is necessary, and that this sixth factor has been replicated "in eight independent lexical studies of personality structure conducted in seven languages: Dutch, French, German, Hungarian, Italian, Korean, and Polish" (p. 1573).

In other words, the number of factors extracted is strongly related to the culture in which the analyses are done. This has major implications—not only for a comprehensive inductive-factor model of personality—but also for the future of the Alternative Model, which has adopted a set of pathological personality domains loosely coordinated to the FFM. Apparently, the FFM and the Big Five model contain a significant cultural bias that results in a missing factor. If the aspiration of the DSM is to be cross-culturally valid, then logically, the DSM should adopt a six-factor instead of a five-factor model. This is not hair-splitting. Ethics require that clinicians determine the cultural frame of reference that is most appropriate for their clients. An FFM model put forward as a universal framework for personality pathology may conceal important dimensions of individual differences and therefore be implicitly unethical.

A related problem is inconsistency between the FFM and the Hexaco models at the level of their facet traits. Are the facets chosen to represent each factor of the model essentially arbitrary, or can some facets be shown to have some special status that makes them better than others? Inspection of the Hexaco model shows that most of the facets are different from those in the FFM. The FFM facets were chosen by Costa and McCrae (Costa, McCrae, & Dye, 1991) based on their appraisal of the importance and precedence of these factors in the personality questionnaire literature. In contrast, Lee and Ashton (2004) chose their facets explicitly because of their lexical roots. The Hexaco model, therefore, has stronger lexical credentials than the FFM. However, it is a more recent development and does not yet have the momentum of the FFM within the PD community.

How do we deal with the inconsistency between the FFM and the Hexaco model? One counterargument is that disagreement at the level of facet traits is unimportant. What is important is that the models agree on five of the six factors. Given that Widiger and associates have translated the PDs into the FFM facets, however, the arrival of another inductive model with stronger lexical roots than the FFM raises an important question: Are there facets of the Hexaco model that appear to be more strongly related than FFM facets to the PDs? The answer to this question is "yes." Research seeking the so-called "Dark Triad" traits—Psychopathy, Machiavellianism, and Narcissism—in the FFM and in the Hexaco model has shown the utility of the Honesty–Humility factor. Lee and Ashton (2005) concluded (p. 1571) that "correlations among the Dark Triad variables were explained satisfactorily by the HEXACO variables, but not by the Five-Factor Model." Thus, the Hexaco model shows that the FFM, for all its putative breadth of content, remains incomplete. A single example is not a gaping hole, but the fact that there is so little overlap between the FFM and Hexaco facets suggests that (1) additional factor models have much to add to contemporary trait models of the PDs, and (2) it would be premature to argue that any factor-analytic model of personality explains the PDs, since several factor-analytic models may be necessary simply to describe them. This further suggests that Widiger and Mullins-Sweatt's (2009) important research translating the PDs into FFM facets is incomplete and that an adequate description of the PDs requires that facets from a variety of factor models be pooled in order to eventually arrive at an adequate description. Paradoxically, it is important to apply the inductive method to the results of various inductive models in order to ensure we have an adequate description of the PDs, an ironic outcome considering all the methodological rigor that supposedly accompanies factor analysis. Perhaps the relevance of the Hexaco Dark Triad derives from the fact that Costa and McCrae (1992) cherry-picked the traits that were relevant in the literature at the time they created the FFM. Times change and other traits appear relevant now. Perhaps pooling the FFM and Hexaco traits could also shed light on whether six factors have more predictive power than five. The Dark Triad does seem to be an important component of personality pathology. As such, clinical significance argues that Honesty–Humility and its constituent traits deserve their own factor. This is not just a nuance or a tweak of the FFM. Instead, it is potentially a Pandora's Box that warns the field against prematurely settling on the FFM as an adequate description of abnormal personality. After all, the FFM is a "Big Five-ish" model that sought to supplement the lexical naiveté of the Big Five with the psychological sophistication of Costa and McCrae, who chose the facets for the FFM. Nevertheless, there is an important need to be as "purely lexical" as possible in order to determine (1) whether Costa and McCrae inadvertently omitted further PD content, as occurred with the Dark Triad traits, and (2) whether the Hexaco model might be better overall, simply because it is cross-cultural.

A related question is: Why six facets per factor or four facets per factor? In factor analysis, the first factor is always the largest. Each successive factor is somewhat smaller. A more scientifically accurate approach would be to abandon concerns with symmetry and make the number of facets within a factor proportional to its lexical importance. The factor that consumes the most lexical variance should have the most facets. The factor that consumes the least lexical variance should have the least facets. This suggests that in the FFM and Hexaco models, the larger factors—particularly Neuroticism—may be underpopulated with facets, while the smaller factors may be overpopulated with facets. Underrepresentation is the greater problem, since facets important in describing the PDs may currently be omitted from the larger factors. By presenting the number of facet traits as equal across factors, this important problem of inductive models is hidden beneath a façade of symmetry.

And finally, it is not clear that lexical models have converged on a cross-culturally valid representation of personality. When presenting the advantages of the FFM for personality disorders, cross-cultural validity is frequently cited. However, it appears that this may be more myth than reality. De Raad, Barelds, Timmerman, De Roover, Mlačić, and Church (2014) merged data from 11 lexical studies of personality. They judged only three factors as being cross-cultural, namely, dynamism, affiliation, and order. The authors offer the following definitions (p. 499). Dynamism refers to "the condition of being a competent individual, and it is manifested in determined action, versatility, effective communication, and entrepreneurship." This factor includes traits such as "dynamic, sociable, enterprising, and extraverted versus withdrawn, timid, taciturn, and introverted." Affiliation refers to "the condition of being part of a larger social entity or group, [as] manifested in strivings for intimacy, union, and solidarity within that larger entity," and includes traits such as "kind, helpful, sympathetic, peaceful, and compassionate versus egoistic, quarrelsome, domineering, and aggressive." Order refers to "the condition to disambiguate the mind and the environment, and it is manifested in striving for order, stability, regulations, and precision"; it includes traits such as "thorough, consistent, organized, and conscientious versus unsystematic rebellious, lazy, illogical, and chaotic."

Saucier (2009) noted that lexical studies in Chinese, English, Filipino, Greek, Hebrew, Spanish, and Turkish appeared to converge on six recurrent factors using a relatively narrow sample of lexical attributes. Sampling a broader range of attributes that included evaluative terms (e.g., "great," "awful"), Saucier found a "wideband cross-language six" (WCL6) structure, which outperformed the Big Five in predicting dissociative tendencies, obsessive–compulsive symptoms, borderline personality, self-assessed health status, depression, mental health history and medical history, compulsive drinking, risk-taking after drinking, law breaking, and phobias. Smoking was the only criterion variable not better predicted by the WCL6. The WCL6 includes Conscientiousness, Honesty (or Propriety/Non-Violativeness), Agreeableness, Resiliency (or if reversed, Emotionality), Extraversion, and Intellect/Openness (or Originality/Talent). Since "carving nature at its joints" necessarily involves predicting external criteria, it would seem that Saucier's WCL6 structure comes closer to carving nature than does the Big Five, and by implication, the FFM. If the DSM-5 Alternative Model seeks to be cross-cultural, then logically, the WCL6 may provide an excellent point of departure. Perhaps the 25 Alternative Model traits can be fit within the WCL6 structure.

## Where Do the PDs Come From?

If we assume that factor analysis has already revealed the major dimensions of normal and abnormal personality, then why is it that the PDs, considered dimensionally, do not line up neatly with the factors? For each factor in both the FFM and the Hexaco model, one pole is considered more adaptive and the other pole is considered more maladaptive. Neuroticism (vs. Emotional Stability), Introversion (vs. Extraversion), Antagonism (vs. Agreeableness), Disinhibition (vs. Conscientiousness) and Rigidity (vs. Openness to Experience) represent acceptable names for the maladaptive poles in the FFM. To this, the Hexaco model would add the Dark Trial traits as the maladaptive pole of Honesty–Humility. Why is it that the various DSM Work Groups have not identified a Neurotic personality, an Introverted personality, an Antagonistic personality, a Disinhibited and Overconscientious personality, and a Rigid (from the FFM perspective) or Uncultured (from a Big Five perspective) personality? As world experts in abnormal personality, surely the members of the various Work Groups from DSM-II through DSM-5 were clinically sensitive enough to these "main effects" to recognize their pathological influence. Or, are we required to believe that factor analysis exceeds human clinical intuition, to the extent that even our best experts have ignored the most obvious dimensions of human nature as extracted by factor analysis, and have done so for many decades? This seems impossible, if not absurd, but if it is indeed the case, then it requires an explanation. Perhaps all clinical taxonomies should be created methodologically. Perhaps human beings are just not up to the task of constructing taxonomies with the scope and depth of the DSMs.

## The Lexical Hypothesis: Inspiration and Limitation

The lexical hypothesis states that all important dimensions of individual differences are already encoded in the language (Pervin, 1994). As such, the dictionary provides the greatest reservoir of personality trait terms, and sampling traits from the dictionary becomes the primary means of constructing a pool of trait adjectives. Induction first asks what the world has in it.

Preconceived notions are rejected. The results are thus mostly a product of our sampling methods, and it is by copious and comprehensive sampling that we obtain the intellectual security that nothing has been left out, that every aspect of the subject domain has been scrutinized, and that the factor-analytic results represent truth. Factor analysis provides the means to systematize or categorize these observations, and the extracted factors are assumed to represents the fundamental dimensions of personality.

However, factor models typically rely on self-report, and as such, are limited by the average ability of subjects in the sample to reflect on their characteristics and report accurately. Could the degree to which the self-schema is elaborated moderate the results of lexical studies? The idea that complexity of self-representation is important in personality is by no means new. Linville (1985, 1987) showed that less complex representations of the self construct were associated with greater emotional lability and indicated greater vulnerability to depression, as shown by subjects' reactions to success and failure experiences. Self-complexity was interpreted as a buffer against the effects of stressful life events. A simplistic self-concept leads to more extreme evaluations. A complex self-concept leads to more nuanced evaluations, which protect mood against the "totalizing effects" of global interpretations. Complexity of self-representation is therefore related to at least two DSM-5 alternative model traits, namely, Emotional Lability and Depressivity. Research in cognitive complexity proposes that the ability to make psychological distinctions mediates the number of factors extracted in a lexical analysis. If the five factors are "out there" in reality, then samples of individuals capable of making fine distinctions should return a cleaner five-factor structure rather than more factors. This is not what happens. Bowler, Bowler, and Phillips (2009) administered Goldberg's 100 unipolar Big Five markers (20 per factor) along with the computer version of the Construct Repertory Test (CRT). In the CRT, subjects identity 10 people who correspond to 10 life roles (e.g., yourself, a person you dislike, your mother, your father). Each person is then rated on 10 adjectives, each on a 6-point Likert scale. The number of matching ratings is multiplied by 2 points. This is added to the number of ratings within 1 point, yielding a measure of cognitive complexity. The underlying idea is that more nuanced perceptions indicate complexity and should yield more diverse ratings. Factor analyses of the low-complexity, average-complexity, and high-complexity groups yielded three, five, and seven factors, respectively. Pressed to its logical conclusion, cognitive complexity argues that subjects incapable of making important personality-related distinctions "have a three-factor mind," while subjects exceptionally capable of making such distinctions "have a seven-factor mind."

Moreover, these results were obtained with Big Five markers, explicitly chosen to reproduce the Big Five. If factor analysis is the "lexical telescope" that it is intended to be, subjects capable of making fine distinctions should be able to discern significant dimensions of individual differences that, for most people, would simply be lost in the background noise. To the naked eye, a faint star becomes lost in the heavens that surround it. Hence, the telescope. As such, it is necessary to identify such subjects who possess seven- or even eight-factor minds, then repeat large-scale lexical studies in order to determine the last meaningful distinction that these cognitively complex and psychologically minded individuals are able to make. That becomes the last significant personality factor. These factors can then be given facets in proportion to the amount of variance they represent, thereby disclosing the limitations of their inductive origins. Otherwise, there is a legitimate possibility that the field will continue to standardize on five factors, while neglecting at least two additional and independent domains of content. If that sounds absurd, it probably is. At the same time, it is a conclusion consistent with the overarching philosophy of the inductive approach, whereby stopping rules should be derived from considerations internal to the data alone.

## The Causal Status of the Factors

Imagine that your car needs servicing. Arriving at the mechanic shop, you see three lines, one with red cars of various shades, one with blue cars of various shades, and one with yellow cars of various shades. A man greets you. "Sir, please wait your turn in the red line to receive the red treatment." Seeing your astonishment, the man elaborates, "You have a red car, and therefore you will receive the red treatment." "But I think it's the engine," you protest, "Perhaps we should lift the hood." "No," he says, "We've never been able to figure out what's in there . . . it's much better that we group cars in terms of their color. We've looked at cars in every culture, and they are mainly red, yellow, and blue." "But that's silly, there's a noise coming from the engine," you say. The man shrugs. "It's the best we can do." This little parable captures the main criticism of induction: that it yields clusters or dimensions of superficial similarities, without capturing the inner causative structures that actually compose personality. To what extent is Introversion–Extraversion causative of behavior? To what extent is Honesty–Humility causative of behavior? Presumably, psychotherapy based on the FFM or the Hexaco model, then, would be like receiving the "red treatment."

## Rebuttals to Criticism

Our purpose in this chapter is to understand the structure of argumentation between various personality models. At the beginning of the chapter, we argued that the strengths and weaknesses of various models of personality sort together according to epistemic assumptions made along three dimensions. We also argued that much of what happens in contemporary debates about abnormal personality is not about empirical evidence, but instead about making arguments that accord with paradigmatic assumptions. The idea that personality traits should be dimensional, and, therefore, that the DSM should embrace a dimensional model is one such example. One might say that because personality is composed of traits, personality pathology should be concerned with pathological traits. There is nothing empirical about this argument.

An important problem of inductive models is the absence of stopping rules. A few major dimensions are extracted, after which the significance of additional dimensions wanes dramatically. From the perspective of deductive models of personality, such as the interpersonal circle and Millon's model, the FFM and the Hexaco model contain too many dimensions.

Even if we believe that factor models of personality are purely descriptive—that they never successfully make the transit from description to explanation—they nevertheless provide an important threshold against which the success of theory should be evaluated. Earlier, we cited

Saucier's work with the WCL6, which showed that the WCL6 substantially increments the FFM in predicting a variety of important external criteria. The WCL6 therefore makes a more convincing claim to "carve nature at its joints" than does the FFM. If a theory is to be explanatory rather than descriptive, shouldn't the theory prove its mettle by showing its greater predictive power relative to the best descriptive models considered as a baseline? By this reasoning, even if we reject factor models of personality as carving nature, they nevertheless serve as an important gadfly for theory, which has as one of its own shortcomings a tendency to degenerate into self-satisfied delusion.

Another important thrust of the inductive agenda could be to question the strategy of identifying latent variables. All approaches to personality described in this chapter have in common the desire to explain a great variety of manifest observations with some small number of latent variables at all. Science typically assumes that the number of latent variables is smaller than the number of manifest variables, parsimony being an important scientific value. What happens if the number of latent variables (e.g., gene combinations interacting with parenting styles interacting with peer influences interacting with random events) is actually equal to or larger than the number of manifest variables? What if the interactions are so diverse that the impact of the original latent variables is highly diluted, or completely obscured? In this case, there are no explanations in the traditional scientific sense because there are no joints in nature to be carved (effect sizes in published research are typically small). There is only cataloguing and organizing observations, which factor analysis readily accomplishes. If we accept that description is the best we can do, then what is important is not explaining but modeling. Chemistry has as its taxonomy the Periodic Table, the structure of which is dictated by electrons in their quantum orbitals. Step up to biology, and there is the Tree of Life, which has no necessary structure. Historical contingency becomes paramount. Without any particular asteroid, comet, or volcanic eruption to wipe out the dinosaurs and cause other mass extensions, the structure of the Tree of Life would look far different. Step up another level to psychology. Surely whatever taxonomy is appropriate for personality has an even more contingent and arbitrary structure than biology's Tree of Life. A factor-analytic model that at least structures the data into more or less orthogonal dimensions is at least as convenient as any other taxonomy.

## Conclusion

Personality, both normal and abnormal, is awash in models. Fortunately, theoretical models can at least be grouped in terms of various domains—biophysical, interpersonal, cognitive, psychodynamic, existential, evolutionary, and so on. Because the purpose of science is to test models against reality in order to better approximate the truth, an overabundance of models is discouraging. Moreover, recent attempts to replicate the findings of 100 studies published in three leading psychology journals suggests that empirical research is misleading at least as often as it is clarifying. Accordingly, it is necessary to understand the underlying properties of the paradigms that spawn empirical studies in the first place.

Millon's (1990) evolutionary model provides one way of generating the classical personality disorders of DSM-III through DSM-IV-TR. The various perspectives on personality—biophysical, cognitive, psychodynamic, and interpersonal—suggest content domains through which the PDs can be described in accordance with the theory. A table of descriptors was provided for narcissistic PD.

The promise of the lexical factor models was to bypass theoretical models by identifying cross-culturally valid dimensions of personality through more pure science methods. Unfortunately, the cross-cultural generalizability of the Big Five model seems to have been exaggerated. With the Big Five now surpassed by the cross-cultural generalizability of the Hexaco and other models, the Big Five—and by extension, the FFM—seem inappropriate for abnormal personality as well. Since translations of the PDs into the language of the FFM is a direction with enormous momentum, it is important to reconsider the PDs in terms of more purely lexical perspective. Hierarchical lexical models such as the Hexaco include facet traits that differ dramatically from the FFM. As such, the adoption of five trait domains in the alternative model, loosely coordinated to the FFM, may be premature and culturally biased.

Theory and induction are complementary. Both seek to determine "the truth," but their methods are different. Ideally, theory-driven (top-down) and observation-driven (bottom-up) approaches would converge on some single result. Unfortunately, this has not yet happened. Because paradigms determine what counts as evidentiary, it appears that personality follows more the philosophy of science of Thomas Kuhn than it does that of Karl Popper (1959), who advocated falsifying theories. Both theoretical and inductive approaches appear to have a large enough ratio of advantages to disadvantages to weather many cycles of criticism and sustain themselves indefinitely. Nevertheless, we argue that this criticism will possess a structure determined by certain epistemic choices, as we have described in this chapter.

## REFERENCES

Allport, G. W., & Odbert, H. S. (1936). Trait-names: A psycho-lexical study. *Psychological Monographs, 47*(1), i–171.

Beck, A. T., Davis, D. D., & Freeman, A. (2014). *Cognitive therapy of personality disorders* (3rd ed.). New York: Guilford Press.

Benjamin, L. S. (1974). Structured analysis of social behavior. *Psychological Review, 81,* 392–425.

Benjamin, L. S. (1986). Adding social and intrapsychic descriptors to Axis I of DSM-III. In T. Millon & G. Klerman (Eds.), *Contemporary directions in psychopathology: Toward the DSM-IV.* New York: Guilford Press.

Benjamin, L. S. (1996). *Interpersonal diagnosis and treatment of personality disorders.* New York: Guilford Press.

Block, J. (1995). A contrarian view of the five-factor approach to personality description. *Psychological Bulletin, 117,* 187–215.

Bornstein, R. F. (1993). *The dependent personality.* New York: Guilford Press.

Bowler, M. C., Bowler, J. L., & Phillips, B. C. (2009). The Big-5 ± 2?: The impact of cognitive complexity on the factor structure of the five-factor model. *Personality and Individual Differences, 47*(8), 979–984.

Cattell, R. B. (1966). The scree test for the number of factors. *Multivariate Behavioral Research, 1*(2), 245–276.

Cattell, R. B., Eber, H. W., & Tatsuoka, M. M. (1970). *Handbook for the Sixteen Personality Factor Questionnaire (16 PF): In clinical, educational, industrial, and research psychology, for use with all forms of the test.* Savoy, IL: Institute for Personality and Ability Testing.

Costa, P. T., Jr., & McCrae, R. R. (1978). Objective personality assessment. In M. Storandt, I. C. Siegler, & M. F. Elias (Eds.), *The clinical psychology of aging* (pp. 119–143). New York: Plenum Press.

Costa, P. T., Jr., & McCrae, R. R. (1980). Still stable after all these years: Personality as a key to some issues in adulthood and old age. In P. B. Baltes & O. G. Brim, Jr. (Eds.), *Life span development and behavior* (Vol. 3, pp. 65–102). New York: Academic Press.

Costa, P. T., Jr., & McCrae, R. R. (1985). *The NEO personality inventory: Manual, form S and form R.* Odessa, FL: Psychological Assessment Resources.

Costa, P. T., Jr., & McCrae, R. R. (1992). The five-factor model of personality and its relevance to personality disorders. *Journal of Personality Disorders, 6*(4), 343–359.

Costa, P. T., Jr., McCrae, R. R., & Dye, D. A. (1991). Facet scales for agreeableness and conscientiousness: A revision of the NEO Personality Inventory. *Personality and Individual Differences, 12*(9), 887–898.

De Raad, B., Barelds, D. P., Timmerman, M. E., De Roover, K., Mlačić, B., & Church, A. T. (2014). Towards a pan-cultural personality structure: Input from 11 psycholexical studies. *European Journal of Personality, 28*(5), 497–510.

Dougherty, J. W. D. (1978). Salience and relativity in classification. *American Ethnologist, 5,* 66–80.

Fabrigar, L. R., Wegener, D. T., MacCallum, R. C., & Strahan, E. J. (1999). Evaluating the use of exploratory factor analysis in psychological research. *Psychological Methods, 4*(3), 272–299.

Freedman, M. B., Leary, T., Ossorio, A. G., & Coffey, H. S. (1951). The interpersonal dimension of personality. *Journal of Personality, 20,* 143–161.

Galton, F. (1884). Measurement of character. *Fortnightly Review, 36,* 179–185.

Gilligan, C. (1981). *In a different voice.* Cambridge, MA: Harvard University Press.

Goldberg, L. R. (1993). The structure of phenotypic personality traits. *American Psychologist, 48,* 26–34.

Hempel, C. G. (1965). *Aspects of scientific explanation.* New York: Free Press.

Hogan, R. (1986). *Manual for the Hogan Personality Inventory.* Minneapolis, MN: National Computer Systems.

Horowitz, M. J. E. (1991). *Hysterical personality style and the histrionic personality disorder* (rev. ed.). Northvale, NJ: Jason Aronson.

Ioannidis, J. P. A. (2005). Why most published research findings are false. *PLOS Medicine, 2,* 696–701.

John, O. P., Naumann, L. P., & Soto, C. J. (2008). Paradigm shift to the integrative Big Five trait taxonomy. In O. P. John, R. W. Robins, & L. A. Pervin (Eds.), *Handbook of personality: Theory and research* (3rd ed., pp. 114–158). New York: Guilford Press.

Kohut, H. (1971). *The analysis of self.* New York: International Universities Press.

Kuhn, T. S. (1975). *The structure of scientific revolutions* (2nd ed.). Chicago: University of Chicago Press.

Leary, T. (1957). *Interpersonal diagnosis of personality: A functional theory and methodology for personality evaluation.* New York: Ronald Press.

Lee, K., & Ashton, M. C. (2004). Psychometric properties of the HEXACO Personality Inventory. *Multivariate Behavioral Research, 39,* 329–358.

Lee, K., & Ashton, M. C. (2005). Psychopathy, Machiavellianism, and narcissism in the five-factor model and the HEXACO model of personality structure. *Personality and Individual Differences, 38*(7), 1571–1582.

Lieb, K., Zanarini, M. C., Schmahl, C., Linehan, M. M., & Bohus, M. (2004). Borderline personality disorder. *Lancet, 364,* 453–461.

Linehan, M. M. (1993). *Cognitive-behavioral treatment of borderline personality disorder.* New York: Guilford Press.

Linville, P. W. (1985). Self-complexity and affective extremity: Don't put all of your eggs in one cognitive basket. *Social Cognition, 3*(1), 94–120.

Linville, P. W. (1987). Self-complexity as a cognitive buffer against stress-related illness and depression. *Journal of Personality and Social Psychology, 12*(4), 663–676.

McCrae, R. R. (1994). Openness to experience: Expanding the boundaries of Factor V. *European Journal of Personality, 8*(4), 251–272.

McCrae, R. R., Costa, Jr., P. T., & Martin, T. A. (2005). The NEO–PI–3: A more readable Revised NEO Personality Inventory. *Journal of Personality Assessment, 84*(3), 261–270.

McCrae, R. R., & John, O. P. (1998). An introduction to the five-factor model and its applications. *Personality: Critical Concepts in Psychology, 60,* 175–215.

McWilliams, N. (2011). *Psychoanalytic diagnosis: Understanding personality structure in the clinical process* (2nd ed.). New York: Guilford Press.

Meehl, P. E. (1978). Theoretical risks and tabular asterisks: Sir Karl, Sir Ronald, and the slow progress of soft psychology. *Journal of Consulting and Clinical Psychology, 46*(4), 806–834.

Millon, T. (n.d.). Domains of the confident-narcissistic personality. Retrieved September 7, 2017, from *www.millonpersonality.com/theory/diagnostic-taxonomy/narcissistic.htm.*

Millon, T. (1981). *Disorders of personality: DSM-III, Axis II.* New York: Wiley-Interscience.

Millon, T. (1990). *Toward a new personology: An evolutionary model.* New York: Wiley.

Millon, T. (2011). *Disorders of personality.* Hoboken, NJ: Wiley.

Millon, T., with Davis, R. D. (1996). *Disorders of personality.* Hoboken, NJ: Wiley.

Norman, W. T. (1963). Toward an adequate taxonomy of personality attributes: Replicated factor structure in peer nomination personality ratings. *Journal of Abnormal and Social Psychology, 66,* 574–583.

Open Science Collaboration. (2012). An open, large-scale, collaborative effort to estimate the reproducibility of psychological science. *Perspectives on Psychological Science, 7*(6), 657–660.

Open Science Collaboration. (2015). Estimating the reproducibility of psychological science. *Science, 349,* No. 6251.

Pervin, L. A. (1994). A critical analysis of current trait theory. *Psychological Inquiry, 5*(2), 103–113.

Popper, K. R. (1959). *The logic of scientific discovery.* New York: Routledge.

Quine, W. V. O. (1977). Natural kinds. In S. P. Schwartz (Ed.), *Naming, necessity, and natural groups* (pp. 155–175). Ithaca, NY: Cornell University Press.

Ronningstam, E. F. (2005). *Identifying and understanding the narcissistic personality.* New York: Oxford University Press.

Rounsaville, B. J., Alarcon, R. D., Andrews, G., Jackson, J. S., Kendell, R. E., & Kendler, K. (2002). Basic nomenclature issues for DSM-5. In D. J. Kupfer, M. B. First, & D. E. Regier (Eds.), *A research agenda for DSM-5* (pp. 1–29). Washington, DC: American Psychiatric Association.

Rushton, J. P. (1985). Differential K theory: The sociobiology of individual and group differences. *Personality and Individual Differences, 6,* 441–452.

Saucier, G. (2009). Recurrent personality dimensions in inclusive lexical studies: Indications for a Big Six structure. *Journal of Personality, 77*(5), 1577–1614.

Schaefer, E. (1965). Configurational analysis of children's report of parent behavior. *Journal of Consulting Psychology, 29,* 552–557.

Schroeder, M. L., Wormworth, J. A., & Livesley, W. J. (1992). Dimensions of personality disorder and their relationships to the Big Five dimensions of personality. *Psychological Assessment, 4*(1), 47–53.

Tversky, A. (1977). Features of similarity. *Psychological Review, 84,* 327–352.

Widiger, T. A. (1993). The DSM-III-R categorical personality disorder diagnoses: A critique and an alternative. *Psychological Inquiry, 4*(2), 75–90.

Widiger, T. A., & Mullins-Sweatt, S. N. (2009). Five-factor model of personality disorder: A proposal for DSM-V. *Annual Review of Clinical Psychology, 5,* 197–220.

Wilson, E. O. (1978). *On human nature.* Cambridge, MA: Harvard University Press.

Zachar, P., & Kendler, K. S. (2010). Philosophical issues in the classification of psychopathology. In T. Millon, R. F. Krueger, & E. Simonsen (Eds.), *Contemporary directions in psychopathology: Scientific foundations of the DSM-V and ICD-11* (pp. 126–148). New York: Guilford Press.

# CHAPTER 3

# Official Classification Systems

Thomas A. Widiger

Disorders of personality are of a concern to many different professions and agencies, whose participants hold an equally diverse array of beliefs regarding etiology, pathology, and treatment. It is imperative that these persons be able to communicate meaningfully with one another. Markon (2013) argued against the existence of a uniform, authoritative diagnostic system, but imagine if clinicians were free to use whatever personality disorder (PD) classification they preferred. Even if in some cases they used the same diagnosis (which is unlikely), they would probably use very different criteria to determine its presence. The primary purpose of an official classification system is to provide a common language of communication (Kendell, 1975; Sartorius et al., 1993; Widiger, 2001). The current languages of modern psychiatry are the fifth edition of the American Psychiatric Association's (APA) *Diagnostic and Statistical Manual of Mental Disorders* (DSM-5; 2013) and the 10th edition of the World Health Organization's (WHO) *International Classification of Diseases* (ICD-10; 1992) (albeit by the time this book is published there will likely be an 11th edition of the ICD; Tyrer et al., 2011, 2014).

A common language of PD classification is also necessary for scientific research. It would be difficult to accumulate a body of knowledge regarding respective PDs if each researcher used his or her own idiosyncratic system. Of course, an authoritative diagnostic nomenclature, such as DSM-5 or ICD-11, might in principle hinder creativity, innovation, and scientific progress to the extent that it stifled the consideration of alternative conceptualizations.

Hyman (2010), past Director of the National Institute of Mental Health (NIMH), indeed argued that the existing APA nomenclature was hindering productive research because of the perceived necessity of studies to adhere to its structure and content. However, it would appear that NIMH was not so much against requiring a common language of communication. NIMH just did not care for the language of DSM-IV. NIMH has now produced its own authoritative nomenclature, strongly encouraging persons who wish to receive funding to adhere to their Research Domain Criteria (Insel, 2013).

It is in fact debatable whether the APA or forthcoming ICD-11 diagnostic nomenclatures will actually stifle scientific research concerning alternative nomenclatures and constructs. The APA nomenclature has largely served as a useful foil, a point of common comparison. Researchers have been free to assert through argument and research that their own version of a respective diagnostic construct is preferable to that provided within the manual. For example, there has clearly been quite a bit of productive research on psychopathy, much of which has been in direct contrast with the APA diagnosis of antisocial personality disorder (ASPD) (Crego & Widiger, 2015; Hare & Neumann, 2008). There is also now a considerable body of research on alternative dimensional trait models that have been effectively compared to the APA diagnostic categories (Widiger & Simonsen, 2005). It would even appear that the ICD-11 personality disorder nomenclature may not include any of the ICD-10 (or DSM-IV) diagnostic categories (Tyrer et al., 2011, 2014), hardly a suggestion of a hegemonic APA or ICD-10 stifling alternative systems.

My purpose in this chapter is to describe and discuss the historical development of the DSM and ICD official classifications of PD. The chapter begins with an historical overview, followed by a discussion of the controversies that beset the development of DSM-5, as well as a comparison with the likely ICD-11. The chapter ends with suggestions for future research.

## Historical Overview

PD classifications have been evident throughout the history of psychology, psychiatry, and medicine (Millon, 2011). The impetus for the development of an official, uniform nomenclature was the crippling confusion that existed as a result of the absence of any such authoritative system (Widiger, 2001). "For a long time confusion reigned. Every self-respecting alienist [the 19th-century term for a psychiatrist], and certainly every professor, had his own classification" (Kendell, 1975, p. 87). The production of a new system for classifying psychopathology was essentially a rite of passage for the young, aspiring professor.

> To produce a well-ordered classification almost seems to have become the unspoken ambition of every psychiatrist of industry and promise, [just] as it is the ambition of a good tenor to strike a high C. This classificatory ambition was so conspicuous that the composer Berlioz was prompted to remark that after their studies have been completed a rhetorician writes a tragedy and a psychiatrist a classification. (Zilboorg, 1941, p. 450)

Initial efforts to develop a uniform language, though, did not meet with much success. The Statistical Committee of the British Royal Medico-Psychological Association had produced a classification in 1892, and conducted formal revisions in 1904, 1905, and 1906. However, "the Association finally accepted the unpalatable fact that most of its members were not prepared to restrict themselves to diagnoses listed in any official nomenclature" (Kendell, 1975, p. 88). The Association of Medical Superintendents of American Institutions for the Insane (the forerunner to the APA) adopted a slightly modified version of the British nomenclature in 1886, but it was no more successful in getting its membership to use it.

The U.S. Bureau of the Census struggled to obtain national statistics in the absence of an officially recognized nomenclature (Grob, 1991). In 1908, it asked the American Medico-Psychological Association (which changed its name to the American Psychiatric Association in 1921) to appoint a Committee on Nomenclature of Diseases to develop a standard nosology. This committee affirmed in 1917 the need for an authoritative diagnostic system.

> The importance and need of some system whereby uniformity in reports would be secured have been repeatedly emphasized by officers and members of this Association, by statisticians of the United States Census Bureau, by editors of psychiatric journals. . . . The present condition with respect to the classification of mental diseases is chaotic. Some states use no well-defined classification. In others the classifications used are similar in many respects but differ enough to prevent accurate comparisons. Some states have adopted a uniform system, while others leave the matter entirely to the individual hospitals. This condition of affairs discredits the science of psychiatry. (Salmon, Copp, May, Abbot, & Cotton, 1917, pp. 255–256)

The American Medico-Psychological Association, in collaboration with the National Committee for Mental Hygiene, issued a nosology in 1918, titled *Statistical Manual for the Use of Institutions for the Insane* (Grob, 1991; Menninger, 1963). The National Committee for Mental Hygiene—formed by Clifford Beers (a Wall Street financier who had suffered from bipolar mood disorder), psychologist Williams James, and psychiatrist Adolf Meyer—published and distributed the nosology. This nomenclature was of use to the census, but many hospitals failed to adopt the system for clinical practice, in part because of its narrow representation. There were only 22 diagnoses, and they were confined largely to psychoses with a presumably neurobiological pathology (the closest to PDs were conditions within the category of "not insane," which included drug addiction without psychosis and constitutional psychopathic inferiority without psychosis; Salmon et al., 1917). Confusion continued to be the norm (Blashfield, Keeley, Flanagan, & Miles, 2014). "In the late twenties, each large teaching center employed a system of its own origination, no one of which met more than the immediate needs of the local institution. . . . There resulted a polyglot of diagnostic labels and systems, effectively blocking communication" (APA, 1952, p. v).

A conference was held at the New York Academy of Medicine in 1928, with representatives from a number of different mental health professions as well as governmental agencies. A trial edition of a proposed nomenclature (modeled after the *Statistical Manual*) was distributed to hospitals in 1932 within the American Medical Association's *Standard Classified Nomenclature of Disease*. Most hospitals and teaching centers used this system, or at least a modified version that was compatible with the perspectives of the clinicians at a particular center.

However, the *Standard Nomenclature* proved to be grossly inadequate when the attention of mental health professionals expanded beyond the severe "organic" psychopathologies to address the many casualties of the World War II (Grob, 1991). "Military psychiatrists, induction station psychiatrists, and Veterans Administration psychiatrists, found themselves operating within the limits of a nomenclature specifically not designed for 90% of the cases handled" (APA, 1952, p. vi). Of particular importance was the inadequate coverage of somatoform, stress reaction, and PDs. As a result, the Navy, the Army, the Veterans Administration, and the Armed Forces each developed their own nomenclatures during World War II.

## ICD-6 and DSM-I

Two medical statisticians, William Farr in London and Jacques Bertillon in Paris, had convinced the International Statistical Congress in 1853 of the importance to produce a uniform classification of causes of death. A classification system was eventually developed by Farr, Bertillon, and Marc d'Espine (of Geneva). The benefits of the *Bertillon Classification of Causes of Death* became immediately evident to many public health care agencies. In 1889, the International Statistical Institute urged that the task of sponsoring and revising this nomenclature be accepted by a more official governing agency. The French government therefore convened a series of international conferences in Paris in 1900, 1920, 1929, and 1938, producing successive revisions to the *International List of Causes of Death*.

The WHO accepted the authority to produce the sixth edition of the International List, renamed in 1948 as the *International Statistical Classification of Diseases, Injuries, and Causes of Death* (Kendell, 1975). It was no coincidence that this occurred soon after World War II, during which it had become very apparent that clinicians from different countries needed to be using a common nomenclature, including one for the classification and communication of psychopathology. It is at times stated that this sixth edition was the first to include mental disorders. However, mental disorders had been included within the 1938 fifth edition within the section for Diseases of the Nervous System and Sense Organs (Kramer, Sartorius, Jablensky, & Gulbinat, 1979). Within this section were the four subcategories of dementia praecox, manic–depressive psychosis, mental deficiency, and other mental disorders. Several other mental disorders (e.g., alcoholism) were also included within other sections of the manual. The ICD-6, though, was the first to include a specific (and greatly expanded) section devoted to the diagnosis of mental disorders (Kendell, 1975; Kramer et al., 1979). However, the "mental disorders section [of ICD-6] failed to gain acceptance and eleven years later was found to be in official use only in Finland, New Zealand, Peru, Thailand, and the United Kingdom" (Kendell, 1975, p. 91).

The ICD-6 had attempted to be responsive to the needs of the war veterans. As acknowledged by the APA (1952), the ICD-6 "categorized mental disorders in rubrics similar to those of the Armed Forces nomenclature" (p. vii). One specific absence from the ICD-6, though, was a diagnosis for passive–aggressive PD, which was the most frequently diagnosed PD by American psychiatrists during the war, accounting for 6% of all admissions to Army hospitals (Malinow, 1981; Wetzler & Jose, 2012).

The U.S. Public Health Service commissioned a committee, chaired by George Raines, with representation from a variety of professional and public health associations, to develop a variant of ICD-6 for use within the United States. This nomenclature was coordinated with ICD-6, but it resembled more closely the Veterans Administration system developed by William Menninger. Although a number of different professional agencies were involved in its development, responsibility for publishing and distributing the nosology was provided to the APA (1952) under the title, *Diagnostic and Statistical Manual: Mental Disorders* (hereafter referred to as DSM-I).

Disorders of personality were organized into three sections (see Table 3.1). There were the personality pattern disturbances (e.g., schizoid,

**TABLE 3.1. PD Diagnoses in Each Edition of the APA's DSM**

| DSM-I | DSM-II | DSM-III | DSM-III-R | DSM-IV-TR | DSM-5 proposals |
|---|---|---|---|---|---|
| **Personality pattern disturbance** | | | | | |
| Inadaquate | Inadaquate | | | | |
| Schizoid | Schizoid | Schizoid | Schizoid | Schizoid | |
| Cyclothymic | Cyclothymic | | | | |
| Paranoid | Paranoid | Paranoid | Paranoid | Paranoid | |
| | | Schizotypal | Schizotypal | Schizotypal | Schizotypal |
| **Personality trait disturbance** | | | | | |
| Emotionally unstable | Hysterical | Histrionic | Histrionic | Histrionic | |
| | | Borderline | Borderline | Borderline | Borderline |
| Compulsive | Obsessive–compulsive | Compulsive | Obsessive–compulsive | Obsessive–compulsive | Obsessive–compulsive |
| Passive–aggressive | | | | | |
| Passive–dependent subtype | | Dependent | Dependent | Dependent | |
| Passive–aggressive subtype | Passive–aggressive | Passive–aggressive | Passive–aggressive | | |
| Aggressive subtype | | | | | |
| | Explosive | | | | |
| | Aesthenic | | | | |
| | | Avoidant | Avoidant | Avoidant | Avoidant |
| | | Narcissistic | Narcissistic | Narcissistic | |
| **Sociopathic personality disturbance** | | | | | |
| Antisocial reaction | Antisocial | Antisocial | Antisocial | Antisocial | Antisocial Psychopathic |
| Dyssocial reaction | | | | | |
| Sexual deviation | | | | | |
| Addiction | | | | | |
| | | | _Appendix_ | _Appendix_ | |
| | | | Self-defeating | Negativistic | |
| | | | Sadistic | Depressive | |

cyclothymic, and paranoid); the personality trait disturbances (e.g., emotionally unstable, compulsive, and passive–aggressive); and the sociopathic personality disturbance (e.g., antisocial reaction, sexual deviation, and addiction).

DSM-I was more successful than the previously published *Standard Classified Nomenclature of Disease* in obtaining acceptance across a wide variety of clinical settings, due in large part to its inclusion of the many new psychological (rather than neurobiological) diagnoses of considerable interest to practicing clinicians. In addition, DSM-I, unlike ICD-6, included brief narrative descriptions of each condition, which facilitated a uniform understanding of the meaning, intention, and application of the diagnoses.

DSM-I, however, was not without significant opposition. The New York State Department of Mental Hygiene, which had been influential in the development of the original standard nomenclature, continued for some time to use its own classification. Fundamental objections and criticisms regarding the reliability and validity of psychiatric diagnoses were also being raised (e.g., Zigler & Phillips, 1961). For example, in a widely cited reliability study, Ward, Beck, Mendelson, Mock, and Erbaugh (1962) concluded that most of the poor agreement among psychiatrists' diagnoses was due largely to inadequacies of DSM-I rather than to idiosyncracies of the clinical interview or inconsistent patient reporting. "Two thirds of the disagreements were charged to inadequacies of the nosological system itself" (p. 205). The largest single disagreement was determining "whether the neurotic symptomatology or the characterological pathology is more extensive or 'basic'" (p. 202). Ward and colleagues criticized the DSM-I apparent requirement that clinicians choose between a neurotic condition and a PD when in fact both might be present. The second most frequent cause of disagreement was said to be unclear diagnostic criteria.

The WHO was also concerned with the failure of its member countries to adopt the ICD-6 and therefore commissioned a review by the English psychiatrist, Erwin Stengel. Stengel (1959) reiterated the importance of establishing an official diagnostic nomenclature.

> A . . . serious obstacle to progress in psychiatry is difficulty of communication. Everybody who has followed the literature and listened to discussions concerning mental illness soon discovers that psychiatrists, even those apparently sharing the same basic orientation, often do not speak the same language. They either use different terms for the same concepts, or the same term for different concepts, usually without being aware of it. It is sometimes argued that this is inevitable in the present state of psychiatric knowledge, but it is doubtful whether this is a valid excuse. (p. 601)

Stengel (1959) attributed the failure of clinicians to accept ICD-6 to three problems, all of which he felt needed to be addressed: (1) the presence of theoretical biases within the nomenclature that were inconsistent with the diverse array of perspectives within the profession; (2) cynicism regarding psychiatric diagnoses within some theoretical perspectives, opposing the use of any diagnostic terms; and (3) the absence of specific, explicit diagnostic criteria (complicating the obtainment of agreement among clinicians who were actually attempting to use the manual). Stengel recommended that future nomenclatures be shorn of their theoretical and etiological assumptions, and base the diagnosis on more behaviorally specific descriptions.

## ICD-8 and DSM-II

Work began on ICD-8 soon after Stengel's (1959) report (ICD-6 had been revised to ICD-7 in 1955, but there had been no revisions to the section for mental disorders). The first meeting of the Subcommittee on Classification of Diseases of the WHO Expert Committee on Health Statistics was held in Geneva in 1961. It was evident to all participants that there would be closer adherence by the member countries of the WHO to the ICD-8 than had been the case for ICD-6. Considerable effort was made to develop a system that would be usable by all countries. The United States collaborated with the United Kingdom in developing a common, unified proposal; additional proposals were submitted by Australia, Czechoslovakia, the Federal Republic of Germany, France, Norway, Poland, and the Soviet Union. These alternative proposals were considered within a joint meeting in 1963. The most controversial points of disagreement concerned mental retardation with psychosocial deprivation, reactive psychoses, and antisocial PD (Kendell, 1975). The final edition of ICD-8 was approved by the WHO in 1966 and became effective in 1968. A companion glossary, in the spirit of Stengel's (1959) recommendations, was to be published conjointly, but work did not begin on the glossary until 1967, and it was not completed until 1972. "This delay greatly reduced [its] usefulness, and also [its] authority" (Kendell, 1975, p. 95).

In 1965, the APA appointed the Committee on Nomenclature and Statistics, chaired by Ernest M. Gruenberg, to revise DSM-I to be compatible with ICD-8, yet also be suitable for use within the United States (a technical consultant to DSM-II was the young psychiatrist, Robert Spitzer). A draft was circulated in 1967 to 120 psychiatrists with a special interest in diagnosis for their review of the proposals, and the final version was approved in 1967, with publication in 1968.

Spitzer and Wilson (1968) summarized the changes to DSM-I (see Table 3.1). Deleted from the PDs were the substance dependencies and sexual deviations. Deleted as well was the passive–dependent variant of the passive–aggressive personality trait disturbance. New additions were the explosive, hysterical, and asthenic PDs. Spitzer and Wilson (1975) subsequently criticized the absence of a diagnosis for depressive PD: "No adequate classification is furnished for the much larger number of characterologically depressed patients" (p. 842). They also objected to the inclusion of other diagnoses. "In the absence of clear criteria and follow-up studies, the wisdom of including such categories as explosive personality, asthenic personality, and inadequate personality may be questioned" (p. 842).

The time period in which DSM-II and ICD-8 were published was again highly controversial for mental disorder diagnoses (e.g., Rosenhan, 1973; Szasz, 1961). A fundamental problem continued to be the absence of empirical support for the reliability, let alone the validity, of mental disorder diagnosis (e.g., Blashfield & Draguns, 1976). Spitzer and Fleiss (1974) reviewed nine major studies of interrater reliability. Kappas for PD diagnoses ranged from .11 to .56, with a mean of only .29. DSM-II was blamed for much of this poor reliability, although concerns were also raised with respect to idiosyncratic clinical interviewing (Spitzer, Endicott, & Robins, 1975).

Many researchers had by now taken to heart the recommendations of Stengel (1959), developing more specific and explicit diagnostic criteria. The most influential effort was provided by Feighner and colleagues (1972), who developed criteria for 14 conditions (as well as secondary depression), one of which was ASPD.

Many other researchers followed the lead of Feighner and colleagues, most notably Spitzer and colleagues (1975). Research has since indicated that mental disorders can be diagnosed reliably with explicit, specific criterion sets assessed via semistructured interviews, resulting in a considerable body of reliable information concerning etiology, pathology, course, and treatment (Kendler, Muñoz, & Murphy, 2010).

## ICD-9 and DSM-III

By the time Feighner and colleagues (1972) was published, work was nearing completion on the ninth edition of the ICD. Representatives from the APA were involved, particularly Henry Brill, Chairman of the Task Force on Nomenclature, and Jack Ewalt, past president of the APA (Kramer et al., 1979). A series of international meetings were held, each of which focused on a specific problem area (the 1971 meeting in Tokyo focused on PDs and drug addiction). It was decided that ICD-9 would include a narrative glossary describing each of the conditions, but it was apparent that ICD-9 would not include the more specific and explicit criterion sets being developed by many research programs (Kendell, 1975).

In 1974, the APA appointed a Task Force on Nomenclature and Statistics to revise DSM-II in a manner that would be compatible with ICD-9 but also incorporate many of the innovations that were currently being developed. By the time this Task Force was appointed, ICD-9 was largely completed (the initial draft of ICD-9 was published in 1973). Spitzer and Williams (1985) described the mission of the DSM-III Task Force more with respect to developing an alternative to ICD-9 than with developing a manual that would coordinate well with ICD-9.

> As the mental disorders chapter of the ninth revision of the *International Classification of Diseases* (ICD-9) was being developed, the American Psychiatric Association's Committee on Nomenclature and Statistics reviewed it to assess its adequacy for use in the United States. . . . There was some concern that it had not made sufficient use of recent methodological developments, such as specified diagnostic criteria and multiaxial diagnosis, and that, in many specific areas of the classification, there was insufficient subtyping for clinical and research use. . . . For those reasons, the American Psychiatric Association in June 1974 appointed Robert L. Spitzer to chair a Task Force on Nomenclature and Statistics to develop a

new diagnostic manual. . . . The mandate given to the task force was to develop a classification that would, as much as possible, reflect the current state of knowledge regarding mental disorders and maximize its usefulness for both clinical practice and research studies. Secondarily, the classification was to be, as much as possible, compatible with ICD-9. (Spitzer & Williams, 1985, p. 604)

DSM-III was published by the APA in 1980 and did indeed include many innovations and significant revisions (Blashfield et al., 2014; Decker, 2013; Spitzer, Williams, & Skodol, 1980). Four of the PDs that had been included in DSM-II were deleted (i.e., aesthenic, cyclothymic, inadequate, and explosive) and four were added (i.e., avoidant, dependent, borderline, and narcissistic) (Frances, 1980; Spitzer et al., 1980; see Table 3.1). Equally important, each of the PDs was now provided with more specific and explicit diagnostic criteria, with the expectation, or at least hope, that they would now be diagnosed reliably in general clinical practice.

Field trials indicated that the criterion sets of DSM-III were indeed helpful in improving reliability (e.g., Spitzer, Forman, & Nee, 1979; Williams & Spitzer, 1980). "In the DSM-III field trials over 450 clinicians participated in the largest reliability study ever done, involving independent evaluations of nearly 800 patients. . . . For most of the diagnostic classes the reliability was quite good, and in general it was much higher than that previously achieved with DSM-I and DSM-II" (Spitzer et al., 1980, p. 154). However, there was less success with the PDs. Spitzer and colleagues (1979) reported a kappa of only .61 for the agreement regarding the presence of any PD for jointly conducted interviews. "Although Personality Disorder as a class is evaluated more reliably than previously, with the exception of Antisocial Personality Disorder . . . the kappas for the specific Personality Disorders are quite low" (Williams & Spitzer, 1980, p. 468).

The inadequate reliability was attributed largely to the difficulty in developing behavioral indicators. "For some disorders . . . particularly the Personality Disorders, a much higher order of inference is necessary" (APA, 1980, p. 7). Mellsop, Varghese, Joshua, and Hicks (1982) reported the agreement for individual DSM-III PDs in general clinical practice, with kappa ranging in value from a low of .01 (schizoid) to a high of .49 (ASPD). The relative "success" obtained for the ASPD diagnosis was attributed to the greater specificity of its diagnostic criteria, a finding that has since been frequently replicated (Widiger & Boyd, 2009; Zimmerman, 1994).

However, it should also be emphasized that poor reliability was attributed by Mellsop and colleagues (1982) to idiosyncratic biases among the clinicians rather than to inadequate criterion sets. They noted how one clinician diagnosed 59% of patients as borderline, whereas another diagnosed 50% as antisocial. Mellsop and colleagues concluded that "Axis II of DSM-III represents a significant step forward in increasing the reliability of the diagnosis of personality disorders in everyday clinical practice" (p. 1361). They acknowledged that further specification of the diagnostic criteria might be helpful, but they emphasized instead the development of more standardized and structured interviewing techniques to address idiosyncratic clinical interviewing and biased clinical assessments. In other words, clinicians needed to be encouraged to assess the specific diagnostic systematically rather than rely on their subjective impressions and quick, hasty judgments.

Another innovation of DSM-III was the placement of the PDs and some of the developmental disorders on a separate "axis" to ensure that they would not be overlooked in the presence of more florid and immediate conditions, and to emphasize that a diagnosis of a PD was not mutually exclusive with the diagnosis of an anxiety, mood, or other mental disorder (Frances, 1980; Spitzer et al., 1980). The effect of this placement was indeed a boon to the diagnosis of PDs, dramatically increasing the frequency of their recognition (Loranger, 1990).

## DSM-III-R

A limitation of DSM-III, however, was the absence of adequate research to support many of the revisions. Errors were quickly discovered soon after its publication. "Criteria were not entirely clear, were inconsistent across categories, or were even contradictory" (APA, 1987, p. xvii). The APA therefore authorized the development of a revision to DSM-III to correct these errors, as well as to provide a few additional refinements and clarifications. A more fundamental revision to the manual was to be tabled until work began on ICD-10. The criteria were only to be "reviewed for consistency, clarity, and conceptual accuracy, and revised when necessary" (APA, 1987, p. xvii). However, it was perhaps unrealistic to expect the authors of DSM-III-R to confine their efforts to simply refinement and clarification given the impact, success, and importance of DSM-III.

> The impact of DSM-III has been remarkable. Soon after its publication, it became widely accepted in the United States as the common language of mental health clinicians and researchers for communicating about the disorders for which they have professional responsibility. Recent major textbooks of psychiatry and other textbooks that discuss psychopathology have either made extensive reference to DSM-III or largely adopted its terminology and concepts. In the seven years since the publication of DSM-III, over two thousand articles that directly address some aspect of it have appeared in the scientific literature. (APA, 1987, p. xviii)

It was not difficult to find persons who wanted to be part of DSM-III-R, and most work group members wanted to have a significant impact. Substantially more persons were assigned to make the corrections to DSM-III than had been involved in its original construction. The DSM-III Personality Disorders Advisory Committee included just 10 persons, whereas the DSM-III-R Advisory Committee had 38. Not surprisingly, there were many proposals for significant additions, revisions, and deletions. Work began on DSM-III-R in 1983, with an anticipated publication date of 1985, but DSM-III-R was not published until 1987, and the final edition included major revisions to the section on PDs (Widiger, Frances, Spitzer, & Williams, 1988).

The threshold for the inclusion of new diagnoses in DSM-III and DSM-III-R was rather liberal. As expressed by Spitzer, Sheehy, and Endicott (1977), "If there is general agreement among clinicians, who would be expected to encounter the condition, that there are a significant number of patients who have it and that its identification is important in their clinical work, it is included in the classification" (p. 3). One proposal for DSM-III-R was the inclusion of a new diagnosis, masochistic PD (MPD).

MPD was included in DSM-III, albeit as just one example for the possible application of atypical, mixed, or other PD (APA, 1980, p. 329); this diagnosis became "not otherwise specified" in DSM-III-R (APA, 1987). Its interest was driven in part by the desire to include some variant of a depressive personality disorder. As expressed by Frances (1980), there was a need to include a PD for those who have "psychological conflicts that make them pessimistic, self-defeating, and unhappy" (p. 1052). The concept of a masochistic–depressive personality was fairly common in the existing psychoanalytic literature (Kass, Spitzer, Williams, & Widiger, 1989). A proposal was generated for its inclusion in DSM-III-R with relatively more emphasize on the construct of masochism rather than depressiveness in order to minimize opposition to its inclusion by the mood disorders work group (Kass, MacKinnon, & Spitzer, 1986).

However, the proposal generated considerable opposition, in part because of the perception that it was resurrecting archaic psychoanalytic theory that women who were victims of abuse were at least partially responsible for their victimization (Fiester, 1991; Widiger, 1995). The name was eventually changed to self-defeating PD in part to distance the proposal from analytical theories concerning masochism, but this did not end the controversy (Caplan, 1991). In the meantime, a proposal for a complementary diagnosis of sadistic PD (SPD) was generated. SPD would apply to some men who were victimizing women with MPD, and there was suspicion that the proposal was generated in part as an effort to mollify opposition to the MPD/self-defeating PD (Fiester & Gay, 1991). Data were obtained in support of both proposals (including a survey of forensic psychiatrists; Fiester, 1991; Fiester & Gay, 1991). Both proposals were approved by the Personality Disorders Advisory Committee and by the DSM-III-R Work Group (the central committee was titled Work Group rather than Task Force, consistent with its limited mandate). However, both proposals were rejected by the APA Board of Trustees due to their controversial nature and questionable empirical support (Widiger, 1995; Widiger et al., 1988).

Most of the sets of criteria were revised substantially in an effort to improve their discriminant validity. One of the more significant revisions was the conversion of the schizoid, avoidant, dependent, and compulsive monothetic criterion sets (all of the criteria are required) to polythetic criterion sets (only a specified subset of optional criteria are required). The monothetic criterion sets were successful in describing a prototypical case, but the typical case was not prototypical. Persons who were thought to share the same PD did not necessarily have or share all of the same features (Widiger et al., 1988).

## ICD-10 and DSM-IV

By the time work was completed on DSM-III-R, work had already begun on ICD-10. The decision of the authors of DSM-III to develop an alternative to ICD-9 was instrumental in developing a highly innovative manual (Kendell, 1991; Spitzer & Williams, 1985; Spitzer et al., 1980). However, this was also at the cost of decreasing compatibility with the nomenclature being used throughout the rest of the world, and contrary to the stated purpose of providing a common language of communication. International compatibility would only be achieved by a more cooperative, joint construction.

The APA Committee on Psychiatric Diagnosis and Assessment recommended in 1987 that work begin on the development of DSM-IV in collaboration with the development of ICD-10, and in May 1988, the APA Board of Trustees appointed a DSM-IV Task Force, chaired by Allen Frances (Frances, Widiger, & Pincus, 1989). John Gunderson was appointed to be the Chair of the Personality Disorders Work Group (Robert Spitzer chaired all of the work groups of DSM-III and DSM-III-R). Mandates for this Task Force were to revise DSM-III-R in a manner that would be more compatible with ICD-10, more user-friendly to the practicing clinician, and more explicitly empirically based (Frances, Pincus, Widiger, Davis, & First, 1990).

### ICD-10 and DSM-IV Compatibility

Members of the ICD-10 and DSM-IV committees began meeting soon after the DSM-IV Task Force was formed (the PD representatives from ICD-10 were Alv Dahl, Armand Loranger, and Charles Pull). These joint meetings were successful in increasing the congruency of the two nomenclatures. For example, a borderline subtype was added to the ICD-10 emotionally unstable PD that was closely compatible with DSM-IV borderline PD (BPD). The DSM-IV Personality Disorders Work Group recommended that a diagnosis for the ICD-10 personality change after catastrophic experience be included in DSM-IV (Shea, 1996) but this recommendation was not approved by the Task Force (Gunderson, 1998). Many revisions to DSM-III-R criterion sets were also implemented to increase the congruency of the two nomenclatures (Widiger, Mangine, Corbitt, Ellis, & Thomas, 1995). For example, the DSM-IV obsessive–compulsive criterion of rigidity and stubbornness and many of the DSM-IV criteria for schizoid PD were obtained from the ICD-10 research criteria.

### Clinical Utility

A difficulty shared by the authors of DSM-IV and ICD-10 was the development of criterion sets that would maximize reliability without being overly cumbersome for clinical practice. Maximizing the feasibility of the diagnostic criteria for the practicing clinician had been an important concern for the authors of DSM-III and DSM-III-R, but it did appear that priority had been given to the needs of the researcher over the clinician (Frances et al., 1990). This was particularly evident in the lengthy and detailed criterion sets. Researchers can devote more than 2 hours to assess PD diagnostic criteria, but this is grossly unrealistic for the general practitioner. The WHO, therefore, provided separate versions of ICD-10 for the researcher and the clinician (Sartorius, 1988; Sartorius et al., 1993). The researcher's version included relatively specific and explicit criterion sets, whereas the clinician's version included only narrative descriptions. The DSM-IV Task Force considered this option but decided that it would complicate the generalization of research findings to clinical practice, and vice versa (Frances et al., 1990). One might also question the implications of providing more detailed, reliable criterion sets for the researcher and simpler, less reliable criterion sets for clinical practice. The DSM-IV Task Force decided instead to simplify the most cumbersome and lengthy criterion sets, the best example of which for the PDs was the criterion set for ASPD (Widiger et al., 1996; Widiger & Corbitt, 1995).

A potential innovation of DSM-IV to help improve clinical utility was the presentation of the criterion sets in a descending order of diagnostic value (Gunderson, 1998; Widiger et al., 1995). Clinicians often fail to systematically consider all of the diagnostic criteria given the limited amount of time available. Research concerning how clinicians diagnose PDs suggests that they emphasize a subset of the criteria that they feel are especially diagnostic (Blashfield & Flanagan, 1998; Herkov & Blashfield, 1995; Miller, 2008). If clinicians are not going to consider all of the criteria, then it would be useful if they were informed as to which criteria are most diagnostic (Mullins-Sweatt & Widiger, 2009). The existence of this information, however, was never noted within DSM-IV, in part because there was insufficient research concerning the new diagnostic criteria (all of which were therefore placed at the bottom of the list).

## Empirical Support

One of the more common concerns regarding DSM-III and DSM-III-R was empirical support. It was often suggested that the decisions were more consistent with the a priori wishes of Work Group or Advisory Committee members than with the published research. "For most of the personality disorder categories there was either no empirical base (e.g., avoidant, dependent, passive–aggressive, narcissistic) or no clinical tradition (e.g., avoidant, dependent, schizotypal); thus their disposition was much more subject to the convictions of individual Advisory Committee members" (Gunderson, 1983, p. 30). Millon (1981) criticized the DSM-III criteria for ASPD for being too heavily influenced by Robins (1966), a member of the DSM-III Personality Disorders Advisory Committee. Gunderson (1983) and Kernberg (1984), on the other hand, criticized the inclusion of AVPD as being too heavily influenced by Millon, another member of the same committee.

The development of DSM-IV proceeded through three stages of empirical review, including systematic and comprehensive reviews of the research literature, reanalyses of multiple datasets, and field trials, all of which would be published in a series of archival texts (Frances et al., 1990). It was emphasized that the intention of the literature reviews was not simply to make the best case for a respective proposal (Widiger, Frances, Pincus, Davis, & First, 1991). The authors were required to acknowledge and address findings inconsistent with their proposals (Frances & Widiger, 2012). An explicit method of literature search was required to maximize the likelihood that it would be objective and systematic, including the specification of the criteria for study inclusion and exclusion, thereby making it difficult to confine the review to a limited set of studies that were most consistent with the viewpoints of the authors (Widiger et al., 1991). Each review was also submitted for critical review by persons likely to oppose the suggested proposals.

Also conducted was a field trial of the proposed revisions to ASPD criteria that included four sites, two of which involved competing viewpoints (i.e., a site for which the Principal Investigator was Robert Hare, and another for which the Principal Investigator was Lee Robins). The study compared the DSM-IV proposal with the existing criterion set with respect to a number of external validators, including clinicians' diagnostic impression of the patient using whatever construct they preferred (at the drug addicted–homeless, methadone maintenance, and inpatient sites); interviewers' diagnostic impressions at all four sites; criminal history; and self-report measures of empathy, Machiavellianism, perspective taking, antisocial personality, and psychopathy (Widiger et al., 1996).

Only one new diagnosis was considered: depressive personality disorder. As noted earlier, Spitzer and Wilson (1975) lamented the absence of a diagnosis for depressive personality disorder in DSM-II. It was proposed for inclusion in DSM-III but opposed by the Mood Disorders Work Group who was proposing a new diagnosis of dysthymia, the literature review for which though was based heavily on the research and literature concerning depressive personality (i.e., Keller, 1989). In their presentation of the primary achievements of DSM-III, Spitzer and colleagues (1980) acknowledged that "dysthymia is roughly equivalent to the concept of depressive personality" (p. 159). DSM-III-R even expanded the construct of dysthymia to include an early-onset variant. It was acknowledged in the text of DSM-III-R that "this disorder usually begins in childhood, adolescence, or early adult life and for this reason has often been referred to as Depressive Personality" (APA, 1987, p. 231).

The proposal to include a diagnosis of depressive personality disorder was again made for DSM-IV (Phillips, Gunderson, Hirschfeld, & Smith, 1990). Phillips, Hirschfeld, Shea, and Gunderson (1993) developed a criterion set that emphasized cognitive and interpersonal features that they hoped would identify a group of persons who did not meet criteria for early-onset dysthymia, a rather difficult task given that early-onset dysthymia was largely equivalent to depressive personality (APA, 1987). If a distinction could be made, then presumably its inclusion in DSM-IV would not be opposed by the Mood Disorders Work Group. The criterion set was provided to the Mood Disorders Work Group for inclusion in its field trial. The proposed criterion set was successful in identifying a different set of persons (Phillips et al., 1998). However, the Mood Disorders Work Group was equally impressed with the criterion set and revised the criterion set for dysthymia to incorporate some of these new features (Keller et al., 1995). The DSM-IV Task Force recognized that it would not really be fair to allow mood disorders to annex these new features. The final decision was to include both the depressive PD (DPD) and the new proposal for dysthymia within an appendix to DSM-IV. In the text discussion for DPD, it was stated that "it remains controversial whether the distinction between depressive personality and Dysthymic Disorder is useful" (APA, 1994, p. 732). No discussion or consideration of this diagnosis appeared to occur for DSM-5, and it is no longer even in an appendix to the diagnostic manual (Bagby, Watson, & Ryder, 2012).

In the end, no new PD diagnoses were added to DSM-IV. The self-defeating and sadistic PDs, approved for inclusion by the DSM-III-R Advisory Committee, were deleted entirely from the manual (Widiger, 1995). The PD that was the most frequently diagnosed by clinicians during World War II (passive–aggressive) was downgraded to an appendix (Wetzler & Jose, 2012). DSM-IV, however, did include some substantive revisions. Extensive revisions were made to the criterion sets. Only 10 of the 93 DSM-III-R PD diagnostic criteria were left unchanged, 21 received minor revisions, 10 were deleted, 9 were added, and 52 received a significant revision (Widiger et al., 1995). In addition, reference was made in the text of DSM-IV to the existence of an alternative dimensional trait model of PD.

## DSM-IV-TR

The APA diagnostic manual includes a considerable amount of information beyond simply the criterion sets, such as prevalence, course, cross-cultural presentation, impact of age and gender, familiar pattern, and associated features. This information can change over just a few years, and the APA concluded that it would be useful to update the text. Harold Pincus was appointed the Chair for the DSM-IV Text Revision; Michael First was appointed to be Vice Chair (First & Pincus, 2002).

Consistent with the goals for DSM-IV-TR, no substantive changes were made to the PD diagnoses (APA, 2000). The text for some of the PDs (e.g., ASPD) was indeed updated. However, the text for other PDs was not revised. There was also an intention to publish and/or distribute documentation of the empirical support for the statements made in the text. Documentation for the text was obtained for some of the PDs but, again, not for all of them. In the end, it was decided not to publish or distribute this documentation, perhaps because it was incomplete and/or inconsistent in its coverage.

## ICD-11 and DSM-5

The authors of DSM-5 wanted to implement a "paradigm shift" (Kupfer, First, & Regier, 2002, p. xix); more specifically, toward a dimensional classification. "We have decided that one, if not the major difference, between DSM-IV and DSM-V will be the more prominent use of dimensional measures" (Regier, Narrow, Kuhl, & Kupfer, 2009, p. 649). The development of DSM-5 was preceded by a series of preparatory conferences, most of which focused on this intended shift to a dimensional model. The first "DSM-V Research Planning Conference" was held in October 1999. The Nomenclature Work Group concluded that it would be "important that consideration be given to advantages and disadvantages of basing part or all of DSM-V on dimensions rather than categories" (Rounsaville et al., 2002, p. 13). This work group suggested that the section of the diagnostic manual for which this shift would be most clearly suited was the PDs. It was now readily apparent that the DSM-IV-TR PDs were not categorically distinct entities or homogeneous conditions, with specific etiologies, pathologies, or treatments (Clark, 2007; Livesley, 2007; Widiger & Trull, 2007). The PDs are instead overlapping constellations of maladaptive traits that not only shade into one another but also into normal personality functioning (Widiger & Costa, 1994).

The Personality Disorders and Relational Disorders Work Group from this first conference summarized the research in support of shifting the PDs section to a dimensional trait model and identified the primary alternative proposals (First et al., 2002). They recommended that DSM-5 revise "the classification of personality disorders using a dimensional approach that avoids the artificiality of the current categorical approach and facilitates the identification and communication of the patient's clinical relevant personality traits" (p. 179).

This initial DSM-5 preparatory conference was followed by a series of international conferences. The first, "Dimensional Models of Personality Disorder: Etiology, Pathology, Phenomenology, and Treatment," was held in December 2004. Its purpose was to review the literature and set a research agenda "that would be most effective in leading the field toward a dimensional classification of personality disorder" (Widiger, Simonsen, Krueger, Livesley, & Verheul, 2005, p. 315). A proposed dimensional PD model that was an integration of existing models consisted of the four domains: emotional dysregulation versus emotional stability, extraversion versus introversion, antagonism versus compliance, and constraint versus impulsivity. The authors of this integrative model suggested that a fifth broad domain, unconventionality versus closed to experience, would also be necessary to account fully for all of the maladaptive trait scales included within the alternative dimensional models.

The seventh conference of this series was devoted to shifting the entire diagnostic manual to dimensional models (Helzer et al., 2008). One section of this conference was concerned with the PDs (Krueger, Skodol, Livesley, Shrout, & Huang, 2008). The dimensional model of Livesley (2007) was provided as an illustration for the PDs.

Andrew Skodol was appointed Chair of the DSM-5 Personality and Personality Disorders Work Group (PPDWG), which began meeting in 2007 (Krueger & Markon, 2014). Skodol, Morey, Bender, and Oldham (2013, p. 344) indicated that "for the first year or so [in the development of DSM-5], 'everything was on the table,' with no a priori limitations on the extent of changes that DSM-5 could incur. . . . Work group members were encouraged to 'think outside the box.'"

## Initial DSM-5 PD Proposals

The initial proposals by the DSM-5 PPDWG were indeed quite extensive. As indicated by Skodol (2010) in the first posting on the DSM-5 website, approximately 3 years after work had begun, "the work group recommends a major reconceptualization of personality psychopathology" ("Reformulation of personality disorders in DSM-5," para. 1). The proposals included a level of personality functioning, along with a significant revision to the definition of PD; the replacement of the specific and explicit criterion sets with narrative paragraphs; deletion of half of the diagnoses; and the inclusion of a supplementary dimensional trait model (APA, 2010; Skodol, 2010). Perhaps not surprisingly, given the extensive nature of the revisions, the proposals were met with substantial opposition. A special section of the *Journal of Personality Disorders* included six critical reviews (i.e., Bornstein, 2011; Clarkin & Huprich, 2011; Paris, 2011; Ronningstam, 2011; Widiger, 2011a; Zimmerman, 2011); a special section of *Personality Disorders: Theory, Research, and Treatment* included three critical reviews (Pilkonis, Hallquist, Morse, & Stepp, 2011; Pincus, 2011; Widiger, 2011b). Additional critical reviews were published, independent of these special sections (e.g., Gunderson, 2010a; Shedler et al., 2010; Miller, Widiger, & Campbell, 2010; Zimmerman, 2012). There was even a critical review published by a work group member (i.e., Livesley, 2010). Each proposal is discussed in turn.

### Level of Personality Functioning

DSM-IV included a brief set of criteria for the presence of a PD, consisting of deviations from expectations with respect to cognition, affectivity, interpersonal functioning, and/or impulse control (any two of which were required). The DSM-5 PPDWG proposed a substantial shift in the PD definition, coordinating it with a long and complex assessment of level of personality functioning tied to deficits in the sense of self (with respect to identity and self-regulation) and interpersonal relatedness (with respect to empathy and intimacy). Each of the four components was to be assessed along a 5-point scale, from *little to no impairment,* to *some, moderate, severe,* and *extreme impairment,* with each level defined by a brief paragraph.

The proposal was criticized in part for its complexity (Clarkin & Huprich, 2011; Pilkonis et al., 2011; Widiger, 2011b). One might also question the decision to align the definition and level of a PD to constructs of self and interpersonal deficits proposed from the perspective of the psychodynamic theoretical model of PD. One of the innovations of DSM-III was a shift away from any particular theoretical model toward a more neutral perspective, one that can be comfortably used across persons who vary in their theoretical model (Spitzer et al., 1980). Yet the DSM-5 PPDWG proposed shifting the definition of PD toward psychodynamic constructs. This proposal was well received by persons who shared this theoretical perspective (e.g., Bender, Morey, & Skodol, 2011; Kernberg, 2012; Pincus, 2011) but it would be problematic for the rest of persons in psychiatry and psychology who work from an alternative theoretical model. It was also somewhat anachronistic, as the rest of psychiatry was shifting toward a neurobiological perspective (Hyman, 2010; Insel, 2009, 2013; Insel & Quirion, 2005).

## Narrative Prototype Matching

Another proposal was to abandon the well-established specific and explicit criterion sets for lengthy narrative paragraphs. As noted earlier, one of the major innovations of DSM-III (APA, 1980) was the provision of specific and explicit criterion sets (Spitzer et al., 1980; Zimmerman, 1994). As expressed by Kendler and colleagues (2010), the "interest in diagnostic reliability in the early 1970s—substantially influenced by the Feighner criteria—proved to be a critical corrective and was instrumental in the renaissance of psychiatric research witnessed in the subsequent decades" (p. 141). One of the beneficiaries of this renaissance was the well-published Collaborative Longitudinal Study of Personality Disorders (CLPS), which used as its primary measure a semistructured interview that systematically assessed the DSM-IV-TR PDs' specific and explicit criterion sets (Skodol et al., 2005). CLPS would likely never have even been funded if the investigators had proposed abandoning the criterion sets for subjective matching to narrative paragraphs.

There was certainly support among some PD clinicians and researchers for narrative prototypes (e.g., First & Westen, 2007; Huprich, Bornstein, & Schmitt, 2011; Shedler et al., 2010). One of the attractive features of this form of prototype matching is its simplicity. "Clinicians could make a complete Axis II diagnosis in 1 or 2 minutes" (Westen, Shedler, & Bradley, 2006, p. 855) because they would no longer have to assess systematically each of the sentences included within a diagnostic criterion set or a narrative description. "Diagnosticians rate the overall similarity or 'match' between a patient and the prototype . . . considering the prototype as a whole rather than counting individual symptoms" (p. 847).

It seems self-evident though that clinicians would not likely provide reliable diagnoses if they could in fact assess (for instance) a lengthy, three paragraph description of BPD in just 1 to 2 minutes through their subjective impression of the entire gestalt (Livesley, 2010; Pilkonis et al., 2011). There was one study that supported the reliability of narrative prototype matching (Westen & Muderrisoglu, 2003) and another that supported its validity (Westen et al., 2006), but significant concerns were raised with respect to the methodology of these two studies (Widiger, 2011b; Zimmerman, 2011). Research with DSM-I and DSM-II had also repeatedly demonstrated the failings of this approach (Spitzer & Fleiss, 1974; Spitzer et al., 1975). In addition, it does not in fact appear to be the case that clinicians match their impression to an entire gestalt. Most clinicians probably could not even repeat or recall what is contained within the lengthy narrative paragraphs. Research has indicated that clinicians are unable to recall even the simpler and more straightforward criterion sets of DSM-III and DSM-III-R (Blashfield & Breen, 1989; Morey & Ochoa, 1989). Clinicians appear instead to focus on a particular subset of criteria that they feel is most diagnostic (Blashfield & Flanagan, 1998; Herkov & Blashfield, 1995; Miller, 2008). The narratives proposed for DSM-5 would likely have been even less reliable than had been the case for DSM-II (APA, 1968), as they were considerably longer and more complex, allowing for even more variation across clinicians in the selection of which features to consider and emphasize.

## Deletion of Five Diagnoses

There is compelling empirical support for the lack of construct validity for PD diagnostic categories (Clark, 2007; Livesley, 2012, 2013; Widiger & Trull, 2007). In that regard, perhaps all of the categories should be replaced by a dimensional trait model. This is precisely the recommendation from the ICD-11 work group (Tyrer et al., 2011). However, a different question is which of the 10 DSM-IV-TR personality syndromes should be retained if only a subset of them is to be retained.

The DSM-5 PPDWG proposed to delete half of the PD diagnoses: histrionic, narcissistic, dependent, paranoid, and schizoid (Skodol, 2010). The rationale for their removal was not that dependent, histrionic, or narcissistic traits are not important to recognize. On the contrary, some of the traits from the deleted diagnoses were to be retained within the dimensional trait model (Clark & Krueger, 2010). For example, included within the initial (and final) dimensional trait model were submissiveness (a dependent trait), attention seeking (histrionic), anhedonia (schizoid), and grandiosity (narcissistic). However, considerably less coverage in the dimensional trait model was given to the five PDs slated for deletion than to the diagnoses being retained (Samuel, Lynam, Widiger, & Ball, 2012).

The rationale provided for the deletions was to reduce problematic diagnostic co-occurrence (Skodol, 2010, 2012). Diagnostic co-occurrence has been a significant problem (Clark, 2007; Trull & Durrett, 2005; Widiger & Trull, 2007) but sacrificing fully half of the PDs to address this problem would seem to be a rather draconian solution (Widiger, 2011b). Lack of adequate coverage has also been a problem of comparable magnitude (Verheul & Widiger, 2004). With the removal of the histrionic and dependent PDs, essentially half of all manner of maladaptive interpersonal relatedness would no longer have been recognized (Pincus & Hopwood, 2012; Widiger, 2010). The credibility of the PD field might also have suffered from the fact that the DSM-5 PPDWG decided that literally half of the disorders that have been recognized, discussed, and treated over the past 30 years lacked sufficient utility or validity to remain within the diagnostic manual (Pilkonis et al., 2011; Widiger, 2011b).

Skodol and colleagues (2011) suggested that the narcissistic, dependent, histrionic, schizoid, and paranoid diagnoses had less empirical support for their validity and/or clinical utility than the avoidant, obsessive–compulsive, borderline, schizotypal, and antisocial PDs. There is clearly much less research on the histrionic, paranoid, and schizoid PDs than for borderline, antisocial, and schizotypal PDs (Blashfield & Intoccia, 2000; Blashfield, Reynolds, & Stennett, 2012; Boschen & Warner, 2009; Hopwood & Thomas, 2012). Shedler and colleagues (2010) responded that "absence of evidence is not evidence of absence" (p. 1027). A dearth of research can reflect a failure of PD researchers rather than an absence of the clinical importance of a respective PD. Nevertheless, it is evident that the histrionic, paranoid, and schizoid PDs have not been generating much interest among researchers (Blashfield & Intoccia, 2000; Blashfield, Reynolds, & Stennett, 2012).

The proposals to delete the dependent and narcissistic PDs was more difficult to defend (Bornstein, 2011, 2012a, 2012b; Gore & Pincus, 2013; Ronningstam, 2011; Widiger, 2011b). As suggested by Livesley (2010), a work group member, "the criteria for deciding which PD diagnoses to delete are not explicit and the final selection appears arbitrary" (p. 309). There might in fact be as much, if not more, research to support the validity and utility of the dependent and narcissistic PDs than for the avoidant and obsessive–compulsive PDs (Bornstein, 2011, 2012a, 2012b; Gore & Pincus, 2013; Miller et al., 2010; Mullins-Sweatt, Bernstein, & Widiger, 2012; Ronningstam, 2011; Widiger, 2011b). As expressed by Livesley (2010), "Well-studied conditions that represent important clinical presentations, such as dependent and narcissistic personality disorders, are slated for elimination, whereas obsessive–compulsive personality disorder, which is often associated with less serious pathology, will be retained" (p. 309).

Bornstein (2011) suggested that the decision about which diagnoses to retain was biased in favor of the PDs studied within the heavily funded and widely published CLPS (Skodol et al., 2005), perhaps thereby providing a distinct advantage to these diagnoses. The CLPS project was confined largely to the avoidant, schizotypal, obsessive–compulsive, and borderline diagnoses. Zimmerman (2012) suggested further that the DSM-5 PPDWG may have even felt obligated to retain the avoidant and obsessive–compulsive PDs because they were the focus of CLPS. It would indeed have been difficult to delete from the diagnostic manual the disorders that were the focus of over 10 years of NIMH-funded research.

However, CLPS did not actually yield much research concerned with issues of specific or unique importance for the understanding and validation of the avoidant and obsessive–compulsive PDs. The typical CLPS publication was concerned with generic issues that were applicable to all of the PDs (e.g., course, factor structure, temporal stability, differential diagnosis, and external correlates). This is not the case for a good part of the research concerning the dependent and narcissistic PDs, both of which have generated considerable findings devoted to questions and issues specific to them (Bornstein, 2011, 2012a; Campbell & Miller, 2011; Ronningstam, 2010, 2011).

### Dimensional Trait Model

Krueger, Derringer, Markon, Watson, and Skodol (2012) stated that in the development of the dimensional trait model, "our focus was initially on identifying and operationalizing specific maladaptive personality falling within five broad domains" (p. 1880). "If the work group members had ample opportunity to contribute (e.g., in describing a wide range of personality disorder characteristics), and the data pointed to the well-replicated structure of personality pathology, it would be hard for work group members to argue that somehow the empirical model was imposed from the outside by persons who know nothing about what these patients are really like" (Krueger, 2013, p. 359). In other words, using the work group members' own nominations, "one hope was that . . . we would arrive at essentially the same well-replicated empirical structure of personality pathology delineated by Widiger and Simonsen (2005)" (Krueger, 2013, p. 350).

However, the initial proposal was for a six-domain model (i.e., negative emotionality, introversion, antagonism, disinhibition, compulsivity, and schizotypy) that was explicitly distinguished from the five-factor model (FFM); more specifically, that compulsivity and schizotypy did not align with any FFM domain (i.e., Clark & Krueger, 2010). In the end, the dimensional trait model was said to be aligned with the FFM (Krueger & Markon, 2014), but it was presented in its initial years as if it was created de novo, with no alignment with any established model (Livesley, 2013). This provided considerable fuel to those who opposed the dimensional trait perspective (Miller & Lynam, 2013; Widiger, 2013). As expressed by Shedler and colleagues (2010) in their *American Journal of Psychiatry* editorial, "the resulting model no longer rests on decades of research, which had been the chief rationale for including it" (p. 1027).

The dimensional trait proposal did indeed meet with considerable opposition. Gunderson (2010a), the Chair of the DSM-IV Personality Disorders Work Group, argued that the trait-based system has an "(1) unfamiliarity to clinicians (and possibly unfeasibility), (2) lack of clinical utility, (3) preliminary quality to the science upon which the proposed change is based, and (4) harmful effects on the diagnosis of borderline personality disorder" (p. 119). In the editorial coauthored by esteemed psychoanalytic clinicians, Shedler and colleagues (2010) further asserted that "clinicians find dimensional trait approaches significantly less relevant and useful, and consider them *worse,* than the current DSM-IV system" (p. 1027; original emphasis). There is a considerable body of research to counter these charges (Widiger, Samuel, Mullins-Sweatt, Gore, & Crego, 2012) but very little of this research was included in the PPDWG literature review. In fact, the review (i.e., Skodol, 2010) cited clinical studies that were critical of the trait-based approach, neglecting to acknowledge the clinical utility studies that countered this research and supported the trait approach (Widiger, 2011a).

### Final DSM-5 Proposals

All of the proposals were eventually revised, some quite significantly (Skodol, 2012). The proposal to delete narcissistic PD (NPD) was withdrawn. Some suggest that this reversal was due to external, political pressure (Livesley, 2013). Livesley points out that the initial review by the PPDWG suggested inadequate empirical support (Skodol et al., 2011), and no subsequent review was generated to question this initial conclusion. "The only thing that seems to have changed was the power of the lobby for including narcissistic personality disorder" (Livesley, 2013, p. 213). There may have indeed been a considerable amount of backchannel communication and pressure, and it is regrettable that "behind the scenes" politicking can indeed exert a significant influence. However, there was also a substantial body of research to support the validity of narcissistic personality (NPD) disorder that would appear to be equal to and perhaps considerably stronger than the research specific to the avoidant and obsessive–compulsive PDs (Campbell & Miller, 2011; Miller et al., 2010; Ronningstam, 2005, 2010, 2011) that did not seem to be appreciated or acknowledged by the PPDWG (e.g., Skodol et al., 2011).

Dependent personality disorder (DPD), though, remained slated for deletion (APA, 2012) despite a comparable body of research that would appear to be equal to that in support of NPD and, again, greater than the research specific to the avoidant or obsessive–compulsive PDs (Bornstein, 2012a, 2012b; Gore & Pincus, 2013; Mullins-Sweatt, Bernstein, & Widiger, 2012). DPD, though may not have had the lobbying power that was available for NPD.

The six-domain, 37-trait model was reduced to a five-domain, 25-trait model on the basis of a factor analysis (Krueger et al., 2012). In the final posting on the DSM-5 website, there was no longer an effort to distinguish the model from the FFM (APA, 2012). It was stated instead that "the proposed model represents an extension of the Five-Factor Model (Costa & Widiger, 2002) of personality that specifically delineates and encompasses the more extreme and maladaptive personality variants" (APA, 2012, p. 7).

The narrative prototype-matching proposal was dropped, likely due to questions concerning the empirical support for its reliability and validity (Livesley, 2010; Pilkonis et al., 2011; Widiger, 2011b; Zimmerman, 2011). Nevertheless, the PPDWG did not return to the specific and explicit criterion sets of DSM-IV-TR. Instead, with relatively little time remaining, it cobbled together a new hybrid model of PD diagnosis (Skodol, 2012) combining psychodynamically oriented deficits in self- and interpersonal functioning obtained from the level of personality functioning proposal (Bender et al., 2011; Kernberg, 2012; Pincus, 2011) with maladaptive personality traits obtained from the dimensional trait proposal (Krueger et al., 2012).

## Final DSM-5 Decisions

Kendler, Kupfer, Narrow, Phillips, and Fawcett (2009) developed guidelines for the degree of empirical support needed for the approval of respective proposals. These guidelines were quite demanding and conservative. For example, any change to the diagnostic manual had to be accompanied by "a discussion of possible unintended negative effects of this proposed change, if it is made, and a consideration of arguments against making this change should also be included" (p. 2). They further stated that "the larger and more significant the change, the stronger should be the required level of support" (p. 2).

Skodol and colleagues (2013) acknowledged an awareness of the Kendler and colleagues (2009) guidelines, but suggested that the PPDWG had not expected that they would actually have to adhere to them. "The problems with the existing 10-category system for diagnosing PDs seemed so severe, and the advantages of a hybrid system as gauged against . . . traditional validity markers . . . so substantial, that a reduced threshold for change seemed warranted" (Skodol et al., 2013, p. 345). Proposals from other work groups that had marginal empirical support were indeed approved, such as mood dysregulation disorder (originally titled temper dysregulation disorder of childhood) and somatic symptom disorder (Frances & Widiger, 2012; Widiger & Crego, 2015).

By the time DSM-5 was completed, three oversight committees had been formed. There was the Oversight Committee (chaired by Dr. Carolyn Robinowitz), which served largely as an advisor, keeping the APA Board of Trustees informed of the nature and progress of the DSM-5 effort. All of the proposals of the DSM-5 Task Force must be approved by the APA Board of Trustees. There was also the Clinical and Public Health Review Committee (CPHC; chaired by Drs. Jack MacIntyre and Joel Yager), which was concerned with implications of a respective proposal for public health care. Finally, there was the Scientific Review Committee (SRC; chaired by Drs. Kenneth Kendler and Robert Freedman) which was concerned with the extent of empirical support for the respective proposals.

The final literature review by the PPDWG was submitted to the DSM-5 Task Force, which approved the proposals. Their review was then forward to the CPHC and the SRC. As indicated by Skodol and colleagues (2013, p. 348), "the review by the CPHC primarily raised concerns about the decision . . . not to specify four of the DSM-IV PDs" that the CPHC felt were in fact of importance to clinicians. The CPHC also felt that the new method proposed for diagnosing the PDs was "too complicated and unfamiliar for immediate use by psychiatrists" (p. 348). Skodol and colleagues also summarized the conclusions of the SRC: "Predictive validators and familial aggregation were given special weight. Because such data had not been gathered on the specific model proposed by the [work group] . . . the proposal was viewed as not strongly supported by the published research at the time" (p. 347). In summary, the CPHC and SRC recommended to the APA Board of Trustees to reject all of the proposals by the PPDWG. The DSM-5 Task Force argued for their approval, but the Board of Trustees agreed with the SRC and CPHC, and rejected all of the recommendations of the Task Force and the PPDWG. None of the proposals was approved. No other work group met with such a wholesale dismissal.

DSM-5 retained the PD categories and criterion sets of DSM-IV-TR. Gunderson (2010b) had offered suggestions for improving the criterion set for BPD. Regrettably, nobody on the PPDWG was given the responsibility of improving the criterion sets on the basis of what was likely to be a considerable body of existing research. The PD diagnostic criterion sets have remained unchanged since 1994.

Krueger and Markon (2014) suggest that rejection of the PPDWG's proposals was the result of "political processes" (p. 482). As suggested earlier, there may indeed have been a considerable amount of backchannel communication and backroom pressure. However, as indicated by First (2014) and Skodol and colleagues (2013), it was the opinion of the SRC (Kendler, 2013) that the PPDWG proposals lacked adequate empirical support. Blashfield and Reynolds (2012) systematically reviewed the reference list provided in the final PPDWG review, and concluded that it was slanted heavily toward papers and studies published by the work group members and/or their close colleagues, neglecting a considerable body of additional research. For example, Blashfield and Reynolds noted that there was only one reference to FFM research despite it being the "dominant dimensional approach in the personality literature. . . . Cleckley and Hare are well-known authors who defined how psychopathy is currently conceptualized; neither was referenced in the DSM-5 rationale" (p. 826). And, it should be noted, Blashfield and Reynolds had reviewed the final version of the literature review that could have benefited from the critiques of the original reviews. The critique of Blashfield and Reynolds would surely have been even stronger if they had reviewed the initial PPDWG literature reviews (i.e., Clark & Krueger, 2010; Skodol, 2010), which were even more narrow and circumscribed. It was these reviews that helped to generate the objections and controversy (i.e., Bornstein, 2011; Clarkin & Huprich, 2011; Gunderson, 2010a, 2010b; Paris, 2011; Pilkonis et al., 2011; Pincus, 2011; Ronningstam, 2011; Shedler et al., 2010; Widiger, 2011a, 2011b; Zimmerman, 2011, 2012). Two work group members even resigned in frustration over the process and content of the PPDWG proposals and process (Livesley, 2012; Verheul, 2012). A special section of *Personality Disorders: Theory, Research, and Treatment* was devoted to a postmortem review of what went wrong and what should perhaps happen next (i.e., Gunderson, 2013; Krueger, 2013; Skodol et al., 2013; Widiger, 2013).

## Future Editions

The PPDWG proposals were placed in Section III of DSM-5 to stimulate research, as well as to set the stage perhaps for the next edition. As expressed in DSM-5, dimensional approaches will "supersede current categorical approaches in coming years" (AMA, 2013, p. 13). However, what is in store for the future is not really clear.

DSM-5 shifted from Roman numeric (e.g., DSM-IV) to Arabic (i.e., DSM-5) because it is anticipated that future revisions will occur more frequently and at times be confined to one or more particular sections of the manual (First, 2014). However, the timetable has not been specified and will likely be at the discretion of the APA Committee on Diagnosis and Assessment. The future PD work group will face a number of issues. A few of these are discussed in turn.

### DSM-IV-TR Diagnostic Categories

One might say that many of the DSM-IV-TR PD diagnostic categories obtained a stay of execution. The death of four had been scheduled, but with the dismissal of virtually all of the proposals, dependent, histrionic, paranoid, and schizoid PDs managed to avoid the executioner. However, it would appear that their existence lies on thin ice. Some persons came to the defense of DPD (Bornstein, 2011; Gore & Pincus, 2012; Widiger, 2010), but the schizoid (Hopwood & Thomas, 2012; Hummelen, Pedersen, Wilberg, & Karterud, 2015; Triebwasser, Chemerinski, Roussos, & Siever, 2012), paranoid (Hopwood & Thomas, 2012; Triebwasser, Chemerinski, Roussos, & Siever, 2013), and histrionic (Blashfield et al., 2012) PDs have received little defense.

Shedler and colleagues (2010) argued against the deletion of any PD diagnosis, suggesting that the absence of research does not imply an absence of clinical utility. The DSM-5 CPHC appeared to agree with them (Skodol et al., 2013). If deleted, they might indeed be missed. There is little direct research concerning the histrionic, schizoid, and paranoid PDs, but they do cover important areas of maladaptive personality functioning. For example, the histrionic and schizoid PDs anchor the opposite poles of FFM Extraversion and Introversion (Lynam & Widiger, 2001); their deletion would lose a considerable body of relatively unique maladaptive personality functioning. In any case, it will be important for researchers who want this content to be retained to conduct studies demonstrating their specific and/or incremental importance relative to the other PDs.

The other six PDs are not really safe from potential termination. The schizotypal and antisocial PDs are cross-listed within the schizophrenia and disruptive behavior disorder sections of the diagnostic manual, as one step toward their potential removal from the PDs section. A proposal considered at the first DSM-5 research planning conference, co-chaired by Steven Hyman, was to reformulate many of the PDs as early-onset, chronic variants of an Axis I disorder (e.g., BPD becomes mood dysregulation disorder and AVPD becomes a variant of generalized phobia). The only PDs that appeared to be difficult to change into an Axis I disorder were NPD, DPD, and histrionic PD, and these were proposed for deletion by the DSM-5 PPDWG. Dr. Hyman was Chair of the DSM-5 Diagnostic Spectra and DSM/ICD Harmonization Study Group, and he continued to lobby for the reformulations of the PDs as variants of Axis I disorders. He met with little success, but the cross-listing for two of them is one clear step in this direction. It will be important for future research to address the question of whether the borderline, antisocial, schizotypal, avoidant, and obsessive–compulsive PDs (along with the NPD and DPD) are best understood as disorders of personality if this section of the diagnostic manual is to survive (Links & Eynan, 2013; Widiger, 2003, 2012).

### The Hybrid Model

The hybrid model appears to have been a last-minute compromise among work group members after the rejection of the prototype narratives (Livesley, 2013). A useful focus of future research will be a comparison of the hybrid and DSM-IV criterion sets, whose focus should be to demonstrate improvement rather than just agreement. It was the intention of the authors of DSM-5 to address the limitations of DSM-IV-TR, such as the excessive co-occurrence and heterogeneity (APA, 2012; Skodol, 2010). However, it is not clear how the hybrid model criterion sets offer any improvement. The focus of the existing research has been on the extent to which the hybrid model reproduces DSM-IV-TR (e.g., Morey & Skodol, 2013) as if that were actually the goal of DSM-5. What is needed is research indicating that the hybrid model provides an improvement in discriminative validity, homogeneity of membership, and/or any other stated failing of the DSM-IV-TR.

For example, Skodol, Bender, and Morey (2014) present the DSM-5 Section III hybrid model diagnostic criteria for NPD, which includes four deficits in sense of self and interpersonal relatedness (any two of which are required) and the maladaptive traits of grandiosity and attention seeking (both of which are required). They stated that "the Section III representation of narcissistic phenomena using dimensions of self and interpersonal functioning and relevant traits offers a significant improvement over Section II NPD, which continues to perpetuate all of the shortcomings associated with the diagnosis since DSM-III" (p. 426). However, they did not present any findings that indicated or even suggested an improvement. This appears to be simply an assumption. No study has yet demonstrated an improvement of the hybrid model criterion sets with respect to the failings that have been evident for the DSM-IV criterion sets. In fact, the research has been confined to how the hybrid criteria replicate DSM-IV-TR diagnoses. If the goal were to reproduce DSM-IV-TR, then the optimal revision would have been simply to make no changes whatsoever.

Another area of useful research will be the extent to which the self–interpersonal deficits (Criterion A) and the maladaptive personality traits (Criterion B) within the hybrid model are actually both necessary. In theory, they cover different aspects of personality pathology; otherwise, there would be no need for both to be present. However, they have the appearance of simply two different perspectives being cobbled together (Livesley, 2013). The limited research to date suggests that there is little to distinguish them (e.g., Bastiaansen, De Fruyt, Rossi, Schotte, & Hofmans, 2013; Berghuis, Kamphuis, & Verhuel, 2014).

### NIMH Research Domain Criteria

As the construction of DSM-5 was drawing to a close, Thomas Insel, the Director of NIMH, announced that the agency no longer wished to fund studies that used the APA nomenclature. "It is critical to realize that we cannot succeed if we use DSM categories" (Insel, 2013). NIMH has become frustrated with the (presumably inadequate) rate at which researchers have been able to identify specific etiologies, pathologies, and treatments. NIMH blames much of this on a diagnostic system that relies on overt features rather than assessing for the underlying pathology. NIMH appears to be embracing one particular model of psychopathology: the neurobiological (i.e., clearly not the psychodynamic). "Mental disorders are biological disorders involving brain circuits that implicate specific domains of cognition, emotion, or behavior"

(Insel, 2013). NIMH is likely to give preference in future funding to its own neurobiologically oriented nomenclature, the Research Domain Criteria (RDoC), consisting of five broad domains: negative valence, positive valence, cognitive systems, social processes, and arousal/modulatory systems (Insel, 2013).

Skodol (2014) suggests that the DSM-5 hybrid diagnostic categories are consistent with the RDoC social processes domain. This might be a bit optimistic given the explicit rejection of DSM-IV-TR constructs by Insel (2013). However, the DSM-5 Section III negative affectivity domain from the dimensional trait model does appear to align well with RDoC negative valence, and the psychoticism domain may align with RDoC cognitive systems. RDoC positive valence (reward, approach) might align well with FFM Extraversion as positive affectivity is the driving temperament for extraversion (Clark & Watson, 2008). RDoC arousal regulatory systems may in turn align well with FFM Conscientiousness, as this domain concerns regulatory constraint (Clark & Watson, 2008). The Section III DSM-5 dimensional trait model domains of detachment and disinhibition would then, in turn, align with RDoC positive valence and RDoC arousal regulatory systems, albeit reverse-keyed. The dimensional trait dimensions of antagonism and detachment concern matters of interpersonal relatedness and might then align with RDoC social processes. In summary, it would be of interest for future research to test empirically the congruency of the hybrid model, Section III level of personality functioning, and the dimensional trait model with the RDoC domains.

## ICD-11

As the DSM-5 PPDWG struggled with dissension, controversy, and pushback, the ICD-11 PD work group has progressed without a comparable level of attention or apparent controversy, yet an even more radical proposal for ICD-11 has been put forward (Tyrer et al., 2011). The official proposal for ICD-11 is to delete all of the categories, including BPD and ASPD, and replace them with a global rating of level of severity and a five-domain dimensional trait model.

The severity rating concerns four levels: personality difficulty, PD, complex PD, and severe PD (Tyrer et al., 2011). The proposed severity rating aligns conceptually with the DSM-5 level of personality functioning but it is considerably less complex and does not include inferences with respect to deficits in the sense of self (Tyrer, 2014).

The ICD-11 dimensional trait model has varied. One version consisted of four domains: internalization, externalization, schizoid, and compulsivity (Mulder, Newton-Howes, Crawford, & Tyrer, 2011). A subsequent version consisted of five domains: emotionally unstable, anxious/dependent, asocial/schizoid, dissocial, and obsessional/anankastic (Tyrer et al., 2011). The latest version (to date) consists of a revised set of five domains: negative emotionality, schizoid/detached, dissocial/externalizing, obsessional/anankastic, and disinhibition that resulted from "negotiations" (Tyrer et al., 2014) and is more closely aligned with the DSM-5 trait model, albeit without including psychoticism (the WHO [1992] considers schizotypal PD to be a form of schizophrenia rather than a PD), and has disinhibition and obsessional/anakastic as independent domains, consistent with the original Clark and Krueger (2010) proposal.

One distinction between the ICD-11 dimensional trait model and the DSM-5 proposal is that the former does not include lower-order facet scales. A significant focus of the existing research concerning the DSM-5 dimensional trait is its ability to recover the DSM-IV-TR personality syndromes (Krueger & Markon, 2014). Being able to recover the DSM-IV and ICD-10 syndromes with the dimensional trait models should be reassuring to persons who still wish to conceptualize PDs in terms of these syndromes. However, the absence of lower-order trait scales will make it difficult for the ICD-11 trait model to provide this information. The names for two of the ICD-10 syndromes do appear in the titles of the ICD-11 domains (i.e., anankastic and dissocial), but these domains may not actually be entirely equivalent to any particular ICD-10 syndrome. It might be useful for future research to compare not only the DSM-5 dimensional trait model with the ICD-11 dimensional trait model but also their relative ability to recover DSM-IV and/or ICD-10 personality syndromes.

## Conclusions

The construction of a diagnostic manual is a difficult task, in large part because it represents simply the opinions of its authors (Frances & Widiger, 2012). There is no "gold standard" for determining whose opinion is correct and whose is incorrect (Widiger & Crego, 2015). It has been suggested that there is actually a consensus within the PD field (i.e., Skodol, 2014), but there may instead be sharply divided factions (Widiger, 2013). Kendler and colleagues (2009) had suggested that any revision should represent a consensus view. This might not be realistic for the field of PD. One only has to read the critiques of the PPDWG proposals to appreciate that there is not much of a consensus (i.e., Bornstein, 2011; Clarkin & Huprich, 2011; Gunderson, 2010a, 2010b; Livesley, 2010, 2013; Paris, 2011; Pilkonis et al., 2011; Pincus, 2011; Ronningstam, 2011; Shedler et al., 2010; Widiger, 2011a, 2011b; Zimmerman, 2011, 2012). All of these authors disagree strongly with the views of the DSM-5 PPDWG, but they also disagree strongly with one another. It may take a strong hand and brave soul to achieve innovation in the presence of this diversity of opinion.

## REFERENCES

American Psychiatric Association. (1952). *Diagnostic and statistical manual of mental disorders.* Washington, DC: Author.
American Psychiatric Association. (1968). *Diagnostic and statistical manual of mental disorders* (2nd ed.). Washington, DC: Author.
American Psychiatric Association. (1980). *Diagnostic and statistical manual of mental disorders* (3rd ed.). Washington, DC: Author.
American Psychiatric Association. (1987). *Diagnostic and statistical manual of mental disorders* (3rd ed., rev.). Washington, DC: Author.
American Psychiatric Association. (1994). *Diagnostic and statistical manual of mental disorders* (4th ed.). Washington, DC: Author.
American Psychiatric Association. (2000). *Diagnostic and statistical manual of mental disorders* (4th ed., text rev.). Washington, DC: Author.
American Psychiatric Association. (2010, February 10). Personality disorders. Retrieved February 12, 2010, from *www.dsm5.org/proposedrevisions/pages/personalityandpersonalitydisorders.aspx.*
American Psychiatric Association. (2012). *Rationale for the proposed changes to the personality disorder classification in DSM-5.* Unpublished manuscript, American Psychiatric Association, Washington, DC.
American Psychiatric Association. (2013). *Diagnostic and statistical manual of mental disorders* (5th ed.). Arlington, VA: Author.
Bagby, R. M., Watson, C., & Ryder, A. G. (2012). Depressive personality disorder. In T. A. Widiger (Ed.), *The Oxford handbook of personality disorders* (pp. 628–647). New York: Oxford University Press.

Bastiaansen, L., De Fruyt, F., Rossi, G., Schotte, C., & Hofmans, J. (2013). Personality disorder dysfunction versus traits: Structural and conceptual issues. *Personality Disorders: Theory, Research, and Treatment, 4,* 293–303.
Bender, D. S., Morey, L. C., & Skodol, A. E. (2011). Toward a model for assessing level of personality functioning in DSM-5: Part I. A review of theory and methods. *Journal of Personality Assessment, 93,* 332–346.
Berghuis, H., Kamphuis, J. H., & Verheul, R. (2014). Specific personality traits and general personality dysfunction as predictors of the presence and severity of personality disorders in a clinical sample. *Journal of Personality Assessment, 96,* 410–416.
Blashfield, R. K., & Breen, M. (1989). Face validity of the DSM-III-R personality disorders. *American Journal of Psychiatry, 146,* 1575–1579.
Blashfield, R. K., & Draguns, J. G. (1976). Evaluative criteria for psychiatric classification. *Journal of Abnormal Psychology, 85,* 140–150.
Blashfield, R. K., & Flanagan, E. (1998). A prototypic nonprototype of a personality disorder. *Journal of Nervous and Mental Disease, 186,* 244–246.
Blashfield, R. K., & Intoccia, V. (2000). Growth of the literature on the topic of personality disorders. *American Journal of Psychiatry, 157,* 472–473.
Blashfield, R. K., Keeley, J. W., Flanagan, E. H., & Miles, S. R. (2014). The cycle of classification: DSM-I through DSM-5. *Annual Review of Clinical Psychology, 10,* 25–51.
Blashfield, R. K., & Reynolds, S. M. (2012). An invisible college view of the DSM-5 personality disorder classification. *Journal of Personality Disorders, 26,* 821–829.
Blashfield, R. K., Reynolds, S. M., & Stennett, B. (2012). The death of histrionic personality disorder. In T. A. Widiger (Ed.), *The Oxford handbook of personality disorders* (pp. 603–627). New York: Oxford University Press.
Bornstein, R. F. (2011). Reconceptualizing personality pathology in DSM-5: Limitations in evidence for eliminating dependent personality disorder and other DSM-IV syndromes. *Journal of Personality Disorders, 25,* 235–247.
Bornstein, R. F. (2012a). From dysfunction to adaptation: An interactionist model of dependency. *Annual Review of Clinical Psychology, 8,* 291–316.
Bornstein, R. F. (2012b). Illuminating a neglected clinical issue: Societal costs of interpersonal dependency and dependent personality disorder. *Journal of Clinical Psychology, 68,* 766–781.
Boschen, M. J., & Warner, J. C. (2009). Publication trends in individual DSM personality disorders: 1971–2015. *Australian Psychologist, 44,* 136–142.
Campbell, W. K., & Miller, J. D. (Eds.). (2011). *Handbook of narcissism and narcissistic personality disorder: Theoretical approaches, empirical findings, and treatments.* New York: Wiley.
Caplan, P. J. (1991). How do they decide who is normal?:

The bizarre, but true, tale of the DSM process. *Canadian Psychology, 32,* 162–170.

Clark, L. A. (2007). Assessment and diagnosis of personality disorder: Perennial issues and an emerging reconceptualization. *Annual Review of Psychology, 57,* 227–257.

Clark, L. A., & Krueger, R. F. (2010). Rationale for a six-domain trait dimensional diagnostic system for personality disorder. Retrieved February 10, 2010, from *www.dsm5.org/proposedrevisions/pages/rationaleforasix-domaintraitdimensionaldiagnosticsystemforpersonalitydisorder.aspx.*

Clark, L. A., & Watson, D. (2008). Temperament: An organizing paradigm for trait psychology. In O. P. John, R. W. Robins, & L. A. Pervin (Eds.), *Handbook of personality: Theory and research* (3rd ed., pp. 265–286). New York: Guilford Press.

Clarkin, J. F., & Huprich, S. K. (2011). Do DSM-5 personality disorder proposals meet criteria for clinical utility? *Journal of Personality Disorders, 25,* 192–205.

Costa, P. T., Jr., & Widiger, T. A. (Eds.). (2002). *Personality disorders and the five factor model of personality* (2nd ed.). Washington, DC: American Psychological Association.

Crego, C., & Widiger, T. A. (2015). Psychopathy and the DSM. *Journal of Personality, 83*(6), 665–677.

Decker, H. S. (2013). *The making of DSM-III: A diagnostic manual's conquest of American psychiatry.* New York: Oxford University Press.

Feighner, J. P., Robins, E., Guze, S. B., Woodruff, R. A., Winokur, G., & Muñoz, R. (1972). Diagnostic criteria for use in psychiatric research. *Archives of General Psychiatry, 26,* 57–63.

Fiester, S. J. (1991). Self-defeating personality disorder: A review of data and recommendations. *Journal of Personality Disorders, 5,* 194–209.

Fiester, S. J., & Gay, M. (1991). Sadistic personality disorder: A review of data and recommendations for DSM-IV. *Journal of Personality Disorders, 5,* 376–385.

First, M. B. (2014). Empirical grounding versus innovation in the DSM-5 revision process: Implications for the future. *Clinical Psychology: Science and Practice, 21,* 262–268.

First, M. B., Bell, C. B., Cuthbert, B., Krystal, J. H., Malison, R., Offord, D. R., et al. (2002). Personality disorders and relational disorders: A research agenda for addressing crucial gaps in DSM. In D. J. Kupfer, M. B. First, & D. A. Regier (Eds.), *A research agenda for DSM-V* (pp. 123–199). Washington, DC: American Psychiatric Association.

First, M. B., & Pincus, H. A. (2002). The DSM-IV Text Revision: Rationale and potential impact on clinical practice. *Psychiatric Services, 53,* 288–292.

First, M. B., & Westen, D. (2007). Classification for clinical practice: How to make ICD and DSM better able to serve clinicians. *International Review of Psychiatry, 19,* 473–481.

Frances, A. J. (1980). The DSM-III personality disorders section: A commentary. *American Journal of Psychiatry, 137,* 1050–1054.

Frances, A. J., Pincus, H. A., Widiger, T. A., Davis, W. W., & First, M. B. (1990). DSM-IV: Work in progress. *American Journal of Psychiatry, 147,* 1439–1448.

Frances, A. J., & Widiger, T. A. (2012). Psychiatric diagnosis: Lessons from the DSM-IV past and cautions for the DSM-5 future. *Annual Review of Clinical Psychology, 8,* 109–130.

Frances, A. J., Widiger, T. A., & Pincus, H. A. (1989). The development of DSM-IV. *Archives of General Psychiatry, 46,* 373–375.

Gore, W. L., & Pincus, A. L. (2013). Dependency and the five-factor model. In T. A. Widiger & P. T. Costa, Jr. (Eds.), *Personality disorders and the five-factor model* (3rd ed., pp. 163–177). Washington, DC: American Psychological Association.

Grob, G. N. (1991). Origins of DSM-I: A study in appearance and reality. *American Journal of Psychiatry, 148,* 421–431.

Gunderson, J. G. (1983). DSM-III diagnoses of personality disorders. In J. Frosch (Ed.), *Current perspectives on personality disorders* (pp. 20–39). Washington, DC: American Psychiatric Press.

Gunderson, J. G. (1998). DSM-IV personality disorders: Final overview. In T. A. Widiger, A. J. Frances, H. A. Pincus, R. Ross, M. B. First, W. Davis, & M. Kline (Eds.), *DSM-IV sourcebook* (Vol. 4, pp. 1123–1140). Washington, DC: American Psychiatric Association.

Gunderson, J. G. (2010a). Commentary on "Personality traits and the classification of mental disorders: Toward a more complete integration in DSM-5 and an empirical model of psychopathology." *Personality Disorders: Theory, Research, and Treatment, 1,* 119–122.

Gunderson, J. G. (2010b). Revising the borderline diagnosis for DSM-V: An alternative proposal. *Journal of Personality Disorders, 24,* 694–708.

Gunderson, J. G. (2013). Seeking clarity for future revisions of the personality disorders in DSM-5. *Personality Disorders: Theory, Research, and Treatment, 4,* 368–378.

Hare, R. D., & Neumann, C. S. (2008). Psychopathy as a clinical and empirical construct. *Annual Review of Clinical Psychology, 4,* 217–246.

Helzer, J. E., Kraemer, H. C., Krueger, R. F., Wittchen, H.-U., Sirovatka, P. J., & Regier, D. A. (Eds.). (2008). *Dimensional approaches to diagnostic classification: Refining the research agenda for DSM-V.* Washington, DC: American Psychiatric Association.

Herkov, M. J., & Blashfield, R. K. (1995). Clinicians' diagnoses of personality disorder: Evidence of a hierarchical structure. *Journal of Personality Assessment, 65,* 313–321.

Hopwood, C. J., & Thomas, K. M. (2012). Paranoid and schizoid personality disorders. In T. A. Widiger (Ed.), *The Oxford handbook of personality disorders* (pp. 582–602). New York: Oxford University Press.

Hummelen, B., Pedersen, G., Wilberg, T., & Karterud, S. (2015). Poor validity of the DSM-IV schizoid personality disorder construct as a diagnostic category. *Journal of Personality Disorders, 29*(3), 334–346.

Huprich, S. K., Bornstein, R. F., & Schmitt, T. A. (2011). Self-report methodology is insufficient for improving the assessment and classification of Axis II personality disorders. *Journal of Personality Disorders, 23,* 557–570.

Hyman, S. E. (2010). The diagnosis of mental disorders: The problem of reification. *Annual Review of Clinical Psychology, 6,* 155–179.

Insel, T. R. (2009). Translating scientific opportunity into public health impact: A strategic plan for research on mental illness. *Archives of General Psychiatry, 66,* 128–133.

Insel, T. R. (2013). Director's blog: Transforming diagnosis. Retrieved from www.nimh.nih.gov/about/director/2013/transforming-diagnosis.shtml.

Insel, T. R., & Quirion, R. (2005). Psychiatry as a clinical neuroscience discipline. *Journal of the American Medical Association, 294,* 2221–2224.

Kass, F., MacKinnon, R. A., & Spitzer, R. L. (1986). Masochistic personality disorder: An empirical study. *American Journal of Psychiatry, 143,* 216–218.

Kass, F., Spitzer, R. L., Williams, J. B., & Widiger, T. (1989). Self-defeating personality disorder and DSM-III-R: Development of the diagnostic criteria. *American Journal of Psychiatry, 146,* 1022–1026.

Keller, M. (1989). Current concepts in affective disorders. *Journal of Clinical Psychiatry, 50,* 157–162.

Keller, M. B., Klein, D. N., Hirschfeld, R., Kocsis, J. H., McCullough, J. P., Miller, I., et al. (1995). Results of the DSM-IV mood disorders field trial. *American Journal of Psychiatry, 152,* 843–869.

Kendell, R. E. (1975). *The role of diagnosis in psychiatry.* London: Blackwell Scientific.

Kendell, R. E. (1991). Relationship between the DSM-IV and the ICD-10. *Journal of Abnormal Psychology, 100,* 297–301.

Kendler, K. S. (2013). A history of the DSM-5 scientific review committee. *Psychological Medicine, 43,* 1793–1800.

Kendler, K. S., Kupfer, D., Narrow, W., Phillips, K., & Fawcett, J. (2009). *Guidelines for making changes to DSM-V.* Unpublished manuscript, American Psychiatric Association, Washington, DC.

Kendler, K., Muñoz, R. A., & Murphy, G. (2010). The development of the Feighner criteria: A historical perspective. *American Journal of Psychiatry, 167,* 134–142.

Kernberg, O. F. (1984). Problems in the classification of personality disorders. In O. F. Kernberg (Ed.), *Severe personality disorders: Psychotherapeutic strategies* (pp. 77–94). New Haven, CT: Yale University Press.

Kernberg, O. F. (2012). Overview and critique of the classification of personality disorders proposed for DSM-V. *Swiss Archives of Neurology and Psychiatry, 163,* 234–238.

Kramer, M., Sartorius, N., Jablensky, A., & Gulbinat, W. (1979). The ICD-9 classification of mental disorders: A review of its development and contents. *Acta Psychiatrica Scandinavica, 59,* 241–262.

Krueger, R. F. (2013). Personality disorders are the vanguard of the post-DSM-5.0 era. *Personality Disorders: Theory, Research, and Treatment, 4,* 355–362.

Krueger, R. F., Derringer, J., Markon, K. E., Watson, D., & Skodol, A. E. (2012). Initial construction of a maladaptive personality trait model and inventory for DSM-5. *Psychological Medicine, 42,* 1879–1890.

Krueger, R. F., & Markon, K. E. (2014). The role of the DSM-5 personality trait model in moving toward a quantitative and empirically based approach to classifying personality and psychopathology. *Annual Review of Clinical Psychology, 10,* 477–501.

Krueger, R. F., Skodol, A. E., Livesley, W. J., Shrout, P. E., & Huang, Y. (2008). Synthesizing dimensional and categorical approaches to personality disorders: Refining the research agenda for DSM-V Axis II. In J. E. Helzer, H. C. Kraemer, R. F. Krueger, H.-U. Wittchen, P. J. Sirovatka, & D. A. Regier (Eds.), *Dimensional approaches to diagnostic classification: Refining the research agenda for DSM-V* (pp. 85–100). Washington, DC: American Psychiatric Association.

Kupfer, D. J., First, M. B. & Regier, D. A. (2002). Introduction. In D. J. Kupfer, M. B. First, & D. A. Regier (Eds.), *A research agenda for DSM-V* (pp. xv–xxiii). Washington, DC: American Psychiatric Association.

Links, P. S., & Eynan, R. (2013). The relationship between personality disorders and Axis I psychopathology: Deconstructing comorbidity. *Annual Review of Clinical Psychology, 9,* 529–554.

Livesley, W. J. (2007). A framework for integrating dimensional and categorical classifications of personality disorder. *Journal of Personality Disorders, 21,* 199–224.

Livesley, W. J. (2010). Confusion and incoherence in the classification of personality disorder: Commentary on the preliminary proposals for DSM-5. *Psychological Injury and Law, 3,* 304–313.

Livesley, W. J. (2012). Tradition versus empiricism in the current DSM-5 proposal for revising the classification of personality disorders. *Criminal Behavior and Mental Health, 22,* 81–90.

Livesley, W. J. (2013). The DSM-5 personality disorder proposal and future directions in the diagnostic classification of personality disorder. *Psychopathology, 46,* 207–216.

Loranger, A. W. (1990). The impact of DSM-III on diagnostic practice in a university hospital. *Archives of General Psychiatry, 47,* 672–675.

Lynam, D. R., & Widiger, T. A. (2001). Using the five factor model to represent the DSM-IV personality disorders: An expert consensus approach. *Journal of Abnormal Psychology, 110,* 401–412.

Malinow, K. (1981). Passive–aggressive personality. In J. Lion (Ed.), *Personality disorders* (2nd ed., pp. 121–132). Baltimore: Williams & Wilkins.

Markon, K. (2013). Epistemological pluralism and scientific development: An argument against authoritative nosologies. *Journal of Personality Disorders, 27,* 554–579.

Mellsop, G., Varghese, F., Joshua, S., & Hicks, A. (1982). Reliability of Axis II of DSM-III. *American Journal of Psychiatry, 139,* 1360–1361.

Menninger, K. (1963). *The vital balance.* New York: Viking Press.

Miller, J. D., & Lynam, D. R. (2013). Missed opportunities in the DSM-5 Section III personality disorder model. *Personality Disorders: Theory, Research, and Treatment, 4,* 365–366.

Miller, J. D., Widiger, T. A., & Campbell, W. K. (2010). Narcissistic personality disorder and the DSM-V. *Journal of Abnormal Psychology, 119,* 640–649.

Miller, P. R. (2008). Inpatient diagnostic assessments: 3. Causes and effects of diagnostic imprecision. *Psychiatry Research, 111,* 191–197.

Millon, T. (1981). *Disorders of personality: DSM-III: Axis II.* New York: Wiley.

Millon, T. (2011). *Disorders of personality: Introducing a DSM/ICD spectrum from normal to abnormal* (3rd ed.). New York: Wiley.

Morey, L., & Ochoa, E. (1989). An investigation of adherence to diagnostic criteria: Clinical diagnosis of the DSM-III personality disorders. *Journal of Personality Disorders, 3,* 180–192.

Morey, L. C., & Skodol, A. E. (2013). Convergence between DSM-IV-TR and DSM-5 diagnostic models for personality disorder: Evaluation of strategies for establishing diagnostic thresholds. *Journal of Psychiatric Practice, 19,* 179–193.

Mulder, R. T., Newton-Howes, G., Crawford, M. J., & Tyrer, P. J. (2011). The central domains of personality pathology in psychiatric patients. *Journal of Personality Disorders, 25,* 364–377.

Mullins-Sweatt, S. N., Bernstein, D. P., & Widiger, T. A. (2012). Retention or deletion of personality disorder diagnoses for DSM-5: An expert consensus approach. *Journal of Personality Disorders, 26,* 689–703.

Mullins-Sweatt, S. N., & Widiger, T. A. (2009). Clinical utility and DSM-V. *Psychological Assessment, 21,* 302–312.

Paris, J. (2011). Endophenotypes and the diagnosis of personality disorders. *Journal of Personality Disorder, 25,* 260–268.

Phillips, K. A., Gunderson, J. G., Hirschfeld, R. M., & Smith, L. E. (1990). A review of the depressive personality. *American Journal of Psychiatry, 147,* 830–837.

Phillips, K. A., Gunderson, J. G., Triebwasser, J., Kimble, C. R., Faedda, G., Lyoo, I. K., et al. (1998). Reliability and validity of depressive personality disorder. *American Journal of Psychiatry, 155*(8), 1044–1048.

Phillips, K. A., Hirschfeld, R. M., Shea, M. T., & Gunderson, J. G. (1993). Depressive personality disorder: Perspectives for DSM-IV. *Journal of Personality Disorders, 7,* 30–42.

Pilkonis, P., Hallquist, M. N., Morse, J. Q., & Stepp, S. D. (2011). Striking the (im)proper balance between scientific advances and clinical utility: Commentary on the DSM-5 proposal for personality disorders. *Personality Disorders: Theory, Research, and Treatment, 2,* 68–82.

Pincus, A. L. (2011). Some comments on nomology, diagnostic process, and narcissistic personality disorder in the DSM-5 proposal for personality and personality disorders. *Personality Disorders: Theory, Research, and Treatment, 2,* 41–53.

Pincus, A. L., & Hopwood, C. J. (2012). A contemporary interpersonal model of personality pathology and personality disorder. In T. A. Widiger (Ed.), *The Oxford handbook of personality disorders* (pp. 372–388). New York: Oxford University Press.

Regier, D. A., Narrow, W. E., Kuhl, E. A., & Kupfer, D. J. (2009). The conceptual development of DSM-V. *American Journal of Psychiatry, 166,* 645–655.

Robins, L. N. (1966). *Deviant children grown up.* Baltimore: Williams & Wilkins.

Ronningstam, E. (2005). Narcissistic personality disorder: A review. In M. Maj, H. Akiskal, J. Mezzich, & A. Okasha (Eds.), *Evidence and experiences in psychiatry: Personality disorders* (Vol. 8, pp. 277–327). Chichester, UK: Wiley.

Ronningstam, E. (2010). Narcissistic personality disorder—A current review. *Current Psychiatry Reports, 12,* 68–75.

Ronningstam, E. (2011). Narcissistic personality disorder in DSM-V: In support of retaining a significant diagnosis. *Journal of Personality Disorders, 25,* 248–259.

Rosenhan, D. L. (1973). On being sane in insane places. *Science, 179,* 250–258.

Rounsaville, B. J., Alarcon, R. D., Andrews, G., Jackson, J. S., Kendell, R. E., Kendler, K. S., et al. (2002). Toward DSM-V: Basic nomenclature issues. In D. J. Kupfer, M. B. First, & D. A. Regier (Eds.), *A research agenda for DSM-V* (pp. 1–30). Washington, DC: American Psychiatric Press.

Salmon, T. W., Copp, O., May, J. V., Abbot, E. S., & Cotton, H. A. (1917). Report of the committee on statistics of the American Medico-Psychological Association. *American Journal of Insanity, 74,* 255–260.

Samuel, D. B., Lynam, D. R., Widiger, T. A., & Ball, S. (2012). An expert consensus approach to relating the proposed DSM-5 types and traits. *Personality Disorders: Theory, Research, and Treatment, 3,* 1–16.

Sartorius, N. (1988). International perspectives of psychiatric classification. *British Journal of Psychiatry, 152*(Suppl.), 9–14.

Sartorius, N., Kaelber, C. T., Cooper, J. E., Roper, M., Rae, D. S., Gulbinat, W., et al. (1993). Progress toward achieving a common language in psychiatry. *Archives of General Psychiatry, 50,* 115–124.

Shea, M. T. (1996). Enduring personality change after catastrophic experience. In T. A. Widiger, A. J. Frances, H. A. Pincus, R. Ross, M. B. First, & W. W. Davis (Eds.), *DSM-IV sourcebook* (Vol. 2, pp. 849–860). Washington, DC: American Psychiatric Association.

Shedler, J., Beck, A., Fonagy, P., Gabbard, G. O., Gunderson, J. G., Kernberg, O., et al. (2010). Personality disorders in DSM-5. *American Journal of Psychiatry, 167,* 1027–1028.

Skodol, A. (2010). Rationale for proposing five specific personality types. Retrieved February 10, 2010, from www.dsm5.org/proposedrevisions/pages/rationale-forproposingfivespecificpersonalitydisordertypes.aspx.

Skodol, A. (2012). Diagnosis and DSM-5: Work in progress. In T. A. Widiger (Ed.), *The Oxford handbook of personality disorders* (pp. 35–57). New York: Oxford University Press.

Skodol, A. (2014). Personality disorder classification: Stuck in neutral, how to move forward? *Current Psychiatry Reports, 16*(10), 480.

Skodol, A. E., Bender, D. S., & Morey, L. C. (2014). Narcissistic personality disorder in DSM-5. *Personality Disorders: Theory, Research, and Treatment, 5*(4), 422–427.

Skodol, A. E., Bender, D. S., Morey, L. C., Clark, L. A., Oldham, J. M., Alarcon, R. D., et al. (2011). Personality disorder types proposed for DSM-5. *Journal of Personality Disorders, 25,* 136–169.

Skodol, A. E., Gunderson, J. G., Shea, M. T., McGlashan, T. H., Morey, L. C., Sanislow, C. A., et al. (2005). The Collaborative Longitudinal Personality Disorders Study (CLPS): Overview and implications. *Journal of Personality Disorders, 19,* 487–504.

Skodol, A. E., Morey, L. C., Bender, D. S., & Oldham, J. M. (2013). The ironic fate of the personality disorders in DSM-5. *Personality Disorders: Theory, Research, and Treatment, 4,* 342–349.

Spitzer, R. L., Endicott, J., & Robins, E. (1975). Clinical criteria for psychiatric diagnosis and DSM-III. *American Journal of Psychiatry, 132,* 1187–1192.

Spitzer, R. L., & Fleiss, J. L. (1974). A re-analysis of the reliability of psychiatric diagnosis. *British Journal of Psychiatry, 125,* 341–347.

Spitzer, R. L., Forman, J. B., & Nee, J. (1979). DSM-III field trials: I. Initial diagnostic reliability. *American Journal of Psychiatry, 136,* 815–817.

Spitzer, R. L., Sheehy, M., & Endicott, J. (1977). DSM-III: Guiding principles. In V. Rakoff, H. Stancer, & H. Kedward (Eds.), *Psychiatric diagnosis* (pp. 1–24). New York: Brunner/Mazel.

Spitzer, R. L., & Williams, J. B. W. (1985). Classification of mental disorders. In H. Kaplan & B. Sadock (Eds.), *Comprehensive textbook of psychiatry* (4th ed., Vol. 1, pp. 591–613). Baltimore: Williams & Wilkins.

Spitzer, R. L., Williams, J. B. W., & Skodol, A. E. (1980). DSM-III: The major achievements and an overview. *American Journal of Psychiatry, 137,* 151–164.

Spitzer, R. L., & Wilson, P. T. (1968). A guide to the American Psychiatric Association's new diagnostic nomenclature. *American Journal of Psychiatry, 124,* 1619–1629.

Spitzer, R. L., & Wilson, P. T. (1975). Nosology and the official psychiatric nomenclature. In A. M. Freedman, H. I. Kaplan, & B. J. Sadock (Eds.), *Comprehensive textbook of psychiatry* (2nd ed., Vol. 1, pp. 826–845). Baltimore: Williams & Wilkins.

Stengel, E. (1959). Classification of mental disorders. *Bulletin of the World Health Organization, 21,* 601–663.

Szasz, T. S. (1961). *The myth of mental illness.* New York: Hoeber-Harper.

Triebwasser, J., Chemerinski, E., Roussos, P., & Siever, L. J. (2012). Schizoid personality disorder. *Journal of Personality Disorders, 26,* 919–926.

Triebwasser, J., Chemerinski, E., Roussos, P., & Siever, L. J. (2013). Paranoid personality disorder. *Journal of Personality Disorders, 27,* 795–805.

Trull, T. J., & Durrett, C. A. (2005). Categorical and dimensional models of personality disorder. *Annual Review of Clinical Psychology, 1,* 355–380.

Tyrer, P. (2014). The likely classification of borderline personality disorder in adolescents in ICD-11. In C. Sharp & J. Tackett (Eds.), *Handbook of borderline personality disorder in children and adolescents* (pp. 451–457). New York: Springer.

Tyrer, P., Crawford, M., Mulder, R., Blashfield, R., Farnam, A., Fossati, A., et al. (2011). The rationale for the reclassification of personality disorder in the 11th revision of the International Classification of Diseases (ICD-11). *Personality and Mental Health, 5,* 246–259.

Tyrer, P., Crawford, M., Sanatinia, R., Tyrer, H., Cooper, S., Muller-Pollard, C., et al. (2014). Preliminary studies of the ICD-11 classification of personality disorder in practice. *Personality and Mental Health, 8,* 254–263.

Verheul, R. (2012). Personality disorder proposal for DSM-5: A heroic and innovative but nevertheless fundamentally flawed attempt to improve DSM-IV. *Clinical Psychology and Psychotherapy, 19,* 369–371.

Verheul, R., & Widiger, T. A. (2004). A meta-analysis of the prevalence and usage of the personality disorder not otherwise specified (PDNOS) diagnosis. *Journal of Personality Disorders, 18,* 309–319.

Ward, C. H., Beck, A. T., Mendelson, M., Mock, J. E., & Erbaugh, J. K. (1962). The psychiatric nomenclature: Reasons for diagnostic disagreement. *Archives of General Psychiatry, 7,* 198–205.

Westen, D., & Muderrisoglu, S. (2003). Assessing personality disorders using a systematic clinical interview: Evaluation of an alternative to structured interviews. *Journal of Personality Disorders, 17,* 351–369.

Westen, D., Shedler, J., & Bradley, R. (2006). A prototype approach to personality disorder diagnosis. *American Journal of Psychiatry, 163,* 846–856.

Wetzler, S., & Jose, A. (2012). Passive–aggressive personality disorder: The demise of a syndrome. In T. A. Widiger (Ed.), *The Oxford handbook of personality disorders* (pp. 674–693). New York: Oxford University Press.

Widiger, T. A. (1995). Deletion of the self-defeating

and sadistic personality disorder diagnoses. In W. J. Livesley (Ed.), *The DSM-IV personality disorders* (pp. 359–373). New York: Guilford Press.

Widiger, T. A. (2001). Official classification systems. In W. J. Livesley (Ed.), *Handbook of personality disorders* (pp. 60–83). New York: Guilford Press.

Widiger, T. A. (2003). Personality disorder and Axis I psychopathology: The problematic boundary of Axis I and Axis II. *Journal of Personality Disorders, 17,* 90–108.

Widiger, T. A. (2010). Personality, interpersonal circumplex, and DSM-5: A commentary on five studies. *Journal of Personality Assessment, 92,* 528–532.

Widiger, T. A. (2011a). The DSM-5 dimensional model of personality disorder: Rationale and empirical support. *Journal of Personality Disorders, 25,* 222–234.

Widiger, T. A. (2011b). A shaky future for personality disorders. *Personality Disorders: Theory, Research, and Treatment, 2,* 54–67.

Widiger, T. A. (2012). Future directions of personality disorder. In T. A. Widiger (Ed.), *The Oxford handbook of personality disorder* (pp. 797–810). New York: Oxford University Press.

Widiger, T. A. (2013). A postmortem and future look at the personality disorders in DSM-5. *Personality Disorders: Theory, Research, and Treatment, 4,* 382–387.

Widiger, T. A., & Boyd, S. (2009). Personality disorders assessment instruments. In J. N. Butcher (Ed.), *Oxford handbook of personality assessment* (pp. 336–363). New York: Oxford University Press.

Widiger, T. A., Cadoret, R., Hare, R., Robins, L., Rutherford, M., Zanarini, M., et al. (1996). DSM-IV antisocial personality disorder field trial. *Journal of Abnormal Psychology, 105,* 3–16.

Widiger, T. A., & Corbitt, E. M. (1995). Antisocial personality disorder in DSM-IV. In W. J. Livesley (Ed.), *The DSM-IV personality disorders* (pp. 103–126). New York: Guilford Press.

Widiger, T. A., & Costa, P. T. (1994). Personality and personality disorders. *Journal of Abnormal Psychology, 103,* 78–91.

Widiger, T. A., & Crego, C. (2015). Process and content of DSM-5. *Psychopathology Review, 2*(1), 162–176.

Widiger, T. A., Frances, A. J., Pincus, H., Davis, W., & First, M. (1991). Toward an empirical classification for DSM-IV. *Journal of Abnormal Psychology, 100,* 280–288.

Widiger, T. A., Frances, A. J., Spitzer, R. L., & Williams, J. B. W. (1988). The DSM-III-R personality disorders: An overview. *American Journal of Psychiatry, 145,* 786–795.

Widiger, T. A., Mangine, S., Corbitt, E. M., Ellis, C. G., & Thomas, G. V. (1995). *Personality Disorder Interview–IV: A semistructured interview for the assessment of personality disorders.* Odessa, FL: Psychological Assessment Resources.

Widiger, T. A., Samuel, D. B., Mullins-Sweatt, S., Gore, W. L., & Crego, C. (2012). Integrating normal and abnormal personality structure: The five-factor model. In T. A. Widiger (Ed.), *The Oxford handbook of personality disorders* (pp. 82–107). New York: Oxford University Press.

Widiger, T. A., & Simonsen, E. (2005). Alternative dimensional models of personality disorder: Finding a common ground. *Journal of Personality Disorders, 19,* 110–130.

Widiger, T. A., Simonsen, E., Krueger, R., Livesley, W. J., & Verheul, R. (2005). Personality disorder research agenda for the DSM-V. *Journal of Personality Disorders, 19,* 315–338.

Widiger, T. A., & Trull, T. J. (2007). Plate tectonics in the classification of personality disorder: Shifting to a dimensional model. *American Psychologist, 62,* 71–83.

Williams, J. B. W., & Spitzer, R. L. (1980). DSM-III field trials: Interrater reliability and list of project staff and participants. In *Diagnostic and statistical manual of mental disorders* (3rd ed., pp. 467–469). Washington, DC: American Psychiatric Association.

World Health Organization. (1992). *The ICD-10 classification of mental and behavioural disorders: Clinical descriptions and diagnostic guidelines.* Geneva, Switzerland: Author.

Zigler, E., & Phillips, L. (1961). Psychiatric diagnosis: A critique. *Journal of Abnormal and Social Psychology, 63,* 607–618.

Zilboorg, G. (1941). *A history of medical psychology.* New York: Norton.

Zimmerman, M. (1994). Diagnosing personality disorders: A review of issues and research methods. *Archives of General Psychiatry, 51,* 225–245.

Zimmerman, M. (2011). A critique of the proposed prototype rating system for personality disorders in DSM-5. *Journal of Personality Disorders, 25,* 206–221.

Zimmerman, M. (2012). Is there adequate empirical justification for radically revising the personality disorders section for DSM-5? *Personality Disorders: Theory, Research, and Treatment, 3,* 444–445.

# CHAPTER 4

# Dimensional Approaches to Personality Disorder Classification

Shani Ofrat, Robert F. Krueger, and Lee Anna Clark

This chapter serves as an overview of various issues, points of contention, costs, and benefits of a dimensional approach to personality disorder (PD) in authoritative classification systems (e.g., DSM), research, and clinical practice. First, we provide a summary of the well-documented limitations of categorical PD systems, followed by some advantages of a dimensional diagnostic system. Next, we review the five-factor model (FFM) of personality in relation to existing dimensional models of normal and abnormal personality, their points of convergence and divergence, how this research led to the development of a trait-dimensional model in DSM5, and the current state of research investigating the model. Last, we describe the alternative DSM-5 model for PDs in DSM-5 Section III (DSM-5-III) as a whole and consider future directions.

## Limitations of Categorical Approaches to PD

Categorical diagnoses have a long tradition in psychiatry, one that is rooted in psychiatry's adherence to an older medical model of clinical diagnosis (see Blashfield, 1984). As a reaction to the psychoanalytic tradition and DSM-II, which suffered from weak diagnostic reliability (Kirk & Kutchins, 1994), psychiatrists in the late 20th century made the shift to operationally defined diagnoses with strict diagnostic criteria (Regier, Narrow, Kuhl, & Kupfer, 2009). This shift was an important event in the history of psychiatry, but it was not sufficient to produce a valid diagnostic system, especially for PD. Specifically, the shift improved PD diagnostic reliability, but lack of structural validity, that is, the extent to which the diagnostic system mapped onto the way personality pathology is organized in nature (Jacobs & Krueger, 2013; Loevinger, 1957), persisted. For example, data do not support the validity of the DSM-IV model, which posits 10 PD diagnostic categories, nor do they support the clinical utility of that system, as described below. The next step in the evolution of psychiatric classification is imminent, and PD is in a position to be the vanguard of that evolution (Krueger, 2013).

Readers most likely are already familiar with the limitations of categorical diagnostic systems for PD in psychiatry, through either their own clinical experiences or reading the many thorough criticisms of that approach (e.g., Clark, Livesley, & Morey, 1997; Cloninger, 2000; Livesley, 2003, 2012; Oldham & Skodol, 2000; Tyrer, 2001). Briefly, those problems are comorbidity, heterogeneity within PD categories, temporal instability, arbitrary diagnostic thresholds, widespread use of the "not otherwise specified" (NOS) designation that signifies poor coverage of personality pathology, and limited clinical utility.

## Comorbidity

Despite the idea that diagnostic categories are intended to be discrete entities, research tells us that comorbidity across PD categories is the rule rather than the exception, with point estimates of PD co-occurrence (odds ratios) ranging from 2.8 (Zanarini, Frankenburg, Chauncey, & Gunderson, 1987) to 4.6 (Skodol, Rosnick, Kellman, Oldham, & Hyler, 1988). These data strongly indicate that the DSM PD categories have blurred, rather than distinct, boundaries. Additionally, research examining PD comorbidity in more detail has failed to demonstrate clear distinctions among the DSM PDs (e.g., Oldham et al., 1992).

## Heterogeneity

Since DSM-III, PD categories have been defined "polythetically," which means that a certain number of criteria from within a longer list are required for diagnosis and that patients with the same PD diagnosis actually can share zero criteria from within the larger list. For example, in obsessive–compulsive PD (OCPD), only four of eight criteria are required, allowing diagnosis via nonoverlapping criterion subsets. For antisocial PD (ASPD), although childhood conduct disorder must be shared, only three of seven adult criteria are required, and for all other PDs, it is possible to share only one criterion. Obviously, in cases of minimal overlap, the diagnostic label that is supposed to describe features in common between patients ceases to be descriptive, as the categories are too heterogeneous to be of much clinical utility.

## Temporal Instability

PD is conceptualized as a lifetime diagnosis possessing temporal stability. But work since DSM-IV was published has shown that patients frequently slip below the diagnostic threshold of required criteria in as little as 6 months to 1 year. One study indicated that fewer than half of patients with PD remained at or above full criteria for a particular PD over intervals of 1–2 years, and more than half the patients were in remission within 2 years (Grilo et al., 2004). However, when PD diagnoses were assessed as dimensions instead of categories, there was a high correlation between initial assessment and 2-year follow-up (Samuel et al., 2011), indicating rank-order stability in patients' PD profiles; that is, although their manifest level of personality pathology may have diminished, their overall personality profiles remained intact.

## Arbitrary Thresholds

No study has ever shown a "zone of rarity" between the presence and absence of PD, as there are subclinical manifestations of PD that fall all along the continuum from PD to healthy personality (e.g., Zimmerman & Coryell, 1990). Additionally, the arbitrary number of criteria required for diagnoses (e.g., five of nine criteria for borderline PD [BPD]) are not based on empirical evidence; rather, they were chosen as a cutoff simply because they were half or more of the criteria. Moreover, if a patient falls short of the number of criteria required for diagnosis, the information about subdiagnostic criteria is rarely utilized in treatment planning, even though the features that are present may be extremely impairing.

## Poor Coverage

Patients who do not meet criteria for a specific PD diagnosis may be given a diagnosis of PD not otherwise specified (PD NOS), which indicates the presence of personality dysfunction but typically lacks any description of the nature of that dysfunction. Although clinicians may record the PD features that underlie the PD NOS designation, they seldom do. PD NOS is the most frequent clinical PD diagnosis (Verheul & Widiger, 2004), which seems the clearest evidence that extant PD categories fail to describe personality dysfunction as it presents clinically.

## Clinical Utility

Last, there is direct evidence that clinicians find the PD categories to have limited clinical utility. Bernstein, Iscan, Maser, Boards of Directors of the Association for Research in Personality Disorders, and International Society for the Study of Personality Disorders (2007) asked 400 members of two professional associations, the Association for Research on Personality Disorders, and the International Society for the Study of Personality Disorders, to answer a 78-item Web survey about the clinical utility of the DSM-IV PDs. Of the 96 who completed the survey, 74% found categories to be ineffective in describing PD and 80% felt that personality dimensions or illness spectra better characterized

PD than diagnostic categories. There is clearly room for extensive growth in this area.

Categorical diagnoses, when applied to phenomena that are in reality categorical, have clear advantages over dimensional models. When categories separate patients into meaningfully distinct groups, with different implications for treatment and research for each group, categories are useful distinctions. However, based on accumulated evidence described earlier, the structure of personality dysfunction and, by extension, specific PD diagnoses, do not lend themselves to categorical conceptualization.

## Advantages Provided by Dimensional Models

In contrast to categorical approaches, dimensional approaches to personality and PD are based on continuous spectra of dispositions along which people fall. As documented by Widiger and Simonsen (2005), there are various dimensional approaches to PD classification, including, for example, simply dimensionalizing the existing diagnostic categories—assessing the degree to which individuals meet the diagnostic criteria rather than making a presence–absence judgment. However, in this chapter, we focus on trait-dimensional models, in which individuals are described by their relative standing on a number of dimensions measuring trait components of personality (e.g., Extraversion or Agreeableness).

One significant advantage of a trait-dimensional approach is that it replaces the uninformative and commonly used PD NOS diagnosis with a trait-dimensional profile. It can also address issues related to comorbidity by characterizing maladaptive personality using trait spectra that cross categorical boundaries. Dimensional approaches can also describe within-diagnostic heterogeneity and subclinical presentations of PD that do not meet diagnostic criteria but nonetheless affect case conceptualization. Additionally, trait-dimensional models allow for assessment of both normal and abnormal personality, facilitating providers and researchers attending to the ways in which personality—normal as well as abnormal—relates to treatment response, outcome, and diagnostic course. Indeed, dimensional personality models have demonstrated utility in important treatment considerations such as choice of therapeutic model, duration of treatment, frequency of appointments, and medication selection (e.g., see Harkness, 2007; Harkness & Lilienfeld, 1997; Sanderson & Clarkin, 2002).

## The FFM and Its Relations to PD

### Overview and Historical Summary

The most widely studied dimensional model of personality is the FFM—originally, and often still called the Big Five. It has been replicated in many languages and cultures across the world, and has robust empirical support (McCrae & Costa, 2010). The five factors are most commonly known as Neuroticism (N), Extraversion (E), Agreeableness (A), Conscientiousness (C), and Openness to Experience (O). These factors have been shown to relate reliably to psychopathology (e.g., Kotov, Gamez, Schmidt, & Watson, 2010; Malouff, Thorsteinsson, Rooke, & Schutte, 2007; Ruiz, Pincus, & Schinka, 2008), except for O, as described below. Across the life course, all five factors show increasing rank-order stability and clear nomothetic mean-level changes (e.g., N declines, whereas A and C increase; Roberts & DelVecchio, 2000; Roberts, Walton, & Viechtbauer, 2006).

Early Big Five research was based on ratings of descriptive terms, such as "irritable," "friendly," and "cooperative" (for a history, see Goldberg, 1993). It was not until the late 1980s that the current, more frequently used questionnaire method of assessing the FFM was introduced by McCrae and Costa (1987) and the advent of the Revised NEO Personality Inventory (NEO PI-R; Costa & McCrae, 1992). Questionnaire methods had been widely used for many years to assess personality and related constructs (e.g., the Eysenck Personality Questionnaire: Eysenck & Eysenck, 1975; the Millon instruments: Millon, 1997; and the Minnesota Multiphasic Personality Inventory [MMPI]: Hathaway & McKinley, 1940). In this work, personality and psychopathology were typically studied together but, in contrast, the Big Five/FFM tradition focused almost exclusively on the normal-personality-slanted proportion of the personality space rather than its pathological variations, so when the Big Five/FFM came to dominate personality assessment, the fields of personality and psychopathology largely diverged. In recent years, however, we have come full circle, as subsequent research has demonstrated that normal and abnormal personality intersect at many points, and lie along many of the same continua, differing primarily in severity (Livesley & Jang, 2005; Markon, Krueger, & Watson, 2005; O'Connor, 2002), a point to which we return later.

## Limitations of Normal-Range FFM Measures for Assessing PD

Although the FFM conceptual framework is a strong candidate for a dimensional approach to PD, there are several limitations when using FFM *instruments* developed to measure normal-range personality when the goal is to assess dysfunctional personality. First, there are clinically relevant pathological traits that are "missing" from most measures of normal personality, for example, dependency; nevertheless, such characteristics can be placed into the FFM framework (Morgan & Clark, 2010). Similarly, some report data showing that psychoticism is missing from the FFM and that a sixth factor is needed to incorporate it (e.g., Watson, Clark, & Chmielewski, 2008; Watson, Stasik, Ro, & Clark, 2013), whereas others argue that psychoticism is an extreme version of O (Gore & Widiger, 2013; Wiggins & Pincus, 1989).

DeYoung, Grazioplene, and Peterson (2012) have argued that these two views are reconciled by conceptualizing O as having two subdomains, one that includes facets such as fantasy proneness, which converges better with psychoticism, and another that includes aspects such as curiosity, and artistic and intellectual interests: Differences in domain characteristics occur because various O measures assess these facets differentially. In particular, normal-range personality measures may emphasize the more positively valenced content in O (e.g., the item content of the Big Five Inventory), whereas measures of personality pathology largely assess the more negatively valenced content relevant to psychopathology, such as problems with fantasy intruding on waking life (for discussion, see Watson et al., 2013). In any case, the FFM clearly can be expanded to include a more thorough assessment of the personality facets that assess schizotypy.

An additional issue is that measures of normal-range personality assess traits at the "mild" end of the continuum, and often do not assess more extreme or severe variants of personality. For example, Morey and colleagues (2002) were able to use the NEO PI-R to differentiate personality-disordered patients from community norms but were unable distinguish among personality-disordered patients with different diagnoses because each shared the configuration of high N, low A, and low C. Measures designed to assess the high extreme of N and the low extremes of A and C more thoroughly are better able to parse disorders that broadly share that configuration of traits, but they differ in nuanced ways from one another.

## Extending the FFM

### Pathological FFM Scales

Subsequent studies compared the performance of three PD assessment methods in predicting relevant clinical variables at baseline and at years 2 and 4 (Morey et al., 2007), and again at years 6, 8, and 10 (Morey et al., 2011): a dimensional version of DSM-IV; the FFM using the NEO PI-R (Costa & McCrae, 1992); and the SNAP (Schedule for Nonadaptive and Adaptive Personality; Clark, 1993), a dimensional measure of maladaptive traits. All three dimensional models consistently outperformed DSM-IV categorical PD diagnoses in predicting external variables, such as hospitalizations and suicidal gestures. Additionally, the dimensional DSM-IV PD model was superior in its ability to capture concurrent, but not to predict future, functional impairment; the SNAP provided advantages when predicting external markers of construct validity and other clinically relevant external criteria, and both the SNAP and the NEO PI-R were able to predict enduring aspects of personality with more stability over time. Given the different advantages of the models, the authors concluded that any dimensional PD model should have two components; one that assesses stable components of normal personality variants (e.g., the SNAP and the NEO PI-R), that might be extreme in patients with PDs, and another that reflects the less stable attempts to adapt to, cope with, or compensate for those extreme traits (e.g., the SNAP and the DSM-IV dimensions).

Work by other researchers has also suggested that there is a place for maladaptive trait variants within an expanded conceptualization of the NEO model. In a series of articles, Lynam, Miller, Widiger, and colleagues showed the FFM's conceptual flexibility by augmenting the NEO's survey space to sample maladaptive variants of NEO traits, which still fit within the normal personality factor structure. They developed NEO-derived pathological-range measures for schizotypal, borderline, narcissistic, avoidant, dependent, and obsessive–compulsive PDs, and also psychopathy, with each scale's facets reflecting maladaptive traits, such as perfectionism as a maladaptive variant of the NEO facet of Competence. They further showed convergent validity between each new measure and both traditional measures of the FFM and the targeted PD. These measures are discussed in more detail by Clark and colleagues (Chapter 20, this volume).

### The FFM as a Broad Conceptual Framework

In addition to measures explicitly developed as FFM measures, virtually all other "objective" personality measures (i.e., questionnaires and rating forms) used today can be organized within the FFM framework. Thus, the FFM can be measured by many different instruments, each of which, through its item pool, length, and emphasis, samples a slightly different portion of the personality space. To measure the entire range of personality with reliability and validity at a lower-order "facet" level with traditional questionnaires would require an instrument too long to have practical utility and it might even be impossible, if one considers personality traits in all their possible variations and nuances. But such an instrument also is not necessary to gain a clear picture of an individual's prominent traits, which emerge with any measure that has established reliability and broad construct validity. Table 4.1 lists the current most widely used personality measures, each with its relevant scales organized by the FFM, with schizotypy included within O, and with the additional dimension of compulsivity. Some argue that compulsivity simply reflects extreme C or the opposite of disinhibition (e.g., Haigler & Widiger, 2001), but it has proven difficult to develop measures without introducing additional variance, typically variance correlated with the N domain. For example, in the Haigler and Widiger study, the NEO PI-R Conscientiousness item "I think things through before coming to a decision," was modified to "I think about things too much before coming to a decision," which introduced the element of self-criticism, a hallmark of N.

### Development of a Trait Model for DSM-5

Members of the DSM-5 Personality and Personality Disorders Work Group were well aware that the field of personality assessment had converged on the FFM with respect to both normal- and pathological-range traits. At the same time, they were aware of clinical tradition in PD assessment and that, as mentioned earlier, certain clinically relevant personality traits were not typically well represented in existing FFM measures. And finally, they were aware that every existing instrument represented a particular "version" of the personality trait space, and most were copyrighted. Therefore, it was not feasible simply to select an existing instrument to be the DSM-5 trait model, and members of the Work Group decided that the best course was to develop a clinically relevant, empirically based personality trait model and questionnaire measure for DSM-5 (see Krueger et al., 2011; Krueger, Derringer, Markon, Watson, & Skodol, 2012). The result was a model with 25 facet traits, organized into five broad domains, similar to those of the well-replicated FFM: (1) Negative Affectivity (NA) versus emotional stability; (2) Detachment (DET) versus E; (3) Antagonism (ANT) versus A; (4) Disinhibition (DIS) versus C; and (5) Psychoticism (PSY) versus lucidity. Each facet and domain was considered bipolar theoretically, but emphasis was placed on the extreme end that was more typically pathological for each of the dimensions (see American Psychiatric Association [APA], 2013, p. 773). For example, the DSM-5 model emphasizes *callousness* as a facet within the broader FFM, and notes that this facet can be described more fully as *callousness versus kind-heartedness*.

### Research Integrating Traits Described in DSM-5 within the FFM Framework

When the decision was made to include the alternative DSM-5 model for PDs in DSM-5-III, the self-report measure developed to assess its trait system, the Personality Inventory for DSM5 (PID-5; Krueger et al., 2012) was made freely available online as both a self-report and informant-report measure (*www.psychiatry. org/practice/dsm/dsm5/online-assessment- measures#personality*), in the hope that research on the DSM-5 dimensional traits would accumulate. And, indeed, initial investigations have continued to document that the DSM-5 PD traits, as measured by the PID-5, represent maladaptive extremes of the FFM (e.g., Few et al., 2013; Gore & Widiger, 2013; Wright et al., 2012).

**TABLE 4.1. Mapping Domains and Facets of Personality Models and Measures**

| Measure/model | Common domains | | | | | Domains needing further study | |
|---|---|---|---|---|---|---|---|
| | Negative affectivity | Detachment | Antagonism | Disinhibition | Psychoticism | Schizotypy/openness | Compulsivity |
| EPI/EPQ | Neuroticism | (low) Extraversion | Aggression–Hostility | Impulsive sensation seeking | | | |
| Alternative Five | Neuroticism/Anxiety | (low) Sociability and Activity | Disagreeableness | Impulsive sensation seeking | | | Activity |
| MIPS | Maladaptation | (low) Surgency | Disagreeableness | (low) Conscientiousness | | Closed mindedness | |
| HEXACO | Emotionality | (low) Extraversion | (low) Agreeableness and Honesty–Humility | (low) Conscientiousness | | | |
| PAS | Passive dependence | Schizoid | | Sociopathy | | Anankastic | |
| ICD-11 | Negative affectivity | Detachment | Dissocial | Disinhibition | | (Schizotypy classified with schizophrenia) | Anankastic |
| DAPP | Emotional Instability | Inhibitedness | Dissocial | (low) Compulsivity | | Cognitive distortion[a] | |
| PSY-5 (MMPI-2) | Negative emotionality/neuroticism | (low) Positive emotionality/introversion | Aggressiveness | Disconstraint | | Psychoticism | |
| SNAP | Negative emotionality | (low) Positive emotionality | Aggression,[a] manipulativeness[a] | Disinhibition | | Eccentric perceptions[a] | Workaholism,[a] propriety[a] |
| MCMI[b] | Borderline/dependent | Schizoid vs. histrionic | Narcissistic, sadistic | Antisocial vs. compulsive | | | Antisocial vs. compulsive |
| TCI[c] | Harm Avoid. vs. Self-direct. | (low) Reward seeking + HA | (low) Cooperativeness | Novelty seeking | | Self-transcendence | Persistence, self-transcendence |
| DIPSI | Emotional instability | Introversion | Disagreeableness (dominance–egocentrism) | Disagreeableness (impulsivity, disorderliness) | | | Compulsivity |
| 5DPT | Neuroticism | (low) Extraversion | Insensitivity | (low) Orderliness | | Absorption | |

*Note.* This Table draws from, integrates, and extends/updates Widiger and Simonsen's (2005) Table 1 and Krueger et al.'s (2011) Table 1; see also Tyrer (2009), Table 2. Cell entries are domain labels unless otherwise indicated. Labels are the authors' own. Empty cells represent domains that do not emerge within data obtained from a specific assessment model and for which the model does not contain a lower order facet. Measure abbreviations and sources for the table's data (not necessarily the reference for the instrument): EPQ, Eysenck Personality Questionnaire (Markon et al., 2005); Alternative Five (Rossier et al., 2007); MIPS, Millon Inventory of Personality Style (Weiss, 1997); HEXACO, Honesty–Humility, Emotionality, Extraversion, Agreeableness, Conscientiousness, Openness (to Experience) (Ashton & Lee, 2008; Gaughan, Miller, & Lynam, 2012); PAS, Personality Assessment Schedule (Tyrer, 2009; Tyrer & Alexander, 1979); DAPP, Dimensional Assessment of Personality Pathology (Livesley & Jackson, 2010); PSY-5, Personality Psychopathology Five (via MMPI-2) (Harkness, Finn, McNulty, & Shields, 2012); SNAP, Schedule for Nonadaptive and Adaptive Personality (Clark, Simms, Wu, & Casillas, 2014); MCMI, Millon Clinical Multiaxial Inventory (Aluja, Garcia, Cuevas, & Garcia, 2007); TCI, Temperament and Character Inventory (Clark & Ro, 2014; De Fruyt, Van De Wiele, & Van Heeringen, 2000); Harm Avoid. and HA, Harm Avoidance; DIPSI, Dimensional Personality Symptom Item Pool (De Clercq, De Fruyt, Van Leeuwen, & Mervielde, 2006); 5DPT, Five Dimensional Personality Test (Van Kampen, 2012).

[a]A lower facet whose content fits well within a domain. Listed here typically when there is too little of the factor's content in the measure as having factors. Cell entries are the primary scales loading on the factors.

[b]Factors are based on the work of researchers other than the author, who does not identify the measure as having factors. Cell entries are the primary scales loading on the factors.

[c]The TCI, having only seven scales, does not have factors per se. Thus, scale placement is based on analyses with other personality trait scales.

Wright and colleagues (2012) factor-analyzed the PID-5, beginning with its 25 traits and deriving a trait hierarchical model, depicted in Figure 4.1. This model is theoretically salient because it intersects with, and serves to organize and unify, several models in the psychopathology diagnostic literature. At the five-factor level, the model resembles a maladaptive version of the FFM, as well as the Personality Psychopathology Five (PSY-5) dimensions (Harkness & McNulty, 1994). At the four-factor level, the psychoticism factor collapses back into other domains, and the model resembles the "pathological Big Four" models of personality (Livesley & Jackson, 2010; Watson, Clark, & Harkness, 1994; Widiger & Simonsen, 2005). At the three-factor level, antagonism and disinhibition collapse into an externalizing domain. The authors interpret this level of the structure to be a pathological manifestation of the "Big Three" of the temperament literature (Clark & Watson, 2008; Eysenck, 1994; Tellegen, 1985), in which NA is similar to the Big Three's Negative Temperament, Withdrawal is the inverse of Positive Temperament, and the Externalizing factor is a broader representation of the reverse-scored Constraint domain of the Big Three. At the two-factor level, the internalizing–externalizing (Achenbach, 1966; Kendler, Prescott, Myers, & Neale, 2003; Kessler et al., 2005; Krueger, 1999, 2002) structure seen across domains of common psychopathology emerges. At this level, the DSM-5 PD traits cut across even broad diagnostic groupings to inte-

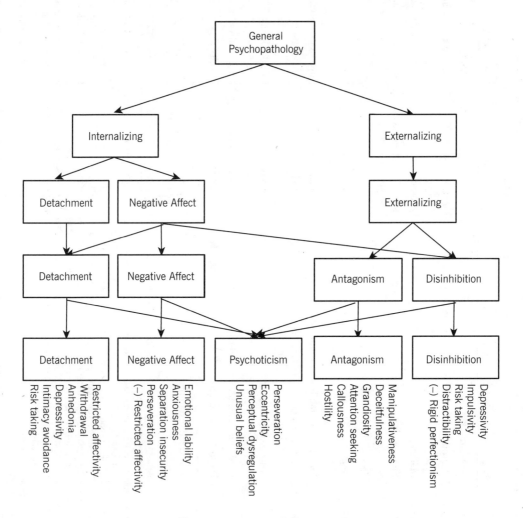

**FIGURE 4.1.** Factor hierarchy resulting from factor analysis of 25 PID-5 traits. From Wright et al. (2012). Copyright © 2012 American Psychological Association. Reprinted by permission.

grate syndromes formerly housed under different axes, now under a common, integrated hierarchy. Finally, in the one-factor solution, 21 of the primary facets loaded > .40, with four facets loading between .21 and .39, suggesting that this single factor captures overall "personality pathology" relatively well.

Furthermore, the PID-5 has been shown to share factor structure with a number of other personality trait measures. A list of such studies is shown in Table 4.1. These analyses show substantial convergence between the five-factor structure that emerges using various extant measures and the DSM-5-III PD model (usually operationalized by the PID-5, except in the Few et al. [2013] study, in which interviewers simply rated each DSM-5-III facet on a 0- to 3-point scale), and also reveal specific points of divergence. For example, when DSM-5-III measures are correlated with FFM domain or factor scores, DET relates primarily to low E but also projects onto N/NA. However, when the researchers factor-analyze each instrument they used, extract five factors and create factor scores for each, then finally factor-analyze the resulting factors, this cross-loading disappears, and DET cleanly marks low E. Similarly, in *correlational* studies, O does not, but PSY-5 Psychoticism does, correlate with DSM-5-III PSY, whereas when factors are factored, then a joint O–PSY factor emerges. However, if a sixth factor is extracted, then O and PSY split into two factors (e.g., De Fruyt et al., 2013; Watson et al., 2013).

What the differences between these correlational and factor analyses indicate is that individual measures contain some specific variance that can be seen at the level of simple zero-order correlations, but when the focus is shifted to higher-order factors, this specific variance is subsumed by the broad dimensions. Thus, to a certain extent, the question of whether Psychoticism is a maladaptive variant of O does not have a simple "yes" or "no" answer, but rather is measure-specific and level-specific. Some measures of Psychoticism and O are not related, whereas others are, and at the broad higher-order level, Psychoticism and O do form a factor, until a sixth factor is extracted, in which case they separate out again.

As noted in Table 4.2, a number of studies have examined the lower-level facets of the DSM-5-III model in relation to a number of other faceted models, revealing a relatively clear higher-order factor structure of the DSM-5-III model. Summary data from six such studies are shown in Table 4.3. Specifically, three studies each reported factor analyses and correlations of the PID-5 with the domains and/or facets of one or more measures of the FFM. The numbers in the tables are medians of these studies' results. When a study reported more than one analysis on the sample, the median result was used, so each study contributed only one sample to Table 4.2.

Overall, the structure of the DSM-5-III alternative emerges fairly clearly from these analyses, with the factor analyses again yielding somewhat cleaner results than the correlations. Specifically, although most scales mark the same factor in both sets of analyses, a few show divergent relations. For example, somewhat surprisingly, Risk Taking marks the O factor in the factor analyses but is related negatively with A and C in the correlational analyses. Impulsivity relates to DIS versus C in both sets of analyses but also has correlations with low A and with PSY in the correlational analyses.

Furthermore, 11 versus five scales have notable cross loadings (≥ .35) in the correlational versus factor analyses, respectively. Four scales (Submissiveness, Restricted Affectivity, Intimacy Avoidance, and Rigid Perfectionism) have no clear FFM counterpart in the correlational analyses, yet all but Submissiveness have a notable loading in the factor analyses. Suspiciousness fails to load on any factor in the factor analyses.

Nine of the scales show particularly clean patterns in both sets of analyses: Anxiousness, Emotional Lability, and Separation Insecurity mark only NA/N; Withdrawal marks only DET (low E); Manipulativeness, Callousness, and Grandiosity mark only ANT (low A); and Unusual Beliefs and Experiences, and Eccentricity mark only O in the five-factor solutions and only PSY in the six-factor solutions. Finally, three scales clearly assess "interstitial" traits; that is, they cross-load in both analyses: Depressivity marks both NA/N and DET (vs. E), as does Anhedonia, though the former is tipped toward NA/N and the latter toward DET, whereas Hostility marks both ANT (vs. A) and NA/N. Although, together, these studies represent almost 2,500 individuals, further replication and research would be valuable. For example, precise patterns of loadings depend on a host of both empirical (e.g., precision of estimation of interscale correlations; source of sample) and methodological (e.g., method of factor extraction and rotation) aspects of a specific study.

**TABLE 4.2. Studies Examining the Factor Structure and Correlational Relations of the DSM-5-III Trait Model to Other Personality Model Measures**

| Study | N, type of sample | Analysis level | FFM measure |
|---|---|---|---|
| Anderson et al. (2013) | 403 undergraduates | Domain, facet[b] | PSY-5 (Harkness, Finn, McNulty, & Shields, 2012; Harkness & McNulty, 1994) |
| Ashton, Lee, de Vries, Hendrickse, & Born (2012) | 378 undergraduates 476 Dutch adults | Domain, facet | HEXACO (Ashton et al., 2004) |
| De Fruyt et al. (2013) | 240 Belgian undergraduates | Domain, facet[c] | NEO-PI-3 (Flemish/Dutch authorized experimental version; Hoekstra & De Fruyt, 2013) |
| Few et al. (2013)[a] | 109 outpatients | Domain | NEO PI-R (Costa & McCrae, 1992) |
| Gore & Widiger (2013) | 585 undergraduates | Domain | NEO PI-R (Costa & McCrae, 1992) IPC-7 (Tellegen & Waller, 1987) 5DPT (Von Kampen, 2012) |
| Quilty, Ayearst, Chmielewski, Pollack, & Bagby (2013) | 201 outpatients | Domain, facet[b] | NEO PI-R (Costa & McCrae, 1992) |
| Thomas et al. (2013) | 963 undergraduates | Domain, facet[c] | FFM-Rating Form (Mullins-Sweatt, Jamerson, Samuel, Oldson, & Widiger, 2006) |
| Watson, Stasik, Ro, & Clark (2013) | 335 community adults | Domain, facet[b] | BFI (John & Srivastava, 1999), FI-FFM (Simms, 2009; see also Naragon-Gainey, Watson, & Markon, 2009) SNAP (Clark, 1993) |
| Wright & Simms (2014) | 628 outpatients | Facet[c] | NEO PI-3FH (McCrae & Costa, 2010) CAT-PD-SF (Simms et al., 2011) |

*Note.* The DSM-5-III (*Diagnostic and Statistical Manual of Mental Disorders,* 5th Edition, Section III; American Psychiatric Association, 2013) measure was the Personality Inventory for DSM-5 (Krueger, Derringer, Markon, Watson, & Skodol, 2012) unless otherwise noted. FFM, five-factor model; PSY-5, Personality Psychopathology Five; NEO PI-3, NEO Personality Inventory–3 (McCrae, Costa, & Martin, 2005); IPC, Inventory of Personal Characteristics; 5DPT, Five Dimensional Personality Test; BFI, Big Five Inventory; FI-FFM, Faceted Inventory of the Five-Factor Model; SNAP, Schedule for Nonadaptive and Adaptive Personality; NEO PI-3FH, NEO PI-3 First Half (McCrae & Costa, 2010); CAT-PD-SF, Computerized Adaptive Test of Personality Disorder—Static Form.
[a]Also used the DSM-5-III Clinician Rating Form.
[b]Correlational data are used in Table 4.3.
[c]Factor data are used in this table.

## Guide to the Alternative DSM-5 Model for PDs

### PD Diagnostic Assessment in DSM-5

Diagnostic assessment in the new dimensional system begins with assessment of impairment in personality functioning. This reflects the DSM-5 position that mental disorder, including PD, must "reflect a dysfunction in the psychological, biological, or developmental processes underlying mental functioning" (APA, 2013, p. 20). Simply exhibiting extreme personality traits is not necessarily pathological. Because extremity on a personality trait may indicate only that an individual falls on the extreme end of a trait's normal distribution, to diagnose a PD, personality dysfunction must accompany the pattern of extreme traits. Thus, the first criterion for a DSM-5 Section III PD is "moderate or greater impairment in personality (self/interpersonal) functioning," with self functioning encompassing identity and self-direction, and interpersonal functioning encompassing empathy and intimacy.

The Level of Personality Functioning Scale (LPFS), designed to operationalize Criterion A, assesses disturbances in each of four subareas of self and interpersonal functioning (identity

TABLE 4.3. Median Factor Loadings and Correlations of DSM-5-III Facets with Five-Factor Model Factors

| DSM-5-III facet | N/NA Fac | N/NA Corr | DET/E Fac | DET/E Corr | ANT/A Fac | ANT/A Corr | DIS/C Fac | DIS/C Corr | O Fac | O Corr | PSY[a] Fac | PSY[a] Corr |
|---|---|---|---|---|---|---|---|---|---|---|---|---|
| Anxiousness | **.70** | **.79** | .03 | −.22 | .01 | −.15 | .14 | −.10 | .10 | .06 | .27 | .29 |
| Emotional lability | **.73** | **.69** | .12 | −.09 | .05 | −.14 | .05 | −.27 | .16 | .14 | .15 | .31 |
| Separation insecurity | **.61** | **.46** | .17 | −.04 | .10 | −.13 | .02 | −.21 | .05 | .00 | .05 | .18 |
| Perseveration | **.39** | **.54** | .10 | −.26 | .07 | −.25 | .10 | −.19 | .31 | .16 | **.36** | .34 |
| Suspiciousness | .32 | **.42** | .25 | −.11 | .30 | −.47 | .00 | −.29 | .18 | −.01 | .28 | **.33** |
| Rigid perfectionism | **.44** | .34 | .09 | −.13 | .13 | −.13 | **.56** | .13 | .16 | .15 | .23 | .12 |
| Submissiveness | .29 | .32 | .03 | −.17 | −.15 | .16 | .08 | −.01 | .05 | −.12 | .15 | −.03 |
| Depressivity | **.44** | **.65** | **.42** | **−.41** | −.01 | −.19 | .20 | −.22 | .09 | .01 | .21 | .26 |
| Anhedonia | **.39** | **.53** | **.57** | **−.50** | −.04 | −.22 | .01 | −.21 | −.08 | −.11 | .21 | .22 |
| Withdrawal | .23 | .29 | **.70** | **−.58** | .07 | −.28 | .08 | −.09 | .24 | −.10 | .29 | .21 |
| Restricted affectivity | −.22 | −.01 | **.57** | −.23 | .22 | −.29 | .08 | −.15 | .24 | .01 | .33 | .06 |
| Intimacy avoidance | .15 | .08 | **.44** | −.26 | .14 | −.02 | .08 | −.10 | .21 | −.11 | .23 | .11 |
| Attention seeking | .08 | .19 | **−.34** | **.38** | **.47** | **−.39** | .08 | −.27 | .13 | .18 | .28 | .10 |
| Hostility | **.48** | **.54** | .02 | −.10 | **.56** | **−.58** | .06 | −.27 | −.04 | .00 | .01 | .22 |
| Deceitfulness | .03 | .26 | .13 | .05 | **.67** | **−.58** | .14 | **−.39** | .06 | .00 | .22 | .16 |
| Manipulativeness | .03 | .11 | −.17 | .20 | **.67** | **−.47** | .07 | −.21 | .03 | .10 | .21 | .14 |
| Callousness | −.03 | .16 | .28 | −.02 | **.64** | **−.61** | .02 | −.26 | .05 | −.03 | .16 | .18 |
| Grandiosity | −.05 | .07 | −.02 | .17 | **.57** | **−.48** | .21 | .00 | .25 | .05 | .17 | .05 |
| Risk taking | −.27 | −.08 | −.14 | .33 | .32 | **−.36** | .09 | **−.37** | **.40** | .27 | .31 | .26 |
| Irresponsibility | −.01 | .27 | .10 | −.05 | .31 | **−.40** | **.53** | **−.61** | .16 | .04 | .22 | .34 |
| Impulsivity | .04 | .24 | .11 | .11 | .22 | **−.35** | **.43** | **−.51** | .23 | .08 | .19 | **.36** |
| Distractibility | .19 | **.43** | .10 | −.23 | .02 | −.14 | **.53** | **−.54** | .30 | .07 | .24 | **.35** |
| Cog & perceptual dysreg | .17 | **.41** | .10 | −.07 | .03 | −.26 | .15 | −.31 | **.61** | .03 | **.70** | **.72** |
| Unusual beliefs & expers | .02 | .22 | .00 | .00 | .10 | −.22 | .10 | −.13 | **.63** | .20 | **.67** | **.72** |
| Eccentricity | .20 | .30 | .26 | −.08 | .13 | −.33 | .14 | −.32 | **.60** | .16 | **.60** | **.46** |

*Note.* NA/N, Negative Affectivity/Neuroticism; DET/E, Detachment/Extraversion; ANT/A, Antagonism/Agreeableness; DIS/C, Disinhibition/Conscientiousness; O, Openness to Experience; P, Psychoticism; DSM-5-III, *Diagnostic and Statistical Manual of Mental Disorders*, 5th Edition, Section III Alternative Model for Personality Disorder (American Psychiatric Association, 2013); Fac, Factor loadings; Corr, Correlations; Cog & perceptual dysreg, cognitive and perceptual dysregulation; expers, experiences. Factor loadings are median loadings from the following studies: De Fruyt et al. (2013), Thomas et al. (2013), Wright and Simms (2014). Correlations are median correlations from the following studies: Anderson et al. (2013); Quilty, Ayearst, Chmielewski, Pollack, and Bagby (2013); Watson, Stasik, Ro, and Clark (2013). Loadings ≥|.35| are shown in **bold**.
[a]Psychoticism results are from De Fruyt et al. (2013) for the factor loadings and Watson et al. (2013) for the correlations.

and self-direction for self; empathy and intimacy for interpersonal, respectively). These subareas are rated on continua ranging from 0 (healthy, adaptive functioning) to level 4 (extreme impairment), then aggregated by the clinician or researcher into a single rating, using the same 0- to 4-point severity scale, with a moderate level (a rating of 2) or greater of personality impairment required for PD diagnosis. Patients who have at least moderate impairment in personality functioning are then assessed in terms of traits. Each of the six specific PD diagnoses in DSM-5 is defined by a particular configuration of impaired personality functioning and a set of pathological traits. For example, ASPD is diagnosed when there are elevations on any six of seven traits of manipulativeness, deceitfulness, callousness, hostility, irresponsibility, impulsivity, and risk taking, in addition to a specific pattern of maladaptive personality functioning.

Extrapolating from the high prevalence of DSM-IV PD NOS (Verheul, Bartak, & Widiger, 2007; Verheul & Widiger, 2004), it is unlikely that patients with PD personality trait profiles will cleanly match only one or two PD trait profiles. Instead, most patients with PD have trait profiles that match either none or three or more specific PD trait profiles, and/or they have multiple elevated traits in addition those required for specific PDs (Clark et al., 2014). Thus, in the DSM-5-III model, rather than the problematic NOS category (slightly revised as "Not Elsewhere Classified" in DSM-5 Section II), patients whose personality pathology does not fit into the hybrid diagnostic system receive a diagnosis of PD–trait specified (PD-TS) and are described by a list of their pathological traits. Thus, PD-TS is used when patients have at least moderate personality pathology as measured by the LPFS dimension and have a maladaptive trait profile but do not meet the criteria for a specific PD. We further recommend that it be used also when patients (1) meet the criteria for multiple PD types because in such cases their psychopathology is better defined globally than by several separate diagnoses, or (2) meet criteria for a specific PD but have additional pathological traits that are important to describe the clinical picture. Clark and colleagues (2014) found that 88% of patients meeting Criterion A and having at least two personality traits in the pathological range met one of the three conditions described earlier. Thus, the vast majority of patients with PD are best diagnosed with PD-TS rather than one of the specific PD types.

## Research Support

The DSM-5-III model is a hybrid in that it allows for the recapture of the PD categories of DSM-IV/DSM-5 Section II (DSM-IV/5-II) using trait dimensions. This was done to smooth the transition between DSMs and to preserve the research literature on specific PD categories. Hopwood, Thomas, Markon, Wright, and Krueger (2012) showed that the PID-5 explained substantial proportions of the variance in DSM-IV PDs in a sample of undergraduates. Samuel, Hopwood, Krueger, Thomas, and Ruggero (2013) demonstrated that when a trait sum score was computed from traits assigned to represent each DSM-IV/5-II PD by the DSM-5 work group (as posted on the DSM-5 development website), the PID-5 traits produced large convergent correlations (median = .61) with the PDQ-4 (Hyler, 1994), an extant DSM-IV/5-II PD self-report measure. The convergent correlations in some cases (i.e., schizoid, schizotypal, histrionic, and obsessive–compulsive PDs) were higher than the internal consistency of the scales within the measure. Morey and Skodol (2013) investigated convergence between DSM-IV/5-II and DSM-5-III PDs by asking clinicians to rate one of their patients using both systems (final $N = 337$), and reported that correspondence was quite high for all PDs (borderline [BPD], .80, antisocial [ASPD], .80; avoidant [AVPD], .77; narcissistic [NPD], .74; schizotypal [STPD], .63; and obsessive–compulsive [OCPD], .57). Skodol, Morey, Bender, and Oldham (2013) pointed out that these figures are actually higher than the usual test–retest reliabilities of DSM-IV PD criteria themselves (Clark et al., 1997).

The dimensional PD model in Section III extends beyond the specifiers in Criterion B, in that it requires that a PD also be described using Criterion A, personality functioning impairment, which has been shown empirically to be the most informative indicator of overall personality pathology (Morey, Berghuis, et al., 2011; Morey & Skodol, 2013). This is congruent with the proposed ICD-11 conceptualization of PD as first and foremost reflecting a dimension of personality dysfunction severity (e.g., Crawford, Koldobsky, Mulder, & Tyrer, 2011; Tyrer et al., 2011). Few and colleagues (2013) studied the performance of the entire DSM-5-III dimensional model, including both the impairment criterion and the trait rating system, in a sample of community adults currently receiving outpatient mental health treatment, and compared its performance to the categorical PD classification system. Interrater reliabilities for clinicians' ratings of impairment and the pathological traits were fair. Impairment ratings were highly correlated with depression and anxiety symptoms, as well as DSM-5 PD symptoms and pathological traits. The clinicians' ratings of PD traits, and participants' self-reported personality trait scores using the PID-5, demonstrated good convergence with one another; furthermore, both accounted for substantial variance in DSM-IV/5-II PD constructs and showed convergence with relevant external criteria. In addition, Miller, Few, Lynam, and MacKillop (2014) found high correlations ($r = .63$) between interview-based PD scores derived from DSM-IV/5-II to DSM-5 trait counts for those PD diagnoses based on mappings posted by the DSM-5 PD Work Group on the DSM-5 development website. DSM-IV PD scores and DSM-5 traits showed a good convergent–discriminant pattern and similar patterns of correlations to FFM traits, demonstrating that the alternative DSM-5 PD diagnostic approach is capable of capturing the same features as the DSM-IV diagnostic system. These findings are very similar to those described earlier by Samuel and colleagues (2013), who used self-report data in an undergraduate study, providing corroborating evidence of the DSM-5 PD traits' validity across samples.

Responding to concerns that the LPFS rating system was too complex and would be difficult to use reliably, Zimmermann and colleagues (2014) tested reliability in untrained undergraduate students viewing expert interviews and provided LPFS ratings. They found the LPFS total score demonstrated an intraclass correlation of .51 for a single rater, and .96 when aggregated across the 22 raters. Zimmermann and colleagues also found that LPFS global ratings were significantly higher in patients with a DSM-IV PD diagnosis than in those without, and positively associated with the number of PD diagnoses, supporting the idea that the LPFS construct captures variance associated with DSM-IV comorbidity. Most recently, Morey, Benson, Busch, and Skodol (2015) summarized research on the DSM-5 Section III PD dimensional classification system, concluding that early results are promising, and suggesting the alternative classification system is at least as, if not more, useful and valid than the DSM-IV categorical approach.

## Next Steps in Research

There is substantial research documenting the problems of categorical PD classification and the advantages of dimensional approaches, and although a growing literature supports the clinical utility and reliability of the alternative dimensional system for diagnosing PDs, more work remains to be done. In terms of next research steps, Widiger, Simonsen, Krueger, Livesley, and Verheul (2005) provide specific suggestions regarding the research questions that must be answered before an alternative dimensional PD system can fully replace the current system. Specifically, they suggested further research that investigates (1) the alternative system's coverage of clinical presentations of PD, (2) consistency with developmental and etiological models, (3) consistency with models of course and change, (4) effects on professional communication, (5) interrater reliability, (6) improvements to subtlety of diagnosis, and (7) clinical decision making. They also suggested clinician comfort and perceived utility, but this can be effected through education, which is a necessary part of change in any system. Moreover, frontline clinicians find the alternative DSM-5 PD model superior to the DSM-IV PD model in numerous aspects of clinical utility, particularly the trait specifiers (Morey, Skodol, & Oldham, 2014).

Some of this work, as discussed earlier, has already been done, and has established the ability of the DSM-5-III dimensional approach to recreate traditional PD categories (e.g., Miller et al., 2014; Morey & Skodol, 2013) and also demonstrated improvements in diagnostic subtlety, by providing a reliable and valid method of characterizing the adaptive and maladaptive personality trait profile of all patients—whether they have multiply comorbid PD, a single PD diagnosis with additional pathological traits beyond those subsumed by the diagnosis, or do not meet criteria for PD but have several pathological personality traits that are important to consider in the course of treating whatever other psychiatric diagnoses they may have. Importantly, with regard to clinical utility, over 80% of clinicians (both psychologists and psychiatrists) in a recent survey conducted by Morey and colleagues (2014) rated the new system, including Criteria A and B as "moderately" to "extremely" more useful than the DSM-IV approach (Skodol et al., 2013).

## *PD as the Vanguard of Empirically Supported Diagnosis*

Even more than its predecessors, DSM5 is intended to undergo revisions more frequently to reflect evolving diagnostic considerations. As such, it should be conceptualized more as a living document, with planned revisions along the way to its next iteration, than as the psychiatric bible, written in stone. Because of the deeply flawed PD diagnostic system in DSM-IV and DSM-5-II, and because of the availability of the DSM-5-III PD model, the PD field is in a position to lead the development of DSM toward empirically supported diagnostic systems guided by research rather than solely clinical intuition.

## REFERENCES

Achenbach, T. M. (1966). The classification of children's psychiatric symptoms: A factor-analytic study. *Psychological Monographs: General and Applied, 80*(7), 1.

Aluja, A., Garcia, L. F., Cuevas, L., & Garcia, O. (2007). The MCMI-III personality disorders scores predicted by the NEO-FFI-R and the ZKPQ-50-CC: A comparative study. *Journal of Personality Disorders, 21*(1), 58–71.

American Psychiatric Association. (2013). *Diagnostic and statistical manual of mental disorders* (5th ed). Arlington, VA: Author.

Anderson, J. L., Sellbom, M., Bagby, R. M., Quilty, L. C., Veltri, C. O., Markon, K. E., et al. (2013). On the convergence between PSY-5 domains and PID-5 domains and facets: Implications for assessment of DSM5 personality traits. *Assessment, 20*, 286–294.

Ashton, M. C., & Lee, K. (2008). The prediction of honesty–humility-related criteria by the HEXACO and five-factor models of personality. *Journal of Research in Personality, 42*, 1216–1228.

Ashton, M. C., Lee, K., de Vries, R. E., Hendrickse, J., & Born, M. P. (2012). The maladaptive personality traits of the Personality Inventory for DSM-5 (PID-5) in relation to the HEXACO personality factor and schizoypy/dissociation. *Journal of Personality Disorder, 26*(5), 641–649.

Ashton, M. C., Lee, K., Perugini, M., Szarota, P., De Vries, R. E., Di Blas, L., et al. (2004). A six-factor structure of personality-descriptive adjectives: Solutions from psycholexical studies in seven languages. *Journal of Personality and Social Psychology, 86*, 356–366.

Bernstein, D. P., Iscan, C., & Maser, J., Association for Research in Personality Disorders, & International Society for the Study of Personality Disorders. (2007). Opinions of personality disorder experts regarding the DSMIV personality disorders classification system. *Journal of Personality Disorders, 21*, 536–551.

Blashfield, R. K. (1984). *The classification of psychopathology: Neo-Kraepelinian and quantitative approaches*. New York: Plenum Press.

Clark, L. A. (1993). *Schedule for Nonadaptive and Adaptive Personality (SNAP)*. Minneapolis: University of Minnesota Press.

Clark, L. A., Livesley, W. J., & Morey, L. (1997). Personality disorder assessment: The challenge of construct validity. *Journal of Personality Disorders, 11*, 205–231.

Clark, L. A., & Ro, E. (2014). Three-pronged assessment and diagnosis of personality disorder and its consequences: Personality functioning, pathological traits, and psychosocial disability. *Personality Disorder: Theory, Research, and Treatment, 5*(1), 55–69.

Clark, L. A., Simms, L. J., Wu, K. D., & Casillas, A. (2014). *Manual for the Schedule for Nonadaptive and Adaptive Personality (SNAP–2)*. Minneapolis: University of Minnesota Press.

Clark, L. A., Vanderbleek, E. N., Shapiro, J. L., Nuzum, H., Allen, X., Daly, E., et al. (2014). The brave new world of personality disorder-trait specified: Effects of additional definitions on coverage, prevalence, and comorbidity. *Psychopathology Review, 2*(1), 52–82.

Clark, L. A., & Watson, D. (2008). Temperament: An organizing paradigm for trait psychology. In O. P. John, R. W. Robins, & L. A. Pervin (Eds.), *Handbook of personality: Theory and research* (3rd ed., pp. 265–286). New York: Guilford Press.

Cloninger, C. R. (2000). A practical way to diagnosis personality disorders: A proposal. *Journal of Personality Disorders, 14*, 99–108.

Costa, P. T., Jr., & McCrae, R. R. (1992). *NEO PI-R professional manual*. Odessa, FL: Psychological Assessment Resources.

Crawford, M. J., Koldobsky, N., Mulder, R., & Tyrer, P. (2011). Classifying personality disorder according to severity. *Journal of Personality Disorder, 25*(3), 321–330.

De Clercq, B., De Fruyt, F., Van Leeuwen, K., & Mervielde, I. (2006). The structure of maladaptive personality traits in childhood: A step toward an integrative developmental perspective for *DSM5*. *Journal of Abnormal Psychology, 115*, 639–657.

De Fruyt, F., De Clercq, B., Bolle, M., Wille, B., Markon, K., & Krueger, R. F. (2013). General and maladaptive traits in a five factor framework for DSM5 in a university student sample. *Assessment, 20*, 295–307.

De Fruyt, F., Van De Wiele, L., & Van Heeringen, C. (2000). Cloninger's psychobiological model of temperament and character and the five-factor model of personality. *Personality and Individual Differences, 29*(3), 441–452.

DeYoung, C. G., Grazioplene, R. G., & Peterson, J. B. (2012). From madness to genius: The Openness/Intellect trait domain as a paradoxical simplex. *Journal of Research in Personality, 46*, 63–78.

Eysenck, H. J. (1994). Normality–abnormality and the three-factor model of personality. In S. Strack & M. Lorr (Eds.), *Differentiating normal and abnormal personality* (pp. 3–25). New York: Springer.

Eysenck, H. J., & Eysenck, S. B. G. (1975). *Manual of the Eysenck Personality Questionnaire*. San Diego, CA: Educational and Industrial Testing Service.

Few, L. R., Miller, J. D., Rothbaum, A. O., Meller, S., Maples, J., Terry, D. P., et al. (2013). Examination of the Section III DSM-5 diagnostic system for personality disorders in an outpatient clinical sample. *Journal of Abnormal Psychology, 122*(4), 1057–1069.

Gaughan, E. T., Miller, J. D., & Lynam, D. R. (2012). Examining the utility of general models of personality in the study of psychopathy: A comparison of the HEXACO-PI-R and NEO PI-R. *Journal of Personality Disorders, 26,* 513–523.

Goldberg, L. R. (1993). The structure of phenotypic personality traits. *American Psychologist, 48*(1), 26.

Gore, W. L., & Widiger, T. A. (2013). The DSM-5 dimensional trait model and five factor models of general personality. *Journal of Abnormal Psychology, 122,* 816–821.

Grilo, C. M., Shea, M. T., Sanislow, C. A., Skodol, A. E., Stout, R. L., Gunderson, J., et al. (2004). Two year stability and change in schizotypal, borderline, avoidant, and obsessive–compulsive personality disorders. *Journal of Consulting and Clinical Psychology, 72,* 767–775.

Haigler, E. D., & Widiger, T. A. (2001). Experimental manipulation of NEO-PI-R items. *Journal of Personality Assessment, 77*(2), 339–358.

Harkness, A. R. (2007). Personality traits are essential for a complete clinical science. In S. O. Lilienfeld & W. T. O'Donohue (Eds.), *The great ideas of clinical science: 17 principles that every mental health professional should understand* (pp. 263–290). New York: Routledge/Taylor & Francis Group.

Harkness, A. R., Finn, J. A., McNulty, J. L., & Shields, S. M. (2012). The Personality Psychopathology–Five (PSY-5): Recent constructive replication and assessment literature review. *Psychological Assessment, 24,* 432–443.

Harkness, A. R., & Lilienfeld, S. O. (1997). Individual differences science for treatment planning: Personality traits. *Psychological Assessment, 9,* 349–360.

Harkness, A. R., & McNulty, J. L. (1994). The Personality Psychopathology Five (PSY-5): Issue from the pages of a diagnostic manual instead of a dictionary. In S. Strack & M. Lorr (Eds.), *Differentiating normal and abnormal personality* (pp. 291–315). New York: Springer.

Hathaway, S. R., & McKinley, J. C. (1940). A multiphasic personality schedule (Minnesota): I. Construction of the schedule. *Journal of Psychology, 10,* 249–254.

Hoekstra, H. A., & De Fruyt, F. (2013). *NEO-PI-3 Persoonlijkheidsvragenlijst [NEO-PI-3 Personality Inventory].* Manuscript in preparation.

Hopwood, C. J., Thomas, K. M., Markon, K. E., Wright, A. G., & Krueger, R. F. (2012). DSM-5 personality traits and DSM-IV personality disorders. *Journal of Abnormal Psychology, 121,* 424–432.

Hyler, S. E. (1994). *Personality Diagnostic Questionnaire, 4+.* New York: New York State Psychiatric Institute.

John, O. P., & Srivastava, S. (1999). The Big Five trait taxonomy: History, measurement, and theoretical perspectives. In L. A. Pervin & O. P. John (Eds.), *Handbook of personality: Theory and research* (2nd ed., pp. 102–138). New York: Guilford Press.

Kendler, K. S., Prescott, C. A., Myers, J., & Neale, M. C. (2003). The structure of genetic and environmental risk factors for common psychiatric and substance use disorders in men and women. *Archives of General Psychiatry, 60,* 929–937.

Kessler, R. C., Berglund, P., Demler, O., Jin, R. Merikangas, K. R., & Walters, E. F. (2005). Lifetime prevalence and age-of-onset distributions of DSM-IV disorders in the National Comorbidity Survey Replication. *Archives of General Psychiatry, 62,* 593–602.

Kirk, S. A., & Kutchins, H. (1994). The myth of the reliability of DSM [Electronic version]. *Journal of Mind and Behavior, 15,* 71–86.

Kotov, R., Gamez, W., Schmidt, F., & Watson, D. (2010). Linking "big" personality traits to anxiety, depressive, and substance use disorders: A metaanalysis. *Psychological Bulletin, 136,* 768–821.

Krueger, R. F. (1999). The structure of common mental disorders. *Archives of General Psychiatry, 56,* 921–926.

Krueger, R. F. (2002). Psychometric perspectives on comorbidity. In J. E. Helzer & J. J. Hudziak (Eds.), *Defining psychopathology in the 21st century: DSM-V and beyond* (pp. 41–54). Washington, DC: American Psychiatric Publishing.

Krueger, R. F. (2013). Personality disorders are the vanguard of the post-DSM-5.0 era. *Personality Disorder, 4,* 355–362.

Krueger, R. F., Derringer, J., Markon, K. E., Watson, D., & Skodol, A. E. (2012). Initial construction of a maladaptive personality trait model and inventory for DSM5. *Psychological Medicine, 42,* 1879–1890.

Krueger, R. F., Eaton, N. R., Clark, L. A., Watson, D., Markon, K. E., Derringer, J., et al. (2011). Deriving an empirical structure of personality pathology for DSM5. *Journal of Personality Disorders, 25*(2), 170–191.

Livesley, W. J. (2003). Diagnostic dilemmas in classifying personality disorder. In K. A. Phillips, M. B. First, & H. A. Pincus (Eds.), *Advancing DSM: Dilemmas in psychiatric diagnosis* (pp. 153–190). Washington, DC: American Psychiatric Association.

Livesley, W. J. (2012). Tradition versus empiricism in the current DSM-5 proposal for revising the classification of personality disorders. *Criminal Behaviour and Mental Health, 22,* 81–90.

Livesley, W. J., & Jackson, D. (2010). *Dimensional Assessment of Personality Pathology—Basic Questionnaire.* Port Huron, MI: Sigma.

Livesley, W. J., & Jang, K. L. (2005). Differentiating normal, abnormal, and disordered personality. *European Journal of Personality, 19,* 257–268.

Loevinger, J. (1957). Objective tests as instruments of psychological theory. *Psychological Reports, 3,* 635–694.

Malouff, J. M., Thorsteinsson, E. B., Rooke, S. E., & Schutte, N. S. (2007). Alcohol involvement and the five-factor model of personality: A meta-analysis. *Journal of Drug Education, 37,* 277–294.

Markon, K. E., Krueger, R. F., & Watson, D. (2005).

Delineating the structure of normal and abnormal personality: An integrative hierarchical approach. *Journal of Personality and Social Psychology, 88*(1), 139–157.

McCrae, R. R., & Costa, P. T., Jr. (1987). Validation of the five-factor model of personality across instruments and observers. *Journal of Personality and Social Psychology, 52*(1), 81–90.

McCrae, R. R., & Costa, P. T., Jr. (2010). The five-factor theory of personality. In O. P. John, R. W. Robins, & L. A. Pervin (Eds.), *Handbook of personality: Theory and research* (3rd ed., pp. 159–181). New York: Guilford Press.

McCrae, R. R., Costa, P. T., Jr., & Martin, T. A. (2005). The NEO-PI-3: A more readable revised NEO Personality Inventory. *Journal of Personality Assessment, 84,* 261–270.

Miller, J. D., Few, L. R., Lynam, D. R., & MacKillop, J. (2014). Pathological personality traits can capture DSM-IV personality disorder types. *Personality Disorders: Theory, Research, and Treatment, 6*(1), 32–40.

Millon, T. (1997). *The Millon Inventories: Clinical and Personality Assessment.* New York: Guilford Press.

Morey, L. C., Benson, K. T., Busch, A. J., & Skodol, A. E. (2015). Personality disorders in DSM-5: Emerging research on the alternative model. *Current Psychiatry Reports, 17*(4), 24.

Morey, L. C., Berghuis, H., Bender, D. S., Verheul, R., Krueger, R. F., & Skodol, A. E. (2011). Toward a model for assessing level of personality functioning in DSM-5: Part II. Empirical articulation of a core dimension of personality pathology. *Journal of Personality Assessment, 93,* 347–353.

Morey, L. C., Gunderson, J. G., Quigley, B. D., Shea, M. T., Skodol, A. E., McGlashan, T. H., et al. (2002). The representation of borderline, avoidant, obsessive–compulsive, and schizotypal personality disorders by the five-factor model. *Journal of Personality Disorders, 16,* 215–234.

Morey, L. C., Hopwood, C. J., Gunderson, J. G., Skodol, A. E., Shea, M. T., Yen, S., et al. (2007). Comparison of alternative models for personality disorders. *Psychological Medicine, 37,* 983–994.

Morey, L. C., & Skodol, A. E. (2013). Convergence between DSM-IV-TR and DSM-5 diagnostic models for personality disorder: Evaluation of strategies for establishing diagnostic thresholds. *Journal of Psychiatric Practice, 19,* 179–193.

Morey, L. C., Skodol, A. E., & Oldham, J. M. (2014). Clinician judgments of clinical utility: A comparison of DSM-IV-TR personality disorders and the alternative model for DSM-5 personality disorders. *Journal of Abnormal Psychology, 123,* 398–405.

Morgan, T. A., & Clark, L. A. (2010). Passive–submissive and active–emotional trait dependency: Evidence for a two-factor model. *Journal of Personality, 78,* 1325–1352.

Mullins-Sweatt, S. N., Jamerson, J. E., Samuel, D. B., Olson, D. R., & Widiger, T. A. (2006). Psychometric properties of an abbreviated instrument of the five-factor model. *Assessment, 13*(2), 119–137.

Naragon-Gainey, K., Watson, D., & Markon, K. E. (2009). Differential relations of depression and social anxiety symptoms to the facets of extraversion/positive emotionality. *Journal of Abnormal Psychology, 118*(2), 299.

O'Connor, B. P. (2002). The search for dimensional structure differences between normality and abnormality: A statistical review of published data on personality and psychopathology. *Journal of Personality and Social Psychology, 83*(4), 962–982.

Oldham, J. M., & Skodol, A. E. (2000). Charting the future of Axis II. *Journal of Personality Disorders, 14,* 17–29.

Oldham, J. M., Skodol, A. E., Kellman, H. D., Hyler, S. E., Rosnick, L., & Davies, M. (1992). Diagnosis of DSMIII-R personality disorders by two structured interviews: Patterns of comorbidity. *American Journal of Psychiatry, 149,* 213–220.

Quilty, L. C., Ayearst, L., Chmielewski, M., Pollock, B. G., & Bagby, R. M. (2013). The psychometric properties of the Personality Inventory for *DSM-5* in an APA *DSM-5* field trial sample. *Assessment, 20*(3), 362–369.

Regier, D. A., Narrow, W. E., Kuhl, E. A., & Kupfer, D. J. (2009). The conceptual development of *DSMV*. *American Journal of Psychiatry, 166,* 645–650.

Roberts, B. W., & DelVecchio, W. F. (2000). The rank-order consistency of personality traits from childhood to old age: A quantitative review of longitudinal studies. *Psychological Bulletin, 126,* 3–25.

Roberts, B. W., Walton, K. E., & Viechtbauer, W. (2006). Patterns of mean-level change in personality traits across the life course: A meta-analysis of longitudinal studies. *Psychological Bulletin, 132,* 1–25.

Rossier, J., Aluja, A., García, L. F., Angleitner, A., De Pascalis, V., Wang, W., et al. (2007). The cross-cultural generalizability of Zuckerman's alternative five-factor model of personality. *Journal of Personality Assessment, 89*(2), 188–196.

Ruiz, M. A., Pincus, A. L., & Schinka, J. A. (2008). Externalizing pathology and the fivefactor model: A metaanalysis of personality traits associated with antisocial personality disorder, substance use disorder, and their cooccurrence. *Journal of Personality Disorders, 22,* 365–388.

Samuel, D. B., Hopwood, C. J., Ansell, E. B., Morey, L. C., Sanislow, C. A., Markowitz, J. C., et al. (2011). Comparing the temporal stability of self-report and interview assessed personality disorder. *Journal of Abnormal Psychology, 120,* 670–680.

Samuel, D. B., Hopwood, C. J., Krueger, R. F., Thomas, K. M., & Ruggero, C. (2013). Comparing methods for scoring personality disorder types using maladaptive traits in DSM5. *Assessment, 20*(3), 353–361.

Sanderson, C. J., & Clarkin, J. F. (2002). Further use of the NEO PI-R personality dimensions in differential treatment planning. In P. T. Costa, Jr., & T. A. Widiger (Eds.), *Personality disorders and the Five-Factor*

*Model of Personality* (2nd ed., pp. 351–376). Washington, DC: American Psychological Association.

Simms, E. E. (2009). *Assessment of the facets of the five factor model: Further development and validation of a new personality measure.* Ames: University of Iowa.

Simms, L. J., Goldberg, L. R., Roberts, J. E., Watson, D., Welte, J., & Rotterman, J. H. (2011). Computerized adaptive assessment of personality disorder: Introducing the CAT–PD project. *Journal of Personality Assessment, 93*(4), 380–389.

Skodol, A. E., Morey, L. C., Bender, D. S., & Oldham, J. M. (2013). The ironic fate of the personality disorders in DSM-5. *Personality Disorders: Theory, Research, and Treatment, 4,* 342–349.

Skodol, A. E., Rosnick, L., Kellman, H. D., Oldham, J., & Hyler, S. E. (1988). Validating structures DSMIII-R personality disorder assessments with longitudinal data. *American Journal of Psychiatry, 145,* 1297–1299.

Tellegen, A. (1985). Structures of mood and personality and their relevance to assessing anxiety, with an emphasis on self-report. In A. H. Tuma & J. D. Maser (Eds.), *Anxiety and the anxiety disorders* (pp. 681–706). Hillsdale, NJ: Erlbaum.

Tellegen, A., & Waller, N. G. (1987). *Exploring personality through test construction: Development of the Multidimensional Personality Questionnaire.* Unpublished manuscript, Minneapolis, MN.

Thomas, K. M., Yalch, M. M., Krueger, R. F., Wright, A. G., Markon, K. E., & Hopwood, C. J. (2013). The convergent structure of DSM5 personality trait facets and five-factor model trait domains. *Assessment, 20*(3), 308–311.

Tyrer, P. (2001). Personality disorder. *British Journal of Psychiatry, 179,* 81–84.

Tyrer, P. (2009). Why borderline personality disorder is neither borderline nor a personality disorder. *Personality and Mental Health, 3*(2), 86–95.

Tyrer, P., & Alexander, J. (1979). Classification of personality disorder. *British Journal of Psychiatry, 135,* 163–167.

Tyrer, P., Crawford, M., Mulder, R., Blashfield, R., Farnam, A., Fossati, A., et al. (2011). The rationale for the reclassification of personality disorder in the 11th revision of the *International Classification of Diseases* (ICD-11). *Personality and Mental Health, 5,* 246–259.

Van Kampen, D. (2000). Idiographic complexity and the common personality dimensions insensitivity, extraversion, neuroticism, and orderliness. *European Journal of Personality.* Retrieved from http://onlinelibrary.wiley.com/doi/10.1002/1099-0984(200005/06)14:3%3C217::AID-PER374%3E3.0.CO;2-G/abstract.

Van Kampen, D. (2012). The 5-Dimensional Personality Test (5DPT): Relationships with two lexically based instruments and the validation of the absorption scale. *Journal of Personality Assessment, 94,* 92–101.

Verheul, R., Bartak, A., & Widiger, T. A. (2007). Prevalence and construct validity of personality disorder not otherwise specified (PDNOS). *Journal of Personality Disorders, 21*(4), 359–370.

Verheul, R., & Widiger, T. A. (2004). A meta-analysis of the prevalence and usage of the personality disorder not otherwise specified (PDNOS) diagnosis. *Journal of Personality Disorders, 18*(4), 309–319.

Watson, D., Clark, L. A., & Chmielewski, M. (2008). Structures of personality and their relevance to psychopathology: II. Further articulation of a comprehensive unified trait structure. *Journal of Personality, 76*(6), 1485–1522.

Watson, D., Clark, L. A., & Harkness, A. R. (1994). Structures of personality and their relevance to psychopathology. *Journal of Abnormal Psychology, 103,* 18–31.

Watson, D., Stasik, S., Ro, E., & Clark, L. A. (2013). Integrating normal and pathological personality: Relating the DSM-5 trait dimensional model to general traits of personality. *Assessment, 20,* 312–326.

Weiss, L. G. (1997). The MIPS: Gauging the dimensions of normality. In T. Millon (Ed.), *The Millon Inventories: Clinical and personality assessment* (pp. 498–522). New York: Guilford Press.

Widiger, T. A., & Simonsen, E. (2005). Alternative dimensional models of personality disorder: Finding a common ground. *Journal of Personality Disorders, 19,* 110–130.

Widiger, T. A., Simonsen, E., Krueger, R., Livesley, J. W., & Verheul, R. (2005). Personality disorder research agenda for the DSMV. *Journal of Personality Disorders, 19,* 315–338.

Wiggins, J., & Pincus, A. (1989). Conceptions of personality disorders and dimensions of personality. *Psychological Assessment, 1,* 305–316.

Wright, A. G., & Simms, L. J. (2014). On the structure of personality disorder traits: Conjoint analyses of the CAT-PD, PID-5, and NEO-PI-3 trait models. *Personality Disorders: Theory, Research, and Treatment, 5*(1), 43.

Wright, A. G. C., Thomas, K. M., Hopwood, C. J., Markon, K. E., Pincus, A. L., & Krueger, R. F. (2012). The hierarchical structure of DSM-5 pathological personality traits. *Journal of Abnormal Psychology, 121,* 951–957.

Zanarini, M., Frankenburg, F., Chauncey, D., & Gunderson, J. (1987). The Diagnostic Interview for Personality Disorders: Interrater and test–retest reliability. *Comprehensive Psychiatry, 28,* 467–480.

Zimmerman, M., & Coryell, W. H. (1990). DSMIII personality disorder dimensions. *Journal of Nervous and Mental Disease, 178,* 686–692.

Zimmermann, J., Benecke, C., Bender, D. S., Skodol, A. E., Schauenburg, H., Cierpka, M., et al. (2014). Assessing DSM-5 level of personality functioning from videotaped clinical interviews: A pilot study with untrained and clinically inexperienced students. *Journal of Personality Assessment, 96,* 397–409.

# CHAPTER 5

# Cultural Aspects of Personality Disorder

Roger T. Mulder

Any discussion relating to culture and personality needs to consider the possibility that there are different self-concepts in different cultures. There is general acceptance of the notion that people everywhere are likely to understand themselves as physically distinct and separate from others. Beyond this physical sense of self, each person has some awareness of internal activity, including thoughts and feelings that cannot directly be known to others, a sense of an inner, private self. Some understanding and some representation of the private, inner-self may be universal but other aspects may be specific to particular cultures. In addition, the nature of the outer or public self that derives from relations with other people and social institutions may also vary by culture (Markus & Kitayama, 1991). For example, what is seen as social withdrawal or shyness in one culture may be seen as courtesy or gentleness in another (Lee & Oh, 1999).

In Western cultures, the significance assigned to the private, inner aspects of self compared with the public, relational aspects of behavior is high. The self is seen as an object separate from the world, located in an inner compartment and comprised of distinctive properties, including habits, emotions, behaviors, intentions, and conflicts (Fabrega, 1994). These internal attributes are seen as the universal reference for behavior. In some non-Western cultures, the individual may not be the primary unit of consciousness, since the sense of belongingness to a social relationship is so strong that the relationship may be seen as the functional unit of conscious reflection (Triandis, 1989). Individuals are attentive and responsive to others to maintain and further interpersonal relationships. Ways of thinking are more context-dependent and occasion-bound concepts that also link with the status the person occupies.

Therefore, it is not surprising that several conceptual models have developed relating personality and culture. The models include evolutionary psychology, cultural trait psychology, the individualism–collectivism model and the independent–interdependent self-models. What is surprising is how little these models have been discussed in relation to the current personality disorder (PD) classification system. While the fifth edition of the *Diagnostic and Statistical Manual of Mental Disorders* (DSM-5) PD classification states that "a personality disorder is an enduring pattern of inner experience and behavior that deviates markedly from the expectations of the individual's culture" (American Psychiatric Association [APA], 2013, p. 645), there is little guidance on how or when to apply this statement. The manual simply states that "personality disorders should not be confused with problems associated with acculturation following immigration or with the expression of habits, customs, or religious and political values professed by the individual's culture of origin" (p. 648)

This chapter considers the relationship between culture and PDs in five ways. The first section focuses on the cultural assumptions behind the classification of PDs as medical entities in the DSM. The second section takes the logic and theory of DSM PDs as given and considers the relevance of cultural factors on PD presentation and prevalence. The third section considers alternative models, including personality trait models and higher-order PD domains. The fourth section focuses on interactions between personality pathology, culture, and environment, including the so-called "personality culture clash" hypothesis. Finally, consideration of the potential impact of culture on the treatment of PD is discussed.

## The Culture of PD Classification

Pre-Enlightenment medical traditions incorporated ways of behaving (personalities) as being directly implicated in the cause of illnesses. The most well known is the Galenic theory of the four humors, which explicitly linked personality to diseases of the body and mind (Mulder, 1992a). However, while these traditions medically pathologized certain types of emotions and ways of behaving, they did so as part of a "holistic" medical tradition. There is little evidence that specific personalities, irrespective of their ties to illness, were singled out as pathological entities. Personality theory was part of the system of explanations for general medical problems (Fabrega, 1994). Both non-Western societies and pre-Enlightenment Western traditions did not offer specific pathological types based on behavioral deviance from standards of social conduct.

Fabrega (1994) and Berrios (1984) have described the historical developments leading to the current conceptions of PDs as clinical entities. The modern concept of disease was applied to psychiatric phenomena in the 19th century. Descriptions of psychiatric disorders produced distinctive concepts around the behavior and disposition of people who were suffering from these mental disorders. As psychiatric disorders became further refined and developments continued in the fields of psychoanalysis and the concept of neurosis, ideas about personality malformation began to take place (Berrios, 1984). Eventually, the concept of personality as a functional system developed, and PD was referred to as a specific "thing," independent of other psychiatric disorders (Fabrega, 1994). The development of PDs as medical entities is virtually confined to the Western medical tradition. As Fabrega (1994) noted, "From a culture and personality perspective, it is reasonable to claim that many of the characteristics of the various personality disorders constitute deviations in experiences and behavior that are calibrated purely in terms of contemporary Western or Anglo-American norms of personality function" (p. 159). Behavior is therefore normal when it follows accepted ways of behaving in Western capitalist societies. Abnormal behavior is contrasted to this "normal" script of behavior and this "abnormality" is codified in DSM PD checklists (Fabrega, 1994).

However, the cultural bias of these descriptions of PDs appears to have been ignored or, more probably, not recognized. Persons describing PDs assumed that, like other medical disorders, PD symptoms and signs were based on deviance from medical scientific norms rather than social or cultural values. Western conceptions of behavioral normality and abnormality were considered universal and pancultural, not to mention superior. As Fabrega (2001) noted, the rationale behind the classification was rooted in Western middle-class values and standards, and consisted of a mix of ideas about normality and deviance based on these standards.

This problem has been exacerbated by the DSM's explicit attempts to medicalize and naturalize its descriptive systems and to render mental disorders impersonal, technical, and most importantly, from this chapter's perspective, pancultural and universal. DSM diagnostic entities, including PDs, are objectified as impersonal phenomena separate from social and cultural values. The PD symptom descriptions are mechanical and theoretically pancultural across different societies.

In summary, PDs do not readily conform to definitions of illness. When behaviors and emotions were encompassed in traditional medical descriptions, they were seen as part of a system of explanation for general medical problems. In non-Western societies, deviation from behavioral norms generally requires civil or familial modes of resolution rather than medical ones. The development of PDs as medical entities arose almost exclusively within the Western medical tradition and the deviations in behavior described in DSM are calibrated largely in terms of contemporary Western norms. The globalization of psychiatric diagnoses, particularly since DSM-III (APA, 1980), has resulted in the export of PD clinical entities to most other societies.

## DSM PDs across Cultures

While acknowledging the historical–cultural boundedness of DSM PD descriptions, it would be useful to test their universality in a range of cultures. Studies comparing community prevalence rates, types of symptoms, and cohort effects in different countries would help to demonstrate the influence (or not) of social and cultural factors. Such studies have proved invaluable in other mental disorders—notably schizophrenia and mood disorders. Unfortunately the only disorder to merit serious epidemiological study is antisocial personality disorder (ASPD) or psychopathy (Paris, 1998). All other PDs have minimal or indirect cross-cultural data, which I briefly summarize.

### PDs Other Than ASPD

Loranger and colleagues' (1994) International Personality Disorder Examination (IPDE) reliability study is frequently cited in discussions of cross-cultural PD studies but, as the authors note, it was not intended to be an epidemiological survey. Although 11 countries were involved, the 421 subjects were all nonrandomly selected patients. Loranger and colleagues did note that the majority of PD subtypes were diagnosed in most countries. The exceptions were in the two developing countries included in the study; India reported no avoidant personality disorder (AVPD) diagnoses and Kenya reported no borderline personality disorder (BPD) diagnoses.

The most extensive epidemiological data on PDs comes from the United States. The National Comorbidity Survey Replication (Lenzenweger, Lane, Loranger, & Kessler, 2007) used PD screening questions from the IPDE and reported prevalence rates of 5.7% Cluster A, 1.5% Cluster B, 6.0% Cluster C, and 9.1% overall. Similar questions were used in the DSM-IV PD World Health Organization (WHO) survey of eight countries, which reported rates of 3.6% Cluster A, 1.5% Cluster B, 3.7% Cluster C, and 6.1% overall. They reported no particular cultural patterns or differences in developing and developed countries, with estimates lowest in Nigeria (2.7%) and Western Europe (2.4%) and highest in the United States (7.6%) and Colombia (7.9%).

There is indirect evidence, derived from cross-cultural differences in the prevalence of symptoms such as parasuicidality and substance abuse that BPD may be more common in Western societies (Millon, 1987; Paris, 1991). Parasuicidial behaviors are more likely to go unreported in non-Western countries than in Western countries, but there does truly appear to be a true lower prevalence, particularly of repeated self-harm, in non-Western societies (Paris, 1991). There may also have been a cohort effect, especially in the 1980s and 1990s, when young people's parasuicide and suicide rates in Western countries were significantly increasing (Paris, 1998). The few epidemiological studies performed more recently in Western countries report a range of prevalence figures for BPD within these societies. A recent U.S. study reported the lifetime prevalence of BPD to be 5.9% (Grant et al., 2008) compared to a prevalence estimate of 1.6% in the U.S. National Comorbidity Study (Lenzenweger et al., 2007). Point prevalence rates of BPD in European national community samples were around 0.7 (Coid, Yang, Tyrer, Roberts, & Ullrich, 2006; Torgersen, Kringlen, & Cramer, 2001). This variation in prevalence across the same and different countries suggests that measurement issues, as well as social and cultural factors, may play a role in determining rates and presentations of BPD.

A large Chinese study assessed DSM-IV PDs in psychiatric patients using the Personality Diagnostic Questionnaire–4 (PDQ-4) and the Personality Inventory for DSM-IV (PID-IV). They reported all 10 DSM-IV diagnoses; the most common were obsessive–compulsive PD (OCPD), AVPD, paranoid PD (PPD), and BPD (all at rates over 40%) (Yang et al., 2000). The sample consisted of psychiatric patients, so all prevalence data need to be interpreted cautiously (although rates are similar to those in Western patient samples). However, the study does support the possibility that all DSM PDs may be present in China even if their prevalence may differ from Western countries. A recent Jamaican study reported an overall population prevalence of 41.4% PDs using their own Jamaican Personality Inventory (Hickling & Walcott, 2013) the highest rate in any population.

### Antisocial Personality Disorder

As noted earlier, ASPD provides the most reliable evidence for the effects of culture on PD. There are three major findings. In the first, there appears to be a universal or pancultural propensity toward antisocial behavior. Psychopaths have been described throughout history and across cultures (Cleckley, 1988). Murphy (1976) reported that groups as different as the Inuit of Alaska and the Yoruba of Nigeria have a concept of psychopathy. Both societies distinguished psychopathy from other forms of medical disorder; they had specific terms for the disorder—*Kulangeta* and *Aranakan,* respectively—as well as specific management strategies (Cooke, 2009).

The second major finding is that the prevalence of antisocial behavior varies in different social groups. Murphy (1976) also observed that psychopathy was rare in both Inuit and Yoruba peoples. The first study in which two cultures could be directly compared used methodology taken from the Epidemiologic Catchment Area Study (ECA) to conduct a survey of antisocial personality symptoms in Taiwan. The lifetime prevalence of ASPD in Taiwan was around 0.2% compared to nearly 3% in United States (Compton et al., 1991). Similar low rates were reported in a Japanese primary care setting (Sato & Takeichi, 1993). Even with comparable methodologies, it remains uncertain that these data represents actual differences in prevalence. It is possible that the Taiwanese and Japanese offered socially desired answers due to cultural negation of antisocial behaviors (Calliess, Sieberer, Machleidt, & Ziegenbein, 2008). However, the fact that a higher prevalence was reported in South Korea (Lee et al., 1987), which has similar cultural attitudes, suggests that there is likely to be a real difference in the prevalence of ASPD.

The third major finding is that ASPD appears to be increasing in North America, nearly doubling in frequency since World War II (Kessler et al., 1994). This strong cohort effect suggests that social and cultural factors make a significant contribution to rates of ASPD. Reasons proposed for the change include increasing frequency of family breakdown and a dramatic increase in the prevalence of substance abuse (Paris, 1998). Whether a similar increase is present in other cultures has not been studied. It is possible that factors such as high family cohesion and deference to elders, which are more common in East Asian families, may be protective.

In summary, we lack well designed epidemiological studies that would help determine cross-cultural differences in the community prevalence of PDs. Measures are not standardized; most studies use screening instruments or idiosyncratic questionnaires, which lead to widely varying population estimates even in samples from the same population. From the limited available data, three issues emerge. First, DSM PDs appear to exist in most cultures, albeit at different rates. Second, ASPD and possibly BPD are more common in Western cultures. Third, rates of ASPD and possibly other PDs are increasing, which suggests that social and cultural factors play a significant role in determining these behaviors.

## Personality Traits and Culture

The limited utility of the current DSM-5 and *International Classification of Diseases* (ICD-10) PD classification systems is related not only to cultural studies but also to general studies of personality pathology (Bernstein, Iscan, & Maser, 2007). Only ASPD, BPD, and PD not otherwise specified (PD NOS) are utilized in most countries (Tyrer, Crawford, & Mulder, 2011). The multiple diagnostic categories make designing epidemiological studies so cumbersome and time consuming that few are performed, and almost never in developing countries. Alternative models include grouping personality pathology symptoms into latent dimensions or clusters, or using a dimensional approach based on normal personality traits. These models have been more widely used in different cultures.

When using PD latent dimensions, most researchers report four higher-order dimensions. There are loosely called antisocial or dissocial, asocial or inhibited, asthenic or neurotic, and anankastic or compulsive (Livesley, Jackson, & Schroeder, 1989; Mulder & Joyce, 1997). Similar dimensions have been reported in Chinese population samples (Zheng et al., 2002) and Swiss and African groups (Rossier & Rigozzi, 2008) suggesting that such dimensions may have more pan-cultural validity than current classifications.

The most well-known dimensional personality trait models contain the five dimensions—Neuroticism, Extraversion, Openness, Agreeableness, Conscientiousness—called the Big Five or five-factor model (FFM) (Costa & McCrae, 1990). These dimensions, which are derived from English descriptive personality terms, have been translated into other languages and measured in different cultural contexts. There are significant methodological concerns about whether descriptions conceived in English can be translated into different languages (what Church [2000] called the "transport and test" variety of research). Nevertheless, studies using the Big Five generally demonstrate some consistency in different cultures, therefore supporting the concept of at least some pancultural validity for underlying personality traits (McCrae, Yik, Trapnell, Bond, & Paulhus, 1998). Not surprisingly there are cultural mean differences in trait scores but these need to be interpreted carefully due to problems with cross-cultural measurement equivalence (Church, 2000). The findings tend to reinforce ethnic group stereotypes; the Japanese show greater restraint, less extraversion, and greater self-effacement when compared to Americans, for example, while Hong Kong Chinese, relative to Canadians, have less imaginative fantasy, need for variety, and cheerful optimism (McCrae et al., 1998). Japanese students have significantly higher neuroticism and introversion scores than do English students (Iwawaki, Eysenck, & Eysenck, 1977).

Perhaps more persuasive evidence of cross-cultural comparability of personality traits come from studies that search for indigenous dimensions first. In a similar manner to that in which the English language Big Five was derived, investigators have compiled indigenous trait terms, assuming that the most salient behavioral traits will be encoded in local language. The Big Five have been reasonably replicated in several European languages, including Dutch, German and Russian (MacDonald, 1998). The Big Five have also been replicated with moderate consistency in Asian lexical studies, including Chinese (Church, 2000). Church summarized the data by stating, "In sum, the replication of fairly comparable personality dimensions, using both imported and indigenous approaches in a wide variety of cultures, provides one source of evidence for the viability of the trait concept across cultures" (p. 656).

Evolutionary psychologists have also tended to support a personality trait approach to provide an evolutionary perspective on cross-cultural variation in personality. They argue that the universality of underlying traits reflect a fundamental similarity of human interests related to negotiating status hieratics, affiliations including sexual partners, perseverance, and so on. Cultures evolving under differing ecological conditions may develop different mean levels of these universal traits, reflecting different contexts for pursuing the universal interests of status and reproduction. Cultures may manipulate the environmental influences to affect the mean level of personality traits, so that cultures may differ on which traits are valued most highly (MacDonald, 1998). Extremes in trait measures might be viewed as a type of PD. Some evolutionary psychologists argue that even culturally disvalued behavioral traits such as those found in ASPD constitute an alternative evolutionarily derived strategy that may be adaptive given a social ecology of stress and deprivation. This does not imply that antisocial behavior in some societies should mitigate social responsibility and accountability. However, it does suggest that the derivation of such behaviors is complex and prone to expression under some ecological conditions more than others (Fabrega, 2006).

By far the largest study examining the generalizability of behavioral traits across societies was by Ivanova and colleagues (2007). The Youth Self-Report (YSR) was completed by 30,243 youth in 23 countries. An eight-syndrome taxonomic model was derived. The syndromes were labeled anxious/depressed, withdrawn/depressed, somatic complaints, social problems, thought problems, attention problems, rule-breaking behavior, and aggressive behavior. Countries included Ethiopia, Japan, Korea, Puerto Rico, and Jamaica, in addition to Western counties. The authors reported that the eight behavioral syndromes were closely replicated across all 23 countries. In addition, differences in scores in the eight scales were small to medium, and the within-society variances greatly exceeded the between-societies variance in youth self-ratings of their behavior, emotional, and social problems (Ivanova et al., 2007).

In summary, while there are concerns that measuring personality traits assumes a Western perspective on behavioral classification, there appear to be broadly comparable traits and behaviors across different societies. These may reflect fundamental human propensities toward survival and reproduction. It seems likely that the expression of these traits and behaviors is shaped by social facilitation and cultural sanctions leading to group differences in their prevalence and manifestations. The larger and better designed studies report the least societal differences and reinforce the idea that personality traits vary more within cultures than across them.

## Personality and Individualism–Collectivism

The individualism–collectivism cultural syndrome has been called the most significant culture difference among societies (Triandis, 2001). The individualism–collectivism model proposes that collectivistic cultures are interdependent within groups (usually family or tribe), shape their behavior primarily on the basis of ingroup norms, and behave in a communal way (Mills & Clark, 1982). In contrast, individualist cultures encourage members to be autonomous and independent of their ingroups. These respective imperatives are likely to have a significant influence on the expression of behavior and personality within these cultures. In the collectivist construct of self, both the expression and the experience of emotions and motives are strongly shaped by a consideration of the reactions of others. In contrast, the individualist construct of self concerns an individual whose behavior is organized and made meaningful largely by reference to his or her own internal thoughts and feelings rather than the thoughts and feelings of the group (Markus & Kitayama, 1991).

The consequences of such differences are readily discerned and well summarised by Oyserman, Coon, and Kemmelmeier (2002). In collectivistic cultures, group membership is a central aspect of identity, and valued personal traits reflect the goals of the group. Life satisfaction derives from successfully carrying out social roles and obligations. Restraint in emotional expression, rather than open and direct expression of personal feelings, is likely to be valued, since it promotes ingroup harmony. Social context and status roles figure prominently in a person's perception and causal reasoning. In contrast, individualistic cultures encourage the creation and maintenance of a positive sense of self as a basic endeavor. Having unique or distinctive personal attitudes and opinions is valued and central to self-definition. Individualism implies open emotional expression and striving to attain personal goals. Judgment, reasoning, and causal inference are generally orientated toward the person rather than the situation or social context (Oyserman et al., 2002).

On the face of it, individualism–collectivism would appear to have a profound influence on the expression and classification of personality abnormality in different cultures. Yet there are virtually no studies of the relationship between PD and individualism–collectivism. The literature on the measurement of individualism–collectivism in different cultures includes rating scales, the so-called "Hofstede approach" and "priming studies" (for a detailed analysis, see Oyserman et al., 2002). Most studies contrast European Americans with other ethnic groups both within North America and across countries. A meta-analysis reported large and stable cross-cultural differences in individualism–collectivism. However, the differences were neither as large nor as systemic as often believed. European Americans were more individualistic and less collectivistic than others. However, they were not more individualistic than African American or Latino cultures and not less collectivistic than Japanese or Korean cultures. Only the Chinese, who are both less individualistic and more collectivistic, show large effects (Oyserman et al., 2002).

One study has attempted to relate the Big Five to an individualism–collectivism model. Realo, Allik, and Vadi (1997) developed a measure of collectivism in Estonia and reported a negative correlation between Openness and collectivism, and positive correlations between Agreeableness and Conscientiousness and collectivism. These relationships at least demonstrate face validity.

The domain relating individualism–collectivism to personality that has received most study is the relationship between social withdrawal or shyness in individualistic and collectivistic cultures. In Western, individualistic societies, social withdrawal in adolescents has been found to correlate with poor social and emotional status (Kim, Rapee, Oh, & Moon, 2008). In contrast to data from Western cultures, data on social withdrawal among Asian collectivistic populations has produced mixed results. Studies have reported that shy Chinese adolescents were not viewed as incompetent but considered well behaved and easily accepted by their peers (Chen & Stevenson, 1995). One study comparing Australian and South Korean students reported that shy and less sociable individuals in Korea showed better social and emotional adjustment than comparable shy Australian students. The authors pointed out that reserved and reticent attitudes are more valued than outspoken behavior in Korea, and that rather than being viewed negatively, shyness is associated with virtues such as courtesy, gentleness, and consideration for others.

Social phobia may be viewed as overlapping with AVPD traits. The lifetime prevalence of social phobia in Korea is lower than that in Western countries (approximately 2 vs. 7–13%; Furmark, 2002). However, symptoms of social anxiety are as prevalent in the general Korean population as in Western cultures (Lee & Lee, 1984). It therefore appears that the lower prevalence of clinical cases might be due to the higher threshold at which social anxiety is defined as a disorder in a collectivistic society such as Korea (Rapee & Spence, 2004).

In summary, the evidence suggests that not all cultures consider positive self-regard or high self-esteem to be desirable. Well-being may be related to attaining culturally valued outcomes rather than personal ones. At the societal level, collectivistic societies are likely to promote obligation to groups and punish those who do not promote ingroup harmony. Societies that focus on individualism promote personal uniqueness and punish those who do not separate themselves from others. However, societal differences in individualism and collectivism may be less pronounced than is generally believed based on Oyserman and colleagues' (2002) exhaustive meta-analysis. At an individual level, there is likely to be greater variability in individualism and collectivism, with some arguing that differences in interdependent and independent self-concepts may vary as much within individualistic and collectivistic cultures as between them. There is a need for research to identify what happens when people from different cultures are encouraged to change behavior toward an individualistic or collectivistic manner when moving between different cultures.

## Personality and Cultural Interactions

Collectivism and individualism may have adaptive advantages or disadvantages in promoting psychological health and well-being. For example, individualism fosters the pursuit of self-actualization, but this may come at the expense of social isolation (Triandis, 2001). Collectivism provides a sense of belonging and social support, but it may also bring anxiety about not meeting social obligations (Caldwell-Harris & Aycicegi, 2006). People with individualist traits value completion, self-reliance, and hedonism. Individuals with a collectivist orientation value tradition, social values, and cooperation.

Extreme independence or interdependence might be risk factors for personality pathology regardless of the society an individual finds him- or herself. High individualistic values that result in placing personal goals above group harmony may underlie antisocial and narcissistic behavior. This may be particularly so when indulgence and lack of parental control mean that children have little practice in impulse control (Cooke, 1996). Similarly, high interdependent values may result in more internalizing disorders such as fearfulness and avoidance, leading to compliant but not innovative adults. Unfortunately, there are no data on the effects of extreme individualistic or collectivistic orientations and their relationship to PDs (Caldwell-Harris & Aycicegi, 2006).

The data on the concept of "person–environment fit" suggest that individuals whose characteristics fit well with a given cultural concept tend to show better adaptation than those whose characteristics do not fit cultural demands. For example, in a comparison of Anglo American and Mexican American U.S. schoolchildren, Triandis (2001) reported that students with the highest self-esteem were independent Anglo American children and cooperative Mexican-American children. Caldwell-Harris and Aycicegi (2006) contrasted students residing in an individualistic society (Boston) with those in a collectivistic society (Istanbul, Turkey). They reported that in Boston, collectivism scores were positively correlated with social anxiety and dependent personality (as well as depression and OCPD). High collectivism scores also correlated with the more positive personality trait of empathy. In contrast, high scores on individualism were associated with self-reports of low psychological distress. In Istanbul, a completely different pattern emerged. High individualism scores were correlated with paranoid and narcissistic features, impulsivity, antisocial, and borderline personality features. Collectivism was associated with low scores on these scales and less psychological distress (Caldwell-Harris & Aycicegi, 2006). These differing patterns of association support the personality–culture clash hypothesis. The idea that individualism is associated with disorders of impulse control (Cooke, 1996) was supported in the Turkish sample but not the American sample. On the other hand, high collectivism scores were associated with dependence and social anxiety in the U.S. but not the Turkish sample. An interdependent personality style appears to be healthier for individuals living in Turkey.

Why a person's individualistic or collectivistic orientation clashes with a culture's values is a risk factor for personality pathology or psychiatric syndromes is not clear. Two major possibilities exist. First, having a personality that is discrepant with prevailing social values is a stressor, leading to peer rejection and punishment by adults. A collectivistic orientation in collectivistic cultures may result in positive feelings about accepting ingroup norms. An individualistic orientation may result in ambivalence or even bitterness and feelings of estrangement. In contrast, a collectivistic orientation in individualistic cultures may result in feelings of personal failure with social withdrawal and low self-esteem. An alternative explanation is that those individuals with a flexible and healthy personality may be more equipped during socialization and development to internalize cultural values and adapt their style accordingly. Regardless of causality, the personality–culture clash hypothesis appears to have some support and may be seen to extend the "goodness-of-fit" model from developmental psychology into the realm of personality and culture.

## Immigration and Modernization

An increasing proportion of populations in Western countries are immigrants, often from non-Western societies. The association between migration and PDs has received little study. Surveys in forensic and nonforensic psychiatric services have reported lower PD rates among black and ethnic-minority patients compared with white patients (Coid, et al., 2006; McGilloway, Hall, Lee, & Bhui, 2010). Similarly, studies reporting on the relationship between ethnicity and PDs in patients presenting at emergency services have also noted a lower incidence of PDs in immigrant groups compared to indigenous patients (Baleydier, Damsa, Schutzbach, Stauffer, & Glauser, 2003; Pascual et al., 2008; Tyrer, Merson, Onyett, & Johnson, 1994). This is in contrast to other mental health disorders, such as psychosis, which are often reported to be higher in immigrant groups (Cantor-Graae & Selten, 2005).

The reason for the lower rate of PD diagnosis among immigrant groups is uncertain. Most immigrant groups come from traditional collectivistic cultures that may provide rules, values, and roles that inhibit emotional expression and increase community expectations (Pascual et al., 2008). Such cultural practices appear to be associated with lower rates of Cluster B PDs (Paris, 1998), with the type of individuals most likely to present to psychiatric emergency services and in forensic settings. It may be that as cultures interact, acculturation only occurs in some domains, such as job behavior and socializing, but not in domains such as religious or family life (Triandis, 2001), so that the protective effects remain. Alternatively, the findings may be influenced by cross-cultural bias, including methods bias and item bias. However, most groups reporting the findings believe that they reflect genuinely lower rates of PDs. It is also possible that immigration is too recent to significantly influence behaviors, and comparable or even higher PD rates may be found in the next generation of families of immigrants.

"Modernization" is defined in a variety of ways, but it usually involves transformation of a society, leading to a breakdown of traditional roles and values, changes in childrearing patterns, urbanization, and job specialization. Some definitions include specific reference to role changes, noting that the individual becomes increasingly important, gradually replacing the family, community, occupational group, or the basic unit of society.

The implication is that modernization requires a transformation of self from one suited to prescriptive action and ascribed social roles to one who adjusts to social environments dominated by choice, achievement, and competition. Collectivistic societies provide relatively secure roles for most individuals. Even vulnerable members of a society have some function that protects them from feeling useless and socially isolated. In contrast, individualistic societies provide less secure social roles and expect individuals to find or create their own. Collectivist societies are less tolerant of deviance and tend to promote behavioral patterns characterized by inhibition and constriction of emotion. Modernization rewards active and expressive personality styles and is more tolerant of deviance, although it may reject those who are less autonomous and successful (Paris, 1998).

Increased immigration and accelerated rates of social change might be expected to have significant effects on patterns of behavior and personality pathology over the past few decades. However, there is surprisingly few data about these effects. Some have suggested that neurotic and somatic symptoms may be diminishing, but personality pathology is increasing in modernizing societies (Paris, 1991). In an Indian village clinic studied in the 1960s and again in the 1980s, Nandi, Banerjee, Nandi, and Nandi (1992) reported that conversion symptoms had waned during the 20 years but self-harm was much more frequent. High suicide rates among young Inuit males have been linked with the breakdown of a traditional way of life, and similar findings have been reported in other modernizing cultures (Jilek-Aall, 1988). It seems reasonable to suggest that rapid social change makes forging a personal identity without clear models or pathways more stressful, but there is little evidence one way or the other.

In addition to the effects of modernization, Western culture has also aggressively promoted a pancultural model of mental illness across the world. The belief that DSM and ICD classification systems provide a guide to real illnesses relatively unaffected by culture is presented with similar confidence to those who believed in 19th-century Western mental illness descriptions. The disorders described, as previously discussed, are based on a questionable model of pancultural universality. Despite this, there is increasing evidence that syndromes such as depression, anorexia, and posttraumatic stress disorder have been successfully exported to developing countries (Watters, 2010). Some argue that this cultural influence goes beyond PD categories. The diagnoses promote a theory of human nature, a definition of personhood and self, and even a source of moral authority that reflects core components of Western culture (Summerfield, 2006). Western cultures highly value at least an illusion of self-control and the ability to exert some control over circumstances. They promote a high level of individualization and autonomy. Some even suggest that autonomy is a prevalent human trait regardless of culture and society (Chirkov, Ryan, Kim, & Kaplan, 2003).

In addition, Western cultures encourage the belief that the mind is fragile and that difficult behaviors or problems in living may be conceived as illness requiring professional interventions (Mulder, 1992b, 2008). It has been suggested that this medicalization of larger areas of human behavior and experience is itself a cultural response, reflecting the loss of older belief systems that once gave meaning and context to mental suffering (Watters, 2010).

## Summary

Discussing the relationship between PDs and culture is limited by current diagnostic formulations of PDs and poor integration among conceptual models. DSM PDs are based on Western models of an individualistic self and assume the perspective of an individual within Western culture. Contemporary psychiatry has attempted to render PDs, along with other disorders, as impersonal, mechanical, pancultural entities. There is little recognition that certain personality traits may have different meanings in different cultures and little acknowledgment of the personality–culture clash that may result in behaviors being judged pathological in one culture but reasonable, or even valued, in another. There have been few cross-cultural epidemiological studies on the existing personality diagnoses and almost no attempt to integrate cultural concepts such as individual–collectivism or trait psychology with personality behaviors.

Any conclusions must therefore be very tentative. First, ASPD or psychopathy is found in all cultures in which these behaviors have been studied, although the prevalence may vary. While the data are less consistent for the other PDs, studies suggest that these disorders are also found in most cultures. There is more consistent evidence that higher-order domains of personality pathology based on DSM symptoms are reproducible across different cultural groups. Second, personality traits most commonly measured using the FFM are reported reasonably consistently across different cultures. Lexical studies using different languages also report personality traits closely related to the Big Five. Most studies report differences in mean trait scores across cultures. However, the largest and best designed studies report that the within-society variances exceed the between-society variances. Third, the psychological distress caused by PDs is significantly influenced by the culture in which these behaviors are expressed. Simplistically, the more the behavior is congruent with social and cultural values, the less psychological distress an individual reports. Behavior and culture appear to interact in a way that is similar to the "goodness of fit" described in development psychology.

Fourth, minority and immigrant cultures in Western countries may have lower rates of PDs than the indigenous population. This may reflect the fact that the most studied PDs are ASPD and BPD, and that most minority groups come from collectivistic cultures. There is some evidence that factors associated with collectivistic cultures, such as high family cohesion and discouragement of emotional expression, may protect against the "externalizing" PDs. Whether these protective factors remain relevant in succeeding generations is yet to be seen. There are also no reliable data that allow comparison of PD rates in these "minority" groups within their home cultures prior to immigration. It is possible that PD rates in individuals from immigrant cultures who have moved to the West are higher than rates for those who remain in their own countries but still lower than the indigenous Western population.

Fifth, Western cultural values including mental illness diagnostic systems are spreading throughout the world. Accelerating rates of social change and modernization are likely to change behaviors and self-concepts. The breakdown of some social norms may be associated with an increased propensity for expression of psychological distress as externalizing behaviors—currently measured using concepts such as ASPD and BPD.

## Clinical Considerations

There are no studies evaluating whether better assessment or knowledge of the cultural background of individuals receiving treatment for their PD results in better treatment outcomes. Nor are there studies evaluating whether treatment by someone with a similar cultural background results in any difference in outcome. However, it seems reasonable that consideration of cultural factors in the assessment and treatment of individuals with PDs is likely to be valuable in understanding and managing the patient.

The practical reality of achieving this is more complex. It requires the clinician to gauge the social appropriateness of behaviors in individuals who come from cultural groups with which the clinician may have little or no acquaintance. Clinicians are naturally likely to judge behavior based on their own reference culture rather than the patient's cultural conventions. However, such conventions, by definition, are central to conceptions of normality, deviance, and PD (Fabrega, 1994).

The most obvious way around this dilemma is to have someone who is familiar with the patient's cultural conventions be part of the assessment team. However, often this is not possible. Fabrega (1994) has proposed a set of criteria that clinicians should consider when deciding on a diagnosis of PD in an individual from a different culture. The clinician needs to keep separate the following issues: (1) whether the personality traits or behaviors are manifest in a prominent way and persistent; (2) whether they are part of the "normal" accepted patterns in an individual's culture; (3) whether the individual and/or his or her reference group judge the behaviors as pathological; (4) whether the behaviors constitute requirements of the role the individual is expected to perform; and (5) whether they are part of a reaction to the changed social situation.

As an example, Chen, Nettles, and Chen (2009) considered how dependent personality disorders might be seen within Chinese culture. They point out that acting submissively and dependently may be a healthy coping strategy and a sign of emotional regulation rather than features of a PD. Manifesting dependence and obedience based on Confucianism is considered proper, required behavior for some social roles. Dependence and obedience in Chinese culture are not only a manifestation of personality but they also reflect standards of social relationships and contexts.

## Conclusions and Future Directions

Personality diagnoses are derived from the concept of an individualistic, independent self. PD symptoms are based on Western middle-class norms. Despite this culturally bound derivation of PDs, diagnostic categories appear to exist in most cultures, although their prevalence and severity varies. Such variation may be partially related to different values in individualistic versus collectivistic cultures, although the empirical bases of these differences may not be as strong as is often assumed. While there is evidence of some commonality of underlying personality traits across cultures, there is also evidence that in some societies, behavior may be more interdependent within the sociocultural context. However, personality differences in individuals within a society appear to be as great or greater than the differences in personality styles among societies.

Research on cultural aspects of PDs is hampered by a diagnostic system with multiple complex, overlapping categories, as well as a lack of integration among PD research, cultural trait psychology, evolutionary psychology, and individualism–collectivism and related models. Despite cultural aspects of personality sometimes being overplayed, it is clear that PDs are much more than the developmental outcomes of neurobiological and psychological processes. Ongoing research needs to take into account the ethnic and cultural background of individuals, integrating knowledge from cultural psychology and sociology in the study of PDs.

## REFERENCES

American Psychiatric Association. (1980). *Diagnostic and statistical manual of mental disorders* (3rd ed.). Washington, DC: Author.

American Psychiatric Association. (2013). *Diagnostic and statistical manual of mental disorders* (5th ed.). Arlington, VA: Author.

Baleydier, B., Damsa, C., Schutzbach, C., Stauffer, O., & Glauser, D. (2003). Comparison between Swiss and foreign patients characteristics at the psychiatric emergencies department and the predictive factors of their management strategies. *Encephale, 29*(3, Pt. 1), 205–212.

Bernstein, D. P., Iscan, C., & Maser, J. (2007). Opinions of personality disorder experts regarding the DSM-IV personality disorders classification system. *Journal of Personality Disorders, 21*(5), 536–551.

Berrios, G. E. (1984). Descriptive psychopathology: Conceptual and historical aspects. *Psychological Medicine, 14*(2), 303–313.

Caldwell-Harris, C. L., & Ayicegi, A. (2006). When personality and culture clash: The psychological distress of allocentrics in an individualist culture and idiocentrics in a collectivist culture. *Transcultural Psychiatry, 43*(3), 331–361.

Calliess, I. T., Sieberer, M., Machleidt, W., & Ziegenbein, M. (2008). Personality disorders in a cross-cultural perspective: Impact of culture and migration on diagnosis and etiological aspects. *Current Psychiatry Reviews, 4*(1), 39–41.

Cantor-Graae, E., & Selten, J. P. (2005). Schizophrenia and migration: A meta-analysis and review. *American Journal of Psychiatry, 162*(1), 12–24.

Chen, C., & Stevenson, H. W. (1995). Motivation and mathematics achievement: A comparative study of Asian-American, Caucasian-American, and east Asian high school students. *Child Development, 66*(4), 1214–1234.

Chen, Y., Nettles, M. E., & Chen, S. W. (2009). Rethinking dependent personality disorder: Comparing different human relatedness in cultural contexts. *Journal of Nervous and Mental Disease, 197*(11), 793–800.

Chirkov, V., Ryan, R. M., Kim, Y., & Kaplan, U. (2003). Differentiating autonomy from individualism and independence: A self-determination theory perspective on internalization of cultural orientations and well-being. *Journal of Personality and Social Psychology, 84*(1), 97–110.

Church, A. T. (2000). Culture and personality: Toward an integrated cultural trait psychology. *Journal of Personality, 68*(4), 651–703.

Cleckley, H. (1988). *The mask of sanity* (5th ed.). St. Louis, MO: Mosby.

Coid, J., Yang, M., Tyrer, P., Roberts, A., & Ullrich, S. (2006). Prevalence and correlates of personality disorder in Great Britain. *British Journal of Psychiatry, 188*, 423–431.

Compton, W. M., III, Helzer, J. E., Hwu, H. G., Yeh, E. K., McEvoy, L., Tipp, J. E., et al. (1991). New methods in cross-cultural psychiatry: Psychiatric illness in Taiwan and the United States. *American Journal of Psychiatry, 148*(12), 1697–1704.

Cooke, D. J. (1996). Psychopathic personality in different cultures: What do we know? What do we need to find out? *Journal of Personality Disorders, 10*, 23–40.

Cooke, D. J. (2009). Understanding cultural variation in psychopathic personality disorder: Conceptual and measurement issues. *Neuropsychiatrie, 23*, 1–5.

Costa, P., & McCrae, R. (1990). Personality disorders and the five-factor model of personality. *Journal of Personality Disorders, 4*, 362–371.

Fabrega, H., Jr. (1994). Personality disorders as medical entities: A cultural interpretation. *Journal of Personality Disorders, 8*(2), 149–167.

Fabrega, H., Jr. (2001). Culture and history in psychiatric diagnosis and practice. *Psychiatric Clinics of North America, 24*(3), 391–405.

Fabrega, H., Jr. (2006). Why psychiatric conditions are special: An evolutionary and cross-cultural perspective. *Perspectives in Biology and Medicine, 49*(4), 586–601.

Furmark, T. (2002). Social phobia: Overview of community surveys. *Acta Psychiatrica Scandinavica, 105*(2), 84–93.

Grant, B. F., Chou, S. P., Goldstein, R. B., Huang, B., Stinson, F. S., Saha, T. D., et al. (2008). Prevalence, correlates, disability, and comorbidity of DSM-IV borderline personality disorder: Results from the Wave 2 National Epidemiologic Survey on Alcohol and Related Conditions. *Journal of Clinical Psychiatry, 69*(4), 533–545.

Hickling, F. W., & Walcott, G. (2013). Prevalence and correlates of personality disorder in the Jamaican population. *West Indian Medical Journal, 62*(5), 443–447.

Ivanova, M. Y., Achenbach, T. M., Rescorla, L. A., Dumenci, L., Almqvist, F., Bilenberg, N., et al. (2007).

The generalizability of the Youth Self-Report syndrome structure in 23 societies. *Journal of Consulting and Clinical Psychology, 75*(5), 729–738.

Iwawaki, S., Eysenck, S. B., & Eysenck, H. J. (1977). Differences in personality between Japanese and English. *Journal of Social Psychology, 102,* 27–33.

Jilek-Aall, L. (1988). Suicidal behavior among youth: A cross-cultural comparison. *Transcultural Psychiatric Research Review, 25,* 87–105.

Kessler, R. C., McGonagle, K. A., Zhao, S., Nelson, C. B., Hughes, M., Eshleman, S., et al. (1994). Lifetime and 12-month prevalence of DSM-III-R psychiatric disorders in the United States: Results from the National Comorbidity Survey. *Archives of General Psychiatry, 51*(1), 8–19.

Kim, J. J., Rapee, R. M., Oh, K. J., & Moon, H.-S. (2008). Retrospective report of social withdrawal during adolescence and current maladjustment in young adulthood: Cross-cultural comparisons between Australian and South Korean students. *Journal of Adolescence, 31,* 543–563.

Lee, C. K., Kwak, Y. S., Rhee, H., Kim, Y. S., Han, J. H., Choi, J. O., et al. (1987). The nationwide epidemiological study of mental disorders in Korea. *Journal of Korean Medical Science, 2*(1), 19–34.

Lee, S. H., & Lee, C. L. (1984, May). The social anxiety in Korean student population. In *Proceedings of the Third Pacific Congress of Psychiatry,* Seoul, South Korea.

Lee, S. H., & Oh, K. S. (1999). Offensive type of social phobia: Cross-cultural perspectives. *International Medical Journal, 6,* 271–279.

Lenzenweger, M. F., Lane, M. C., Loranger, A. W., & Kessler, R. C. (2007). DSM-IV personality disorders in the National Comorbidity Survey Replication. *Biological Psychiatry, 62*(6), 553–564.

Livesley, W. J., Jackson, D. N., & Schroeder, M. L. (1989). A study of the factorial structure of personality pathology. *Journal of Personality Disorders, 3,* 292–306.

Loranger, A., Sartorius, N., Andreoli, A., Berger, P., Buchheim, P., Channabasavanna, S., et al. (1994). The International Personality Disorder Examination: The World Health Organization/Alcohol, Drug Abuse, and Mental Health Administration International Pilot Study of Personality Disorders. *Archives of General Psychiatry, 51,* 215–224.

MacDonald, K. (1998). Evolution, culture, and the five-factor model. *Journal of Cross Cultural Psychology, 29,* 119–149.

Markus, H. R., & Kitayama, S. (1991). Culture and the self: Implications for cognition, emotion and motivation *Psychological Review, 98*(2), 224–253.

McCrae, R. R., Yik, M. S., Trapnell, P. D., Bond, M. H., & Paulhus, D. L. (1998). Interpreting personality profiles across cultures: Bilingual, acculturation, and peer rating studies of Chinese undergraduates. *Journal of Personality and Social Psychology, 74*(4), 1041–1055.

McGilloway, A., Hall, R. E., Lee, T., & Bhui, K. S. (2010). A systematic review of personality disorder, race and ethnicity: Prevalence, aetiology and treatment. *BMC Psychiatry, 10*(33), 1–14.

Millon, T. (1987). On the genesis and prevalence of borderline personality disorders: A social learning thesis. *Journal of Personality Disorders, 1,* 354–372.

Mills, J., & Clark, M. S. (1982). Exchange and communal relationships. In L. Wheeler (Ed.), *Review of personality and social psychology* (Vol. 3, pp. 121–144). Beverly Hills, CA: SAGE.

Mulder, R. T. (1992a). The biology of personality. *Australian and New Zealand Journal of Psychiatry, 26*(3), 364–376.

Mulder, R. T. (1992b). Boundaries of psychiatry. *Perspectives in Biology and Medicine, 35,* 443–459.

Mulder, R. T. (2008). An epidemic of depression or the medicalization of distress? *Perspectives in Biology and Medicine, 51*(2), 238–250.

Mulder, R. T., & Joyce, P. R. (1997). Temperament and the structure of personality disorder symptoms. *Psychological Medicine, 27*(1), 99–106.

Murphy, J. M. (1976). Psychiatric labeling in cross-cultural perspective. *Science, 191,* 1019–1028.

Nandi, D. N., Banerjee, G., Nandi, S., & Nandi, P. (1992). Is hysteria on the wane?: A community survey in West Bengal, India. *British Journal of Psychiatry, 160,* 87–91.

Oyserman, D., Coon, H. M., & Kemmelmeier, M. (2002). Rethinking individualism and collectivism: Evaluation of theoretical assumptions and meta-analyses. *Psychological Bulletin, 128*(1), 3–72.

Paris, J. (1991). Personality disorders, parasuicide and culture. *Transcultural Psychiatric Research Review, 28,* 25–39.

Paris, J. (1998). Personality disorders in sociocultural perspective. *Journal of Personality Disorders, 12*(4), 289–301.

Pascual, J. C., Malagon, A., Corcoles, D., Gines, J. M., Soler, J., Garcia-Ribera, C., et al. (2008). Immigrants and borderline personality disorder at a psychiatric emergency service. *British Journal of Psychiatry, 193*(6), 471–476.

Rapee, R. M., & Spence, S. H. (2004). The etiology of social phobia: Empirical evidence and an initial model. *Clinical Psychology Review, 24*(7), 737–767.

Realo, A., Allik, J., & Vadi, M. (1997). The hierarchical structure of collectivism. *Journal of Research in Personality, 31,* 93–116.

Rossier, J., & Rigozzi, C. (2008). Personality disorders and the five-factor model among French speakers in Africa and Europe. *Canadian Journal of Psychiatry, 53*(8), 534–544.

Sato, T., & Takeichi, M. (1993). Lifetime prevalence of specific psychiatric disorders in a general medicine clinic. *General Hospital Psychiatry, 15*(4), 224–233.

Summerfield, D. (2006). Depression: Epidemic or pseudo-epidemic? *Journal of the Royal Society of Medicine, 99*(3), 161–162.

Torgersen, S., Kringlen, E., & Cramer, V. (2001). The

prevalence of personality disorders in a community sample. *Archives of General Psychiatry, 58*(6), 590–596.

Triandis, H. C. (1989). The self and social behavior in differing cultural contexts. *Psychological Review, 96*(3), 506–520.

Triandis, H. C. (2001). Individualism–collectivism and personality. *Journal of Personality, 69*(6), 907–924.

Tyrer, P., Crawford, M., & Mulder, R. (2011). Reclassifying personality disorders. *Lancet, 377,* 1814–1815.

Tyrer, P., Merson, S., Onyett, S., & Johnson, T. (1994). The effect of personality disorder on clinical outcome, social networks and adjustment: A controlled clinical trial of psychiatric emergencies. *Psychological Medicine, 24*(3), 731–740.

Watters, E. (2010, January 8). The Americanization of mental illness. *New York Times,* p. MM40.

Yang, J., McCrae, R. R., Costa, P. T., Jr., Yao, S., Dai, X., Cai, T., et al. (2000). The cross-cultural generalizability of Axis-II constructs: An evaluation of two personality disorder assessment instruments in the People's Republic of China. *Journal of Personality Disorders, 14*(3), 249–263.

Zheng, W., Wang, W., Huang, Z., Sun, C., Zhu, J., & Livesley, W. J. (2002). The structure of traits delineating personality disorder in a Chinese sample. *Journal of Personality Disorders, 16*(5), 477–486.

# PART II

# PSYCHOPATHOLOGY

## INTRODUCTION

The chapters in Part II address the psychopathology of personality disorder (PD), a somewhat neglected topic. The four chapters in this section address issues that are central to formulating a psychopathology of PD and the construction of a cogent conceptual framework to guide research and clinical practice: self and identity; the interplay between self and attachment system; cognitive structures and processes; and the relationship between PD and other mental disorders. It is fitting to begin the section with a chapter on identity. The centrality of the self to understanding and defining PD is highlighted by the DSM-5 decision to adopt self pathology and chronic interpersonal dysfunction as defining features of PD. However, the DSM-5 decision evoked criticism from some who thought the concept of self was too psychoanalytic and others who considered the very idea unscientific, which are concerns that seem to be shared by the architects of the forthcoming *International Classification of Diseases* (ICD-11), who define PD only in terms of chronic interpersonal dysfunction. However, the DSM-5 definition drew on the conception of PD as adaptive failure that was formulated on the basis of philosophical and evolutionary analyses of the self and psychological research, not on psychoanalytic thinking (Livesley, 1998, 2003).

Psychological research on the self (see Leary & Tangney, 2012, for an overview of this work) is largely guided by a three-component model: (1) the ontological self—the self as experiencing subject or knower; (2) self as a body of self-referential knowledge; and (3) the agentic self—the self as agent and center of self-regulation. The distinction between self as knower and the self as known originated with William James (1890) and it remains a central organizing construct. We need to discuss these ideas a little because they provide context for the chapters by Carsten René Jørgensen (Chapter 6), Peter Fonagy and Patrick Luyten (Chapter 7), and Arnoud Arntz and Jill Lobbestael (Chapter 8).

The self as knower—the experiential or ontological self—refers to the person's experience of him- or herself. This has largely been the preserve of philosophers concerned with the nature of self-knowledge and whether this knowledge differs from other forms of knowledge. However, this aspect of the self is also central to understanding the core impairments of PD. At least four aspects of self-experience (self as knower) seem important for mental well-being, and all seem to be impaired with PD: (1) personal unity—a sense of wholeness, coherence, and integration; (2) continuity and historicity—a sense of temporal continuity with recognition that one has a past and an anticipated future; (3) clarity and certainty about self-knowledge; and (4) authenticity—the conviction that immediate experiences are "real" or genuine. The latter is probably the most fundamental feature because other aspects of the ontological self require a sense of certainty about basic self states.

The philosophical literature distinguishes between self-knowledge about particular mental states and knowledge about the attributes of a persisting self. Certainty about the first kind of self-knowledge, that is, knowledge of the more immediate mental states that Descartes referred to as "sensations, emotions, and appetites," seems especially important for adaptive functioning. It also forms the basis for other aspects of self as knower and for constructing a cognitive representation of the self—what James referred to as "self as known." The impairments to this basic form of self-knowledge in individuals with PDs is shown by the tendency to question the genuineness of emotions and wants. Patients often wonder whether their feelings are real or genuine, and whether they "are really upset," and how it is possible to know whether they are in fact really upset, and whether the word "upset" could be substituted with "angry," "anxious," "depressed," or "despondent." This lack of experienced authenticity about basic experiences creates uncertainty about how to respond to situations and impedes self-development.

Certainty about basic emotions is also important from an evolutionary perspective. When our ancestors roamed the savannas of East Africa, certainty about feelings was important to survival. When they suddenly felt fear, signaling the possible presence of a predator, doubt about whether they really felt that way was inconsistent with survival. The importance of certainty and authenticity raises the question of why the mechanism involved is impaired in persons with PDs. This question is addressed by Peter Fonagy and Patrick Luyten (Chapter 7) in their discussion of existential distrust, an issue to which we return to after considering other components of the self.

The second component of the self—the self as known—is essentially a knowledge system composed of self-referential knowledge that develops through simultaneous differentiation of self-understanding and integration of this knowledge into a hierarchical structure. Self-referential knowledge is organized into self-schemas (see the Chapter 8 by Arnoud Arntz and Jill Lobbestael) that become organized into different representations of the self, culminating in an autobiographical self that provides a narrative account of the person's major qualities and life experiences. This narrative gives meaning and structure to experience and plays a crucial role in directing and coordinating goal-directed action. The self-knowledge constituting the self as known is more inferential than the knowledge referred to when discussing the self as knower. It is also constructed and reconstructed during development. What seems to be important for effective adaptation is a kind of qualified certainty about this knowledge that involves acceptance that this how one thinks, feels, and sees him- or herself and his or her world, which is also accompanied by the understanding that alternative interpretations and constructions are possible. It is important to note that this conception of the self as a knowledge system does not imply a fixed structure, as so often seems to be implied by clinical concepts of self and identity, an issue also discussed by Fonagy and Luyten in Chapter 7. Rather, self-referential knowledge is best represented by the analogy of the self as a matrix, with the different elements of self-knowledge forming nodes within the matrix. The more extensive the connections between nodes, the greater the sense of personal coherence and integration. This structure is used to generate different presentations of the self in the different situations the individual encounters. These momentary working selves are tailored to the situation and help to organize the resources needed to adapt to and manage the situation, an ability that is often impaired in persons with PDs (Livesley, 2017).

The cognitive or inferred self is the most studied component of the self system by both psychology and clinical psychiatry. Psychoanalysis in particular has been concerned with the integrative aspects of the self: Kohut (1971) described problems with the cohesiveness associated with naricissistic conditions, and Kernberg (1984) described the identity diffusion associated with borderline personality organization.

However, PD also seems to involve problems with the differentiation of the self system: Self-knowledge is often limited to relatively few general self-schemas, leading to an impoverished sense of self, and the self–other boundary is often poorly developed.

Interest in the third component of the self—the self as agent and center of self-regulation—really emerged only in the 1970s and was largely made possible by substantial developments in cognitive psychology. This aspect of the self has largely been neglected by psychiatry (Livesley 1998); an exception is Cloninger's (2000) inclusion of self-directedness in the definition of PD. However, goals are important to personality functioning. They energize and give meaning, purpose, and direction to lives (Baumeister, 1989; Carver, 2012; Carver & Scheier, 1998), and as Allport (1937, 1961) noted over half a century ago, striving to attain goals helps to integrate personality functioning by drawing together different resources, talents, and abilities needed to attain a goal. As with other aspects of the self, the motivational or conative aspect is impaired in PD: Most persons with the condition find it difficult to set and consistently work toward attaining long-term goals.

Turning to specific chapters, Jørgensen (Chapter 6) discusses a core issue—the problem of identity and identity problems. As Jørgensen notes, a person's identity is largely revealed by his or her response to the question "Who am I?" Within the previously described tripartite framework for conceptualizing the self, identity is a key component of the self-referential knowledge that constitutes the inferred or cognitive self. "Identity" refers to people's knowledge of their position in the world—who they are, how they see themselves in relation to others, and their roles and relationships. However, the term is often used in psychiatry in a way that is synonymous with the term "self." Consequently, Jørgensen discusses the relationship between self and identity from different conceptual positions. This discussion also addresses two important issues. First, a strong case is made that self/identity is an important organizing factor that contributes to the coherence of personality functioning, and that persons with identity problems lack an essential resource that impedes self-regulation and personal autonomy. Second, a comprehensive and clinically useful account of identity requires a variety of explanatory frameworks drawn from diverse disciplines. The chapter concludes with a discussion of the development of the self and treatment of identity problems that link nicely with the theme of the next chapter. Overall, Jørgensen makes a strong case that identity is basic to understanding self-regulation, and that the construct is a necessary part of a comprehensive account of the psychopathology of PD.

In Chapter 7, Fonagy and Luyten analyze the complex relationships between attachment and mentalization, and their contribution to the formation of the self. They begin by outlining their views on the role of mentalizing in the development of PD and how mentalizing develops in the context of the attachment relationship, most notably how emotional neglect and abuse impair the acquisition of mentalizing capacity. The authors' previous discussions of these issues are extended by considering what it is about emotional neglect that impedes the acquisition of these abilities. The explanation offered is that problems with the attachment relationship, most notably emotional neglect, lead to epistemic distrust. By this, they mean distrust of the individual's experience of communications from others; in other words, information gained through interaction with attachment figures is not considered trustworthy. This recalls Erikson's (1950) proposal that identity in its earliest form rests on "basic trust" in attachment figures. The idea of epistemic distrust also offers a possible explanation for the previously discussed uncertainty about the authenticity of basic emotions and needs seen in individuals with PD. In subsequent sections of the chapter, the authors discuss the multifaceted nature of mentalizing before describing the role of mentalizing in the formation and functioning of the self system. The authors offer a conceptualization of the self that differs from the static model that often underlies clinical concepts but is similar to the model we discussed earlier. They adopt the view emerging from psychological research that representations of the self, like representations of others, are constructed in the moment to meet the demands of the situation. This where the authors consider mentalizing capacity important: It allows individuals to construct and maintain a consistent sense of the self across different situations of their lives.

In Chapter 8, Arntz and Lobbestael review the substantial progress being made in explicating the cognitive structures and process associated with PD. Much of the earlier part of the chapter is a discussion of schemas—the factors influencing their development, their effect on information processing and responses to specific events, and factors contributing to schema change. The focus is understandable given that the schema is the basic unit of description and explanation in cognitive therapy. The interesting feature of their exposition—unusual in descriptions of clinical phenomena—is the extent to which their position is supported by empirical research. An important feature of this work is also the extent to which these studies lay the foundation for the systematic evaluation of the mechanisms of therapeutic change. The authors also discuss another clinically useful idea—the concept of "schema mode," which is a combination of an activated early maladaptive schema and a specific coping style, a concept that the authors suggest is useful in understanding the different and sometimes sudden changes in state observed in many patients. This provides a cognitive formulation of a common feature of severe PD—the occurrence of different, and often poorly integrated, mental states. These are often described in very different language across the different schools of thought: Psychoanalytic theory refers to the fragmentation of the self, and elsewhere these states are described as mental states (Horowitz, 1979) and self-states (Ryle, 1997; Ryle & Kellett, Chapter 27, this volume). The concept of schema mode provides an additional perspective on a common but poorly understood clinical phenomenon and an additional treatment method.

An interesting question prompted by Arntz and Lobbestael (Chapter 8) is the extent to which the developments described could contribute to a transtheoretical conceptualization of the psychopathology of PD. We noted earlier the apparent similarity between the concept of schema mode and the concepts used by other theoretical models. Also, as several authors have noted, although theories of PD are at an early stage of construction, many of these theories share the idea that cognitive structures are the basic building blocks of personality, and that in the final analysis, most therapies seek to bring about changes in these structures and processes. Given the progress being made in explicating the schemas and schema function noted in Chapter 8, the idea seems to offer a productive path to a more integrated approach.

Chapter 9, the final entry in this section, by Merav H. Silverman and Robert F. Krueger, deals with a very different aspect of psychopathology: the relationships among PDs and the relationship of PD and other forms of psychopathology. These are complex and thorny issues that date to the very beginning the field. As discussed in Chapter 1, the idea that PDs are attenuated versions of other mental disorders was a major theme in early 20th-century nosology, and the idea still continues to surface despite evidence to the contrary. This idea was replaced in the mid-20th century by interest in the relationship between mental disorders and personality, influenced especially by Eysenck's theory of personality. Multiple studies documented the predisposing and alloplastic effects of personality traits on psychopathology. Subsequently, as the authors note, researchers' interest began to focus more on diagnostic co-occurrence. When describing the history of research on the co-occurrence of PD and other mental disorders, the authors describe how research has changed from a focus on the co-occurrence of two conditions to the development of more comprehensive models that seek to describe the extensive patterns of diagnostic co-occurrence among mental disorders.

The first step beyond bivariate studies was the construction of spectrum models that sought to explain the relationship among multiple disorders in terms of a common spectrum, the best known of which is the schizophrenia spectrum. However, the model most pertinent to PD was Siever and Davis's (1991) suggestion that four broad dimensions underlie both the PDs and many other mental disorders: cognitive/perceptual organization, impulsivity/aggression, affective instability, and anxiety/inhibition. This helped to explain some relationships among PDs and some other major mental disorders, but it did not provide a comprehensive account of diagnostic co-occurrence. For this, multivariate models are needed, such as the one the authors discuss: the internalizing–externalizing model that offers a systematic account of the extensive covariation among mental disorders. The internalizing and externalizing factors are also correlated, explaining the occurrence of conditions showing features of both.

Silverman and Krueger (Chapter 9) offer a different way to understand the relationships among PDs and other mental disorders that also constitutes a very different way to think about psychopathology. Rather than conceptualizing mental disorder in terms of large set of discrete diagnostic entities—the framework proposed by the neo-Kraepelinians that was the foundation of DSM—they propose an overarching model that describes all forms of psychopathology in terms of a hierarchical structure of dimensions culminating in general factors of psychopathology.

**REFERENCES**

Allport, G. W. (1937). *Personality: A psychological interpretation*. New York: Holt, Rinehart & Winston.

Allport, G. W. (1961). *Pattern and growth in personality*. New York: Holt, Rinehart & Winston.

Baumeister, R. F. (1989). Social intelligence and the construction of meaning in life. In R. S. Wyer, Jr., & T. K. Srull (Eds.), *Social intelligence and cognitive assessments of personality: Advances in social cognition* (Vol. 2, pp. 71–80). Hillsdale, NJ: Erlbaum.

Carver, C. S. (2012). Self-awareness. In M. R. Leary & J. P. Tangney (Eds.), *Handbook of self and identity* (2nd ed., pp. 50–68). New York: Guilford Press.

Carver, C. S., & Scheier, M. F. (1998). *On the self-regulation of behavior*. Cambridge, UK: Cambridge University Press.

Cloninger, C. R. (2000). A practical way to diagnosis personality disorders: A proposal. *Journal of Personality Disorders, 14*, 99–108.

Erikson, E. (1950). *Childhood and society*. New York: Norton.

Horowitz, M. J. (1979). *States of mind*. New York: Plenum Press.

James, W. (1890). *The principles of psychology*. New York: Holt.

Kernberg, O. F. (1984). *Severe personality disorders*. New Haven, CT: Yale University Press.

Kohut, H. (1971). *The analysis of the self*. New York: International Universities Press.

Leary, M. R., & Tangney, J. P. (Eds.). (2012). *Handbook of self and identity* (2nd ed.). New York: Guilford Press.

Livesley, W. J. (1998). Suggestions for a framework for an empirically based classification of personality disorder. *Canadian Journal of Psychiatry, 43*, 137–147.

Livesley, W. J. (2003). Diagnostic dilemmas in the classification of personality disorder. In K. Phillips, M. First, & H. A. Pincus (Eds.), *Advancing DSM: Dilemmas in psychiatric diagnosis* (pp. 153–189). Arlington, VA: American Psychiatric Association Press.

Livesley, W. J. (2017). *Integrated modular treatment for borderline personality disorder*. Cambridge, UK: Cambridge University Press.

Ryle, A. (1997). *Cognitive analytic therapy and borderline personality disorder*. Chichester, UK: Wiley.

Siever, J., & Davis, K. L. (1991). A psychobiological perspective on the personality disorders. *American Journal of Psychiatry, 148*, 1647–1658.

# CHAPTER 6

# Identity

Carsten René Jørgensen

*My facade is all I have. Without it, I don't know who I am. How sad being halfway through one's life, not knowing who one is or should be.*
—24-YEAR-OLD WITH BORDERLINE PERSONALITY DISORDER

Development of a normal, coherent identity is an essential precondition for psychological functioning, including normal self-esteem, realistic appraisal of self and others, and the capacity to do well (Crawford, Cohen, Johnson, Snead, & Brook, 2004). "Once an identity has been formed, it constitutes a powerful organiser of experience and a lens through which reality is made meaningful" (Marcia, 2006, p. 585). Identity integration is an important element in psychological resilience. A stable, flexible, and coherent identity constitutes an inner resource that is important for self-regulation and the ability to navigate in a complex social world; it can provide predictability and continuity in psychological and interpersonal functioning, enabling autonomous functioning and efficacious exchange with others. Conversely, people with diffuse identity lack an essential inner resource, with severe implications for self-regulation and the ability to experience life and the world as meaningful. Disturbed identity is a defining characteristic of severe personality disorder (PD), with important implications for psychotherapeutic treatment.

Phenomenologically, normal identity is manifested in more or less explicit (conscious), subtle, and realistic answers to the fundamental question "Who am I?" and associated questions such as "How am I different from real or imagined others?"; "What are my basic goals and needs?"; and "How does my past, present, and future life constitute a meaningful whole?" The normal developed and mature identity is a precondition for our essential inner subjective sense of personal sameness and continuity over time, in the midst of change and across different contexts, and for the ability to make stable commitment to and identify with specific social roles and groups and their accompanying ideals, norms, and values as self-defining. People without this sense of a stable inner core, people with destabilized identity and deep-seated doubts about who they really are and how to understand others, such as people with severe PDs, find it difficult to anticipate and invest themselves in their own future. They live in the here and now, unable to really learn from their past experiences and to plan how to realize future goals, make long-term commitments, and avoid repeating past mistakes.

The term "identity" is located in the borderland between several scientific disciplines, including developmental, clinical, and personality psychology, and sociology, philosophy, anthropology, and political science. Identity is often seen as a feature of the clearly delimited individual, reflecting processes of individual self-definition, but identity development is also associated with interpersonal processes, social reality, and contemporary culture. Identity formation occurs at the intersection of the individual, the group, and society. In Western culture, collective support for identity formation has waned, and the individual is expected to develop an adult identity with limited institutional guidance (Schwartz, 2002). Bauman (2004, p. 33; 2005) has suggested that contemporary Western culture or "liquid modernity," characterized by continuous change, contributes to the development of a "permanently impermanent self." Thus, changes in late modern culture could increase the risk for development of identity disturbance (Jørgensen, 2006). Since the modern identity concept was first introduced by Erikson in the 1950s it has changed from a primarily inner emergent property of the clearly delimited individual (one-person psychology) to an inner intersubjectively constituted and process-related entity (two-person psychology) (Blatt, 2008; Bohleber, 2012), and we still lack a concise and universally accepted definition of "identity." Some definitions refer to clearly different phenomena; some theoreticians use the term ambiguously, and it is used in "so many ways that it is not possible simply to say what it refers to" (Schafer, 1968, p. 39). Numerous schools and traditions in psychology and sociology have focused on human identity, and one might argue that efforts to integrate the many existing definitions and approaches to identity, identity development, and identity disturbance, including empirical research, and apply them to PDs "is a difficult and somewhat scientifically dubious endeavour, given their differing origins and purposes" (Marcia, 2006, p. 577). Identity is often considered confusing, especially by persons who adopt a natural science perspective. From a positivist perspective, one might argue that the concept is unscientific because the phenomena it represents are difficult to operationalize, unobservable, and therefore unknowable. On the other hand, it has the potential to enrich our understanding of essential aspects of human existence, including how psychology and psychopathology are embedded in interpersonal relations and contemporary culture (see Jørgensen, 2006; 2008). Hence, the identity concept is important for dynamic, hermeneutic, and phenomenological approaches to psychology and psychopathology. Moreover, identity and other aspects of human subjectivity should not be excluded from psychology and psychiatry just because they are difficult to operationalize and research using traditional quantitative methods. To understand identity, we need to focus on subjective experience and how to interpret subjective experience and mental states using hermeneutic methods.

The prevailing confusion regarding how to define identity is related to research from different theoretical traditions (psychoanalysis, cognitive theory, theories of normal development) and disciplinary traditions (psychology, sociology, political science, anthropology), using different research methods and focusing on different layers or aspects of identity (Vignoles, Schwartz, & Luyckx, 2011). The field is characterized by substantial disagreement concerning questions such as whether identity should be seen as a relatively stable or constantly changing phenomenon (process), is best researched using quantitative or qualitative methods, and should be viewed as individually discovered, personally or socially constructed, or developed in interpersonal relationships (Vignoles et al., 2011). From a psychological perspective, normal identity (especially normal ego-identity, see below) is a relatively stable inner core primarily developed in exchanges with others.

Identity disturbance is suggestive of a poorly integrated personality and considered a core characteristic of severe PDs related to what Kernberg (1984) has called "borderline personality organization." In his structural diagnostic approach, Kernberg (2004) proposed that identity diffusion is the crucial criterion in differentiating severe character pathology from milder PDs and neurotic personality organization. Others have argued that a well-consolidated identity rules out more severe character pathology (Samuel & Akhtar, 2009); however, empirical data are sparse and inconsistent (Hörz et al., 2010; Modestin, 1987; Sollberger et al., 2012; Stern et al., 2010; Wilkinson-Ryan & Westen, 2000). Identity disturbance is primarily discussed in relation to borderline personality disorder (BPD), but there is reason to believe that it is also a feature of other severe PDs (Kernberg & Caligor, 2005). According to DSM-5, "identity disturbance: markedly and persistently unstable self-image or sense of self" is a diagnostic criterion for BPD (American Psychiatric Association [APA], 2013, p. 663). Identity disturbance is manifested in "sudden and dramatic shifts in self-image, characterised by shifting goals, values, and vocational aspirations. There may be sudden changes in opinions and plans about career, sexual identity, values, and types of friends" and individuals with BPD "may at times have feelings that they do not exist at all" (APA, 2013, p. 664). Several empirical studies have evaluated the predictive value of identity disturbance in diagnosing BPD and differentiating BPD from other PDs and non-PDs (Becker, Grilo, Edell, & McGlashan, 2002; Clarkin, Hull, & Hurt, 1993; Clarkin, Widiger, Frances, Hurt, & Gilmore, 1983; Fossati et al., 1999; Modestin, Oberson, & Erni, 1998; Pfohl, Zimmerman, & Strengl, 1986; Widiger, Frances, Warner, & Bluhm, 1986). The findings are inconsistent, but generally the predictive value of identity disturbance is high in diagnosing BPD, which implies that disturbed identity is an important aspect of BPD (Jørgensen, 2006). In the promising and ambitious alternative DSM-5 classification of PD, "identity diffusion" is defined as one of the central features of PD in general, not just a core symptom of BPD (APA, 2013).

## The Self

Terms related to identity and the self ("self-image," "self-esteem," "self-concept," etc.) are often used synonymously, which can give rise to confusion. The concepts of self and identity have a long and controversial history in philosophy and psychology (Jørgensen, 2006; Levin, 1992; Sollberger, 2013; Sorabji, 2006). In philosophy, the "self" typically refers to the person as agent, knower, and subject of mental states and conscious experience; it is an integral part of subjective experience itself as defined by phenomenology. Following Leary and Tangney (2003), the possession of a self allows us to direct our conscious attention toward, think consciously about, and regulate ourselves. In psychology, the concepts self and identity are often used for the set of attributes or characteristics a person consciously or unconsciously attaches to him- or herself (Perry 2002). Some writers use the term "self" more or less synonymously with the person as a whole, but in most conceptions the self is related to self-reflexive processes, the individual's conception of him- or herself, and the ability to look at the self from an outside perspective. One might even argue that the self is constituted by self-reflective thinking, and that severe self-pathology is intimately related to severe deficits in self-reflective thinking (mentalization, etc.). Basically, the "self" refers to the more experiential side of personhood, of being a person, and it has been argued that the core self represents an elementary form of self-awareness and self-relatedness manifested in sensations, feelings, images, and a sense of personal continuity (Glas, 2006).

William James (1890) differentiated between four levels of the self: (1) the material self, primarily the body and one's physical existence and appearance; (2) the spiritual self, the individual's "inner or subjective being, his psychic faculties" (p. 296); (3) "the pure ego," related to one's sense of personal sameness over time and across different contexts; and (4) the social self, related to each individual's social relationships and received recognition from others. James argued that "a man has as many social selves as there are individuals who recognize him and carry an image of him in their mind. . . . He has as many different social selves as there are discrete groups of persons about whose opinion he cares. He generally shows a different side of himself to each of these different groups" (p. 294). The individual has to integrate and create a meaningful whole out of these many selves, a task that has become even more complicated in modern culture in which the Internet and other electronic media have multiplied the number of potential (virtual and "real-life") relationships. People with severe PDs often experience great difficulties in creating a stable and integrated self out of the many different selves related to various relationships and social contexts; as formulated by a young woman with BPD: "I have so many different selves and I am a different person, depending on who I am with at the moment. I don't know who 'I' really am, but you know me so well, please tell me who I am."

Following James, the self has been conceptualized as the center of human agency (the source of action), as an object (the self as known, object of reference and mental representations), as the core of subjectivity (the self as knower and center of experience), and as an embodied entity or the self as equated with the physical body (Meissner, 2009). The philosopher Søren Kierkegaard (1849) defined the "self" as a relation that relates to itself, and in relating to itself is associated with something outside itself (ultimately God). Thus, as argued by Glas (2006, p. 133), being oneself is responding to a difference in oneself between "who I am and was in the past," between "who I am and could become in the future," and between "how I see myself and [how I am] seen by significant others." The self is therefore a responding and self-reflective agency, and it is relational; it is constituted and continuously stabilized in dialogue with significant others. Self-reflection presupposes and is developed in relationships in which the self is mirrored and validated by others.

One can differentiate a number of contemporary approaches to the self (Glas, 2006, p. 130), including (1) a meta-psychical approach, focusing on the self as a substance; (2) empirical approaches, which deny the existence of such a thing as the self and reduce the self to a series of perceptions, sensations, and feelings; (3) a hermeneutic approach, which is understanding the self as a narrative construction; and (4) a phenomenological approach, in which the self is seen as an experiencing subject that reveals an elementary form of self-relatedness. From a clinical point of view, the self is best understood as an experiencing subject, and a subject constructing narratives about itself. To minimize conceptual confusion, I suggest that the term "self" be used primarily to denote the conscious, self-reflective agent, subject, or person. And the identity concept should be used to refer to essential defining characteristics of the self that influence the person's level of agency. No matter how we choose to define the self, PDs involve disturbances in the self, including deficits in self-reflection and autonomous agency.

## Definitions of Identity

Most definitions of identity are rooted in Erikson's classical understanding of identity and it has been seen as a shortcoming of most identity theories that identity is primarily conceptualized in terms of Western individualistic values and ideals, making it difficult to generalize all aspects of the identity concept to more collectivistic cultures (Berman et al., 2014, p. 288). Erikson approached human identity from several perspectives and never arrived at an unequivocal definition. Modern psychoanalytic theorists (Kernberg & Caligor, 2005, p. 121) primarily understand identity as an inner psychic structure, intimately related to the internalization of object relationships. In normal development, internalized object relations are synthesized and "reflected in an internal sense and an external appearance of self-coherence" (p. 121). Based on contemporary personality research and narrative psychology, McAdams, Diamond, Aubin, and Mansfield (1997, p. 678) view identity as "an internalized and evolving life story, a way of telling the self to the self and others." Identity is understood as—some might say, reduced to—a narrative that the individual constructs to make sense and create a sense of meaning in life (McAdams, 1989, 1996), a narrative that organizes life in time, and "the stories people construct and tell about themselves to define who they are for themselves and others" (McAdams, 2006, p. 4). Following this conception of identity, severe identity disturbance is manifested in the inability to construct a coherent self-narrative and a painful experience of meaningless confusion (concerning "who I am," "what I want/need," etc.), and emptiness, often seen in patients with PDs, particularly BPD. In persons with PDs, deficits in the self-narrative create gaps and discontinuities in self-experience and behavior (see Dimaggio, Semerari, Carcione, Nicolo, & Procacci, 2007). One might argue that severe deficits in personal narratives can only be understood with reference to underlying deficits in the structural organization of personality, including insufficient integration of representations of the self and others (Bohleber, 1999; Jørgensen, 2010). The construction of a coherent self-narrative and autobiographical sense of self is one of the ultimate achievements of development of the personality or self-system (Stern, 1985; McAdams, 2015), and deficits in the identity narrative are an important manifestation of a failure to integrate salient aspects of the self. Inability to construct a coherent self-narrative is associated with deficits in the ability to mentalize (Bateman & Fonagy, 2004), insufficient assimilation of problematic experiences (painful memories and feelings, destructive behavior, etc.) into cognitive self-schemas (Stiles et al., 1990), and with insufficient integration of inner object relationships (Kernberg, 1984).

In social and cognitive psychology, identity is primarily understood as a mental construct that refers to "the traits and characteristics, social relations, roles, and social group memberships that define who one is" (Oyserman, Elmore, & Smith, 2012, p. 69). It is associated with one's primarily cognitive self-concept, including one's past (remembered), present (experienced), and imagined future life: the person one is trying to become and tries to avoid becoming. Normally, we assume that people have a stable core or essence that defines who they are and makes their behavior predictable and understandable. "Experienced stability allows people to make predictions based on their sense that they know themselves and increases their willingness to invest in their own futures"

(Oyserman et al., 2012, p. 94). This experienced stability is absent or substantially compromised in severe PDs. Similarly, PD is often associated with experienced confusion regarding the self's social relations, roles, and group membership.

In defining human identity, one has to differentiate between structural and more phenomenological aspects of identity. Structural aspects of identity are defined in accordance with Kernberg's (1984) psychodynamic model, whereas phenomenological aspects of identity primarily are associated with more specific contents or qualitative aspects of identity (explicit, cognitive, and conscious ideas of "who one is"), including subjective manifestations of structural identity: an experienced and more emotionally accessed "sense of identity." Jørgensen (2010) has suggested four descriptive layers of identity: ego-identity and personal, social, and collective identity, related to the concept of identity used in parts of psychoanalytic theory, personality theory, social psychology, and sociology, respectively.

1. The first layer, ego-identity, is associated with intrapsychic personality structure, the integration of internalized object relationships and temporal continuity of personal character, as defined by Kernberg. Ego-identity is not primarily defined by a specific and conscious "content"; it is not a "substance" but a capacity to experience inner coherence and self-sameness, a capacity to create "continuity in the persistent self-consciousness over space and time" (Sollberger, 2013, p. 3), and the development of a clear sense of how the individual self is differentiated from others. Ego-identity therefore refers to the core, most basic and structural aspects of identity that are diffused and disturbed in severe PD. The other three layers, personal, social, and collective identity, primarily denote more phenomenological aspects or specific manifestations of identity.
2. Personal identity is associated with individual attributes and characteristics, and reflects one's basic traits, goals, values, characteristics, and way of being in the world.
3. Social identity involves a sense of identification and inner solidarity with—a sense belonging and emotional attachment to—specific social groups. One's social identity is related to the self as object, the self as a known me-self, and what we might call the outer side of identity, including how the self is seen and reflected by others. Social identity is associated with "categorizations of the self into more inclusive social units that depersonalize the self-concept, where I becomes we" (Brewer, 1991, p. 476); the self is no longer primarily understood as a distinct individual entity but in terms of characteristics that the individual shares with others, with members of a social group.
4. Finally, collective identity is grounded in one's membership in larger social groups and one's inclination to identify with a specific religion, nation, or ethnic group.

The four layers of identity are intimately related, and dysfunctions in one layer, particularly diffusions in the ego-identity, typically cause and are manifested in problems in one or more of the others. People with severe deficits in identity experience painful misgivings concerning "who they really are"; they are unable to make long-term commitments and to identify with specific social groups, alternating between mutually incompatible identifications and social affinities. They have trouble handling ambivalence and complex self-representations that are based on the ability to contain and integrate contradictory identity fragments, emotions, and other mental states without having to evacuate these or resort to denial.

Preliminarily, one can define the normally developed identity as a stable, flexible, and coherent sense of the self ("myself" as a person, as an experiencing and acting subject); as a distinct center of understandable affects, mental states, and autonomous acts; a sense of the self as a person (subject or agent) with specific, distinct, and stable characteristics and an elaborated life story (self-narrative), who belongs to and identifies with one or more social groups and their norms, values, ideals and worldviews (Jørgensen, 2010, p. 347).

Some of the essential subjective experiences and psychological functions that have been associated with normal identity are listed in Table 6.1. Normal identity development is an important precondition for the development of mature agency and personal autonomy, or what the DSM work group on PD has called "self-direction" (APA, 2013, p. 775); it is the ability to "set and attain satisfying and rewarding personal goals that give direction, meaning and purpose to life" (Skodol et al., 2011, p. 18). It is therefore essential for actual and personally experienced

**TABLE 6.1. Selected Manifestations of Mature Personal Identity and Identity Diffusion**

| Normal (mature) identity | Pathological (diffuse) identity |
|---|---|
| Stable, nuanced and realistic sense of "who I am" and "how I am similar to/different from others" | Deep-seated insecurity and confusion concerning "who I really am," "what I have in common with others," and "how I am different from others" |
| Displays roughly similar character traits and behavior in different contexts and in interaction with different others; genuineness and authenticity of character and behavior | Exhibits highly contradictory character traits; behavior and self-representations are difficult to integrate; manifests in inauthentic, chameleon-like identity, shifts in identity depending on who one is with and on shifting affective states; behavior has an "as if" quality, at times dominated by "false" or "alien" self-parts |
| Subjective sense of personal sameness, coherence, and continuity over time and across different situations/contexts, despite perpetual change; temporal continuity in self-experience | Impaired capacity to experience the self as being the same amid change and over time; one's own past, present and imagined future is not integrated into continuous self-experience; a sense of life lived in fragments or disconnected/isolated pieces; no or severely impaired sense of coherence and continuity |
| Stable emotional sense of inner core, enjoys being alone from time to time | Feelings of inner emptiness accompanied by fear of being alone/abandoned; needs others to continuously define, "fill in"/complete, and stabilize the self |
| Ongoing awareness of having a unique self; stable and clear boundaries between the self and others | Experience of having a unique self is severely compromised; unstable, poorly, and/or rigidly defined boundaries between the self and others; overidentification with others and/or overemphasis on independence from others |
| Enjoys physical and emotional intimacy | Difficulties handling emotional and physical intimacy, fear of "losing the self" in intimate relationships (increased risk of sexual problems) |
| Realistic and adaptive sense of one's own body | Disturbed body image (increased risk of eating disorder) |
| Subjective clarity regarding one's own gender, gender identity, and sexual orientation | Gender dysphoria manifested in confusion regarding sexual orientation and gender-specific expectations |
| Consistent positive self-esteem, supported by accurate self-appraisal | Highly fragile self-esteem, easily influenced by immediate interactions with others and associated with un-nuanced, confused, or distorted self-appraisal |
| Subjective confidence that one's identity is acknowledged and recognized by significant others | Deep-seated fear of being faulty, a fraud, not real; diffusive sense of inner lack, of personal insufficiency |
| Goal-directed behavior, well-developed ability to hold on to and carry out long-term goals | Unable to cling to long-term goals, lacks a sense of direction; behavior is determined by immediate and quickly alternating impulses |
| Realistic and stable sense of personal agency (autonomy) and experience of oneself as a coherent unit with one's own thoughts and feelings | Sense of agency (autonomy) is compromised or alternates between unrealistic ideas about one's own effectiveness |
| Continuous personal commitments and attachment to significant others, which are seen as self-defining | Deficits in the ability to make commitments, often related to insecure or disorganized attachment |

*(continued)*

**TABLE 6.1.** *(continued)*

| Normal (mature) identity | Pathological (diffuse) identity |
|---|---|
| Inner solidarity and continuous identification with one's social group | "Lone wolf" or perpetually alternating identifications with different social groups, no deeper sense of belonging |
| Stable commitment to coherent and socially accepted set of norms, values, ideals, and a valid worldview that gives meaning to one's life | Contradictions in value system, significant moral relativism; life is experienced as meaningless; in some cases, counteridentification with prevailing norms, values, and ideals (negative identity) |
| Shifts easily between different social roles and contexts | Rigid adherence to narrowly defined social roles, difficulties in adapting to different social contexts |

*Note.* Partially adapted from Akhtar (1984, 1992), Akhtar and Samuel (1996), American Psychiatric Association (2013, p. 775.f), Jørgensen (2006, 2010), and Westen and Heim (2003).

agency that "the person" or one's identity is unified, that we experience our actions as authentic expressions of ourselves, rather than as product of forces at work in or on us, outside our control (Korsgaard, 2009, p. 18). Autonomous actions, unlike impulsive behavior determined by insufficient self-regulation, require agency, and agency requires unity (integration), stability, and coherence in one's identity and self. "An action is a movement attributable to an agent considered as an integrated whole, not a movement attributable merely to a part of an agent, or to some force working in or on her" (Korsgaard, 2009, p. 45). When aspects of the self (including traumatic experiences) are dissociated or shut out, "what is left" and accessible can be felt as "false," inauthentic or incomplete (Bromberg, 2001, p. 197). In the face of strong affects and impulses, patients with PDs often are unable to experience themselves as authors of their own behavior, and their sense of agency and autonomy is impaired, which is associated with identity diffusion and painful experiences of incoherence and inauthenticity. Trait impulsivity in itself is not pathological, nor is it directly associated with identity diffusion except when it is accompanied by a lack of inner continuity and painful experience of incoherence. Based on self-report data from a small group of adolescents, it has been suggested that adolescents with externalizing disorders (attention-deficit/hyperactivity disorder [ADHD], conduct disorders) do not have elevated levels of identity diffusion, possibly because they are able to stabilize their identity and boost their self-esteem by externalizing their problems (Jung, Pick, Schlüter-Müller, Schmeck, & Goth, 2013). Similarly, the manifested level of identity diffusion may be lower in patients with PD and severe externalizing behavior and salient dissocial traits.

## Identity Diffusion

Identity disturbance must be understood as a broad continuum of severity and duration, from normal and provisional identity conflicts and confusion in an otherwise consolidated identity in one end, to severe and prolonged, in some cases chronic, identity diffusion seen in severe character disorders in the other end (Akhtar & Samuel, 1996; Akhtar, 1984; Dammann, Hügli, et al., 2011; Foelsch et al., 2010). In addition to this, some psychotic disorders (schizophrenia) are associated with actual identity fragmentation, involving bizarre changes in self-concept, severely compromised boundaries between the self and others (reality testing), and complete breakdown of (numeric) identity. "The greater the identity disturbance, the more severe the underlying psychopathology" (Akhtar & Samuel, 1996, p. 260), including ego-impairment, compromised agency (autonomy), and interpersonal problems. Identity disturbance might to some extent constitute an essential psychological impairment underlying a broader range of severe psychopathological conditions, including not only PD but also bipolar disorder and eating disorders (Neacsiu, Herr, Fang, Rodriguez, & Rosenthal, 2015; Stein & Corte, 2007). What differentiates more "normal" and transient identity crises in adolescence from severe identity diffusion is that the better functioning adolescent with momentary identity problems has a fundamentally secure sense of self and the structural basis for eventually forming a stable identity, and the stable inner core (ego-identity) that is an important precondition for eventually making long-term commitments (Jørgensen, 2006, 2009b).

Most theorists agree that pathology of self and identity is one of the defining characteristics of BPD and is associated with most other PDs. Plutchik (1980) described the development of a coherent sense of identity as an essential task in personality development, and Livesley (2003) suggested that enduring failure to establish stable and integrated representations of the self and others, starting in adolescence or early adulthood, is one of the defining characteristics of PD in general. PDs generally involve problems in the sense of self or identity (Livesley, 2003). More specifically, Hurt, Clarkin, Munroe-Blum, and Marzialli (1992) defined problems relating to identity as one of three core problem areas presented by individuals with BPD. Similarly, Linehan (1993) argued that dysregulation of the sense of self, including not knowing who one really is, feelings of inner emptiness, and having no sense of self, is one of four essential pathological domains in BPD. In Linehan's cognitive-behavioral model of BPD, emotional dysregulation, impulsive and unpredictable behavior, cognitive dysregulation, and inability to establish a coherent and stable sense of identity are closely associated problem areas (see also Levy, Edell, & McGlashan, 2007). Empirical studies has related emotional dysregulation to identity disturbance (Neacsiu et al., 2015). Some of the core subjective experiences associated with identity diffusion are listed in Table 6.1.

Informed by contemporary object relations theory, Kernberg (1995, 2006) has linked identity diffusion and severe character pathology with a fundamental inability to integrate or synthesize different aspects of self and others into stable and coherent representations, and an inability to tolerate both positive and negative (good and bad) aspects of self and others, involving poorly integrated images of self and others. As a result, the experience of self and others, and interpersonal behavior, is dominated by constant shifts between insufficiently integrated, inflexible, and undifferentiated mental representations. The self is continually experienced in shifting positions, and identity is chameleon-like, marked by sharp discontinuities; unrealistic and crude images of the self as omnipotent and idealized are suddenly replaced by images of the self as worthless and devalued.

The person is fundamentally unable to answer the question "Who am I, really?" and is lacking an inner sense of meaning and direction in life (see Dammann, Walter, & Benecke, 2011). In Ryle's (1997) multiple states model, borderline pathology is associated with abrupt switches between mutually dissociated self-states, leading to experienced confusion and identity diffusion. Some have even suggested that PDs in general represent the characterological outcome of ego-syntonic dissociation (Bromberg, 2001). Similarly, Young, Klosko, and Weishaar (2003) have related BPD to continuous switches between different maladaptive cognitive schemas or schema modes in response to life events and subjective experiences, switches leading to diffusion in the patient's self-concept and to incoherent behavior.

A strong sense of self and identity has been associated with (1) stable and secure feelings of self-worth; (2) having a strong sense of agency, reflected in one's actions; and (3) a clearly and confidently defined self-concept (Kernis, Paradise, Whitaker, Wheatman, & Goldman, 2000). Conversely, severe identity diffusion typically implies unstable feelings of self-worth, often accompanied by feelings of insecurity; a strong need for continuous validation from others; impaired sense of agency; and a diffuse, nebulous or vague sense of self and identity. The structure and specific manifestations of identity diffusion possibly change in the natural course of PD, but further research is necessary to clarify this.

In patients with PD and identity diffusion, the use of dissociation, denial, projective identification, and other primitive defense mechanisms organized around splitting can be motivated by an urgent need to create a stable and coherent sense of identity. Fragments of identity are evacuated or denied in order to stabilize and create a coherent (albeit illusionary and momentary) sense of identity. Severe deficits in the patient's sense of identity and related painful feelings of inner emptiness may also result in various forms of impulsive (or obsessive–compulsive) and self-destructive behaviors such as cutting, misuse of drugs or alcohol, disordered eating, compulsive socializing, and promiscuous sexual behaviors—all motivated by an urgent need to delineate and stabilize identity.

To some extent, understanding identity and identity diffusion allows us to differentiate more severe PDs from higher-level PDs, making identity-related issues important for the PD field. On the other hand, identity and identity diffusion are complex constructs that so far have been difficult to operationalize. Paucity of empirical studies on identity diffusion in PD therefore stems from difficulties in defining and operationalizing the concept. In clinical practice, it can be difficult to identify identity diffusion correctly using patient self-report and without prolonged observation or contact with the patient. Even individuals with highly developed mentalization skills are only partly able to verbalize and report aspects of their identity. Hence, important aspects of identity, including the ability to construct coherent and stable representations of the self and others, "exist" outside consciousness and are primarily "lived" or manifested in one's way of interpreting experience, descriptions of the self and others, and behavioral patterns, rather than being actively chosen (Jørgensen, 2010).

When people are asked to describe themselves, what they typically provide is conscious, cognitive, and explicit self-representations or self-concepts, including specific manifestations of (personal and social) identity, not deeper (structural) aspects or layers of (ego) identity. Mental representations of the self as a person (identity), related to the self-as-object, can be implicit or explicit, conscious or unconscious. A person's explicit self-concept, activated when he or she is asked to answer a questionnaire, does not necessarily correspond with his or her implicit self-concept or with the self-concept that is activated when he or she is emotionally aroused or in an intimate relationship. These possible inconsistencies pose some problems for the use of self-report questionnaires in trying to understand the self, identity, and other aspects of self-representations and how they influence mental functioning, psychopathology, and behavior. Thus, a person's explicit and conscious self-representation can be a defensively transformed edition of implicit and unconscious self-representations (Westen & Cohen, 1993; Westen & Heim, 2003). Unconscious, nonintegrated, and implicit self-representations may be disavowed and evacuated in an effort to avoid anxiety, shame, or other painful mental states.

A number of instruments have been developed to measure the level of identity functioning and manifestations of identity diffusion, using different formats: self-report questionnaires (Adams, 1998; Berzonsky, 1989; Clarkin, Foelsch, & Kernberg, 2001; Goth et al., 2012; Kaufman, Cundiff, & Crowell, 2015; Samuel & Akhtar, 2009; Verheul et al., 2008), therapist ratings (Wilkinson-Ryan & Westen, 2000), and structured interviews (Clarkin, Caligor, Stern, & Kernberg, 2006). The validity and reliability of these instruments have received some empirical support but are still issues of concern. To some extent, the instruments capture different aspects and layers of identity, and some of them (Adams, 1998; Berzonsky, 1989) appear less suitable in diagnosing severe identity diffusion. The two most promising instruments are the Structured Interview of Personality Organization (STIPO; Clarkin et al., 2006) and the Self-Concept and Identity Measure (SCIM; Kaufman et al., 2015). It has been argued that studies of self-narratives and structural aspects of autobiographical memories have great potential in understanding identity disturbance in people with PD (Adler, Chin, Kilisetty, & Oltmanns, 2012; Jørgensen et al., 2012). When people with deficits in identity integration are asked to describe themselves or significant others, they are inclined to give one-dimensional, global, and minimizing descriptions, often heavily colored by their current affective state and revealing their inabililty to grasp the complexity of human personality. Kernberg (1984 p. 12) has suggested that, diagnostically, "identity diffusion appears in the patient's inability to convey significant interactions with others to an interviewer, who thus cannot emotionally empathize with the patient's conception of himself and others in such interactions." When listening to the patient's interpersonal and self-narratives, "one should look for consistency versus contradiction, clarity versus confusion, solidity versus emptiness" (Akhtar, 1999, p. 72) and the ability to provide subtle, realistic, and coherent descriptions of the self and others. The patient's level of intelligence, age, mentalizing capacity, and situational factors must also be taken into account when evaluating the quality of his or her descriptions of the self, significant others, and interpersonal relationships.

Studies have investigated the relationship between severe identity diffusion and other aspects of PD, almost exclusively focusing on identity diffusion in BPD. Wilkinson-Ryan and Westen (2000) asked a group of experienced clinicians to rate one of their adult patients (approximately one-third with BPD) using a specially designed identity disturbance questionnaire. Based on factor analyses of the collected data, they identified four factors of identity disturbance:

- Role absorption, a tendency to define the self in terms of a single social role or cause that can help the person create a sense of order and meaningfulness rather than chaos, meaninglessness, or emptiness
- A painful subjective sense of self-incoherence and distress/concern about lack of coherence of the self
- Inconsistencies in thoughts, feelings, and behavior—grossly contradictory beliefs and actions, and other manifestations of instability (incoherence), including difficulties constructing a coherent and meaning-generating life narrative that link one's past, present, and imagined future self;
- Lack of commitment to jobs, relationships, and values.

All four factors, particularly painful incoherence, distinguished BPD from patients with no PD and to some extent from patients with other PDs, suggesting that identity diffusion is most severe in patients with BDP. A later study, using a sample of adolescents, confirmed the four factors (Westen, Betan, & Defife, 2011). In addition to this, sexual abuse was strongly associated with painful incoherence, and one could argue that this factor includes aspects of identity disturbance related to dissociation or traumatization (Westen et al., 2011).

Other studies support the notion that identity diffusion correlates with BPD (Fossati, Borroni, Feeney, & Maffei, 2012) and differentiates patients with BPD from nonclinical adults (Jørgensen, 2009a; Verheul et al., 2008). In addition to this, a number of studies have associated the presence and severity of identity diffusion with higher levels of various psychiatric symptoms (depression, anxiety, self-mutilation, lower level of global function, higher level of self-criticism, the use of primitive defense mechanisms, and compromised reality testing) in patients with BPD (Hörz et al., 2010; Leichsenring, Kunst, & Hoyer, 2003; Lenzenweger, Clarkin, Kernberg, & Foelsch, 2001; Levy et al., 2007; Sollberger et al., 2012), partially supporting the notion that identity diffusion is associated with more severe pathology. However, most of these studies have a number of limitations (based on small or nonclinical samples, etc.) and the direction of causality between identity diffusion and symptom severity is unclear. Thus, identity diffusion could exacerbate other manifestations of psychopathology; alternatively, various other aspects of PD (emotional instability, behavioral dysregulation, etc.) could give rise to disintegration of identity (Sollberger et al., 2012). Finally, an older study (Hull, Clarkin, & Kakuma, 1993) found that the presence of severe identity diffusion in patients with BPD was associated with less than favorable results of 6 months of inpatient psychotherapy, possibly indicating that identity diffusion is associated with more severe pathology that is harder to treat successfully. At present it is unclear whether identity diffusion is associated with less than favorable results of psychotherapy in general, but there is reason to assume that severe identity diffusion must be taken into account if psychotherapy is to be effective (Clarkin, Yeomans, & Kernberg, 2006).

### Development of Identity and Identity Diffusion

Erikson, Kernberg, and other psychoanalysts (e.g., Akhtar, 1992; Jacobson, 1964) have written extensively about the development of identity and identity diffusion, primarily from the point of view of ego psychology and object relations theory. Identity development and consolidation are important psychological themes in adolescence, when the individual has to struggle with issues related to emotional disengagement from significant others (and their internalized representations); the development of autonomy, sexual, and gender identity, and how to establish mature adult relationships; and finding the right balance between self-distinction (separateness, distance) and relatedness (emotional attachment and commitment). But "identity development neither begins nor ends with adolescence: it is a lifelong development, largely unconscious to the individual and his society. Its roots go back all the way to the first self-recognition" (Erikson, 1959, p. 113). Identity development is a never-ending process (Kroger, 2007). Similarly, although severe identity diffusion is often manifested in adolescence and early adulthood, its development typically goes back to early childhood.

Erikson (1968, p. 159) argued that identity formation "arises from the selective repudiation and mutual assimilation of childhood identifications and their absorption in a new configuration." Following Erikson, psychoanalytic theory has described three phases of identity development, all associated with the internalization and gradual integration of early object relationships (Kernberg, 1966, 1995). These developmental phases imply (1) introjection of early memory traces involving images of the self and others; (2) identification with significant others, including the internalization of role relationships; and (3) proper identity formation, in which earlier introjections and identifications are depersonified and synthesized into more integrated and extensive representations of the self and others. The normal separation and individuation process in early childhood (Mahler, Pine, & Bergman, 1975) and the second individuation process in adolescence (Blos, 1979) implies that the self is differentiated from significant others and their internal mental representations, resulting in the creation of a personal or individuated identity. Masterson (2000) and other psychoanalysts (e.g., Blos, 1979) have conceptualized identity diffusion as the result of severe disruptions of normal separation and particularly normal individuation processes in early childhood and adolescence. Kernberg (1984, 2006) understands identity diffusion as a derivative of pathology in internalized object relations, in which insecure attachment is seen as an important risk factor for the development of identity diffusion and disorganized inner working models.

Development of the ability to mentalize is invaluable in one's effort to integrate early introjections and identifications into coherent representations of the self and others, including the construction of a self-narrative that generates meaning. Bateman and Fonagy (2006, p. 4) have argued that mentalization "gives us the sense of continuity and control that generates the subjective experience of agency or 'I-ness' which is at the very core of a sense of identity." Normally, when states of mind are not felt to fit coherently into our dominant sense of self or identity, they "are nevertheless integrated into it by the capacity for mentalization. We smooth the discontinuities by creating an intentional narrative" (p. 15). Conversely, in PD, prementalistic modes of functioning (psychic equivalence, teleological and pretend mode) often disorganize relationships and "destroy the coherence of self-experience that the narrative provided by normal mentalisation generates" (Bateman & Fonagy, 2008, p. 183). Deficits in the development of mentalization and of identity diffusion are therefore intimately related. Accurate, validating, and clearly "marked" mirroring of the self from significant others contribute to normal identity development (Bateman & Fonagy, 2004). "The earliest sense of identity may be induced by the experience of the child perceiving its mother's face responding to it. The child sees itself reflected in its mother's face" (Modell, 1968, p. 49). If these important interpersonal processes are disrupted, normal identity development may fail. Inaccurate, invalidating, inconsistent, and insufficiently marked mirroring of the self can compromise the development of a stable and coherent identity that is clearly differentiated from others. Discontinuity in identity is associated with unstable and unpredictable behavior that often evokes similarly unpredictable, alienating, and distancing reactions in others, leading to unstable interpersonal feedback and insufficient mirroring from others, which can cause further destabilization of identity. A self-perpetuating process is therefore established, with potentially aggravating identity diffusion and maladaptive relationships (see Figure 6.1). When one feels lonely, unable to connect with other people, unable to "read" and understand what others think about one, there is a heightened risk of developing identity diffusion and relational problems.

Blatt and Luyten (2009) argue that personality development proceeds in dialectic interaction between two dimensions: (1) the development of self-definition or identity and (2) the development of interpersonal relatedness, related to a fundamental tension between the need for uniqueness and individuation on the one hand, and for validation from, and similarity with others, on the other (Brewer, 1991). Normally, these two developmental dimensions are integrated during adolescence, an integration that is lacking in most PDs, with one of the two polarities developing at the expense of the other. Identity is developed in dialogue and exchange with others, and if one's identity is to remain stable and coherent, one should receive continued recognition from significant others. Hence, the development and maintenance of self-definition and interrelatedness are intimately related processes. Blatt (2008, p. 160) has suggested that "personality disorders are organised into two primary configurations: one around issues of relatedness and the other around issues of self-definition or distinctiveness. Both issues are intimately related to identity, and findings suggest that particularly patients with BPD have severe problems with both configurations (p. 161).

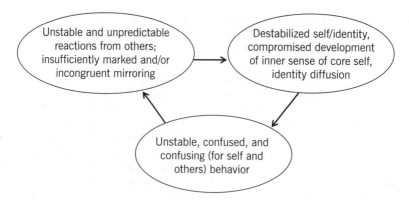

**FIGURE 6.1.** Self-perpetuating processes involving insufficient mirroring, identity diffusion, and unstable behavior. From Jørgensen (2009b, p. 77).

## Psychotherapeutic Implications

The existence of identity diffusion has a number of implications for treatment in that patients with severe identity diffusion require the predominance of different therapeutic strategies compared with patients with well-consolidated and coherent identities. Transference-focused psychotherapy was specifically developed for the treatment of patients with severe identity diffusion (Yeomans, Clarkin, & Kernberg, 2015) and has been shown to have significant impact on the level of identity diffusion in patients with BPD (Sollberger et al., 2015; see also Feenstra, Hutsebaut, Verheul, & Van Limbeek, 2014) In general, persons with a coherent identity are able to relate to others as separate and autonomous subjects, a capacity that is highly important for the ability to develop and sustain a good working alliance based on some measure of basic trust and to profit from focused short-term therapy (Akhtar, 1999; Akhtar & Samuel 1996). In contrast, patients with severe identity diffusion lack the stabilizing inner core and coherent self-experience that is necessary for short-term therapy and more explorative and confrontational interventions to be effective. These patients typically need long-term treatment and, in some cases, treatment dominated by more supportive, validating, mirroring, and affirmative interventions, particularly in the early phases of treatment. Pathology manifests itself in how the patient relates to the therapist in the here and now. Patients with severe identity diffusion experience great difficulties in establishing mature relationships with others that they recognize as autonomous individuals; others are primarily seen as objects that can be used to stabilize the self and to satisfy various needs—and the therapist's ability to handle conflict, confusion, and substantial fluctuations in the relationship will be extremely important for the therapeutic process and outcome. Identity diffusion can also be observed in the therapeutic transference "as a form of interpersonal manifestation of intrapsychic conflicts amongst different internal states" (Sollberger et al., 2015, p. 560) or insufficiently integrated part-identities that alternately dominates how the patient relates to the therapist. An important aspect of psychotherapy with patients with PD with severe identity diffusion is that the patient, over time, will internalize, mentalize, and integrate prominent elements of the interaction with the therapist in his or her inner object relations, including his or her conceptualization of the self and others (ego identity). In addition to this, development of the patient's ability to mentalize and self-reflective capacity will improve the ability to construct a coherent and meaningful self-narrative and therefore help the patient reach a higher level of identity integration; the patient's access to, and understanding of, his or her inner world will be improved. Impairment in the patient's self-regulation and ability to hold on to long-term goals, such as coming to treatment every week for months or years in order to get better, implies that it is part of the therapist's job to insist that the patient come to treatment, even when the patient apparently has changed his or her mind concerning therapy. In addition, the therapist's continuous mirroring, recognition, and validation of the patient's self and subjective experience will invigorate the patient's fragile self-esteem, contribute to the definition and stabilization of the patient's identity, and reduce the painful inner confusion and emptiness often seen in patients with severe PD.

## REFERENCES

Adams, G. R. (1998). *The objective measure of ego identity status: A reference manual* (2nd ed.). Unpublished manuscript, University of Guelph, Guelph, ON, Canada.

Adler, J. M., Chin, E. D., Kolisetty, A. P., & Oltmanns, T. F. (2012). The distinguishing characteristics of narrative identity in adults with features of borderline personality disorder: An empirical investigation. *Journal of Personality Disorders, 26,* 498–512.

Akhtar, S. (1984). The syndrome of identity diffusion. *American Journal of Psychiatry, 141,* 1381–1385.

Akhtar, S. (1992). *Broken structures: Severe personality disorders and their treatment.* New York: Jason Aronson.

Akhtar, S. (1999). *Immigration and identity: Turmoil, treatment, and transformation.* New York: Jason Aronson.

Akhtar, S., & Samuel, S. (1996). The concept of identity: Developmental origins, phenomenology, clinical relevance, and measurement. *Harvard Review of Psychiatry, 3,* 254–267.

American Psychiatric Association. (2013). *Diagnostic and statistical manual of mental disorders* (5th ed.). Arlington, VA: Author.

Bateman, A., & Fonagy, P. (2004). *Psychotherapy for borderline personality disorder: Mentalization-based treatment.* Oxford, UK: Oxford University Press.

Bateman, A., & Fonagy, P. (2006). *Mentalization-based treatment for borderline personality disorder: A practical guide.* Oxford, UK: Oxford University Press.

Bateman, A., & Fonagy, P. (2008). Comorbid antisocial and borderline personality disorders: Mentalization-based treatment. *Journal of Clinical Psychology: In Session, 64,* 181–194.

Bauman, Z. (2004). *Identity.* London: Polity Press.

Bauman, Z. (2005). *Liquid life.* London: Polity Press.

Becker, D., Grilo, C., Edell, W., & McGlashan, T. (2002). Diagnostic efficacy of borderline personality disorder criteria in hospitalized adolescents: Comparison with hospitalized adults. *American Journal of Psychiatry, 159,* 2042–2046.

Berman, S. L., Ratner, K., Cheng, M., Li, S., Jhingon, G., & Sukumaran, N. (2014). Identity distress during the era of globalization: A cross-national study of India, China, and United States. *Identity: An International Journal of Theory and Research, 14,* 286–296.

Berzonsky, M. D. (1989). Identity style: Conceptualization and measurement. *Journal of Adolescent Research, 4,* 268–282.

Blatt, S. J. (2008). *Polarities of experience: Relatedness and self-definition in personality development, psychopathology, and the therapeutic process.* Washington, DC: American Psychological Association.

Blatt, S. J., & Luyten, P. (2009). A structural-developmental psychodynamic approach to psychopathology: Two polarities of experience across the life span. *Development and Psychopathology, 21,* 793–814.

Blos, P. (1979). *The adolescent passage: Developmental issues.* New York: International Universities Press

Bohleber, W. (1999). Psychoanalyse, Adoleszenz und das Problem der Identity [Psychoanalysis, adolescence, and the problem of identity]. *Psyche, 53,* 507–529.

Bohleber, W. (2012). Adoleszenz und Identität: Psychoanalytische Persönlichkeitstheorien und das Problem der Identität in der Spätmoderne [Adolescense and identity: Psychoanalytic theories of personality and the problem of identity in late modernity]. In W. Bohleber (Ed.), *Was psychoanalyse heute leistet* [Destructiveness, intersubjectivity, and trauma: The identity crisis of modern psychoanalysis] (pp. 61–85). Stuttgart, Germany: Klett-Cotta.

Brewer, M. B. (1991). The social self: On being the same and different at the same time. *Psychological Bulletin, 17,* 475–482.

Bromberg, P. M. (2001). *Standing in the spaces: Essays on clinical process, trauma and dissociation* (rev. ed.). Hillsdale, NJ: Analytic Press.

Clarkin, J. F., Caligor, E., Stern, B., & Kernberg, O. F. (2006). *Structured Interview of Personality Organization (STIPO).* Unpublished manuscript, Weill Medical College, Cornell University, White Plains, NY.

Clarkin, J. F., Foelsch, P. A., & Kernberg, O. F. (2001). *The Inventory of Personality Organization.* Unpublished manuscript, Weill Medical College, Cornell University, White Plains, NY.

Clarkin, J. F., Hull, J. W., & Hurt, S. W. (1993). Factor structure of borderline personality disorder criteria. *Journal of Personality Disorders, 7,* 137–143.

Clarkin, J. F., Widiger, T. A., Frances, A., Hurt, S. W., & Gilmore, M. (1983). Prototypic typology of the borderline personality disorder. *Journal of Abnormal Psychology, 92,* 263–275.

Clarkin, J. F., Yeomans, F. E., & Kernberg, O. F. (2006). *Psychotherapy for borderline personality: Focusing on object relations.* Washington, DC: American Psychiatric Publishing.

Crawford, T. N., Cohen, P., Johnson, J. G., Sneed, J. R., & Brook, J. S. (2004). The course and psychosocial correlates of personality disorder symptoms in adolescence: Erikson's developmental theory revisited. *Journal of Youth and Adolescence, 33,* 373–387.

Dammann, G., Hügli, C., Selinger, J., Gremaud-Heitz, D., Sollberger, D., Wiesbeck, G. A., et al. (2011). The self-image of borderline personality disorder: A in-depth qualitative research study. *Journal of Personality Disorders, 25,* 517–527.

Dammann, G., Walter, M., & Benecke, C. (2011). Identität und Identitätsstörungen bei Borderline-Persönlichkeitsstörungen [Identity and identity disturbance in borderline personality disorder]. In B. Dulz, S. C. Herpertz, O. F. Kernberg, & U. Sachsse (Eds.), *Handbuch der Borderline-Störungen* [*Handbook for borderline disorders*] (pp. 275–285). Stuttgart, Germany: Schattauer.

Dimaggio, G., Semerari, A., Carcione, A., Nicolo, G., & Procacci, M. (2007). *Psychotherapy of personality disorders*. London: Routledge.

Erikson, E. H. (1959). *Identity and the life cycle*. New York: International Universities Press.

Erikson, E. H. (1968). *Identity: Youth and crisis*. New York: Norton.

Feenstra, D. J., Hutsebaut, J., Verheul, R., & Van Limbeek, J. (2014). Changes in the identity integration of adolescents in treatment for personality disorders. *Journal of Personality Disorders, 28*, 101–112.

Foelsch, P. A., Odom, A., Arena, H., Krischer, M. K., Schmeck, K., & Schlüter-Müller, S. (2010). Differenzierung zwichen Identitätskrise und Identitätsdiffusion und ihre Bedeutung für die Behandlung [Differentiating identity crisis and identity diffusion and implications for treatment]. *Praxis Kinderpsychologie und Kinderpsychiatrie, 59*, 418–434.

Fossati, A., Borroni, S., Feeney, J., & Maffei, C. (2012). Predicting borderline personality features from personality traits, identity orientation, and attachment style in Italian non-clinical adults: Issues of consistence across age ranges. *Journal of Personality Disorders, 26*, 280–297.

Fossati, A., Maffei, C., Bagnato, M., Donati, D., Nambia, C., & Novella, L. (1999). Latent structure analysis of DSM-IV borderline personality disorder criteria. *Comprehensive Psychiatry, 40*, 72–79.

Glas, G. (2006). Person, personality, self, and identity: A philosophically informed conceptual analysis. *Journal of Personality Disorders, 20*, 126–138.

Goth, K., Foelsch, P., Schlüter-Müller, S., Birkhölzer, M., Jung, E., Pick, O., et al. (2012). Assessment of identity development and identity diffusion in adolescence—Theoretical basis and psychometric properties of the self-report questionnaire AIDA. *Child and Adolescent Psychiatry and Mental Health, 6*, 27.

Hörz, S., Rentrop, M., Fischer-Kern, M., Schuster, P., Kapusta, N., Buchheim, P., et al. (2010). Strukturniveau in klinischer Schweregrad der Borderline-Persönlichkeitsstörung [Structural level of functioning and severity of borderline personality disorder]. *Zeitschrift für Psychosomatische Medicin und Psychotherapie, 56*, 136–149.

Hull, J. W., Clarkin, J. F., & Kakuma, T. (1993). Treatment response of borderline patients: A growth curve analysis. *Journal of Nervous and Mental Disease, 181*, 503–509.

Hurt, S. W., Clarkin, J. F., Munroe-Blum, H., & Marzialli, E. (1992). Borderline behavioural cluster and different treatment approaches. In J. F. Clarkin, E. Marziali, & H. Munroe-Blum (Eds.), *Borderline personality disorder: Clinical and empirical perspectives* (pp. 199–219). New York: Guilford Press.

Jacobson, E. (1964). *The self and the object world*. New York: International Universities Press.

James, W. (1890). *The principles of psychology* (Vols. 1–2). Boston: Dover.

Jørgensen, C. R. (2006). Disturbed sense of identity in borderline personality disorder. *Journal of Personality Disorders, 20*, 618–644.

Jørgensen, C. R. (2008). *Identitet: Psykologiske og kulturanalytiske perspektiver* [*Identity: Psychological and cultural-analytic perspectives*]. Copenhagen, Denmark: Hans Reitzels Forlag

Jørgensen, C. R. (2009a). Identity style in patients with borderline personality disorder and normal controls. *Journal of Personality Disorders, 23*, 101–112.

Jørgensen, C. R. (2009b). *Personlighedsforstyrrelser: Moderne relational forståelse og behandling af borderline-lidelser* [*Personality disorders: Modern relational understanding and treatment of borderline disorders*]. Copenhagen, Denmark: Hans Reitzels Forlag.

Jørgensen, C. R. (2010). Invited essay: Identity and borderline personality disorder. *Journal of Personality Disorders, 24*, 344–364.

Jørgensen, C. R., Berntsen, D., Bech, M., Kjølbye, M., Bennedsen, B. E., & Ramsgaard, S. B. (2012). Identity-related autobiographical memories and cultural life scripts in patients with borderline personality disorder. *Consciousness and Cognition, 21*, 788–798.

Jung, E., Pick, O., Schlüter-Müller, S., Schmeck, K., & Goth, K. (2013). Identity development in adolescents with mental problems. *Child and Adolescent Psychiatry and Mental Health, 7*, 26.

Kaufman, E., Cundiff, J. M., & Crowell, S. E. (2015). The development, factor structure, and validation of the self-concept and identity measure (SCIM): A self-report assessment of clinical identity disturbance. *Journal of Psychopathology and Behavioural Assessment, 37*, 122–133.

Kernberg, O. F. (1966). Structural derivatives of object relationships. *International Journal of Psychoanalysis, 47*, 236–252.

Kernberg, O. F. (1984). *Severe personality disorders: Psychotherapeutic strategies*. New Haven, CT: Yale University Press.

Kernberg, O. F. (1995). *Object relations theory and clinical psychoanalysis* (rev. ed.). New York: Jason Aronson.

Kernberg, O. F. (2004). *Aggressivity, narcissism, and self-destructiveness in the therapeutic relationship*. New Haven, CT: Yale University Press.

Kernberg, O. F. (2006). Identity: Recent findings and clinical implications. *Psychoanalytic Quarterly, 65*, 969–1004.

Kernberg, O. F., & Caligor, E. (2005). A psychoanalytic theory of personality disorders. In M. F. Lenzenweger & J. F. Clarkin (Eds.), *Major theories of personality disorder* (2nd ed., pp. 114–156). New York: Guilford Press.

Kernis, M. H., Paradise, A. W., Whitaker, D. J., Wheatman, S. R., & Goldman, B. N. (2000). Master of one's psychological domain?: Not likely if one's self-esteem is unstable. *Personality and Social Psychologial Bulletin, 26,* 1297–1305.

Kierkegaard, S. (1849). *Sygdommen til døden* [Sickness unto death]. Copenhagen, Denmark: Borgen.

Korsgaard, C. M. (2009). *Self-constitution: Agency, identity and integrity.* Oxford, UK: Oxford University Press.

Kroger, J. (2007). *Identity development: Adolescence through adulthood* (2nd ed.). London: SAGE.

Leary, M. R., & Tangney, J. P. (2003). The Self as an organizing construct in the behavioral and social sciences. In M. R. Leary & J. P. Tangney (Eds.), *Handbook of self and identity* (pp. 3–14). New York: Wiley.

Leichsenring, F., Kunst, H., & Hoyer, J. (2003). Borderline personality organization in violent offenders: Correlations of identity diffusion and primitive defense mechanisms with antisocial features, neuroticism, and interpersonal problems. *Bulletin of the Menninger Clinic, 67,* 314–327.

Lenzenweger, M. F., Clarkin, J. F., Kernberg, O. F., & Foelsch, P. A. (2001). The Inventory of Personality Organization: Psychometric properties, factorial composition, and criterion relations with affect, aggressive dyscontrol, psychotic proneness, and self-domains in a nonclinical sample. *Psychological Assessment, 13,* 577–591.

Levin, J. D. (1992). *Theories of the self.* Washington, DC: Hemisphere.

Levy, K. N., Edell, W. S., & McGlashan, T. H. (2007). Depressive experiences in inpatients with borderline personality disorder. *Psychiatric Quarterly, 78,* 129–143.

Linehan, M. M. (1993). *Cognitive-behavioral treatment of borderline personality disorder.* New York: Guilford Press.

Livesley, W. J. (2003). *Practical management of personality disorder.* New York: Guilford Press.

Mahler, M., Pine, F., & Bergman, A. (1975). *The psychological birth of the human infant.* New York: Basic Books.

Marcia, J. E. (2006). Ego identity and personality disorders. *Journal of Personality Disorders, 20,* 577–596.

Masterson, J. F. (2000). *The personality disorders.* Phoenix, AZ: Zeig, Tucker, & Theisan.

McAdams, D. P. (1989). The development of a narrative identity. In D. M. Buss & N. Cantor (Eds.), *Personality psychology: Recent trends and emerging directions* (pp. 160–175). New York: Springer.

McAdams, D. P. (1996). Personality, modernity, and the storied self: A contemporary framework for studying persons. *Psychological Inquiry, 7,* 295–321.

McAdams, D. P. (2006). Introduction. In D. P. McAdams, R. Josselson, & A. Lieblich (Eds.), *Identity and story: Creating self in narrative* (pp. 3–12). Washington, DC: American Psychological Association.

McAdams, D. P. (2015). *The art and science of personality development.* New York: Guilford Press.

McAdams, D. P., Diamond, A., Aubin, E., & Mansfeld, E. (1997). Stories of commitment: The psychosocial construction of generative lives. *Journal of Personality and Social Psychology, 72,* 678–694.

Meissner, S. J. (2009). The genesis of the self: I. The self and its parts. *Psychoanalytic Review, 96,* 187–217.

Modell, A. H. (1968). *Object love and reality.* New York: International Universities Press.

Modestin, J. (1987). Quality of interpersonal relationships: The most characteristic DSM-III BPD criterion. *Comprehensive Psychiatry, 28,* 397–402.

Modestin, J., Oberson, B., & Erni, T. (1998). Identity disturbance in personality disorders. *Comprehensive Psychiatry, 39,* 352–357.

Neacsiu, A. D., Herr, N. R., Fang, C. M., Rodriguez, M. A., & Rosenthal, M. Z. (2015). Identity disturbance and problems with emotion regulation are related constructs across diagnoses. *Journal of Clinical Psychology, 71,* 346–361.

Oyserman, D., Elmore, K., & Smith, G. (2012). Self, self-concept, and identity. In M. R. Leary & J. P. Tangney (Eds.), *Handbook of self and identity* (2nd ed., pp. 69–104). New York: Guilford Press.

Perry, J. (2002). *Identity, personal identity and the self.* Indianapolis, IN: Hackett.

Pfohl, B., Zimmerman, M., & Strengl, D. (1986). DSM-III personality disorders: Diagnostic overlap and internal consistency of individual DSM-III criteria. *Comprehensive Psychiatry, 29,* 21–34.

Plutchik, R. (1980). A general psychoevolutionary theory of emotion. In R. Plutchik & H. Kellerman (Eds.), *Emotion, psychopathology, and psychopathology* (pp. 3–33). New York: Guilford Press.

Ryle, A. (1997). *Cognitive analytic therapy and borderline personality disorder: The model and the method.* New York: Wiley.

Samuel, S., & Akhtar, S. (2009). The identity consolidation inventory (ICI): Development and application of a questionnaire for assessing the structuralization of individual identity. *American Journal of Psychoanalysis, 69,* 53–61.

Schafer, R. (1968). *Aspects of internalization.* New York: International Universities Press.

Schwartz, S. J. (2002). In search of mechanisms of change in identity development. *Identity: An International Journal of Theory and Research, 2,* 317–339.

Skodol, A. E., Clark, D. S., Bender, J. M., Krueger, L. A., Morey, L. C., Verheul, R., et al. (2011). Proposed changes in personality and personality disorder assessment and diagnosis for DSM-5: Part I. Description and rationale. *Personality Disorders: Theory, Research, and Treatment, 2,* 4–22.

Sollberger, D. (2013). On identity: From a philosophical point of view. *Child and Adolescent Psychiatry and Mental Health, 7* (29), 1–10.

Sollberger, D., Gremaud-Heitz, D., Riemenschneider, A., Agarwalla, P., Benecke, C., Schwald, O., et al. (2015). Change in identity diffusion and psychopathology in a specialized inpatient treatment for borderline personality disorder. *Clinical Psychology and Psychotherapy, 22,* 559–569.

Sollberger, D., Gremaud-Heitz, D., Riemenschneider, A., Küchenhoff, J., Dammann, G., & Walter, M. (2012). Associations between identity diffusion, Axis II disorder, and psychopathology in inpatients with borderline personality disorder. *Psychopathology, 45,* 15–21.

Sorabji, R. (2006). *Self: Ancient and modern insights about individuality, life, and death.* Oxford, UK: Oxford University Press.

Stein, K. F., & Corte, C. (2007). Identity impairment and the eating disorders: Content and organization of the self-concept in women with anorexia nervosa and bulimia nervosa. *European Eating Disorders Review, 15,* 58–69.

Stern, D. N. (1985). *The interpersonal world of the infant.* New York: Basic Books.

Stern, B. L., Caligor, E., Clarkin, J. F., Critscfield, K. L., Horz, S., MacCornack, V., et al. (2010). Structured Interview of Personality Organization (STIPO): Preliminary psychometrics in a clinical sample. *Journal of Personality Assessment, 92,* 35–44.

Stiles, W. B., Elliott, R., Llewelyn, S. P., Firth-Cozens, J. A., Marginson, F. R., Shapiro, D. A., et al. (1990). Assimilation of problematic experiences by clients in psychotherapy. *Psychotherapy, 27,* 411–420.

Verheul, R., Andrea, H., Berghout, C., Dolan, C. C., van Busschbach, J. J., van der Croft, P. J. A., et al. (2008). Severity Indices of Personality Problems (SIPP-118): Development, factor structure, reliability, and validity. *Psychological Assessment, 20,* 23–34.

Vignoles, V. L., Schwartz, S. J., & Luyckx, K. (2011). Introduction: Toward an integrative view of identity. In S. J. Schwartz, K. Luycks, & V. L. Vignoles (Eds.), *Handbook of identity theory and research* (pp. 1–30). New York: Springer Verlag.

Westen, D., Betan, E., & Defife, J. A. (2011). Identity disturbance in adolescence: Associations with borderline personality disorder. *Development and Psychopathology, 23,* 305–313.

Westen, D., & Cohen, R. P. (1993). The self in borderline personality disorder: A psychodynamic perspective. In Z. V. Segal & S. J. Blatt (Eds.), *The self in emotional distress: Cognitive and psychodynamic perspectives* (pp. 334–360). New York: Guilford Press.

Westen, D., & Heim, A. K. (2003). Disturbances of self and identity in personality disorders. In M. R. Leary & J. P. Tangney (Eds.), *Handbook of self and identity* (pp. 643–666). New York: Guilford Press.

Widiger, T. A., Frances, A., Warner, L., & Bluhm, C. (1986). Diagnostic criteria for the borderline and schizotypal personality disorders. *Journal of Abnormal Psychology, 95,* 43–51.

Wilkinson-Ryan, T., & Westen, D. (2000). Identity disturbance in borderline personality disorder: An empirical investigation. *American Journal of Psychiatry, 157,* 528–541.

Yeomans, F., Clarkin, J. F., & Kernberg, O. F. (2015). *Transference-focused psychotherapy for borderline personality disorder.* Washington, DC: American Psychiatric Publishing.

Young, J. E., Klosko, J. S., & Weishaar, M. E. (2003). *Schema therapy: A practitioner's guide.* New York: Guilford Press.

# CHAPTER 7

# Attachment, Mentalizing, and the Self

Peter Fonagy and Patrick Luyten

Mentalizing is often simplistically understood to be synonymous with the capacity for empathy toward other people. In fact, mentalizing comprises a spectrum of capacities that critically involve the ability to see one's own behavior as coherently organized by mental states, and to differentiate oneself psychologically from others. It is these capacities that tend to be noticeably absent in individuals with a personality disorder (PD), particularly at moments of interpersonal stress. In this chapter, we attempt to demonstrate that such impairments in mentalizing are at the heart of our explanatory framework for conceptualizing PDs. The foundations of our thinking lie in attachment theory, but, according to our most recent formulation, the heart of the relationship between mentalizing and personality pathology lies in the capacity to engage productively in communication, and more specifically, in the quality of *epistemic trust* the individual possesses in relationships and, formatively, in the relationship between the child and his or her primary caregivers. "Epistemic trust" is defined in terms of an individual's experience of communication from others, specifically, the ability to receive and treat new knowledge from others as personally relevant and therefore to be capable of modifying durable representational structures pertaining to self, others, and interpersonal relationships. Underpinning this capability is the consideration of the informant as a "trustworthy" source likely to communicate information that is generalizable and relevant to the self (Fonagy & Luyten, 2016).

PDs are often defined in terms of enduring interpersonal difficulties (Higgitt & Fonagy, 1992). We argue that these difficulties are generated by the rigidity of the patient's thinking about his or her subjective experience, and an inability to engage in authentic communication about the causes of his or her own or others' actions, and therefore to modify his or her behavior in response to such communications, in particular. It is this impervious and inflexible quality that has, in the past, made patients with PD so conspicuously "hard to treat." We therefore argue that the psychological mechanism behind the rigidity associated with PD is driven by the deep epistemic mistrust that has been generated in the patient—whether through environmental adversity, genetic vulnerability, or, most likely, a complex combination of these factors—which interferes with social learning and creates an overreliance on unhelpful forms of mentalizing, or outright failures in mentalizing at moments of attachment arousal.

The mentalizing approach was originally formulated in the context of treating patients with borderline personality disorder (BPD; Bateman & Fonagy, 2004), and has developed into a more comprehensive approach to the understanding and treatment of (severe) PD (Bateman & Fonagy, 2012). More recently, we have moved this thinking a little further to consider the role of epistemic attitudes and epistemic trust in relation to social learning. These recent formulations have taken us into an even broader integrative theory about normal and disrupted personality development rooted in evolutionary considerations concerning the role of social cognition and the intergenerational transmission of knowledge about the (social) world. Three related features are considered to be central to PD and the typical distortions in self-experience and relationships in patients with PD: (1) disruptions in attachment experiences, (2) associated impairments in mentalizing, and (3) epistemic mistrust and hypervigilance. In this chapter, we direct our argument in relation to attachment, mentalizing, and epistemic trust to focus on the concept of self—a concept that, historically, has been central to thinking about personality pathology, and is notably central to the thinking on PD adopted in proposals to reconceptualize the concept of PD in DSM (Skodol, 2012).

## The Mentalizing Approach to PD

### Attachment Relationships and the Development of Mentalizing

Mentalizing, like language, is a constitutional propensity, largely a developmental achievement made over the early years of life. The optimal development of mentalizing depends on the quality of attachment relationships, and early attachments in particular. The latter reflect the extent to which subjective experiences were adequately mirrored by a trusted other, that is, the extent to which attachment figures were able to respond with contingent and marked affective displays of their own experience in response to the infant's subjective experience, thus enabling the child to develop second-order representations of his or her own subjective experiences. The quality of affect mirroring by attachment figures plays a major role in the development of affect regulative processes and self-control (including attention mechanisms and effortful control), laying the groundwork for mentalizing capacity in the individual. Mentalizing is fundamentally interactive, in that it develops in the context of interactions with others and is continually influenced by others' levels of mentalizing (i.e., good mentalizing promotes good mentalizing, while poor mentalizing engenders poor mentalizing).

### The Multidimensional Nature of Mentalizing

Mentalizing is not unidimensional. It can be organized around four dimensions, each with its own relatively distinct underlying neural circuits (Fonagy & Luyten, 2009): (1) *automatic* versus *controlled* mentalizing, (2) mentalizing with regard to *self* or *others,* (3) mentalizing based on *external* or *internal* features of self and others, and (4) *cognitive* versus *affective* mentalizing. Automatic mentalizing refers to fast, parallel reflexive processes that require little consciousness or effort, whereas controlled mentalizing involves more conscious, deliberate, and serial reflective processes. The focus in mentalizing can be the self (including one's embodied experiences) or others, and can involve inferences based on external features of others (e.g., facial expressions) or direct assumptions about one's own mind or the mind of others (externally–internally-based mentalizing). Finally, full mentalizing involves the integration of both cognitive knowledge (i.e., agent–attitude–propositions) and affective input (i.e., affective–state propositions).

Normally, these dimensions are in balance and may be used flexibly, depending on the processing demands of a particular social context or setting. The persistent dominance of one end (or *pole*) of a dimension over another signals a potential failure of accurate mental-state understanding. Specific forms of psychopathology may be understood on the basis of different combinations of impairments along the mentalizing dimensions (Bateman, Bolton, & Fonagy, 2013; Fonagy, Bateman, & Bateman, 2011; Fonagy et al., 2010). Different types of psychopathology are characterized by different patterns of inappropriate domination of one or another pole of one or more mentalizing dimensions, with the imbalances generating apparent failures of mentalizing in the individual. Patients with BPD, for example, may typically give a misleading appearance of sophisticated insight or remarkable intuitive empathy based on the dominance of external, automatic, and affective mentalizing over internal, reflective, and cognitive processing of mental states. This imbalanced structure breaks down at moments of interpersonal stress or attachment arousal (Figure 7.1), when the capacity for reflective mentalizing and cognitive flexibility about the possible motivation or intentions of other people (or indeed the self) is called for (Figure 7.2).

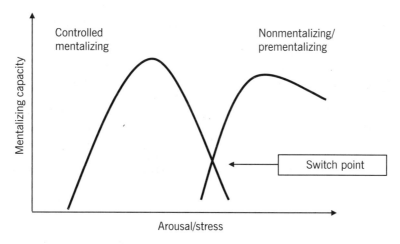

**FIGURE 7.1.** Switch from controlled mentalizing to nonmentalizing/pre-mentalizing modes under conditions of high arousal. From Fonagy and Luyten (2009, Figure 1, p. 1367), by permission of Cambridge University Press.

Understanding mentalizing as being constituted of several subprocesses organized along dimensions, rather than a single capacity, is essential in preventing the iatrogenic effects of therapy for patients with BPD that can arise if the therapist overestimates the patient's overall mentalizing capacity based on having identified conspicuous, isolated strengths.

### The Context/Relationship-Specific Nature of Mentalizing

Furthermore, the capacity to mentalize has both "trait" and "state" aspects that may vary in quality in relation to emotional arousal and interpersonal context (e.g., an individual's mentalizing levels may differ considerably when reflecting on his or her relationship with his or her mother

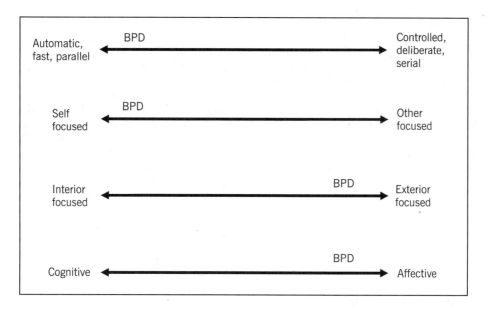

**FIGURE 7.2.** Mentalizing profile of BPD across the four polarities that underlie mentalizing. note. Adapted from Bateman and Fonagy (2016, Figure 2.1, p. 49), by permission of Oxford University Press.

compared with his or her father, or when reflecting on these relationships "offline" versus "online" in the course of a real-life interaction). Typically, with increasing arousal, the capacity for controlled mentalizing is likely to become (for the context) inappropriately dominated by automatic and often unreflective mentalizing as the balance between the two poles is lost.

## Attachment Strategies, Mentalizing, and PD

Attachment hyperactivating and deactivating strategies play a key role in explaining the relationships among stress/arousal and mentalizing in different interpersonal/arousal contexts. This explains in part some of the heterogeneity observed in patients with BPD and those with PDs more generally (Fonagy & Luyten, 2009). The relationship between attachment and imbalances in mentalizing in the context of BPD rests on the way in which attachment hyperactivating or deactivating strategies trigger overreliance on particular forms of mentalizing, obstructing the ability to call on a wider and more balanced range of mentalizing skills.

Most patients with BPD, for example, are typically characterized by an excessive use of attachment hyperactivating strategies, often in the context of disorganized attachment. At least two strands of research support the link between hyperactivating strategies and disorganized attachment and mentalizing impairments in BPD. The first strand has provided direct evidence for such a link by showing that BPD is associated with increased levels of insecure attachment styles, by using both interview-based assessment of attachment such as the Adult Attachment Interview (AAI), and self-report measures (Steele & Siever, 2010). The second strand relates to attachment trauma (Allen, 2013), which we discuss later in this chapter. These views are congruent with general biopsychosocial models of BPD (Oldham, 2009), which assume that adverse childhood experiences and genetic factors interact to create a particular combination of biological factors (neurobiological structures and dysfunctions) and psychosocial factors (personality traits and personality functioning) that underpins BPD pathology (affective and behavioral dysregulation and disturbed relatedness).

Some time ago, Fonagy and colleagues (Fonagy & Higgitt, 1990; Fonagy, Target, & Gergely, 2000) suggested that hyperactivation of the attachment system may be a core aspect of BPD. When exposed to threat and experiencing fear and distress that activates the attachment system, young children are biologically predisposed to seek proximity to their caregiver. If the caregiver is optimally sensitive and responsive to the distressed child, a down-regulation of the child's emotion and deactivation of his or her attachment system occurs, and a lasting bond is formed to the caregiver who was attentive to the child's need (Bowlby, 1969, 1973). However, in circumstances in which early relationships are disrupted, whether for reasons of biology, circumstance, or a combination of the two, the proximity seeking that is triggered by activation of the child's attachment system is anticipated to lead to further adverse emotional experience. This negative experience generates the same emotional response of fear and distress that triggers the attachment system, which then inevitably stimulates further proximity seeking by the child, in the hope of achieving down-regulation (Main, 2000). Within this model there is considerable room for individual differences to emerge; these differences are affected by genetic predisposition (Fearon, Shmueli-Goetz, Viding, Fonagy, & Plomin, 2013) and formative psychosocial experience (e.g., Fraley, Roisman, Booth-LaForce, Owen, & Holland, 2013; Repetti, Taylor, & Seeman, 2002).

There is now a rich body of empirical data to support these speculations about the relationship between attachment and BPD. For example, in a large investigation with over 1,400 participants, Scott, Levy, and Pincus (2009) compared competing multivariate models of adult attachment patterns, impulsivity, and trait negative affect as these related to borderline features. The relationship between attachment anxiety and features of BPD was most effectively modeled when considered to generate negative affectivity and impulsivity. This provided a better fit than the alternative model of impulsivity or negative affectivity generating attachment anxiety. This study suggested that impulsivity and negative affect can lead to BPD when they occur in the context of high levels of attachment anxiety. In a review, Agrawal, Gunderson, Holmes, and Lyons-Ruth (2004) considered 13 empirical studies of the adult attachment styles of individuals with BPD; all the studies showed an association between BPD and insecure attachment. These findings were subsequently confirmed in comparisons with groups of people with other PDs (Aaronson, Bender, Skodol, & Gunderson, 2006; Barone, Fossati, & Guiducci, 2011; Fossati et al., 2005;

Meyer, Ajchenbrenner, & Bowles, 2005; Scott et al., 2013).

A further cross-sectional study reported by Choi-Kain, Fitzmaurice, Zanarini, Laverdiere, and Gunderson (2009) differentiated patients with mood disorder from patients with BPD on the basis of attachment style. While both depressed patients and patients with BPD showed greater preoccupation and fearfulness than did control individuals (although patients with BPD were more severely affected for both traits), only patients with BPD simultaneously showed preoccupation *and* fearfulness. This study confirmed, as a number of attachment theorists have suggested, that the key marker of BPD is a lack of a functional regulation strategy to reduce attachment distress (Fonagy & Bateman, 2008; Main, 2000).

## Childhood Adversity, Mentalizing, and PD

In drawing up a mentalizing, developmental model of PD in relation to childhood adversity, we suggest that two processes unfold, which have a cumulative effect.

1. We assume that the development of mentalizing depends on the social co-construction of internal states between the child and his or her parents. Following from this, we hypothesize that early neglect and an early emotional environment that is incompatible with the normal acquisition of understanding self and others creates vulnerability to PD.
2. Furthermore, we hypothesize that subsequent neglect and abuse in an attachment context can disrupt mentalizing as part of an adaptive adjustment to adversity when a child whose early experiences of neglect have left him or her less resilient to deal with trauma is in a state of helplessness in relation to the responsible individuals (Fonagy, Steele, Steele, Higgitt, & Target, 1994; Stein, Fonagy, Ferguson, & Wisman, 2000).

In summary, we (Fonagy & Luyten, 2009) propose that early emotional neglect, more so than physical or sexual abuse, predisposes individuals to developing PD, and specifically BPD, by limiting their opportunity to acquire the full spectrum of mentalizing skills, leaving their capacity to mentalize vulnerable to being disrupted under the influence of later stress.

We further contend that childhood environments that are emotionally abusive, or in which discussion and validation of mental states do not occur, lead to the generation of coping strategies that favor rapid, intuitive (as opposed to more deliberate and reflective), emotion-focused (as opposed to cognition-focused) mentalizing—particularly in individuals who have been primed by experiences of early neglect to identify risk rapidly. This intuitive state is dominated by mental-state attributions based on external observable cues (as opposed to the inference of internal states, which may be unreliable in a maltreating environment). In addition, such individuals may need to develop a strategy of being highly sensitive to and readily influenced by (mirroring) mental states in others (at the cost of achieving a clear differentiation of "self" and "other" mental states) (Fonagy, 2000; Fonagy & Luyten, 2009; Luyten, Fonagy, Lowyck, & Vermote, 2012).

We wish to emphasize that while this approach may appear to suggest a deficit theory, our emphasis is on adaptation. For instance, the specific configuration of mentalizing capacities that characterizes individuals with BPD may be conceived of as that most likely to favor survival under conditions of significant adversity (Frankenhuis, Panchanathan, & Clark Barrett, 2013). Our model is fully compatible with Linehan's (1993) original biosocial theory of the development of BPD and its later elaboration (Crowell, Beauchaine, & Linehan, 2009), which emphasizes that an invalidating childhood environment can serve to undermine the understanding, regulation, and toleration of affect states, leading the child to adapt by displaying more extreme emotions to achieve a contingent response from caregivers, that is, the intermittent reinforcement of extreme emotional outbursts.

In line with these assumptions, many studies support the suggestion that secure children perform better than insecure children at mentalizing tasks (see, e.g., de Rosnay & Harris, 2002). In the first of these studies, from the London Parent–Child Project, Fonagy, Steele, Steele, and Holder (1997) reported that 82% of children who were securely attached to their mothers in the Strange Situation passed Harris's Belief–Desire Reasoning Task at age 5.5 years, compared with 50% of those who showed an avoidant attachment style and 33% of the few children with preoccupied attachment. As we describe in more detail later, findings along these lines are not always consistent (see, e.g.,

Meins et al., 2002), but in general, it appears that secure attachment and mentalizing are affected by similar social influences.

It is necessary to identify what it is about emotional abuse and neglect that can render the child increasingly vulnerable to disrupted mentalizing. We (Fonagy & Luyten, 2009) have stressed the importance of secure attachment in providing a context within which the child can develop the ability to mentalize and regulate his or her own emotions. Clearly, in an environment that is invalidating and emotionally abusive, an insecure and disorganized attachment pattern is likely to develop (Fonagy, 2000; Fonagy & Luyten, 2009). We contend that it is the absence of a "safe base", from which the child can learn the capacity to mentalize and self-regulate, that can create a greater vulnerability for developing PD (and BPD in particular) in later life.

For instance, emotional dysregulation (Gratz, Tull, Baruch, Bornovalova, & Lejuez, 2008), schema modes (particularly disconnection/rejection and impaired limits; Specht, Chapman, & Cellucci, 2009), and distorted self-representation in middle childhood (Carlson, Egeland, & Sroufe, 2009) have all been shown to mediate the relationship between childhood abuse and BPD. However, these studies used a composite score of maltreatment rather than focusing on particular aspects of emotional abuse and/or neglect. Rogosch and Cicchetti (2005) found that attentional networks and processes did not mediate the precursors to BPD in children who had been abused. The formation of schemas and the representation of the self, which are often conspicuously impoverished in individuals with BPD, are themselves mediated by the selective disruption of social cognition (Carlson et al., 2009). These studies point to the importance of these key psychological processes in mediating the impact of childhood experience of trauma on the development of BPD symptoms in later life. More work is needed in this area, but the research to date suggests that the psychological processes that make the impact of trauma on personality development so harmful and enduring relate to the emergence of the concept of self and identity.

Patients with BPD have also been found to exhibit high levels of alexithymia (i.e., impairments in mentalizing with regard to the self) and to have difficulty in describing their emotions in social situations (New et al., 2012)—features that have both been related to trauma. In samples containing a majority of patients reporting early trauma, patients showed amygdala hyperreactivity in response to viewing emotional or neutral images, combined with blunted subjective appraisals of these same stimuli (Hazlett et al., 2012; Minzenberg, Fan, New, Tang, & Siever, 2007). Considered in relation to attachment, the mentalizing deficits associated with childhood maltreatment may be a form of decoupling, inhibition, or even a phobic reaction to mentalizing: (1) The experience of adversity may undermine cognitive development in general (Cicchetti, Rogosch, & Toth, 2000; Crandell & Hobson, 1999; Stacks, Beeghly, Partridge, & Dexter, 2011); (2) the mentalizing problems may reflect arousal problems associated with exposure to chronic stress (see Cicchetti & Walker, 2001); and (3) the child may avoid mentalizing to avoid perceiving the abuser's hostile and malevolent thoughts and feelings about him or her (e.g., Fonagy, 1991; Goodman, Quas, & Ogle, 2010). These potential problems all have a significant negative impact on a child's psychological, emotional, social, and educational development.

Maltreatment can contribute to an acquired partial "mind-blindness" by compromising open, reflective communication between parent and child. It may undermine the benefit derived from learning about the links between internal states and actions in attachment relationships (e.g., the child may be told that he or she "deserves," "wants," or even "enjoys" the abuse to which he or she is being subjected). This is more likely to be harmful if the maltreatment is being perpetrated by a family member. In cases where the maltreatment is taking place outside the home, the parents' lack of awareness of it may serve to invalidate the child's communications with the parents about his or her feelings. In such a situation, the child finds that reflective discourse does not correspond to his or her feelings—a consistent misunderstanding that could reduce the child's ability to understand and mentalize verbal explanations of other people's actions. In such circumstances, the child is likely to struggle to detect the mental states behind people's actions and tends to see these actions as inevitable rather than intended.

Taken together, these views clearly imply that the foundations of subjective selfhood will be less robustly established in individuals who have experienced early neglect. These individuals find it more difficult to learn about how subjective experiences inevitably vary between people and about the need for flexibility in relation to the relative merits of one's own and alternative perspectives. As we have described, in some longitudinal investigations, low parental affection or nurturing in early childhood appears to be more strongly associated with elevated risk for antisocial, paranoid, and schizotypal PDs and BPD than physical or sexual abuse in adolescence (Afifi et al., 2011; Gao, Raine, Chan, Venables, & Mednick, 2010; Hengartner, Ajdacic-Gross, Rodgers, Müller, & Rossler, 2013; Johnson, Cohen, Kasen, Ehrensaft, & Crawford, 2006; Powers, Thomas, Ressler, & Bradley, 2011; Tyrka, Wyche, Kelly, Price, & Carpenter, 2009; Widom, Czaja, & Paris, 2009), again pointing to the importance of neglect, low parental involvement, and emotional maltreatment in undermining the normally biologically predetermined learning and communication processes involved in the healthy development of perspective taking.

### The Reemergence of Nonmentalizing Modes

Modes of experiencing the self and others that are characteristic of the prementalizing child tend to reemerge whenever we lose the ability to mentalize, as typically happens in individuals with PD, particularly in high arousal contexts (Fonagy & Target, 1997). According to our conceptualization of mentalizing as consisting of four dimensions, we understand the emergence of these nonmentalizing modes as indications of imbalances in mentalizing, in which one extreme form of mentalizing has come to dominate. We have described these nonmentalizing modes as falling into three distinct categories (Fonagy, Gergely, Jurist, & Target, 2002) as a way of understanding the subjective mentalizing experience of the individual and providing a formulation that is useful for clinicians, particularly when they are responding to highly affect-driven, nonmentalizing behavior on the part of the patient.

1. In the *psychic equivalence mode,* thoughts and feelings become overwhelmingly real, allowing for no alternative perspectives or doubt. This mode reflects the domination of self–affect state thinking with limited internal focus.
2. In the *teleological mode,* there is only a recognition of real, observable goal-directed behavior and objectively discernible events that may potentially constrain these goals. Hence, there is a recognition of the existence and potential role of mental states, but limited to very concrete and observable goals. This mode reflects an extreme exterior focus and the momentary loss of controlled mentalizing.
3. In the *pretend mode,* thoughts and feelings become severed from reality ("hypermentalizing" or "pseudomentalizing"), which, in the extreme, may lead to feelings of derealization and dissociation. This reflects the domination of controlled mentalizing by an implicit but inadequately internal focus, combined with poor belief–desire reasoning and a consequent sense of vulnerability to fusion with others.

Understanding and recognizing the prementalizing modes is important because they often appear alongside a pressure to externalize unmentalized and self-hating aspects of the self (so-called "alien-self" parts). Torturing feelings of badness, possibly linked to experiences of abuse that are felt to be part of the self but are not integrated with it (the "alien-self" parts), can come to dominate self-experience. We assume that these discontinuities in internal experience (when one feels aspects of one's self-experience to be of oneself or one's own, yet also to be alien) generate a sense of incongruence, which is dealt with through externalizing. For example, the individual may attempt to dominate the mind-states of others by behaving toward others as though others own the unmentalized self-experiences, and on occasion may even be successful in generating these experiences in them (Fonagy & Target, 2000). This brings about relief, even if the immediate impact of externalizing a torturing part of the self in this way is to manipulate the other person into punitive persecutory behavior toward the self. Attempts to adapt to these torturing internal experiences may also manifest as attacks on the self (e.g., self-harming behaviors) or other types of behavior that in the teleological mode are expected to relieve tension and arousal (Fonagy & Target, 2000).

### Mentalizing and the Self

How do these considerations help us to understand the subjective experience of patients with PD, and in particular the feelings of identity diffusion that are typical of many of these patients? We approach this question from a developmental psychopathology perspective in line with the more general mentalizing approach. Most modern psychological approaches assume that "self-coherence" (the sense that one has continuity and consistency in thought and behavior) is something of an illusion (Bargh, 2011, 2014). Thought of in this way, there can be no such thing as self-coherence, identity, or self; these are constructs referring to a self-generated feeling or a subjective state of coherence. This is not to deny the importance of self-coherence. On the contrary, we submit that a feeling or state of self-coherence is at the heart of mental health and is associated with feelings of agency and autonomy.

How then can we understand individuals with PD from this perspective? Identity diffusion, that is, a lack of self-coherence, has notably been central to many theoretical formulations of serious PD. A *disturbed sense of identity*, or "failure to establish stable and integrated representations of self and others" (Livesley, 2003, p. 19), is frequently described as characteristic of BPD (e.g., Blatt & Auerbach, 1988; Bradley & Westen, 2005; Jørgensen, 2010; Kernberg, 1975, 1984) and was a core part of the reformulation of PD proposed for DSM-5, which was criticized by many (Shedler et al., 2010, 2011), and found its way into Section III of DSM-5 (American Psychiatric Association, 2013). Rooted in a dysfunction or deficit in a sense of agency or self-directedness, this characteristic has also been identified in empirical clinical studies (e.g., Adler, Chin, Kolisetty, & Oltmanns, 2012; Barnow, Ruge, Spitzer, & Freyberger, 2005; Bender & Skodol, 2007; Jørgensen et al., 2012).

We argue that it is the capacity for mentalizing that enables us to create and maintain this consistent sense of the self across different contexts. Mental-state language and the experience of being "mind-minded" (Meins et al., 2002) construct the narrative around one's thoughts and feelings, which in turn helps us continuously to construct a benign and coherent self-structure. When mentalizing impairments weaken this integrative process, an experience of incoherence in self-representation is likely to emerge. Rather than seeing personality impairments as classically defined—as impairments in the self or rigidity in representations—we thus postulate that PD in fact involves failures of this building process and generates a sense of epistemic rigidity, which inhibits the dynamic and ongoing construction of the self. Rigidity is often invoked in discussions of the phenomenology of PD (Beck, Freeman, & Davis, 2004; Caligor, Kernberg, & Clarkin, 2007; McWilliams, 2011; Mikulincer & Shaver, 2016; Rogers & Dymond, 1954). "Rigidity," as we use the term here, describes a state of being closed to social learning, which requires being comfortable in taking knowledge from others as relevant to oneself—what we might refer to as a sense of *epistemic trust*. As we explain in more detail in the next section, we see rigidity as indicating the absence of a willingness to fully engage in social learning, and PD as reflecting impairments in mentalizing that are associated with an exaggeration of *epistemic vigilance* (being on the lookout for the possibility of being misled): It signifies epistemic mistrust of the interpersonal world. If we conceptualize our sense of self as a consequence of a process of mentalizing rather than as a fixed representation, then exaggerated vigilance or *epistemic hypervigilance* will inhibit the internalization of social knowledge and the reflection on this knowledge that is necessary for the healthy maintenance of the social learning process.

This more dynamic approach to the ongoing relationship among mentalizing, the social environment, and the construction of the self is at odds with the traditional tendency to reify the notion of representation or internal working models of self and other. This inclination is best exemplified by theoretical writings and empirical studies on the (hierarchical) organization of object or attachment representations, descriptions of splitting of object representations, and even studies on the activation of object representations commonly present in traditional psychodynamic formulations (Fonagy & Target, 2003).

These can be clinically useful descriptions, but they are no longer in line with what we now know about representational processes: Representations do not exist; therefore, they cannot be split or integrated, and they cannot be hierarchically or even nonhierarchically organized (see Fonagy, 1982, for an early exposition of this point of view). A more parsimonious way of describing these processes, which is also in line with our growing knowledge of representational processes in the brain (Fonagy & Luyten, 2009; Luyten & Blatt, 2013), is to conceptualize them in terms of *states of mind* that, for instance, are created by the capacity for mentalizing, which itself is subserved by different neural circuits (Luyten et al., 2012). It would therefore be more accurate to say that we generate a representation of ourselves and others, rather than to say we "have" representations that are stored somewhere and are hierarchically organized and can be activated, changed, or structurally modified. What is assumed to be a trait-like quality of representations (e.g., self-representation) is better described as stability in the capacity for generating such representations, or even better as states of mind that bring some stability in our experience of self.

Furthermore, in the context of this notional representation that is stable, differentiated, and integrated, there is little space for the reality that we all sometimes feel inferior, fragmented, or isolated. Traditionally, such states are understood as reflecting the activation of split-off or repressed representations, perhaps because of defensive processes, or as regression. But, again, do we really believe that we have stored somewhere various representations of ourselves and others that can be (re)activated? We can explain these same phenomena much more parsimoniously by arguing that in particular circumstances (i.e., when arousal/conflict is high), we are unable to create a feeling of stability, agency, and positive self-regard; we do not need to assume more.

This has important clinical and research implications. It means that patients do not "change" their self- (and object) representations as a result of treatment or experiences (and therefore we should not try to assess these changes in their representations); rather, they have acquired the capacity to think and feel differently about themselves and others, and therefore to think, reflect, and narrate differently about themselves and others. Hence, the primary focus in treatment (and in outcome studies) should be on these capacities and not on changes in object representations per se, which are a secondary consequence ("the fruit on the tree," so to speak) of a growing capacity for social cognition.

Indeed, when one considers the human ability to reflect on self-experience in relation to others, it naturally follows that this capacity shows features of both stability and change over time, as it is likely to be influenced by context (and particularly attachment contexts) (Luyten et al., 2012). Similarly, demanding that the self, identity, or personality should be highly stable across the lifespan makes little sense from this perspective, as people do not *have* a self, identity, or personality; rather, they have the ability, to a greater or lesser extent, to activate a more or less consistent, coherent, and differentiated *feeling* or *experience* of coherence and stability. It is this reflective function that creates a feeling of coherence in the moment, rather than it being the case that there *is* a feeling of coherence. This is also congruent with findings from neuroscience suggesting that a cortical midline system is responsible for generating the experience of self as distinct from others (Fonagy & Luyten, 2016; Luyten & Blatt, 2013; Northoff, Qin, & Feinberg, 2011).

This idea of the self as a work in progress also allows us to take into account a way of accommodating the role of the social environment in the sense of self. A long-standing critique of psychoanalytic thinking and psychology more broadly is that both fail to take into account the effects of how the socioeconomic environment might buffet the individual psyche (Fonagy, Target, & Gergely, 2006). Given the evidence accruing that increasing levels of social inequality are connected with an increased prevalence of BPD (Fonagy & Luyten, 2016), an approach to PD that understands the mechanism between personality pathology and the social context of the self is even more pertinent (Grant et al., 2008; Wilkinson & Pickett, 2009). An explanation of psychopathology relating to the self that allows for the impact of the environment in an evolutionarily convincing manner is made possible by this dynamic interpretation of our self-representations. If we consider that the evolutionary drive behind mentalizing was to enable human survival in increasingly complex social situations involving matters of hierarchy, cooperation, exclusion, and inclusion, it makes eminent sense that representations of ourselves and those around us should calibrate the extent to which we may be experiencing social isolation, alienation, or inferiority.

Psychological resilience enables an individual to resist these pressures to some degree. By contrast, individuals with PD are often conspicuously reactive to such pressures, while to be wholly impervious to their effects suggests mentalizing impairments of a different nature altogether. Both extremes, however, derive from a lack of capacity to absorb information from the social environment in a way that is compatible with the construction of a normatively coherent sense of self. This ability, or inability, to take in social data, and to be able to reflect on it with some coherence and pragmatism, is key to understanding PD, with its phenomenology of enduring interpersonal difficulties and troubled sense of self. It is the second-order developmental constructs of flexibility and rigidity that determine how individuals respond to the aspects of their environment or themselves that constitute what we might call personality—whether we term these cognitive schemas, internal object relationships, interpersonal expectations, or intersubjective concerns. Rigidity points to an individual's inability to progress fluidly, flexibly, and adaptively across the phases of individual development; it is a metaconstruct associated with personality functioning. According to this thinking, the concept of rigidity encapsulates an understanding of PD as the failure of appropriate responsiveness to information within a system at the interface of the person and his or her social environment.

The three prementalizing modes, discussed earlier, are significant here; they constitute forms of mentalizing that make the individual appear difficult or even impossible to reach, rendering him or her potentially impervious to meaningful social influence. Rigidity, or the inability to adjust to other, more reflective forms of mentalizing, breaks down the individual's ability to form a stable self-structure, creating the fragmented sense of self often experientially associated with BPD. Rigidity is perhaps greatest in individuals who show both the high level of avoidance and intense attachment anxiety that is so typical of patients with BPD (e.g., Choi-Kain et al., 2009): An irresolvable dilemma is created by an intense desire for reassurance from an attachment figure if the individual is also unable to fully accept this reassurance owing to a mistrust of the attachment figure's motives. Thus, while security is buttressed by flexibility, which derives from refusing to consider closeness and autonomy as antagonistic and irreconcilable goals, insecurity and partial rigidity arise when an individual is unable to relocate on the closeness–distance dimension without fearing either a permanent loss of autonomy or the loss of affection of his or her attachment figure. The key here is the invalidation of interpersonal information that arises from any encounter, regardless of the nature of the information. Even a positive response from the attachment figure will, in the context of epistemic mistrust, be discounted by assumptions about the person's motives. But dismissal or closing of the flow of information is also unsustainable because of the overriding need for reassurance. Let us now scrutinize further this concept of trust as it applies to socially transmitted information.

## Mentalizing and Epistemic Trust

Studies of attachment have confirmed that secure attachment is driven by sensitive responsivity of the caregiver, contingent upon the infant's reaction (Belsky & Fearon, 2008; Marvin & Britner, 2008). In addition, we have maintained that attachment experiences also provide the context in which the caregiver's mentalizing can influence the security of attachment and mentalizing in the child (Arnott & Meins, 2007; Fonagy, Steele, Steele, Moran, & Higgitt, 1991; Grienenberger, Kelly, & Slade, 2005; Meins, Fernyhough, Fradley, & Tuckey, 2001; Meins et al., 2002; Slade, Grienenberger, Bernbach, Levy, & Locker, 2005). Recently, we have added a third consideration: Secure attachment is created by a system that simultaneously generates a sense of epistemic trust.

Looked at from a distance, microanalytic (e.g., Beebe et al., 2010) and more global (e.g., DeWolf & van IJzendoorn, 1997; Isabella, Belsky, & von Eye, 1989; Kiser, Bates, Maslin, & Bayles, 1986; Mills-Koonce et al., 2007) ratings of sensitive caregiving may in essence be seen as recognizing the child's agentive self. We believe that through the down-regulation of affect that results from successful proximity seeking in the distressed infant, attachment not only establishes a lasting bond but also opens a channel for information that can be used for the transfer of knowledge between the generations. Given that the infant needs to overcome the self-preservative barrier created by natural epistemic vigilance (Sperber et al., 2010; Wilson & Sperber, 2012) and open his or her mind to acquiring the myriad pieces of culturally relevant information on which his or her survival will ultimately depend, it is fortunate that nature (evolution) has provided us with a mechanism of deferential knowledge transmission that can create an "epistemic superhighway" between learners and teachers, who normally share genetic material (Hamilton, 1964). It is this openness to information transfer that we believe offers the cognitive advantage to secure attachment that has been fairly consistently noted, although not, to our knowledge, systematically studied (e.g., Crandell & Hobson, 1999; Jacobsen & Hofmann, 1997; Moss, Rousseau, Parent, St.-Laurent, & Saintong, 1998). Although still somewhat speculative, evidence for these assumptions comes from two strands of research that are increasingly becoming intertwined: (1) developmental studies and (2) evolutionary approaches concerning the development of social cognition (for a detailed discussion, see Fonagy & Allison, 2014; Fonagy & Luyten, 2016; Fonagy, Luyten, & Allison, 2015).

As we suggested elsewhere (Fonagy et al., 2015), building on pioneering work by Dan Sperber (Sperber et al., 2010; Wilson & Sperber, 2012) and accumulating developmental evidence (e.g., Corriveau et al., 2009), secure attachment experiences pave the way for the acquisition of mentalizing and at the same time foster epistemic trust. In other words, natural selection may have hit upon attachment as a means to mediate the reliable transmission of "memes" from one generation to the next. Secure attachment helps to create a benign condition for the relaxation of epistemic vigilance, and sensitive and appropriate ostensive cueing is a key constituent element of sensitivity on the part of the primary caregiver. Attachment is a much older instinct, in evolutionary terms, than the imperative to generate epistemic trust for the safe transmission of "memes"; in that sense, the two processes are distinct. In terms of the phenomenology of child development, however, they are closely interwoven, and it seems likely that in human evolution, epistemic trust piggybacked onto preexisting attachment processes.

However, we suggest that while attachment may be a key mechanism for mediating epistemic trust, it is secondary to an underlying biological process preserved by evolution. In other words, secure attachment is unlikely to be *necessary* for generating epistemic trust, but it may be *sufficient* to do so; furthermore, it is the most *pervasive* mechanism in early childhood because it is a highly evolutionarily effective indicator of trustworthiness.

## Implications for the Treatment of PD

### The Mentalization-Based Treatment Approach

Mentalization-based treatment (MBT) is firmly grounded in the theoretical model we outlined in the early sections of this chapter. The approach regards imbalances in mentalizing as the core of the enduring difficulties of BPD and other types of personality pathology; therefore, the aim of treatment is the restoration of more balanced mentalizing (Bateman & Fonagy, 2010). MBT was initially devised for the treatment of patients with BPD in a partial hospital setting. More recently, it has developed into a more comprehensive approach to the understanding and treatment of PDs in a range of clinical contexts, including patients with antisocial PD (ASPD; Bateman & Fonagy, 2008, 2016), patients with BPD and marked comorbid eating disorders (Robinson et al., 2014), and patients with less marked personality pathology (Allen, Fonagy, & Bateman, 2008).

The theoretical model implies that in order to maximize the effect on the patient's ability to think about thoughts and feelings in the context of relationships, especially in the early phases of treatment, the therapist is probably most helpful when his or her interventions (1) are simple and easy to understand, (2) are affect focused, (3) actively engage the patient, (4) focus on the patient's mind rather than on his or her behavior, (5) relate to a current event or activity—that is, whatever is the patient's currently felt mental reality (in working memory), (6) make use of the therapist's mind as a model (by disclosing his or her expected reaction in response to the event being discussed, by explaining to the patient how he or she anticipates reacting in that situation), and (7) are flexibly adjusted in terms of their complexity and emotional intensity in response to the patient's level of emotional arousal (i.e., withdrawing when arousal and attachment are strongly activated).

The key task of therapy is therefore to promote curiosity about the way mental states motivate and explain the actions of the self and others. MBT therapists achieve this through the judicious use of an *inquisitive stance,* highlighting their own interest in the mental states underpinning behavior, qualifying their own understanding and inferences (in that mental states are opaque), and showing how such information can help the patient make sense of his or her own experiences. Pseudomentalizing and other fillers that replace genuine mentalizing (as described earlier in this chapter) should be explicitly identified by the therapist and the lack of practical success associated with them clearly explained. In this way, therapists can help their patients to learn about how they think and feel about themselves and others, how those thoughts and feelings shape their responses to others, and how "errors" in understanding self and others may lead them to inappropriate actions. Conversely, it is not useful for the therapist to tell patients how they feel, what they think, how they should behave, or what the underlying (conscious or unconscious) reasons for their difficulties may be. In fact, any approach that tends toward claiming to "know" how or why patients "are" the way they are, or to dictate how they should behave and think, is likely to be iatrogenic in individuals whose capacity to mentalize is vulnerable.

While the MBT model has a reasonable evidence base (Bateman & Fonagy, 2009, 2013), it makes the strong and so far almost unwarranted assumption that the increasing capacity to mentalize drives improvement in BPD symptoms such as self-harming behavior or suicidality. Furthermore, focusing on the concept of epistemic trust enables us to reconceptualize the importance of mentalizing as a key part of therapeutic effectiveness.

### Reconceptualization of Treatment: Three Systems

Our thinking in relation to the role of rigidity and epistemic mistrust in PD has led us to reconceptualize treatment and the purported mechanisms of change in the treatment of these patients. We believe there is a case to be made for understanding the underlying processes at work for all therapeutic interventions that have been found to be effective in PDs. In the case of BPD, for instance, a considerable number of different therapies have now been found to be effective (for a review, see Leichsenring, Leibing, Kruse, New, & Leweke, 2011) Such forms of treatment all benefit from a well-articulated theoretical framework and a reliable model for delivery of treatment. However, other than this, it is not possible to isolate a factor common to all these therapies that can explain their effectiveness, and that can be pinpointed as missing from less effective interventions. A single model that accounts for how the effective therapies work while accommodating their theoretical specificities is one that accounts for the process that underpins them. In light of our argument about epistemic trust, outlined earlier, we posit that in fact three different processes are necessarily undergone across successful treatments.

### Communication System 1: The Teaching and Learning of Content and the Increase in Epistemic Openness

All evidence-based psychotherapies provide a coherent, consistent, and continuous framework that enables the patient to examine the issues that are deemed to be central to him or her according to a particular theoretical approach (e.g., early schemas, invalidating experiences, object relations, current attachment experiences) in a safe and low-arousal context. These psychotherapies therefore provide the patient with helpful skills or knowledge, such as strategies to handle emotional dysregulation or restructured interpersonal relationship schemas. Perhaps more importantly however, all *evidence-based* psychotherapies implicitly provide for the patient a model of mind and an understanding of his or her disorder, as well as a hypothetical appreciation of the process of change, *that are accurate enough to enable the patient to feel recognized as agentive,* empowered to make decisions and alter the course of his or her path through life. The conceptual model of each treatment contains considerable personally relevant information, so that the patient experiences feeling markedly mirrored or "understood." Helpful, directive approaches may be more likely than a generic exploratory style to communicate a clear recognition of the patient's position (McAleavey & Castonguay, 2014). The idea that psychotherapies have in common the creation of a sense of being understood while differing in the understandings they provide has been part of integrative approaches to psychotherapy since common factor approaches were first proposed (e.g., Frank & Frank, 1991; Prochaska & Norcross, 2013; Rogers, 1951). We know that without a coherent body of knowledge based on a systematically established set of principles, psychological therapy is of little value (Benish, Imel, & Wampold, 2008). Even in large cohort study meta-analyses, therapies without a credible and tight intellectual frame are observed to fail (Abbass, Rabung, Leichsenring, Refseth, & Midgley, 2013).

The fact that so many different therapies, using so many different theoretical models, have been found to be of some benefit indicates that the significance of Communication System 1 lies perhaps not only in the essential truth of the "wisdom" of the specific approach but also in that it causes the patient to give weight to communication from the social world (Ahn & Wampold, 2001; Paris, 2013). This brings us to the second communication system at work in psychotherapy.

### Communication System 2: The Reemergence of Robust Mentalizing

As noted earlier, through passing on knowledge and skills that feel appropriate and helpful to the patient, the therapist implicitly recognizes the patient's agency. The therapist's presentation of information that is relevant to the patient serves as a form of ostensive cue that conveys the impression that the therapist seeks to understand the patient's perspective; this in turn enables the patient to listen and to hear. In effect, the therapist is modeling how he or she engages in mentalizing in relation to the patient. It is important that, in this process, both patient and therapist come to see each other more clearly as intentional agents. It is not sufficient for the therapist to present his or her "mentalizing wisdom" to the patient if the therapist is not clearly seen as an agentive actor whose actions are predictable given the principles of theoretical rationality (Kiraly, Csibra, & Gergely, 2013). The context of an open and trustworthy social situation helps to achieve a better understanding of the beliefs, wishes, and desires underpinning the actions of others and of the self. This in turn allows for a more trusting relationship in the consulting room. Ideally, the patient's feeling of being responded to sensitively by the therapist opens a second virtuous cycle in interpersonal communication *in which the patient's own capacity to mentalize is regenerated.*

However, the mentalizing of patients—that is, acting in accordance with the patient's perspective—may be a common factor across psychotherapies not because patients need to learn about the contents of their minds or those of others, but because mentalizing may be a generic way of increasing epistemic trust and therefore achieving change in mental *function*.

We would like to underline a point that initially may seem puzzling given our own declared commitment to mentalization-based psychotherapy: *Mentalizing in itself is only an intermediate step and is not the ultimate therapeutic objective.* True and lasting improvement, we believe, rests on a third communication system: learning from experience beyond therapy.

## Communication System 3: The Reemergence of Social Learning with Improved Mentalizing and Epistemic Trust

We hypothesize that feeling understood, just as in normal psychological development, opens a key biological route to information transmission and the possibility of taking in knowledge that is felt to be personally relevant and generalizable; this is what brings about change in previously rigidly held beliefs. In essence, the experience of feeling thought about enables us to learn new things about our social world.

We hypothesize that as the patient's state of epistemic hypervigilance relaxes, he or she develops a greater capacity to trust and begins to discover new ways of learning about others. This facilitates an increase in the patient's willingness to modify his or her cognitive structures for interpreting the behavior of others. Positive social experiences that in the past were discounted as a result of the patient's epistemic hypervigilance now have the potential to have a positive impact. This is the third system of communication, which becomes available once the second system, which is specific to the therapeutic situation, has enhanced the patient's capacity to mentalize. As the patient begins to experience social interactions in a more benign way and to view his or her social situations more accurately (e.g., not seeing an experience of temporary social disappointment as a complete rejection), he or she can update his or her knowledge of both self and others.

It is the recovery of the capacity for social information exchange that, we feel, may be at the heart of all effective psychotherapies. These therapies impart an ability to benefit from benign social interactions, and to update and build on knowledge about the self and others in social situations. The improved sense of epistemic trust derived from mentalizing enables one to learn from social experience; in this way, the third virtuous cycle is maintained beyond therapy.

As therapists we often assume that the process in the consulting room is the primary driver of change, but experience has shown us that change is also brought about by what happens beyond therapy, in the patient's social environment. Empirical evidence from studies employing session-by-session monitoring of change suggests that the therapeutic alliance in one session foretells change in the next (Falkenstrom, Granstrom, & Holmqvist, 2013; Tasca & Lampard, 2012). This suggests that the change that occurs is a consequence of changed attitudes to learning, engendered by therapy, modifying behavior *between* sessions. The implication is that the extent to which a patient derives benefit from therapy also depends on what he or she encounters in his or her particular social world during and after treatment—that is, the changes in person–environment exchanges that result from the patient's increased openness to the evolutionarily determined and rehabilitated capacity for social learning. We predict that psychotherapy for PD is therefore much more likely to be beneficial if the individual's social environment at the time of treatment is largely benign, or becomes more benign. Although we do not know of any systematic studies that have explored this moderator, clinical experience suggests that there is likely to be some validity to this assertion.

## Summary and Conclusions

Patients with PDs are often notoriously difficult to treat. The often paradoxical combination of marked rigidity and the fluidity of their self-experiences and relationships may confuse clinicians and give them the feeling that they have no grip on what is happening in these patients and in their therapeutic relationships. Patients with PDs often have considerable difficulty in developing a working alliance because they distrust what the clinician is offering them; this may even lead to a simple refusal to be treated. Even when these patients accept treatment, they almost invariably face the therapist's suggestions and interpretations with distrust; this situation frequently persists for a very long time, and change typically happens only slowly as they become more trusting of their treating clinician.

This chapter reflects our evolving attempt to understand these phenomena from a mentalizing perspective. Our previous views focused primarily on disruptions in attachment relationships and associated mentalizing impairments in explaining the typical features of patients with (severe) PD. Specifically, we have consistently argued that early attachment disruptions, likely often in combination with biological vulnerability, give rise to often severe mentalizing impairments that lead to serious discontinuity in the self and associated relational problems. This inconsistency in self-experience, which we conceptualize as resulting from an incapacity to generate a more coherent sense of self because of impairments in mentalizing capacity, leads to a constant pressure to externalize "alien self" parts, which may be expressed in a tendency to dominate the mental states of others and/or (particularly in BPD, but also, for instance, in paranoid PD and ASPD) self-harm. More recently, we have drawn attention to a third, closely related factor, the *epistemic mistrust* or *epistemic hypervigilance* that results from attachment disruptions. This inhibits openness to social knowledge and the reflection on this knowledge that is necessary for the healthy maintenance of the evolutionarily rooted social learning process that is typical of human beings.

These formulations are likely to have important implications for the treatment of patients with PDs, and particularly in relation to the discussion of the role of so-called "specific" versus "common" factors in the treatment of these patients, and our continuous efforts to develop interventions for these "hard to reach" patients.

## REFERENCES

Aaronson, C. J., Bender, D. S., Skodol, A. E., & Gunderson, J. G. (2006). Comparison of attachment styles in borderline personality disorder and obsessive–compulsive personality disorder. *Psychiatric Quarterly, 77,* 69–80.

Abbass, A. A., Rabung, S., Leichsenring, F., Refseth, J. S., & Midgley, N. (2013). Psychodynamic psychotherapy for children and adolescents: A meta-analysis of short-term psychodynamic models. *Journal of the American Academy of Child and Adolescent Psychiatry, 52,* 863–875.

Adler, J. M., Chin, E. D., Kolisetty, A. P., & Oltmanns, T. F. (2012). The distinguishing characteristics of narrative identity in adults with features of borderline personality disorder: An empirical investigation. *Journal of Personality Disorders, 26,* 498–512.

Afifi, T. O., Mather, A., Boman, J., Fleisher, W., Enns, M. W., Macmillan, H., et al. (2011). Childhood adversity and personality disorders: Results from a nationally representative population-based study. *Journal of Psychiatric Research, 45,* 814–822.

Agrawal, H. R., Gunderson, J., Holmes, B. M., & Lyons-Ruth, K. (2004). Attachment studies with borderline patients: A review. *Harvard Review of Psychiatry, 12,* 94–104.

Ahn, H., & Wampold, B. E. (2001). Where oh where are the specific ingredients?: A meta-analysis of component studies in counseling and psychotherapy. *Journal of Counseling Psychology, 48,* 251–257.

Allen, J. G. (2013). *Mentalizing in the development and treatment of attachment trauma.* London: Karnac Books.

Allen, J. G., Fonagy, P., & Bateman, A. W. (2008). *Mentalizing in clinical practice.* Washington, DC: American Psychiatric Publishing.

American Psychiatric Association. (2013). *Diagnostic and statistical manual of mental disorders* (5th ed.). Arlington, VA: Author.

Arnott, B., & Meins, E. (2007). Links among antenatal attachment representations, postnatal mind-mindedness, and infant attachment security: A preliminary study of mothers and fathers. *Bulletin of the Menninger Clinic, 71,* 132–149.

Bargh, J. A. (2011). Unconscious thought theory and its discontents: A critique of the critiques. *Social Cognition, 29,* 629–647.

Bargh, J. A. (2014). Our unconscious mind. *Scientific American, 310,* 30–37.

Barnow, S., Ruge, J., Spitzer, C., & Freyberger, H. J. (2005). Temperament und Charakter bei Personen mit Borderline-Persönlichkeitsstorung [Temperament and character in persons with borderline personality disorder]. *Nervenarzt, 76,* 839–840, 842–834, 846–838.

Barone, L., Fossati, A., & Guiducci, V. (2011). Attachment mental states and inferred pathways of development in borderline personality disorder: A study using the Adult Attachment Interview. *Attachment and Human Development, 13,* 451–469.

Bateman, A., Bolton, R., & Fonagy, P. (2013). Antisocial personality disorder: A mentalizing framework. *FOCUS: The Journal of Lifelong Learning in Psychiatry, 11,* 178–186.

Bateman, A. W., & Fonagy, P. (2004). Mentalization-based treatment of BPD. *Journal of Personality Disorders, 18,* 36–51.

Bateman, A., & Fonagy, P. (2008). Comorbid antisocial and borderline personality disorders: Mentalization-based treatment. *Journal of Clinical Psychology, 64,* 181–194.

Bateman, A., & Fonagy, P. (2009). Randomized controlled trial of outpatient mentalization-based treatment versus structured clinical management for borderline personality disorder. *American Journal of Psychiatry, 166,* 1355–1364.

Bateman, A., & Fonagy, P. (2010). Mentalization based treatment for borderline personality disorder. *World Psychiatry, 9,* 11–15.

Bateman, A. W., & Fonagy, P. (Eds.). (2012). *Handbook of mentalizing in mental health practice.* Washington, DC: American Psychiatric Publishing.

Bateman, A., & Fonagy, P. (2013). Impact of clinical severity on outcomes of mentalisation-based treatment for borderline personality disorder. *British Journal of Psychiatry, 203,* 221–227.

Bateman, A., & Fonagy, P. (2016). *Mentalization-based treatment for personality disorders: A practical guide.* Oxford, UK: Oxford University Press.

Beck, A. T., Freeman, A., & Davis, D. D. (2004). *Cognitive therapy of personality disorders.* New York: Guilford Press.

Beebe, B., Jaffe, J., Markese, S., Buck, K., Chen, H., Cohen, P., et al. (2010). The origins of 12-month attachment: A microanalysis of 4-month mother–infant interaction. *Attachment and Human Development, 12,* 3–141.

Belsky, J., & Fearon, P. R. M. (2008). Precursors of attachment security. In J. Cassidy & P. R. Shaver (Eds.), *Handbook of attachment theory and research* (2nd ed., pp. 295–316). New York: Guilford Press.

Bender, D. S., & Skodol, A. E. (2007). Borderline personality as a self-other representational disturbance. *Journal of Personality Disorders, 21,* 500–517.

Benish, S. G., Imel, Z. E., & Wampold, B. E. (2008). The relative efficacy of bona fide psychotherapies for treating post-traumatic stress disorder: A meta-analysis of direct comparisons. *Clinical Psychology Review, 28,* 746–758.

Blatt, S. J., & Auerbach, J. S. (1988). Differential cognitive disturbances in three types of borderline patients. *Journal of Personality Disorders, 2,* 198–211.

Bowlby, J. (1969). *Attachment and loss: Vol. 1. Attachment.* London: Hogarth Press and Institute of Psycho-Analysis.

Bowlby, J. (1973). *Attachment and loss: Vol. 2. Separation: Anxiety and anger.* London: Hogarth Press and Institute of Psycho-Analysis.

Bradley, R., & Westen, D. (2005). The psychodynamics of borderline personality disorder: A view from developmental psychopathology. *Development and Psychopathology, 17,* 927–957.

Caligor, E., Kernberg, O. F., & Clarkin, J. F. (2007). *Handbook of dynamic psychotherapy for higher level personality pathology.* Washington, DC: American Psychiatric Press.

Carlson, E. A., Egeland, B., & Sroufe, L. A. (2009). A prospective investigation of the development of borderline personality symptoms. *Development and Psychopathology, 21,* 1311–1334.

Choi-Kain, L. W., Fitzmaurice, G. M., Zanarini, M. C., Laverdiere, O., & Gunderson, J. G. (2009). The relationship between self-reported attachment styles, interpersonal dysfunction, and borderline personality disorder. *Journal of Nervous and Mental Disease, 197,* 816–821.

Cicchetti, D., Rogosch, F. A., & Toth, S. L. (2000). The efficacy of toddler–parent psychotherapy for fostering cognitive development in offspring of depressed mothers. *Journal of Abnormal Child Psychology, 28,* 135–148.

Cicchetti, D., & Walker, E. F. (2001). Editorial: Stress and development: Biological and psychological consequences. *Development and Psychopathology, 13,* 413–418.

Corriveau, K. H., Harris, P. L., Meins, E., Fernyhough, C., Arnott, B., Elliott, L., et al. (2009). Young children's trust in their mother's claims: Longitudinal links with attachment security in infancy. *Child Development, 80,* 750–761.

Crandell, L. E., & Hobson, R. P. (1999). Individual differences in young children's IQ: A social-developmental perspective. *Journal of Child Psychology and Psychiatry, 40,* 455–464.

Crowell, S. E., Beauchaine, T. P., & Linehan, M. M. (2009). A biosocial developmental model of borderline personality: Elaborating and extending Linehan's theory. *Psychological Bulletin, 135,* 495–510.

de Rosnay, M., & Harris, P. L. (2002). Individual differences in children's understanding of emotion: The roles of attachment and language. *Attachment and Human Development, 4,* 39–54.

DeWolf, M. S., & van IJzendoorn, M. H. (1997). Sensitivity and attachment: A meta-analysis on parental antecedents of infant attachment. *Journal of Marriage and the Family, 68,* 571–591.

Falkenstrom, F., Granstrom, F., & Holmqvist, R. (2013). Therapeutic alliance predicts symptomatic improvement session by session. *Journal of Counseling Psychology, 60,* 317–328.

Fearon, P., Shmueli-Goetz, Y., Viding, E., Fonagy, P., & Plomin, R. (2013). Genetic and environmental influences on adolescent attachment. *Journal of Child Psychology and Psychiatry, 55,* 1033–1041.

Fonagy, P. (1982). The integration of psychoanalysis and empirical science: A review. *International Review of Psychoanalysis, 9,* 125–145.

Fonagy, P. (1991). Thinking about thinking: Some clinical and theoretical considerations in the treatment of a borderline patient. *International Journal of Psycho-Analysis, 72*(4), 639–656.

Fonagy, P. (2000). Attachment and borderline personality disorder. *Journal of the American Psychoanalytic Association, 48,* 1129–1146.

Fonagy, P., & Allison, E. (2014). The role of mentalizing and epistemic trust in the therapeutic relationship. *Psychotherapy, 51,* 372–380.

Fonagy, P., & Bateman, A. (2008). The development of borderline personality disorder: A mentalizing model. *Journal of Personality Disorders, 22,* 4–21.

Fonagy, P., Bateman, A., & Bateman, A. (2011). The widening scope of mentalizing: A discussion. *Psychology and Psychotherapy: Theory, Research and Practice, 84,* 98–110.

Fonagy, P., Gergely, G., Jurist, E., & Target, M. (2002). *Affect regulation, mentalization, and the development of the self.* New York: Other Press.

Fonagy, P., & Higgitt, A. (1990). A developmental perspective on borderline personality disorder. *Revue Internationale de Psychopathologie, 1,* 125–159.

Fonagy, P., & Luyten, P. (2009). A developmental, mentalization-based approach to the understanding and treatment of borderline personality disorder. *Development and Psychopathology, 21,* 1355–1381.

Fonagy, P., & Luyten, P. (2016). A multilevel perspective on the development of borderline personality disorder. In D. Cicchetti (Ed.), *Development and psychopathology* (3rd ed., Vol. 3, pp. 726–792). New York: Wiley.

Fonagy, P., Luyten, P., & Allison, E. (2015). Epistemic petrifaction and the restoration of epistemic trust: A new conceptualization of borderline personality disorder and its psychosocial treatment. *Journal of Personality Disorders, 29,* 575–609.

Fonagy, P., Luyten, P., Bateman, A., Gergely, G., Strathearn, L., Target, M., et al. (2010). Attachment and personality pathology. In J. F. Clarkin, P. Fonagy, & G. O. Gabbard (Eds.), *Psychodynamic psychotherapy for personality disorders: A clinical handbook* (pp. 37–88). Washington, DC: American Psychiatric Publishing.

Fonagy, P., Steele, H., Steele, M., & Holder, J. (1997). Attachment and theory of mind: Overlapping constructs? *Association for Child Psychology and Psychiatry Occasional Papers, 14,* 31–40.

Fonagy, P., Steele, M., Steele, H., Higgitt, A., & Target, M. (1994). The Emanuel Miller Memorial Lecture 1992: The theory and practice of resilience. *Journal of Child Psychology and Psychiatry, 35,* 231–257.

Fonagy, P., Steele, M., Steele, H., Moran, G. S., & Higgitt, A. C. (1991). The capacity for understanding mental states: The reflective self in parent and child and its significance for security of attachment. *Infant Mental Health Journal, 12,* 201–218.

Fonagy, P., & Target, M. (1997). Attachment and reflective function: Their role in self-organization. *Development and Psychopathology, 9,* 679–700.

Fonagy, P., & Target, M. (2000). Playing with reality: III. The persistence of dual psychic reality in borderline patients. *International Journal of Psychoanalysis, 81,* 853–874.

Fonagy, P., & Target, M. (2003). *Psychoanalytic theories: Perspectives from developmental psychopathology.* London: Whurr.

Fonagy, P., Target, M., & Gergely, G. (2000). Attachment and borderline personality disorder: A theory and some evidence. *Psychiatric Clinics of North America, 23,* 103–122.

Fonagy, P., Target, M., & Gergely, G. (2006). Psychoanalytic perspectives on developmental psychopathology. In D. Cicchetti & D. J. Cohen (Eds.), *Developmental psychopathology: Vol. 1. Theory and method* (2nd ed., pp. 701–749). Hoboken, NJ: Wiley.

Fossati, A., Feeney, J. A., Carretta, I., Grazioli, F., Milesi, R., Leonardi, B., et al. (2005). Modeling the relationships between adult attachment patterns and borderline personality disorder: The role of impulsivity and aggressiveness. *Journal of Social and Clinical Psychology, 24,* 520–537.

Fraley, R. C., Roisman, G. I., Booth-LaForce, C., Owen, M. T., & Holland, A. S. (2013). Interpersonal and genetic origins of adult attachment styles: A longitudinal study from infancy to early adulthood. *Journal of Personality and Social Psychology, 104,* 817–838.

Frank, J. D., & Frank, J. B. (1991). *Persuasion and healing: A comparative study of psychotherapy.* Baltimore: Johns Hopkins University Press.

Frankenhuis, W. E., Panchanathan, K., & Clark Barrett, H. (2013). Bridging developmental systems theory and evolutionary psychology using dynamic optimization. *Developmental Science, 16,* 584–598.

Gao, Y., Raine, A., Chan, F., Venables, P. H., & Mednick, S. A. (2010). Early maternal and paternal bonding, childhood physical abuse and adult psychopathic personality. *Psychological Medicine, 40,* 1007–1016.

Goodman, G. S., Quas, J. A., & Ogle, C. M. (2010). Child maltreatment and memory. *Annual Review of Psychology, 61,* 325–351.

Grant, B. F., Chou, S. P., Goldstein, R. B., Huang, B., Stinson, F. S., Saha, T. D., et al. (2008). Prevalence, correlates, disability, and comorbidity of DSM-IV borderline personality disorder: Results from the Wave 2 National Epidemiologic Survey on Alcohol and Related Conditions. *Journal of Clinical Psychiatry, 69,* 533–545.

Gratz, K. L., Tull, M. T., Baruch, D. E., Bornovalova, M. A., & Lejuez, C. W. (2008). Factors associated with co-occurring borderline personality disorder among inner-city substance users: The roles of childhood maltreatment, negative affect intensity/reactivity, and emotion dysregulation. *Comprehensive Psychiatry, 49,* 603–615.

Grienenberger, J. F., Kelly, K., & Slade, A. (2005). Maternal reflective functioning, mother–infant affective communication, and infant attachment: Exploring the link between mental states and observed caregiving behavior in the intergenerational transmission of attachment. *Attachment and Human Development, 7,* 299–311.

Hamilton, W. D. (1964). The genetic evolution of social behaviour. *Journal of Theoretical Biology, 7,* 1–52.

Hazlett, E. A., Zhang, J., New, A. S., Zelmanova, Y., Goldstein, K. E., Haznedar, M. M., et al. (2012). Potentiated amygdala response to repeated emotional pictures in borderline personality disorder. *Biological Psychiatry, 72,* 448–456.

Hengartner, M. P., Ajdacic-Gross, V., Rodgers, S., Müller, M., & Rössler, W. (2013). Childhood adversity in association with personality disorder dimensions: New findings in an old debate. *European Psychiatry, 28,* 476–482.

Higgitt, A., & Fonagy, P. (1992). Psychotherapy in borderline and narcissistic personality disorder. *British Journal of Psychiatry, 161,* 23–43.

Isabella, R. A., Belsky, J., & von Eye, A. (1989). Origins of infant–mother attachment: An examination of interactional synchrony during the infant's first year. *Developmental Psychology, 25,* 12–21.

Jacobsen, T., & Hofmann, V. (1997). Children's attachment representations: Longitudinal relations to school behavior and academic competency in middle childhood and adolescence. *Developmental Psychology, 33,* 703–710.

Johnson, J. G., Cohen, P., Kasen, S., Ehrensaft, M. K., & Crawford, T. N. (2006). Associations of parental personality disorders and Axis I disorders with childrearing behavior. *Psychiatry (Edgmont), 69,* 336–350.

Jørgensen, C. R. (2010). Invited essay: Identity and borderline personality disorder. *Journal of Personality Disorders, 24,* 344–364.

Jørgensen, C. R., Berntsen, D., Bech, M., Kjolbye, M., Bennedsen, B. E., & Ramsgaard, S. B. (2012). Identity-related autobiographical memories and cultural life scripts in patients with borderline personality disorder. *Consciousness and Cognition, 21,* 788–798.

Kernberg, O. F. (1975). *Borderline conditions and pathological narcissism.* New York: Jason Aronson.

Kernberg, O. F. (1984). *Severe personality disorders: Psychotherapeutic strategies.* New Haven, CT: Yale University Press.

Kiraly, I., Csibra, G., & Gergely, G. (2013). Beyond rational imitation: Learning arbitrary means actions from communicative demonstrations. *Journal of Experimental Child Psychology, 116,* 471–486.

Kiser, L. J., Bates, J. E., Maslin, C. A., & Bayles, K. (1986). Mother–infant play at six months as a predictor of attachment security of thirteen months. *Journal of the American Academy of Child Psychiatry, 25,* 68–75.

Leichsenring, F., Leibing, E., Kruse, J., New, A. S., & Leweke, F. (2011). Borderline personality disorder. *Lancet, 377,* 74–84.

Linehan, M. M. (1993). *Cognitive-behavioral treatment of borderline personality disorder.* New York: Guilford Press.

Livesley, W. J. (2003). *Practical management of personality disorder.* New York: Guilford Press.

Luyten, P., & Blatt, S. J. (2013). Interpersonal relatedness and self-definition in normal and disrupted personality development: Retrospect and prospect. *American Psychologist, 68,* 172–183.

Luyten, P., Fonagy, P., Lowyck, B., & Vermote, R. (2012). Assessment of mentalization. In A. W. Bateman & P. Fonagy (Eds.), *Handbook of mentalizing in mental health practice* (pp. 43–65). Washington, DC: American Psychiatric Publishing.

Main, M. (2000). The organized categories of infant, child, and adult attachment: Flexible vs. inflexible attention under attachment-related stress. *Journal of the American Psychoanalytic Association, 48,* 1055–1096; discussion 1175–1187.

Marvin, R. S., & Britner, P. A. (2008). Normal development: The ontogeny of attachment. In J. Cassidy & P. R. Shaver (Eds.), *Handbook of attachment theory and research* (2nd ed., pp. 269–294). New York: Guilford Press.

McAleavey, A. A., & Castonguay, L. G. (2014). Insight as a common and specific impact of psychotherapy: Therapist-reported exploratory, directive, and common factor interventions. *Psychotherapy, 51,* 283–294.

McWilliams, N. (2011). *Psychoanalytic diagnosis: Understanding personality structure in the clinical process* (2nd ed.). New York: Guilford Press.

Meins, E., Fernyhough, C., Fradley, E., & Tuckey, M. (2001). Rethinking maternal sensitivity: Mothers' comments on infants' mental processes predict security of attachment at 12 months. *Journal of Child Psychology and Psychiatry, 42,* 637–648.

Meins, E., Fernyhough, C., Wainwright, R., Das Gupta, M., Fradley, E., & Tuckey, M. (2002). Maternal mind-mindedness and attachment security as predictors of theory of mind understanding. *Child Development, 73,* 1715–1726.

Meyer, B., Ajchenbrenner, M., & Bowles, D. P. (2005). Sensory sensitivity, attachment experiences, and rejection responses among adults with borderline and avoidant features. *Journal of Personality Disorders, 19,* 641–658.

Mikulincer, M., & Shaver, P. R. (2016). *Attachment in adulthood: Structure, dynamics, and change* (2nd ed.). New York: Guilford Press.

Mills-Koonce, W. R., Gariepy, J. L., Propper, C., Sutton, K., Calkins, S., Moore, G., et al. (2007). Infant and parent factors associated with early maternal sensitivity: A caregiver-attachment systems approach. *Infant Behavior and Development, 30,* 114–126.

Minzenberg, M. J., Fan, J., New, A. S., Tang, C. Y., & Siever, L. J. (2007). Fronto-limbic dysfunction in response to facial emotion in borderline personality disorder: An event-related fMRI study. *Psychiatry Research, 155,* 231–243.

Moss, E., Rousseau, D., Parent, S., St.-Laurent, D., & Saintong, J. (1998). Correlates of attachment at school-age: Maternal reported stress, mother–child interaction and behavior problems. *Child Development, 69,* 1390–1405.

New, A. S., aan het Rot, M., Ripoll, L. H., Perez-Rodriguez, M. M., Lazarus, S., Zipursky, E., et al. (2012). Empathy and alexithymia in borderline personality disorder: Clinical and laboratory measures. *Journal of Personality Disorders, 26,* 660–675.

Northoff, G., Qin, P., & Feinberg, T. E. (2011). Brain imaging of the self-conceptual, anatomical and methodological issues. *Consciousness and Cognition, 20,* 52–63.

Oldham, J. M. (2009). Borderline personality disorder comes of age. *American Journal of Psychiatry, 166,* 509–511.

Paris, J. (2013). How the history of psychotherapy interferes with integration. *Journal of Psychotherapy Integration, 23,* 99–106.

Powers, A. D., Thomas, K. M., Ressler, K. J., & Bradley, B. (2011). The differential effects of child abuse and posttraumatic stress disorder on schizotypal personality disorder. *Comprehensive Psychiatry, 52,* 438–445.

Prochaska, J. O., & Norcross, J. C. (2013). *Systems of psychotherapy: A transtheoretical analysis* (8th ed.). Belmont, CA: Brooks/Cole Cengage Advantage Books.

Repetti, R. L., Taylor, S. E., & Seeman, T. E. (2002). Risky families: Family social environments and the mental and physical health of offspring. *Psychological Bulletin, 128,* 330–366.

Robinson, P., Barrett, B., Bateman, A., Hakeem, A., Hellier, J., Lemonsky, F., et al. (2014). Study protocol for a randomized controlled trial of mentalization based therapy against specialist supportive clinical management in patients with both eating disorders and symptoms of borderline personality disorder. *BMC Psychiatry, 14,* 51.

Rogers, C. R. (1951). *Client-centered therapy.* Boston: Houghton Mifflin.

Rogers, C. R., & Dymond, R. F. (1954). *Psychotherapy and personality change: Coordinated research studies in the client-centered approach.* Chicago: University of Chicago Press.

Rogosch, F. A., & Cicchetti, D. (2005). Child maltreatment, attention networks, and potential precursors to borderline personality disorder. *Development and Psychopathology, 17,* 1071–1089.

Scott, L. N., Kim, Y., Nolf, K. A., Hallquist, M. N., Wright, A. G., Stepp, S. D., et al. (2013). Preoccupied attachment and emotional dysregulation: Specific aspects of borderline personality disorder or general dimensions of personality pathology? *Journal of Personality Disorders, 27,* 473–495.

Scott, L. N., Levy, K. N., & Pincus, A. L. (2009). Adult attachment, personality traits, and borderline personality disorder features in young adults. *Journal of Personality Disorders, 23,* 258–280.

Shedler, J., Beck, A., Fonagy, P., Gabbard, G. O., Gunderson, J., Kernberg, O., et al. (2010). Personality disorders in DSM-5. *American Journal of Psychiatry, 167,* 1026–1028.

Shedler, J., Beck, A. T., Fonagy, P., Gabbard, G. O., Kernberg, O., Michels, R., et al. (2011). Revision of the Personality Disorder Model for DSM-5: Response to Skodol letter. *American Journal of Psychiatry, 168,* 97–98.

Skodol, A. E. (2012). Personality disorders in DSM-5. *Annual Review of Clinical Psychology, 8,* 317–344.

Slade, A., Grienenberger, J., Bernbach, E., Levy, D., & Locker, A. (2005). Maternal reflective functioning, attachment, and the transmission gap: A preliminary study. *Attachment and Human Development, 7,* 283–298.

Specht, M. W., Chapman, A., & Cellucci, T. (2009). Schemas and borderline personality disorder symptoms in incarcerated women. *Journal of Behavior Therapy and Experimental Psychiatry, 40,* 256–264.

Sperber, D., Clement, F., Heintz, C., Mascaro, O., Mercier, H., Origgi, G., et al. (2010). Epistemic vigilance. *Mind and Language, 25,* 359–393.

Stacks, A. M., Beeghly, M., Partridge, T., & Dexter, C. (2011). Effects of placement type on the language developmental trajectories of maltreated children from infancy to early childhood. *Child Maltreatment, 16,* 287–299.

Steele, H., & Siever, L. (2010). An attachment perspective on borderline personality disorder: Advances in gene–environment considerations. *Current Psychiatry Reports, 12,* 61–67.

Stein, H., Fonagy, P., Ferguson, K. S., & Wisman, M. (2000). Lives through time: An ideographic approach to the study of resilience. *Bulletin of the Menninger Clinic, 64,* 281–305.

Tasca, G. A., & Lampard, A. M. (2012). Reciprocal influence of alliance to the group and outcome in day treatment for eating disorders. *Journal of Counseling Psychology, 59,* 507–517.

Tyrka, A. R., Wyche, M. C., Kelly, M. M., Price, L. H., & Carpenter, L. L. (2009). Childhood maltreatment and adult personality disorder symptoms: Influence of maltreatment type. *Psychiatry Research, 165,* 281–287.

Widom, C. S., Czaja, S. J., & Paris, J. (2009). A prospective investigation of borderline personality disorder in abused and neglected children followed up into adulthood. *Journal of Personality Disorders, 23,* 433–446.

Wilkinson, R., & Pickett, K. (2009). *The spirit level: Why equality is better for everyone.* London: Penguin Books.

Wilson, D., & Sperber, D. (2012). *Meaning and relevance.* Cambridge, UK: Cambridge University Press.

# CHAPTER 8

# Cognitive Structures and Processes in Personality Disorders

### Arnoud Arntz and Jill Lobbestael

Cognitive theories of personality disorders (PDs) are built on models that were originally formulated for syndromal disorders such as depression and anxiety disorders. Similar to these models, it is assumed that cognitive structures and processes underlie PDs. In contrast to the models formulated for syndromal disorders, it is assumed that the structures and processes in patients with PDs have a more pervasive and permanent character because they are assumed to emerge early in development from the interaction between temperament and environmental influences, including attachment, parenting styles, modeling by others, and adversity.

The most important cognitive structure conceptualized by cognitive theories is the "schema," which can be defined as a generalized knowledge structure that is represented in memory and governs information processing, including attention (what to focus on), interpretation (what meaning is given to stimuli), and memory (what implicit or explicit memories are triggered by specific cues). Schemas can consist of verbal and nonverbal knowledge, and the verbal parts are sometimes called "beliefs" or "assumptions." Some texts equate schemas with beliefs, which is confusing, given that a schema is a more general psychological concept. Schemas mainly operate automatically and help humans to efficiently deal with an otherwise overwhelming and meaningless amount of information: They filter what to attend to and automatically attach meaning to sensory information. On the one hand, most of the available information is not processed further by selective attentional processes; on the other hand, a lot of meaning is added to the raw data when a schema is activated. The automatic and nonreflective nature of the information processing by schemas offers a powerful explanation of the ego-syntonic, pervasive, and persistent nature of PDs. This is because schemas and information processing constitute the basis for our subjective experience. For human beings it is extremely difficult, if not impossible, to describe only what is observable without adding interpretations. Selective information processes and interpretative processes color our experience, without our being aware of it. Thus, for many people, the experienced emotions and cognitions *are* the truth, and not the result of selective processes governed by schemas.

To understand PDs, it is helpful to distinguish three layers of the beliefs that are part of schemas central to PDs (see Figure 8.1). At the core are unconditional beliefs, which represent basic assumptions about the self, others, and the world. Examples are "I am bad"; "I am superior"; "Others are irresponsible"; "Other people are good", and "The world is a jungle." The first layer around the core consists of conditional assumptions, which are beliefs about conditional

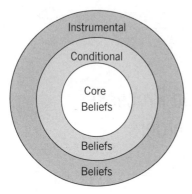

**FIGURE 8.1.** Structure of beliefs.

relationships that can be formulated in "if . . . , then . . ." terms. Examples are "If I let other people discover who I really am, they will reject me"; "If I get attached to other people, they will abandon me"; "If I show weak feelings, others will denigrate me and I will lose respect"; "If I don't check whether everything is done perfectly, it will get a mess"; and so forth. The outer layer is constituted by so-called "instrumental" beliefs about how to act to avoid bad things and acquire good things. Examples include "Check the hidden motives of others"; "Find a strong person to make decisions"; "Avoid emotions"; and "Be the boss." This structure not only reflects different types of beliefs but also distinguishes what is apparent at the "surface" (observable behaviors reflecting instrumental beliefs) and what is behind the "surface." Note that many DSM-5 (American Psychiatric Association, 2013) diagnostic criteria of PDs reflect coping behaviors—in other words, the behavioral manifestations of instrumental beliefs.

Empirical research has demonstrated that patients with PD report elevated levels of specific maladaptive beliefs, and that dimensional measures of PD pathology are associated with increasing levels of such beliefs. There is evidence for specificity of beliefs; that is, although some beliefs are general across all PDs, others are more specific (e.g., Arntz, Dreessen, Schouten, & Weertman, 2004; Beck et al., 2001; Fournier, DeRubeis, & Beck, 2012). For instance, beliefs related to low self-esteem are more general, whereas the belief that one deserves to be punished because one is a bad person is specific to borderline PD (BPD).

Although the study of beliefs relates directly to Beckian formulations of PDs (Beck, 2015; Beck et al., 2001), recently attention has also been given to early maladaptive schemas (EMSs) proposed by Young, Klosko, and Weishaar (2003). They hypothesized that PD-related schemas arise from experiences during early childhood when basic needs are not met. Unlike the Beckian assumptions about the relationship of beliefs to specific disorders, EMSs are not considered to be related to specific DSM-5 PDs. Nonetheless, some schemas show specific associations with disorders (e.g., *abandonment* with BPD, *subjugation* and *emotional inhibition* with avoidant PD [AVPD], *unrelenting standards* with obsessive–compulsive PD [OCPD], *entitlement* with narcissistic PD [NPD], and *social isolation with* schizoid and schizotypal PDs; Ball & Cecero, 2001; Carr & Francis, 2010b; Jovev & Jackson, 2004; Reeves & Taylor, 2007; Zeigler-Hill, Green, Arnau, Sisemore, & Myers, 2011). In a sense, Young and colleagues' (2003) schema theory is a dimensional alternative for the DSM-5 diagnoses, although they also suggested that a full understanding of PD pathology also requires the concept of coping style. Coping styles reflect the way individuals deal with activation of a schema. Young and colleagues hypothesized that EMS-related coping styles are built on primitive responses that animals (and humans) exhibit under high levels of threat: fight, flight, and freeze. Thus, coping responses are grouped into three clusters: overcompensation (the analogue of fight); avoidance (the analogue of flight); and surrender (the analogue of freeze).

In the case of overcompensation, the person behaves and thinks in a way that is the opposite of the triggered EMS. The function of overcompensation is to fight the triggered EMS and to keep it out of awareness as much as possible. In case of strong and successful overcompensation, the person is not aware of the underlying EMS. An example is a narcissistic person with underlying inferiority and loneliness schemas, who acts as if he or she is superior and popular. The function of avoidant coping strategies is to prevent triggering of EMSs, or when an EMS is triggered, to avoid the emotions and thoughts that are aroused. Examples of typical avoidant coping are detachment from emotions and situational avoidance, which involves not getting involved in situations where EMSs might be triggered. The function of surrendering coping strategies is to survive by submitting to what the EMSs dictate. An example would be somebody who completely believes he or she is inferior and has given up any attempt to change these feelings.

An important feature of Young and colleagues' (2007) schema theory is the concept of "schema mode," which refers to the emotional–cognitive-behavioral state of the person, in contrast to the schema concept, which is a trait-like concept. Some schema modes show a specific relationship to certain PDs; for example, BPD is characterized by "detached protector," "abandoned and abused child," and "punitive parent" modes, whereas the "avoidant protector" mode is specific to AVPD, and the "suspicious overcontroller" to paranoid PD (PPD), etc. (Bamelis, Renner, Heidkamp, & Arntz, 2011; Lobbestael, van Vreeswijk, & Arntz, 2008). Theoretically, a schema mode is a combination of an activated specific EMS and a specific coping style, an assumption supported by empirical research (van Wijk-Herbrink et al., in press).

The schema mode concept helps patients and therapists to understand the different, and sometimes conflicting behaviors, and the sudden changes in the state of patients. These sudden changes are referred to as "mode switches." Empirical studies supported this idea. For instance, anger-related modes increase in patients with PD after anger is elicited (Lobbestael, Arntz, Cima, & Chakhssi, 2009), and patients with BPD switch into the detached protector mode after observing movie scenes depicting abuse (Arntz, Klokman, & Sieswerda, 2005). Moreover, schema modes steer the application of schema therapy for PDs, an important extension of cognitive-behavioral therapy (CBT), with increasing evidence for its effectiveness (Bamelis, Bloo, Bernstein, & Arntz, 2012; Bamelis, Evers, Spinhoven, & Arntz, 2014; Giesen-Bloo et al., 2006). In schema therapy, therapist and patient make an idiosyncratic case conceptualization that explains the problems with which the patient is struggling and links these, through these modes, to the early experiences that lie at their root. Moreover, during the session, the therapist tries to detect what mode is activated, and next chooses among a specific set of techniques developed to deal with that mode. That is, for each schema mode a set of techniques is available from which the therapist should choose. For example, the detached protector mode might be dealt with by investigating why it was triggered, reassuring the patient that it is safe in therapy to address difficult feelings and inviting the patient to share the problems that gave rise to the activation of the detached protector; the punitive parent mode might be dealt with by symbolically putting this mode on an empty chair and combating it until its power is diminished; and the abandoned-abused child mode might be met by experiential techniques like imagery rescripting that help the patient to emotionally process childhood abuse or abandonment experiences.

## Origins and Content of Schemas

Schemas that are central to PDs are assumed to develop during childhood from the interaction of biological and environmental influences. Children are assumed to differ in their innate sensitivity to environmental influences such as attachment security, bad parenting, and traumatic experiences, and in how they respond to stressors, for example, with internalizing or externalizing responses. These responses in turn are likely to evoke responses in parents and others that either foster adaptation to the stressor or exacerbate the problem (e.g., when emotional responses and the need for emotional support are punished by parents). Interestingly, some genetic influences that increase the likelihood of superior outcomes when the child is raised in good circumstances also increase the likelihood of poor outcomes under adverse circumstances (e.g., Bakermans-Kranenburg & van IJzendoorn, 2007). The environmental influences on the development of PDs are broad and include maltreatment, especially emotional, sexual and physical abuse, and emotional and physical neglect (e.g., Lobbestael, Arntz, & Bernstein, 2010), as well as parenting practices (e.g., Johnson, Cohen, Chen, Kasen, & Brook, 2006) and lack of parental supervision (Holmes, Slaughter, & Kashani, 2003). In contrast to other PDs, the evidence for such etiological factors in OCPD is less clear, however (Birgenheir & Pepper, 2011).

During development, schematic representations of the world and other people, the self, and the meaning of needs and emotions, and about strategies to avoid negative and attain positive experiences are formed. These schemas are strongly influenced by the relationships of the child with caregivers, and later peers, and by emotional experiences and how they are processed. Important aspects of schemas related to PDs include how the self is experienced (e.g., as basically good or bad), how others are viewed, and how the person thinks that others view him or her (e.g., as welcome or as a nuisance), and how emotional needs are understood (e.g., as something that is bad and should be suppressed, avoided, or compensated for, or as something that is acceptable and can be shared with others). In this sense, cognitive theory shows similarities with object relations theory, although less attention is given to internal conflicts based on sexual and aggressive drives and more attention is paid to biologically determined emotional needs, including dependence on the caregivers, and to cognitive development as studied in empirical developmental psychology.

An important question is whether schemas do in fact mediate the relationship between early events and PDs. Evidence that this is the case is provided by a study showing that specific beliefs statistically mediate the association between reports of childhood abuse and BPD (Arntz, Dietzel, & Dreessen, 1999). Similarly, Young and colleagues' (2003) EMSs mediate between retrospective reports of parenting, childhood abuse, and rejection and PDs (Carr & Francis, 2010a; Specht, Chapman, & Cellucci, 2009; Thimm, 2010).

In summary, schemas assumed to underlie PDs are hypothesized to develop during childhood as a result of the interaction between biological factors and environmental influences. Early experiences shape the development of schemas about the world, other people, the self, the meaning of needs and emotions, and the best survival strategies. Often these schemas were adaptive given the child's development circumstances and his or her capacities and dependence on caregivers, but they may become dysfunctional when the child has become an adult and environmental circumstances change.

### Schema Activation

Specific stimuli, which may be internal (e.g., an emotional need) or external (e.g., the way somebody else behaves), are needed to trigger a schema that then influences information processing and coping. *Schema activation* is important in clinical practice—to understand the patient's responses and to understand why corrective experiences are not effective without schema activation—and in research: Without adequate schema activation, schema processes cannot be studied. In one study, the degree to which EMSs were activated was measured before and after a neutral, happy, and depressed mood induction (Stopa & Waters, 2005). Results showed that some EMSs, such as deprivation and defectiveness, increased after the depressive mood induction, while other EMSs remained stable, which suggests that specific moods can lead to activation of specific, but not all, schemas.

An important characteristic of schemas in PDs is that they are relatively inflexible and remain activated even if they lead to problems. It is often the lack of alternative, functional schemas and/or the overwhelming strength of the activated schema that leads to problems. Once activated, schemas govern information processing, often causing biased information processing. Biased information processing, or "cognitive bias," refers to systematic deviations from the norm (what people usually display) or from what is logical, and may be manifest in perceptual distortion, inaccurate judgment, illogical interpretation, and the consequent irrational emotional and behavioral responses. Cognitive biases are common human phenomena and may have functional aspects (e.g., fast and efficient information processing), but they can also cause problems when the distortion is serious and hinders adaptation. The cognitive model of PDs states that *dysfunctional* cognitive biases play an important role in causing and maintaining the disorder because they create the subjective reality for the individual that underlies the dysfunctional patterns. The main cognitive biases that appear to play a role in PDs are discussed in the following sections.

### Cognitive Biases

Figure 8.2 illustrates the different phases of information processing and the cognitive biases influencing each phase. First, from the usually overwhelming amount of available information, people have to select what is important for them. Attentional processes govern this process, and these can be biased in the sense that priority is given to specific stimuli even when this does not seem to be functional. In a later stage, meaning is given to the information, and automatic (unconscious) associations may play a role. Interpretational and associative biases may influence this process. In the next step, an evaluation is made, which can be influenced by evaluative biases. Then, a coping response (overt behavioral responses and covert internal responses such as ruminating or cognitive avoidance) is chosen, which is influenced by preferred coping styles. Cognitive theory also

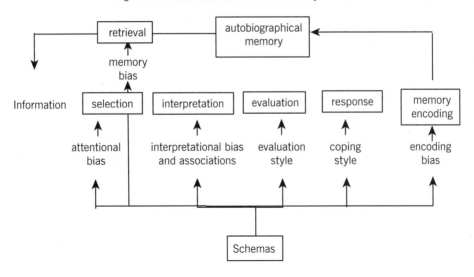

**FIGURE 8.2.** Stages in information processing and cognitive processes, and the structures involved.

assumes that with PDs, cognitive biases influence the final phase of information encoding into autobiographical memory. Similarly, when memories are retrieved, there might be retrieval bias for specific memories or specific aspects of the memory. For example, patients with BPD tend to show a memory bias in the sense that they are more likely to remember being abandoned and that others are untrustworthy.

### Attentional Bias

"Attentional bias" is the process in which attentional resources are allocated to specific classes of stimuli consistent with existing schemas at the expense of other stimuli. A form of attention bias relevant to psychopathology is the way emotions linked to immediate action tendencies, such as fear (fight-or-flight actions) and strong desire (approach actions), increase sensitivity in detecting relevant cues and a focus on these cues. Thus, threats tend to be detected quickly and hold the attention of people who are sensitive to a given kind of threat (Bar-Haim et al., 2007). A similar process is active for signs of reward for those with a strong need for reward. For example, hungry people show an attentional bias for food-related stimuli (Lavy & van den Hout, 1993; Mogg, Bradley, Hyare, & Lee, 1998). Attentional bias is prominent in syndromal disorders such as anxiety disorders and addictions (e.g., persons dependent on alcohol show attentional bias toward alcoholic drinks). One can easily understand the mechanism's survival value (e.g., early detection of threat and keeping it central in the information-processing system increases chance of escape), but in psychopathology, attentional biases are dysfunctional and are hypothesized to contribute to maintenance of the disorder.

Given the central role of emotions and wants in PDs, it is conceivable that attentional biases also play an important role in personality pathology. Pretzer (1990), for instance, suggested that BPD is characterized by hypervigiliance for signs of threat. If so, one would expect that attentional resources would automatically be captured by threatening stimuli—in other words, BPD should be characterized by an attentional bias for threat. Kaiser, Jacob, Domes, and Arntz (2016) conducted a meta-analysis of studies testing attentional bias in BPD and found evidence that, over studies that used the "emotional Stroop paradigm," people with BPD were characterized by attentional bias for negative (threatening) words, and that this bias was stronger than that in clinical controls. The evidence was less clear from studies using the "dot-probe task" (employing emotional vs. neutral faces as stimuli), which may have to do with the difference in stimulus type (words vs. faces) and/or the difference in type of attention (processing resources vs. focus of visual attention) that are involved in the tasks. Nevertheless, research supports Pretzer's hypothesis that BPD is characterized by hypervigilance for threatening stimuli.

One might expect attentional bias also to play a role in other PDs (e.g., in Cluster C PDs and in

PPD), as facilitated detection of signs of threat would follow from cognitive formulations of these disorders. These PDs have been relatively understudied, though at least two studies found positive evidence for attentional bias in Cluster C PDs (Arntz, Appels, & Sieswerda, 2000; Sieswerda, Arntz, Mertens, & Vertommen, 2006). But in these emotional Stroop studies, the Cluster C sample was a clinical control group for the borderline group, while stimuli were not specifically selected to match the concerns typical for Cluster C patients. Clearly, more research is needed here.

## Interpretational Bias

Interpretational biases are manifested when information is systematically interpreted in a way that differs from what is usual in a specific culture. With normal human information processing, preexisting schemas attach meaning to what is perceived. When dysfunctional schemas govern this interpretive process, their effects should become apparent by comparing the interpretations made by people with such schemas and those with more functional schemas. In a typical interpretational bias experiment, participants are invited to interpret a series of ambiguous stimuli that might trigger dysfunctional schemas.

Although relatively few studies have been reported, they involve a wide range of PDs and generally show disorder-specific effects. For example, people with AVPD, BPD, and dependent PD (DPD) showed characteristic interpretations of ambiguous events described in short vignettes that participants had to imagine (Arntz, Weertman, & Salet, 2011). AVPD was for instance characterized by interpreting emotions as threatening and seeing the self as inferior; dependent PD as seeing the self as incapable; and borderline PD by viewing other people as rejecting and abandoning them. No evidence for a characteristic interpretation bias for OCPD was found, leading to the speculation that perhaps implicit interpretations (see below) or cognitive styles rather than schemas are central to OCPD. Using a similar approach, Lobbestael, Cima, and Arntz (2013) demonstrated that antisocial PD (ASPD) is characterized by a hostile interpretation bias involving a tendency to infer hostile intentions in the actions of others.

Weertman, Arntz, Schouten, and Dreessen (2006) assessed interpretational bias related to DPD and PPD traits by asking participants to tell stories in response to ambiguous pictures from the Thematic Apperception Test (TAT). A mediation analysis yielded evidence that specific beliefs (assessed with the Personality Disorder Beliefs Questionnaire [PDBQ]; Arntz et al., 2004) underlie the meaning given to the ambiguous TAT pictures. Also using short vignettes, Moritz and colleagues (2011) found evidence for interpretational and evaluation biases in patients with BPD, reminiscent of those observed in psychosis. Patients with BPD showed elevated levels of catastrophizing, jumping to conclusions, and emotion-based reasoning, similar to what is shown by patients with psychosis. However, the study lacked a clinical control group, so it is not clear to what degree the biases might be characteristic for any severe form of psychopathology. Another paradigm to assess interpretation bias is the thin-slice judgment paradigm, wherein participants are asked to rate personalities of persons they see in a film clip entering a room and taking a seat (Barnow et al., 2009). Patients with BPD evaluated the depicted persons as more aggressive than did depressive patients and nonpatient controls.

The tendency to infer malevolence in others by people with BPD (Pretzer, 1990) is evident not only from vignettes and movie fragments but also from the evaluation of ambiguous emotional faces: When the emotional signs are very weak or mixed, patients with BPD show a bias to interpret anger in the facial expression (Domes et al., 2008; Domes, Schulze, & Herpertz, 2009). Similarly, when playing a virtual ball-tossing game, patients with BPD reported that they were disproportionally excluded by the other players even in the condition in which inclusion was equal across players (Staebler et al., 2011).

Interpretations might be related to implicit and explicit associations that people make when confronted with specific stimuli. *Implicit processes* may be of interest, since they result from automatic and not strategic processes, and may reflect otherwise unobservable schemas. It has been suggested that implicit processes are not influenced by strategic attempts to present oneself positively or to comply with socially desirable norms (Gawronski, LeBel, & Peters, 2007). Especially PDs that are characterized by overcompensating strategies may obscure true interpretations by reporting the opposite (Young et al., 2003). One study found that OCPD traits were related to the tendency to associate the self with characteristics that could be described as based on a responsibility–conscientiousness schema, whereas others tend to be viewed on the basis of an irresponsibility–sloppiness schema. Importantly, no association with OCPD traits was found on the tasks when implicit self- and other-esteem were assessed. Thus, the biases are specific for OCPD schemas and are not found for more general schemas. Both in an implicit association task and in a priming task, OCPD traits were associated with the assumed automatic processes, indicating that OCPD traits are associated with self- and other-schemas of the type described (Weertman, Arntz, de Jong, & Rinck, 2008). Interestingly, both implicit indices contributed independently and additively to explicit beliefs to the prediction of OCPD traits, indicating that explicit beliefs only partially cover the cognitive characteristics of OCPD.

Implicit associations have been examined in NPD. Although people with narcissistic traits show increased self-esteem, on a more implicit level, self-esteem is fragile or poor. This "masking" idea stems from early psychodynamic visions and has mostly been tested with the Implicit Association Test (IAT; Greenwald, McGhee, & Schwartz, 1998). In this task, participants are presented with words on a PC screen that they have to categorize by pressing either the right or left button of a response box. These words are either self-related, non-self-related, positive, or negative. A positive-self association is reflected by a more rapid classification of both positive and self-related words when they are assigned to a similar response button. Early studies did indeed show that NPD was related to low levels of implicit self-esteem as opposed to high levels of self-reported explicit self-esteem (e.g., Jordan, Spencer, Zanna, Hoshino-Browne, & Correll, 2003). However, several studies failed to replicate this finding, and later findings revealed that the level of implicit self-esteem in NPD is not a uniform concept. Instead, narcissism appeared to be related to high implicit positive levels in the agentic domain (e.g., status, intelligence) but not necessarily to favorable communal self-views (e.g., kindness, morality) (Campbell et al., 2007).

Implicit associations have also been investigated in ASPD. Individuals with this disorder tend to show quasi-normal, healthy responses, often to an exaggerated level—a self-representational strategy that has been labeled as "supernormality" (Cima et al., 2003). Lobbestael and colleagues (2009) experimentally induced an angry state in participants and demonstrated that on an implicit level, the association between self and anger increased significantly more in participants with ASPD than in participants with BPD and Cluster C PD or in nonpatients, despite participants with ASPD not reporting on an explicit level a higher anger increase than the other groups. This study suggests that while, at an explicit level, participants with ASPD pretended to be "normal" by reporting a nondeviant anger response, at an implicit level, which they could not control, there is a higher level of anger activation. The discrepancy between the explicit and the implicit levels might point at a conscious "denial" strategy used by these participants, or at an uncontrolled mechanism by which they "fool" even themselves by really believing themselves not to be overly angry. In both cases, the increased association between self and anger indicates an implicit (unconscious) level of deviant anger that relates to both the planned aggression and unplanned (provoked) anger outbursts so common in ASPD.

To summarize, research so far generally has supported the notion that specific PDs are characterized by specific interpretational biases. When interpretations are assessed on an explicit level, they are evident in many but not all PDs. But sometimes important interpretational content only becomes evident when assessments are made at an implicit level, where it is difficult for participants to strategically control responses. This suggests that cognitive schemas rule interpretational processes even when participants cannot explicitly access the content or deny the content for strategic reasons. The implication of this is that we cannot always rely on what patients with PDs report when it comes to how they interpret events. Especially patients with PDs that are characterized by overcompensating strategies, such as ASPD, OCPD, and NPD, might be unable or unwilling to report what interpretations underlie their problematic responses, and we can only infer their interpretations from what we know about the situation and the responses they made. A treatment implication might be that the overcompensation should first diminish, before the patient is able or willing to share what we would like to know about what specific events really meant for them.

### Evaluation Biases

Cognitive theories describe several evaluation styles (e.g., overgeneralization, dichotomous thinking, and negativity). Research has yielded evidence that BPD is characterized by dichotomous thinking in emotional situations, which refers to the tendency to evaluate others in extreme terms, more than Cluster C PD patients do (Arntz & ten Haaf, 2012; De Bonis, De Boeck, Lida-Pulik, Hourtane, & Feline, 1998; Moritz et al., 2011; Napolitano & McKay, 2007; Veen & Arntz, 2000; but for negative findings, see Sieswerda, Barnow, Verheul, & Arntz, 2013). Interestingly, these studies also assessed to what degree evaluations were not only extreme but also "all negative *or* all positive," as psychodynamic theory of splitting would predict. However, none found evidence for splitting in BPD. Thus, these studies found that despite the extremity of the judgments of patients with BPD, the judgments are mixed in terms of emotional valence, and not just negative or just positive.

Another evaluation characteristic studied in BPD is negativistic thinking. Several studies found evidence of more negative evaluations of others by these patients (e.g., when they had to rate faces or film characters—Arntz & Veen, 2001; Barnow et al., 2009; Dyck et al., 2008; Meyer, Pilkonis, & Beevers, 2004; Sieswerda et al., 2013).

### Response Styles

When confronted with stressful events that activate relevant schemas, people may respond in specific ways that reflect their habitual coping, in other words, their instrumental beliefs. Many of these are reflected in the diagnostic criteria of DSM-5 PDs. For example, AVPD is characterized by the tendency to respond to stressful events with avoidant strategies that may be covert, such as avoiding thinking about problems and making decisions. Another example is the use of perfectionistic strategies by people with OCPD. Several studies report that OCPD is characterized by a style dominated by attention to details and a need for information, especially when there is uncertainty, even if this interferes with the task (Aycicegi-Dinn, Dinn, & Caldwell-Harris, 2009; Gallagher, South, & Oltmanns, 2003; Maynard & Meyer, 1996; Yovel, Revelle, & Mineka, 2005). It has been hypothesized that this is an attempt to compensate for cognitive disorganization caused by executive control deficits (Aycicegi-Dinn et al., 2009). Still another example is the tendency of people with ASPD to respond to frustrations caused by others by using reactive aggression, and using proactive aggression to get their self-serving goals met (Lobbestael et al., 2013). Research has indicated that response styles can be reliably distinguished when assessed by self-report and that these response styles (or "coping modes" in schema therapy terms) are related in meaningful ways to different PDs (Bamelis et al., 2011; Lobbestael et al., 2008).

### Memory Bias

Two paradigms have been used to assess memory bias associated with PD. The first is retrieving autobiographical memory. Studies show that depressed patients report less specific memories when presented with a negative cue word (Goddard, Dritschel, & Burton, 1996). Studies assessing autobiographical memory are inconclusive on whether patients with BPD display such an overgeneral memory (Arntz, Meeren, & Wessel, 2002; Jones et al., 1999; Kremers, Spinhoven, & Van der Does, 2004; Renneberg, Theobald, Nobs, & Weisbrod, 2005). This inconsistency may be due to the fact that borderline-specific cues were mostly not included in these studies.

Memory bias is also assessed using directed forgetting paradigms. In this task, participants are presented with a list of words, each followed with the instruction either to forget or to remember the word. Usually, people are able to comply with both instructions, which requires intentional, resource-dependent inhibition of irrelevant information. One study showed that patients with BPD were not able to forget negative words when instructed to do so (Domes et al., 2006), which is suggestive of a negative memory bias. Two other studies found that patients with BPD were unable to suppress borderline-specific words (Korfine & Hooley, 2000) or they more often remembered these words (McClure, 2005), evidencing a borderline-specific memory bias. The inability of patients with BPD to forget negative stimuli, especially when they have a specific relevance for their disorder (e.g., have to do with abandonment, rejection, and abuse) contributes to selective memory: Events that were specifically negative are not forgotten, whereas other events are. As memories of specific events form a fundament for making inferences, this memory bias therefore contributes to interpretations and expectations that are overly pessimistic in people with BPD.

In a sense, these patients' suffering is threefold: memory bias from the past (overrepresentation of negative memories), in the present (negative inferences), and in the future (negative expectations).

Biased memory encoding and retrieval is related to schemas relevant for PDs. One study found that avoidant beliefs predicted a bias to remember explanations that are typical for people with avoidant schema. Participants imagined events that were described to them; the description, however, did not give any explanation for a central part of the event. At a later memory test, participants with high avoidant beliefs reported more memories of explanations in the story read to them that matched avoidant interpretations than did participants scoring low in avoidant beliefs. For example, highly avoidant participants reported that the reason nobody greeted them when entering a room where a party took place was that the guests preferred to talk to each other, and not to them; however, the story read to them did not contain any explanation. With this story, participants with low avoidance more often said that the reason was that it was so crowded that nobody saw them enter (Dreessen, Arntz, Hendriks, Keune, & van den Hout, 1999). In a study examining the relationship between rejection sensitivity (relevant for BPD) and memory bias, Mor and Inbar (2009) found rejection sensitivity to be related to a disproportional recall of rejection-related words but not of other emotional words that people with BPD had to process in a prior task. However, these studies were not done on samples with PD, and the first study failed to demonstrate that AVPD features were associated with attributional memory bias, which may suggest that sometimes associations between schemas and information-processing biases might be stronger than those between DSM-IV/5-based PD features that may reflect coping styles more than core schemas. We return to this issue later in the discussion.

## Causal Status of Cognitive Processes

Tests of the causal status of cognitive processes in the origin and maintenance of psychopathology involve demonstrating that when the pertinent process is manipulated by the experimenter, psychopathology changes in accord with theoretical predictions. Thus, training nonpatients to attend to stimuli related to threat should lead to an acquired attentional bias toward threat and subsequently increase the vulnerability to respond with increased fear to stressful events. Conversely, training to divert attention away from threatening stimuli should result in an attentional bias away from threat, and reduced stress and fear responsivity to stressful events. Similarly, training to interpret ambiguous events into a dysfunctional versus functional direction should lead to opposite interpretational biases, and these should lead to differential responses to stressful events. Recent research confirms that attentional and interpretational biases are causal with regard to responses to stressful events (Beard, Sawyer, & Hofmann, 2012; Hallion & Ruscio, 2011; MacLeod & Mathews, 2012). We are not aware of experiments that trained nonpatients in attentional, interpretational, and evaluative biases that mimic those prominent in PDs, and subsequently tested whether such induced biases led to phenomena similar to what is shown by the pertinent PD. Nevertheless, given that the proof of principle has a solid empirical basis, it is to be expected that such studies would also demonstrate that such cognitive processes are causal.

Another way to test causality is to demonstrate that direct experimental manipulation of the cognitive process in patients with a given disorder leads to changes in the pathology. Although such studies have not been conducted on patients with PDs, one study is now in the pilot phase (van Vreeswijk, Spinhoven, Arntz, & Eureligs-Bontekoe, 2014), and studies on syndromal disorders indicate that directly reducing attentional or interpretational biases reduces psychopathology (MacLeod & Mathews, 2012); thus, it seems likely that the same can be demonstrated in patients with PDs. For instance, the fact that attentional bias reduces to normal levels in (former) borderline patients who recovered with psychological treatment (whereas those who did not recover maintained attentional bias at the level they displayed at baseline) also suggests that successful psychological treatment involves reducing cognitive biases (Sieswerda, Arntz, & Kindt, 2007).

## Clinical Implications

The cognitive model of PDs offers clinicians a framework for understanding the problems with which patients with PDs suffer, by linking the patients' developmental history to dysfunctional schemas, to biased information processing, and to coping strategies. The model can help in formulating individual case conceptualizations and helps to steer the treatment. Various elements of the model may be a focus of treatment, for example, memories of childhood experiences that have contributed to the formation of dysfunctional schemas; attentional and interpretational biases; evaluation styles; and typical responses (both covert and overt behavior). Various forms of CBT, including schema therapy, are based on the model and often used in clinical practice. The model can also be quite easily explained in lay terms to patients, increasing their commitment to treatment. Moreover, the "translation" of terms from the personality (disorder) area with their connotation of unchangeability to cognitive structures and processes normalizes the underlying reasons for the problems and offers hope for good outcome. Last, it should be noted that the cognitive model, in contrast to some other models, is not based not on hypothesized deficits but on normal learning and information processes that because of specific circumstances have become biased.

## Discussion

Cognitive models of PDs are rooted in a psychological paradigm that has received considerable empirical support and is one the most prominent current scientific models in the field of psychology. The model also makes sense intuitively to both clinicians and patients. Nevertheless, research evaluating specific hypotheses derived from cognitive models is relatively scarce, especially compared to that for depression and anxiety disorders. There is a clear need for more studies that assess cognitive structures and processes in detail and promote understanding of their relationship to various forms of PD. Research is also limited due to the failure to use study designs that include a clinical control group, so it is unclear to what degree the phenomenon investigated is specific to a given disorder.

An important difference with other approaches is that cognitive models of PDs explain psychopathology from content (schemas, beliefs) and content-related biases, instead of from deficits and other structural abnormalities; that is, given the unfortunate circumstances the patient was faced with during childhood, it is "normal" that the typical schema's information-processing biases and coping strategies that constitute the PD developed. For example, many patients with BPD were confronted during childhood with a lack of secure attachment, and with emotional and sometimes sexual abuse. Typically, there was a high level of threat and no possibility to find safety. Moreover, expression of needs, emotions, and opinions was often punished. Thus, the patients developed schemas representing the expectation that other people will abuse, reject, or abandon them; that emotions and needs are "bad"; and that they are bad people. Their hypervigilance for signs of threat was probably functional during childhood, as was their detachment from inner needs and from other people. In other words, we can understand BPD with cognitive models without needing to hypothesize structural deficits.

As an example, cognitive models assume that patients with BPD make biased interpretations of other people's intentions, but not that they have a mentalization deficit. The deviating interpretation of other people's intentions is therefore not explained by structural deficits in information-processing capacities, but by the content of activated schemas and by associated cognitive biases. Research indeed shows no consistent evidence for basic mentalization deficits in BPD (e.g., Arntz, Bernstein, Oorschot, & Schobre, 2009; Franzen et al., 2011; Schilling et al., 2012; Tolfree, 2012), although the debate is not yet resolved (Herpertz & Bertsch, 2014). The degree to which the approach directed by cognitive models will be successful is an empirical issue, but it is important to point out this difference with other models. It should also be noted that the cognitive model might be more successful with some, but not all, PDs. For example, structural deficits might be more prominent in schizotypal and schizoid PDs than in other PDs.

A general finding in studies of cognitive models of PDs is that associations of information-processing biases with measures of content of schemas is stronger than those with DSM-IV/5-based PD features. From a cognitive-theoretical point of view, schemas are therefore much more central to PDs than the features described by the DSM-IV/5 criteria. It is striking that many DSM PD criteria seem to reflect coping styles rather than core schemas. As explained, in a cognitive model, coping should be viewed as an individual's way to deal with circumstances to which he or she is sensitive to given his or her schemas, but it is not identical to the schema; that is, one and the same schema can be dealt with by different ways of coping, previously grouped into avoidant, surrender, and overcompensating variants. The consequence of the strong reliance of the DSM operationalization of classification criteria for PDs on coping is that the association of the cognitive processes and content with specific PDs is limited. If diagnostic criteria were based on schemas, a system of classification of PDs could be constructed that would be more coherent from a cognitive-theoretical point of view.

A last important challenge is to test the causal status of the key aspects of the model. Although, as mentioned, general proofs of principle have been successful, it is important to assess to what degree similar proofs can be produced in the area of PDs; that is, it would be important to test whether the experimental induction of specific information-processing biases or beliefs in nonpatients would produce phenomena that are similar to those seen in patients with PDs. For instance, an interpretation training paradigm could be used to induce a tendency in nonpatients to interpret others' as rejecting (vs. the opposite in a control condition) and subsequently test whether the participants are increasingly sensitive to ambiguous rejection situations to infer rejection and to show increased disappointment and anger, similar to how patients with BPD respond. Similarly, it is important to study on a more microscopic level whether experimentally influencing cognitive biases or beliefs in patients with PD leads to changes in their sensitivity to specific situations and to changes in their problems. Although such studies are a challenge for researchers, we believe they are necessary to further the development of cognitive models of PDs.

## REFERENCES

American Psychiatric Association. (2013). *Diagnostic and statistical manual of mental disorders* (5th ed.). Arlington, VA: Author.

Arntz, A., Appels, C., & Sieswerda, S. (2000). Hypervigilance in borderline disorder: A test with the emotional Stroop paradigm. *Journal of Personality Disorders, 14,* 366–373.

Arntz, A., Bernstein, D., Oorschot, M., & Schobre, P. (2009). Theory of mind in borderline and cluster-C personality disorder. *Journal of Nervous and Mental Disease, 197*(11), 801–807.

Arntz, A., Dietzel, R., & Dreessen, L. (1999). Assumptions in borderline personality disorder: Specificity, stability and relationship with etiological factors. *Behaviour Research and Therapy, 37,* 545–557.

Arntz, A., Dreessen, L., Schouten, E., & Weertman, A. (2004). Beliefs in personality disorders: A test with the personality disorder belief questionnaire. *Behaviour Research and Therapy, 42*(10), 1215–1225.

Arntz, A., Klokman, J., & Sieswerda, S. (2005). An experimental test of the schema mode model of borderline personality disorder. *Journal of Behavior Therapy and Experimental Psychiatry, 36,* 226–239.

Arntz, A., Meeren, M., & Wessel, I. (2002). No evidence for overgeneral memories in borderline personality disorder. *Behaviour Research and Therapy, 40,* 1063–1068.

Arntz, A., & ten Haaf, J. (2012). Social cognition in borderline personality disorder: Evidence for dichotomous thinking but no evidence for less complex attributions. *Behaviour Research and Therapy, 50,* 707–718.

Arntz, A., & Veen, G. (2001). Evaluations of others by borderline patients. *Journal of Nervous and Mental Disease, 189,* 513–521.

Arntz, A., Weertman, A., & Salet, S. (2011). Interpretation bias in Cluster-C and borderline personality disorders. *Behaviour Research and Therapy, 49,* 472–481.

Aycicegi-Dinn, A., Dinn, W. M., & Caldwell-Harris, C. L. (2009). Obsessive–compulsive personality traits: Compensatory response to executive function deficit? *International Journal of Neuroscience, 119*(4), 600–608.

Bakermans-Kranenburg, M. J., & van IJzendoorn, M. H. (2007). Research review: Genetic vulnerability or differential susceptibility in child development: The case of attachment *Journal of Child Psychology and Psychiatry, 48,* 1160–1173.

Ball, S. A., & Cecero, J. J. (2001). Addicted patients with personality disorders: Traits, schemas, and presenting problems. *Journal of Personality Disorders, 15,* 72–83.

Bamelis, L. L. M., Bloo, J., Bernstein, D., & Arntz, A. (2012). Effectiveness studies. In M. Van Vreeswijk, J. Broersen, & M. Nadort (Eds.), *The Wiley-Blackwell handbook of schema therapy: Theory, research and practice* (pp. 495–510). Chichester, UK: Wiley-Blackwell.

Bamelis, L. L. M., Evers, S. M. A. A., Spinhoven, P., & Arntz, A. (2014). Results of a multicentered randomised controlled trial of the clinical effectiveness of schema therapy for personality disorders. *American Journal of Psychiatry, 171,* 305–322.

Bamelis, L. L. M., Renner, F., Heidkamp, D., & Arntz, A. (2011). Extended schema mode conceptualizations for specific personality disorders: An empirical study. *Journal of Personality Disorders, 25,* 41–58.

Bar-Haim, Y., Lamy, D., Pergamin, L., Bakermans-Kranenburg, M. J., & van IJzendoorn, M. H. (2007). Threat related attentional bias in anxious and nonanxious individuals: A meta-analytic study. *Psychological Bulletin, 133*(1), 1–24.

Barnow, S., Stopsack, M., Grabe, H. J., Meinke, C., Spitzer, C., Kronmüller, K., et al. (2009). Interpersonal evaluation bias in borderline personality disorder. *Behaviour Research and Therapy, 47,* 359–365.

Beard, C., Sawyer, A. T., & Hofmann, S. G. (2012). Efficacy of attention bias modification using threat and appetitive stimuli: A meta-analytic review. *Behavior Therapy, 43,* 724–740.

Beck, A. T. (2015). Theory of personality disorders. In A. T. Beck, D. D. Davis, & A. Freeman (Eds.), *Cognitive therapy of personality disorders* (pp. 19–62). New York: Guilford Press.

Beck, A. T., Butler, A. C., Brown, G. K., Dahlsgaard, K. K., Newman, C. F., & Beck, J. S. (2001). Dysfunctional beliefs discriminate personality disorders. *Behaviour Research and Therapy, 39,* 1213–1225.

Birgenheir, D. G., & Pepper, C. M. (2011). Negative life experiences and the development of cluster C personality disorders: A cognitive perspective. *Cognitive Behaviour Therapy, 40,* 190–205.

Campbell, W. K., Bosson, J. K., Coheen, T. W., Lakey, C. E., & Kernis, M. H. (2007). Do narcissists dislike themselves "deep down inside"? *Psychological Science, 18,* 227–229.

Carr, S. N., & Francis, A. J. (2010a). Do early maladaptive schemas mediate the relationship between childhood experiences and avoidant personality disorder features?: A preliminary investigation in a non-clinical sample. *Cognitive Therapy and Research, 34,* 343–358.

Carr, S. N., & Francis, A. J. (2010b). Early maladaptive schemas and personality disorder symptoms: An examination in a non-clinical sample. *Psychology and Psychotherapy: Theory, Research, and Practice, 83*(4), 333–349.

Cima, M., Merckelbach, H., Hollnack, S., Butt, C., Kremer, K., Schellbach-Matties, R., et al. (2003). The other side of malingering: Supernormality. *The Clinical Neuropsychologist, 17,* 235–243.

De Bonis, M., De Boeck, P., Lida-Pulik, H., Hourtane, M., & Feline, A. (1998). Self-concept and mood: A comparative study between depressed patients with and without borderline personality disorder. *Journal of Affective Disorders, 48,* 191–197.

Domes, G., Czieschnek, D., Weidler, F., Berger, C., Fast, K., & Herpertz, S. C. (2008). Recognition of facial affect in borderline personality disorder. *Journal of Personality Disorders, 22,* 135–147.

Domes, G., Schulze, L., & Herpertz, S. C. (2009). Emotion recognition in borderline personality disorder: A review of the literature. *Journal of Personality Disorders, 23,* 6–19.

Domes, G., Winter, B., Schnell, K., Vohs, K., Fast, K., & Herpertz, S. C. (2006). The influence of emotions on inhibitory functioning in borderline personality disorder. *Psychological Medicine, 36,* 1163–1172.

Dreessen, L., Arntz, A., Hendriks, T., Keune, N., & van den Hout, M. A. (1999). Avoidant personality disorder and implicit schema-congruent information processing bias: A pilot study with a pragmatic inference task. *Behaviour Research and Therapy, 37,* 619–632.

Dyck, M., Habel, U., Slodczyk, J., Schlummer, J., Backes, V., Schneider, F., et al. (2008). Negative bias in fast emotion discrimination in borderline personality disorder. *Psychological Medicine, 39,* 855–864.

Fournier, J. C., DeRubeis, R. J., & Beck, A. T. (2012). Dysfunctional cognitions in personality pathology: The structure and validity of the Personality Belief Questionnaire. *Psychological Medicine, 42,* 795–805.

Franzen, N., Hagenhoff, M., Baer, N., Schmidt, A., Mier, D., Sammer, G., et al. (2011). Superior "theory of mind" in borderline personality disorder: An analysis of interaction behavior in a virtual trust game. *Psychiatry Research, 187*(1), 224–233.

Gallagher, N. G., South, S. C., & Oltmanns, T. F. (2003). Attentional coping style in obsessive–compulsive personality disorder: A test of the intolerance of uncertainty hypothesis. *Personality and Individual Differences, 34,* 41–57.

Gawronski, B., LeBel, E. P., & Peters, K. R. (2007). What do implicit measures tell us?: Scrutinizing the validity of three common assumptions. *Perspectives on Psychological Science, 2,* 181–193.

Giesen-Bloo, J., van Dyck, R., Spinhoven, P., van Tilburg, W., Dirksen, C., van Asselt, T., et al. (2006). Outpatient psychotherapy for borderline personality disorder: Randomized trial of schema-focused therapy versus transference-focused psychotherapy. *Archives of General Psychiatry, 63,* 649–658.

Goddard, L., Dritschel, B., & Burton, A. (1996). Role of autobiographical memory in social problem solving and depression. *Journal of Abnormal Psychology, 105,* 609–616.

Greenwald, A. G., McGhee, D. E., & Schwartz, J. L. K. (1998). Measuring individual differences in implicit cognition: The Implicit Association Test. *Journal of Personality and Social Psychology, 74,* 1464–1480.

Hallion, L. S., & Ruscio, A. M. (2011). A meta-analysis of the effect of cognitive bias modification on anxiety and depression. *Psychological Bulletin, 137,* 940–958.

Herpertz, S. C., & Bertsch, K. (2014). The social-cognitive basis of personality disorders. *Current Opinion in Psychiatry, 27*(1), 73–77.

Holmes, S. E., Slaughter, J. R., & Kashani, J. (2003). Risk factors in childhood that lead to the development of conduct disorder and antisocial personality disorder. *Child Psychiatry and Human Development, 31,* 183–193.

Johnson, J. G., Cohen, P., Chen, H., Kasen, S., & Brook, J. S. (2006). Parenting behaviors associated with risk for offspring personality disorder during adulthood. *Archives of General Psychiatry, 63,* 579–587.

Jones, B., Heard, H., Startup, M., Swales, M., Williams,

J. M. G., & Jones, R. S. P. (1999). Autobiographical memory and dissociation in borderline personality disorder. *Psychological Medicine, 29,* 1397–1404.

Jordan, C. H., Spencer, S. J., Zanna, M. P., Hoshino-Browne, E., & Correll, J. (2003). Secure and defensive self-esteem. *Journal of Personality and Social Psychology, 85,* 969–978.

Jovev, M., & Jackson, H. J. (2004). Early maladaptive schemas in personality disordered individuals. *Journal of Personality Disorders, 18,* 467–478.

Kaiser, D., Jacob, G. A., Domes, G., & Arntz, A. (2016). Attentional bias for emotional stimuli in borderline personality disorder: A meta-analysis. *Psychopathology, 49*(6), 383–396.

Korfine, L., & Hooley, J. M. (2000). Directed forgetting of emotional stimuli in borderline personality disorder. *Journal of Abnormal Psychology, 109,* 214–221.

Kremers, I. P., Spinhoven, P., & Van der Does, A. J. W. (2004). Autobiographical memory in depressed and nondepressed patients with borderline personality disorder. *British Journal of Clinical Psychology, 43,* 17–29.

Lavy, E., & van den Hout, M. A. (1993). Attentional bias for appetitive cues: Effects of fasting in normal subjects. *Behavioural and Cognitive Psychotherapy, 21,* 297–310.

Lobbestael, J., Arntz, A., & Bernstein, D. P. (2010). Disentangling the relationship between different types of childhood maltreatment and personality disorders. *Journal of Personality Disorders, 24*(3), 285–295.

Lobbestael, J., Arntz, A., Cima, M., & Chakhssi, F. (2009). Effects of induced anger in patients with antisocial personality disorder. *Psychological Medicine, 39,* 557–568.

Lobbestael, J., Cima, M., & Arntz, A. (2013). The relationship between adult reactive and proactive aggression, hostile interpretation bias, and antisocial personality disorder. *Journal of Personality Disorders, 27,* 53–66.

Lobbestael, J., van Vreeswijk, M., & Arntz, A. (2008). An empirical test of schema mode conceptualizations in personality disorders. *Behaviour Research and Therapy, 46,* 854–860.

MacLeod, C., & Mathews, A. (2012). Cognitive bias modification approaches to anxiety. *Annual Review of Clinical Psychology, 8,* 189–217.

Maynard, R. E., & Meyer, G. E. (1996). Visual information processing with obsessive–compulsive and hysteric personalities. *Personality and Individual Differences, 20*(3), 389–399.

McClure, M. M. (2005). Memory bias in borderline personality disorder: An examination of directed forgetting of emotional stimuli. *Dissertation Abstracts International B: The Sciences and Engineering, 66,* 1727.

Meyer, B., Pilkonis, P. A., & Beevers, C. G. (2004). What's in a (neutral) face?: Personality disorders, attachment styles, and the appraisal of ambiguous social cues. *Journal of Personality Disorders, 18,* 320–336.

Mogg, K., Bradley, B. P., Hyare, H., & Lee, S. (1998). Selective attention to food-related stimuli in hunger: Are attentional biases specific to emotional and psychopathological states, or are they also found in normal drive states? *Behaviour Research and Therapy, 36*(2), 227–237.

Mor, N., & Inbar, M. (2009). Rejection sensitivity and schema-congruent information processing biases. *Journal of Research in Personality, 43,* 392–398.

Moritz, S., Schilling, L., Wingenfeld, K., Köther, U., Wittekind, C., Terfehr, K., et al. (2011). Psychotic-like cognitive biases in borderline personality disorder. *Journal of Behavior Therapy and Experimental Psychiatry, 42,* 349–354.

Napolitano, L., & McKay, D. (2007). Dichotomous thinking in borderline personality disorder. *Cognitive Therapy and Research, 31,* 717–726.

Pretzer, J. (1990). Borderline personality disorder. In T. A. Beck, A. Freeman, & Associates (Eds.), *Cognitive therapy of personality disorders* (pp. 176–207). New York: Guilford Press.

Reeves, M., & Taylor, J. (2007). Specific relationships between core beliefs and personality disorder symptoms in a non-clinical sample. *Clinical Psychology and Psychotherapy, 104,* 96–104.

Renneberg, B., Theobald, E., Nobs, M., & Weisbrod, M. (2005). Autobiographical memory in borderline personality disorder and depression. *Cognitive Therapy and Research, 29,* 343–358.

Schilling, L., Wingenfeld, K., Löwe, B., Moritz, S., Terfehr, K., Köther, U., et al. (2012). Normal mind-reading capacity but higher response confidence in borderline personality disorder patients. *Psychiatry and Clinical Neurosciences, 66*(4), 322–327.

Sieswerda, S., Arntz, A., & Kindt, M. (2007). Successful psychotherapy reduces hypervigilance in borderline personality disorder. *Behavioural and Cognitive Psychotherapy, 35,* 387–402.

Sieswerda, S., Arntz, A., Mertens, I., & Vertommen, S. (2006). Hypervigilance in patients with borderline personality disorder: Specificity, automaticity, and predictors. *Behaviour Research and Therapy, 45*(5), 1011–1024.

Sieswerda, S., Barnow, S., Verheul, R., & Arntz, A. (2013). Neither dichotomous nor split, but schema-related negative interpersonal evaluations characterize borderline patients. *Journal of Personality Disorders, 27,* 36–52.

Specht, M. W., Chapman, A., & Cellucci, T. (2009). Schemas and borderline personality disorder symptoms in incarcerated women. *Journal of Behavior Therapy and Experimental Psychiatry, 40,* 256–264.

Staebler, K., Renneberg, B., Stopsack, M., Fiedler, P., Weiler, M., & Roepke, S. (2011). Facial emotional expression in reaction to social exclusion in borderline personality disorder. *Psychological Medicine, 41,* 1929–1938.

Stopa, L., & Waters, A. (2005). The effect of mood on responses to the Young Schema Questionnaire: Short form. *Psychology and Psychotherapy: Theory, Research, and Practice, 78,* 45–57.

Thimm, J. C. (2010). Mediation of early maladaptive schemas between perceptions of parental rearing style and personality disorder symptoms. *Journal of Behavior Therapy and Experimental Psychiatry, 41,* 52–59.

Tolfree, R. J. (2012). *Do difficulties in mentalizing correlate with severity of borderline personality disorder?* Doctoral dissertation, University College London, London, UK.

van Vreeswijk, M. F., Spinhoven, P., Arntz, A., & Eurelings-Bontekoe, E. (2014). *Cognitive bias modification for patients with cluster-C personality disorder (CBM-IST) a pre-therapy.* Manuscript in preparation.

van Wijk-Herbrink, M. F., Bernstein, D. P., Broers, N. J., Roelofs, J., Rijkeboer, M. M., & Arntz, A. (in press). Internalizing and externalizing behaviors share a common predictor: The effects of early maladaptive schemas are mediated by coping responses and schema modes. *Journal of Abnormal Child Psychology.*

Veen, G., & Arntz, A. (2000). Multidimensional dichotomous thinking characterizes borderline personality disorder. *Cognitive Therapy and Research, 24*(1), 23–45.

Weertman, A., Arntz, A., de Jong, P. J., & Rinck, M. (2008). Implicit self- and other-associations in obsessive–compulsive personality disorder traits. *Cognition and Emotion, 22*(7), 1253–1275.

Weertman, A., Arntz, A., Schouten, E., & Dreessen, L. (2006). Dependent personality traits and information processing: Assessing the interpretation of ambiguous information using the Thematic Apperception Test. *British Journal of Clinical Psychology, 45,* 273–278.

Young, J. E., Arntz, A., Atkinson, T., Lobbestael, J., Weishaar, M. E., van Vreeswijk, M. F., et al. (2007). *The Schema Mode Inventory.* New York: Schema Therapy Institute.

Young, J. E., Klosko, J. S., & Weishaar, M. E. (2003). *Schema therapy: A practitioner's guide.* New York: Guilford Press.

Yovel, I., Revelle, W., & Mineka, S. (2005). Who sees trees before forest?: The obsessive–compulsive style of visual attention. *Psychological Science, 16*(2), 123–129.

Zeigler-Hill, V., Green, B. A., Arnau, R. C., Sisemore, T. B., & Myers, E. M. (2011). Trouble ahead, trouble behind: Narcissism and early maladaptive schemas. *Journal of Behavior Therapy and Experimental Psychiatry, 42,* 96–103.

# CHAPTER 9

# Taking Stock of Relationships among Personality Disorders and Other Forms of Psychopathology

Merav H. Silverman and Robert F. Krueger

When the first edition of *Handbook of Personality Disorders: Theory, Research, and Treatment* was published in 2001, Dolan-Sewell, Krueger, and Shea reviewed a relatively new but growing body of research on the relationships among personality disorders (PDs) and other forms of psychopathology. In particular, they focused on the high rates of comorbidity among these clinical phenomena and the philosophical and practical implications of psychiatric comorbidity. Around this same time, several reviews of comorbidity emerged (Clark, Watson, & Reynolds, 1995; Mineka, Watson, & Clark, 1998), similarly highlighting the prevalence of psychiatric comorbidity across the range of clinical disorders and the impact of comorbidity on conceptualization, treatment, and research on psychopathology. In synthesizing the literature on the comorbidity between PDs and what were then called Axis I disorders, the authors underscored the uneasy relationship between these two categories of psychopathology, which, though presented as unrelated in DSM-III, DSM-III-R, DSM-IV, and DSM-IV-TR seemed to co-occur at rates that were far too high to call them truly distinct.

In the subsequent decade and a half since that publication, the structure of psychopathology and the relationship between personality, PDs, and psychiatric syndromes have become more focal, definitional questions, impacting the ways that psychopathology is researched, treated, funded, and diagnosed. Amid these changing ideas about personality, PDs, and other psychopathology, the largest political organizations in the psychological and psychiatric community, the NIMH (National Institute of Mental Health) and the American Psychiatric Association (APA), have endorsed differing views of psychopathology, impacting the rate and direction of associated changes. The APA, in the classification system presented in DSM-5 (APA, 2013), presents a primarily categorical view of psychopathology, where diagnoses represent putatively distinct categorical clinical phenomena. NIMH, on the other hand, has articulated a new funding rubric, the Research Domain Criteria (RDoC), rejecting the DSM model and advocating for a dimensional view of psychopathology, in which dysfunctions are understood to exist within domains based in neuroscience (Cuthbert, 2014; Insel et al., 2010; Sanislow et al., 2010).

In this chapter, we outline the history of comorbidity research between PDs and other psychiatric disorders. In particular, we focus on the shift from research on bivariate models of comorbidity to the development of a more comprehensive, multivariate metastructure for understanding the interrelated nature of various psychiatric disorders. Next, we explore efforts to employ novel research approaches to help explain the biological bases of observed phenotypic relationships between PDs and other forms of psychopathology. This research has utilized various methodologies, including twin studies, electroencephalography (EEG), and neuroimaging, and these available genetic and neurobiological research strategies are being brought to bear on our understanding of the structure of psychopathology. Last, we briefly discuss the impact of political processes, including the preparation of DSM-5 and RDoC (*www.nimh.nih.gov/about/strategic-planning-reports/index.shtml#strategic-objective1*), on our understanding of the relationships between various psychiatric disorders.

## Placing Comorbidity in Context

The term "comorbidity" is a medical term originally introduced by Feinstein (1970) to describe "any distinct additional clinical entity that has existed or that may occur during the clinical course of a patient who has the index disease under study" (pp. 457). This definition of comorbidity presumes an understanding that illnesses are categorical, that different diseases represent putatively different categories, and membership in a category is determined by having a certain number of prescribed symptoms. Though the concept entered the medical literature in the 1970s, its salience in the psychiatric literature was not realized until the "neo-Kraepelinian" revolution (Blashfield, 1984; Lillienfeld, Waldman, & Israel, 1994), which occurred with the publication of DSM-III (American Psychiatric Association, 1980) and was then further reified in DSM-III-R (American Psychiatric Association, 1987), DSM-IV (American Psychiatric Association, 1994), and DSM-IV-TR (American Psychiatric Association, 2000).

For the past 30 years, the neo-Kraepelinian approach has been dominant, undergirding psychiatric classification, primarily due to the ubiquity of the DSM, both in America and internationally. The neo-Kraepelinian tradition posits that there exist discrete mental illnesses that can be differentiated from one another based on observations of symptoms and signs (Klerman, 1978). DSM-III embodied this model and was distinguished from previous DSMs by introducing empirical rules for diagnoses. This change enabled the development of clinical interviews to assess the presence of psychiatric disorders. In the diagnostic criteria, DSM-III included many exclusionary criteria, operating under the assumption that the presence of a disorder higher on a hierarchy of psychiatric disorders could cause manifestations of lower ranked disorders, and would therefore preclude the diagnosis of a lower disorder. With no known theoretical justification for these rules (Boyd et al., 1984), DSM-III-R dropped these exclusionary criteria. One important outcome of this change was increasing research on the phenomenon of comorbidity, in large part due to the surprisingly high rates of co-occurring psychiatric disorders (Clark, 2005; Clark et al., 1995).

For PDs, the problem of comorbidity with other psychiatric disorders became even more pronounced with DSM-III, which introduced a multi-axial diagnostic system. At the time that DSM-III appeared (1980), the multiaxial system was viewed as a novel way to highlight various aspects of psychopathology that were receiving insufficient attention. It is stated in DSM-III, and repeated in the introduction to DSM-IV (which maintained the multiaxial organization), that "listing of personality disorders . . . on a separate axis ensures that consideration will be given to the possible presence of personality disorders . . . that might otherwise be overlooked when attention is directed to the more florid Axis I disorders" (American Psychiatric Association, 2000, p. 28). Guiding this decision to place PDs on a separate axis was the idea that clinicians doing a patient assessment would be encouraged to go through the five axes, therefore making sure to also assess for PDs (Frances, 1980; Loranger, 1990). While one of the primary goals of this change was to highlight PDs, the multiaxial manual created a system that inherently promoted the diagnosis of both common mental disorders and PDs.

Additionally, DSM-III ushered in a new era in which it became possible to systematically study the rates, prevalence, and co-occurrence of psychiatric disorders (Robins, 1994). Clinical interviews developed using the standardized criteria sets for psychiatric disorders found in DSM made it possible to systematically study the rates of psychiatric diagnoses (Spitzer, Williams, & Skodol, 1980). Large-scale, national studies on psychiatric diagnoses, including the National Comorbidity Survey (based on DSM-III-R categories) (Kessler et al., 1994) and the National Comorbidity Survey Replication (based on DSM-IV) (Kessler et al., 2005), evidenced exceptionally high rates of co-occurrence among psychiatric disorders.

Yet the meaning of these high rates of co-occurrence was not immediately clear. For example, the term "comorbidity" might simply refer to the chance that two disorders co-occur at a certain rate, based on the base rates of both disorders. Hypothetically, if the base rate of borderline personality disorder (BPD) is 50% and the base rate of major depression is 50%, then by chance alone, one would expect that 25% of patients would present with both disorders (50% × 50% = 25%). But research was showing that psychiatric disorders were co-occurring at rates much higher than would be expected by chance alone, indicating that psychiatric disorders were not only co-occurring but were also correlated (Krueger & Markon, 2006).

In the PD literature, the rates of comorbidity were found to be particularly high. Research frequently indicated that most patients with PD met criteria for multiple PDs and typically at least one additional clinical syndrome (Oldham et al., 1995). These results have been replicated a number of times in other clinical (e.g., McGlashan et al., 2000; Widiger & Rogers, 1989), community (Samuels, Nestadt, Romanoski, Folstein, & McHugh, 1994), and epidemiological (Grant et al., 2004) samples, indicating that this finding is not likely a function of sampling from a specific population (e.g., clinical vs. community). It was the rare patient with PD patient who did not meet criteria for a PD and either a second PD or a common mental disorder, calling into question the distinctions between the various PDs and between what was then the Axis I–Axis II divide.

The theoretical implications of these high rates of comorbidity were also concerning. Lilienfeld and colleagues (1994) argued that the term itself was inappropriate given that psychiatric diagnoses often exist as syndromes and rarely are distinct diseases (in the sense of having identified, discrete, and readily distinguished etiologies and pathophysiologies). Accordingly, they argued, our knowledge of psychiatric disorders remains too imprecise to state with certainty that what we call comorbidity is not simply varied manifestations of a latent clinical entity. Maj (2005) noted this problem as well, and added that comorbidity was exacerbated by the rate of proliferation of discrete psychiatric diagnoses in each subsequent edition of the DSM. In many ways, the issue of comorbidity became more than just one of many concerns with DSM, becoming the Achilles heel of the neo-Kraepelinian model articulated in it. As Mineka and colleagues (1998, p. 380) wrote: "The greatest challenge that the extensive comorbidity data pose to the current nosological system concerns the validity of diagnostic categories themselves—do these disorders constitute distinct clinical entities?"

Within the PD literature, people have struggled to understand the implications of comorbidity and polymorbidity (or the co-occurrence of more than just two disorders concurrently). If a person can have only one personality, what does it mean that the modal patient with PD has between two and four PDs (Widiger et al., 1991; Zanarini et al., 1998)? The high rates of co-occurrence of PD and common mental disorders raised the question of what actually differentiates these disorders to warrant separate axes for assessing them. Krueger (2005) evaluated the purported distinctions between the axes, including supposed differences in stability, age of onset, treatment response, insight, and etiology. Reviewing the literature revealed that most of these distinctions were either not supported by research or they lacked the necessary research to establish them.

In addition to the philosophical questions inherent in comorbidity between PDs and other psychiatric disorders, other, more practical concerns arose from the classification system. For example, if a researcher was conducting a treatment study for major depressive disorder (MDD), and wanted to know if a treatment was suitable for treating depression, would it be best to use a sample of "pure" patients (i.e., patients with only a diagnosis of depression; Zimmerman, Mattia, & Posternak, 2002)? Or, given that such patients would be the exception and not the rule, would it be best to use polymorbid patients in treatment studies? Conceptual challenges in classification, therefore, created problems for developing protocols designed to study interventions for categorical diagnoses (Westen, Novotny, & Thompson-Brenner, 2004).

From a clinical standpoint, clinicians have little guidance in how to approach the treatment of a patient with two disorders, let alone three or four disorders, a common clinical phenomenon (Batstra, Box, & Neeleman, 2002; Boyd et al., 1984). In the cases of polymorbid patients, which disorder becomes the focus of treatment (Clarkin & Kendall, 1992) and which treatment is most applicable? Even if there are answers to these questions for specific pairings of disorders (e.g., certain treatments have been developed to target both BPD and substance abuse concurrently; Bohus et al., 2013; Steil, Dyer, Priebe, Kleindienst, & Bohus, 2011), it would be impossible to develop a rubric for treating the multitude of possible comorbidity and polymorbidity patterns between PDs and other psychiatric disorders. Furthermore, despite a robust research literature on treating BPD, there is relatively little evidence-based treatment research on the other PDs (Matusiewicz, Hopwood, Banducci, & Lejuez, 2010). This makes it challenging to think about treating a single PD from an evidence-based perspective, let alone multiple PDs concurrently.

## Bivariate Models of Psychopathology

Several models have been proposed to help explain the excessive comorbidity between PDs and common mental disorders. These models are not necessarily mutually exclusive, but together they have offered compelling explanations for the co-occurrence of PDs and other psychiatric disorders. At least four different explanations of the relationship between personality pathology and other psychiatric disorders have been articulated (Table 9.1; for a longer discussion, see, e.g., Dolan-Sewell et al., 2001; Krueger & Tackett, 2003). These include the predisposition/vulnerability model, the complication/scar model, the pathoplasty/exacerbation model, and the spectrum model. For example, using the spectrum model, Siever and Davis (1991) argued that there are four dimensions to clinical syndromes and personality pathology: cognitive/perceptual organization, impulsivity/aggression, affective instability, and anxiety/inhibition. Extreme abnormalities and discrete symptoms in one of these dimensions might result in diagnosis of a clinical syndrome, whereas a more persistent but perhaps milder disturbance in one of these dimensions might crystallize into a long-standing behavioral and cognitive pattern, which might result in a PD.

Spectral models have been useful for explaining the relationship between a number of PDs and clinical syndromes, outlined by First and colleagues (2002). For example, studies have evidenced a dimensional relationship between schizotypal PD (STPD) and schizophrenia. Paul Meehl suggested this in 1962, when he articulated his model of schizotaxia, in which he argued for a spectrum of psychotic-like behaviors that were familial in nature and had common pathogenetic origins. This finding has received substantial support from genetic, biological, phenomenological, and treatment research confirming the existence of a spectral relationship between STPD and schizophrenia (see First et al., 2002). Similar work has connected social phobia with avoidant PD (AVPD) along a spectrum, with particular evidence from treatment studies and from family studies that suggest higher rates of both social phobia and AVPD among family members of those with social anxiety (Reich, Noyes, & Yates, 1989; Tillfors, Furmark, Ekselius, & Fredrikson, 2001).

Though a spectrum model can help account for the interrelationships between individual PDs and common mental disorders, these bivariate models often fail to explain the complete patterns of comorbid or polymorbid diagnoses with which patients present. For example, where does a patient with depression, social phobia, AVPD, and dependent PD (DPD) fit on a spectrum, and how would these models help one to understand or treat that patient? Thus, despite the importance of bivariate models for adding to our understanding of comorbidity, recent years have seen the growth and proliferation of research on a multivariate model of psychopathology, in which disorders are no longer dis-

**TABLE 9.1. Bivariate Models of PD Comorbidity with Other Psychiatric Disorders**

Predisposition/vulnerability

Presence of a PD or maladaptive traits increase the probability of developing other forms of psychopathology or an additional PD.

Complication/scar

Presence of a psychiatric disorder can serve to "scar" an individual's personality, thereby increasing the likelihood that he or she will develop maladaptive traits or a PD.

Pathoplasty/exacerbation

Presence of a PD, even if it has a distinct etiology or age of onset, can complicate the course, presentation, and treatment of other psychiatric disorders.

Spectrum

PDs and other psychiatric disorders represent different manifestations of the same latent processes and exist along continua with one another.

tinguished by an arguably arbitrary Axis I/Axis II differentiation (indeed, a distinction that was abandoned in the DSM-IV to DSM-5 transition), nor are individual disorders understood along single spectrum. Rather, a multivariate model is useful because it can help explain the ways that multiple disorders cluster together.

## Multivariate Models of Psychopathology

Much of the research on multivariate models of psychopathology has been data-driven and has utilized (and spurred the development of) statistical models capable of accounting for the interrelationships among numerous psychiatric disorders (Krueger & Piasecki, 2002). The liability spectrum model of psychopathology posits that various disorders are understood to stem from a unified, underlying latent factor. This structural model of psychopathology is dimensional, with hierarchical liabilities, internalizing, and externalizing, which together can help explain the systematic covariation among disorders that we refer to as comorbidity (Achenbach, 1966; Krueger, 1999; Krueger, Caspi, Moffitt, & Silva, 1998; Krueger, McGue, & Iacono, 2001; Lahey et al., 2004; Vollebergh et al., 2001). The internalizing and externalizing factors are themselves correlated, explaining the comorbidity between disorders falling in both factors. This gives rise to a general factor of psychopathology, similar to the concept of *g*, for general intelligence. Individuals who score high on this dimension are at a heightened risk for all psychiatric disorders, with differentiation into internalizing or externalizing presentations stemming from factors more specific in their influence (Caspi et al., 2014; Lahey et al., 2012). This general factor of psychopathology is significantly correlated with dispositional negative emotionality in children and adolescents, both genetically and phenotypically, providing a developmental link between personality and the structure of psychopathology (Tackett et al., 2013).

The internalizing factor has been associated with neuroticism/negative emotionality and certain psychiatric disorders including MDD, generalized anxiety disorder (GAD), panic disorder, and phobias. Research indicates that the internalizing factor can be further subdivided into two factors, distress and fear, further distinguishing between disorders such as MDD and GAD and more fear-based disorders, such as phobias, obsessive–compulsive disorder (OCD), and panic disorder (Clark & Watson, 2006; Watson, 2005). The externalizing factor has also been associated with neuroticism/negative emotionality (helping to explain the correlations between internalizing and externalizing disorders), but is also characterized by disinhibitory personality traits. The externalizing factor includes substance abuse disorders, attention-deficit/hyperactivity disorder (ADHD), oppositional defiant disorder (ODD), antisocial personality disorder (ASPD), and conduct disorder.

While this model of psychopathology was originally limited to disorders that occurred frequently enough in the population to be included in quantitative models, recent years have seen both the replication (Slade & Watson, 2006) and expansion of the model to include a third dimension of psychosis or thought disorder, which has helped to account for phenotypic correlations between STPD and schizophrenia (Kotov et al., 2011). This structural model of psychopathology has accommodated other, less frequent disorders, such as such as eating disorders, which seem to fall as subfactors within the internalizing factor (Forbush et al., 2010). In addition to encompassing a wide array of psychiatric disorders and helping to explain the phenotypic presentation of comorbidity, this structural model of psychopathology has been found to be applicable cross-culturally, underscoring its utility as a model for classification (Krueger, Chentsova-Dutton, Markon, Goldberg, & Ormel, 2003). The flexibility of the model has meant that, to date, with sufficient observations in a given sample, a number of psychiatric disorders have successfully been located within the structure.

Instead of attempting to explain the interrelationship between distinct categorical diagnoses that are comorbid, this structural model of psychopathology argues that comorbidity in fact stems from common psychopathological processes. This has been particularly useful in explaining the interrelationships between various PDs and common mental disorders. Using a novel, symptom-level analysis of PDs and clinical syndromes, Markon (2010) found replication of the internalizing–externalizing metastructure, with two other factors, thought disorder and pathological introversion. Various symptoms of PDs and other forms of psychopathology fit into the same superordinate structure, providing evidence for the close structural relationship between symptoms of PDs and symptoms of other psychiatric disorders.

Furthermore, this structural model of psychopathology maps onto what we know about the basic structure of personality and helps to better integrate personality and psychopathology, both of which have historically operated in separate research traditions (Clark, 2005; O'Connor, 2002). Continuity between normal and abnormal personality has been shown in a number of ways, but one important example includes the continuum of the Big Five personality traits (Neuroticism, Agreeableness, Conscientiousness, Extraversion, and Openness) across normal and abnormal personality (Markon, Krueger, & Watson, 2005). This Big Five model proved important for the development of the DSM-5 trait model, which we discuss later. While a further exploration of the role of basic personality in psychopathology and PDs is beyond the scope of this chapter, it is important to state briefly the utility of the structural model in tying together these literatures, helping to enrich the conversation about abnormal functioning, using the wealth of research on normal personality (Harkness, Reynolds, & Lilienfeld, 2014; Widiger, 2011; Widiger & Costa, 2002, 2012).

## Reframing PDs and Clinical Syndromes Using Biological Evidence

In addition to quantitative evidence for a hierarchical model of psychopathology, a number of useful biological methods have been applied to better understand the structure of psychopathology, and continue to enrich this field. The search for endophenotypes (Gottesman & Gould, 2003) has helped to strengthen the argument for latent liabilities underlying broad aspects of personality and psychopathology. The discovery of shared biological liabilities has helped to better explain the relationship between PDs and common mental disorders.

One fruitful area of research has been the use of event-related potentials (ERPs), measured using EEG, to identify shared pathophysiology across multiple disorders. Certain ERPs have been identified as potential endophenotypes and are therefore useful for studying psychiatric disorders. For example, individuals with a broad range of behaviors and traits characterized by behavioral disinhibition, such as substance abuse, conduct disorder, and antisocial behavior (captured in ASPD), evidence reduced P300 amplitude in response to visual oddball tasks (Iacono, Malone, & McGue, 2008; Patrick et al., 2006). Research indicates that the P300 ERP, in general, is related to attention, memory, and inhibition of superfluous brain activation, thereby serving as a marker of efficient processing (Polich, 2007). This shared reduction in the P300 ERP serves as a biomarker across psychiatric conditions, providing biological evidence for a common neural deficit spanning disorders across the externalizing spectrum.

Similarly, altered error-related negativity (ERN), an ERP related to performance errors on speeded tasks, has been found across a number disorders. The ERN is believed to measure brain activation in the anterior cingulate cortex in response to error processing. During speeded up tasks, where subjects are bound to make errors (e.g., the color Stroop task, the go/no-go task), the ERN is detected immediately following an error. Spanning a number of internalizing disorders, research has shown an increased ERN peak, whereas reduced ERN has been found in certain externalizing disorders, such as substance use and impulsive personality traits (Hall, Bernat, & Patrick, 2007; Olvet & Hajcak, 2008). Evidence suggests increased ERN might be associated with nonphobic anxiety disorders, such as OCD or GAD, but not with phobic anxiety disorders (Vaidyanathan, Nelson, & Patrick, 2012). This may provide biological support for the differentiation of the fear and distress subfactors found within the internalizing factor. Using biomarkers found in EEG studies, it is possible to gain information about the quantitative and dimensional model of psychopathology, and to help better locate personality traits in the context of other features of psychopathology, such as maladaptive behaviors and cognitions.

Research on the etiology of psychiatric disorders, using twin studies, has been useful in confirming aspects of the dimensional model of psychopathology, by showing that genetic liabilities for psychiatric disorders align with the metastructure of psychopathology. With a twin study design, it is possible to model patterns of psychopathology among individuals with different levels of relatedness (i.e., monozygotic [MZ] vs. dyzygotic [DZ] twins). For example, if features of ASPD and alcohol dependence are more likely to co-occur in MZ twins than in DZ twins, controlling for potential environmental differences, it becomes possible to argue that externalizing disorders, regardless of the specific categorical diagnosis, are likely to some degree genetic in origin (Krueger & Markon, 2006). This method has been particularly useful in establishing a genetic component of the internalizing and externalizing spectra.

Kendler, Prescott, Myers, and Neale (2003) found that genetic influences replicate the dimensional, quantitatively derived internalizing–externalizing structure of psychopathology, which is seen phenotypically. Thus, if one twin has an internalizing disorder, the co-twin is more likely to also be diagnosed with a disorder from the internalizing spectrum. Furthermore, an MZ co-twin would have a higher likelihood of having an externalizing diagnosis than would a DZ co-twin, indicating a genetic contribution beyond their shared environment. A general vulnerability for externalizing disorders indicates that an underlying pathological process, likely characterized by behavioral undercontrol, confers high and shared vulnerability across a number of externalizing disorders (substance abuse, conduct disorder, and antisocial behavior; Hicks, Krueger, Iacono, McGue, & Patrick, 2004).

Twin studies also help explain the high rates of comorbidity seen among PDs and between PDs and other forms of psychopathology. Studies have found shared genetic risk for negative emotionality underlying all PDs, regardless of what cluster (A, B, or C) and shared risk for PDs and other common disorders (Kendler et al., 2008; Reichborn-Kjennerud et al., 2010). In a large-scale analysis including 22 psychiatric disorders from the Axis I and Axis II sections of DSM-IV-TR, Kendler and colleagues (2011) found evidence for genetic risk for PDs and for other psychiatric disorders that reflected the internalizing–externalizing structure. These findings indicate that the etiology of psychiatric disorders follows the same organization as that obtained from the hierarchical structural model of psychopathology found using data-driven, quantitative modeling. Furthermore, these results from twin study designs support the idea that the underlying liability for PDs and other psychiatric disorders is shared genetically, with specific personality traits, such as neuroticism, at the core of many forms of psychopathology (Livesley & Jang, 2008).

Larger sample sizes and emerging neuroimaging techniques provide promise for better understanding the relationships between various psychiatric diagnoses. Historically, most of the functional neuroimaging research in psychopathology has been task-based, generally involving a single disorder, with a single functional task meant to highlight altered functioning in a specific patient group during that task. In many ways, this primarily has allowed for the use of univariate models (using regression) to explain relationships between psychopathology and brain function, but it has not been as useful in shedding light on the interrelationships between psychiatric diseases and varied aspects of brain activation.

Furthermore, usage of tasks to learn about diseases, and even specific symptoms, has not allowed us to articulate the diversity of a single deficit. For example, in schizophrenia, even a single symptom, such as auditory hallucinations, is not specific to a single brain area (Jardri, Pouchet, Pins, & Thomas, 2011). Thus, while functional magnetic resonance imaging (fMRI) during tasks has shed light on the nature of psychopathology, there are limitations in our ability to understand the structure of symptoms and single disorders, as well as the larger interrelationships between disorders.

Developments in clinical neuroscience have opened the doors to using a multivariate approach to studying the relationship between brain activation patterns and psychopathology (Hyman, 2007). With novel methods for studying connectivity in the absence of a specific task, for example, using functional scans during rest, larger sample sizes can be accrued across multiple sites, not requiring the same task be administered to all subjects. This helps circumvent the current high cost of neuroimaging. This is a similar strategy to that employed in genetics research, in which large-scale collaborations allow for the sample sizes necessary for conducting relevant and well-powered research (Ioannidis, Trikalinos, Ntzani, & Contopoulos-Ioannidis, 2003). Integrated neuroimaging projects, such as the Human Connectome Project (Barch et al., 2013; Van Essen et al., 2013), have enabled the development of collaborative, large-scale studies. Using these larger datasets, it is possible to use neuroimaging to study multivariate models, enabling further testing of these theories. Using connectivity methods in neuroimaging, it is possible to break down complicated interrelationships into component pieces, allowing better understanding of the patterns of neural connectivity underlying the internalizing and externalizing spectra.

## Give Change a Chance

Given the quantitative and biological evidence, the theoretical difficulties, and the practical challenges for treatment and research engendered by the classification system in previous DSMs, DSM-5 has provided an opportunity for redrawing the lines in psychiatric classification in a way that better reflects nature. At the outset of the DSM-5 process, there was openness to novel approaches to classification. In *A Research Agenda for DSM-V,* Rounsaville and colleagues (2002) noted that research called into question the idea that there are natural boundaries between psychiatric disorders and normal functioning, The authors suggested the importance of developing dimensional systems of classification for certain psychiatric disorders. In 2009, as research for DSM-5 was well under way, this sentiment was reiterated by the chair and vice-chair of the task force for DSM-5, David Kupfer and Darrel Regier, when they wrote that "the single most important precondition for moving forward to improve the clinical and scientific utility of DSM-V will be the incorporation of simple dimensional measures for assessing syndromes within broad diagnostic categories and supraordinate dimensions that cross current diagnostic boundaries" (Regier, Narrow, Kuhl, & Kupfer, 2009, p. 649)

The area of PDs was ripe for reexamination, with additional conceptual problems aside from pervasive comorbidity, including arbitrary criteria cutoffs, instability in the diagnoses over time, and confusion as to the Axis I–Axis II distinction (Widiger & Trull, 2007). As a result of these classification issues, the DSM-5 PD development process began with a focus on dimensional alternatives to the DSM-IV categorical model (Widiger & Simonsen, 2005). As time progressed and the official DSM-5 Personality and PD Work Group was appointed in 2007, there continued to be a willingness to consider new ideas. This openness, though, ultimately resulted in a somewhat chaotic process that was amplified by its availability to the public online, at *www.dsm5.org.* At varying points during the process, there were proposals for a purely dimensional model of PDs, a hybrid model between dimensions and categories, a model that utilized narrative prototypes of PDs, and a model that maintained only specific categorical PD diagnoses, with the specific retained diagnoses varying in different iterations.

Amid this confusion, there were efforts to operationalize core elements of PD, resulting in the DSM-5 trait model (APA, 2013, p. 773; Krueger, Derringer, Markon, Watson, & Skodol, 2012). This model was developed iteratively, using data collected from both community and clinical samples. The data-derived trait model reiterated what had been captured in earlier research, replicating the continuum between abnormal and normal personality traits. Specifically, the five domains of maladaptive personality that were derived (negative affect, detachment, antagonism, disinhibition, and psychoticism), mapped onto the five-factor model, as well as the maladaptive variants of the Big Five (the Personality Psychopathology Five [PSY-5]— Anderson et al., 2013; Harkness & McNulty, 1994; Widiger & Costa, 2012) and the Big Four of personality pathology, measured using the Dimensional Assessment of Personality Pathology—Basic Questionnaire (DAPP-BQ—Livesley, Jang, & Vernon, 1998; Van den Broeck et al., 2014).

Along with the trait model presented in DSM-5 is an assessment instrument (the Personality Inventory for DSM-5 [PID-5]; Krueger et al., 2012; available at *www.psychiatry.org/practice/dsm/dsm5/online-assessment-measures#level2*) that has since become freely available to clinicians and researchers. The availability of the PID-5 distinguishes it from other personality inventories, such as the NEO Five-Factor Inventory (NEO-FFI), many of which belong to specific test publishers (Costa & McCrae, 1992) and makes it possible for researchers and clinicians to assess dimensions of personality using a freely available instrument.

The work group ultimately proposed a hybrid model for DSM-5, which included six specific PDs and could account for other personality pathology beyond these six in the context of the trait model. The hybrid model has two criteria: Criterion A requires problems in functioning ("difficulties establishing coherent working models of self and others"), and Criterion B requires the presence of maladaptive personality traits, which are described in the trait model and assessed using the PID-5. This hybrid approach was designed to preserve features of DSM-IV and to allow for an easier transition between a categorical and a dimensional model. Ultimately, the DSM-5 Task Force supported inclusion of the hybrid model in Section II of DSM-5, but the APA Board of Trustees overruled the Task

Force, deciding to maintain the DSM-IV-TR PD section verbatim in Section II (Diagnostic Criteria and Codes). The "hybrid model" developed for DSM-5 is described in Section III (consisting of Emerging Measures and Models).

A dimensional, trait model of PDs helps to provide a framework for accommodating comorbidity among various forms of psychopathology. Better understanding of personality functioning in all psychiatric patients is useful for case conceptualization and treatment of all forms of psychopathology (Krueger, Hopwood, Wright, & Markon, 2014). For example, the relationship between neuroticism and psychopathology has been well documented. Research indicates that knowledge of an individual's level of neuroticism can be predictive of new onsets of psychiatric disorders, treatment utilization, and treatment outcome (Lahey, 2009; Ormel et al., 2013). Personality traits have been shown to modify the length and severity of depression and treatment response in social phobia (Cain, Pincus, & Grosse Holtforth, 2010; Cain et al., 2012). Notably, personality traits are even more highly correlated with common mental disorders than with PDs, partially due to the heterogeneous nature of PD criteria, but also due to the strong relationship between personality traits and clinical disorders (Kotov, Gamez, Schmidt, & Watson, 2010).

Despite concern that moving to a trait model would transform PDs, so as to make PDs assessed using a trait model entirely different than those assessed using the categorical model (Gunderson, 2010), early research evidences a large degree of overlap and high correlations between these diagnostic methods (Miller, Few, Lynam, & MacKillop, 2014; Samuel, Hopwood, Krueger, Thomas, & Ruggero, 2013). Furthermore, examining just BPD and ASPD (the two most heavily researched PDs), Yalch, Thomas, and Hopwood (2012) found good convergent validity with the categorical approach currently found in DSM-5 Section II and better criterion-related validity to other measures of functioning. Furthermore, the trait model reproduces the interrelationships between PDs seen using categorical assessment, indicating that the trait model captures not only the PDs themselves but also the network of PDs.

In addition to the inclusion of a dimensional model of PDs, another major change in DSM-5 was the discontinuation of the multiaxial system, placing PDs and intellectual disabilities among the other clinical syndromes. Responding to the limited research supporting the multiaxial system and the high rates of comorbidity that this system fostered, the DSM-5 Task Force changed the organization to make it more consistent with research on the metastructure of psychopathology. Thus, chapters consisting of internalizing disorders are grouped together, as are chapters consisting of externalizing disorders. Chapter layout and order, therefore, reflects the rates of comorbidity and premorbid risk factors for developing clusters of psychopathology (Regier, Kuhl, & Kupfer, 2013).

Coinciding with the preparation of DSM-5, and in large part resulting from the widely acknowledged shortcomings of the classification system presented by DSM, the NIMH articulated its own model for how it would evaluate psychiatric research for funding moving forward. In 2008, the NIMH presented its new aims, specifically, to "develop, for research purposes, new ways of classifying mental disorders based on dimensions of observable behavior and neurobiological measures (*www.nimh.nih.gov/about/strategic-planning-reports/index.shtml#strategic-objective1*). This became the basis for the RdoC, which aims to fund research that is not tethered by the faulty, categorical disease constructs presented in DSM (Insel et al., 2010). RDoC delineates five domains of functioning, including positive valence, negative valence, cognition, social processes, and arousal/regulatory systems, all of which are conceptualized dimensionally and based in concepts from cognitive neuroscience. Instead of focusing on disorders, or even on specific clinical phenomena, RDoC appears to catalogue our understanding of psychiatric illness in terms of genes, neural systems, cognitive and affective systems, and symptoms (Cuthbert & Kozak, 2013). In particular, though, RDoC has emphasized research on neural circuits as the basis for psychiatric disorders.

Inasmuch as RDoC has tried to address the shortcomings of the DSM classification system by developing a model for research based on dimensions and domains, it has been criticized for going too far in the other direction, and for being overly reductionistic, to the detriment of other important psychological indicators. For one thing, the domains and dimensions on which RDoC focuses are essentially areas of research for cognitive neuroscientists. Though these are important research areas, they lack a clear connection to clinical phenomena (Fava, 2014; First, 2014; Jablensky & Waters, 2014; Weinberger & Goldberg, 2014). In an explicit attempt not to mention DSM constructs, RDoC precludes important avenues of research pertaining to concrete manifestations of mental illness. For example, a study on suicide or self-injury, though obviously a necessary area of study for mental health and a cross-cutting symptom of both PDs and common mental disorders, does not necessarily fit within the RDoC rubric.

To date, the evidence does not suggest that psychopathology can easily be reduced to one level of analysis, namely, neurobiology, as RDoC seems to propose. As Berenbaum (2013, p. 894) says, "Etiological factors (e.g., genetic, neural, cognitive, interpersonal, and sociocultural) all appear to account for at least moderate proportions of variance" in psychopathology. Unlike other medical diseases, such as cystic fibrosis, in which the etiology can be reduced to mutation at the gene level, Kendler (2012) argues that the etiology and course of psychopathology is "fuzzy," with various cross-level mechanisms operating. Thus, while RDoC encourages movement in the right direction, with the benefit of being outside of the politicized DSM process, there are costs associated with the RDoC approach, including no direct connections to concepts with which people are familiar (e.g., DSM rubrics) and an emphasis on neurobiology to the relative exclusion of other aspects.

So where does this leave us? In many ways, it seems like we are getting closer to an understanding of the latent constructs of psychopathology with sophisticated statistical and biological methods at our disposal. Yet the field seems more fractured than before, particularly with NIMH and APA heading in different directions. Reminiscent of the mood at the opening of *The Divine Comedy*, "Midway along the journey of our life, I woke to find myself in a dark wood, for I had wandered off from the straight path." The path from here is not straight and the future for psychopathology research, treatment, and classification is not readily apparent.

And yet, this moment does not augur an ominous future for the field. Rather, at a point of midlife crisis for the relatively new science of psychopathology, there are many things to be excited and optimistic about. Now is a time when people are actively thinking about these basic questions about psychopathology and personality, and what it means to study mental illness and to suffer from mental illness. People are tackling these questions from a philosophical level, as well as from quantitative and biological perspectives. The issue of comorbidity has evolved from a single conceptual hurdle to our classification system, to a rallying cry for devoting more time and energy to understanding psychopathology. Thus, while the future is somewhat unclear, it is also a moment in time when renewed energy and thought about the classification of PDs, personality, and psychopathology more generally can help shape our conceptions of these constructs moving forward. PDs represent the forefront of this vibrant moment in the field of psychopathology. Integrative research has brought together scholars from a wide array of disciplines; by including psychology, statistics, and neuroscience, and using a variety of methodologies, they are shedding light on our understanding of the nature of these disorders.

# REFERENCES

Achenbach, T. M. (1966). The classification of children's psychiatric symptoms: A factor-analytic study. *Psychological Monographs, 80,* 1–37.

American Psychiatric Association. (1980). *Diagnostic and statistical manual of mental disorders* (3rd ed.). Washington, DC: Author.

American Psychiatric Association. (1987). *Diagnostic and statistical manual of mental disorders* (3rd ed., rev.). Washington, DC: Author.

American Psychiatric Association. (1994). *Diagnostic and statistical manual of mental disorders* (4th ed.). Washington, DC: Author.

American Psychiatric Association. (2000). *Diagnostic and statistical manual of mental disorders* (4th ed., text rev.). Washington, DC: Author.

American Psychiatric Association. (2013). *Diagnostic and statistical manual of mental disorders* (5th ed.). Arlington, VA: Author.

Anderson, J. L., Sellbom, M., Bagby, R. M., Quilty, L. C., Veltri, C. O., Markon, K. E., et al. (2013). On the convergence between PSY-5 domains and PID-5 domains and facets implications for assessment of DSM-5 personality traits. *Assessment, 20,* 286–294.

Barch, D. M., Burgess, G. C., Harms, M. P., Petersen, S. E., Schlaggar, B. L., Corbetta, M., et al. (2013). Function in the human connectome: Task-fMRI and individual differences in behavior. *NeuroImage, 80,* 169–189.

Batstra, L., Bos, E. H., & Neeleman, J. (2002). Quantifying psychiatric comorbidity: Lessons from chronic disease epidemiology. *Social Psychiatry and Psychiatric Epidemiology, 37,* 105–111.

Berenbaum, H. (2013). Classification and psychopathology research. *Journal of Abnormal Psychology, 122,* 894–901.

Blashfield, R. K. (1984). *Classification of psychopathology: Neo-Kraepelinian and quantitative approaches.* New York: Plenum Press.

Bohus, M., Dyer, A. S., Priebe, K., Krüger, A., Kleindienst, N., Schmahl, C., et al. (2013). Dialectical behaviour therapy for post-traumatic stress disorder after childhood sexual abuse in patients with and without borderline personality disorder: A randomised controlled trial. *Psychotherapy and Psychosomatics, 82,* 221–233.

Boyd, J. H., Burke, J. D., Jr., Gruenberg, E., Holzer, C. E., III, Rae, D. S., George, L. K., et al. (1984). Exclusion criteria of DSM-III: A study of co-occurrence of hierarchy-free syndromes. *Archives of General Psychiatry, 41,* 983–989.

Cain, N. M., Ansell, E. B., Wright, A. G. C., Hopwood, C. J., Thomas, K. M., Pinto, A. N., et al. (2012). Interpersonal pathoplasticity in the course of major depression. *Journal of Consulting and Clinical Psychology, 80,* 78–86.

Cain, N. M., Pincus, A. L., & Grosse Holtforth, M. (2010). Interpersonal subtypes in social phobia: Diagnostic and treatment implications. *Journal of Personality Assessment, 92,* 514–527.

Caspi, A., Houts, R. M., Belsky, D. W., Goldman-Mellor, S. J., Harrington, H., Israel, S., et al. (2014). The p factor: One general psychopathology factor in the structure of psychiatric disorders. *Clinical Psychological Science, 2,* 119–137.

Clark, L. A. (2005). Temperament as a unifying basis for personality and psychopathology. *Journal of Abnormal Psychology, 114,* 505–521.

Clark, L. A., & Watson, D. (2006). Distress and fear disorders: An alternative empirically based taxonomy of the "mood" and "anxiety" disorders. *British Journal of Psychiatry, 189,* 481–483.

Clark, L. A., Watson, D., & Reynolds, S. (1995). Diagnosis and classification of psychopathology: Challenges to the current system and future directions. *Annual Review of Psychology, 46,* 121–153.

Clarkin, J. F., & Kendall, P. C. (1992). Comorbidity and treatment planning: Summary and future directions. *Journal of Consulting and Clinical Psychology, 60,* 904–908.

Costa, P. T., & McCrae, R. R. (1992). Normal personality assessment in clinical practice: The NEO Personality Inventory. *Psychological Assessment, 4,* 5–13.

Cuthbert, B. N. (2014). The RDoC framework: Facilitating transition from ICD/DSM to dimensional approaches that integrate neuroscience and psychopathology. *World Psychiatry, 13,* 28–35.

Cuthbert, B. N., Kozak, M. J. (2013). Constructing constructs of psychopathology: The NIHM Research Domain Criteria. *Journal of Abnormal Psychology, 122,* 928–937.

Dolan-Sewell, R. T., Krueger, R. F., & Shea, M. T. (2001). Co-occurrence with syndrome disorders. In W. J. Livesley (Ed.), *Handbook of personality disorders: Theory, research, and treatment* (pp. 84–104). New York: Guilford Press.

Fava, G. A. (2014). Road to nowhere. *World Psychiatry, 13,* 49–50.

Feinstein, A. R. (1970). The pre-therapeutic classification of co-morbidity in chronic disease. *Journal of Chronic Diseases, 23,* 455–468.

First, M. B. (2014). Preserving the clinician-researcher interface in the age of RDoC: The continuing need for DSM-5/ICD-11 characterization of study populations. *World Psychiatry, 13,* 53–54.

First, M. B., Bell, C. C., Cuthbert, B., Krystal, J. H., Malison, R., Offord, D. R., et al. (2002). Personality disorders and relational disorders: A research agenda for addressing crucial gaps in DSM. In D. J. Kupfer, M. B. First, & D. A. Regier (Eds.), *A research agenda for DSM-V* (pp. 123–200). Washington, DC: American Psychiatric Publishing.

Forbush, K. T., South, S. C., Krueger, R. F., Iacono, W. G., Clark, L. A., Keel, P. K., et al. (2010). Locating eating pathology within an empirical diagnostic taxonomy: Evidence from a community-based sample. *Journal of Abnormal Psychology, 119,* 282–292.

Frances, A. (1980). The DSM-III personality disorders section: A commentary. *American Journal of Psychiatry, 137,* 1050–1054.

Gottesman, I. I., & Gould, T. D. (2003). The endophenotype concept in psychiatry: Etymology and strategic intentions. *American Journal of Psychiatry, 160,* 636–645.

Grant, B. F., Stinson, F. S., Dawson, D. A., Chou, S. P., Ruan, W. J., & Pickering, R. P. (2004). Co-occurrence of 12-month alcohol and drug use disorders and personality disorders in the United States. *Archives of General Psychiatry, 61,* 361–368.

Gunderson, J. (2010). Revising the borderline diagnosis for DSM-V: An alternative proposal. *Journal of Personality Disorders, 24,* 694–708.

Hall, J. R., Bernat, E. M., & Patrick, C. J. (2007). Externalizing psychopathology and the error-related negativity. *Psychological Science, 18,* 326–333.

Harkness, A. R., & McNulty, J. L. (1994). The Personality Psychopathology Five (PSY-5): Issue from the pages of a diagnostic manual instead of a dictionary. In S. Strack & M. Lorr (Eds.), *Differentiating normal and abnormal personality* (pp. 291–315). New York: Springer.

Harkness, A. R., Reynolds, S. M., & Lillienfeld, S. O. (2014). A review of systems for psychology and psychiatry: Adaptive systems, Personality and Psychopathology Five (PSY-5), and the DSM-5. *Journal of Personality Assessment, 96,* 121–139.

Hicks, B. M., Krueger, R. F., Iacono, W. G., McGue, M., & Patrick, C. J. (2004). Family transmission and heritability of externalizing disorders: A twin-family study. *Archives of General Psychiatry, 61,* 922–928.

Hyman, S. E. (2007). Can neuroscience be integrated into the DSM-V? *Nature Reviews Neuroscience, 8,* 725–732.

Iacono, W. G., Malone, S. M., & McGue, M. (2008). Behavioral disinhibition and the development of early-onset addition: Common and specific influences. *Annual Reviews of Clinical Psychology, 4,* 325–348.

Insel, T., Cuthbert, B., Garvey, M., Heinssen, R., Pine, D. S., Quinn, K., et al. (2010). Research domain criteria (RDoC): Toward a new classification framework for research on mental disorders. *American Journal of Psychiatry, 167,* 748–751.

Ioannidis, J. P. A., Trikalinos, T. A., Ntzani, E. E., & Contopoulos-Ioannidis, D. G. (2003). Genetic associations in large versus small studies: An empirical assessment. *Lancet, 361,* 567–571.

Jablensky, A., & Waters, F. (2014). RDoC: A roadmap to pathogenesis? *World Psychiatry, 13,* 43–44.

Jardri, R., Pouchet, A., Pins, D., & Thomas, P. (2011). Cortical activations during auditory verbal hallucinations in schizophrenia: A coordinate-based meta-analysis. *American Journal of Psychiatry, 168*(1), 73–81.

Kendler, K. S. (2012). Levels of explanation in psychiatric and substance use disorders: Implications for the development of an etiologically based nosology. *Molecular Psychiatry, 17,* 11–21.

Kendler, K. S., Aggen, S. H., Czajkowski, N., Røysamb, E., Tambs, K., Torgersen, S., et al. (2008). The structure of genetic and environmental risk factors for DSM-IV personality disorders: A multivariate twin study. *Archives of General Psychiatry, 65,* 1438–1446.

Kendler, K. S., Aggen, S. H., Knudsen, G. P., Rysamb, E., Neale, M. C., & Reichborn-Kjennerud, T. (2011). The structure of genetic and environmental risk factors for syndromal and subsyndromal common DSM-IV Axis I and Axis II disorders. *American Journal of Psychiatry, 168,* 29–39.

Kendler, K. S., Prescott, C. A., Myers, J., & Neale, M. C. (2003). The structure of genetic and environmental risk factors for common psychiatric and substance use disorders in men and women. *Archives of General Psychiatry, 60,* 929–937.

Kessler, R. C., Berglund, P., Demler, O., Jin, R., Merikangas, K. R., & Walters, E. E. (2005). Lifetime prevalence and age-of-onset distributions of DSM-IV disorders in the National Comorbidity Survey Replication. *Archives of General Psychiatry, 62,* 593–602.

Kessler, R. C., McGonagle, K. A., Zhao, S., Nelson, C. B., Hughes, M., Eshleman, S., et al. (1994). Lifetime and 12-month prevalence of DSM-III-R psychiatric disorders in the United States: Results from the National Comorbidity Survey. *Archives of General Psychiatry, 51*(1), 8–19.

Klerman, G. L. (1978). The evolution of a scientific nosology. In J. C. Shershow (Ed.), *Schizophrenia: Science and practice* (pp. 99–121). Cambridge, MA: Harvard University Press.

Kotov, R., Chang, S. W., Fochtmann, L. J., Mojtabai, R., Carlson, G. A., Sedler, M. J., et al. (2011). Schizophrenia in the internalizing–externalizing framework: A third dimension. *Schizophrenia Bulletin, 37,* 1168–1178.

Kotov, R., Gamez, W., Schmidt, F., & Watson, D. (2010). Linking "big" personality traits to anxiety, depressive, and substance use disorders: A meta-analysis. *Psychological Bulletin, 136,* 768–821.

Krueger, R. F. (1999). The structure of common mental disorders. *Archives of General Psychiatry, 56*(10), 921–926.

Krueger, R. F. (2005). Continuity of Axes I and II: Toward a unified model of personality, personality disorders, and clinical disorders. *Journal of Personality Disorders, 19,* 233–261.

Krueger, R. F., Caspi, A., Moffitt, T. E., & Silva, P. A. (1998). The structure and stability of common mental disorders (DSM-III): A longitudinal-epidemiological study. *Journal of Abnormal Psychology, 107*(2), 216–227.

Krueger, R. F., Chentsova-Dutton, Y. E., Markon, K. E., Goldberg, D., & Ormel, J. (2003). A cross-cultural study of the structure of comorbidity among common psychopathological syndromes in the general health care setting. *Journal of Abnormal Psychology, 112,* 437–447.

Krueger, R. F., Derringer, J., Markon, K. E., Watson, D., & Skodol, A. E. (2012). Initial construction of a maladaptive personality trait model and inventory for DSM-5. *Psychological Medicine, 42*(9), 1879–1890.

Krueger, R. F., Hopwood, C. J., Wright, A. G. C., Markon, K. E. (2014). DSM-5 and the path toward empirically based and clinically useful conceptualization of personality and psychopathology. *Clinical Psychology: Science and Practice, 21*(3), 245–261.

Krueger, R. F., & Markon, K. E. (2006). Reinterpreting comorbidity: A model-based approach to understanding and classifying psychopathology. *Annual Review of Clinical Psychology, 2,* 111–133.

Krueger, R. F., McGue, M., & Iacono, W. G. (2001). The higher-order structure of common DSM mental disorders: Internalization, externalization, and their connections to personality. *Personality and Individual Differences, 30*(7), 1245–1259.

Krueger, R. F., & Piasecki, T. M. (2002). Toward a dimensional and psychometrically-informed approach to conceptualizing psychopathology. *Behaviour Research and Therapy, 40*(5), 485–499.

Krueger, R. F., & Tackett, J. L. (2003). Personality and psychopathology: Working toward the bigger picture [Special issue]. *Journal of Personality Disorders, 17*(2), 109–128.

Lahey, B. B. (2009). Public health significance of neuroticism. *American Psychologist, 64*(4), 241–256.

Lahey, B. B., Applegate, B., Hakes, J. K., Zald, D. H., Hariri, A. R., & Rathouz, P. J. (2012). Is there a general factor of prevalent psychopathology during adulthood? *Journal of Abnormal Psychology, 121,* 971–977.

Lahey, B. B., Applegate, B., Waldman, I. D., Loft, J. D., Hankin, B. L., & Rick, J. (2004). The structure of child and adolescent psychopathology: Generating new hypotheses. *Journal of Abnormal Psychology, 113,* 358–385.

Lilienfeld, S. O., Waldman, I. D., & Israel, A. C. (1994). A critical examination of the use of the term and concept of comorbidity in psychopathology research. *Clinical Psychology: Science and Practice, 1,* 71–83.

Livesley, W. J., & Jang, K. L. (2008). The behavioral genetics of personality disorder. *Annual Review of Clinical Psychology, 4,* 247–274.

Livesley, W. J., Jang, K. L., & Vernon, P. A. (1998). Phenotypic and genetic structure of traits delineating personality disorder. *Archives of General Psychiatry, 55,* 941–948.

Loranger, A. W. (1990). The impact of DSM-III on diagnostic practice in a university hospital: A comparison of DSM-II and DSM-III in 10,914 patients. *Archives of General Psychiatry, 47*(7), 672–675.

Maj, M. (2005). "Psychiatric comorbidity": An artefact of current diagnostic systems? *British Journal of Psychiatry, 186,* 182–184.

Markon, K. E. (2010). Modeling psychopathology structure: A symptom-level analysis of Axis I and II disorders. *Psychological Medicine, 12,* 273–288.

Markon, K. E., Krueger, R. F., & Watson, D. (2005). Delineating the structure of normal and abnormal personality: An integrative hierarchical approach. *Journal of Personality and Social Psychology, 88*(1), 139–157.

Matusiewicz, A. K., Hopwood, C. J., Banducci, A. N., & Lejuez, C. W. (2010). The effectiveness of cognitive behavioral therapy for personality disorders. *Psychiatric Clinics of North America, 33,* 657–685.

McGlashan, T. H., Grilo, C. M., Skodol, A. E., Gunderson, J. G., Shea, M. T., Morey, L. C., et al. (2000). The Collaborative Longitudinal Personality Disorders Study: Baseline Axis I/II and II/II diagnostic co-occurrence. *Acta Psychiatrica Scandinavica, 102,* 256–264.

Meehl, P. E. (1962). Schizotaxia, schizotypy, schizophrenia. *American Psychologist, 17,* 827–838.

Miller, J. D., Few, L. R., Lynam, D. R., & MacKillop, J. (2014). Pathological personality traits can capture DSM-IV personality disorder types. *Personality Disorders: Theory, Research, and Treatment, 6*(1), 32–40.

Mineka, S., Watson, D., & Clark, L. A. (1998). Comorbidity of anxiety and unipolar mood disorders. *Annual Review of Psychology, 49,* 377–412.

O'Connor, B. P. (2002). The search for dimensional structure differences between normality and abnormality: A statistical review of published data on personality and psychopathology. *Journal of Personality and Social Psychology, 83,* 962–982.

Oldham, J. M., Skodol, A. E., Kellman, H. D., Hyler, S. E., Doidge, N., Rosnick, L., et al. (1995). Comorbidity of Axis I and Axis II disorders. *American Journal of Psychiatry, 152,* 571–578.

Olvet, D. M., & Hajcak, G. (2008). The error-related negativity (ERN) and psychopathology: Toward an endophenotype. *Clinical Psychology Review, 28,* 1343–1354.

Ormel, J., Jeronimus, B. F., Kotov, R., Riese, H., Bos, E. H., Hankin, B., et al. (2013). Neuroticism and common mental disorders: Meaning and utility of a complex relationship. *Clinical Psychology Review, 33,* 686–697.

Patrick, C. J., Bernat, E. M., Malone, S. M., Iacono, W. G., Krueger, R. F., & McGue, M. (2006). P300 amplitude as an indicator of externalizing in adolescent males. *Psychophysiology, 43*(1), 84–92.

Polich, J. (2007). Updating P300: An integrative theory of P3a and P3b. *Clinical Neuropsychology, 118,* 2128–2148.

Regier, D. A., Kuhl, E. A., & Kupfer, D. J. (2013). The DSM-5: Classification and criteria changes. *World Psychiatry, 12,* 92–98.

Regier, D. A., Narrow, W. E., Kuhl, E. A., & Kupfer, D. J. (2009). The conceptual development of DSM-V. *American Journal of Psychiatry, 166,* 645–650.

Reich, J., Noyes, R., & Yates, W. (1989). Alprazolam treatment of avoidant personality traits in social phobic patients. *Journal of Clinical Psychiatry, 50,* 91–95.

Reichborn-Kjennerud, T., Czajkowski, N., Røysamb, E., Ørstavik, R. E., Neale, M. C., Torgersen, S., et al. (2010). Major depression and dimensional representations of DSM-IV personality disorders: A population-based twin study. *Psychological Medicine, 40,* 1475–1484.

Robins, L. N. (1994). How recognizing "comorbidities" in psychopathology may lead to an improved research nosology. *Clinical Psychology: Science and Practice, 1,* 93–95.

Rounsaville, B. J., Alarcón, R. D., Andrews, G., Jackson, J. S., Kendell, R. E., & Kendler, K. (2002). Basic nomenclature issues for DSM-V. In D. J. Kupfer, M. B. First, & D. A. Regier (Eds.), *A research agenda for DSM-V* (pp. 1–30). Washington, DC: American Psychiatric Publishing.

Samuel, D. B., Hopwood, C. J., Krueger, R. F., Thomas, K. M., & Ruggero, C. (2013). Comparing methods for scoring personality disorder types using maladaptive traits in DSM-5. *Assessment, 20,* 353–361.

Samuels, J. F., Nestadt, G., Romanoski, A. J., Folstein, M. F., & McHugh, P. R. (1994). DSM-III personality disorders in the community. *American Journal of Psychiatry, 151,* 1055–1062.

Sanislow, C. A., Pine, D. S., Quinn, K. J., Kozak, M. J., Garvey, M. A., Heinssen, R. K., et al. (2010). Developing constructs for psychopathology research: Research domain criteria. *Journal of Abnormal Psychology, 119,* 631–639.

Siever, L. J., & Davis, K. L. (1991). A psychobiological perspective on the personality disorders. *American Journal of Psychiatry, 148,* 1647–1658.

Slade, T., & Watson, D. (2006). The structure of common DSM-IV and ICD-10 mental disorders in the Australian general population. *Psychological Medicine, 36,* 1593–1600.

Spitzer, R. L., Williams, J. B., & Skodol, A. E. (1980). DSM-III: The major achievements and an overview. *American Journal of Psychiatry, 137,* 151–164.

Steil, R., Dyer, A., Priebe, K., Kleindienst, N., & Bohus, M. (2011). Dialectical behavior therapy for posttraumatic stress disorder related to childhood sexual abuse: A pilot study of an intensive residential treatment program. *Journal of Traumatic Stress, 24,* 102–106.

Tackett, J. L., Lahey, B. B., van Hulle, C., Waldman, I., Krueger, R. F., & Rathouz, P. J. (2013). Common genetic influences on negative emotionality and a general psychopathology factor in childhood and adolescence. *Journal of Abnormal Psychology, 122,* 1142–1153.

Tillfors, M., Furmark, T., Ekselius, L., & Fredrikson, M. (2001). Social phobia and avoidant personality disorder as related to parental history of social anxiety: A general population study. *Behaviour Research and Therapy, 39,* 289–298.

Vaidyanathan, U., Nelson, L. D., & Patrick, C. J. (2012). Clarifying domains of internalizing psychopathology using neurophysiology. *Psychological Medicine, 42*(3), 447–459.

Van den Broeck, J., Bastiaansen, L., Rossi, G., Dierckx, E., De Clercq, B., & Hofmans, J. (2014). Hierarchical structure of maladaptive personality traits in older adults: Joint factor analysis of the PID-5 and the DAPP-BQ. *Journal of Personality Disorders, 28*(2), 198–211.

Van Essen, D. C., Smith, S. M., Barch, D. M., Behrens, T. E., Yacoub, E., Ugurbil, K., et al. (2013). The WU-MINN Human Connectome Project: An overview. *NeuroImage, 15,* 62–79.

Vollebergh, W. A. M., Iedema, J., Bijl, R. V., de Graaf, R., Smit, F., & Ormel, J. (2001). The structure and stability of common mental disorders: The NEMESIS Study. *Archives of General Psychiatry, 58,* 597–603.

Watson, D. (2005). Rethinking the mood and anxiety disorders: A quantitative hierarchical model for DSM. *Journal of Abnormal Psychology, 114,* 522–536.

Weinberger, D. R., & Goldberg, T. E. (2014). RDoCs redux? *World Psychiatry, 13,* 36–38.

Westen, D., Novotny, C. M., & Thompson-Brenner, H. (2004). The empirical status of empirically supported psychotherapies: Assumptions, findings, and reporting in controlled clinical trials. *Psychological Bulletin, 130,* 631–663.

Widiger, T. A. (2011). Integrating normal and abnormal personality structure: A proposal for DSM-V. *Journal of Personality Disorders, 25,* 338–363.

Widiger, T. A., & Costa, P. T., Jr. (2002). Five-factor model personality disorder research. In P. T. Costa, Jr., & T. A. Widiger (Eds.), *Personality disorders and the five-factor model of personality* (2nd ed., pp. 57–89). Washington, DC: American Psychological Assocation.

Widiger, T. A., & Costa, P. T., Jr. (2012). Integrating normal and abnormal personality structure: The five-factor model. *Journal of Personality, 80,* 1471–1506.

Widiger, T. A., Frances, A. J., Harris, M., Jacobsberg, L. B., Fyer, M., & Manning, D. (1991). Comorbidity among Axis II disorders. In J. M. Oldham (Ed.), *Personality disorders: New perspectives on diagnostic validity* (pp. 163–194). Washington, DC: American Psychiatric Publishing.

Widiger, T. A., & Rogers, J. H. (1989). Prevalence and comorbidity of personality disorders. *Psychiatric Annals, 19,* 132–136.

Widiger, T. A., & Simonsen, E. (2005). Alternative dimensional models of personality disorder: Finding a common ground. *Journal of Personality Disorders, 19,* 110–130.

Widiger, T. A., & Trull, T. J. (2007). Plate tectonics in the classification of personality disorder: Shifting to a dimensional model. *American Psychologist, 62,* 71–83.

Yalch, M. M., Thomas, K. M., & Hopwood, C. J. (2012). The validity of the trait, symptom, and prototype approaches for describing borderline personality disorder and antisocial personality disorders. *Personality and Mental Health, 6,* 207–216.

Zanarini, M. C., Frankenburg, F. R., Dubo, E. D., Sickel, A. E., Trikha, A., Levin, A., et al. (1998). Axis II comorbidity of borderline personality disorder. *Comprehensive Psychiatry, 39,* 296–302.

Zimmerman, M., Mattia, J. I., & Posternak, M. A. (2002). Are subjects in pharmacological treatment trials of depression representative of patients in routine clinical practice? *American Journal of Psychiatry, 159,* 469–473.

# PART III

# EPIDEMIOLOGY, COURSE, AND ONSET

## INTRODUCTION

This section of the *Handbook* covers topics that have been the subject of extensive research since the first edition was published, resulting in findings that have challenged traditional assumptions. The first chapter, by Theresa Morgan and Mark Zimmerman on epidemiology (Chapter 10), deals with what is probably the least controversial issue, but even here some findings are subject to discussion, if not dispute. The paucity of epidemiological research noted in the first edition has partly been addressed by some larger scale studies, although knowledge of personality disorders (PDs) remains limited compared with that available for other mental disorders. The chapter provides a comprehensive review of current knowledge based not only on the results of formal epidemiological surveys but also data obtained from large-scale studies conducted for other purposes that included a normal control or family groups that provided additional epidemiological data.

The authors conclude that accumulated data suggests that the prevalence of at least one PD ranges from 5 to 15% (median = 11.5%), with the prevalence of specific disorders ranging from 0.5 to 3%. There is also extensive co-occurrence among specific diagnoses and extensive comorbidity with other mental disorders. Prevalence rates for any disorder seem similar in males and females, although gender differences occur for some disorders, most notably increased prevalence of antisocial personality disorder in men. Other consistent findings are increased prevalence in younger adults and an association with marital and occupational functioning. As the authors suggest, the marked differences in prevalence across studies probably reflect differences in samples and measurement instruments. Some studies have used measures known to substantially overdiagnose. There is also a more troublesome possibility: DSM criteria sets themselves may contribute to overdiagnosis. Concern has repeatedly been expressed that the DSM pathologizes normal variation, a concern that may also apply to PD. The median reported prevalence of about 10% is often interpreted as indicating how common the disorder is; hence, the need to expand treatment services. However, this may simply be an overestimate. Although one could debate what level of prevalence would be more appropriate, 1 out of every 10 persons in the population seems to be a lot. In this connection, recall that the diagnostic thresholds are arbitrary and based not on a systematic evaluation of risk or established clinical criteria but rather on committee opinion. Hence, the results of epidemiological studies, no matter how rigorous, need to be interpreted in the context of documented problems with the taxonomy used.

The longitudinal course of PD, the subject of the chapter by Mark F. Lenzenweger, Michael N. Hallquist, and Adian G. C. Wright (Chapter 11), has received even more attention than epidemiology over the last two decades. These studies have also produced findings that many consider to have changed our understanding of diagnostic stability because they show that endorsement of DSM criteria tends to decrease over time. The chapter focuses both on the conclusions reached by longitudinal studies, the challenges they confronted, and the implications of these challenges for evaluating findings. The authors meticulously document the methodological strengths and liabilities of four current studies and draw attention to issues that are not always considered when focusing on specific findings. The consistent finding across studies that promises to change the way PD is conceptualized concerns the stability of PD criteria. It was noted in Chapter 1 that temporal stability was used in the 19th and early 20th centuries to differentiate PD from other mental disorders, an assumption that was held until recently. However, clinical tradition also noted that some of these disorders tended to "burn out" with age, and follow-up studies also provided evidence of improvement without treatment (Paris, 2003). Nevertheless, the predominant assumption was that PD showed temporal stability, an assumption that is challenged by the robust finding of longitudinal studies that the number of diagnostic criteria endorsed tends to decrease over time, over and above that explained by regression to the mean.

This finding paints a more optimistic picture of prognosis than previous assumptions, one that is consistent with the results of treatment outcome studies. However, this conclusion, and the implications commonly drawn from it, warrant further consideration. Earlier, we raised the issue of whether the high prevalence of PD occurred because DSM criteria sets overdiagnose PD. This could also account for at least some of the improvement recorded by longitudinal studies: Overdiagnosis would lead to some participants having less pervasive and more circumscribed personality dysfunction rather than actual PD. This possibility is consistent with the remarkable changes in criteria over relatively short periods of time noted in some reports. A second issue raised by these studies is the apparent disconnect between DSM criteria sets and measures of social adjustment. Much has been made in the literature about the fact that many participants show a decrease in symptoms over time and, as a result, no longer meet the threshold for diagnosing the disorder in question. This phenomenon is usually referred to as "diagnostic remission" or simply "remission." In medicine, the term "remission" is used to describe the disappearance of active signs or symptoms of a condition. However, this is not how the term is used in some reports of longitudinal studies. Rather, it is applied to cases that no longer meet DSM diagnostic thresholds. Thus, someone with borderline personality disorder, who originally met the threshold for diagnosis and when reassessed met only four diagnostic criteria, is said to have "remitted" even if these criteria were identity disturbance, unstable relationships, affective instability, and abandonment fears. There are two aspects to this interpretation that are problematic. First, it implies that diagnostic thresholds are invariant and that they validly divide individuals into two distinct groups—those with the disorder and those without. However, as noted earlier, thresholds are arbitrary. Moreover, they do not signify a discontinuity in the dysfunction or impairment associated with the diagnosis. In fact, the impairments associated with PD are continuously distributed. Moreover, as these studies also note (often in the same article that claims the disorder has "remitted"), even those said to be in remission (no longer meeting the threshold for diagnosis) show significant impairment in social adjustment. This latter finding raises a second, and more troublesome, issue. In these situations, the DSM criteria set does not seem to reflect impaired social adjustment. Since impaired social adjustment is a defining feature of PD (Is it possible for someone with PD to have good social adjustment?), the finding suggests serious problems with DSM criteria sets. Hence, the findings of longitudinal studies, far from supporting DSM diagnoses, as often claimed, actually reveal substantial problems.

It is also interesting to note in this connection that although DSM criteria vary over time, personality as assessed by trait measures is more stable (see Clark and colleagues, Chapter 20).

The final chapter in this section (Chapter 12) by Andrew Chanen, Jennifer L. Tackett, and Katherine Thompson explores the important issue of PD and pathology in children and adolescents; hence, it addresses an issue that has been part of the traditional assumptions about personality disorder for some time—whether PD should only be diagnosed in adulthood. Originally, it was assumed that adolescence is a period of turmoil; hence, it was inappropriate to diagnose PD when the condition in question may merely be a transient manifestation of this turmoil. As an aside, it is interesting to note that this assumption is merely one of a long list of assumptions—including the medical model is the basis for classification, disorders are discrete, and PD is stable—that have shaped contemporary conceptions and classifications of PD, unfettered by evidence. Chanen and colleagues marshal several lines of evidence to build an irrefutable case for recognizing PD in childhood and youth. They make the case that youth is a distinct and extended developmental phase that lays the foundation for adult functioning; hence, it has major implications for understanding PD. They then turn to the substantial research collected over the last decade or so, showing that robust evidence of continuity between normal and disordered personality in adults also applies to earlier stages of development, and that the factorial structure of PD traits in younger samples is similar to that identified in adult samples. These findings are consistent with longitudinal studies showing continuity of individual differences in personality from early childhood to young adulthood in the general population. Interestingly, while longitudinal clinical studies in adults show evidence of change in DSM diagnostic criteria, studies of children, youth, and young adults are providing strong evidence of stability. However, these results are consistent with evidence emerging from longitudinal studies on adults that traits are more stable than DSM diagnoses. Subsequently, the authors review the literature on developmental experiences that are risk factors for developing PD and conclude that there is general agreement that PD has its roots in childhood and adolescence, and that the evidence indicates the relevance of the diagnosis to younger age groups. Although sensitive to the issues of stigma and labeling, they also note the value of early diagnosis and intervention.

## REFERENCE

Paris, J. (2003). *Personality disorders over time.* Washington, DC: American Psychiatric Publishing.

# CHAPTER 10

# Epidemiology of Personality Disorders

Theresa A. Morgan and Mark Zimmerman

In the previous edition of this volume, Mattia and Zimmerman (2001, p. 107) noted that "while specific constellations of traits, behavior, and self-perception represented as disordered have been defined, modified, included, or excluded across successive generations of the diagnostic nomenclature, the epidemiology of personality disorders (PDs) still remains somewhat elusive." Indeed, prevalence estimates provided in DSM-III and DSM-III-R were essentially "informed speculation" based on clinical experience, community surveys from the 1950s, and observed rates of PD in specific samples (e.g., patients and their biological relatives), rather than on carefully conducted population sampling (see Lenzenweger, Loranger, Korfine, & Neff, 2008). Although important, such studies provided little guidance for estimates of PDs occurring in modern, community-based samples. In contrast, larger, community-based studies not only address prevalence but also provide information about public health costs, risk factors, patterns of comorbidity, and other variables necessary for case identification and treatment. Nonetheless, considerable work has been done on the epidemiology of PDs using DSM-III, DSM-III-R, and DSM-IV diagnostic criteria in samples ranging from less than 100 to over 40,000. Although a large proportion of PD epidemiological studies have been conducted in the United States and Great Britain, at least one worldwide, international study exists, sampling over 20,000 community members. Large epidemiological studies also frequently include, at a minimum, data on demographics, Axis I comorbidity, and other risks factors.

Despite this, relatively few epidemiological data are available on PDs versus the majority of Axis I disorders, which may in part be due to the comparatively limited time in which these diagnoses have existed in their present form. Lyons (1995) noted that with the possible exception of antisocial personality disorder (ASPD), the systematic study of PDs did not begin until the publication of DSM-III (American Psychiatric Association [APA], 1980). Prior epidemiological efforts were hampered by a lack of explicit criteria sets and, consequently, limited availability of standardized assessment tools. Current research continues to be hindered by methodological limitations, cost of conducting broadband PD investigations, and ongoing disagreement within the field as to how PDs should be defined (see Trull & Durrett, 2005).

Although DSM-IV (APA, 1994) has been available since 1994, most epidemiological surveys have been conducted using DSM-III and DSM-III-R diagnoses. Although small differences in nosology exist between these texts, the PD section is broadly consistent throughout DSM-III, DSM-III-R, and DSM-IV; a notable exception is passive–aggressive PD, which was dropped from DSM-IV. Other, smaller changes to diagnostic criteria were also made, and are discussed, with results for each PD, later in this chapter. As such, in this review, we report on the prevalence and clinical correlates as defined in DSM-III, DSM-III-R, and DSM-IV PDs.

Merikangas and Weissman (1986) and Weissman (1993) have published excellent reviews, including information regarding the epidemiology of PDs prior to the advent of DSM-III.

DSM-5 (2013) also incorporates a hybrid trait/categorical system in Section III, "Emerging Measures and Models." A similar, trait-based model that includes a severity index has been proposed for the *International Classification of Diseases* (ICD-11; see Tyrer et al., 2011). However, the proposed changes proved controversial, primarily because of lack of empirical support, possible bias toward retention of particular disorders over others, and failure to demonstrate superiority over the categorical system with respect to comorbidity and diagnostic stability (see Zimmerman, 2012). Nonetheless, an alternative form of diagnosing PD based on a hybrid trait-categorical model appears in the current DSM-5 and is discussed briefly in this chapter. However, because these diagnoses are considered provisional, and because their application outside of research laboratories may take multiple forms (trait-specified, use of constructs, or broad PD diagnosis only), we elected to defer detailed discussion of these diagnoses until more research is available.

## Overview of Studies Included in the Review

We describe in this first section the studies included in the review (see Table 10.1 for a summary). We then reference these studies in the second and third sections when reporting PD prevalences and clinical/demographic correlates, respectively. Of course, diagnosis in mental health is inextricably nested within assessment methodology. The most common instruments used for epidemiological investigations are structured and semistructured interviews. Similarly, experimental investigations assessing PDs also used some sort of structured or semistructured measure, although some have used self-report questionnaires instead. These measures are described elsewhere in this book and are mentioned only briefly here.

Multiple epidemiological surveys of the full range of PDs have been conducted for DSM-IV, using a variety of measures and samples. As described below, several epidemiological studies of Axis I syndromes also included DSM-III ASPD in their assessment batteries. A reanalysis of these data or reexamination of participating subjects has provided some information regarding the prevalence of other PDs. Because of the relative paucity of formal epidemiological data, quasi-epidemiological data based on studies of nonpatient samples are included in this review. Some of these were studies of first-degree family members of healthy control probands, and others were studies of control samples whose selection was not based on the sophisticated sampling methods of epidemiological investigations.

## Epidemiological Studies

### DSM-III and DSM-III-R

The two largest epidemiological efforts in the United States using DSM-III or DSM-III-R criteria were the National Institute of Mental Health's Epidemiologic Catchment Area study (ECA; Regier et al., 1988) and the National Comorbidity Survey (NCS; Kessler et al., 1994). The ECA was the largest effort in the United States to derive population estimates of DSM-III psychiatric disorders. Over 18,000 subjects were interviewed across five sites (New Haven, CT; Baltimore; St. Louis; North Carolina; and Los Angeles) with the Diagnostic Interview Schedule (DIS; Robins, Helzer, Croughan, & Ratcliff, 1981), a fully structured interview designed to be administered by lay interviewers. Results were weighted both to account for nonresponse and to approximate national population distributions of age, gender, and ethnicity. DSM-III ASPD was the only PD included in the ECA assessment battery.

Swartz, Blazer, George, and Winfield (1990) reanalyzed data for the 1,541 subjects from the ECA–North Carolina site to estimate the prevalence of DSM-III borderline PD (BPD). Although BPD was not included in the DIS, an algorithm was constructed to use information from the DIS interview to estimate prevalence. At the Baltimore site, Nestadt and colleagues (1990, 1991, 1992) reported the results of a second-stage clinical reappraisal of subjects who participated in the ECA. All subjects considered to have filtered-positive for a DSM-III psychiatric disorder and a 17% random subsample of filtered-negative subjects were reassessed. In all, 1,086 subjects were selected for reappraisal, and 810 subjects (or 759 subjects; the reported final sample varies across publications) completed this assessment. The reappraisal was completed by psychiatrists administering the Standardized Psychiatric Examination (Romanoski et

TABLE 10.1. Overview of Studies Included in the Review

| Study | N | Sample type | Criteria used | Axis II measure | Disorders assessed |
|---|---|---|---|---|---|
| Baron et al. (1985) | 374 | Control-Exp | DSM-III | SIB-SADS | Par Szoid Stypl Bord Anti Avoid Dep |
| Black et al. (1993) | 127 | Control-Fam | DSM-III | SIDP | All |
| Blanchard et al. (1995) | 93 | Control-Exp | DSM-III-R | SCID-II | Par Anti Bord Avoid Dep OC |
| Bland et al. (1988)[a] | 3,258 | Epidemiology | DSM-III | DIS | Anti |
| Coid et al. (2006)[a] | 8.886 | Epidemiology | DSM-IV | SCID-II | All |
| Coryell & Zimmerman (1989) | 185 | Control-Fam | DSM-III | SIDP | All |
| Crawford et al. (2005) | 644 | Community | DSM-IV | SCID-II; CIS-SR | All |
| Drake & Vaillant (1985) | 369 | Control-Exp | DSM-III | unspecified | Cluster A Cluster B Avoid Dep |
| Erlenmeyer-Kimling et al. (1995) | 93 | Control-Fam | DSM-III-R | PDE | Cluster A |
| Grant, Hasin, et al. (2004) | 43,093 | Epidemiology | DSM-IV | AUDADIS-IV | Avoid Dep OC Par Szoid Hist Anti |
| Huang et al. (2009)[a] | 21,162 | Epidemiology | DSM-IV | IPDE | Cluster A Cluster B Cluster C |
| Kendler et al. (1989)[a] | 580 | Control-Fam | DSM-III-R | SIS | Par Szoid[b] Stypl Bord[b] Avoid[b] |
| Kessler et al. (1994) | 8,098 | Epidemiology | DSM-III-R | CIDI | Anti |
| Lenzenweger et al. (1997) | 810 | Undergrads | DSM-III-R | IPDE | Presence of at least one PD |
| Lenzenweger et al. (2007) | 5,692 | Epidemiology | DSM-IV | IPDE | Cluster A Cluster B Cluster C Anti Bord |
| Maier et al. (1992, 1995)[a] | 320 | Control-Fam | DSM-III-R | SCID-II | All |
| Nestadt et al. (1990, 1991, 1992) | 810 | Epidemiology | DSM-III | SPE | Hist OC |
| Regier et al. (1988) | 18,571 | Epidemiology | DSM-III | DIS | Anti |
| Reich et al. (1989) | 235 | Community | DSM-III | PDQ | All |
| Samuels et al. (2002) | 742 | Community | DSM-IV | IPDE | All |
| Swartz et al. (1990) | 1,541 | Epidemiology | DSM-III | DIB-DIS | Bord |
| Torgersen et al. (2001)[a] | 2,053 | Epidemiology | DSM-III-R | SIDP-R | All |
| Trull et al. (2010) | 43,093 | Epidemiology | DSM-IV | AUDADIS-IV | All |
| Wells et al. (1989)[a] | 1,498 | Epidemiology | DSM-III | DIS | Anti |

*Note.* Exp, experimental study with a control group; Fam, family study of control probands; CIDI, Composite International Diagnostic Interview (World Health Organization, 1990); DIS, Diagnostic Interview Schedule (Robins, Helzer, Croughan, & Ratcliff, 1981); IPDE, International Personality Disorders Examination (Loranger et al., 1994; Loranger, Sartorious, & Janca, 1996); PDQ, Personality Diagnostic Questionnaire (Hyler et al., 1983; Hyler, Lyons, et al., 1990; Hyer, Skodol, et al., 1990); PDE, Personality Disorder Examination (Loranger, Susman, Oldham, & Russakoff, 1987), SADS-L, Schedule for Affective Disorders and Schizophrenia—Lifetime Version (Endicott & Spitzer, 1979); SPE, Standardized Psychiatric Examination (Nestadt et al., 1992); SCID-II, Structured Clinical Interview for DSM-III-R Personality Disorders (Spitzer, Williams, Gibbon, & First, 1990b); SIDP, Structured Interview for DSM-III Personality Disorders (Pfohl, Stangl, & Zimmerman, 1982); SIS, Structured Interview for Schizotypy (Kendler, Lieberman, & Walsh, 1989); AUDADIS-IV, Alcohol Use Disorder and Associated Disabilities Interview Schedule–DSM-IV (Grant, Dawson & & Hasin, 2001); CIS-SR, Children in the Community Self-Report Scales (Crawford et al., 2005); PD, personality disorder; Par, paranoid PD; Szoid, schizoid PD; Stypl, schizotypal PD; Hist, histrionic PD; Anti, antisocial PD; Bord, borderline PD; Avoid, avoidant PD; Dep, dependent PD; OC, obsessive–compulsive PD; All, all DSM PDs for version indicated.
[a]Non-U.S. sample.
[b]All criteria not assessed.

al., 1988), and interview results were used to estimate the prevalence of histrionic PD (HPD) and obsessive–compulsive PD (OCPD).

The second national study, the NCS, assessed 8,098 individuals ages 15–54 years. In contrast to the ECA, which drew subjects from five discrete catchment areas, the NCS selected subjects from the 48 contiguous states. As such, the NCS was designed to estimate the prevalence, comorbidity, and risk factors of DSM-III-R psychiatric disorders in a representative national sample. Participants were interviewed with the Composite International Diagnostic Interview (CIDI; World Health Organization [WHO], 1990), a structured interview based on the DIS and administered by trained nonclinician interviewers. As in the ECA study, ASPD was the only PD assessed, and results were weighted both to account for nonresponse and to approximate national population characteristics of gender, ethnicity, marital status, education, living arrangements, region, and urbanicity.

Two epidemiological studies conducted outside of the United States also confined assessment of PDs to ASPD. Bland, Orn, and Newman (1988) reported the results of an epidemiological investigation in Edmonton, Canada. Over 3,000 randomly selected residents were interviewed with the DIS. Wells, Bushnell, Hornblow, Joyce, and Oakley-Browne (1989) reported the results of an epidemiological study in Christchurch, New Zealand. A sample of 1,498 residents were randomly selected and interviewed with the DIS. Both investigations used DSM-III criteria, and both investigations weighted their results according to age and sex distributions of their respective populations. The Christchurch group later replicated its efforts in a prison sample (Brinded et al., 1999), finding prevalence as high as 71% for ASPD in 146 prisoners. Other international efforts (e.g., Torgersen, Kringlen, & Cramer, 2001) assessed PDs by cluster only, using the Structured Interview for DSM-III-R Personality Disorders—Revised (SIDP-R; Pfohl, Blum, & Zimmerman, 1997). These authors selected a representative sample of 2,053 Norwegian adults ages 18–65, and all assessments were administered by trained psychiatric nurses, primarily in participants' homes.

## DSM-IV

Several studies have examined the epidemiology of PDs using DSM-IV nosology. In the United States, one of the largest such studies, the National Comorbidity Survey Replication (NCS-R), entailed face-to-face interviews with 9,282 adults between February 2001 and December 2003 (Kessler & Merikangas, 2004). Lenzenweger, Lane, Loranger, and Kessler (2007) reported on two NCS-R subsamples ($n = 9,282$ adults in the full sample, of whom 70.9% participated): (1) 5,692 respondents who met criteria for a "core" Axis I disorder in an initial screening, and (2) a probability subsample of 214 respondents who did not initially participate but later were offered an incentive to complete a "nonresponse" survey. Methods broadly replicated those from the original NCS (described earlier), using the International Personality Disorder Examination (IDPE) and DSM-IV criteria. As in the original NCS, survey respondents were identified based on self-reported PD characteristics over the past 12 months. Importantly, the full sample assessed only Clusters A, B, and C, as well as ASPD and BPD. Prevalence estimates were then predicted based on previous sampling and the much smaller ($n = 214$) subsample. Because prevalence estimates for specific PDs other than BPD and ASPD are based on multiple imputation and not on observed cases, we included only the cluster, BPD, and ASPD findings in our tables. However, we included some discussion of the multiply imputed data in the text, to provide additional context to the discussion.

Also in the United States, Samuels and colleagues (2002) reported PD prevalence rates in a sample of 742 adults from the Baltimore, Maryland, area using the IPDE. Subjects were samples from the Baltimore ECA follow-up survey (see Eaton et al., 1997), and included 3,481 adult household residents who were sampled probabilistically using the DIS. Subsequently, a subsample was identified, based on positive interview results for lifetime Axis I pathology, as well as a random sample of the remaining subjects. Master's-level clinicians administered both diagnostic and demographic interviews to this group.

Crawford and colleagues (2005) used the Structured Clinical Interview for DSM-IV Axis II (SCID-II; First et al., 1997) to assess PDs in 644 United States adult community members. Individuals were first screened using the Children in the Community Self-Report Scales (CIS-SR), which assessed self-reported DSM-IV PDs longitudinally as part of the Children in the Community Study (see Cohen & Cohen, 1996). Axis II diagnostic assessments were conducted by trained interviewers, and participants' mean age was 33 years. Importantly, despite being an unvalidated measure, the CIS-SR did not appear to overestimate diagnoses when results were directly compared to the SCID-II in this sample. Results reported in this study are based on SCID-II diagnoses, with the exception of HPD and ASPD, which were based on the CIS-SR.

The National Epidemiologic Survey on Alcohol and Related Conditions (NESARC) is a large, community-based survey of U.S. adults ages 18 and over from all 50 states and the District of Columbia. Face-to-face interviews were conducted with over 40,000 respondents, and the overall survey response rate was predictably high at 81%. Data were weighted to account for selection of only one person per household, oversampling of young adults, and nonresponse at the household and person level. Importantly, the NESARC results for PDs have been criticized for the use of census workers with minimal experience who administered an unvalidated Axis II diagnostic instrument, the Alcohol Use Disorder and Associated Disabilities Interview Schedule—DSM-IV (AUDADIS-IV; Grant, Dawson, & Hasin, 2001). Importantly, the NESARC sample reported on lifetime prevalence of PD characteristics, and participants responses were not validated by reinterview as in the NCS-R.

We included two studies that analyzed the original NESARC results. First, Grant, Hasin, and colleagues (2004) reported on raw AUDADIS scores, which were based primarily on the presence/absence of PD symptoms. To be included as having a PD, participants had to indicate that they experienced significant distress, impairment, or dysfunction for one of the required PD items per disorder. Seven PDs were assessed and reported (see Table 10.1). However, some authors criticized this report as being overly inclusive, and resulting in exaggerated PD prevalence estimates. Trull, Jahng, Tomko, Wood, and Sher (2010) revised the original NESARC scoring to require significant distress or impairment be present to count each PD criterion individually rather than cumulatively. The authors then applied this revision to original NESARC algorithms, reporting revised prevalence rates for the seven PDs reported. Because these methods yielded somewhat different estimations of PD prevalence in the same population, we included both the original (Grant, Hasin, et al., 2004) and revised (distress/impairment weighted; Trull et al., 2010) data in our review.

Several studies have also assessed PDs internationally using DSM diagnostic categories, one of the largest being the WHO World Mental Health (WMH) Survey Initiative (Huang et al., 2009; also see Kessler & Üstün, 2008), which reported estimated prevalence and correlates of DSM-IV clusters across 13 countries from Asia, Africa, the Americas, the Middle East, and Western Europe using items from the IPDE (Loranger 1999; Loranger et al., 1994). Interviews were conducted in two parts: (1) All respondents completed a "core diagnostic assessment" consisting of primarily Axis I disorders and demographic questions; (2) any individual who met criteria for any anxiety, mood, externalizing, or substance use disorders—as well as a probability subsample of other part 1 participants—completed part 2, which assessed PDs. In total, 21,162 respondents completed questions about PDs, and the data were weighted based on government census data to account for differential probability of selection and other possible discrepancies between sample and population variables (see Heeringa et al., 2008, for a detailed description of sample weighting).

Coid, Yang, Tyrer, Roberts, and Ullrich (2006) reported a national PD survey of adult community members in Great Britain. Similar to the NCS-R, a two-step procedure was used, consisting of (1) Axis II screening within the British National Survey of Psychiatric Morbidity, which had an approximately 70% response rate, and (2) follow-up interviews for patients who screened positive for PD in stage 1 and agreed to continue participation (~7.2% of all respondents). The sample consisted of 8,886 adults completing the first-wave interview, and 626 completers who were assessed at both stages. Second-stage assessments were conducted by trained interviewers using the SCID-II. Unlike the majority of other studies, this sample also assessed PD not otherwise specified (PD NOS), which was the most commonly diagnosed PD in their sample at 5.7%.

*DSM-5*

As noted, Section III, "Emerging Measures and Models" of DSM-5 contains a proposed, hybrid trait-categorical model for diagnosing PD that includes five broad personality domains—Negative Affectivity, Detachment, Antagonism, Disinhibition, and Psychoticism—comprised of 25, specific, pathological personality trait dimensions (APA, 2013). PD diagnosis is subsequently rendered through combinations of core personality dysfunctions (five broad domains) and related configurations of the 25 specific traits. The Personality Inventory for DSM-5 (PID-5) was based on this model (Krueger et al., 2011), and a number of formats were designed, including self- and clinician-report scales. However, PID-5 research primarily concerned itself with reliability and concordance with existing trait models, and it has yet to be established what (if any) differences exist with respect to PD prevalence using this measure.

A limited number of PDs appear specifically in the published DSM-5 field trials, in part due to limited sample sizes and because the reports included only those diagnoses "that were considered to be of high public health importance or were proposed for new additions" (Regier et al., 2013, p. 61). Thus, because several specific PDs were proposed for deletion, the deleted PDs were not specifically assessed or reported, nor was "PD-trait specified" which could have approximated DSM-IV categories. Seven adult and four child/adolescent sites were selected as representative samples of patients in typical clinical settings, using "usual clinical interviewing" methods. Results showed prevalence of .06–.13 for DSM-IV and .04–.08 for DSM-5 (kappas from .34 to .75) for BPD. For ASPD, prevalence was .05 and .03 for DSM-IV and -5, respectively (kappa = .21). Rates of obsessive–compulsive PD (OCPD; .07 vs. .02) and STPD (.03 vs. .00) were also reported, but with insufficient sample sizes to determine reliability. Similarly, data on narcissistic PD (NPD) were gathered at one site, but results were not reported due to insufficient sample size. The authors specifically note this as a limitation of the field trials, and suggest that PDs specifically would benefit from additional field trial evidence including disorder-specific pilot studies. Thus, the effect of the new, proposed system on epidemiology of PDs remains unclear.

### Controlled Studies

Because epidemiological investigations have been narrowly focused in terms of PD assessment, the most information regarding the prevalence and clinical/demographic correlates of PDs obtained prior to DSM-IV was from experimental normal control or family study normal control groups. Results derived from experimental control groups are included here provided that potential control subjects were not screened and excluded for psychopathology. Family study control groups were similarly included, regardless of whether their corresponding control probands were screened to exclude individuals with psychopathology. While these controlled studies can provide valuable information, they fall short of the selection rigor and sampling representation found in epidemiological investigations and should be interpreted in that light.

### Experimental Studies with Control Groups

Baron and colleagues (1985) interviewed 374 normal controls with the Schedule for Affective Disorders and Schizophrenia—Lifetime Version (SADS-L; Endicott & Spitzer, 1979) and the Schedule for Interviewing Borderlines (SIB; Baron & Gruen, 1980). Additional questions were included as a supplement to assess DSM-III criteria for paranoid, schizoid, and schizotypal PD, and BPD, ASPD, AVPD, and DPD. The normal control sample was obtained by randomly selecting acquaintances of the non-ill relatives (although not confirmed with a diagnostic interview) of patients with schizophrenia. This normal control sample was part of a larger study examining the risk of Axis I and Axis II disorders in the relatives of individuals with schizophrenia.

Blanchard, Hickling, Taylor, and Loos (1995) recruited a sample of normal controls through advertisements, from staff at referral sources, and some were friends of the motor vehicle accident (MVA) subjects for comparison to a group of individuals with posttraumatic stress disorder (PTSD) secondary to an MVA. Controls were screened only to be MVA free within the prior 12 months and were matched on age and gender distribution with the MVA group. The 93 individuals in the control group were interviewed with the Structured Clinical Interview for DSM-III-R (SCID; Spitzer, Williams, Gibbon, & First, 1990a) and the Structured Clinical Interview for DSM-III-R Personality Disorders (SCID-II; Spitzer, Williams, Gibbon, & First, 1990b). Although the SCID-II assesses all DSM-III-R Axis II diagnoses, only the prevalences of PPD, ASPD, BPD, AVPD, DPD, and OCPD were reported.

Drake and Vaillant (1985) followed 369 (80%) of 456 men who were originally recruited as normal control probands in a study of juvenile delinquency (Glueck & Glueck, 1950). Subjects were interviewed with an unspecified 2-hour interview by experienced clinicians and included ratings of health, social competence, alcoholism, and criteria for all of the DSM-III PDs. Clinicians who did the ratings and the interviews were blind to information gathered on subjects when they were adolescents.

## Family Studies of Normal Control Probands

Coryell and Zimmerman (1989; see also Zimmerman & Coryell, 1989) interviewed 185 first-degree relatives of normal control probands with the DIS and the Structured Interview for DSM-III Personality (SIDP; Pfohl, Stangl, & Zimmerman, 1982). Probands were recruited with advertisements targeting hospital personnel, and only individuals who were interviewed with the SADS-L and the SIDP and not diagnosed with either an Axis I or Axis II disorder were included. The normal control group of family members was part of a larger study examining the relative risk of DSM-III psychiatric disorders in family members of probands with depression or schizophrenia. Other reviews of PD epidemiology (e.g., Lyons, 1995; Weissman, 1993) report prevalences based on all family members in the larger investigation (i.e., first-degree relatives of normal control probands *and* first-degree relatives of psychiatric probands). Because this might inflate prevalence estimates, we report only results derived from the assessment of normal probands' family members (*n* = 185; Coryell & Zimmerman, 1989). It is possible, however, that results based on these family members may underestimate true population prevalences given that probands were screened to exclude individuals with any psychiatric difficulties. Data regarding the demographic/clinical correlates of PD diagnoses in normal control family members were not reported. For the purposes of this review, we discuss these correlates based on *all* family members in the study (i.e., 185 first-degree relatives of control probands *and* the 612 first-degree relatives of psychiatric probands; Zimmerman & Coryell, 1989). Black, Noyes, Pfohl, Goldstein, and Blum (1993) used similar methodology to that of Coryell and Zimmerman (1989) to ascertain a second normal control group at the same site to serve as a comparison group in a family study of obsessive–compulsive disorder (OCD). The resulting 127 family members of similarly screened hypernormal probands were interviewed with the DIS and the SIDP. Again, it is possible that results based on these family members may underestimate true population prevalences given that probands' were screened to exclude individuals with psychiatric difficulties.

Erlenmeyer-Kimling and colleagues (1995) gathered a control group as a part of a larger study comparing the offspring of probands with schizophrenia or a mood disorder. Normal probands were parents identified through two large school districts in the New York City metropolitan area, screened to have had no psychiatric treatment history and to have at least one child age 7–12 years, without current symptoms or a history of psychiatric disturbance. Normal probands were also matched on demographic characteristics to psychiatric probands, and the offspring of both groups were followed and compared. Ninety-three of the original 100 children in the normal control group were contacted approximately two decades later (mean age 30.84 ± 1.83). This normal control group was interviewed with the SADS-L and the Personality Disorder Examination (PDE; Loranger, Susman, Oldham, & Russakoff, 1987).

Kendler, McGuire, Gruenberg, and Walsh (1994) assessed 580 relatives of 150 unscreened control subjects selected from an electoral registry in a rural county in the west of Ireland as part of a larger family study of probands with schizophrenia or a mood disorder. The 150 control probands were matched for age and sex to two other study groups comprised of individual with schizophrenia or mood disorder. One first-degree relative, the informant, of control probands was questioned regarding other first-degree relatives' possible symptoms of paranoid PD (PPD) and schizotypal PD (STPD) and assessed with the SCID for Axis I disorders, and the Structured Interview for Schizotypy (SIS; Kendler, Lieberman, & Walsh, 1989). The SIS assesses the schizotypal signs and symptoms relevant to the identification of nonpsychotic but symptomatic relatives of individuals with schizophrenia and DSM-III-R criteria for STPD and PPD, five criteria for each of SPD, AVPD, and BPD. Psychiatric hospital records, if available, were also used.

Maier, Minges, Lichtermann, and Heun (1995) randomly recruited 109 control subjects from the community as part of a larger family study of DSM-III-R schizophrenia and mood disorders. Control probands were recruited from the Rhein-Main area and were not screened for psychiatric status. All available first-degree relatives of the 109 control probands were interviewed by physicians and research assistants using the SADS-L and the SCID-II, yielding a sample of 320 subjects. For the purposes of this review, only results derived from the assessment of normal probands' family members will be reported in the PD prevalence section. Data regarding the demographic/clinical correlates of PD diagnoses in normal control family members were not reported. However, reported information regarding correlates of PDs was based on a mixed group of normal control probands, their spouses, and their first-degree relatives (Maier, Lichtermann, Klinger, & Heun, 1992).

### Survey Studies

Two large-scale surveys included assessment of personality traits. The first study examined a fairly specialized population—university undergraduates. Lenzenweger, Loranger, Korfine, and Neff (1997) used a two-stage method to estimate the prevalence of at least one DSM-III-R PD in nonclinical undergraduates. Subjects were recruited from approximately 2,000 incoming freshmen at Cornell University. Fifteen research assistants used a door-to-door epidemiological style survey distribution and collection method, and recruited 1,684 subjects into the first stage of the study. All subjects initially completed the IPDE-S, a self-report version of the IPDE (Loranger et al., 1994; Loranger, Sartorius, & Janca, 1996) that screens for the presence of PDs. Results from the screening questionnaire indicated that 43% screened positive for a probable PD. A subset (n's = 134 and 124, respectively) of the screen-probable and screen-negative groups was randomly selected to be interviewed with the IPDE and the SCID. These sampling procedures resulted in a slight overrepresentation of screen-probables in the final study sample.

Reich, Yates, and Nduaguba (1989) recruited a community sample in a university town in the Midwest by random questionnaire mailings to 401 of approximately 36,697 adults whose names and addresses were listed in the Iowa City directory. Selected subjects were mailed the Personality Diagnostic Questionnaire (PDQ; Hyler, Lyons, et al., 1990; Hyler, Reider, & Spitzer, 1983; Hyler, Skodol, Kellman, Oldham, & Rosnick, 1990), a self-report measure that assesses criteria related to the 11 DSM-III PDs. Approximately 62% (n = 235) of those selected returned the mailing with a completed PDQ.

### Prevalence of PDs

#### Cluster A PDs

*Paranoid*

The median prevalence of PPD across all studies was 1.1% (see Table 10.2). The prevalence rates of DSM-III-defined PPD ranged from 0.5% (Coryell & Zimmerman, 1989) to 2.7% (Baron et al., 1985) with a median of 1.6%. The range according to DSM-III-R criteria was similar, 0.4% (Kendler et al., 1994) to 2.4% (Torgersen et al., 2001), and the median was lower—1.1%. DSM-IV prevalence rates varied considerably more, and ranged from 0.7% (Coid et al., 2006; Samuels et al., 2002) to as high as 5.1% (Crawford et al., 2005) with a median of 1.9%.

The highest overall rates were reported for large epidemiological studies using DSM-IV criteria (5.1%, Crawford et al., 2005; 4.4%, Grant, Hasin, et al., 2004). Importantly, the Trull and colleagues (2010) reanalyses of the NESARC (Grant, Hasin, et al., 2004) data found a much lower prevalence (1.9%) when data were limited by distress/impairment for each criteria. This finding was consistent across all PDs except ASPD and DPD.

For DSM-III and DSM-III-R, the studies reporting both the highest (2.7%; Baron et al., 1985) and lowest (0.4%; Kendler et al., 1994) prevalences in their control groups were investigations of schizophrenia and, in the latter case, also mood disorders. There appeared to be no pattern in prevalences related to methodology or assessment instrument, and the two studies (Black et al., 1993; Coryell & Zimmerman, 1989) with the closest methods showed a threefold difference in rates (0.5 and 1.6%, respectively). This is a consistent pattern that tends to repeat itself for these two investigations with every PD except NPD.

*Schizoid*

The median prevalence of SPD was 0.9% (see Table 10.2). Again, methodology appeared to have no relationship with prevalence, nor did DSM nosology. Median prevalence of SPD for DSM-IV fell exactly between DSM-III and DSM-III-R estimates at 0.8%, with a range of 0.6% (Trull et al., 2010) to 3.1% (Grant, Hasin,

**TABLE 10.2. Prevalence (%) of Cluster A PDs**

| Study | Paranoid | Schizoid | Schizotypal | Any Cluster A |
|---|---|---|---|---|
| Baron et al. (1985)[III] | 2.7 | 0 | 2.1 | — |
| Black et al. (1993)[III] | 1.6 | 0 | 3.9 | 5.5 |
| Blanchard et al. (1995)[III-R] | 1.1 | — | — | — |
| Coid et al. (2006)[a,IV] | 0.7 | 0.8 | 0.1 | 1.6 |
| Coryell & Zimmerman (1989)[III] | 0.5 | 1.6 | 2.2 | 3.8 |
| Crawford et al. (2005)[IV] | 5.1 | 1.7 | 1.1 | 6.8 |
| Drake & Vaillant (1985)[III] | 1.6 | 5.7 | 0.3 | — |
| Erlenmeyer-Kimling et al. (1995)[III-R] | 1.1 | 1.1 | 0 | 2.2 |
| Grant et al. (2004)[IV] | 4.4 | 3.1 | — | — |
| Huang et al. (2009)[a,IV] | — | — | — | 3.6 |
| Kendler et al. (1994)[a,III-R] | 0.4 | 0.2 | 1.4 | — |
| Lenzenweger et al. (2007)[IV] | — | — | — | 5.7 |
| Maier et al. (1995)[a,III-R] | 0.9 | 0.3 | 0.3 | — |
| Reich et al. (1989)[III] | 0.9 | 0.9 | 5.1 | — |
| Samuels et al. (2002)[IV] | 0.7 | 0.9 | 0.6 | 2.1 |
| Torgersen et al. (2001)[a,III-R] | 2.4 | 1.7 | 0.6 | 4.1 |
| Trull et al. (2010)[IV] | 1.9 | 0.6 | 0.6 | 2.1 |
| Median prevalence | 1.1 | 0.9 | 0.6 | 3.8 |
| Median prevalence DSM-III | 1.6 | 0.9 | 2.2 | 4.7 |
| Median prevalence DSM-III-R | 1.1 | 0.7 | 0.5 | 3.2 |
| Median prevalence DSM-IV | 1.9 | 0.8 | 0.6 | 2.9 |

[a]Non-U.S. sample.
[III]DSM-III; [III-R]DSM-III-R; [IV]DSM-IV.

et al., 2010), anchored at both ends by NESARC estimates. The range according to DSM-III criteria was 0% (Baron et al., 1985; Black et al., 1993) to 5.7% (Drake & Vaillant, 1985) with a median of 0.9%. A narrower range appeared to be associated with DSM-III-R criteria—0.2% (Kendler et al., 1994) to 1.7% (Torgersen et al., 2001), and with a slightly lower median of 0.7%. The Kendler and colleagues (1994) data might be a slight underestimate of SPD in their sample given that all criteria were not assessed.

## Schizotypal

The median prevalence of STPD was 0.6% (see Table 10.2). The rates of DSM-IV-defined STPD ranged from 0.1 (Coid et al., 2006) to 1.1% (Crawford et al., 2005), with a median of 0.6%. DSM-III-defined STPD ranged from 0.3 (Drake & Vaillant, 1985) to 5.1% (Reich et al., 1989), with a median of 2.2%. DSM-III-R prevalence ranged more narrowly—0% (Erlenmeyer-Kimling et al., 1995) to 1.4% (Kendler et al., 1994), with a slightly lower median of 0.5%.

## Comment

DSM-IV studies reporting Cluster A prevalence are uniformly community-based epidemiological studies with large samples. The commonest Cluster A PD was STPD for DSM-III criteria and PPD for DSM-IV. Most DSM-III and DSM-III-R Cluster A studies included in this review are part of larger family studies of psychotic probands. However, there was no evidence that the rates of these schizophrenic spectrum PDs were higher in the family studies than in the other studies.

Across clusters, rates of PDs tended to be higher according to DSM-III versus DSM-III-R criteria, although no study directly compared prevalence rates derived from both sets, nor did studies exist comparing DSM-IV to previous diagnostic sets. Rates of PPD and SPD tended to be higher in DSM-IV than in DSM-III or DSM-III-R criteria. The higher rate of PDs in DSM-III would not have been predicted from changes in criteria from DSM-III to DSM-III-R. DSM-III SPD required the presence of three out of three criteria, whereas DSM-III-R employed an easier subset strategy of four out of seven criteria. Likewise, criteria for PPD seemed easier to meet in DSM-IV and DSM-III-R than DSM-III. The schizotypal criteria are essentially the same in all DSM versions we reported. Consequently, it is more likely that the difference in median prevalence rates between DSM-III, DSM-III-R, and DSM-IV is due to methodological differences between studies than to differences in the broadness of criteria sets. For example, the presence of any Cluster A diagnosis yielded a wider range and lower median estimate in DSM-IV as compared to DSM-III and DSM-III-R, which may be due to the use of primarily epidemiological and community samples in the former (vs. family studies in the latter).

### Cluster B Personality Disorders

*Histrionic*

The median prevalence of HPD across all studies was 1.8% (see Table 10.3). The range of DSM-III HPD was 1.6 (Coryell & Zimmerman, 1989) to 3.9% (Black et al., 1993), with a median of 2.1%. The piece of data associated with an epidemiological investigation (Nestadt et al., 1990) reported a rate right at the median of 2.1%. DSM-IV prevalence was narrower than that of DSM-III, and ranged from 0.2% (Samuels et al., 2002) to 1.8% (Grant, Hasin, et al., 2004), with a median of 0.6%. Only two studies reported a prevalence of DSM-III-R-defined HPD, and these found rates of 1.3 (Maier et al., 1995) and 2.0% (Torgersen et al., 2001).

*Antisocial*

ASPD is by far the most studied PD, with 19 reports included in this review. The median overall prevalence of ASPD was 1.2% (see Table 10.3). Using DSM-IV, criteria ranges fell from 0.6 (Coid et al., 2006; Lenzenweger et al., 2007) to 4.1% (Samuels et al., 2002). The median prevalence for DSM-IV ASPD was higher than that for other nosologies, at 2.4%. DSM-III prevalence reflected a similar range to DSM-IV, falling from 0 (Baron et al., 1985) to 3.7% (Bland et al., 1988), but with a slightly lower median of 1.9%. Unlike most other PDs, a similar range appeared to be associated with DSM-III-R criteria—0 (Blanchard et al., 1995) to 3.5% (Kessler et al., 1994), again with a lower median of 0.3%.

Both NESARC reports (Grant, Hasin, et al., 2004; Trull et al., 2010) found ASPD to be nearly 4%, in contrast to the NCS-R estimate at 0.6% (Lenzenweger et al., 2007). These differences may reflect the lifetime assessment of the NESARC versus 12-month time frame for the NCS-R. However, the original NCS—which was also on a 12-month time frame—reported a somewhat higher prevalence of 3.5%, based on DSM-III-R criteria. Regier and colleagues (1988) reported the lifetime prevalence of DSM-III ASPD in the ECA study to be 2.5%, with 1-month and 6-month prevalences of 0.5 and 0.8%, respectively. The two epidemiological studies conducted outside of the United States and using DSM-III criteria reported rates of ASPD similar to that found in the NCS: 3.7% in Edmonton, Canada (Bland et al., 1988) and 3.1% of a New Zealand sample (Wells et al., 1989). DSM-IV ASPD was estimated at 0.6% in a British sample but was not assessed in the larger WHO sample reported by Huang and colleagues (2009).

*Borderline*

BPD was the second most reported PD in our sample, with 15 estimates across the three diagnostic manuals, giving a median prevalence of 1.1% (see Table 10.3). The range of DSM-III BPD was 0.4 (Reich et al., 1989) to 5.5% (Black et al., 1993), with a median of 1.4%. DSM-III-R criteria were associated with a narrower range—0 (Kendler et al., 1994) to 1.3% (Maier et al., 1995), with a median of 0.9%. The Kendler study may be an underestimate given that all criteria were not assessed. DSM-IV criteria resulted in BPD prevalence estimates ranging from 0.5 (Samuels et al., 2002) to 3.9% (Crawford et al., 2005), with a median of 1.4%.

*Narcissistic*

The median prevalence of NPD was 0.4% (see Table 10.3). However, four of nine available es-

**TABLE 10.3. Prevalence (%) of Cluster B PDs**

| Study | Histrionic | Antisocial | Borderline | Narcissistic | Any Cluster B |
|---|---|---|---|---|---|
| Baron et al. (1985)[III] | — | 0 | 1.6 | — | — |
| Black et al. (1993)[III] | 3.9 | 0.8 | 5.5 | 0 | 7.9 |
| Blanchard et al. (1995)[III-R] | — | 0 | 1.1 | — | — |
| Bland et al. (1988)[a][III] | — | 3.7 | — | — | — |
| Coid et al. (2006)[a][IV] | — | 0.6 | 0.7 | — | 1.2 |
| Coryell & Zimmerman (1989)[III] | 1.6 | 1.6 | 1.1 | 0 | 4.3 |
| Crawford et al. (2005)[IV] | 0.9 | 1.2 | 3.9 | 2.2 | 6.1 |
| Drake & Vaillant (1985)[III] | 1.9 | 2.2 | 0.8 | 5.7 | — |
| Grant, Hasin, et al. (2004)[c][IV] | 1.8 | 3.6 | — | — | — |
| Huang et al. (2009)[a][IV] | — | — | — | — | 1.5 |
| Kendler et al. (1994)[III-R] | — | 0.2 | 0 | — | — |
| Kessler et al. (1994)[III-R] | — | 3.5 | — | — | — |
| Lenzenweger et al. (2007)[IV] | — | 0.6 | 1.4 | — | 1.5 |
| Maier et al. (1995)[a][III-R] | 1.3 | 0.3 | 1.3 | 0 | — |
| Nestadt et al. (1990)[III] | 2.1 | — | — | — | — |
| Regier et al. (1988)[III] | — | 2.5 | — | — | — |
| Reich et al. (1989)[III] | 2.1 | 0.4 | 0.4 | 0.4 | — |
| Samuels et al. (2002)[IV] | 0.2 | 4.1 | 0.5 | 0.0 | 4.5 |
| Swartz et al. (1990)[III] | — | — | 1.8 | — | — |
| Torgersen et al. (2001)[a][III-R] | 2.0 | 0.7 | 0.7 | 0.8 | 3.1 |
| Trull et al. (2010)[IV] | 0.3 | 3.8 | 2.7 | 1.0 | 5.5 |
| Wells et al. (1989)[a][III] | — | 3.1 | — | — | — |
| Median prevalence | 1.8 | 1.2 | 1.1 | 0.4 | 3.7 |
| Median prevalence DSM-III | 2.1 | 1.9 | 1.4 | 0.2 | 6.1 |
| Median prevalence DSM-III-R | 1.7 | 0.3 | 0.9 | 0.4 | — |
| Median prevalence DSM-IV | 0.6 | 2.4 | 1.4 | 1.0 | 3.0 |

[a]Non-U.S. sample.
[b]Only prevalence in category.
[c]HPD and APD estimates were based on self-report data in the study.
[III]DSM-III; [III-R]DSM-III-R; [IV]DSM-IV.

timates were 0%. Three investigations reported DSM-IV prevalence estimates ranging from 0 (Samuels et al., 2002) to 2.2% (Crawford et al., 2005), with a median of 1.0% (Trull et al., 2010). Black and colleagues (1993) and Coryell and Zimmerman (1989) reported that none of their subjects met criteria for NPD, which was the only time these two investigations agreed. The other two studies that used DSM-III criteria, Drake and Vaillant (1985) and Reich and colleagues (1989), were quite disparate, with estimates of 5.7 and 0.4%, respectively. The two studies using DSM-III-R criteria reported prevalences of 0 (Maier et al., 1995) and 0.8% (Torgersen et al., 2001). The data together indicate that NPD seems to be the least prevalent PD.

*Comment*

The most common Cluster B PD in DSM-III and DSM-III-R was HPD, although its prevalence declined like all Cluster B PDs when comparing studies using DSM-III-R to DSM-III criteria. However, a shift is notable for DSM-IV estimates, in which ASPD became the most commonly diagnosed Cluster B PD. Relative to DSM-III and DSM-III-R, DSM-IV criteria for ASPD deemphasized criminal behaviors and emphasized psychopathic traits such as poor empathy, inflated self-appraisal, and superficial charm (see Widiger & Corbitt, 1993). This shift to trait-based versus behavior-based diagnosis resulted in a higher rate of diagnosable cases because it does not restrict the diagnosis to only those with a history of criminality.

Because ASPD was examined in all but three of the epidemiological investigations reviewed, it is instructive to compare results from these studies with those obtained from experimental control groups to determine whether methodology systematically biased prevalence estimates. Relative to experimental control research, epidemiological investigations as a group reported the highest prevalence of ASPD. The median epidemiological prevalence of ASPD was 3.1% compared to the median experimental control group prevalence of 0.4%. Looking at this another way, the prevalence of ASPD was less than 1.0% in six of the 10 nonepidemiological studies, and it was 2.5% or higher in six of nine epidemiological studies. The differences in prevalence may reflect differences between studies in the period of assessment: when confined to 1-month and 6-month time periods, the prevalence based on epidemiological data begins to resemble rates from normal control research. However, when Zimmerman and Coryell (1989) suspended the 5-year rule of the SIDP and included any lifetime evidence of the disorder, the prevalence of ASPD in their family study sample increased by a very modest 15% (from 26 subjects to 30). Thus, while time period of assessment may be related to the differences between epidemiological and normal control research, there is sufficient variance for additional methodological factors.

### Cluster C PDs: Anxious/Fearful

### Avoidant

Prevalence estimates of AVPD varied widely across diagnostic systems. The median prevalence across all studies was 1.5% (see Table 10.4). With DSM-IV criteria, prevalence ranged from 0.8 (Coid et al., 2006) to 6.4% (Crawford et al., 2005), with a median of 1.8%. Using DSM-III-R criteria, rates ranged from 0% (Kendler et al., 1994) to 5.0% (Torgersen et al., 2001), although not all criteria were assessed in the Kendler study. Median prevalence for DSM-III-R was 1.2%. Finally, DSM-III AVPD ranged from 0 (Baron et al., 1985; Reich et al., 1989) to 4.6% (Drake & Vaillant, 1985) with a median of 1.6%.

### Dependent

The median prevalence of DPD was 0.8% (see Table 10.4). DSM-IV prevalence estimates had a fairly limited range, from 0.1 (Coid et al., 2006; Samuels et al., 2002) to 0.8% (Crawford et al., 2005), based on five estimates. The median prevalence of DSM-IV dependent PD was 0.3%. Three estimates of DSM-III-R DPD were available, ranging from 1.5 (Torgersen et al., 2001) to 2.2% (Blanchard et al., 1995), with a median of 1.6%. In contrast, rates of DPD varied widely based on DSM-III criteria. Baron and colleagues (1985) reported that no subjects received a diagnosis of AVPD in their sample, and Drake and Vaillant (1985) found that 7.9% of their sample merited the diagnosis. The median prevalence of DSM-III DPD was 2.4%.

### Passive–Aggressive

The median prevalence of passive–aggressive PD (PAPD) was 2.1% (see Table 10.4). Black and colleagues (1993) reported that a high 12.6% of their sample met criteria for PAPD, while the median prevalence was 2.2%. Two studies reported DSM-III-R criteria to assess PAPD, reporting prevalence rates of 1.7 (Torgersen et al., 2001) and 1.9% (Maier et al., 1995). As noted in the introduction, PAPD was subsequently dropped from later DSM editions.

### Obsessive–Compulsive

The median prevalence of OCPD was 3.2% (see Table 10.4). Rates of OCPD varied across diagnostic manuals. DSM-IV prevalences ranged from 1.9 (Coid et al., 2006; Trull et al., 2010) to 7.9% (Grant, Hasin, et al., 2004), and like PPD, was anchored at both ends by NESARC estimates. The median DSM-IV prevalence was 3.3%. Studies using DSM-III-R criteria found OCPD prevalence rates from 2.0 (Torgersen et al., 2001) to 5.4% (Blanchard et al., 1995), with a median of 2.2%. Using DSM-III criteria, prevalence of OCPD ranged from 1.5 (Nestadt et al., 1991) to 7.9% (Black et al., 1993), with a median of 4.8%.

**TABLE 10.4. Prevalence (%) of Cluster C PDs**

| Study | Avoidant | Dependent | Passive–aggressive | Obsessive–compulsive | Any Cluster C |
|---|---|---|---|---|---|
| Baron et al. (1985)[III] | 0 | 0 | — | — | — |
| Black et al. (1993)[III] | 3.2 | 2.4 | 12.6 | 7.9 | 18.1 |
| Blanchard et al. (1995)[III-R] | 1.1 | 2.2 | — | 5.4 | — |
| Coid et al. (2006)[a,IV] | 0.8 | 0.1 | — | 1.9 | 1.6 |
| Coryell & Zimmerman (1989)[III] | 1.6 | 0.5 | 2.2 | 3.2 | 7.0 |
| Crawford et al. (2005)[IV] | 6.4 | 0.8 | — | 4.7 | 10.6 |
| Drake & Vaillant (1985)[III] | 4.6 | 7.9 | — | — | — |
| Grant, Hasin, et al. (2004)[IV] | 2.4 | 0.5 | — | 7.9 | — |
| Huang et al. (2009)[a,IV] | — | — | — | — | 2.7 |
| Kendler et al. (1994)[a,III-R] | 0 | — | — | — | — |
| Lenzenweger et al. (2007)[IV] | — | — | — | — | 6.0 |
| Maier et al. (1995)[a,III-R] | 1.3 | 1.6 | 1.9 | 2.2 | — |
| Nestadt et al. (1991)[III] | — | — | — | 1.5 | — |
| Reich et al. (1989)[III] | 0 | 5.1 | 0 | 6.4 | — |
| Samuels et al. (2002)[IV] | 1.8 | 0.1 | — | — | 2.8 |
| Torgersen et al. (2001)[a,III-R] | 5.0 | 1.5 | 1.7 | 2.0 | 9.4 |
| Trull et al. (2010)[IV] | 1.2 | 0.3 | — | 1.9 | 2.3 |
| Median prevalence | 1.5 | 0.8 | 1.9 | 3.2 | 6.5 |
| Median prevalence DSM-III | 1.6 | 2.4 | 2.2 | 4.8 | 12.6 |
| Median prevalence DSM-III-R | 1.2 | 1.6 | 1.8 | 2.2 | — |
| Median prevalence DSM-IV | 1.8 | 0.3 | — | 3.3 | 2.8 |

[a]Non-U.S. sample.
[III]DSM-III; [III-R]DSM-III-R; [IV]DSM-IV.

## Comment

For DSM-III and DSM-III-R, the Cluster C PDs were the most common of the three clusters. In contrast, median rates for any Cluster A, B, and C PD were approximately equivalent for DSM-IV epidemiological studies, at 2.9, 3.0, and 2.8%, respectively. OCPD was consistently the most common PD across studies and diagnostic systems, although there is some evidence that prevalence rates are lower when based on DSM-III-R criteria. Again, this would not be predicted from the change in diagnostic algorithms from DSM-III to DSM-III-R. Because no study has directly compared prevalence rates between nosological sets, it is not possible to determine the reason for this discrepancy. Importantly, OCPD may differ from the other PDs in that some of the traits of this disorder (e.g., perfectionism and excessive responsibility) are associated with achievement and may be less reflective of functional impairment. Evidence of this can be seen in the significant drop in prevalence using the NESARC data, from 7.9 (Grant, Hasin, et al., 2004) to 1.9% (Trull et al., 2010) when functional impairment or distress was more fully taken into account.

## Prevalence of Any One PD

Fourteen studies reported the prevalence of any PD, and the rates varied nearly eightfold, from a low of 4.4% (Coid et al., 2006) to a high of 33.1% (Black et al., 1993) (see Table 10.5). Using an unstructured clinical interview, Drake and Valliant (1985) found the rate of at least one DSM-III PD in their sample to be 23%. Two

**TABLE 10.5. Prevalence (%) of Any PD**

| Study | Prevalence (%) |
|---|---|
| Black et al. (1993)[III] | 33.1 |
| Coid et al. (2006)[a,b,IV] | 4.4 |
| Coryell & Zimmerman (1989)[III] | 14.6 |
| Crawford et al. (2005)[IV] | 15.7 |
| Drake & Vaillant (1985)[III] | 23.0 |
| Grant, Hasin, et al. (2004)[IV] | 14.8 |
| Huang et al. (2009)[a,b,IV] | 6.1 |
| Lenzenweger et al. (1997)[b,III-R] | 6.7 |
| Lenzenweger et al. (2007)[b,IV] | 11.9 |
| Maier et al. (1995)[a,III-R] | 9.4 |
| Reich et al. (1989)[III] | 11.1 |
| Samuels et al. (2002)[IV] | 9.0 |
| Torgersen et al. (2001)[a,III-R] | 13.4 |
| Trull et al. (2010)[IV] | 9.1 |
| Median prevalence | 11.5 |
| Median prevalence DSM-III | 18.8 |
| Median prevalence DSM-III-R | 9.4 |
| Median prevalence DSM-IV | 9.1 |

[a]Non-U.S. sample.
[b]Including PD NOS.
[III]DSM-III; [III-R]DSM-III-R; [IV]DSM-IV.

family studies, Coryell and Zimmerman (1989) and Maier and colleagues (1995), reported that 14.6 and 9.4%, respectively, of their samples met criteria for at least one PD. The lower rate found in Maier and colleagues study is consistent with the trend for prevalences based on DSM-III-R PD criteria to be lower than those based on DSM-III criteria. In another family study of health probands, Black and colleagues (1993) reported a 33.1% prevalence rate of at least one PD in their sample, approximately two and a half times higher than that in the Coryell and Zimmerman (1989) study. This discrepancy is consistent with the pattern of disagreement between the two research groups out of the same site regarding prevalences of each specific PD. Reich and colleagues (1989), also studying a sample obtained in Iowa, found a prevalence of 11.1% for at least one DSM-III PD. In spite of slightly oversampling the screen-positive PD group, only 6.7% of the college students in the Lenzenweger and colleagues (1997) study came up positive for any definite PD (and 11.0% for any definite/probable PD). Selection for high academic achievement (hence, university admission) may have biased the sample toward less pathology. Also, as university freshmen, the sample members had not yet completed the risk age cohort for developing or manifesting a PD.

The majority of any PD estimates were drawn from DSM-IV-based studies, with estimates ranging from the aforementioned 4.4 to 15.7% (Crawford et al., 2005), with a median estimate of 9.1%. This overall estimate is approximately the same as that found for DSM-III-R but notably lower than that found for DSM-III. The entirety of the DSM-IV sample we report is epidemiological studies, whereas DSM-III and DSM-III-R studies included experimental and student groups. Several of the DSM-IV reports also drew from larger sample sizes as compared to DSM-III and III-R. To date, no study exists that has directly compared PD diagnostic rates for all three criteria sets, so it is unclear whether these discrepancies reflect true differences in PD rates based on criteria differences, or are artifacts of method or sample differences.

## Demographic and Clinical Correlates of PDs

### Clinical Correlates

#### Axis I Comorbidity

PDs appear to be associated with substantial Axis I comorbidity. Maier and colleagues (1995) reported that 63.3% of individuals with a PD diagnosis were also diagnosed with an Axis I disorder. Half or more of those subjects with PPD, HPD, BPD, AVPD, DPD, or OCPD also met criteria for an Axis I disorder. No subjects with SPD or STPD were diagnosed with an Axis I disorder. The Canadian epidemiological data (Swanson, Bland, & Newman, 1994) indicated that subjects with ASPD were three times more likely to merit an Axis I diagnosis that subjects without the diagnosis. Overall, 90.4% of subjects with ASPD were also diagnosed with an Axis I disorder—85.6% with alcohol abuse/dependence, 34.6% with drug abuse/dependence, and 25.0% with depression.

Lenzenweger and colleagues (2007) provide the detailed account of 12-month Axis I comorbidity patterns for DSM-IV PDs reported in the NCS-R. All PDs were consistently, strongly, and positively associated with Axis I pathology. In fact, 88% of odds ratios for individuals with PDs having Axis I diagnoses were statistically significant. In contrast, the proportion of individuals with Axis I disorders who also met criteria for a PD was comparatively low: 25.2% versus 67.0% of patients with PDs who had at least one comorbid Axis I disorder. The range of odds ratios was narrow for Clusters A and C, suggesting little differentiation in Axis I disorders in the strength of association with PD diagnosis. Both Cluster A and Cluster C were most commonly comorbid with specific (14.1 and 22.8%, respectively) and social phobia (11.4 and 21.1%, respectively). Odds ratios were more varied for Cluster B PDs (median OR = 8.3) than for Clusters A (median OR = 2.4) and C (median OR = 3.2). Within Cluster B, odds ratios were highest for dysthymic disorder, bipolar disorder, intermittent explosive disorder, and attention-deficit/hyperactivity disorder. In contrast, lowest odds ratios were observed for specific phobia and nicotine dependence. Of individuals with ASPD and BPD, 73.4 and 84%, respectively, met criteria for an additional Axis I disorder. Cluster B PDs were most commonly comorbid with intermittent explosive disorder (35.0%), alcohol use disorder (26.7%), specific phobia (26.7%), and social phobia (26.4%). The most common comorbidities for ASPD were intermittent explosive disorder (34.2%) and alcohol use disorder (23.9%); for BPD, the most common comorbidities were intermittent explosive disorder (38.0%), specific phobia (30.3%), social phobia (28.4%), and alcohol use disorder (27.0%).

Results from the British National Survey (Coid et al., 2006) showed increased odds of affective/anxiety disorders for Clusters A (OR = 2.7), B (OR = 20.3) and C (OR = 4.2). Psychosis and alcohol dependence were also common in participants meeting criteria for a Cluster B PD. Interestingly, individuals meeting criteria for a Cluster C PD had significantly reduced odds of comorbid alcohol use disorder compared to those without a PD. Lenzenweger and colleagues (2007) reported similar results, finding that nearly all Axis I conditions were commonly comorbid with PDs, and particularly with Cluster B PDs.

All PD clusters were significantly associated with elevated rates of four classes of Axis I disorders assessed in the WHO study, including any anxiety disorder, any mood disorder, any externalizing disorder, and any substance use disorder (Huang et al., 2009). Higher rates of Axis I comorbidity was also noted for Clusters A, B, and C (OR = 9.7, 49.3, and 34.8, respectively, for having three or more Axis I disorders). By comparison, the authors note that only 16.5% of responders with Axis I disorders reported at least one comorbid PD. Coid and colleagues (2006) reported significant incidence of affective/anxiety disorders, functional psychosis, and alcohol dependence (but not substance dependence) for individuals reporting a Cluster B PD, and of anxiety/affective disorders and hazardous drinking among those reporting a Cluster C PD.

Trull and colleagues (2010) reported on a limited number of Axis I disorders, emphasizing alcohol and substance use disorders from the NESARC dataset. Results showed highest comorbidity rates for alcohol and nicotine dependence, with nearly half of those with any PD diagnosis meeting criteria for lifetime dependence on these substances. Participants meeting criteria for any PD diagnosis also had over 12 times the risk of a lifetime diagnosis of substance dependence as compared to participants without PDs. In the original NESARC sample, Grant, Stinson, and colleagues (2004) reported 12-month alcohol use disorder rates at 16.4% and substance use disorder rates at 6.5% for any PD. This is in contrast to the lifetime rates reported by Trull and colleagues. Rates of alcohol use disorder was highest for HPD (29.1%) and ASPD (28.7%), and lowest for SPD (13.7%) and OCPD (12.9%) (Grant, Stinson, et al., 2004). Substance use disorders were highest for DPD (18.5%) and ASPD (15.2%), and lowest for SPD (7.9%) and OCPD (4.3%).

The most detailed examination of the comorbidity between Axis I and Axis II in DSM-III was reported by Zimmerman and Coryell (1989), who examined the demographic and clinical correlates of PDs in their cohort of first-degree relatives of control and psychiatric probands. All 12 Axis I disorders assessed (mania, major depression, dysthymia, alcohol abuse/dependence, drug abuse/dependence, schizophrenia, obsessive–compulsive disorder, phobic disorders, panic disorder, bulimia, tobacco use disorder, and psychosexual dysfunction) were significantly more common in subjects with versus without a PD. Individuals with a PD were also seven times more likely to have made a suicide attempt (14.0 vs. 2.0%).

When examining the individual PDs, Zimmerman and Coryell (1989) used two comparison strategies. First, subjects with each specific PD were compared to the group of subjects who received no PD diagnosis. Second, subjects with each specific PD were compared to subjects who were diagnosed with at least one of the other nine PDs (only 10 PDs were examined with this strategy because NPD was not diagnosed in any subject). Thus, the comparison group using the first strategy always comprised the 654 subjects who received no PD diagnosis of any kind, whereas the comparison group in the latter strategy changed with each analysis (e.g., seven subjects with PPD vs. 136 subjects with a non-paranoid PD; 14 subjects with DPD vs. 129 subjects with a non-dependent PD). Each set of analyses consisted of 120 comparisons (10 PDs × 12 Axis I disorders).

In all, 68 (56.7%) of the 120 comparisons of subjects with a specific PD and subjects with no PD were significant, and 16 (13.3%) of the comparisons of subjects with a specific PD and subjects with any other PD were significant. Individuals with PPD had increased rates of all 12 Axis I disorders compared to individuals without a PD, although only six differences were significant (alcohol abuse/dependence, drug abuse/dependence, schizophrenia, obsessive–compulsive disorder, phobic disorder, and bulimia). There was only one significant difference between individuals with PPD and nonparanoid PDs (higher rate of bulimia in the subjects with PPD), and this was thought to be due to the high comorbidity between PPD and the other PDs (six of the seven subjects with PPD had another Axis II disorder). Individuals with SPD and DPD had the lowest rates of Axis I diagnoses. Individuals with SPD had a significantly lower rate of MDD, and those with DPD had a significantly lower rate of alcohol abuse/dependence compared to subjects with other PDs. Axis I disorder rates were most often elevated in subjects with STPD and BPD. Compared to subjects without a PD, individuals with STPD had significantly higher rates of all disorders except bulimia, and individuals with BPD had significantly higher rates of all Axis I disorders except psychosexual dysfunction. Additionally, those with STPD had significantly higher rates of MDD and obsessive–compulsive disorder compared to subjects with other PDs, and those with BPD had higher rates of alcohol abuse/dependence, schizophrenia, phobic disorder, and tobacco use disorder. The Axis I correlates of HPD and PAPD were very similar. Individuals with each of these PDs had significantly higher rates of eight Axis I disorders (mania, MDD, alcohol abuse/dependence, drug abuse/dependence, schizophrenia, obsessive–compulsive disorder, phobic disorder, and psychosexual dysfunction), and there were no significant differences between subjects with each of these PDs and subjects with other PDs. The only difference in the pattern of Axis I correlates between subjects with HPD and PAPD was that only the former had a significantly higher rate of tobacco use disorder. OCPD had a similar pattern of Axis I correlates to HPD and PAPD except that it was not associated with an increased rate of drug abuse/dependence or schizophrenia. Subjects with ASPD had the highest rates of drug and alcohol abuse/dependence and tobacco use disorder, whereas subjects with AVPD had the highest rate of MDD and dysthymia.

## Axis II Comorbidity

PDs as diagnosed in DSM-III, DSM-III-R, and DSM-IV tend to covary. Whether this is an artifact of symptom overlap or the true co-occurrence of distinct underlying clinical syndromes is beyond the scope of this review and has been discussed in detail elsewhere (e.g., Clark, 2007; Hayward & Moran, 2008; Trull & Durrett, 2005). Nevertheless, epidemiological studies reporting the overlap between PD diagnoses uniformly found high rates of comorbidity. Co-occurrence of PDs was "unexpectedly high" in the NESARC sample (Grant, Hasin, et al. 2004). All associations among PDs were statistically significant, both within and between PD clusters. Coid and colleagues (2006), who also reported high rates of PD comorbidity, found that nearly half those meeting criteria for any PD also met criteria for a second PD diagnosis (mean Axis II diagnoses = 1.92) and 14% of the sample met four or more individual PD diagnoses. Drake and Vaillant (1985) reported similar results.

Lenzenweger and colleagues (2007) also reported high co-occurrence of PDs, with average tetrachoric correlations from .64 to .74 within PD clusters. The authors did not report specific rates of co-occurrence but noted that the sum of prevalence estimates for all individual PDs was nearly twice as large as the prevalence estimate for any PD (22.9 vs. 11.9%), providing additional evidence of high comorbidity rates overall. Additionally, 85% of within-cluster correlations and 62% of between-cluster correlations were significant in this sample. Highest reported correlations were for SPD and STPD (*r* = .96) and PD NOS and ASPD (*r* = .90). Importantly, several significant negative correlations between diagnoses occurred, particularly for SPD (negatively correlated with ASPD, DPD, and PD NOS) and DPD (negatively correlated with SPD, STPD, ASPD, and PD NOS). Importantly, the majority of these results are based on multiply imputed rates for individual PDs, not observed cases.

Maier and colleagues (1992) found that approximately one-fourth of subjects with at least one PD met criteria for more than one PD, similar to the results of Zimmerman and Coryell (1989). Zimmerman and Coryell found that PPD, AVPD, and BPD were most commonly diagnosed with at least one other PD. In contrast, SPD and DPD were most frequently diagnosed as the sole PD. The greatest percentage of overlap was between AVPD and STPD—half of the individuals with AVPD also met criteria for STPD. Also, more than 40% of individuals with PPD received a diagnosis of HPD or BPD.

## Demographic Correlates

### Gender

DSM-IV (APA, 1994) suggested that all three Cluster A PDs are most common among men. Clusters B and C are split, with HPD and BPD characterized as more common among women, ASPD as more common in men (Cluster B), and AVPD and DPD as more common among women, and OCPD as more common in men. Results supporting these suggestions were mixed. The original NESARC study (Grant, Hasin, et al., 2004) found higher rates of PD diagnosis overall in men than in women, and significantly so for ASPD. In contrast, PPD, AVPD, and DPD were significantly more commonly diagnosed in women. Similarly, in the NCS-R data, Lenzenweger and colleagues (2007) reported a trend toward ASPD to be more prevalent in men. However, these authors did not find any significant relations between any PD and gender.

In the revised NESARC data, Trull and colleagues (2010) found that men were more likely to meet diagnostic criteria for PD overall, and for SPD, ASPD, and NPD specifically. Women were more likely to be diagnosed with PPD, BPD, HPD, AVPD, DPD, and OCPD. Coid and colleagues (2006) reported higher weighted prevalence estimates for all PDs assessed except STD, although it should be noted that only one case of SPD was found in each gender.

Sex differences for PDs did not appear to have a clear pattern at the cluster level. At least one study reported that Cluster B PDs were significantly more common in women than in men (Coid et al., 2006). Two samples found both Cluster A and Cluster B PDs to be more common in men than in women (Crawford et al., 2005; Samuels et al., 2002), with the odds of having a Cluster A disorder estimated at four times greater for men than for women in the latter sample. The NCS-R data showed no significant differences for gender and PD clusters (Lenzenweger et al., 2007). Huang and colleagues (2009) reported that Clusters A and C were significantly more prevalent in men than in women. Respondents with any PD were more likely to be male in the British National Survey (Coid et al., 2006).

Receiving a diagnosis of at least one PD does not clearly appear to favor gender using the DSM-III and DSM-III-R systems either. Maier and colleagues (1992) found that approximately 9.6% of males and 10.3% of females were diagnosed with at least one PD. Of those who met criteria for a PD in the Reich and colleagues (1989) study, approximately half (46%) were male. Zimmerman and Coryell (1989) also reported that approximately half (52.4%) of their subjects with a PD were male.

As in DSM-IV, some limited and inconsistent evidence was found, showing differentiation between genders for specific PDs. Maier and colleagues (1992) reported that DPD, PAPD, and HPD tended to be more frequently diagnosed in females, and OCPD, SPD, and ASPD tended to be more frequently diagnosed in males. No statistical tests of these trends were reported. Swartz and colleagues' (1990) reexamination of the ECA data from the North Carolina site indicated that approximately 73% of those categorized as having BPD were female. Zimmerman and Coryell (1989) found that compared to subjects without a PD, subjects with ASPD and OCPD were significantly more likely to be male, and subjects with DPD were significantly more likely to be female. There was a nonsignificant tendency for individuals diagnosed with SPD to be male and individuals diagnosed with AVPD to be female. Of note, there was no association between gender and HPD and BPD. All four epidemiological studies that included assessment of ASPD found higher prevalence among males. In contrast, no sex differences were found at the cluster level in the Torgersen (2001) study. Instead, the authors reported that women were twice as likely as men to have HPD and DPD, and less than half as likely to have SPD.

## Age

It appears that PDs tend to be more common in youth, and rates of PDs may decline with age. This was true across studies and nosologies. Although neither means nor statistical tests were reported, subjects diagnosed with a PD in the Maier and colleagues (1992) study tended to be younger than those without such a diagnosis. Zimmerman and Coryell (1989) found that individuals in all but one PD category (SPD) tended to be younger than individuals without a PD diagnosis. These differences were statistically significant for BPD, ASPD, PAPD, and STPD. Subjects with BPD were the youngest ($M = 30.3$) of all subjects with a PD, followed closely by individuals with ASPD ($M = 32.5$). Individuals with SPD were the oldest ($M = 43.3$). In contrast, Torgersen and colleagues (2001) reported that individuals age 50 or older were twice as likely to have SPD, STPD, and OCPD as individuals age 50+.

Reich, Yates and Nduaguba (1988) found that PD traits and age were significantly and negatively correlated across all PD clusters. Also, the relationship between age and Cluster B and Cluster C traits appeared to follow a J distribution, wherein the mean number of traits declined with age, followed by a slight upturn in the oldest age group. Data from three of the epidemiological studies (Bland et al., 1988; Regier et al., 1988; Wells et al., 1989) indicated that the majority of subjects diagnosed with ASPD were below age of 45, and rates of ASPD appeared to decline with increasing age.

In the NESARC study, nearly all PDs were more common in younger participants (ages 18–29) with the exception of OCPD, which was marginally more common in participants ages 30–44 (prevalence estimates of 8.2 and 9.0%, respectively; Grant, Hasin, et al., 2004). The most prevalent PD in adults aged 65+ was OCPD (see Schuster, Hoertel, Le Strat, Manetti, & Limosin, 2013). Age was also inversely related to PD diagnosis generally in the WHO study (Huang et al., 2009), and to Cluster B diagnoses specifically in the NCS-R report (Lenzenweger et al., 2007). In contrast, Coid and colleagues (2006) reported that only Cluster B disorders were significantly more likely in younger age groups (ages 16–34 and ages 35–54) than in older age groups (ages 54–74). Similarly, Samuels and colleagues (2002) reported that only Cluster B disorders were significantly and inversely related to age.

## Marital Status

Presence of a PD may be associated with lower rates of marriage and higher marital discord. Grant, Hasin, and colleagues (2004) reported that for six of the seven PDs assessed, those who met criteria for PD were more likely to be divorced or never married than currently married except for those with OCPD. Similarly, Trull and colleagues (2010) found that of those meeting criteria for any PD, 7.2% were married, 17.1% were cohabiting, and 35.9% were widowed, separated, or divorced. A history of separation or divorce was also associated with any PD diagnosis in the British National Survey sample, although this finding was only significant for Clusters A and B when broken down by PD cluster (Coid et al., 2006). Similarly, Samuels and colleagues (2002) reported greater prevalence of separation/divorce for those with Cluster A PDs, and of never married for those with Cluster C PDs. In fact, individuals who were never married were more than 20 times more likely to have a Cluster A PD in multivariate analyses for this sample, and this relationship was much greater in men than in women. Few significant findings were reported with respect to marital status in international samples, with the exception that individuals with a Cluster C PD were more likely to present with a history of previous marriage (separation, divorce, or widowed; Huang et al., 2009). No significant findings were reported for marital status and PD measures in the NCS-R sample (Lenzenweger et al., 2007).

In the Zimmerman and Coryell (1989) study, of those who merited a PD diagnosis, 55.9% were married, 3.5% were separated, 13.3% were divorced, 3.5% were widowed, and 23.8% were single. Compared to subjects without a PD diagnosis, individuals with a PD diagnosis were significantly more likely to be single or divorced. Among those who ever married, subjects who merited a PD diagnosis were twice as likely (54.1%) as subjects without a PD diagnosis (25.6%) to have had a lifetime history of separation or divorce. All married subjects with BPD had a lifetime history of being separated or divorced, as did a substantial majority of subjects with DPD (78.6%) or ASPD (70.0%). In contrast, no married subject with SPD had a history of being separated or divorced.

## Education

In general, results suggest that PDs have an inverse relationship with educational attainment. In the NESARC study, participants meeting criteria for any PD except OCPD commonly reported having 12 years or less of education (Grant, Hasin, et al., 2004). All three PD clusters were significantly inversely related to education level internationally (Huang et al., 2009), and Clusters A and B were associated with having no educational qualifications in a British sample (Coid et al., 2006). Similarly, Lenzenweger and colleagues (2007) reported an inverse relation between education and Cluster B diagnoses. Samuels and colleagues (2002) reported that individuals with a high school or higher education were significantly less likely to also report a Cluster B PD. Interestingly, the odds of having a Cluster C PD were highest in those who graduated high school but did not continue their education. Torgersen and colleagues (2001) reported that individuals with 12 or fewer years of education were more likely to present with PPD or STPD, but less likely to present with OCPD.

Importantly, some of the DSM-III studies provide evidence that PDs can be associated with a moderate level of educational achievement. The mean number of years of education for individuals who met criteria for a PD in the Reich and colleagues (1989) study was slightly higher at 14.9 ($SD = 3.0$), and Swartz and colleagues (1990) found that 75% of those categorized as having BPD had graduated from high school.

## Occupation

There are data suggesting that occupational difficulties may be associated with PDs, although no epidemiological study formally compared individuals with and without a PD on occupational functioning. Reich and colleagues (1989) reported that 23% of subjects diagnosed with a PD were unemployed for longer than 6 months in the preceding 5 years. Drake and Vaillant (1985) reported more substantial impairment: 42% of those with an Axis II PD had been unemployed for more than 4 years. Unemployment was also significantly positively related to Cluster B PDs in the NCS-R (Lenzenweger et al., 2007). Although putatively linked to occupation, low socioeconomic status was found to be a significant risk factor for developing any PD in the NESARC study (Grant, Hasin, et al., 2004). Internationally, only Cluster C was notable for elevated levels of unemployment or disability (Huang et al., 2009). Coid and colleagues (2006) reported that individuals with any PD were more likely to report being unemployed or "economically inactive." This finding was consistent for all three PD clusters, which were assessed individually, and individuals meeting criteria for Cluster A PDs specifically reported a significantly higher likelihood of having a low weekly income.

## Race, Class, and Ethnicity

Trull and colleagues (2010) reported that prevalence for any PD was highest among Native Americans/Alaskan Natives (17.4%), and lowest among Asian/Pacific Islanders (5.3%). Rates for European Americans/non-Hispanics (8.9%), African Americans/non-Hispanics (10.3%), and Hispanics (9.4%) were approximately equivalent. Similarly, the original NESARC study characterized being Native American or African American as a general risk factor for PD (Grant, Hasin, et al., 2004). Ethnic origin was not significantly associated with any PD diagnosis in the British sample (Coid et al., 2006), although individuals meeting criteria for Cluster A and Cluster B PDs were more likely to report being in a lower social class.

## Assessment

Who should be questioned when assessing PDs in epidemiological investigations—the target individual or someone who knows the target individual well? The evaluation of PDs presents special problems that may require the use of informants. In contrast to the symptoms of major Axis I disorders, the defining features of PDs are based on an extended longitudinal perspective of how individuals act in different situations, how they perceive and interact with a constantly changing environment, and the perceived reasonableness of their behaviors and cognitions. Only a minority of the PD criteria are discrete, easily enumerated behaviors. For any individual to describe his or her normal personality, he or she must be somewhat introspective and aware of the effect their attitudes and behaviors have on others. But insight is the very thing usually lacking in an individual with a PD. DSM-IV notes that the characteristics defining a PD may not be considered problematic by the affected individual (i.e., ego-syntonic) and suggests that supplemental assessment information be obtained from informants. Research comparing patient and informant report of personality pathology has found rather marked disagreement between the two sources of information (Dowson, 1992a, 1992b; Tyrer, Alexander, Cicchettic, Cohen, & Remington, 1979; Zimmerman, Pfohl, Coryell, Stangl, & Corenthal, 1988). It is probable that a similar discrepancy would be found between the individuals participating in an epidemiological investigation (i.e., a nonpatient sample) and the people who know them well.

So should informants be included in epidemiological assessment for PDs? While it certainly makes empirical sense to obtain as much information as possible, an algorithm regarding how to use that information is needed first. Psychiatric assessment of patients with informants relies on "best clinical judgment" to combine discrepant information, a vague and unsatisfying procedure for an epidemiological approach that tends to use nonclinician interviewers. Even if clinicians are used, the increased personnel cost on top of the added costs of recruiting and interviewing informants makes the value of the extra information somewhat uncertain.

PD assessment in epidemiological investigations also cannot be as flexible as clinical evaluations. Clinicians not only assess for criteria per se but also generally judge the reliability of patients as historians. Depending on a patient's mental status and apparent forthrightness, a clinician can extend the assessment out over subsequent appointments and continue to identify or accumulate evidence of PD characteristics and criteria. Assessment for epidemiological investigations, indeed, for most research efforts, usually is confined to one opportunity. Very clear algorithms deciding "caseness" must be defined *and* implemented uniformly—similarity of methodology and instrument are not enough. For example, in spite of nearly identical methodologies, Black and colleagues (1993) found the prevalence of specific PDs to be two to five times higher than that found in the Coryell and Zimmerman (1989) study.

There are two possible explanations of the interstudy differences in prevalence rates—true sample differences or systematic diagnostic bias. Reich and colleagues' (1989) community survey using the PDQ found that 11.1% of respondents had a PD. Zimmerman and Coryell (1990) compared 697 subjects of their original sample who completed both the PDQ and SIDP. The rate of any PD was 10.3% according to the PDQ, similar to the rate found by Reich and colleagues using the same measure. Black and colleagues (1993) also used the PDQ in their study. In a comparison of the two Iowa family study samples Zimmerman, Coryell, and Black (1993) found that there were no demographic differences between samples. PDQ scores in the Black and colleagues sample also were not different than those in the Coryell and Zimmerman (1989) sample. These data suggest that the discrepancy in prevalence rates between the Zimmerman–Coryell and Black studies was probably due to a systematic diagnostic bias. Diagnostic raters in the two research groups probably held different evidence thresholds to count a symptom as "present" and contributing toward a PD diagnosis.

If investigators from the same institution using similar methodologies can produce such disparate results, epidemiological investigations are at a rather substantial risk of producing inconsistent results across sites. The incurred risk for bias to operate, although not unique to Axis II disorders, is perhaps greater than that for Axis I disorders, as PD criteria rely more heavily on latent constructs rather than overt symptomatology. As such, fully structured interviews such as the DIS may not completely address the problem.

## Conclusion

Due to the relative paucity of national efforts, the epidemiology of PDs in the general population is a difficult issue about which to draw firm conclusions. Although several large, epidemiological samples have been undertaken in recent years, the body of research on PD prevalence as compared to that of Axis I disorders is relatively scant. Moreover, notable differences in results exist across studies with respect to prevalence and correlates of PD diagnoses in these studies. Further complicating matters is that less than half of the studies contained in this review report on the full range of DSM-IV PD diagnoses. The NIMH's ECA study, one of the largest programs estimating the lifetime prevalences of mental disorders in the general population, excluded assessment of all PDs with the exception of ASPD. This was no doubt due in part to a lack of structured instruments for the full range of Axis II PDs. The NCS and NCS-R, another large effort to derive prevalence estimates of psychiatric disorders in the community, followed a similar strategy. Although impressive in sample size and breadth, even the NESARC samples reported here have been criticized for relying on relatively untrained assessors using an insufficiently validated measure. Thus, with the exception of ASPD, the largest epidemiological efforts in the United States have yielded only a small amount of information about the prevalence of these disorders. Even international samples predominantly assess only a limited range of PDs, and the largest such survey conducted by the WHO only reported PD results by cluster. Inquiry into the epidemiology of PDs must rely on evidence derived from an admixture of quasi-epidemiological investigations based on experimental, family, and survey designs.

Based on the accumulated data, the prevalence of at least one PD appears to be approximately 5–15% (median = 11.5%), a significant number when taken in the context that PDs are a source of long-term impairment in both treated and untreated populations (Merikangas & Weissman, 1986). The prevalence of each specific PD tends to vary between 0.5 and 3%. These rates may represent the lower prevalence boundary of PDs; a comparison of experimental and epidemiological research in ASPD suggests that experimental research tended to be lower than rates found in epidemiological research. There appears to be significant comorbidity among the PDs themselves, and a substantial number of individuals with a PD diagnosis also seem to have at least one comorbid Axis I disorder. Overall, males and females may be similar in terms of receiving a diagnosis of at least one PD, although diagnosis of specific PDs may be more common in one gender than in the other. This is particularly true for ASPD, which is consistently higher in men. PDs also seem to favor youth and appear to be associated with disturbances in marital and occupational functioning.

Unfortunately, Axis II disorders are not nearly as well researched as Axis I disorders. While epidemiological data for this disorder class are scarce, demographic characteristics and clinical correlates—important descriptive information of individuals with PDs—are even rarer. Clearly, more research is needed. Of course the largest stumbling block for such a large-scale study has been cost. Because of the low base rates of PDs, it is expensive to recruit and cull the massive sample sizes needed. Interviewer training also affects cost. If lay interviewers are to be used in a large-scale epidemiological study of Axis II (as they were in the ECA, NCS, and NESARC), then it is unlikely that semistructured interviews could be used because of potential for systematic diagnostic biases. Those investigations based on fully structured instruments such as the DIS yielded somewhat similar rates of antisocial PD. Perhaps these instruments can be expanded to include all PDs. Whether or not fully structured PD interviews would be valid is an empirical question. A similar issue is at stake with regard to self-report instruments, which typically are not used in epidemiological research. Nonetheless, Crawford and colleagues (2005) found good concordance between their self-report data and SCID-II interviews, and both Lenzenweger and colleagues (1997) and Reich, Yates, and Nduagba (1989) used self-report scales as part of their assessment battery. Despite this, whether fully self-administered scales alone would provide valid epidemiological estimates remains an empirical issue.

Hand in glove with the fiscal difficulties of such research are nosological considerations: Theoretical conceptualizations have changed, diagnostic specificity has increased in service to assessment reliability, and criteria sets for PDs have evolved. Another source of variability is the differing assessment methodologies among studies. While the SIDP (Pfohl et al., 1982) is a comprehensive instrument, it was perhaps its semistructured nature (rather than being a fully structured instrument) that allowed the widely discrepant findings from the two studies conducted at the same site using similar recruitment strategies. A continuing source of variability among prevalence estimates and the relationships among clinical correlates may come from different criteria sets. This situation is likely to get worse before it gets better given the significant changes to nosology currently proposed for future PD diagnoses.

## ACKNOWLEDGMENT

We would like to acknowledge contributions by Jill Mattia to our chapter in the first edition of the *Handbook*. She has not participated in this revision.

## REFERENCES

American Psychiatric Association. (1980). *Diagnostic and statistical manual of mental disorders* (3rd ed.). Washington, DC: Author.

American Psychiatric Association. (1987). *Diagnostic and statistical manual of mental disorders* (3rd ed., rev.). Washington, DC: Author.

American Psychiatric Association. (1994). *Diagnostic and statistical manual of mental disorders* (4th ed.). Washington, DC: Author.

American Psychiatric Association. (2013). *Diagnostic and statistical manual of mental disorders* (5th ed.). Arlington, VA: Author.

Baron, M., & Gruen, R. (1980). *The schedule for interviewing borderlines (SIB)*. New York: New York Psychiatric Institute.

Baron, M., Gruen, R., Rainer, J. D., Kane, J., Asnis, L., & Lord, S. (1985). A family study of schizophrenic and normal control probands: Implications for the spectrum concept of schizophrenia. *American Journal of Psychiatry, 142*, 447–455.

Black, D. W., Noyes, R., Pfohl, B., Goldstein, R. B., & Blum, N. (1993). Personality disorder in obsessive-compulsive volunteers, well comparison subjects, and their first degree relatives. *American Journal of Psychiatry, 150*, 1226–1232.

Blanchard, E. B., Hickling, E. J., Taylor, A. E., & Loos, W. (1995). Psychiatric morbidity associated with motor vehicle accidents. *Journal of Nervous and Mental Disease, 183*, 495–504.

Bland, R. C., Orn, H., & Newman, S. C. (1988). Lifetime prevalence of psychiatric disorders in Edmonton. *Acta Psychiatrica Scandinavica, 77*(Suppl. 338), 24–32.

Brinded, P. M. J., Stevens, I., Mulder, R., Fairley, N., Malcolm, F., & Wells, E. (1999). The Christchurch prisons psychiatric epidemiology study: Methodology and prevalence rates for psychiatric disorder. *Criminal Behavior and Mental Health, 9*, 131–143.

Clark, L. A. (2007). Assessment and diagnosis of personality disorder: Perennial issues and an emerging reconceptualization. *Annual Review of Psychology, 58*, 227–257.

Cohen, P., & Cohen, J. (1996). *Life values and adolescent mental health*. Mahwah, NJ: Erlbaum.

Coid, J., Yang, M., Tyrer, P., Roberts, A., & Ullrich, S. (2006). Prevalence and correlates of personality disorder in Great Britain. *British Journal of Psychiatry, 188*, 423–431.

Coryell, W. H., & Zimmerman, M. (1989). Personality disorder in the families of depressed, schizophrenic, and never-ill probands. *American Journal of Psychiatry, 146*, 496–502.

Crawford, T. N., Cohen, P., Johnson, J. G., Kasen, S., First, M. B., Gordon, K., et al. (2005). Self-reported personality disorder in the children in the community sample: Convergent and prospective validity in late adolescence and adulthood. *Journal of Personal Disorders, 19*, 30–52.

Dowson, J. H. (1992a). Assessment of DSM-III-R personality disorders by self-report questionnaire: The role of informants and a screening test for comorbid personality disorders (STCPD). *British Journal of Psychiatry, 161*, 344–352.

Dowson, J. H. (1992b). DSM-III-R narcissistic personality disorder evaluated by patients' and informants' self-report questionnaires: Relationships with other personality disorders and a sense of entitlement as an indicator of narcissism. *Comprehensive Psychiatry, 33*, 397–406.

Drake, R. E., & Vaillant, G. E. (1985). A validity study of Axis II of DSM-III. *American Journal of Psychiatry, 142*, 553–558.

Eaton, W. W., Anthony, J. C., Gallo, J., Cai, G., Tien, A., Romanoski, A., et al. (1997). Natural history of the Diagnostic Interview Schedule/DSM-IV major depression: The Baltimore Epidemiological Catchment Area follow-up. *Archives of General Psychiatry, 54*, 993–999.

Endicott, J., & Spitzer, R. L. (1979). Use of the Research Diagnostic Criteria and the Schedule for Affective Disorders and Schizophrenia. *American Journal of Psychiatry, 136*, 52–56.

Erlenmeyer-Kimling, L., Squires-Wheeler, E., Hilldoff Adamo, U., Bassett, A. S., Cornblatt, B. A., Kestenbaum, C. J., et al. (1995). The New York High-Risk Project: Psychoses and Cluster A personality disorders in offspring of schizophrenic parents at 23 years of follow-up. *Archives of General Psychiatry, 52*, 857–865.

First, M. B., Gibbon, M., Spitzer, R. L., Williams, J. B. W., & Janet, B. W. (1997). *Structured Clinical Interview for DSM-IV Axis II Personality Disorders (SCID-II)*. Washington DC: American Psychiatric Press.

Glueck, J., & Glueck, E. (1950). *Unraveling juvenile delinquency*. New York: Commonwealth Fund.

Grant, B. F., Dawson, D. A., & Hasin, D. S. (2001). *The Alcohol Use Disorder and Associated Disabilities Interview Schedule—DSM-IV Version*. Bethesda, MD: National Institute on Alcohol Abuse and Alcoholism.

Grant, B. F., Hasin, D. S., Stinson, F. S., Dawson, D. A., Chou, S. P., Ruan, W. J., et al. (2004). Prevalence, correlates, and disability of personality disorders in the United States: Results from the National Epidemiologic Survey on Alcohol and Related Conditions. *Journal of Clinical Psychiatry, 65*, 948–958.

Grant, B. F., Stinson, F. S., Dawson, D. A., Chou, S. P., Ruan, W. J., & Pickering, M. S. (2004). Co-occurrence of 12-month alcohol and drug use disorders and personality disorders in the United States: Results from the National Epidemiologic Survey on Alcohol and Related Conditions. *Archives of General Psychiatry, 61,* 361–368.

Hayward, M., & Moran, P. (2008). Comorbidity of personality disorders and mental illness. *Psychiatry, 7,* 102–104.

Heeringa, S. G., Wells, J. E., Hubbard, F., Mneimneh, Z., Chiu, W. T., Sampson, N. A., et al. (2008). Sample designs and sampling procedures. In R. C. Kessler & T. B. Üstün (Eds.), *The WHO World Mental Health Surveys: Global perspectives on the epidemiology of mental disorders* (pp. 14–32). New York: Cambridge University Press.

Huang, Y., Kotov, R., de Girolamo, G., Preti, A., Angermeyer, M., Benjet, C., et al. (2009). DSM-IV personality disorders in the WHO World Mental Health Surveys. *British Journal of Psychiatry, 195,* 46–53.

Hyler, S., Lyons, M., Reider, R., Young, L., Williams, J., & Spitzer, R. (1990). The factor structure of self-report DSM-III Axis II symptoms and their relationship to clinician's ratings. *American Journal of Psychiatry, 147,* 751–757.

Hyler, S., Reider, R., & Spitzer, R. (1983). *Personality Diagnostic Questionnaire (PDQ).* New York: New York State Psychiatric Institute.

Hyler, S., Skodol, A., Kellman, D., Oldham, J., & Rosnick, L. (1990). Validity of the Personality Diagnostic Questionnaire—Revised: Comparison with two structured interviews. *American Journal of Psychiatry, 147,* 1043–1048.

Kendler, K. S., Lieberman, J. A., & Walsh, D. (1989). The Structured Interview for Schizotypy (SIS): A preliminary report. *Schizophrenia Bulletin, 15,* 559–571.

Kendler, K. S., McGuire, M., Gruenberg, A. M., & Walsh, D. (1994). Outcome and family study of the subtypes of schizophrenia in the west of Ireland. *American Journal of Psychiatry, 151*(6), 849–856.

Kessler, R. C., McGonagle, K. A., Zhao, S., Nelson, C. B., Hughes, M., Eshleman, S., et al. (1994). Lifetime and 12-month prevalence of DSM-III-R psychiatric disorders in the United States. *Archives of General Psychiatry, 51,* 8–19.

Kessler, R. C., & Merikangas, K. R. (2004). The National Comorbidity Survey Replication (NCS-R): Background and aims. *International Journal of Methods in Psychiatric Research, 13,* 60–68.

Kessler, R. C., & Üstün, T. B. (Eds.). (2008). *The WHO World Mental Health Surveys: Global perspectives on the epidemiology of mental disorders.* New York: Cambridge University Press.

Krueger, R. F., Eaton, N. R., Derringer, J., Markon, K. E., Watson, D., & Skodol, A. E. (2011). Personality in the DSM-5: Helping delineate personality disorder content and framing the meta-structure. *Journal of Personality Assessment, 93,* 325–331.

Lenzenweger, M. F., Lane, M. C., Loranger, A. W., & Kessler, R. C. (2007). DSM-IV personality disorders in the National Comorbidity Survey Replication. *Biological Psychiatry, 62,* 553–564.

Lenzenweger, M. F., Loranger, A. W., Korfine, L., & Neff, C. (1997). Detecting personality disorders in a nonclinical population: Application of a 2-stage procedure for case identification. *Archives of General Psychiatry, 54,* 345–351.

Lenzenweger, M. F., Loranger, A. W., Korfine, L., & Neff, C. (2008). Epidemiology of personality disorder. *Psychiatric Clinics of North America, 31,* 395–403.

Loranger, A. W. (1999). *International Personality Disorder Examination: DSM-IV and ICD-10 interviews.* Odessa, FL: Psychological Assessment Resources.

Loranger, A. W., Sartorius, N., Andreoli, A., Berger, P., Buchheim, P., Channabasavanna, S. M., et al. (1994). The International Personality Disorder Examination (IPDE): The World Health Organization/Alcohol, Drug Abuse, and Mental Health Administration International Pilot Study of Personality Disorders. *Archives of General Psychiatry, 51,* 215–224.

Loranger, A. W., Sartorius, N., & Janca, A. (1996). *Assessment and diagnosis of personality disorders: The International Personality Disorder Examination (IPDE).* New York: Cambridge University Press.

Loranger, A. W., Susman, V. L., Oldham, J. M., & Russakoff, L. M. (1987). The Personality Disorder Examination: A preliminary report. *Journal of Personality Disorders, 1,* 1–13.

Lyons, M. J. (1995). Epidemiology of personality disorders. In M. T. Tsuang, M. Tohen, & G. E. P. Zahner (Eds.), *Textbook in psychiatric epidemiology* (pp. 407–436). New York: Wiley-Liss.

Maier, W., Lichtermann, D., Klinger, T., & Heun, R. (1992). Prevalences of personality disorders (DSM-III-R) in the community. *Journal of Personality Disorders, 6,* 187–196.

Maier, W., Minges, J., Lichtermann, D., & Heun, R. (1995). Personality disorders and personality variations in relatives of patients with bipolar affective disorders. *Journal of Affective Disorders, 53,* 173–181.

Mattia, J. I., & Zimmerman, M. (2001). Epidemiology. In W. J. Livesley (Ed.), *Handbook of personality disorders* (pp. 107–123). New York: Guilford Press.

Merikangas, K., & Weissman, M. (1986). Epidemiology of DSM-III Axis II personality disorders. In A. Frances & R. Hales (Eds.), *Psychiatry update: American Psychiatric Association annual review* (Vol. 5, pp. 258–278). Washington, DC: American Psychiatric Association.

Nestadt, G., Romanoski, A. J., Brown, C. H., Chahal, R., Merchant, A., Folstein, M. F., et al. (1991). DSM-III compulsive personality disorder: An epidemiologic survey. *Psychological Medicine, 21,* 461–471.

Nestadt, G., Romanoski, A. J., Chahal, R., Merchant, A., Folstein, M. F., Gruenberg, E. M., et al. (1990). An epidemiological study of histrionic personality disorder. *Psychological Medicine, 20,* 413–422.

Nestadt, G., Romanoski, A. J., Samuels, J. F., Folstein, M. F., Gruenberg, E. M., McHugh, P. R. (1992). The relationship between personality and DSM-III Axis I disorders in the population: Results from an epidemiological survey. *American Journal of Psychiatry, 149,* 1228–1233.

Pfohl, B., Blum, N., & Zimmerman, M. (1997). *Structured Interview for DSM-IV Personality (SIDP-IV).* Washington, DC: American Psychiatric Press.

Pfohl, B., Stangl, D., & Zimmerman, M. (1982). *The Structured Interview for DSM-III Personality Disorders (SIDP).* Iowa City: Department of Psychiatry, University of Iowa.

Regier, D. A., Boyd, J. H., Burke, J. D., Rae, D. S., Myers, J. K., Kramer, M., et al. (1988). One-month prevalence of mental disorders in the United States. *Archives of General Psychiatry, 45,* 977–986.

Regier, D. A., Narrow, W. E., Clarke, D. E., Kraemer, H. C., Kuramoto, S. J. Kuhl, E. A., et al. (2013). DSM-5 field trials in the United States and Canada: Part II. Test–restest reliability of selected categorical diagnoses. *American Journal of Psychiatry, 170,* 59–70.

Reich, J., Yates, W., & Nduaguba, M. (1988). Age and sex distribution of DSM-III personality cluster traits in a community population. *Comprehensive Psychiatry, 29,* 298–303.

Reich, J., Yates, W., & Nduaguba, M. (1989). Prevalence of DSM-III personality disorders in the community. *Social Psychiatry and Psychiatric Epidemiology, 24,* 12–16.

Robins, L. N., Helzer, J. E., Croughan, J., & Ratcliff, K. S. (1981). National Institute of Mental Health Diagnostic Interview Schedule: Its history, characteristics, and validity. *Archives of General Psychiatry, 38,* 381–389.

Romanoski, A. J., Nestadt, F., Chahal, R., Merchant, A., Folstein, M. F., Gruenberg, E. M., et al. (1988). Interobserver reliability of a Standardized Psychiatric Examination (SPE) for case ascertainment (DSM-III). *Journal of Nervous and Mental Disease, 176,* 63–71.

Samuels, J., Eaton, W. W., Bienvenu, O. J., Brown, C. J., Costa, P. T., & Nestadt, G. (2002). Prevalence and correlates of personality disorders in a community sample. *British Journal of Psychiatry, 180,* 536–542.

Schuster, J. P., Hoertel, N., Le Strat, Y., Manetti, A., & Limosin, F. (2013). Personality disorder in older adults: Findings from the National Epidemiologic Survey on Alcohol and Related Conditions. *American Journal of Geriatric Psychiatry, 21,* 757–768.

Spitzer, R. L., Williams, J. B. W., Gibbon, M., & First, M. (1990a). *Structured Clinical Interview for DSM-III-R Non-patient edition (SCID-NP; Version 1.0).* Washington, DC: American Psychiatric Association.

Spitzer, R. L., Williams, J. B. W., Gibbon, M., & First, M. (1990b). *Structured Clinical Interview for DSM-III-R Personality Disorders (SCID-II; Version 1.0).* Washington, DC: American Psychiatric Association.

Swanson, M. C., Bland, R. C., & Newman, S. C. (1994). Antisocial personality disorder. *Acta Psychiatrica Scandinavica, 376*(Suppl.), 63–70.

Swartz, M., Blazer, D., George, L., & Winfield, I. (1990). Estimating the prevalence of borderline personality disorder in the community. *Journal of Personality Disorders, 4,* 257–272.

Torgersen, S., Kringlen, E., & Cramer, V. (2001). The prevalence of personality disorders in a community sample. *Archives of General Psychiatry, 58,* 590–596.

Trull, T. J., & Durrett, C. A. (2005). Categorical and dimensional models of personality disorder. *Annual Review of Clinical Psychology, 1,* 355–380.

Trull, T. J., Jahng, S., Tomko, R. L., Wood, P. K., & Sher, K. J. (2010). Revised NESARC personality disorder diagnoses: Gender, prevalence, and comorbidity with substance dependence disorders. *Journal of Personality Disorders, 24,* 412–426.

Tyrer, P., Alexander, M. S., Cicchetti, D., Cohen, M. S., & Remington, M. (1979). Reliability of a schedule for rating personality disorders. *British Journal of Psychiatry, 135,* 168–174.

Tyrer, P., Crawford, M., Mulder, R., Blashfield, R., Farnuam, A., Fossati, A., et al. (2011). The rationale for the reclassification of the personality disorder in the 11th revision of the International Classification of Diseases (ICD-11). *Personality and Mental Health, 5,* 246–259.

Weissman, M. M. (1993). The epidemiology of personality disorders: A 1990 update. *Journal of Personality Disorders, 7,* 44–62.

Wells, J. E., Bushnell, J. A., Hornblow, A. R., Joyce, P. R., & Oakley-Browne, M. A. (1989). Christchurch psychiatric epidemiology study: Part I. Methodolgy and lifetime prevalence for specific psychiatric disorders. *Australian and New Zealand Journal of Psychiatry, 23,* 315–326.

Widiger, T. A., & Corbitt, E. M. (1993). Antisocial personality disorder: Proposals for DSM-IV. *Journal of Personality Disorders, 7,* 63–77.

World Health Organization. (1990). *Composite International Diagnostic Interview (CIDI) version 1.0.* Geneva, Switzerland: Author.

Zimmerman, M. (2012). Is there adequate empirical justification for radically revising the personality disorders section for DSM-5? *Personality Disorders: Theory, Research and Treatment, 4,* 444–457.

Zimmerman, M., & Coryell, W. (1989). DSM-III personality disorder diagnoses in a nonpatient sample: Demographic correlates and comorbidity. *Archives of General Psychiatry, 46,* 682–689.

Zimmerman, M., & Coryell, W. (1990). Diagnosing personality disorders in the community: A comparison of self-report and interview measures. *Archives of General Psychiatry, 47,* 527–531.

Zimmerman, M., Coryell, W., & Black, D. W. (1993). A method to detect intercenter differences in the application of contemporary diagnostic criteria. *Journal of Nervous and Mental Disease, 181,* 130–134.

Zimmerman, M., Pfohl, B., Coryell, W., Stangl, D., & Corenthal, C. (1988). Diagnosing personality disorder in depressed patients: A comparison of patient and informant interviews. *Archives of General Psychiatry, 45,* 733–737.

# CHAPTER 11

## Understanding Stability and Change in the Personality Disorders
### Methodological and Substantive Issues Underpinning Interpretive Challenges and the Road Ahead

Mark F. Lenzenweger, Michael N. Hallquist, and Aidan G. C. Wright

This chapter provides an overview and interpretation of the principal findings of the four major longitudinal studies of personality disorder (PD) against a backdrop of methodological and substantive issues and interpretive challenges. Each study has both methodological assets and liabilities; however, overall findings with respect to stability and change in PD over time are remarkably consistent. Our primary intention is to summarize the important findings in a "user-friendly" way for researchers and clinicians. Since hundreds of articles have emerged from these studies, with many more likely in future, we do *not* detail every finding or review the numerous predictor, outcome, and moderating variables that appear to impact longitudinal course, or the statistical procedures that might be applied to the broader data corpus. Besides summarizing key findings, we also seek to caution against simplistic interpretations—the picture harbored within these longitudinal data is far more complex than is suggested in summary statements such as "PDs maintain their rank order stability over time" or "PDs show declines in mean levels of symptoms over time."

A second intention is to inform the reader about dramatic methodological differences among longitudinal studies of PD by reviewing the complex methodological issues involved in longitudinal studies generally, comparing and contrasting the four studies in terms of meaningful methodological differences that qualify the interpretation and generalizability of findings, and pointing the way forward in terms of method-informed statistical treatments of longitudinal data. These goals reflect our concern that many scientists and practitioners are relatively unaware of how methodological differences across studies shape research questions and findings. In our discussions with colleagues and students in various venues, we have been alarmed to hear overly general summaries about the longitudinal course of PDs that referenced study acronyms (LSPD, CIC, MSAD, CLPS), with little awareness of the details of each study or how these details are crucial to an accurate interpretation of the findings. We hope that by highlighting important methodological and conceptual issues, our review will reveal a more nuanced, science-informed view that transcends simplistic summaries such as "Why study the PDs over time? We know they are stable" or "Why study PDs over time? We know they change." This is consistent with the spirit of this handbook, which is to be used by researchers, clinicians, and PhD graduate students/MD psychiatric residents. Finally, we articulate potentially rich future directions in the longitudinal study of PDs that promise to move the field beyond basic concepts of stability and change.

## Background and Context for the Longitudinal Investigation of Personality Pathology

In the mid-1980s, the PD research area was largely concerned with debates regarding the proper definition of PDs (e.g., categories vs. dimensions), as well as the development of diagnostic assessment instruments, because PDs had only recently been defined explicitly (i.e., DSM-III; American Psychiatric Association [APA], 1980) and reliable assessment instrumentation was just emerging (forerunners of the International Personality Disorder Examination [IPDE], Structured Clinical Interview for DSM-IV Axis II [SCID-II], and Structured Interview for DSM-III-R Personality Disorders [SIDP]). At that time, there was also a palpable concern with diagnostic issues, for example, (1) the comorbidity of PDs with Axis I disorders, (2) the challenging reality of multiple PDs in the same individual, (3) the utility of interview versus self-report assessment (Zimmerman, 1994), and (4) possible sex/gender bias in the definition/diagnosis of PDs (for reviews, see Lenzenweger & Clarkin, 1996, 2005). Many of these issues continue to be of concern today, as reflected in the attempted revision of the PDs section of DSM-5. By the end of the 1980s, more substantive and methodological questions had begun to loom large as investigators began to seek answers to the following fundamental questions: (1) Does mental state impact the assessment of PDs, which are putatively more enduring (i.e., a "state–trait" issue)?; (2) Could one develop a reasonably efficient screening instrument for PDs (i.e., generate few false-negative cases) for application in epidemiological studies?; (3) What is the epidemiology of PDs in *nonclinical* community populations?; (4) Can one find DSM-defined PDs in other countries (cultures)?; (5) Are there diagnostic approaches to PDs that might supplement traditional methods and incorporate information from observers other than clinicians?; (6) What would a theory of PD's look like that incorporates contemporary neural science, affective neuroscience, genomics, temperament, personality, and so on?; and (7) What is the precise nature of the natural history and course of personality psychopathology when studied from longitudinal perspective?

## The Emergence of Longitudinal Studies of PD

A final item in the previous list—"Are personality disorders as genuinely stable over time as we assume them to be?"—captured the interest of several researchers, stimulated principally by one glaring but often ignored historical fact: *Although predominant schools of thought in psychiatry and clinical psychology taught for nearly 100 years that personality pathology is stable, trait-like, and enduring, there were essentially no empirical data to support this assertion.* This impression owed much, albeit not often credited in clinical circles, to William James (1890/1950), who suggested that personality is "set like plaster" and unlikely to change after young adulthood. This notion of stability was an assumption gleaned from clinical observations and theoretical discussions, and tenaciously inculcated in generations of clinicians and researchers. To be fair, many clinicians working with patients with PDs (including the authors of this chapter) sensed that there are elements of stability to the dysfunction seen in such patients, such as interpersonal deficits, self-defeating behaviors, problems with intimacy, and impaired work performance (Freud's "love" and "work"). Nevertheless, although the modern editions of DSM consistently defined PDs as "enduring," "stable," "inflexible," and of "long duration," these "official" assumptions were *not* grounded in empirical findings from properly designed longitudinal studies. They reflected the impact of clinical experience and theory on the nomenclature architects and, in some small measure, crude inferences drawn from limited test–retest studies. Even the newly minted DSM-5 still holds that PD is trait-like in nature: The official PD criteria in DSM-5 [Section II] are directly imported from *DSM-IV-TR*, while the much debated "alternative criteria" are in Section III: Emerging Measures and Models of DSM-5. Although empirical studies of the longitudinal course of personality pathology have dramatically advanced knowledge in the past 20 years, these remain "early days" in understanding the stability of PD and we still lack empirical documentation of the *long-term* (30 years or more study duration) course of PDs (comparable to that available for nondisordered personality (McCrae & Costa, 1990, 2002; Ferguson, 2010; Funder, Parke, Tomlinson-Keasey, & Widaman, 1993; Roberts & DelVecchio, 2000; Roberts, Walton, & Viechtbauer, 2006; Robins, Fraley, Roberts, & Trzesniewski, 2001; Srivastava, John, Gosling, & Potter, 2003).

## Matters of Basic Method in Designing Longitudinal Studies of PD

Short-term test–retest studies of PDs, typically of borderline personality disorder (BPD), conducted during the 1980s and early 1990s (e.g., McDavid & Pilkonis, 1996; Perry, 1993) provided some of the context for the development of longitudinal studies. They suggested that some forms of personality pathology exhibited moderate short-term reliability. However, test–retest (time 1–time 2) studies cannot address *long-term* (i.e., periods of years or decades) stability as established by lifespan research (Nesselroade & Baltes, 1979; Nesselroade, Stigler, & Baltes, 1980; Rogosa, 1988; Rogosa et al., 1982). The use of two waves of longitudinal data (even if separated by a long period of time) is a limited design for investigating stability or change because (1) the amount of change between time 1 and time 2 is not informative about the *shape* of each person's individual growth trajectory and (2) valid estimates of the true rate of change cannot be determined with only two waves of data (Singer & Willett, 2003; Willett, 1988). Moreover, two-wave data cannot discern the impact of regression to the mean effects on longitudinal trajectories (Nesselroade et al., 1980), an important issue when interpreting findings (see later discussion of CLPS findings). Test–retest studies, however, are useful in establishing the test–retest reliability of assessment instruments (e.g., Loranger et al., 1994; Trull, 1993), but they have really minimal scientific utility in the study of stability (see Singer & Willett, 2003; Willett, 1988).

In contrast to test–retest studies, the *prospective multiwave* design has many advantages for studying continuity and change in PD that were well known when the four longitudinal studies of PD were designed (Collins & Sayer, 2001; Nesselroade & Baltes, 1979; Nesselroade et al., 1980; Rogosa, 1988; Rogosa, Brandt, & Zimowski, 1982; Singer & Willett, 2003; Willett, 1988). Lifespan developmentalists concerned with the study of cognitive, emotional, behavioral, and educational constructs over time had established that multiwave assessment was necessary to examine stability, change, and growth. Multiwave design permits examination of different aspects of stability, namely, (1) individual differences (rank-order or differential stability), (2) level (mean-level or absolute stability), (3) structural (factorial invariance), and (4) ipsative (intraindividual or profile stability) (Caspi & Roberts, 1999; Kagan, 1980; see also Roberts & DelVecchio, 2000; Roberts et al., 2006; Robins et al., 2001). It also allows for state-of-the-art analysis of individual growth curves within a multilevel or hierarchical linear modeling framework (Bryk & Raudenbush, 1987; Raudenbush & Bryk, 2002; Rogosa et al., 1982; Rogosa & Willett, 1985; Singer & Willett, 2003). Finally, it allows for the identification of more complex growth models that seek to examine the impact of simultaneously changing systems such as personality and on temporal changes in PD.

## The Four Major Studies of PD

We briefly describe in this section the four studies of PD. Table 11.1 presents an overview of the methodological, sampling, and other design features of these four studies. Perhaps the single most important distinction among the four studies is the nature of the populations sampled, namely, nonclinical versus treatment/clinical populations, a factor that constrains the generalizability of findings for each study in different ways. Highly detailed accounts of the design features, study samples, and findings from each of these studies are readily available, and we do not repeat such detail here (Longitudinal Study of Personality: Lenzenweger, 2006; Children in the Community Study: Cohen, Crawford, Johnson, & Kasen, 2005; McLean Study of Adult Development: Zanarini, Frankenburg, Hennen, Reich, & Silk, 2005; Collaborative Longitudinal Personality Disorders Study: Skodol et al., 2005).

### Studies Based on Nonclinical Population Sampling

*Longitudinal Study of Personality Disorders*

The Longitudinal Study of Personality Disorders (LSPD), which commenced in 1990 under the direction of Mark F. Lenzenweger, was the first National Institute of Mental Health (NIMH)–funded, prospective, multiwave longitudinal study focused on all DSM-defined personality pathology. Using a sample of 258 young adult subjects from a nonclinical university undergraduate setting, the LSPD has sought to explore substantive questions regarding the determinants of stability and change in personality pathology. The study sample was obtained by screening a larger population ($N = 1,684$) for PD features. The LSPD contains two groups: a possible personality disorder (PPD) group and

**TABLE 11.1. Overview of Methodological, Sampling, and Other Design Characteristics of the Four Major Longitudinal Studies of PD**

| Feature | LSPD | CLPS | MSAD | CIC |
|---|---|---|---|---|
| Start date | 1990 | 1996 | 1993 | 1990s[a] |
| Funding | NIMH | NIMH | NIMH | NIMH |
| Disorders covered | 11 (all PDs) | 4 PDs | 1 (BPD) | 11 (all PDs) |
| Instrumentation | IPDE/MCMI | DIPD-IV/SNAP | DIB-R/DIPD-R | SCID-II (last wave) |
| Interviewers blind | Yes | Partial (first 4 waves unblinded) | Yes | Yes |
| Untreated and treated cases included | Yes | No (all treated) | No (all treated) | Yes |
| Selection independence | Yes | No | No | Yes |
| Deviance range: Wave 1 | Wide | Narrow (all met DSM threshold) | Narrow (all met DSM threshold) | Wide |
| Possible site effects | No | Yes | No | No |
| Age range at baseline | 18–19 | 18–45 | 18–35 | 9–18 |
| Current status | Continuing | Closed | Continuing | Hiatus |

*Notes.* LSPD, Longitudinal Study of Personality Disorders; CLPS, Collaborative Longitudinal Personality Disorders Study; MSAD, McLean Study of Adult Development; CIC, Children in the Community Study; IPDE, International Personality Disorder Examination; MCMI, Millon Clinical Mutiaxial Inventory; DIPD-IV, Diagnostic Interview for Personality Disorders –IV; SNAP, Schedule for Nonadaptive and Adaptive Personality; DIB-R, Diagnostic Interview for DSM-III-R Borderlines—Revised; SCID-II, Structured Clinical Interview for DSM-III-R Axis II Disorders; Treated and untreated cases, sample included subjects who were seeking treatment of their own accord, as well as those who were not seeking treatment; presence of untreated cases allows for a rigorous evaluation of treatment × time interactions when testing change in PD features; Selection independence, refers to use of a clinical instrument for initial subject selection that differs from the instrument used subsequently in the clinical evaluation of PD features, thus guarding against endogeneity effects in the data; Deviance range, refers to the breadth of personality pathology evident in the sample subjects at baseline assessments; a wide range implies PD deviance extending from relative absence to severe, above DSM-threshold PD; a narrow range refers to the presence of marked deviance in all subjects at baseline assessments; Possible site effects, refers to study design features that might yield different findings within subsamples of subjects owing to being recruited in markedly different contexts (e.g., private psychiatric hospital vs. urban psychiatric clinic in low socioeconomic settings).
[a]Start date for the CIC refers to when PD assessments were begun using an archival case rating system in the ongoing CIC study, which began with different study aims in 1975 (see text for detail).

a no personality disorder (NPD) group. Besides studying PD features, the LSPD included measures of Axis I disorders, normal personality, temperament, and sex role conformity. This array of constructs, assessed at all three study waves to date (Wave I: baseline, Wave II: 1 year later, and Wave III: 3 years later), provides the foundation for all LSPD analyses. Each psychological or psychopathological construct is defined by at least two measures, which facilitates statistical modeling. A rigorous assessment blind was used throughout the study: The same subject was never assessed more than once by the same interviewer, and all interviewers were blind to the initial PPD or NPD status of subjects. The LSPD is now entering its 24th year and planning is under way for assessment Wave IV, which will reexamine subjects as they enter midlife (mid-40s). The inclusion of an NPD group positions the study uniquely to examine the emergence of PD in adulthood and compare trajectories across groups.

## Children in the Community Study

Under the direction of Patricia Cohen and Judith Brook, the Children in the Community Study (CIC) is a prospective study of various forms of psychopathology, including PD symptoms, in a large sample of children followed into adulthood. The children ($N = 800$) were initially sampled from the populations of Albany and

Saratoga counties in Upstate New York. The study began in 1975, with a focus on emotional and behavioral problems in children and how these features impacted family functioning, drug abuse, Axis I psychopathology, and other outcomes in adolescence. In the early 1990s, the study sample was evaluated for PDs by systematically rating participants on each PD criterion based on case history information (supplied principally by the subjects' mothers), but in subsequent assessments a structured clinical interview was used. The first assessments occurred when subjects were approximately 14 years old, with additional waves at the mean ages of 16, 22, and 33 years. The CIC used probability sampling to ensure a demographically representative sample with no preselection for PD. These features have allowed investigation of the emergence of PD over time. Moreover, the CIC may have the greatest generalizability to rural and lower socioeconomic status (SES) populations (Cohen et al., 2008). The CIC is currently on hiatus, but additional work with the sample is possible in the future.

### Studies Based on Treatment-Seeking Clinical (Inpatient, Outpatient) Population Sampling

*Collaborative Longitudinal Personality Disorders Study*

The Collaborative Longitudinal Personality Disorders Study (CLPS), conducted by John Gunderson and colleagues (2000), focused on four specific PDs followed prospectively over a 10-year period: borderline PD (BPD), schizotypal PD (STPD), avoidant PD (AVPD), and obsessive–compulsive PD (OCPD). All subjects had previously received psychiatric services or were recruited from inpatient or outpatient psychiatric clinics from four clinical sites, ranging from a disadvantaged, urban setting to a working-class urban setting, to a private psychiatric hospital. Participants were diagnosed according to DSM-IV using a semistructured interview developed by one of the study investigators (M. Zanarini), with auxiliary input from self-report measures and clinician ratings at entry into the study (Gunderson et al., 2000). The CLPS also included a contrast group of individuals with major depressive disorder (MDD; $n = 95$), who showed minimal PD features. Participants were assessed repeatedly over time. The first four assessments (baseline, 6 month, 12 month, and 24 month), however, were *not* done with a blind in place; therefore, the same interviewer often assessed the same patient. In subsequent assessments (after the 24-month assessment) a blind was instituted such that follow-along interviewers had not previously assessed a given participant. The CLPS is distinguished by the large sample sizes in each of the four PD cells at baseline (BPD $n = 175$, STPD $n = 86$, AVPD $n = 158$, OCPD $n = 154$), as well as a 10-year follow-up assessment. Unfortunately, the study had large attrition: The sample of 668 patients at baseline (573 were PD cases) eroded to only 266 patients at 10-year follow-up (patients lost to follow-up [$n = 237$]; patients lost due to incomplete data [$n = 165$]) (Hopwood et al., 2012). The CLPS study is now closed and no new waves of data will be collected (J. Gunderson, personal communication, November 8, 2011). Although McLean Hospital was one of the recruitment sites for CLPS, the sample does not overlap with that of the MSAD described below (J. Gunderson, personal communication, May 14, 2012).

*McLean Study of Adult Development*

The McLean Study of Adult Development (MSAD), under the direction of Mary Zanarini and conducted at the McLean Hospital (a private psychiatric hospital in Belmont, Massachusetts), focuses exclusively on patients with BPD ($n = 290$) evaluated on a host of constructs considered relevant to the course of the disorder (e.g., abuse history, premorbid psychosocial functioning, Axis I pathology, family history). The study also contains a contrast group of non-BPD patients with other PDs ($n = 72$). All subjects were initially inpatients receiving psychiatric treatment at McLean Hospital. Assessments began in 1993 and have been conducted every 2 years since. The MSAD has made ample use of semistructured clinical interviews and self-report inventories to assess individual-difference variables (e.g., personality) across the study period. The crisp focus on one PD has allowed an in-depth evaluation of stability and change in borderline pathology.

### A Fine-Grained Look at the Major Longitudinal Studies of Personality from a Methodological Vantage Point

In this section we highlight the importance of methodological *differences* among the studies because methodological decisions place constraints on what data from any given study can tell us, how the data are shaped a priori, and, importantly, what issues one needs to bear in mind when interpreting statistical findings. As noted earlier, Table 11.1 highlights several features with respect to these studies. The issue of PD sampling is salient and may be summarized easily: The MSAD focuses only on BPD, the CLPS examined four specific PDs (BPD, STPD, AVPD, and OCPD), whereas the LSPD and the CIC provide a full sampling of all DSM PD diagnoses.

## Primary Clinical Instrumentation

The evaluation of PD varied across all four studies. The LSPD used the IPDE, developed by Armand W. Loranger, throughout. The IPDE is a relatively conservative measure, with a detailed glossary that guides administration and scoring. It was used in the LSPD, in part, because it was used in the World Health Organization (WHO)/Alcohol, Drug Abuse and Mental Health Administration (ADAMHA) International Pilot Study of Personality Disorders (Loranger et al., 1994) to facilitate cross-cultural comparisons. DSM-III-R diagnostic criteria were used in the first three waves. Planned future assessments will also use DSM-III-R criteria to ensure consistency with previous waves of data collection, but DSM-IV/DSM-5 criteria will also be assessed using a hybrid version of the IPDE tailored for use in the LSPD.

The CIC began assessing PD features using a case rating system initially adapted from the Personality Diagnostic Questionnaire (PDQ) and subsequently expanded through incorporation of items from a prototype version of the Structured Clinical Interview for Axis II (SCID-II), with considerable clinical material gleaned from interviews with participants' mothers. Assessments of participants in adulthood (mean age = 33 years) were based on the SCID-II. The CIC team made a considerable effort to ensure that subjects were assessed for PD using a relatively common metric across the study period despite the assessment method switching from case rating/maternal interview methods to semistructured, subject-focused assessments (see Cohen et al., 2005, for details). The CLPS and MSAD both primarily used the semistructured interview developed by Mary Zanarini, known as the Diagnostic Interview for Personality Disorders (DIPD). The MSAD also used the Revised Diagnostic Interview for Borderlines, developed by John Gunderson and Mary Zanarini.

Besides considerable variation across studies in what PDs were assessed, there are also instances in which changes in assessment method were necessary to meet new challenges. For example, in the CIC, assessments based on maternal reports had to change to direct interviews when participants were assessed in adulthood. Although one can assume that all measures tapped a set of common *constructs,* each of the interviews used different diagnostic thresholds for the criteria assessed, were investigated differently for potential artifacts (e.g., state–trait considerations; cf. IPDE; Loranger et al. 1991), and enjoy considerably different levels of use across the field. Thus, there is every reason to believe that these interviews are not fungible and that each places its own unique imprint on the assessment process and results. For example, the IPDE is the most conservative of the semistructured interviews, which may enhance its precision in characterizing more severe pathology, perhaps at the expense of being relatively insensitive to moderate dysfunction. A sobering implication of the variation in the instruments is that the same patient may not have been assessed identically across these various interviews.

## Common Metrics, Ratings, and Use of an Experimenter Blind across PD Assessments

Longitudinal analysis typically requires that a common metric is used over time and, critically, that the instruments used measure constructs of interest in the same way throughout the study (i.e., they retain construct validity over time). With clinical interviews, the assessments (i.e., symptom counts) hail from *ratings* made by human assessors according to metrics of the measures used. Moreover, it should be noted that interview-based ratings are based on clinical *judgments* guided by an interview structure (i.e., they are *not* ratio- or interval-scaled data; rather they reflect ordinal scaling at best). We do not yet have laboratory measures of PD that yield objective data, measured in a ratio-scale manner, that enable the diagnosis of personality pathology (i.e., there are no biomarkers, endophenotypes, or neural circuits that possess high fidelity in identifying personality pathology). Keeping in mind that typical assessments represent interviewer ratings, let us consider how those assessments should be done to avoid potential artifacts that could undermine meaningful results. When studying construct or diagnosis over time, earlier assessments need to be conducted in a manner does *not* influence later assessments. This creates the need for an *experimenter blind,* so that each occasion the experimenter does not have prior information about the person could influence their current assessment. This is an example of the "halo effect," which is well established in the psychological research (Thorndike, 1920). Three of the studies (LSPD, CIC, and MSAD) had an intact complete blind throughout. The CLPS did *not* have a blind during the first four waves of data collection (baseline, 6-month, 12-month, and 24-month assessments) but implemented one for the fifth and subsequent waves. This methodological feature may limit the validity of longitudinal results from the first 2 years of the CLPS study.

In the case of PD assessments done repeatedly on the same subject by the same interviewer, the "halo effect" may operate in at least two ways. First, the assessor may remember broadly what general diagnostic picture was associated with a subject (e.g., "I recall this patient; he was schizotypal PD last time I saw him") and this may activate a schema that could artificially inflate the likelihood of seeing the same features in the patient again, even before an interview begins (what is sometimes called "a logical error in rating"; Rosenthal & Rosnow, 1991). Second, even if the interviewer resists this bias, the assessor may retain specific information regarding prior specific PD diagnostic criteria and may seek evidence that such criteria have changed (or remained the same), which in turn may impact the results of a current assessment differentially (e.g., "I recall this patient burned herself many times at last PD assessment; let me be sure to check whether that has changed").

### Impact of Starting with Treatment-Seeking Patients with PD in a Longitudinal Study

When beginning a longitudinal study, should one start with diagnosed cases receiving treatment and follow them over time (e.g., CLPS, MSAD) or *not* insist on the presence of a diagnosis of PD in study subjects at the outset of the project (e.g., LSPD, CIC)? The impact of including only a clinically diagnosed sample in treatment at the outset of the investigation should be considered in at least two ways. The MSAD and the CLPS began with clinically affected patients who were both formally diagnosed with a PD and were in either outpatient or inpatient psychiatric treatment. The CIC and LSPD did not use treatment-seeking patients who initially met the diagnostic criteria for a specific PD. The CIC was already under way when the PD component was added in the early 1990s, whereas the LSPD was explicitly designed to *not* rely on diagnosed cases for sample composition. That decision was taken in the LSPD because, as of the late 1980s (when the study was designed), it was not known whether diagnosed and treated patients with PD (particularly those presenting at clinics and hospital settings) were representative of the population of individuals affected by PDs.

In light of what is known about Berkson's (1946) bias in the epidemiology literature, it is reasonable to assume that clinic/hospital patients are *unrepresentative* of the population of PD-affected cases (e.g., showing more severe PD impairment, or gender-related artifacts related to treatment-seeking behavior) and likely to have greater pathology of all sorts, such as Axis I psychopathology, medical disorders, and other psychosocial impairment. Second, some patients with PD are likely to present at clinics only during times of crisis (e.g., consider someone with STPD who routinely escape clinical attention except during periods of crisis). Thus, while a diagnosed, treatment-seeking sample could provide useful information about the typical course of PD symptoms in a psychiatric outpatient sample, the results may not generalize or extend to the general population. Hence, CLPS and MSAD have provided useful information about the longitudinal stability of PDs in treated cases, whereas the LSPD and CIC likely provide a better picture of PD symptom stability in the general population.

### Selection of Above-Threshold Diagnosed Cases of PD and the "Law of Initial Values"

Here we consider the impact of selecting subjects that are a priori quantitatively deviant on a clinical measure (e.g., symptom counts). This is a complicated consideration, and fortunately for the field, the available longitudinal studies have been conducted both ways. By definition, individuals meeting diagnostic threshold for a PD at the outset of a study are quantitatively deviant for the PD under consideration (i.e., they have "high" scores). The "law of initial values" (Wilder, 1957) comes into effect in this situation. It basically states that the higher the initial value on a measure of interest, the more rapid its drop on subsequent assessments (Benjamin, 1967). Elevated values (e.g., high symptom counts) typically have only one direction to go, *and that is down,* as demonstrated life-span methods literature (Nesselroade et al., 1980). This reality illustrates the ubiquitous phenomenon of "regression to the mean." However, we note that this phenomenon is also likely to lead to increases in PD features among those sampled to be particularly low in symptoms at baseline. This law of initial values clouds the interpretability of mean-level symptom change in all four studies, but it is especially problematic for the CLPS and MSAD, which required high levels of symptoms for study eligibility.

On the other hand, including subjects *without* clinically significant personality pathology at the beginning of the study is valuable because it allows for the possibility that some unaffected individuals might subsequently develop a PD, thereby providing an opportunity to explore factors associated with the onset of the PD. The LSPD and the CIC designs allow for this possibility (see below). If there is to be a next generation of longitudinal PD studies, larger samples across the full range of symptom severity would be ideal for a detailed study of the longitudinal course. Larger samples would mitigate concerns about floor or ceiling effects, leading to misestimates of the true longitudinal course of PDs. In this context, we would like to state clearly that we do see positive value in some studies beginning with "above-threshold" diagnosed PD cases for study. Such a design allows for meaningful studies of prognosis or the course of clinical cases, which has obvious relevance to treatment and understanding the natural history of diagnosed individuals.

### Selection Independence: Independent Variables versus Dependent Variables

"Selection independence" applies to the use of a different measure to *select* subjects for inclusion in a study from that used to tap the construct during the course of the study. This consideration is important, as it aims to ensure that the independent variable (the selection measure) is not one and the same as the dependent variable (the longitudinal measure). When the selection variable is precisely the same as the variable under study, then the selection variable is not exogenous to the developmental process or construct (i.e., the variable under longitudinal study has also influenced selection for the study). Stated differently, the independent variable and the dependent variable are one and the same. This is a variant of what is often termed the "endogeneity problem" in developmental studies, wherein the same variable cannot be both the independent and the dependent variable simultaneously (Duncan, Magnuson, & Ludwig, 2004). Selection independence occurred with both the LSPD and CIC. The LSPD used a screening instrument to identify "possible PD" versus "no PD" cases for study inclusion, but clinical assessments for specific PDs were based on either a clinician-administered interview (IPDE) or self-report (Millon Clinical Multiaxial Inventory–II [MCMI-II]). In the CIC, subjects were probability sampled for inclusion, and clinical PD measures were only used once subjects had entered the study. It is also important to understand that by virtue of meeting the selection criterion (e.g., a diagnosed PD), all other measures administered to study subjects are ipso facto conditioned on the presence of that disorder, another variant of the endogeneity problem. For example, if a subject is selected for the presence of STPD to enter a study, then responses on a personality measure are necessarily impacted by the presence of that disorder. Hence, the personality disorder measure is not *exogenous* to the system under study, even though one might be tempted to think of one or another component of the measure as useful in "predicting" PD symptoms (e.g., one cannot really claim that low extraversion predicts STPD features in a longitudinal perspective).

### Treatment and Time Intertwined: The Issue of Treatment × Time Interaction in Longitudinal Perspective

All of the longitudinal studies included participants with differing mental health treatment exposure, which raises the issue of whether treatment × time interactions influenced estimates of symptom change. Inclusion of subjects with and without a psychiatric treatment history allows one to evaluate this interaction and separate treatment effects from other processes, something that is more difficult with samples of *only* treated cases. The treatment × time interaction problem can be addressed statistically, by trying to quantify treatment exposure intensity. In the LSPD, for example, the interaction could be incorporated in analyses directly because some subjects had treatment exposure, whereas others did not. With the CLPS, in which treatment × time were conflated, the solution adopted was to parse treatment exposure into meaningful levels of treatment intensity and incorporate intensity × time interactions in analyses. This indicated substantial interaction between treatment intensity and time in relation to PD symptom change. For example, Shea and colleagues (2002) reported that subjects with STPD and BPD who received high-intensity treatments showed *less* change in symptom features over the first year of study. This suggests that treatment was maintaining the mental health of those subjects by preventing deterioration or, more likely, that subjects receiving the most intensive treatment were the most impaired and not likely to change. Both possibilities may also be true within subgroups of the high-intensity treatment group. However, by the 2-year assessments (Grilo et al., 2004), treatment intensity × time interactions disappeared from the CLPS sample. Clearly, the role of treatment in relation to symptom change in PD over time is a complicated matter, and the results of any naturalistic study in which subjects could be exposed to treatment should be evaluated with this in mind. The essential message is to view suggestions regarding stability and/or change in the PDs with caution when treatment effects and time effects, as well as their interaction, are active in a longitudinal study. This is particularly relevant to both the CLPS and MSAD results.

## Consider the Site from Which the Subjects Are Sampled

The site from which the subjects for a longitudinal study are drawn is relevant when considering the nature and pattern of resulting findings. For example, the LSPD subjects were drawn initially from a nonclinical university undergraduate population. As a result, it is possible that the resulting sample did not include the most severe cases of PD deviance simply because individuals with severe PDs might not gain admission to a university. However, we know that the prevalence of PD cases in the LSPD sample (11%) is comparable to that in the U.S. population (9%), as determined by the National Comorbidity Survey Replication (NCS-R; Lenzenweger, Lane, Loranger, & Kessler, 2007). The MSAD drew its subjects from patients admitted to a university-affiliated private psychiatric hospital (McLean Hospital, Belmont, Massachusetts), many of whom were economically advantaged or possess substantial health insurance coverage. In contrast, many CLPS subjects were drawn from clinics affiliated with university-based psychiatry programs situated in (1) an impoverished urban setting with unique demographics and elevated crime levels (Washington Heights, New York City) or (2) a blue-collar, working-class urban environment, where many residents live below the poverty line (Providence, Rhode Island). Finally, the CIC drew its subjects from a largely rural section of New York State, with some subjects coming from the Albany metropolitan region, including especially low SES level subjects. Such variability in the sampling frames underscores the importance of knowing methodological details of the four studies, as the generalizability of findings from each study is greatest for populations that best match the relevant sampling frame. For example, the MSAD probably offers the best characterization of longitudinal change in BPD symptoms among severe psychiatric inpatients, whereas the CIC may offer a better window into the course of PD symptoms in rural general population samples.

## Classic Stability and Change Methodological Approaches: Rank-Order and Mean Levels

Having reviewed the four longitudinal studies, it is fitting to summarize conclusions in terms of stability and change in PD features. Conceptualizing PD features (a symptom count or symptom dimension variable) as the primary unit of analysis makes the most sense given the enhanced sensitivity of dimensional assessment. One could examine the stability of PD diagnoses over time; however, the meaning of such analyses is ambiguous given (1) the arbitrary cutoff scores used to establish diagnostic thresholds (e.g., why five, not six, out of nine criteria for BPD? [see Krueger, 2013]); and (2) the loss of information in reducing a quasi-dimensional measurement (i.e., symptom counts) to a dichotomously scored (present vs. absent) variable (Markon & Krueger, 2006).

Thus, we ask two primary questions:

1. "Do PDs reveal rank-order stability over time?" That is, do the individuals in a sample maintain their relative rank on the variable of interest across time?
2. "Do PDs show evidence of mean level stability over time?" That is, is there evidence of stability or change over time in the group mean for a given PD measure?

The concepts of rank-order and mean-level stability have been used in all four studies. Although each concept has a rich tradition in lifespan developmental research, each has limited information value with respect to stability and change. For example, rank-order stability, assessed with the correlation coefficient, just captures a "snapshot" of the relative ranking of a sample at two arbitrary time points and fails to capture the full picture of change or stability, particularly intraindividual stability or change, whereas mean-level stability ignores individual variation in growth, assumes that the average pattern of change is reasonably representative of all cases samples (which is untenable given what we know about PD change and stability), and constrains all subjects to a common assessment schedule (an unrealistic assumption with longitudinal research Richer measures of stability are available as we discuss later).

### RANK-ORDER (DIFFERENTIAL) STABILITY

Analyses of rank-order stability suggests moderate stability. In their meta-analytic summary, Morey and Hopwood (2013) reported rank-order stability coefficients ranging from .30 to .50 over periods ranging 3–10 years for interview-based assessments. The CIC and LSPD studies reported rank-order stability for PD around .40 (over 2-, 4-, and 10-year time frames) and approximately .50 (over 1- and 3-year time frames), respectively. The CLPS found that rank-order stability declined steeply over time: Short-term rank-order stability (12 month) was high (mean $r$ = .86), but long-term rank-order stability was lower (2-year mean $r$ = .59; 4-year mean $r$ = .47, 10-year mean $r$ = .35) (Morey & Hopwood, 2013). These values are average correlations that have not been statistically adjusted for reliability (e.g., attenuated reliability adjustments). It is interesting to keep in mind that all of these correlations concern interview-based PD assessments. Self-report measures of PD show greater stability. With the LSPD study, for example, median rank-order stability was 0.74 at 1 year and 0.64 at 3 years (Lenzenweger, 1999). The CLPS study reported similar findings. These findings suggest that self-report data may harbor stability characteristics that are not reflected in interview-based PD data, representing a rich area for future research.

Finally, it is important to consider the level of data aggregation when evaluating rank-order stability statistics. For example, with the LSPD, if the PD criteria are aggregated at the level of DSM Clusters A, B, and C or total PD features (all disorders combined), interview-based and self-report data reveal greater rank-order stability than most estimates for specific disorders. This may reflect the increase in reliability gained from using a composite measure of PD rather than criteria counts for specific PDs. The general thrust of the rank-order stability findings across studies is that individuals tend to maintain their rank over time; however, these data also hint at some degree of movement in ranks because the correlations obtained are far from unity.

### MEAN-LEVEL (ABSOLUTE) STABILITY

The *zeitgeist* of the last 100 years or so in psychiatry and clinical psychology has suggested that individuals with PDs reveal a behavioral and psychological profile that is relatively immutable. In some corners of the field, particularly in some treatment venues, this assumption has even led to therapeutic nihilism regarding the ability to effect change in PD-affected individuals. This commitment to stability has been the official position of DSM-III through DSM-5. If individuals do not change, then the mean levels of PD features in a group of individuals should not change either. The results from longitudinal studies have dramatically challenged this view. Lenzenweger (1999) first reported clinically meaningful declines in personality pathology over a multiyear period using data from the LSPD. Consistent results were quickly reported by the CIC, MSAD, and CLPS studies. Additional evidence for change (generally declines) in PD features over time subsequently was reported by other longitudinal studies (Chanen et al., 2004). The CIC reported 28–48% reductions in PD symptoms (continuous dimensional count format) over time across the various PDs, along with substantial and significant declines in the Clusters A, B, and C composite feature counts, and total PD feature count (Johnson et al., 2000).

Moving to the patient-based samples, data from the CLPS study revealed that that 66% of patients dropped below diagnostic thresholds after 1 year (Shea et al., 2002) and 57% at a 2-year follow-up (Grilo et al., 2004). However, direct comparison of these results with the 1-year and 2-year data is difficult because attrition in the CLPS sample was already evident at the 2-year follow-up (consisting of only 499 patients vs. 573 patients with PD enrolled at baseline). Treating the PD feature counts for the four studied PDs as continuous variables, Shea and colleagues (2002) reported statistically significant and substantial mean level declines for all four PDs assessed over a 1-year span. Similar results were reported at the 2-year follow-up (Grilo et al., 2004). Dramatic declines in BPD features were also documented in the CLPS at the 10-year follow-up assessment (Gunderson et al., 2011; Morey & Hopwood, 2013). Finally, the MSAD study also found that nearly 75% of individuals with BPD no longer met the diagnostic threshold for the disorder at a 6-year assessment (Zanarini, Frankenburg, Hennen, & Silk, 2003). This figure increased to 88% at the 10-year follow-up (Zanarini et al., 2006). At the 16-year follow-up, 99% of subjects initially diagnosed as BPD had shown remission for at least 2 years' duration; furthermore, 90% of those initially diagnosed with BPD were found to have been in remission for 6 years (see Zanarini, Frankenburg, Reich, & Fitzmaurice, 2012). In this context, we note that the use of the term "remission" in the Zanarini studies departs from standard medical usage. A patient with BPD might no longer meet the threshold for a BPD diagnosis (five of nine criteria) by presenting three or four criteria, but such a case is not genuinely remitted (i.e., showing no signs/symptoms of disease). Although data on mean-level changes have not been reported for dimensional BPD symptoms in the MSAD study articles, substantial BPD symptom declines must have occurred given the remarkable (really stunning) rates of diagnosis "remission." As articulated earlier, one must bear in mind the sampling frame, treatment effects, and the level of baseline severity when interpreting findings on mean-level change. Nonetheless, the overall picture that emerges from all studies is that PD features tend to decline over time.

### Heterogeneity in Growth and Treating Time in a More Sensitive Manner

Whereas the initial analyses of rank-order and mean-level stability for PD features in the LSPD dataset pointed to appreciable levels of stability when all subjects were taken together, our exploration of the symptom data from the LSPD found remarkable *heterogeneity* among growth curves across individual subjects for all PDs, suggesting considerable variation in longitudinal trajectories. Obscured when only simple group means are used as the unit of statistical aggregation, Figure 11.1 depicts the individual growth trajectories of "total PD features" for

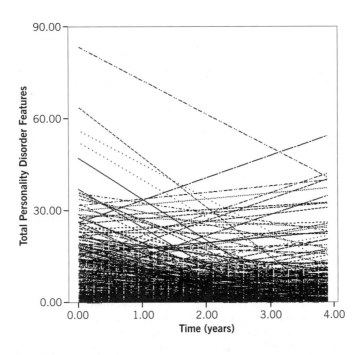

**FIGURE 11.1.** Ordinary least squares individual growth trajectories for total PD features (IPDE) in 250 LSPD subjects over the study period. Time is reported in years, since the beginning of the study, and it is centered for each subject using the subject's age of entry into the study.

each participant in the LSPD, with each line representing a person. The figure plainly shows that there is no obvious consistent growth trajectory followed by all subjects. Change was *not* uniform across all individuals: Despite an overall pattern of symptom decline, some subjects showed declines, others showed increases in pathology, and still others were stable. This impressive degree of interindividual variability in change requires further exploration to discover whether personality features, other psychiatric characteristics, psychological attributes (e.g., ego strength, identity diffusion, defense mechanisms), and/or other factors account for the longitudinal variability (Hallquist & Lenzenweger, 2013; Lenzenweger, Johnson, & Willett, 2004; Wright, Pincus, & Lenzenweger, 2013; cf. Estes, 1956; Grimm, Ram, & Hamagami, 2011).

We could discuss numerous other methodological and substantive issues within the context of research on the longitudinal nature of PDs. At this juncture, however, we depart from that more technical corpus and turn our attention to the future.

## The Road Ahead: Important Opportunities for Understanding Stability and Change

Given the important insights gained from these longitudinal studies, it is useful to reflect on what is next in this arena. We organize our consideration of the design of future longitudinal PD studies around the traditional "W" questions: Who? What? Where? When? and How? We leave aside for the moment the final question: Why? Because we believe the value of longitudinal studies is self-evident, we might first ask, "Who should be included?" As we discussed earlier, sampling issues are of central importance. To maximize the scientific yield, one must be clear about the constructs of interest—for example, whether to select individuals with certain PD features or to sample based on the severity of overall personality dysfunction—as well as the core population of interest (e.g., patients vs. nonpatients), because findings from one population are unlikely to generalize to another. For example, in treatment-seeking samples, BPD is often more prevalent in females than in males, whereas there is little evidence for sex differences in the general population (Lenzenweger, Lane, Loranger, & Kessler, 2007). Moreover, how PD is expressed may differ from one population to another, such as the greater occurrence of self-harm and suicidal behavior in individuals with BPD from a hospital compared to community sample (Korfine & Hooley, 2009). If one's goal is to answer basic questions about the nature of personality pathology writ large, it is important to include individuals who span the full range of severity drawn from the general population, while also ensuring sufficient variability in covariates to avoid inadvertent bias in the sample. More limited sampling strategies may be warranted to answer specific questions of public health interest (e.g., what is the long-term prognosis of psychiatric inpatients with severe PDs? Or what are the most common co-occurring mood and anxiety disorders in individuals with narcissistic PD?), but these necessarily constrain the generalizability of the investigation.

What variables should be assessed? First, one should address the issue of which variables should be used to select participants, which represents the intersection of the "Who?" and "What?" questions. Currently, numerous problems with polythetic threshold definitions of PDs in the DSM, such as poor discriminant validity (Sanislow et al., 2009) and arbitrary diagnostic thresholds (Cooper, Balsis, & Zimmerman, 2010; Krueger, 2013), limit enthusiasm for the system (Pilkonis, Hallquist, Morse, & Stepp, 2011). Moreover, the DSM-5 revision process revealed deep divisiveness about the definition of PD constructs. Some of the tensions can be waved aside as the creaking of wagons circling around protected interests (e.g., research programs founded on the old model), but others reflect thoughtful criticism (e.g., Pilkonis et al., 2011; Pincus, 2011). Moreover, the revision process may have been enfeebled by inadequate consultation (both real and imagined) with the extant corpus of research findings available when revision efforts were made (see Lenzenweger, 2012). Regardless of future changes to official psychiatric nosologies, it is currently unclear whether there is a consensus about the definition of PD. Given the *zeitgeist,* however, it is clear that accruing a fresh longitudinal sample by sampling current diagnostic constructs is probably unwise. Instead, we recommend that future new longitudinal studies study a broader set of variables, including traditional measures of symptomatology and self-report questionnaires, and variables closer to the neurobehavioral core of PDs, such as psychophysiological or neuroimaging indices relevant to key psychological processes. Additionally, greater emphasis should be given to context, including, but not limited to, denser measurement of the social environment, social role, and work functioning (networks), and possibly environmentally sensitive designs that sample physical and social environment features of neighborhoods where individuals live and work. The ultimate goal is to better understand the contextualized individual at multiple levels of analysis, ranging from the biological to the social, setting up networks of variables that can be profitably probed to understand the mechanisms of change underlying individual trajectories of personality pathology.

The foregoing concerns underscore the variety of opinions about how best to define and measure personality pathology, and indeed the ontological status of PDs as an area of research. In psychometric theory, the reliability of an instrument sets the upper bound on the validity of the construct it seeks to measure (Nunnally & Bernstein, 1994). If a construct cannot be measured consistently (Widaman, Ferrer, & Conger, 2010), then resolving meaningful patterns of change will be difficult. Although the internal consistency of personality pathology assessed by interview or self-report is reasonably good for a cross-sectional assessment (e.g., Zimmerman et al., 2005), an important finding of the CLPS study is that the longitudinal stability of individual PD criteria is remarkably heterogeneous, with some features showing more trait-like stability and others marked instability (McGlashan et al., 2005). Conversely, even as clinician-assessed PD symptoms decline with time, self-reported personality pathology and core aspects of psychosocial dysfunction are often more stable (e.g., Gunderson et al., 2011; Lenzenweger, 1999).

Thus, future longitudinal studies need to consider both their definition of personality pathology and means of assessment. In particular, greater emphasis on differentiating acute illness from enduring pathology may help to refine models of PDs (Zanarini et al., 2012). To truly understand the longitudinal course of personality pathology, however, our diagnostic tools must measure the same latent construct at each assessment. This is a problem with current constructs: The temporal heterogeneity among DSM PD criteria suggests that using a threshold for diagnosis or summing individual criteria scores is unlikely to yield a measure of PD that can be trusted to tap into the same construct over time. Thus, the field must be concerned with ensuring that the construct validity of personality pathology, however it is assessed, is consistent over time in order to be confident that changes (or stability) in PDs reflect the dynamics of the underlying constructs, not artifacts of the instrumentation. In this respect, we hope that future research tests the longitudinal measurement invariance of interview-based and self-report PD instruments. At a deeper level, moving forward, the field needs to deepen its focus on the ontology or emergence of PDs to move beyond simplistic accounts of clinical entities versus multidimensional trait profiles. In short, how do PD's come to be or come to exist? What is the process or mechanism by which this domain of psychopathology emerges? It would be beneficial to capitalize on the momentum generated by the passionate arguments about the definition of PDs that occurred during the DSM-5 revision process. Even though a plurality of theories about personality dysfunction are crucial to bootstrap our understanding of PDs, without construct definitions that reflect an empirically derived consensus among researchers, longitudinal research on PDs may become too cacophonous to uncover etiological mechanisms or curative factors.

Where should participants be assessed? Existing longitudinal studies have primarily collected the types of data that populate clinical reports (symptoms, diagnoses, personality scales, etc.). Moving forward, we believe it will be necessary for investigators to include both laboratory and ecological assessments, in addition to conventional assessment methods: If we aim to fully understand the phenomenon of PD, assessments should range from the "synapse to the street." Since the four longitudinal studies were designed, major advances have been made in neuroimaging, portable electronic devices, inexpensive bioassays, and other technologies that allow for a more detailed assessment of the proximal processes underlie the development of PD. Accordingly, the past decade has seen impressive leveraging of this technology, although not in a longitudinal context. For instance, the use of ecological momentary assessments, in which individuals provide momentary ratings of their environment, perceptions of others, and their own behavior *in situ* as they live their lives (Trull & Ebner-Priemer, 2013), have provided a remarkable ability to capture clinically salient phenomena such as hostile outbursts (e.g., Russell, Moskowitz, Zuroff, Sookman, & Paris, 2007; Trull et al., 2008) and to provide new insights into core processes of disorders (e.g., the differential power of interpersonal triggers and emotional responses in PD; Coifman, Berenson, Rafaeli, & Downey, 2012; Sadikaj, Moskowitz, Russell, Zuroff, & Paris, 2013; Sadikaj,

Russell, Moskowitz, & Paris, 2010). Contemporary techniques for collecting data in the lived environment include self-report, bioassays, and even snippets of audio recording that can be coded for behavior and content (Trull & Ebner-Priemer, 2013). Future studies should also consider including informant reports (Oltmans & Turkheimer, 2009) and following target participants, along with significant others, to provide collateral reports. It is now well known in both the assessment of basic personality (Vazire & Carlson, 2010) and PD (Oltmans & Turkheimer, 2009) that informants provide incrementally valid information, with particularly valuable contributions for certain forms of pathology (e.g., narcissism; Klonsky, Oltmanns, & Turkheimer, 2003).

When should assessments occur? This question actually encompasses two considerations: rate of measurement and developmental stage. Each longitudinal study we discussed has adopted (mostly) annual or biannual assessment schedules. These are the "bread and butter" of longitudinal panel study designs that offer many conceptual and statistical advantages. However, moving forward, it is worth considering alternative schedules. For instance, recent research has shown that PD-relevant fluctuations can occur on the order of months (Wright, Hallquist, Beeney, & Pilkonis, 2013). Additionally, as we mentioned in response to the previous question, intensive repeated measurement, on the order of moments and days, holds powerful potential for the study of PD. Although it is clear that understanding macrolevel change on the order of years cannot be accomplished "one day at a time" via daily diary methods, it would be possible to embed momentary, daily, weekly, and monthly assessments within a larger panel study to leverage the ability of these methods to capture key processes at the relevant temporal scale. For example, slow changes in personality traits (Roberts et al., 2006) may be related to the remission of PD symptoms over several years, but momentary outbursts of interpersonal aggression in BPD may be closely related to romantic relationship satisfaction. Indeed, the power of experience sampling methodology could augment a traditional study design in what has been termed a "random burst design." Additionally, with the increasing ubiquity of Internet access, participants could complete modest assessments on a monthly or bimonthly basis to further enrich data collection.

The second consideration is when (or at what point) in the lifespan future studies should focus their efforts? At what age, for example, should subjects be enrolled in long-term developmental longitudinal studies of PD? Although we cannot devote much space to this issue, this does not mean this issue is not important. In our estimation, there remains a need for studies that adopt an earlier focus (e.g., starting in late childhood and early adolescence) and continue on through adulthood if we are to gain a better appreciation of etiological and contributory factors to the onset and development of PD (Tackett, Balsis, Oltmanns, & Krueger, 2009). In this vein, studies should increasingly measure developmentally appropriate constructs that likely will shift over the course of a longitudinal study.

As described earlier, normal-range personality variables are likely to track with PD change; however, the precise nature of these relationships requires considerable illumination (Lenzenweger & Willett, 2007). For instance, in CLPS, the general finding was that the PDs were largely variants of a single exaggerated pattern on the five-factor personality measures of high Neuroticism, low Agreeableness, and low Conscientiousness (Morey et al., 2002). While it is unlikely that PDs can be fully captured using lexically based trait profiles such as five-factor measures (Wright, 2011), it is scientifically problematic if models of PD are not rooted in basic models of personality. Therefore, continued study of the longitudinal links between the two—personality and PD—is important. What do we know already about the connections between normal personality, PD, and psychosocial functioning from the vantage point of change? A number of key findings should be considered. First, personality traits exhibit greater temporal stability than do PD features. Second, psychosocial impairments remain despite PD changes (Gunderson et al., 2011). This suggests the possibility, although circumstantially, that basic personality functioning is responsible for long-term stability of psychosocial functioning, even as PD symptoms wax and wane at a faster rate. Thus, it is important to test whether both PD and basic personality features demonstrate comparable associations with psychosocial functioning change, and whether the change increments each other in the prediction of psychosocial functioning change. In this vein, it may be that certain personality traits (e.g., the triad of neuroticism or negative affectivity, antagonism or low communal positive emotionality, and conscientiousness or nonaffective constraint) capture much of the core variance in measures of psychosocial impairment. Relatedly, it would be interesting to disentangle the variance in PD that can be accounted for by basic personality from the remainder. Stated differently: "Are there aspects of personality disorder that are actually important net of relations with normal personality dimensions?" Clearly, further study of change/growth in personality and PD must be probed more deeply (cf. Lenzenweger & Willett, 2007). This may go a long way toward clarifying which features are related to core personality pathology, and which appear to operate more like symptomatic flare-ups. Furthermore, there is ample room for considering additional models of personality that have not emerged from the trait tradition such as the interpersonal (Hopwood, Wright, Ansell, & Pincus, 2013) and neurobehavioral models (Depue & Lenzenweger, 2005).

Many other fascinating questions about personality pathology remain, and we can only hint at them as we close our chapter. For example, what more needs to be done to make sense of the PD NOS concept, given its ubiquitous nature, in a longitudinal perspective, given that it is associated with a variety of noteworthy demographic, psychosocial, and psychopathological outcomes over the lifespan (cf., Johnson et al., 2005). Furthermore, how do we really understand PD when we see rapid and/or spontaneous recovery in patients whom we presume to have been validly diagnosed with one or another PD (e.g., consider BPD and the 10% recovery rate for this disorder in the first 6 months of the CLPS study or, longer term, consider the nearly complete remission of BPD in the MSAD study over the 16-year study period)? What characterizes the longitudinal course of such persons? How are they different from other, similarly diagnosed patients with PD? The list of interesting topics can only extend, and the powerful method of longitudinal research will continue to inform our understanding of PD in the decades to come. The road ahead is rich with possibilities, but, of course, it will all take time, perhaps the most powerful lever in our research toolbox.

## REFERENCES

American Psychiatric Association. (1980). *Diagnostic and statistical manual of mental disorders* (3rd ed.). Washington, DC: Author.

American Psychiatric Association. (1987). *Diagnostic and statistical manual of mental disorders* (3rd ed., rev.). Washington, DC: Author.

American Psychiatric Association. (1994). *Diagnostic and statistical manual of mental disorders* (4th ed.). Washington, DC: Author.

American Psychiatric Association. (2013). *Diagnostic and statistical manual of mental disorders* (5th ed.). Arlington, VA: Author.

Benjamin, L. S. (1967). Facts and artifacts in using analysis of covariance to "undo" the law of initial values. *Psychophysiology, 4,* 187–206.

Berkson, J. (1946). Limitations of the application of fourfold table analysis to hospital data. *Biometrics, 2,* 339–343.

Bryk, A. S., & Raudenbush, S. W. (1987). Application of hierarchical linear models to assessing change. *Psychological Bulletin, 101,* 147–158.

Caspi, A., & Roberts, B. W. (1999). Personality continuity and change across the life course. In L. A. Pervin & O. P. John (Eds.), *Handbook of personality: Theory and research* (2nd ed., pp. 300–326). New York: Guilford Press.

Chanen, A. M., Jackson, H. J., McGorry, P. D., Allot, K. A., Clarkson, V., & Yuen, H. P. (2004). Two-year stability of personality disorder in older adolescent outpatients. *Journal of Personality Disorders, 18,* 526–541.

Cohen, P., Chen, H., Gordon, K., Johnson, J., Brook, J., & Kasen, S. (2008). Socioeconomic background and developmental course of schizotypal and borderline personality disorder symptoms. *Development and Psychopathology, 20,* 633–650.

Cohen, P., Crawford, T. N., Johnson, J. G., & Kasen, S. (2005). The Children in the Community Study of developmental course of personality disorder. *Journal of Personality Disorders, 19,* 466–486.

Coifman, K. G., Berenson, K. R., Rafaeli, E., & Downey, G. (2012). From negative to positive and back again: Polarized affective and relational experience in borderline personality disorder. *Journal of Abnormal Psychology, 121*(3), 668–679.

Collins, L. M., & Sayer, A. G. (Eds.). (2001). *New methods for the analysis of change.* Washington, DC: American Psychological Association.

Cooper, L. D., Balsis, S., & Zimmerman, M. (2010). Challenges associated with a polythetic diagnostic system: Criteria combinations in the personality disorders. *Journal of Abnormal Psychology, 119*(4), 886–895.

Depue, R. A., & Lenzenweger, M. F. (2005). A neurobehavioral model of personality disturbance. In M. F. Lenzenweger & J. F. Clarkin (Eds.), *Major theories of personality disorder* (2nd ed., pp. 391–453). New York: Guilford Press.

Duncan, G. J., Magnuson, K. A., & Ludwig, J. (2004). The endogeneity problem in developmental studies. *Research in Human Development, 1,* 59–80.

Estes, W. K. (1956). The problem of inference from curves based on group data. *Psychological Bulletin, 53,* 134–140.

Ferguson, C. J. (2010). A meta-analysis of normal and disordered personality across the life span. *Journal of Personality and Social Psychology, 98,* 659–667.

Funder, D. C., Parke, R. D., Tomlinson-Keasey, C., & Widaman, K. (1993). *Studying lives through time: Personality and development.* Washington, DC: American Psychological Association.

Grilo, C. M., Sanislow, C. A., Gunderson, J. G., Pagano, M. E., Yen, S., Zanarini, M. C., et al. (2004). Two-year stability and change of schizotypal, borderline, avoidant, and obsessive–compulsive personality disorders. *Journal of Consulting and Clinical Psychology, 72,* 767–775.

Grimm, K. J., Ram, N., & Hamagami, F. (2011). Nonlinear growth curves in developmental research. *Child Development, 82,* 1357–1371.

Gunderson, J. G., Shea, M. T., Skodol, A. E., McGlashan, T. H., Morey, L. C., Stout, R. L., et al. (2000). The Collaborative Longitudinal Personality Disorders Study: Development, aims, design, and sample characteristics. *Journal of Personality Disorders, 14,* 300–315.

Gunderson, J. G., Stout, R. L., McGlashan, T. H., Shea, M. T., Morey, L. C., Grilo, C. M., et al. (2011). Ten-year course of borderline personality disorder: Psychopathology and function from the Collaborative Longitudinal Personality Disorders Study, *Archives of General Psychiatry, 68,* 827–837.

Hallquist, M. N., & Lenzenweger, M. F. (2013). Identifying latent trajectories of personality disorder symptom change: Growth mixture modeling in the longitudinal study of personality disorders. *Journal of Abnormal Psychology, 122,* 138–155.

Hopwood, C. J., Morey, L. C., Donnellan, M. B., Samuel, D. B., Grilo, C. M., McGlashan, T. H., et al. (2012). Ten-year rank-order stability of personality traits and disorders in a clinical sample. *Journal of Personality, 81,* 335–344.

Hopwood, C. J., Wright, A. G. C., Ansell, E. B., & Pincus, A. L. (2013). The interpersonal core of personality pathology. *Journal of Personality Disorders, 27*(3), 271–295.

James, W. (1950). *Principles of psychology* (Vol. 1). New York: Dover. (Original work published 1890)

Johnson, J. G., Cohen, P., Kasen, S., Skodol, A. E., Hamagan, F., & Brook J. S. (2000). Age-related change in personality disorder trait levels between early adolescence and adulthood: A community-based longitudinal investigation. *Acta Psychiatrica Scandinavica, 102,* 265–275.

Johnson, J. G., First, M. B., Cohen, P., Skodol, A. E., Kasen, S., & Brrok, J. S. (2005). Adverse outcomes associated with personality disorder not otherwise specified in a community sample. *American Journal of Psychiatry, 162,* 1926–1932.

Kagan, J. (1980). Perspectives on continuity. In O. Brim & J. Kagan (Eds.), *Constancy and change in human development* (pp. 26–74). Cambridge, MA: Harvard University Press.

Klonsky, E., Oltmanns, T. F., & Turkheimer, E. F. (2003). Informant reports of personality disorder: Relation to self-reports and future research directions. *Clinical Psychology: Science and Practice, 9,* 300–311.

Korfine, L., & Hooley, J. M. (2009). Detecting individuals with borderline personality disorder in the community: An ascertainment strategy and comparison with a hospital sample. *Journal of Personality Disorders, 23,* 62–75.

Krueger, R. F. (2013). Personality disorders are the vanguard of the post-DSM-5.0 era. *Personality Disorders: Theory, Research, and Treatment, 4*(4), 355–362.

Lenzenweger, M. F. (1999). Stability and change in personality disorder features: The Longitudinal Study of Personality Disorders. *Archives of General Psychiatry, 56,* 1009–1015.

Lenzenweger, M. F. (2006). The Longitudinal Study of Personality Disorders: History, design, and initial findings (Special essay). *Journal of Personality Disorders, 6,* 645–670.

Lenzenweger, M. F. (2008). Epidemiology of personality disorders. *Psychiatric Clinics of North America, 31,* 395–403.

Lenzenweger, M. F. (2012). Facts, artifacts, mythofacts, invisible colleges, illusory colleges: The perils of publication segmentation, citation preference, and megamultiple authorship—A commentary on Blashfield and Reynolds. *Journal of Personality Disorders, 26,* 841–847.

Lenzenweger, M. F., & Clarkin, J. F. (1996). The personality disorders: History, development, and research issues. In J. F. Clarkin & M. F. Lenzenweger (Eds.), *Major theories of personality disorder* (pp. 1–35). New York: Guilford Press.

Lenzenweger, M. F., & Clarkin, J. F. (2005). The personality disorders: History, development, and research issues. In M. F. Lenzenweger & J. F. Clarkin (Eds.), *Major theories of personality disorder* (2nd ed., pp. 1–42). New York: Guilford Press.

Lenzenweger, M. F., Johnson, M. D., & Willett, J. B. (2004). Individual growth curve analysis illuminates stability and change in personality disorder features: The Longitudinal Study of Personality Disorders. *Archives of General Psychiatry, 61,* 1015–1024.

Lenzenweger, M. F., Lane, M., Loranger, A. W., & Kessler, R. C. (2007). DSM-IV personality disorders in the National Comorbidity Survey Replication (NCS-R). *Biological Psychiatry, 62,* 553–564.

Lenzenweger, M. F., & Willett, J. B. (2007). Modeling individual change in personality disorder features as a function of simultaneous individual change in personality dimensions linked to neurobehavioral systems: The Longitudinal Study of Personality Disorders. *Journal of Abnormal Psychology, 116,* 684–700.

Loranger, A., Lenzenweger, M., Gartner, A., Susman, V., Herzig, J., Zammit, G., et al. (1991). Trait–state artifacts and the diagnosis of personality disorders. *Archives of General Psychiatry, 48,* 720–728.

Loranger, A. W., Sartorius, N., Andreoli, A., Berger, P., Buchheim, P., Channabasavanna, S. M., et al. (1994). The International Personality Disorder Examination: The World Health Organization/Alcohol, Drug Abuse and Mental Health Administration International Pilot Study of Personality Disorders. *Archives of General Psychiatry, 51,* 215–224.

Markon, K. E., & Krueger, R. F. (2006). Information-theoretic latent distribution modeling: Distinguishing discrete and continuous latent variable models. *Psychological Methods, 11,* 228–243.

McCrae, R. R., & Costa, P. T. (1990). *Personality in adulthood.* New York: Guilford Press.

McCrae, R. R., & Costa, P. T. (2002). *Personality in adulthood: A five-factor theory perspective* (2nd ed.). New York: Guilford Press.

McDavid, J. D., & Pilkonis, P. A. (1996). The stability of personality disorder diagnoses. *Journal of Personality Disorders, 10,* 1–15.

McGlashan, T., Grilo, C. M., Skodol, E., Gunderson, J. G., Shea, M. T., Morey, L. C., et al. (2005). Two-year prevalence and stability of individual DSM-IV criteria for schizotypal, borderline, avoidant, and obsessive–compulsive personality disorders: Toward a hybrid model of Axis II disorders. *American Journal of Psychiatry, 162,* 883–889.

Morey, L. C., Gunderson, J. G., Quigley, B. D., Shea, M. T., Skodol, A. E., McGlashan, T. H., et al. (2002). The representation of borderline, avoidant, obsessive–compulsive, and schizotypal personality disorders by the five-factor model. *Journal of Personality Disorders, 16*(3), 215–234.

Morey, L. C., & Hopwood, C. J. (2013). Stability and change in personality disorders. *Annual Review of Clinical Psychology, 9,* 499–528.

Nesselroade, J., & Baltes, P. (1979). *Longitudinal research in the study of behavior and development.* New York: Academic Press.

Nesselroade, J., Stigler, S., & Baltes, P. (1980). Regression toward the mean and the study of change. *Psychological Bulletin, 88,* 622–637.

Nunnally, J. C., & Bernstein, I. H. (1994). *Psychometric theory* (3rd ed.). New York: McGraw-Hill.

Oltmanns, T. F., & Turkheimer, E. (2009). Person perception and personality pathology. *Current Directions in Psychological Science, 18,* 32–36.

Perry, J. C. (1993). Longitudinal studies of personality disorders. *Journal of Personality Disorders, 7*(Suppl.), 63–85.

Pilkonis, P. A., Hallquist, M. N., Morse, J. Q., & Stepp, S. D. (2011). Striking the (im)proper balance between scientific advances and clinical utility: Commentary on the DSM-5 proposal for personality disorders. *Personality Disorders: Theory, Research, and Treatment, 2,* 68–82.

Pincus, A. L. (2011). Some comments on nomology, diagnostic process, and narcissistic personality disorder in the DSM-5 proposal for personality and personality disorders. *Personality Disorders: Theory, Research, and Treatment, 2*(1), 41–53.

Raudenbush, S. W., & Bryk, A. S. (2002). *Hierarchical linear models: Applications and data analysis methods* (2nd ed.). Thousand Oaks, CA: SAGE.

Roberts, B. W., & DelVecchio, W. F. (2000). The rank-order consistency of personality traits from childhood to old age: A quantitative review of longitudinal studies. *Psychological Bulletin, 126,* 3–25.

Roberts, B. W., Walton, K. E., & Viechtbauer, W. (2006). Patterns of mean-level change in personality traits across the life course: A meta-analysis of longitudinal studies. *Psychological Bulletin, 132,* 1–25.

Robins, R. W., Fraley, R. C., Roberts, B. W., & Trzesniewki, K. H. (2001). A longitudinal study of personality change in young adulthood. *Journal of Personality, 69,* 617–640.

Rogosa, D. (1988). Myths about longitudinal research. In K. Shaie, R. Campbell, W. Meredith, & S. Rawling (Eds.), *Methodological issues in aging research* (pp. 171–209). New York: Springer.

Rogosa, D., Brandt, D., & Zimowski, M. (1982). A growth curve approach to the measurement of change. *Psychological Bulletin, 90,* 726–748.

Rogosa, D. R., & Willett, J. B. (1985). Understanding correlates of change by modeling individual differences in growth. *Psychometrika, 50,* 203–228.

Rosenthal, R., & Rosnow, R. L. (1991). *Essentials of behavioral research: Methods and data analysis* (2nd ed.). New York: McGraw-Hill.

Russell, J. J., Moskowitz, D. S., Zuroff, D. C., Sookman, D., & Paris, J. (2007). Stability and variability of affective experience and interpersonal behavior in borderline personality disorder. *Journal of Abnormal Psychology, 116*(3), 578–588.

Sadikaj, G., Moskowitz, D. S., Russell, J. J., Zuroff, D. C., & Paris, J. (2013). Quarrelsome behavior in borderline personality disorder: Influence of behavioral and affective reactivity to perceptions of others. *Journal of Abnormal Psychology, 122*(1), 195–207.

Sadikaj, G., Russell, J. J., Moskowitz, D. S., & Paris, J. (2010). Affect dysregulation in individuals with borderline personality disorder: Persistence and interpersonal triggers. *Journal of Personality Assessment, 92*(6), 490–500.

Sanislow, C. A., Little, T. D., Ansell, E. B., Grilo, C. M., Daversa, M., Markowitz, J. C., et al. (2009). Ten-year stability and latent structure of the DSM-IV schizotypal, borderline, avoidant, and obsessive–compulsive personality disorders. *Journal of Abnormal Psychology, 118,* 507–519.

Shea, M., Stout, R., Gunderson, J., Morey, L., Grilo, C., McGlashan, T., et al. (2002). Short-term diagnostic stability of schizotypal, borderline, avoidant, and obsessive–compulsive personality disorders. *American Journal of Psychiatry, 159,* 2036–2041.

Singer, J. D., & Willett, J. B. (2003). *Applied longitudinal data analysis: Modeling change and event occurrence.* New York: Oxford University Press.

Skodol, A. E., Gunderson, J. G., Shea, M. T., McGlashan, T. H., Morey, L. C., Sanislow, C. A., et al. (2005). The Collaborative Longitudinal Personality Disorders Study (CLPS): Overview and implications. *Journal of Personality Disorders, 19,* 487–504.

Srivastava, S., John, O. P., Gosling, S. D., & Potter, J. (2003). Development of personality in early and middle adulthood: Set like plaster or persistent change? *Journal of Personality and Social Psychology, 84,* 1041–1053.

Tackett, J. L., Balsis, S., Oltmanns, T. F., & Krueger, R. F. (2009). A unifying perspective on personality pathology across the life span: Developmental considerations for the fifth edition of the *Diagnostic and Statistical Manual of Mental Disorders. Development and Psychopathology, 21*(3), 687–713.

Thorndike, E. L. (1920). A constant error in psychological ratings. *Journal of Applied Psychology, 4,* 25–29.

Trull, T. J. (1993). Temporal stability and validity of two personality disorder inventories. *Psychological Assessment, 5,* 11–18.

Trull, T. J., & Ebner-Priemer, U. (2013). Ambulatory assessment. *Annual Review of Clinical Psychology, 9,* 151–176.

Trull, T. J., Solhan, M. B., Tragesser, S. L., Jahng, S., Wood, P. K., Piasecki, T. M., et al. (2008). Affective instability: Measuring a core feature of borderline personality disorder with ecological momentary assessment. *Journal of Abnormal Psychology, 117*(3), 647–661.

Vazire, S., & Carlson, E. N. (2010). Self-knowledge of personality: Do people know themselves? *Social and Personality Psychology Compass, 4*(8), 605–620.

Widaman, K. F., Ferrer, E., & Conger, R. D. (2010). Factorial invariance within longitudinal structural equation models: Measuring the same construct across time. *Child Development Perspectives, 4,* 10–18.

Widiger, T. A., & Costa, P. T., Jr. (2012). *Personality disorders and the five-factor model of personality* (3rd ed.). Washington, DC: American Psychological Association.

Wilder, J. (1957). The Law of Initial Values in neurology and psychiatry. *Journal of Nervous and Mental Disease, 13,* 73–86.

Willett, J. B. (1988). Questions and answers in the measurement of change. In E. Rothkopf (Ed.), *Review of research in education (1988–1989)* (pp. 345–422). Washington, DC: American Educational Research Association.

Wright, A. G. C. (2011). Quantitative and qualitative distinctions in personality disorder. *Journal of Personality Assessment, 93*(4), 370–379.

Wright, A. G. C., Hallquist, M. N., Beeney, J. E., & Pilkonis, P. A. (2013). Borderline personality pathology and the stability of interpersonal problems. *Journal of Abnormal Psychology, 122*(4), 1094–1100.

Wright, A. G. C., Pincus, A. L., & Lenzenweger, M. F. (2013). A parallel process growth model of avoidant personality disorder symptoms and personality traits. *Personality Disorders: Theory, Research, and Treatment, 4*(3), 230–238.

Zanarini, M. C., Frankenburg, F. R., Hennen, J., & Silk, K. R. (2003). The longitudinal course of borderline psychopathology: 6-year prospective follow-up of the phenomenology of borderline personality disorder. *American Journal of Psychiatry, 160,* 274–283.

Zanarini, M. C., Frankenburg, F. R., Hennen, J., Reich, D. B., & Silk, K. R. (2005). The McLean Study of Adult Development (MSAD): Overview and implications of the first six years of prospective follow-up. *Journal of Personality Disorders, 19,* 505–523.

Zanarini, M. C., Frankenburg, F. R., Hennen, J., Reich, D. B., & Silk, K. R. (2006). Prediction of the 10-year course of borderline personality disorder. *American Journal of Psychiatry, 163,* 827–832.

Zanarini, M. C., Frankenburg, F. R., Reich, D. B., & Fitzmaurice, G. (2012). Attainment and stability of sustained symptomatic remission and recovery among patients with borderline personality disorder and Axis II comparison subjects: A 16-year prospective follow-up study. *American Journal of Psychiatry, 169,* 476–483.

Zimmerman, M. (1994). Diagnosing personality disorders: A review of issues and research methods. *Archives of General Psychiatry, 51,* 225–245.

Zimmerman, M., Rothschild, L., & Chleminski, I. (2005). The prevalence of DSM-IV personality disorders in psychiatric outpatients. *American Journal of Psychiatry, 162,* 1911–1918.

# CHAPTER 12

# Personality Pathology and Disorder in Children and Youth

Andrew M. Chanen, Jennifer L. Tackett, and Katherine N. Thompson

Individual differences in personality traits develop from birth through the reciprocal interaction of biological and environmental influences over the life course. There is growing understanding that personality pathology can be recognized early in life, is common and clinically significant throughout childhood, adolescence, and emerging adulthood, and is more malleable than previously believed. This makes its recognition and management an important task and offers opportunities to intervene to support more adaptive development. Such prevention and early intervention can be effective but, so far, research is limited to borderline personality disorder (BPD) and antisocial personality disorder (ASPD), which are located at the extreme end of the spectrum of personality disorders (PDs). Further research is needed to improve classification, assessment, and diagnosis of personality pathology in children and youth, to understand the complex interplay between changes in personality traits and clinical presentation over time, and to promote more effective intervention at the earliest possible stage for the full range of maladaptive personality.

## The Extended Developmental Transition from Childhood to Adulthood

The past half-century has seen far-reaching changes in Western culture in the transition from childhood to adulthood (Arnett, 2000). Coupled with new knowledge about the neural substrates underlying cognitive, emotional, and social development (Nelson, Leibenluft, McClure, & Pine, 2005; Paus, 2005; Steinberg, 2005), these discoveries point to an extended and coherent period of development from puberty to around the middle of the third decade of life. This period lays the foundation for the establishment of adult role functioning, the latter part of which is increasingly a period of role exploration and change, in which the goal is to become a self-sufficient person rather than to focus on achieving specific life-stage transitions (Arnett, 2000). The emergence of this period of "youth" as a distinct developmental phase has significant implications for our understanding of the development of PD. It suggests that "adolescent" PD is a relatively uninformative construct (Chanen, 2015) and that more natural developmental periods for consideration are childhood, youth (combining adolescence and emerging adulthood), adulthood, and old age (Tackett, Balsis, Oltmanns, & Krueger, 2009). Accordingly, in this chapter we consider PD across childhood and youth. However, we use the term "adolescence" in relation to studies that have restricted their population of interest to individuals who are 12- to 18-years old.

## Temperament, Personality, and PD

Our understanding of personality across the normal–abnormal range has increased greatly over the past three decades. Normal and abnormal personality are now known to be continuous across the life course (O'Connor, 2002). However, historically, researchers interested in early individual differences often focused on the study of temperament traits, with less emphasis on normal-range personality traits in childhood (Rothbart & Bates, 2006; Tackett, Kushner, De Fruyt, & Mervielde, 2013). Even less attention has been paid to understanding the characteristics of personality pathology in early life. Yet existing research highlights substantial overlap in the content covered across the domains of temperament, normal-range child personality, and child personality pathology (De Clercq, De Fruyt, Van Leeuwen, & Mervielde, 2006; Shiner, 2009; Tackett, Kushner, et al., 2013).

The broader PD literature has largely focused on adult and, to a lesser extent, adolescent populations. Findings indicate that personality pathology is a heterogeneous but nevertheless unitary disorder, comprised of core personality dysfunction, with variability characterized by adaptive and maladaptive personality trait dimensions (Bastiaansen, De Fruyt, Rossi, Schotte, & Hofmans, 2013; Krueger, Skodol, Livesley, Shrout, & Huang, 2007; Tyrer, Crawford, & Mulder, 2011). Also, normal and abnormal personality are now known to change trajectory across the lifespan (Cohen, 2008; Hallquist & Lenzenweger, 2013; Morey et al., 2007), rather than being highly stable. Personality pathology can also change with treatment, with acute manifestations being particularly responsive to intervention (Stoffers et al., 2012). Even characteristic traits can change over time, particularly when facilitated by effective treatments, which may work partly by hastening delayed maturational processes (Newton-Howes, Clark, & Chanen, 2015).

## Convergence between Normal and Abnormal Personality Models across Developmental Periods

The study of normal-range personality has converged on the Big Five, a hierarchical five-factor model (FFM) of personality traits (Markon, Krueger, & Watson, 2005). Measures of these factors have strong psychometric properties and account for a significant amount of the variance in both normal-range personality and personality pathology (Kushner, Quilty, Tackett, & Bagby, 2011; Samuel & Widiger, 2008). Studies have demonstrated a similar higher order structure to these personality dimensions in children, adolescents, and adults (Mervielde, De Clercq, De Fruyt, & Van Leeuwen, 2005; Tackett et al., 2012), and specific measures of personality pathology in children, adolescents, and adults yield consistent findings (Kushner, Tackett, & De Clercq, 2013; Livesley, Jang, & Vernon, 1998). Until recently, most pathological personality trait measures were developed for adults and adapted for use in younger age groups (De Fruyt & De Clercq, 2014; Kushner et al., 2013). Several studies have demonstrated similar associations between normal and pathological personality traits from adolescence through adulthood (and old age), supporting an overarching structural framework across the lifespan (De Fruyt & De Clercq, 2014). Importantly, these shared structures suggest many layers of continuity by demonstrating connections between adult and child trait covariance (Markon et al., 2005; Tackett et al., 2012), connections between normal and pathological personality trait covariance (Markon et al., 2005; Samuel & Widiger, 2008), and overlap between different personality pathology trait measures (Kushner et al., 2013). This set of findings also highlights a major advantage of dimensional approaches to personality pathology, which is to facilitate communication across age and development.

The Big Five traits are observable in early childhood (Tackett et al., 2012) and provide a useful framework for understanding the interrelations between PD and other forms of mental disorder across the lifespan (De Clercq & De Fruyt, 2012; Tackett et al., 2009). For example, conduct disorder is linked to ASPD in adulthood, and Neuroticism in childhood is associated with generalized anxiety disorder (GAD), social phobia, and avoidant personality disorder (AVPD) (De Clercq & De Fruyt, 2012). There is also an observed link between low Conscientiousness and Agreeableness and high Neuroticism and attention-deficit/hyperactivity disorder (ADHD), which might be related to later paranoid PD (PPD), BPD, and ASPD (De Clercq & De Fruyt, 2012). When this system was operationalized, it became clear that it was difficult to distinguish between temperament and personality (De Clercq & De Fruyt, 2012; De Fruyt & De Clercq, 2014). This has also provided impetus for using trait description within the childhood mental health assessment process (De Clercq & De Fruyt, 2012).

Factor-analytic studies have reported that PD traits in childhood overlap substantially with those reported in adults and have similar rank-order stability (Shiner, 2009). The Dimensional Personality Symptom Item Pool (DIPSI) has been used to investigate personality traits in children (De Clercq et al., 2006; Decuyper, De Clercq, & Tackett, 2015), which have been found to be grouped into externalizing and internalizing behaviors that may then be broken down further into four factors: disagreeableness, emotional instability, compulsivity, and introversion (De Clercq et al., 2006; Kushner et al., 2013). When the factor structure of the Structured Interview for DSM-IV Personality was investigated in adolescents with BPD, two main factors were found, one internally oriented (affective instability, paranoid ideation, emptiness, avoidance of abandonment) and the other externally oriented (inappropriate anger, impulsivity, suicidal or self-mutilating behavior, unstable relationships) (Speranza et al., 2012). These findings are comparable to studies in adults using the Dimensional Assessment of Personality Pathology—Basic Questionnaire (DAPP-BQ), which yielded a four-factor structure. They included emotional dysregulation, dissocial behavior, inhibitedness, and compulsivity (Livesley, 1998). Livesley (1998) suggested that this phenotypic approach to PD is advantageous because it results in a large number of building blocks that have specific effects and a few factors with widespread effects, and can explain the complex variation in the structure of personality and PD.

## Stability and Change

Longitudinal studies (Caspi & Silva, 1995) support the continuity of individual differences from early childhood to young adulthood in the general population, although the strength of associations between individual differences in early childhood and adulthood are only weak to moderate. Traits become consistent through genetic influences, psychological makeup, exposure to a consistent environment, goodness of fit between individuals and their environment, and a strong sense of identity (Roberts & DelVecchio, 2000).

The historical separation of the literature examining normal personality development from that examining PD has hampered a lifespan-developmental clinical perspective. More recently, studies across the normal–abnormal range of personality have found that personality traits evident in childhood stabilize throughout life, including into later adulthood (De Fruyt et al., 2006; Roberts & DelVecchio, 2000). Such traits are approximately 50% heritable, with little variance accounted for by shared environmental influences. The remainder are attributable to individuals' unique experiences and the interaction between individuals' biology and their environment (Roberts & DelVecchio, 2000). Genetic factors and environmental consistencies are likely to reinforce the continuity of personality, whereas variable environmental influences are likely to lead to malleability and, consequently, to the opportunity for clinical intervention (Newton-Howes et al., 2015).

Also critical for understanding the development of PD is a better understanding of normal-range personality development. For example, large-scale investigations, particularly in adulthood, have demonstrated that personality trait change tends to develop toward greater maturity across age (i.e., increases in social dominance, conscientiousness, emotional stability, and agreeableness, and decreases in social vitality and openness) (Roberts, Walton, & Viechtbauer, 2006). However, this pattern looks somewhat different across youth development, where some studies have demonstrated a shift toward less maturity (e.g., lower conscientiousness) from childhood to adolescence, with a subsequent upswing in regulation in later adolescence (Soto, John, Gosling, & Potter, 2011). Emotional tendencies and self-regulation capacities are critical for many forms of personality pathology, and by understanding their normal-range development, we are better able to identify pathways to maladaptive personality development.

Consistency in individuals' relative trait levels increases monotonically, beginning in infancy, although the causes of these changes are not clearly understood. Recent meta-analytic data show that personality across the normal–abnormal range is moderately stable during childhood. Rather than "setting like plaster" (James, 1890/1950), personality becomes more "viscous" over time (Ferguson, 2010; Srivastava, John, Gosling, & Potter, 2003). Personality stability increases from the teenage years to emerging adulthood, then the rate of change slows after age 30. Particularly, the Big Five dimensions of personality already show substantial stability across community (De Fruyt et al., 2006) and clinical samples (De Bolle et al., 2009) of children and adolescents. Importantly, for the assessment of personality pathology in adolescence, there is no sudden increase in the stability of traits across the normal–abnormal range during the transition from the teenage years to young adulthood (Roberts & DelVecchio, 2000). Rank-order stability of pathological personality traits is largely identical in adolescence and adulthood (De Clercq, van Leeuwen, van den Noortgate, de Bolle, & de Fruyt, 2009; Johnson et al., 2000), dispelling earlier notions that PD was too capricious in adolescence to systematically diagnose, to study and to treat.

Much of the evidence that personality pathology appears to change from childhood through to adulthood in similar ways to normal-range personality is based on the work of the Children in Community Study (CIC; Cohen, Crawford, Johnson, & Kasen, 2005), which requires replication. The early phases of this study have important methodological limitations with regard to PD assessment, which suggest cautious interpretation of the findings. Remarkably, no well-designed study, using validated measures, has followed the course of personality pathology from childhood to later life. The CIC identified that PD features peak in the early teens and decline linearly from ages 14 to 28 years (Johnson et al., 2000). This decline reflects, in part, normative decreases in impulsivity, attention seeking, and dependency, and normative increases in social competence and self-control. PD features in the CIC were moderately stable, which is remarkably similar to comparable studies in adults over similar time intervals. Adolescents in the CIC with diagnosed PD tended to have elevated PD features during early adulthood. These findings suggest continuity of PD from adolescence to adulthood. Notably, 21% of participants experienced increases in personality pathology during this period. Overall, the CIC's findings show that child and adolescent personality pathology is the strongest predictor, over and above common mental-state disorders, of young adult PD. It is also notable that decreases in PD features are more rapid in individuals who initially had lower levels of PD symptoms (Crawford et al., 2005; De Clercq et al., 2009), giving rise to an increasing gap between individuals scoring high and those scoring low in PD features across adolescent development.

Although traits are largely consistent, they also remain dynamic throughout life. Mean levels of personality traits change across the life course, with the greatest magnitude of change during young adulthood (ages 20–40 years), not during childhood or adolescence (Roberts et al., 2006). Individuals with personality pathology tend to show greater change, which is usually, but not always, in the direction of improvement over time. Despite this waxing and waning picture of acute disturbances (e.g., suicidality) in individuals with PD, psychosocial functioning (e.g., occupational and interpersonal functioning) tends to be poor and relatively stable (Skodol, 2008; Skodol, Gunderson, et al., 2005). Importantly, change in personality traits predicts change in personality pathology, but not vice versa (Warner et al., 2004), which means it is likely that traits more closely resemble the reality of PD (Newton-Howes et al., 2015). It also underscores the importance of devoting greater attention to research on normative child personality emergence and development, as it forms a foundational knowledge base on which a better understanding of personality pathology development must be built.

## Risk Factors and Precursor Signs and Symptoms

Until the late 1990s, most developmental studies of PD focused on early childhood experiences and how they influence later (adult) psychopathology (Newton-Howes et al., 2015). Such childhood effects are important, but they might be mediated and even reversed by later experiences (Schulenberg, Sameroff, & Cicchetti, 2004). A restricted focus on distal factors is arguably "nondevelopmental," because it assumes that the determinants of mental health do not change across the lifespan. Possible mediating mechanisms that might contribute to the continuity or discontinuity in psychopathology between childhood and adult life include genetic mediation, "kindling" effects, environmental influences, coping mechanisms, and cognitive processing of experiences (Rutter, Kim-Cohen, & Maughan, 2006). For example, negative parent–child relationships in youth can exacerbate both internalizing and externalizing symptoms, if an individual is already emotionally dysregulated, whereas warm and accepting parenting can shield a child from negative outcomes (Stepp, Whalen, Pilkonis, Hipwell, & Levine, 2011).

Little is known about perinatal factors associated with PD, except for schizotypal PD (STPD) and schizoid PD (SPD), in which links have been found with influenza and with prenatal exposure to malnutrition and stress (Raine, 2006).

The CIC (Cohen et al., 2005) is the only study that has identified "true" environmental risk factors (i.e., those that prospectively predict PD) for the full range of PDs. These include "distal" factors such as low family-of-origin socioeconomic status, being raised by a single parent, family welfare support, numerous parental conflicts, and parental illness or death (Cohen, 2008; Cohen et al., 2005). Parental dynamics, such as maladaptive family functioning and parenting, including low emotional closeness between parent and child, use of harsh punishment during childhood, maternal overcontrol, and parental psychopathology, have also been found to precede later development of PD (Bezirganian, Cohen, & Brook, 1993; Cohen, 2008; Cohen et al., 2005; Johnson, Cohen, Chen, Kasen, & Brook, 2006), along with adverse childhood experiences such as sexual, physical, and verbal abuse, and childhood neglect (Cohen, 2008; Johnson et al., 2001; Moran et al., 2011). Other strong predictors were poor achievement, school expulsion, lack of goals, and low IQ (Cohen et al., 2005).

In addition, studies have also found that certain temperamental characteristics and early onset mental state or behavioural problems also prospectively predict PD (Chanen & McCutcheon, 2013). These include maternal reports of not only anxiety, depressive symptoms, and conduct problems, along with substance use disorders (especially alcohol use), depression, anxiety disorder, disruptive behavior disorders, especially conduct disorder, but also ADHD and oppositional defiant disorder (ODD) (Bernstein, Cohen, Skodol, Bezirganian, & Brook, 1996; Cohen, 2008; Cohen et al., 2005; Kasen, Cohen, Skodol, Johnson, & Brook, 1999; Kasen et al., 2001; Lewinsohn, Rohde, Seeley, & Klein, 1997; Stepp, Burke, Hipwell, & Loeber, 2012; Thatcher, Cornelius, & Clark, 2005; Zoccolillo, Pickles, Quinton, & Rutter, 1992). Although DSM-5 ASPD requires a diagnosis of conduct disorder before the age of 15, the evidence does not support a unique or specific developmental pathway to ASPD (Frick & Viding, 2009; Rutter, 2012). Rather, conduct disorder is prospectively linked to a range of mental state and PDs (Burke, Waldman, & Lahey, 2010; Helgeland, Kjelsberg, & Torgersen, 2005). Overall, these findings suggest that similar or identical phenomena (e.g., impulsivity and aggression) might be misleadingly characterized as mental-state pathology in children and, in later adult life, redefined as personality pathology (Chanen & Kaess, 2012). In fact, after adjusting for common mental-state pathology (e.g., disruptive behavior disorders, anxiety, and depression), PD features in childhood and adolescence are the strongest long-term predictor of PD diagnoses in adulthood (Cohen et al., 2005; Crawford et al., 2005).

In the CIC, when the cumulative risk of these factors was calculated, risk for BPD was associated with low socioeconomic status, combined with cumulative trauma, stressful life events, low IQ, and paternal and maternal parenting problems, respectively (Cohen et al., 2008). Comparatively, STPD was associated with low socioeconomic status, being male, cumulative trauma, stressful life events, low IQ, and father and mother parenting problems (Cohen et al., 2008). These parenting factors included low closeness to mother and/or father, maternal control through guilt, "power assertive punishment," and parental antisocial behavior (Cohen et al., 2005). Notably, both STPD and BPD personality features significantly contribute to the risk of having depression at any age (Cohen et al., 2008).

The CIC also found that co-occurring mental-state disorder and PD greatly increased the odds of young adult PD relative to the odds of either a mental-state disorder or PD alone (Kasen et al., 1999). For example, when disruptive behavior disorder co-occurred with a Cluster A PD in adolescence, the odds ratio (OR) for persistence of this same PD into adulthood was 24.6 times higher. The same pattern was also found for disruptive behavior co-occurring with a Cluster B PD (OR = 12.5) or C PD (OR = 16.3), for anxiety disorder co-occurring with a Cluster A PD (OR = 16.9), and for major depression co-occurring with a Cluster A (OR = 20.5), B (OR = 19.1), or C (OR = 16.0) PD.

Multilevel frameworks lend themselves particularly well to understanding the emergence and development of personality pathology over time. For example, Shiner and Tackett (2014) described the usefulness of a three-level framework for differentiating early risk and symptomatology characteristics that reflect personality traits, characteristic adaptations (e.g., attachment and emotion regulation), and identity development. All levels are clearly relevant for PD among youth and provide a helpful framework for organizing risk factors, correlates, and early manifestations, while allowing for incorporation of development.

Discontinuities may also provide a window into the mechanisms operating across this period, along with clues for prevention and early intervention, by informing what might protect young people from PD. An example of such research is a study reporting that positive mother parenting behavior during an interaction task was associated with a reduction in BPD pathology over time (Whalen et al., 2014). To date, there are few such studies on protective factors and little is known about the prospective developmental dynamics of resilience for PD (Paris, Perlin, Laporte, Fitzpatrick, & DeStefano, 2014; Skodol et al., 2007).

## PD Begins in Childhood and Adolescence

There is general agreement that PD has its roots in childhood and adolescence, and this was made explicit in the operational definitions of the categorical PDs introduced in DSM-III (American Psychiatric Association [APA], 1980). Nonetheless, the sections on disorders of childhood and adolescence in DSM-5 and the *International Classification of Diseases* (ICD-10) still make no mention of PD, although the forthcoming ICD-11 might acknowledge this (Tyrer, Reed, & Crawford, 2015).

PD commonly becomes clinically apparent during the transition between childhood and adulthood and has the potential to disrupt the complex developmental tasks associated with this phase of life and the achievement of adult role functioning. Yet diagnosing PD prior to age 18 years remains controversial (Chanen & McCutcheon, 2008; De Clercq & De Fruyt, 2012). Although the DSM-5 and ICD-10 advocate caution in doing so, they do not prohibit diagnosis of PD in adolescence, except for ASPD. In fact, DSM-5 still requires that the features of a PD be present for only 1 year, which seems too short a period to accurately distinguish a mental state from a personality trait disorder (Newton-Howes et al., 2015). ICD-10 describes it as "highly unlikely" that PD will be diagnosed before 16–17 years of age, but it offers no scientific justification for this. Nonetheless, accurate diagnosis is also hindered in DSM-5 and ICD-10 by the lack of developmentally appropriate PD criteria or illustrations of current criteria consistent with adolescent behavior (Chanen, Jovev, McCutcheon, Jackson, & McGorry, 2008).

## PD Can Be Diagnosed in Young People

Despite the scientific evidence for the validity of PD in childhood and adolescence, the diagnosis still remains off-limits in this age group for many clinicians (Chanen & McCutcheon, 2008). Clearly, the evidence presented here suggests that such views are no longer justified. However, many clinicians avoid the diagnosis on the grounds of "protecting" patients from the stigma associated with the label (Chanen & McCutcheon, 2013), particularly stigma that is common among health professionals (Newton-Howes, Weaver, & Tyrer, 2008). Although this stigma is undeniable, delaying appropriate diagnosis for this reason risks colluding with the stigmatizers. Delay also carries clinical risks because evidence is accumulating that many of the harms associated with PD emerge early in the course of the disorder, and delay is likely to lead to worse outcomes (Chanen, 2015). Moreover, delay in diagnosis restricts appropriate intervention and risks inappropriate and/or harmful intervention (Newton-Howes et al., 2015). Therefore, it is critical to provide clinicians with information that will help them to stop avoiding the diagnosis of PD in adolescents.

Measurement of early personality pathology is still in the initial stages, although there have been major advances in recent years. Researchers and clinicians hoping to assess early PD characteristics have a number of questionnaire options available to them (e.g., De Clercq et al., 2006; Decuyper et al., 2015; Linde, Stringer, Simms, & Clark, 2013; Tromp & Koot, 2008). These measures capture both overlapping and distinct variance (e.g., Kushner et al., 2013), so attention should be paid to those facets covered in each measure prior to selection. In addition, researchers and clinicians working with youth are largely accustomed to collecting data from multiple informants, and assessment of personality pathology is no exception. Informant differences can also be quantified to better understand differences between reporters (Tackett, Herzhoff, Reardon, Smack, & Kushner, 2013). Another potential option to consider is utilizing a "thin-slice" assessment method to rate traits using available archival video data (Tackett, Herzhoff, Kushner, & Rule, 2016). Specifically, this method harnesses the power inherent in "snap judgments" made by unacquainted individuals (i.e., raters) to measure personality traits, and has been shown to produce reliable and valid personality trait assessments in childhood. Importantly, this method has also been used to leverage existing archival video data (e.g., videos from clinical assessment or intervention) and has been shown to be useful in rating personality traits across the normal–abnormal range (Tackett et al., 2016). Thus, researchers and clinicians have a growing number of options to reliably and validly measure personality pathology characteristics in youth.

DSM-5, Section III Alternative Personality Disorder System has incorporated the evidence for PD in young people, removing age-related caveats for its diagnosis, and the same is proposed for the ICD-11 (Tyrer, Crawford, Mulder, et al., 2011). Both classifications recognize the dimensional nature of PD across the lifespan; furthermore, ICD-11 introduces the term "personality difficulty" to reflect "subthreshold" personality pathology. When clinicians are unsure of or hesitant to use a PD diagnosis with young people, the use of the term "personality difficulty" supports prevention, early identification, and treatment of such problems.

## Prevalence

Although there has been significant progress in the epidemiology of adult PD, data regarding the prevalence PD among children and youth are still limited. Methodological limitations, such as different sampling procedures and lack of psychometrically valid assessment tools, limit the conclusions that can be drawn from these studies.

The prevalence of DSM-5 PD diagnoses in adolescent community and primary care settings generally ranges from 6 to 17% across studies (Kongerslev, Chanen, & Simonsen, 2015), with the exception of one study (Lewinsohn et al., 1997), which reported the prevalence of any PD diagnosis to be 2.8%. This finding was most likely due to methodological differences, which required that a PD feature be present for at least 5 years in order to be rated as present.

The CIC (Bernstein et al., 1993; Cohen et al., 2005) estimated the prevalence of DSM-III-R PD (excluding ASPD) to be 17.2%, with the most prevalent disorder being narcissistic PD (NPD) and the least prevalent being STPD. The prevalence of PD peaked at age 12 for boys and age 13 for girls. Adding waves of data collected through to age 33 years, these researchers estimated the point prevalence of any current DSM-IV (APA, 1994) PD (including depressive PD [DPD] and passive–aggressive PD [PAPD]) to be between 12.7 and 14.6% through adolescence and young adulthood. At mean age 33, the estimated lifetime prevalence of PD was 28.2%.

Prevalence estimates in clinical samples range from 41 to 64% (Feenstra, Busschbach, Verheul, & Hutsebaut, 2011; Grilo et al., 1998), and in youth justice samples from 36 to 88% (Gosden, Kramp, Gabrielsen, & Sestoft, 2003; Kongerslev, Moran, Bo, & Simonsen, 2012; Kongerslev et al., 2015). These prevalence estimates are similar to or slightly higher than those reported for adults (Zimmerman, Chelminski, & Young, 2008), ranking PD among the most common disorders seen in clinical practice in child and youth mental health.

## Prevention and Early Intervention

The recognition of personality pathology in children and youth facilitates prevention and early intervention, which aims to alter the life course trajectory of PD (Chanen & McCutcheon, 2013; Newton-Howes et al., 2015). This was aided by the landmark Institute of Medicine report on the prevention of mental disorders (Mrazek & Haggerty, 1994), based on the work of Robert Gordon (1983), which set out a schema of *universal* (population-based), *selective* (targeting those with risk factors) and *indicated* (targeting those with early/precursor signs and symptoms) prevention, along with *early intervention* for "first-onset" disorders. A particular advantage is that this approach is not specifically concerned with the etiology of disorders, as a complete account of causal mechanisms is unnecessary for prevention. The main requirement is to identify "risk factors" for persistence or deterioration of problems, rather than the "onset" or incidence of disorder per se.

This has been applied to PD (Chanen, Jovev, et al., 2008), but, so far, no study has examined prevention and early intervention across the broad construct of PD. Work in this field is limited to severe (i.e., BPD and ASPD) PD, with a narrow focus on single PD diagnoses, perhaps reflecting clinical and social needs and priorities (Chanen, Jovev, et al., 2008; Chanen & McCutcheon, 2013; National Collaborating Centre for Mental Health, 2009). For example, the large body of knowledge about childhood- and adolescent-onset conduct disorder and the developmental pathways leading to adult PD, along with associated outcomes, such as substance abuse, mental-state disorders, and poor physical health (Moffitt et al., 2008), has given rise to a sizable body of potential universal, selective, and indicated preventive interventions, along with early intervention for the established phenotype (National Collaborating Centre for Mental Health, 2009; Weisz, Hawley, & Doss, 2004; Woolfenden, Williams, & Peat, 2002). However, only a smaller number of these have been studied in randomized controlled trials.

Universal and selective prevention programs include early childhood-, preschool-, and primary school-based programs, along with whole of community universal interventions. These have shown a range of positive maternal and child outcomes, including reductions in offending and related behaviors (Hawkins, Kosterman, Catalano, Hill, & Abbott, 2005; National Collaborating Centre for Mental Health, 2009; Olds, Sadler, & Kitzman, 2007). The Communities That Care system is a prototypical universal preventive intervention for a range of outcomes, including delinquency and antisocial behavior (but not other measures of PD). Controlled trial data indicate that intervention commencing in fifth-grade students yields sustained decreases in the incidence and prevalence of delinquent and violent behavior through to grade 10 (Hawkins et al., 2012), although by grade 12 (8 years after implementation and 3 years after cessation of support for the intervention), there were no significant differences by intervention group in past-year prevalence of delinquency and violence (Hawkins, Oesterle, Brown, Abbott, & Catalano, 2014).

The Nurse Family Partnership program, an exemplar selective intervention program that targets low-income mothers and their newborn to 2-year-old children, has demonstrated sustained benefits with regard to crime (and employment) for both mothers and their children (Olds, 2008). In the United Kingdom, the National Institute for Health and Care Excellence (NICE; National Collaborating Centre for Mental Health, 2009) has recommended selective intervention for children of parents with a history of residential care or who have a mental or substance use disorder, or who have had prior contact with the criminal justice system, or young mothers (under age 18 years). Recommended interventions for these selected groups include nonmaternal care (e.g., well-staffed nursery care) for children younger than age 1 year, or interventions to improve poor parenting skills for the parents of children younger than age 3 years.

A range of indicated prevention and early intervention programs for ASPD targets children with externalizing problems or conduct disorder (Sawyer, Borduin, & Dopp, 2015). Some focus on children or parents, while others are family-based or multisystemic. For example, Fast Track targets kindergarten children assessed by their teachers and parents to have conduct problems. At age 25, 10 years after the end of the intervention, those assigned to Fast Track had lower rates of ASPD, violent crime, and substance abuse convictions (Dodge et al., 2015). Similarly, for those with criminal involvement, multisystemic therapy can have continued effects into adulthood on these youth and their siblings (Dopp, Borduin, Wagner, & Sawyer, 2014).

Compared with ASPD, the prevention and early intervention literature for BPD is meager. There are no universal or selective prevention programs. The first wave of randomized controlled trials of psychosocial treatments for BPD in adolescents has only been published in the past decade (Chanen, 2015; Chanen & Thompson, 2014). These include cognitive analytic therapy (CAT; Ryle, 1997) delivered within the Helping Young People Early (HYPE) program (Chanen et al., 2009), emotion regulation training (ERT; Schuppert et al., 2009, 2012), mentalization-based treatment for adolescents (MBT-A; Rossouw & Fonagy, 2012), and dialectical behavior therapy for adolescents (DBT-A; Mehlum et al., 2014). These trials have used a range of comparison treatments, including manualized good clinical care (GCC; Chanen, Jackson, et al., 2008), nonmanualized treatment as usual (TAU; Rossouw & Fonagy, 2012; Schuppert et al., 2009, 2012), and nonmanualized enhanced usual care (EUC; Mehlum et al., 2014).

Overall, these trials have emphasized the importance of diagnosing and treating BPD in young people. The key findings support the effectiveness of psychosocial treatments for adolescents with either the features of (indicated prevention) or full-syndrome (early intervention) BPD. All treatments were associated with improvement on outcome measures that included internalizing and externalizing psychopathology, depressive symptoms, BPD symptoms, quality of life, deliberate self-harm, and suicidal ideation. However, the structured interventions (CAT, GCC, MBT-A, DBT-A) generally outperformed TAU or EUC, except in the case of ERT. These findings largely echo those for adults with BPD, where various specialist treatments seem to have similar effects despite distinct theories and interventions (Bateman, Gunderson, & Mulder, 2015).

This brief outline shows that prevention and early intervention for PD are possible. However, prevention programs based on nonspecific risk factors and narrowly defined PD categories are unlikely to fully achieve their aims (Chanen & McCutcheon, 2013). In part this is a consequence of the numerous developmental pathways to PD (equifinality) and the wide-ranging outcomes for those with personality pathology (multifinality) (Cicchetti & Crick, 2009). Instead of narrow categories, prevention programs need to measure a range of outcome syndromes, along with functional outcomes. Consequently, they should begin to measure the full range of personality across the normal–abnormal range, using psychometrically valid instruments. However, lingering concerns about early labeling of children and youth must be resolved in order to adopt a comprehensive and developmentally appropriate preventive approach for PD (Chanen & McCutcheon, 2013; Cohen et al., 2005; Newton-Howes et al., 2015).

## Conclusions

The previously discussed knowledge has led to a life course developmental model of PD that recognizes the interactions among a wide variety of biological, psychological, and sociocultural factors (Chanen & Thompson, 2014; Newton-Howes et al., 2015; Tackett et al., 2009). It highlights that PD is a unitary construct, continuous with normal personality, which can be diagnosed in children and youth, and shows both stability and change in the transition from childhood to adulthood and beyond. Such a model underscores the numerous developmental pathways to PD (equifinality) and the wide-ranging outcomes for those with personality pathology (multifinality) (Cicchetti & Crick, 2009). Our current knowledge about risk factors for PD is dependent on a relatively small number of studies, and there is a clear need for more focused empirical attention to this area. In addition, it is clear that personality pathology in children and youth has the potential to disrupt the transition to adult role functioning (Newton-Howes et al., 2015; Shiner, 2009), derailing attainment of vocational and interpersonal goals (Oshri, Rogosch, & Cicchetti, 2013; Skodol, Pagano, et al., 2005). Accordingly, prevention and early intervention have been developed for PD. While effective, prevention programs based on nonspecific risk factors and narrowly defined PD categories are unlikely to fully achieve their aims. Instead, prevention programs need to join with existing programs designed for the full range of mental disorders and should begin to measure the full range of personality across the normal–abnormal range as an outcome.

## REFERENCES

American Psychiatric Association. (1980). *Diagnostic and statistical manual of mental disorders* (3rd ed.). Washington, DC: Author.

American Psychiatric Association. (1994). *Diagnostic and statistical manual of mental disorders* (4th ed.). Washington, DC: Author.

Arnett, J. J. (2000). Emerging adulthood: A theory of development from the late teens through the twenties. *American Psychologist, 55*(5), 469–480.

Bastiaansen, L., De Fruyt, F., Rossi, G., Schotte, C., & Hofmans, J. (2013). Personality disorder dysfunction versus traits: Structural and conceptual issues. *Personality Disorders, 4*(4), 293–303.

Bateman, A. W., Gunderson, J., & Mulder, R. (2015). Treatment of personality disorder. *Lancet, 385*, 735–743.

Bernstein, D. P., Cohen, P., Skodol, A., Bezirganian, S., & Brook, J. (1996). Childhood antecedents of adolescent personality disorders. *American Journal of Psychiatry, 153*(7), 907–913.

Bernstein, D. P., Cohen, P., Velez, C. N., Schwab-Stone, M., Siever, L. J., & Shinsato, L. (1993). Prevalence and stability of the DSM-III-R personality disorders in a community-based survey of adolescents. *American Journal of Psychiatry, 150*(8), 1237–1243.

Bezirganian, S., Cohen, P., & Brook, J. S. (1993). The impact of mother–child interaction on the development of borderline personality disorder. *American Journal of Psychiatry, 150*(12), 1836–1842.

Burke, J. D., Waldman, I., & Lahey, B. B. (2010). Predictive validity of childhood oppositional defiant disorder and conduct disorder: Implications for the DSM-V. *Journal of Abnormal Psychology, 119*(4), 739–751.

Caspi, A., & Silva, P. A. (1995). Temperamental qualities at age three predict personality traits in young adulthood: Longitudinal evidence from a birth cohort. *Child Development, 66*(2), 486–498.

Chanen, A. M. (2015). Borderline personality disorder

in young people: Are we there yet? *Journal of Clinical Psychology, 71*(8), 778–791.

Chanen, A. M., Jackson, H. J., McCutcheon, L., Dudgeon, P., Jovev, M., Yuen, H. P., et al. (2008). Early intervention for adolescents with borderline personality disorder using cognitive analytic therapy: A randomised controlled trial. *British Journal of Psychiatry, 193*(6), 477–484.

Chanen, A. M., Jovev, M., McCutcheon, L., Jackson, H. J., & McGorry, P. D. (2008). Borderline personality disorder in young people and the prospects for prevention and early intervention. *Current Psychiatry Reviews, 4*(1), 48–57.

Chanen, A. M., & Kaess, M. (2012). Developmental pathways toward borderline personality disorder. *Current Psychiatry Reports, 14*(1), 45–53.

Chanen, A. M., & McCutcheon, L. K. (2008). Personality disorder in adolescence: The diagnosis that dare not speak its name. *Personality and Mental Health, 2*(1), 35–41.

Chanen, A. M., & McCutcheon, L. K. (2013). Prevention and early intervention for borderline personality disorder: Current status and recent evidence. *British Journal of Psychiatry, 202*(Suppl. 54), S24–S29.

Chanen, A. M., McCutcheon, L., Germano, D., Nistico, H., Jackson, H. J., & McGorry, P. D. (2009). The HYPE Clinic: An early intervention service for borderline personality disorder. *Journal of Psychiatric Practice, 15*(3), 163–172.

Chanen, A. M., & Thompson, K. (2014). Preventive strategies for borderline personality disorder in adolescents. *Current Treatment Options in Psychiatry, 1*(4), 358–368.

Cicchetti, D., & Crick, N. R. (2009). Precursors and diverse pathways to personality disorder in children and adolescents. *Development and Psychopathology, 21*(3), 683–685.

Cohen, P. (2008). Child development and personality disorder. *Psychiatric Clinics of North America, 31*(3), 477–493.

Cohen, P., Chen, H., Gordon, K., Johnson, J., Brook, J., & Kasen, S. (2008). Socioeconomic background and the developmental course of schizotypal and borderline personality disorder symptoms. *Development and Psychopathology, 20*(2), 633–650.

Cohen, P., Crawford, T. N., Johnson, J. G., & Kasen, S. (2005). The Children in the Community Study of developmental course of personality disorder. *Journal of Personality Disorders, 19*(5), 466–486.

Crawford, T. N., Cohen, P., Johnson, J. G., Kasen, S., First, M. B., Gordon, K., et al. (2005). Self-reported personality disorder in the Children in the Community sample: Convergent and prospective validity in late adolescence and adulthood. *Journal of Personality Disorders, 19*(1), 30–52.

De Bolle, M., De Clercq, B., Van Leeuwen, K., Decuyper, M., Rosseel, Y., & De Fruyt, F. (2009). Personality and psychopathology in Flemish referred children: Five perspectives of continuity. *Child Psychiatry and Human Development, 40*(2), 269–285.

De Clercq, B., & De Fruyt, F. (2012). A five-factor model framework for understanding childhood personality disorder antecedents. *Journal of Personality, 80*(6), 1533–1563.

De Clercq, B., De Fruyt, F., Van Leeuwen, K., & Mervielde, I. (2006). The structure of maladaptive personality traits in childhood: A step toward an integrative developmental perspective for DSM-V. *Journal of Abnormal Psychology, 115*(4), 639–657.

De Clercq, B., van Leeuwen, K., van den Noortgate, W., De Bolle, M., & de Fruyt, F. (2009). Childhood personality pathology: Dimensional stability and change. *Development and Psychopathology, 21*(3), 853–869.

Decuyper, M., De Clercq, B., & Tackett, J. L. (2015). Assessing maladaptive traits in youth: An English-language version of the Dimensional Personality Symptom Itempool. *Personality Disorders, 6*(3), 239–250.

De Fruyt, F., Bartels, M., Van Leeuwen, K. G., De Clercq, B., Decuyper, M., & Mervielde, I. (2006). Five types of personality continuity in childhood and adolescence. *Journal of Personality and Social Psychology, 91*(3), 538–552.

De Fruyt, F., & De Clercq, B. (2014). Antecedents of personality disorder in childhood and adolescence: Toward an integrative developmental model. *Annual Review of Clinical Psychology, 10,* 449–476.

Dodge, K. A., Bierman, K. L., Coie, J. D., Greenberg, M. T., Lochman, J. E., McMahon, R. J., et al. (2015). Impact of early intervention on psychopathology, crime, and well-being at age 25. *American Journal of Psychiatry, 172*(1), 59–70.

Dopp, A. R., Borduin, C. M., Wagner, D. V., & Sawyer, A. M. (2014). The economic impact of multisystemic therapy through midlife: A cost–benefit analysis with serious juvenile offenders and their siblings. *Journal of Consulting and Clinical Psychology, 82*(4), 694–705.

Feenstra, D. J., Busschbach, J. J., Verheul, R., & Hutsebaut, J. (2011). Prevalence and comorbidity of Axis I and axis II disorders among treatment refractory adolescents admitted for specialized psychotherapy. *Journal of Personality Disorders, 25*(6), 842–850.

Ferguson, C. J. (2010). A meta-analysis of normal and disordered personality across the life span. *Journal of Personality and Social Psychology, 98*(4), 659–667.

Frick, P. J., & Viding, E. (2009). Antisocial behavior from a developmental psychopathology perspective. *Development and Psychopathology, 21*(4), 1111–1131.

Gordon, R. S., Jr. (1983). An operational classification of disease prevention. *Public Health Reports, 98*(2), 107–109.

Gosden, N. P., Kramp, P., Gabrielsen, G., & Sestoft, D. (2003). Prevalence of mental disorders among 15–17-year-old male adolescent remand prisoners in Denmark. *Acta Psychiatrica Scandinavica, 107*(2), 102–110.

Grilo, C. M., McGlashan, T. H., Quinlan, D. M., Walker, M. L., Greenfeld, D., & Edell, W. S. (1998). Frequency of personality disorders in two age cohorts of psychiatric inpatients. *American Journal of Psychiatry, 155*(1), 140–142.

Hallquist, M. N., & Lenzenweger, M. F. (2013). Identifying latent trajectories of personality disorder symptom change: Growth mixture modeling in the longitudinal study of personality disorders. *Journal of Abnormal Psychology, 122*(1), 138–155.

Hawkins, J. D., Kosterman, R., Catalano, R. F., Hill, K. G., & Abbott, R. D. (2005). Promoting positive adult functioning through social development intervention in childhood: Long-term effects from the Seattle Social Development Project. *Archives of Pediatrics and Adolescent Medicine, 159*(1), 25–31.

Hawkins, J. D., Oesterle, S., Brown, E. C., Abbott, R. D., & Catalano, R. F. (2014). Youth problem behaviors 8 years after implementing the communities that care prevention system: A community-randomized trial. *JAMA Pediatrics, 168*(2), 122–129.

Hawkins, J. D., Oesterle, S., Brown, E. C., Monahan, K. C., Abbott, R. D., Arthur, M. W., et al. (2012). Sustained decreases in risk exposure and youth problem behaviors after installation of the Communities That Care prevention system in a randomized trial. *Archives of Pediatrics and Adolescent Medicine, 166*(2), 141–148.

Helgeland, M. I., Kjelsberg, E., & Torgersen, S. (2005). Continuities between emotional and disruptive behavior disorders in adolescence and personality disorders in adulthood. *American Journal of Psychiatry, 162*(10), 1941–1947.

James, W. (1950). *The principles of psychology.* New York: Dover. (Original work published 1890)

Johnson, J. G., Cohen, P., Chen, H., Kasen, S., & Brook, J. S. (2006). Parenting behaviors associated with risk for offspring personality disorder during adulthood. *Archives of General Psychiatry, 63*(5), 579–587.

Johnson, J. G., Cohen, P., Kasen, S., Skodol, A. E., Hamagami, F., & Brook, J. S. (2000). Age-related change in personality disorder trait levels between early adolescence and adulthood: A community-based longitudinal investigation. *Acta Psychiatrica Scandinavica, 102*(4), 265–275.

Johnson, J. G., Cohen, P., Smailes, E. M., Skodol, A. E., Brown, J., & Oldham, J. M. (2001). Childhood verbal abuse and risk for personality disorders during adolescence and early adulthood. *Comprehensive Psychiatry, 42*(1), 16–23.

Kasen, S., Cohen, P., Skodol, A. E., Johnson, J. G., & Brook, J. S. (1999). Influence of child and adolescent psychiatric disorders on young adult personality disorder. *American Journal of Psychiatry, 156*(10), 1529–1535.

Kasen, S., Cohen, P., Skodol, A. E., Johnson, J. G., Smailes, E., & Brook, J. S. (2001). Childhood depression and adult personality disorder: Alternative pathways of continuity. *Archives of General Psychiatry, 58*(3), 231–236.

Kongerslev, M. T., Chanen, A. M., & Simonsen, E. (2015). Personality disorder in childhood and adolescence comes of age: A review of the current evidence and prospects for future research. *Scandinavian Journal of Child and Adolescent Psychiatry and Psychology, 3*(1), 31–48.

Kongerslev, M., Moran, P., Bo, S., & Simonsen, E. (2012). Screening for personality disorder in incarcerated adolescent boys: Preliminary validation of an adolescent version of the Standardised Assessment of Personality—Abbreviated Scale (SAPAS-AV). *BMC Psychiatry, 12,* 94.

Krueger, R. F., Skodol, A. E., Livesley, W. J., Shrout, P. E., & Huang, Y. (2007). Synthesizing dimensional and categorical approaches to personality disorders: Refining the research agenda for DSM-V Axis II. *International Journal of Methods in Psychiatric Research, 16*(Suppl. 1), S65–S73.

Kushner, S. C., Quilty, L. C., Tackett, J. L., & Bagby, R. M. (2011). The hierarchical structure of the Dimensional Assessment of Personality Pathology (DAPP-BQ). *Journal of Personality Disorders, 25*(4), 504–516.

Kushner, S. C., Tackett, J. L., & De Clercq, B. (2013). The joint hierarchical structure of adolescent personality pathology: Converging evidence from two approaches to measurement. *Journal of the Canadian Academy of Child and Adolescent Psychiatry, 22*(3), 199–205.

Lewinsohn, P. M., Rohde, P., Seeley, J. R., & Klein, D. N. (1997). Axis II psychopathology as a function of Axis I disorders in childhood and adolescence. *Journal of the American Academy of Child and Adolescent Psychiatry, 36*(12), 1752–1759.

Linde, J. A., Stringer, D., Simms, L. J., & Clark, L. A. (2013). The Schedule for Nonadaptive and Adaptive Personality for Youth (SNAP-Y): A new measure for assessing adolescent personality and personality pathology. *Assessment, 20*(4), 387–404.

Livesley, W. J. (1998). Suggestions for a framework for an empirically based classification of personality disorder. *Canadian Journal of Psychiatry, 43*(2), 137–147.

Livesley, W. J., Jang, K. L., & Vernon, P. A. (1998). Phenotypic and genetic structure of traits delineating personality disorder. *Archives of General Psychiatry, 55*(10), 941–948.

Markon, K. E., Krueger, R. F., & Watson, D. (2005). Delineating the structure of normal and abnormal personality: An integrative hierarchical approach. *Journal of Personality and Social Psychology, 88*(1), 139–157.

Mehlum, L., Tormoen, A. J., Ramberg, M., Haga, E., Diep, L. M., Laberg, S., et al. (2014). Dialectical behavior therapy for adolescents with repeated suicidal and self-harming behavior: A randomized trial. *Journal of the American Academy of Child and Adolescent Psychiatry, 53*(10), 1082–1091.

Mervielde, I., De Clercq, B., De Fruyt, F., & Van Leeuwen, K. (2005). Temperament, personality, and developmental psychopathology as childhood antecedents of personality disorders. *Journal of Personality Disorders, 19*(2), 171–201.

Moffitt, T. E., Arseneault, L., Jaffee, S. R., Kim-Cohen, J., Koenen, K. C., Odgers, C. L., et al. (2008). Research review: DSM-V conduct disorder: research needs for an evidence base. *Journal of Child Psychology and Psychiatry and Allied Disciplines, 49*(1), 3–33.

Moran, P., Coffey, C., Chanen, A. M., Mann, A., Carlin, J. B., & Patton, G. C. (2011). The impact of childhood sexual abuse on personality disorder: An epidemiological study. *Psychological Medicine, 41*(6), 1311–1318.

Morey, L. C., Hopwood, C. J., Gunderson, J. G., Skodol, A. E., Shea, M. T., Yen, S., et al. (2007). Comparison of alternative models for personality disorders. *Psychological Medicine, 37*(7), 983–994.

Mrazek, P. J., & Haggerty, R. J. (1994). *Reducing risks for mental disorders: Frontiers for preventive intervention research*. Washington, DC: National Academy Press.

National Collaborating Centre for Mental Health. (2009). *Antisocial personality disorder: Treatment, management and prevention* (NICE Clinical Guidelines, No. 77). Leichester, UK: National Institute for Health and Clinical Excellence.

Nelson, E. E., Leibenluft, E., McClure, E. B., & Pine, D. S. (2005). The social re-orientation of adolescence: A neuroscience perspective on the process and its relation to psychopathology. *Psychological Medicine, 35*(2), 163–174.

Newton-Howes, G., Clark, L. A., & Chanen, A. M. (2015). Personality disorder across the life course. *Lancet, 385*, 727–734.

Newton-Howes, G., Weaver, T., & Tyrer, P. (2008). Attitudes of staff towards patients with personality disorder in community mental health teams. *Australian and New Zealand Journal of Psychiatry, 42*(7), 572–577.

O'Connor, B. P. (2002). The search for dimensional structure differences between normality and abnormality: A statistical review of published data on personality and psychopathology. *Journal of Personality and Social Psychology, 83*(4), 962–982.

Olds, D. L. (2008). Preventing child maltreatment and crime with prenatal and infancy support of parents: The nurse-family partnership. *Journal of Scandinavian Studies in Criminology and Crime Prevention, 9*(Suppl. 1), 2–24.

Olds, D. L., Sadler, L., & Kitzman, H. (2007). Programs for parents of infants and toddlers: Recent evidence from randomized trials. *Journal of Child Psychology and Psychiatry and Allied Disciplines, 48*(3–4), 355–391.

Oshri, A., Rogosch, F. A., & Cicchetti, D. (2013). Child maltreatment and mediating influences of childhood personality types on the development of adolescent psychopathology. *Journal of Clinical Child and Adolescent Psychology, 42*(3), 287–301.

Paris, J., Perlin, J., Laporte, L., Fitzpatrick, M., & DeStefano, J. (2014). Exploring resilience and borderline personality disorder: A qualitative study of pairs of sisters. *Personality and Mental Health, 8*(3), 199–208.

Paus, T. (2005). Mapping brain maturation and cognitive development during adolescence. *Trends in Cognitive Sciences, 9*(2), 60–68.

Raine, A. (2006). Schizotypal personality: Neurodevelopmental and Psychosocial Trajectories. *Annual Review of Clinical Psychology, 2*(1), 291–326.

Roberts, B. W., & DelVecchio, W. F. (2000). The rank-order consistency of personality traits from childhood to old age: A quantitative review of longitudinal studies. *Psychological Bulletin, 126*(1), 3–25.

Roberts, B. W., Walton, K. E., & Viechtbauer, W. (2006). Patterns of mean-level change in personality traits across the life course: A meta-analysis of longitudinal studies. *Psychological Bulletin, 132*(1), 1–25.

Rossouw, T. I., & Fonagy, P. (2012). Mentalization-based treatment for self-harm in adolescents: A randomized controlled trial. *Journal of the American Academy of Child and Adolescent Psychiatry, 51*(12), 1304–1313.

Rothbart, M. K., & Bates, J. E. (2006). Temperament. In N. Eisenberg, W. Damon, & R. M. Lerner (Eds.), *Handbook of child psychology* (Vol. 3, pp. 99–166). Hoboken, NJ: Wiley.

Rutter, M. (2012). Psychopathy in childhood: Is it a meaningful diagnosis? *British Journal of Psychiatry, 200*(3), 175–176.

Rutter, M., Kim-Cohen, J., & Maughan, B. (2006). Continuities and discontinuities in psychopathology between childhood and adult life. *Journal of Child Psychology and Psychiatry and Allied Disciplines, 47*(3–4), 276–295.

Ryle, A. (1997). *Cognitive analytic therapy of borderline personality disorder: The model and the method*. New York: Wiley.

Samuel, D. B., & Widiger, T. A. (2008). A meta-analytic review of the relationships between the five-factor model and DSM-IV-TR personality disorders: A facet level analysis. *Clinical Psychology Review, 28*(8), 1326–1342.

Sawyer, A. M., Borduin, C. M., & Dopp, A. R. (2015). Long-term effects of prevention and treatment on youth antisocial behavior: A meta-analysis. *Clinical Psychology Review, 42*, 130–144.

Schulenberg, J. E., Sameroff, A. J., & Cicchetti, D. (2004). The transition to adulthood as a critical juncture in the course of psychopathology and mental health. *Development and Psychopathology, 16*(4), 799–806.

Schuppert, H. M., Giesen-Bloo, J., van Gemert, T., Wiersema, H., Minderaa, R., Emmelkamp, P., et al. (2009). Effectiveness of an emotion regulation group training for adolescents—a randomized controlled pilot study. *Clinical Psychology and Psychotherapy, 16*(6), 467–478.

Schuppert, H. M., Timmerman, M. E., Bloo, J., van Gemert, T. G., Wiersema, H. M., Minderaa, R. B., et al. (2012). Emotion regulation training for adolescents with borderline personality disorder traits: A randomized controlled trial. *Journal of the American Academy of Child and Adolescent Psychiatry, 51*(12), 1314–1323.

Shiner, R. L. (2009). The development of personality disorders: Perspectives from normal personality development in childhood and adolescence. *Development and Psychopathology, 21*(3), 715–734.

Shiner, R. L., & Tackett, J. L. (2014). Personality and personality disorders. In E. J. Mash & R. A. Barkley (Eds.), *Child psychopathology* (3rd ed., pp. 848–896). New York: Guilford Press.

Skodol, A. E. (2008). Longitudinal course and outcome of personality disorders. *Psychiatric Clinics of North America, 31*(3), 495–503, viii.

Skodol, A. E., Bender, D. S., Pagano, M. E., Shea, M. T., Yen, S., Sanislow, C. A., et al. (2007). Positive childhood experiences: Resilience and recovery from personality disorder in early adulthood. *Journal of Clinical Psychiatry, 68*(7), 1102–1108.

Skodol, A. E., Gunderson, J. G., Shea, M. T., McGlashan, T. H., Morey, L. C., Sanislow, C. A., et al. (2005). The Collaborative Longitudinal Personality Disorders Study (CLPS): Overview and implications. *Journal of Personality Disorders, 19*(5), 487–504.

Skodol, A. E., Pagano, M. E., Bender, D. S., Shea, M. T., Gunderson, J. G., Yen, S., et al. (2005). Stability of functional impairment in patients with schizotypal, borderline, avoidant, or obsessive–compulsive personality disorder over two years. *Psychological Medicine, 35*(3), 443–451.

Soto, C. J., John, O. P., Gosling, S. D., & Potter, J. (2011). Age differences in personality traits from 10 to 65: Big Five domains and facets in a large cross-sectional sample. *Journal of Personality and Social Psychology, 100*(2), 330–348.

Speranza, M., Pham-Scottez, A., Revah-Levy, A., Barbe, R. P., Perez-Diaz, F., Birmaher, B., et al. (2012). Factor structure of borderline personality disorder symptomatology in adolescents. *Canadian Journal of Psychiatry, 57*(4), 230–237.

Srivastava, S., John, O. P., Gosling, S. D., & Potter, J. (2003). Development of personality in early and middle adulthood: Set like plaster or persistent change? *Journal of Personality and Social Psychology, 84*(5), 1041–1053.

Steinberg, L. (2005). Cognitive and affective development in adolescence. *Trends in Cognitive Sciences, 9*(2), 69–74.

Stepp, S. D., Burke, J. D., Hipwell, A. E., & Loeber, R. (2012). Trajectories of attention deficit hyperactivity disorder and oppositional defiant disorder symptoms as precursors of borderline personality disorder symptoms in adolescent girls. *Journal of Abnormal Child Psychology, 40*(1), 7–20.

Stepp, S. D., Whalen, D. J., Pilkonis, P. A., Hipwell, A. E., & Levine, M. D. (2011). Children of mothers with borderline personality disorder: Identifying parenting behaviors as potential targets for intervention. *Personality Disorders, 3*(1), 76–91.

Stoffers, J. M., Vollm, B. A., Rucker, G., Timmer, A., Huband, N., & Lieb, K. (2012). Psychological therapies for people with borderline personality disorder. *Cochrane Database of Systematic Reviews, 8*, 8, CD005652.

Tackett, J. L., Balsis, S., Oltmanns, T. F., & Krueger, R. F. (2009). A unifying perspective on personality pathology across the life span: Developmental considerations for the fifth edition of the *Diagnostic and Statistical Manual of Mental Disorders*. *Development and Psychopathology, 21*(3), 687–713.

Tackett, J. L., Herzhoff, K., Kushner, S. C., & Rule, N. (2016). Thin slices of child personality: Perceptual, situational, and behavioral contributions. *Journal of Personality and Social Psychology, 110*(1), 150–166.

Tackett, J. L., Herzhoff, K., Reardon, K., Smack, A., & Kushner, S. K. (2013). The relevance of informant discrepancies for the assessment of adolescent personality pathology. *Clinical Psychology: Science and Practice, 20*, 378–392.

Tackett, J. L., Kushner, S. C., De Fruyt, F., & Mervielde, I. (2013). Delineating personality traits in childhood and adolescence: Associations across measures, temperament, and behavioral problems. *Assessment, 20*(6), 738–751.

Tackett, J. L., Slobodskaya, H. R., Mar, R. A., Deal, J., Halverson, C. F., Jr., Baker, S. R., et al. (2012). The hierarchical structure of childhood personality in five countries: Continuity from early childhood to early adolescence. *Journal of Personality, 80*(4), 847–879.

Thatcher, D. L., Cornelius, J. R., & Clark, D. B. (2005). Adolescent alcohol use disorders predict adult borderline personality. *Addictive Behaviors, 30*(9), 1709–1724.

Tromp, N. B., & Koot, H. M. (2008). Dimensions of personality pathology in adolescents: Psychometric properties of the DAPP-BQ-A. *Journal of Personality Disorders, 22*(6), 623–638.

Tyrer, P., Crawford, M., & Mulder, R. T. (2011). Reclassifying personality disorders. *Lancet, 377*, 1814–1815.

Tyrer, P., Crawford, M., Mulder, R. T., Blashfield, R., Farnam, A., Fossati, A., et al. (2011). The rationale for the reclassification of personality disorder in the 11th revision of the *International Classification of Diseases* (ICD-11). *Personality and Mental Health, 5*(4), 246–259.

Tyrer, P., Reed, G. M., & Crawford, M. J. (2015). Classification, assessment, prevalence, and effect of personality disorder. *Lancet, 385*, 717–726.

Warner, M. B., Morey, L. C., Finch, J. F., Gunderson, J. G., Skodol, A. E., Sanislow, C. A., et al. (2004). The longitudinal relationship of personality traits and disorders. *Journal of Abnormal Psychology, 113*(2), 217–227.

Weisz, J. R., Hawley, K. M., & Doss, A. J. (2004). Empirically tested psychotherapies for youth internalizing and externalizing problems and disorders. *Child and Adolescent Psychiatric Clinics of North America, 13*(4), 729–815, v–vi.

Whalen, D. J., Scott, L. N., Jakubowski, K. P., McMakin, D. L., Hipwell, A. E., Silk, J. S., et al. (2014). Affective behavior during mother–daughter conflict and borderline personality disorder severity across adolescence. *Personality Disorders, 5*(1), 88–96.

Woolfenden, S. R., Williams, K., & Peat, J. K. (2002). Family and parenting interventions for conduct disorder and delinquency: A meta-analysis of randomised controlled trials. *Archives of Disease in Childhood, 86*(4), 251–256.

Zimmerman, M. E., Chelminski, I., & Young, D. (2008). The frequency of personality disorders in psychiatric patients. *Psychiatric Clinics of North America, 31*(3), 405–420.

Zoccolillo, M., Pickles, A., Quinton, D., & Rutter, M. (1992). The outcome of childhood conduct disorder: Implications for defining adult personality disorder and conduct disorder. *Psychological Medicine, 22*(4), 971–986.

# PART IV

# ETIOLOGY AND DEVELOPMENT

## INTRODUCTION

This part of the *Handbook* covers a wide range of issues and perspectives linked to the intertwined themes of etiology and development. Chapters on biological contributions to personality disorder (PD) cover genetic factors, neurotransmitter systems, specific mechanisms, and evidence of neuropsychological impairments. Other chapters review research on the associations between early psychosocial adversity and personality pathology from a vulnerability–stress perspective, provide a developmental psychopathology perspective, and suggest new avenues of research from attachment-based perspectives to the origins and expression of personality pathology. Together, these chapters provide an overview of the field that illustrates the extent to which developmental considerations have become progressively integrated with the empirical literature on PDs. We originally thought about dividing the contents into three parts—biological etiology, psychosocial etiology, and development—but this seemed to perpetuate several unhelpful polarities and assumptions about etiology and development. Discussion of etiology has tended to be polarized around matters such as nature versus nurture and genetic versus environmental influences. Although it is now generally accepted that the phenotypic features of PD arise from the interaction of genetic and environmental influences, the debate lingers on in the form of discussion of the relative effects of genes and environment and the search for "genes for" a given mental disorder, including different PDs, and in the priority given to biological mechanisms and explanations. Categorizing etiological influences into biological and psychosocial factors seems to encourage seeing them as having distinct and unrelated contributions to development and seeing some etiological factors as being more fundamental or privileged than others. This is especially apparent in some areas of American psychiatry that advocate a rigid form of reductionism that places emphasis on neurobiological mechanisms and minimizes the contributions of other etiological factors. However, the tendency to adopt a single perspective on etiology and to neglect other viewpoints is not the monopoly of some facets of biological psychiatry. The treatment literature tends to adopt a similar stance. Typical treatment manuals usually note the contribution of what are frequently called "constitutional factors" but then proceed to concentrate on treating the consequences of psychosocial adversity, with scant attention to how biological factors may influence the treatment process.

Construction of a more integrated understanding of etiology and development requires an approach that avoids the extremes of these polar positions and offers a more broadly-based perspective of the biological and psychosocial factors contributing to PD. The perspective of developmental systems theory (Griffiths & Gray, 1994; Oyama, Griffiths, & Gray, 2001a) seems to provide a way to move in this direction. Developmental systems theory is not a theory in the sense that it provides a specific model that can be used to derive testable predictions; rather, it is a general conceptual perspective for understanding development. Some of the major themes of the approach are as follows: (1) Phenotypic features result from the interaction of multiple factors that may be grouped in multiple ways—of which genes versus environment is only one—according to the developmental questions that are being explored; (2) causal factors are sensitive to the state of the rest of the system, and their significance is contingent on the state of the total system at that time; (3) organisms inherit a large number of factors that influence development—the approach defines inheritance widely and recognizes that a wide range of resources besides genes are "passed-on" and may be used to construct developmental outcomes; (4) development is a construction—all features of the individual are constructed during development rather than programmed or preformed in some way; and (5) no single set of factors influencing development controls or directs the process; rather, control is distributed, and the organism influences its own development and helps to determine what additional factors influence its development (Oyama, Griffiths, & Gray, 2001b).

Since PD is clearly a developmental outcome, development systems theory seems relevant to understanding the processes involved. Also, as illustrated by the chapters in Part IV, the general conclusions of etiological and developmental research are consistent with the theory's assumptions. The evidence suggests that PD arises from the interaction of multiple factors, ranging from genes to culture. Each etiological factor appears to have a relatively small effect, and none appear to be either necessary or sufficient to cause disorder. The evidence also suggests that disorder emerges along multiple developmental pathways, with considerable differences across individuals. These conclusions differ from notions that were common only a couple of decades ago when PD was assumed to be largely psychosocial in origin and borderline PD (BPD) was a form of chronic posttraumatic stress disorder caused by childhood sexual abuse. These were common and often strongly held positions. Now, if anything, the pendulum seems to have swung in the opposite direction, leading to an increasing tendency to view PD as a "biological disorder." However, unless some kind of metaphysical assumption of brain–mind dualism is assumed, such statements are empty of meaning, since any psychological event must be associated with some kind of neural event. As Meehl (1972) noted, the important issue for explanation is whether the biological factor is strong or weak. Strong explanations involve specific mechanisms that are found in all individuals with the disorder. Such effects are rare with mental disorders (Turkheimer, 2015) and confined to conditions such as phenylketonuria and Huntington's disease. With PD, as with most mental disorders, specific genetic mechanisms have not been identified. Instead, PD is influenced by multiple genes, each having a small effect. This does not mean that specific genetic mechanisms will not be found, but it is unlikely given the polygenic mode of transmission. Discussion of the biological etiology of PD often confuses weak and strong biological explanation and inappropriately attributes strong causation to what Meehl considered weak explanation. The fact that genetic and other forms of causal influences are likely to be weak does not mean that it is not important to study genetic and other biological influences on PD. It is important to understand the neurobiological mechanisms involved in PD and for treatment to become increasingly informed by this understanding. However, it is also important that biological etiology is understood within a broader conceptual framework that recognizes a plurality of causal perspectives.

Consequently, we thought it important to juxtapose biological factors with psychosocial contributions to the etiology and development of PD. Although, as we have noted, PD is a developmental disorder and the DSM definition of PD suggests a developmental aspect in relation to onset, relatively little empirical research on very early developmental pathways has been conducted (e.g., Venta, Herzhoff, Cohen, & Sharp, 2014) . Also, until recently, research on etiology and course was almost exclusively conducted with adult samples, in part due to long-standing concerns regarding diagnosis of PD in children and adolescents because of assumptions about the malleability of personality in early developmental stages and potential harmful effects associated with the diagnosis (e.g., Kaess, Brunner, & Chanen, 2014). However, there is a growing consensus that developmental considerations are important in conceptualizing PD (Cicchetti & Crick, 2009; Shiner, 2009; Tackett, Balsis, Oltmanns, & Krueger, 2009), that personality pathology exists and can be reliably measured children and youth, that the BPD diagnosis is applicable in adolescence (de Clercq, van Leeuwen, van den Noortgate, De Bolle, & de Fruyt, 2009; de Clercq et al., 2014; Kongerslev, Chanen, & Simonsen, 2015; see also Chanen, Tackett, & Thompson, Chapter 12, this volume), and that pathways to adult PD begin in childhood (e.g., Tackett et al., 2009).

Taken together, this body of work offers an understanding of the development of PD that is more advanced than was the case just a decade ago. The field has progressed beyond investigating explanatory models involving isolated risk and protective factors to begin examining developmental models that incorporate multiple levels of analysis, taking into account genetically based vulnerabilities and resiliencies to disorder (e.g., Foley et al., 2004).

Accompanying this shift is considerable interest in identifying and testing the effects of proximal and intermediate developmental mechanisms that mediate and moderate identified risk factors, including individual-level factors such as genetics, temperament, and adversity, including experiences of maltreatment; family-level factors such as parental psychopathology, and distal contextual influences such as socioeconomic status. This current wave of research is a departure from earlier developmental studies of PD that largely focused on the borderline diagnosis in retrospectively assessing childhood experiences and investigating associations between identified risk factors and BPD in adulthood (e.g., Herman, Perry, & van der Kolk, 1989; Klonsky, Oltmanns, Turkheimer, & Fiedler, 2000). Such foundational research provided evidence showing that specific types and combinations of childhood and adolescent adversities (e.g., different forms of abuse and neglect) are associated with risk for the emergence of PDs in adulthood (see Kongerslev et al., 2015; Lobbestael, Arntz, & Bernstein, 2010). Although retrospective studies supported the generation of developmental hypotheses and considerable information regarding distal correlates of personality pathology, these studies often did not differentiate between experiences that occurred across different developmental periods (i.e., childhood vs. adolescence), and their utility in supporting causal inferences is limited further due to the possibility of recall bias and inaccurate reporting of early experiences (e.g., Johnson et al., 2005; Macfie & Strimpfel, 2014).

The chapters in Part IV amply illustrate the complexity of the etiology and development of PD and diversity of perspectives needed to account for this complexity. The first chapter (Chapter 13) on genetics, by Kerry Jang and Philip A. Vernon, describes the intricacies of genetic influences and documents the successes and the disappointments of genetic research. The results of behavioral genetic studies are robust in showing that the features of PD are heritable and that environmental effects are largely confined to nonspecific influences—that is, influences specific to a given twin—and that common environmental influences have little impact on personality. The evidence is also robust that the structure of genetic influences is highly congruent with the phenotypic structure. In contrast to the consistent findings of behavioral genetic studies, the results of molecular genetic research have been remarkably inconsistent. The contemporary situation contrasts markedly with the optimism of early molecular genetic studies of personality that seemed to identify specific loci associated with some common traits. However, these initial findings were not replicated and, to date, linkage, candidate gene, and association studies have failed to generate consistent findings.

The chapter on neurotransmitter systems by Jennifer R. Fanning and Emil F. Coccaro

(Chapter 14) documents similar complexity. Initial assumptions at the turn of century linked to early molecular genetic studies that posited robust and direct relationships between specific neurotransmitters and specific traits have not been substantiated. The chapter clearly shows that specific components of personality are linked to a cascade of multiple transmitters that interact with each other in complex ways, and that neurotransmitter functioning is affected by multiple variables, including environmental events. The chapter clearly illustrates that the challenge of unraveling this complexity is more difficult when the personality construct being studied is itself complex and comprises different components. This raises the question of what is the best way to characterize personality pathology in order to investigate biological functioning. Fanning and Coccaro suggest that the investigation of specific dimensions may be more productive than studying global diagnoses. This seems to point to the value of a research strategy that focuses on specific mechanisms.

The value of a mechanism-based approach is illustrated by the chapter on emotional regulation and emotional processing by Paul H. Soloff (Chapter 15). Problems with emotion regulation and processing is a transdiagnostic construct that applies to most forms of PD. The chapter begins by examining emotional functioning in healthy individuals. This is makes an important and refreshing point: To understand pathological functioning, we also need to understand normal functioning. Although obvious, normal personality functioning has not had a great impact on the formulation of clinical conceptions of PD: They have largely been developed on the basis of clinical observation of relatively few cases. Normal emotional functioning is examined both in terms of "bottom-up" processes concerned with emotional arousal and "top-down" processes linked to emotion regulation. Subsequently, research on emotion dysregulation in patients with PD is reviewed, and the chapter concludes with a consideration of treatment implications. Much of this work was conducted on patients with BPD, so that in many cases it is not clear whether findings are specific to this disorder, common to all forms of PD with emotional dysregulation as a salient feature, or a consequence of emotional dysregulation generally.

In Chapter 16, Marianne Skovgaard Thomsen, Anthony C. Ruocco, Birgit Bork Mathiesen, and Erik Simonsen review the literature on neuropsychological impairments associated with BPD. Clinicians often note that many patients with PD have a history of mild neurological trauma but do not know what significance it has. Likewise, studies are reported that suggest modest cognitive impairment of some kind and, again, it is difficult to know whether the finding has general clinical significance. This chapter provides a comprehensive account of the literature on neurocognitive functioning in patients with BPD, the only disorder that has been extensively investigated. The review documents somewhat mixed findings. For many cognitive functions studies suggesting an impairment are matched by a similar number of studies failing to find one. It also seems that many early studies were poorly designed, with sample sizes too small to generate generalizable findings. The authors conclude that BPD is not associated with any specific pattern of cognitive deficit. However, a variety of specific impairments have been identified, such as problems with sustained attention, episodic memory, response inhibition, decision making, problem solving, and planning. Also, meta-analyses have identified deficits in attention, cognitive flexibility, learning and memory, planning, processing speed, and visuospatial abilities. What is less clear is whether these deficits are due to neurological impairments or whether they are the functional consequence of emotional dysregulation (see Soloff, Chapter 15). This important issue needs to be addressed by future research.

The chapters with a primary biological focus are followed by the chapter by Joel Paris on the association between childhood adversities and adult PD (Chapter 17). Different forms of childhood adversity have been found to be associated with psychopathology and PD (e.g., see Stepp, Lazarus, & Byrd, 2016). Childhood adversities and traumatic stress are viewed here in the context of a developmental psychopathology model of diathesis–stress that recognizes the proximal and distal interrelationships among child-level characteristics (e.g., temperament; resilience), life events, developmental maturation, and outcomes in adulthood. The diathesis–stress model of mental disorders (see Monroe & Simons, 1991) accounts for the inconsistent associations between childhood adversity and developmental outcomes; furthermore, it explains how some individuals exposed to the same specific risk factors will not develop disorder (i.e., multifinality) whereas other individuals who do develop the disorder may have experienced different risk factors (i.e., equifinality). This perspective raises possibilities for different pathways through which disorder emerges and unfolds.

Similarly, Rebecca L. Shiner and Timothy A. Allen (Chapter 18) articulate a developmental psychopathology framework based on current DSM-5 formulation of PD as consisting of pathological personality traits and impaired personality functioning. They discuss the development and interrelation of normal-range and pathological personality traits across childhood and adolescence by (1) reviewing the current literature articulating a developmental taxonomy of traits from a five-factor model (FFM) perspective; (2) summarizing current work on the development, stability, and change of pathological personality traits in youth; and (3) describing a model for the role of abnormal traits in the development of PD. They conclude by considering the ways in which future research will benefit from further investigation of the expression or form of children's and adolescents' emerging pathological personality traits, examining stability and change in PD symptoms and PD traits; and evaluating pathological traits and impairment in other aspects of personality functioning to determine the ways in which these components may be interrelated and influence each other over time.

In Chapter 19, Roseann Larstone, Stephanie G. Craig, and Marlene M. Moretti explore the idea of developmental pathways by reviewing research on the emergence of callous–unemotional (CU) traits that have been shown to identify a subgroup of aggressive children and youth who are likely to show severe and persistent antisocial behavior, a core component of antisocial PD (ASPD) and psychopathy. They discuss the current literature and present two mutually informative perspectives regarding the etiological and developmental trajectory of CU traits, one from the dominant developmental genetic approach and the other from a developmental model that conceptualizes these traits as acquired adaptations to environmental or contextual influences. These developmental models are useful in conceptualizing the development of "primary" versus what has been recently termed in the literature as "acquired" CU traits, respectively. Recent evidence suggests a two-step developmental process in the case of acquired CU traits that begins with the attachment relationship. The authors review findings on the etiology and development of CU traits and implications for treatment. They conclude that although there is emerging evidence of distinct developmental pathways to development of CU traits, these pathways are not mutually exclusive.

### REFERENCES

Cicchetti, D., & Crick, N. R. (2009). Precursors of and diverse pathways to personality disorder in children and adolescents. *Development and Psychopathology, 21,* 683–685.

de Clercq, B., de Fruyt, F., De Bolle, M., van Hiel, A., Markon, K. E., & Krueger, R. F. (2014). The hierarchical structure and construct validity of the PID-5 trait measure in adolescence. *Journal of Personality, 82,* 158–169.

de Clercq, B., van Leeuwen, K., van den Noortgate, W., De Bolle, M., & de Fruyt, F. (2009). Childhood personality pathology: Dimensional stability and change. *Development and Psychopathology, 21,* 853–869.

Foley, D. L., Eaves, L. J., Wormley, B., Silberg, J. L., Maes, H. H., Kuhn, J., et al. (2004). Childhood adversity, monoamine oxidase A genotype, and risk for conduct disorder. *Archives of General Psychiatry, 61,* 738–744.

Griffiths, P. E., & Gray, R. D. (1994). Developmental systems and evolutionary explanation. *Journal of Philosophy, 91,* 277–304.

Herman, J. L., Perry, J. C., & van der Kolk, B. A. (1989). Childhood trauma in borderline personality disorder. *American Journal of Psychiatry, 146,* 490–495.

Johnson, J. G., McGeoch, P. G., Caske, V. P., Abhary, S. G., Sneed, J. R., & Bornstein, R. F. (2005). The developmental psychopathology of personality disorders. In B. L. Hankin & R. Z. Abela (Eds.), *Development of psychopathology: A vulnerability–stress perspective* (pp. 417–464). Thousand Oaks, CA: SAGE.

Kaess, M., Brunner, R., & Chanen, A. (2014). Borderline personality disorder in adolescence. *Pediatrics, 134*(4), 782–793.

Klonsky, E. D., Oltmanns, T. F., Turkheimer, E., & Fiedler, E. R. (2000). Recollections of conflict with parents and family support in the personality disorders. *Journal of Personality Disorders, 14,* 327–338.

Kongerslev, M. T., Chanen, A. M., & Simonsen, E. (2015). Personality disorder in childhood and adolescence comes of age: A review of the current evidence and prospects for future research. *Scandinavian Journal of Child and Adolescent Psychiatry and Psychology, 3,* 31–48.

Lobbestael, J., Arntz, A., & Bernstein, D. P. (2010). Disentangling the relationship between different types of childhood maltreatment and personality disorders. *Journal of Personality Disorders, 24*(3), 285–295.

Macfie, J., & Strimpfel, J. M. (2014). Parenting and the development of borderline personality disorder. In C. Sharp & J. L. Tackett (Eds.), *Handbook of borderline personality disorder in children and adolescents* (pp. 277–291). New York: Springer Science + Business Media.

Meehl, P. E. (1972). A critical afterword. In I. I. Gottesman & J. Shields (Eds.), *Schizophrenia and genetics* (pp. 367–416). New York: Academic Press.

Monroe, S. M., & Simons, A. D. (1991). Diathesis–stress theories in the context of life stress research: Implications for the depressive disorders. *Psychological Bulletin, 110,* 406–425.

Oyama, S., Griffiths, P. E., & Gray, R. D. (Eds.). (2001a). *Cycles of contingency: Developmental systems and evolution.* Cambridge, MA: MIT Press.

Oyama, S., Griffiths, P. E., & Gray, R. D. (2001b). Introduction: What is developmental systems theory? In S. Oyama, P. E. Griffiths, & R. D. Gray (Eds.), *Cycles of contingency: Developmental systems and evolution* (pp. 1–11). Cambridge, MA: MIT Press.

Shiner, R. (2009). The development of personality disorders: Perspectives from normal personality development in childhood and adolescence. *Development and Psychopathology, 21*(3), 715–734.

Stepp, S. D., Lazarus, S. A., & Byrd, A. L. (2016). A systematic review of risk factors prospectively associated with borderline personality disorder: Taking stock and moving forward. *Personality Disorders: Theory, Research and Treatment, 7,* 316–323.

Tackett, J. L., Balsis, S., Oltmanns, T. F., & Krueger, R. F. (2009). A unifying perspective on personality pathology across the life span: Developmental considerations for the fifth edition of the *Diagnostic and Statistical Manual of Mental Disorders. Development and Psychopathology, 21,* 687–713.

Turkheimer, E. (2015). The nature of nature. In K. S. Kendler & J. Parnas (Eds.), *Philosophical issues in psychiatry III: The nature and sources of historical change* (pp. 227–244). Oxford, UK: Oxford University Press.

Venta, A., Herzhoff, K., Cohen, P., & Sharp, C. (2014). The longitudinal course of borderline personality disorder in youth. In C. Sharp & J. L. Tackett (Eds.), *Handbook of borderline personality disorder in children and adolescents* (pp. 229–245). New York: Springer Science + Business Media.

# CHAPTER 13

# Genetics

Kerry L. Jang and Philip A. Vernon

Although genetic research on personality disorder (PD) remains an active area of research, in the past decade this research has fundamentally changed in terms of the foci of investigation, emerging methods, and the development of novel theoretical frameworks to further our understanding of the role of genes. This shift is interesting because, until recently, much genetic research on personality function yielded a consistently reproducible result: that approximately half of the variability observed in personality function is directly attributable to genetic differences between individuals. This finding, coupled with the availability of increasingly detailed maps of the human genome, suggested that it would be a relatively straightforward task to identify putative genes for personality and its disorders. However, despite intensive undertakings over the last 20 years to identify genes corresponding to specific PDs or aspects of personality pathology, the results have fallen short of this goal and, in contrast to previous research, they are regularly irreproducible. Our aim in this chapter is to review foundational and recent behavior genetics research as applied to personality pathology and to discuss behavior genetics methods, theoretical models, and the challenges associated with each of these in the search for genes associated with personality function. We conclude the chapter with a discussion of emerging methods and recent research that may hold promise in this area.

## The Phenotype

### PD Diagnoses

In the first edition of this volume, it was noted that genetic research requires a clear definition of the phenotype. Although progress has been made in the intervening years, the key problem remains of how disordered personality is measured and incorporated into various genetic methodologies. Classical measurement issues, including discrepancies between self- and other-reports and the operationalization of constructs or categories (e.g., diagnoses), are important considerations.

Any misdiagnosis or inaccuracy in measurement of the phenotype, whether due to unclear, misapplied, or overlapping diagnostic criteria, spuriously alters findings because all genetic methods are predicated on the assumption that if a given disorder has a genetic component, the responsible gene(s) will be passed from parents to offspring with certain probabilities, and that patterns vary under different conditions (e.g., if the gene is autosomal dominant as opposed to recessive), as dictated by the laws of genetic transmission. These laws are expressed as mathematical models that compare or "test" whether the observed probabilities that the phenotype is present in an affected population are not different from those expected by genetic theory. Congruence between observed and predicted probabilities would be provided as evidence for whether specific genetic influences (e.g., a particular gene or broader genetic effect whose probabilities are being tested) are present.

This fundamental measurement problem was recognized nearly 20 years ago by Faraone, Tsuang, and Tsuang (1999):

> A mathematical model will not produce meaningful results if the psychiatric diagnoses it analyzes do not correspond to genetically crisp categories. The dilemma we face is that the diagnoses were developed to serve many masters: clinicians, scientists, insurance companies, and more. There is no a priori reason why these categories would be ideal for genetic studies. (p. 114)

### Dimensional Models of PD

It would be unfair, however, to single out diagnostic categories as being solely unsuitable for genetics research. Dimensional models of personality pathology that are based on normal personality trait scales have inherent challenges similar to those found with diagnostic categories. One such issue is the problem of criterion or exemplar overlap between measures. For example, symptoms and features of anxiety appear in several personality dysfunction measures and scales. It is virtually impossible to isolate and locate a behavioral–affective feature such as anxiety within specific scales. To do so would eliminate any ecological validity of the scale or it would no longer adequately describe observable behavior. To overcome this issue, genetic methods have been developed in an attempt to mitigate and/or accommodate the idiosyncrasies of personality measures.

The basic challenge is illustrated by the following example. Although it may seem unnecessary in the context of this chapter to discuss scale content, it is nonetheless important because scale content determines the precise range of behavior under study. Do the scales, for example, focus on behavior within the normal range, the abnormal range, or the entire distribution (see Figure 13.1)?

Figure 13.1 is instantly recognizable as the basis of the dimensional model of PD that has received a great deal of support in the literature over the past two decades. The distribution of personality function is seen to vary on a continuum that ranges from the normal or not-ill range of functioning (0 to $T_1$) to the spectrum conditions that refer to mild pathology—the interface between normal and disordered personality ($T_1$ to $T_2$)—to an extreme behavior or ill range of functioning ($T_2$ to $\infty$). As Figure 13.1 illustrates, most people have moderate levels of vulnerability, and fewer have very high or very low levels. When a person's vulnerability exceeds the threshold denoted by $T_2$, that person will develop the full disorder; between $T_1$ and $T_2$, the person will develop a spectrum condition; below $T_1$, the individual will be unaffected and not exhibit psychopathology. At the same time, Figure 13.1 can also be seen to define diagnostic categories in which individuals are simply classified as "ill" or "not ill," by removing some of the intermediate thresholds. However one looks at it, the commonality is the notion of an underlying liability to illness and this

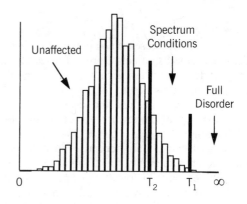

**FIGURE 13.1.** Threshold liability model. The distribution of personality function is seen to vary on a continuum that ranges from a normal or "not ill" range of functioning (0 to $T_1$) to the spectrum conditions that refer to mild pathology—the interface between normal and disordered personality ($T_1$ to $T_2$) to an extreme behavior or ill range of functioning ($T_2$ to $\infty$). When a person's vulnerability exceeds the threshold denoted by $T_2$, he or she will develop the full disorder; if between $T_1$ and $T_2$, he or she will develop a spectrum condition, or if below $T_1$, he or she will be unaffected and will not exhibit psychopathology. The model assumes that multiple genetic and environmental effects combine to create an individual's susceptibility, suggesting, then, that patients differ from nonpatients only in the number of pathogenic genetic and/or environmental events or experiences to which they have been exposed. Adapted from Faraone, Tsuang, and Tsuang (1999). Copyright © 1999 The Guilford Press. Adapted by permission.

*threshold liability model* can be used to conduct genetic studies with distinct populations falling within different distributions of the continuum.

## The Threshold Liability Model

According to the threshold liability model, the number of individuals in a population that fall into each range is determined by the amount, or "dosage," of genetic and environmental influence. The model is multifactorial in nature and assumes that several genes and environmental effects combine to create an individual's susceptibility. This suggests that patients differ from nonpatients only in the number of pathogenic genetic and/or environmental events or experiences to which they have been exposed. The threshold liability model can easily be modified to explain disorders that exhibit clear discontinuities in the expression of pathology. These disorders are typically found with a bimodal distribution (see Figure 13.2). Under this variant of the threshold liability model, the same multifactorial causes are still exerting an influence that creates much of the variability between people, with the addition of one or more significant genetic and/or environmental causes that create the patient group. The threshold liability model is also important because it explains why the pattern of responses of general population subjects to items assessing PD and symptoms of psychopathology is similar to those of clinical samples (e.g., Jackson & Messnick, 1962; Livesley, Jackson, & Schroeder, 1992; Livesley, Jang, & Vernon, 1998).

## Types of Genetic Analyses

Genetic studies of personality function are designed to estimate the extent to which the vulnerability or dosage is attributable to genetic causes. There are several methods available to estimate this dosage, each addressing a different question and using different types of data but all relying on the greater genetic similarity of relatives for a phenotype as compared to unrelated individuals. Much of the work in the broader area of psychiatric genetics has been to develop these methods and understand their strengths and limitations in relation to specific types of data. The evolution and focus of these methods are provided below.

## Family Studies

The first question usually addressed is whether a behavior, regardless of how it is measured, runs in families. A traditional family study uses a case–control methodology to test whether the frequency of diagnosis is greater among genetically related individuals than in a sample of unrelated matched controls. Finding greater similarity or "familiality" does not imply genetic causation because the similarity of related individuals might be attributable to the influence

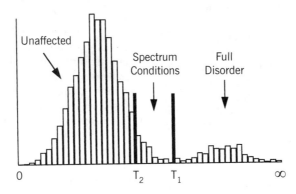

**FIGURE 13.2.** Modified threshold liability model that accounts for discontinuities in the expression of pathology. Under this model, the same multifactorial causes are still exerting an influence that creates much of the variability between people, 0 to $T_1$, $T_1$ to $T_2$, with the addition of one or more significant genetic and/or environmental causes that creates the patient group ($T_2$ to $\infty$). Adapted from Faraone, Tsuang, and Tsuang (1999). Copyright © 1999 The Guilford Press. Adapted by permission.

of a common home environment, experiences, or culture. The family study design is unable to separate the influence of common genes from common environment, and the primary benefit of the design is that it establishes whether additional genetic analyses of a phenotype are warranted.

Family studies have typically been conducted using DSM diagnostic criteria because it is relatively straightforward to ascertain the affected status of individual family members using standard clinical interviews. Moreover, the classification of study participants amounts to little more than a frequency count of the disorder, and the statistical analyses required are a straightforward test of whether the disorder appears more in affected than in nonaffected families. However, if there are errors in diagnosis, the frequencies vary greatly; thus, unsurprisingly, there are virtually no family studies of dimensional or trait models of personality in the literature. To say that "anxiety" runs in families is meaningless because everybody displays anxiety to some degree and there is frequently no clear-cut threshold between normal and abnormal behavior. The usual approach to finding a threshold is to plot the distribution of scores and look for a discontinuity in the distribution, such as bimodality (similar to that illustrated in Figure 13.2).

## Segregation Analysis

Once a disorder or phenotype has been shown to run in families, the next step is usually to determine how the disorder is transmitted from generation to generation. For example, is it transmitted in a dominant, recessive, x-linked, or multifactorial manner? How many genes are implicated—one, two, several, many? The mode of transmission from one generation to the next is studied using "segregation analysis," which translates the laws of genetic transmission into a set of mathematical rules that express the probability that a gene (or a gene variant) will be transmitted from parent to child. The probabilities differ for each mode of inheritance. These theoretical or "predicted" probabilities are compared to the actual transmission rate observed in a sample of affected families. Correspondence between the predicted and observed probabilities supports the presence of particular forms of genetic influence because the disorder is passed on in a manner consistent with genetic theory. This procedure is referred to as "model fitting" or "goodness-of-fit" approach. Like the family study, segregation analysis requires the assignment of affected status, and any misdiagnosis can influence the results.

## Twin Studies

Comparison between identical (monozygotic, or MZ) and fraternal (dizygotic, or DZ) twin pairs on a variable of interest has become probably the most popular method to study the influence of genetics in personality; hence, we discuss this approach in detail. A primary reason for the popularity of twin studies is that this method can handle quantitative measures typical of personality research and uses model fitting to test a broad array of questions. Twin studies use path-analytic techniques (see Neale & Cardon, 1992) to compare the similarities of MZ and DZ twins on a variable of interest, and path analysis allows the separation of genetic and environmental influence. These methods are extremely flexible in that they are able to analyze data from different populations and response formats (including diagnostic categories), and have generated an explosion of studies over the past two decades.

Most twin studies use data obtained from reared-together twins because of the relative ease of finding a large representative sample, although there are several variations of the basic design, such as twins reared apart and family-of-twin designs (see Plomin, DeFries, & McClearn, 1990). The primary statistic used to measure twin similarity is the correlation coefficient such as Pearson's $r$ or intraclass correlation. If greater MZ to DZ similarity is found, this is directly attributable to the twofold greater genetic similarity of MZ to DZ twins, assuming all other things being equal. This is because MZ twins share all of their genes, whereas DZ twins share only half on average.

To understand the logic of the twin study, as an example, if $r_{MZ} = .42$ and $r_{DZ} = .25$, the proportion (%) to which the individual differences observed on a measure is due to genetic differences, or the "heritability coefficient," is estimated as

$$\text{Heritability } (h^2) = 2(r_{MZ} - r_{DZ}) = 2(.42 - .25)$$
$$= .34 \, (100\%) = 34\%$$

The heritability coefficient computed with this formula estimates genetic influences from all sources, such as additive genetic influences (i.e., the extent to which genotypes "breed true" from parent to offspring) and genetic dominance (i.e., genetic effects attributable to the interaction of alleles at the same locus, which results in a phenotype that is not exactly intermediate in expression as would be expected between pure breeding [homozygous] individuals). With twin research, we explain below are a number of issues that are central to the usefulness of the method.

The results of any twin study are predicated on the assumption that the greater observed MZ than DZ twin similarity is not caused by nongenetic factors, such as MZ twins being treated more similarly than DZ twins. Having MZ and DZ twins rate the similarity of their environments on standard measures is a common test of this assumption. For example, twins complete measures that assess the degree to which they were often dressed alike, went to the same schools, and so on. MZ and DZ agreement or concordance rates on these items are then compared. If differences are found (suggesting that the environments of MZ and DZ twins are not the same), then the defaulting twin similarity variables are correlated with the dependent measure(s) to determine whether they account for a significant proportion of the variance. The influence of these variables may be controlled for by computing the standardized residual from the regression of the twin similarity variable on the study variables prior to genetic analyses. To date, the assumption of "equal environments" has been shown to hold across numerous different twin study designs (e.g., Derks, Dolan, & Boomsma, 2006).

Twin studies require a relatively large number of twin pairs to have adequate power to detect genetic and environmental influences with any certainty (see Neale, Eaves, & Kendler, 1994). Unlike studies of normal personality, it is difficult to recruit a large sample of twins who display personality dysfunction. If twins comprise approximately 3% of the general population, and if the prevalence of personality dysfunction is itself no more than 3%, few affected pairs would be captured using conventional recruitment methods such as newspaper advertisements. This problem has been addressed in several ways. The simplest solution has been to develop a population-based twin registry that uses birth records to identify all twins born in a geographic area. Once the twins have been identified, each pair is systematically contacted and recruited into the study. From this huge sample, sufficient numbers of affected twin pairs may be found. However, population-based studies are rare, given their expense, but they are invaluable in terms of the information they yield. Good examples of this type of study are the "Virginia 30,000" (e.g., Eaves et al., 1999) and the well-known Finnish and Swedish studies (e.g., Pedersen, McClearn, Plomin, & Nesselroade, 1991). A listing of the world's major twin studies is described in a recent issue of *Twin Research and Human Genetics* (Hur & Craig, 2013).

The literature contains literally hundreds of twin studies of personality, and the results converge on the findings that between 40 to 50% of the total observed variance is due to additive genetic factors, that none or very little is due to shared environmental factors, and that the remainder of the variance is accounted for by nonshared environmental factors. A full review can be found in Jang (2005) and Johnson, Vernon, and Feiler (2008).

Studies of traits delineating PD have yielded similar results. Early studies, such as that reported by DiLalla, Carey, Gottesman, and Bouchard (1996), estimated the heritability of the Minnesota Multiphasic Personality Inventory (MMPI) scales to be between 28% (Paranoia) and 61% (Schizophrenia). DiLalla and colleagues also estimated the heritability of the Wiggins's Content Scales (see Greene, 1991; Wiggins, 1966), which have demonstrated content validity and no item overlap, and cover a wide range of thoughts, experiences, and behaviors associated with psychopathology. The heritability of these scales was estimated at Social Maladjustment (27%), Depression (44%), Feminine Interests (36%), Poor Morale (39%), Religious Fundamentalism (57%), Authority Conflict (42%), Psychoticism (62%), Organic Symptoms (42%), Family Problems (50%), Manifest Hostility (37%), Phobias (59%), Hypomania (45%), and Poor Health (56%). Across all of these scales, the median heritability was 44%.

Similarly, heritability analyses of the 18 dimensions of the Dimensional Assessment of Personality Pathology (DAPP; Livesley & Jackson, 2009) yielded similar results (Jang, Livesley, Vernon, & Jackson, 1996). The estimates were Affective Lability (45%), Anxiousness (44%), Callousness (56%), Cognitive Distortion (49%), Compulsivity (37%), Conduct Problems (56%), Identity Problems (53%), Insecure Attachment (48%), Intimacy Problems (48%), Narcissism (53%), Oppositionality (46%), Rejection (35%), Restricted Expression (50%), Self-Harm (41%), Social Avoidance (53%), Stimulus Seeking (40%), Submissiveness (45%), and Suspiciousness (45%). The 560-item version of the DAPP divides these 18 basic dimensions into 69 defining facet scales, which were also found to be significantly heritable (0.0 to 58%, median = 45%). In short, the results from these studies are congruent with those obtained with measures of normal personality function.

Unsurprisingly, analyses of higher-order trait domains yield similar estimates. For example, principal component analysis of the 18 DAPP dimensions (e.g., Jang, Livesley, & Vernon, 1999; Livesley et al., 1998; Schroeder, Wormworth, & Livesley, 1992) yields a four-factor structure that broadly resembles some of the DSM-IV/DSM-5 diagnostic categories. The first factor, Emotional Dysregulation, represents unstable and reactive tendencies, dissatisfaction with the self and life experiences, and interpersonal problems. The factor subsumes the personality trait Neuroticism as measured by Costa and McCrae's (1992) Revised NEO Personality Inventory (NEO-PI-R; Schroeder et al., 1992) or the Eysenck Personality Questionnaire (EPQ; Jang et al., 1999). This factor broadly resembles the DSM-IV Cluster B diagnosis of borderline PD (BPD). The second factor, Dissocial Behavior, describes antisocial personality characteristics and clearly resembles the DSM-IV/DSM-5 antisocial PD (ASPD) diagnosis. The third factor is Inhibition or Social Avoidance and is defined by DAPP Intimacy Problems and Restricted Expression, which resembles the DSM-IV/DSM-5 avoidant PD (AVPD) and schizoid PD (SPD). The fourth factor, Compulsivity, clearly resembles DSM-IV/DSM-5 Cluster C obsessive-compulsive PD (OCPD). Additive genetic influences accounted for 52, 50, 50, and 44% of the total variance in Emotional Dysregulation, Dissocial Behavior, Inhibition, and Compulsivity, respectively (Jang, Vernon, & Livesley, 2000).

Similarly, Larsson, Andershed, and Lichtenstein (2006) estimated the heritability of a higher-order psychopathic personality factor derived from the Youth Psychopathic Traits Inventory. Their results showed a strong genetic influence behind the higher-order psychopathic personality factor, which was defined by three lower-order dimensions that measured (1) an interpersonal style of glibness, grandiosity, and manipulation; (2) an affective disposition of callousness, lack of empathy, and unemotionality; and (3) a behavioral/lifestyle dimension of impulsivity, need for stimulation, and irresponsibility, underpinning a higher-order construct of psychopathic personality.

Kendler and colleagues (2008) estimated the heritability of the DSM-IV diagnostic categories in a sample of 2,794 young adult members of the Norwegian Institute of Public Health Twin Panel. Heritability was estimated for paranoid PD (PPD) at 23.4%, STPD at 25.8%, schizotypy at 20.5%, histrionic PD (HPD) at 31.3%, BPD at 37.1%, ASPD at 40.9%, narcissistic PD (NPD) at 25.1%, AVPD at 37.3%, dependent PD (DPD) at 29.6%, and OCPD at 27.3%. Of particular interest in these results is that multivariate genetic analysis shows that the genetic influence underlying each of these diagnoses come from a common set of genetic influences. For example, they showed that 50% of the genetic influence on BPD and 97% of same genes are in common to each diagnosis. Indeed, three distinct sets of genetic factors were found underlying the 10 diagnostic categories. PPD, HPD, and NPD share genes, whereas STPD and AVPD share a common basis. Interestingly the genes underlying schizotypy, OCPD, and DPD are unique to each diagnosis.

As shown in the previous example, one of the most significant contributions of behavior genetics resulted from the development of multivariate methods that permitted evaluation of genetic influences on multiple behaviors simultaneously. Behavior does not occur in isolation, and the fact that we observe stable factor structures in personality indicates that there are consistent and predictable relationships among personality features. Genes can have "pleiotropic effects"; that is, they may influence one or more behaviors and hence account for the consistent relationships observed between behaviors. Twin study methodologies offer one avenue to explore these relationships by estimating the genetic correlation ($r_g$), which estimates the extent to which two variables are influenced by the same genes. Variables may also covary because the same environmental factors influence their development. This is estimated by the environmental correlation ($r_e$). Genetic and environmental correlations yield an index that varies between +1.0 and −1.0, and which is interpretable in the same way as Pearson's $r$.

The logic and method used to estimate the genetic correlation between two variables is similar to that used to estimate heritability. The heritability of a single variable is estimated by comparing the similarity of MZ to DZ twins. A higher within-pair correlation for MZ than DZ twins suggests the presence of genetic influences. In the multivariate case, common genetic influences are suggested when the MZ cross-correlation (i.e., the correlation between one twin's score on one of the variables and the other twin's score on the other variable) exceeds the DZ cross-correlation. Mathematically, the relationship between the observed correlation ($r_p$) between two variables (traits) $x$ and $y$ is explained by

$$r_p = (h_x \cdot h_y \cdot r_g) + (e_x \cdot e_y \cdot r_e)$$

where the observed correlation ($r_p$), is the sum of the extent to which the same genetic ($r_g$) and/or environmental factors ($r_e$) influence each variable, weighted by the overall influence of genetic and environmental causes on each symptom ($h_x$, $h_y$, $e_x$, $e_y$, respectively). The terms $h$ and $e$ are the square roots of the heritability estimates ($h^2$ and $e^2$), for variables $x$ and $y$, respectively. Although genetic and environmental correlations can be estimated separately (Crawford & DeFries, 1978; Neale & Cardon, 1992), they can also be incorporated into two general classes of multivariate genetic models that represent the different ways that genes and the environment can influence multiple symptoms (for detailed discussion, see McArdle & Goldsmith, 1990; Neale & Cardon, 1992).

A useful feature of genetic and environmental correlations is that they are amenable to factor analysis (Crawford & DeFries, 1978). Factor analysis of the matrices of genetic and environmental correlations addresses the question of whether an observed structure reflects an underlying biological structure. If the factor analysis of the genetic correlations yields a solution similar to what is expected, this suggests that an observed structure reflects an underlying biological structure. This approach was used to study the higher-order structure of traits delineating PD assessed by the DAPP (Livesley et al., 1998). The DAPP was administered to three independent samples: 656 patients with PDs, 939 general-population subjects, and a volunteer sample of 686 twin pairs, also recruited from the general population. The phenotypic, genetic, and environmental correlation matrices were computed in all three samples separately and subjected to principal component analysis. In all three samples, four factors were extracted: Emotional Dysregulation, Dissocial Behavior, Inhibitedness, and Conscientiousness. The loadings across all three matrices were remarkably similar: Congruence coefficients ranged from .94 to .99. The congruency coefficients between the genetic and phenotypic factors on Emotional Dysregulation, Dissocial Behavior, Inhibitedness, and Compulsivity were .97, .97, .98, and .95, respectively. The congruence between factors extracted from the phenotypic and nonshared environmental matrices was also very high at .99, .96, .99 and .96, respectively. These data show that the phenotypic structure of PD traits closely reflects the underlying etiological architecture.

Multivariate analyses have also been applied to DSM criteria sets. Kendler, Aggen, and Patrick (2012) examined DSM-IV criteria sets for ASPD. Factor analysis of the criteria sets yielded two correlated factors labeled "Aggressive-Disregard" and "Disinhibition." Multivariate genetic analysis yielded two genetic factors that closely resembled the phenotypic factors and varied in their prediction of a range of relevant criterion variables. Scores on the genetic Aggressive-Disregard factor score were more strongly associated with risk for conduct disorder, early and heavy alcohol use, and low educational status, whereas scores on the genetic Disinhibition factor score were more strongly associated with younger age, novelty seeking, and major depression. From a genetic perspective, the DSM-IV criteria for ASPD *do not* reflect a single dimension of liability but rather are influenced by two dimensions of genetic risk reflecting Aggressive-Disregard and Disinhibition. Moreover, the phenotypic structure of the ASPD criteria results largely from genetic and not from environmental influences.

Multivariate analyses have also been used to investigate the etiology of the DSM-IV PD clusters. For example, DSM-IV Cluster B PD diagnoses (ASPD, HPD, NPD, and BPD) demonstrate comorbidity. Torgersen and colleagues (2008) assessed these diagnoses using the Structured Interview for DSM-IV Personality Disorders (SIDP-IV) with 1,386 Norwegian twin pairs between ages 19 and 35 years. Multivariate analyses were conducted to estimate the degree to which genetic and/or environmental factors influence their observed co-occurrence. The authors found that the best-fitting model included common genetic and environmental factors influencing all four PD diagnoses (not including sex or shared environmental effects), and factors influencing only ASPD and BPD. Heritability was estimated at 38% for ASPD traits, 31% for HPD traits, 24% for NPD traits, and 35% for BPD traits. BPD traits had the lowest and ASPD traits had the highest disorder-specific genetic variance. Torgersen and colleagues concluded that the frequently observed comorbidity between Cluster B PDs results from both common genetic and common environmental influences. Etiologically, Cluster B has a "substructure" in which ASPD and BPD are more closely related to each other than to the other Cluster B disorders.

The literature is replete with multivariate genetic analyses that evaluate why two variables frequently co-occur. For example, Hettema, Neale, Meyers, Prescott, and Kendler (2006) studied why anxiety and depressive disorders exhibit high comorbidity. In a sample of over 9,000 twin pairs, the degree to which trait neuroticism covaried with "internalizing disorders" (i.e., major depression, generalized anxiety disorder, panic disorder, agoraphobia, social phobia, animal phobia, and situational phobia) was found to be one-third to one-half attributable to genetic factors. The authors concluded that there is substantial, but not complete, overlap between genetic influences on individual variation in neuroticism and those increasing the liability for internalizing disorders, helping to explain the high rates of comorbidity among them.

## Environmental Influences on Personality

Within the social sciences, the term "environmental factors" usually refers the social environment of the family, extrafamilial factors such as the social environment of the classroom (e.g., peers), and factors unique to each person (e.g., traumatic events). The term "environmental influences" usually refers to objectively measured circumstances, such as socioeconomic status and physical factors (e.g., temperature and degree of sunlight exposure), which are important in the etiology of some forms of psychopathology (e.g., depression). Operationalization of the concept of environment also includes *perceptions* of the environment. These perceptions may be poor representations of reality, but these are typically the features to which individuals respond. Despite the importance of social and physical environments, attempts to identify specific environmental factors, like the search for specific genes, has had limited success.

## Environmental Influences on the Personality Trait Variance

Several studies have computed genetic correlations between measures of the nonshared environment and personality. Nonshared environmental influences are important because they are similar in magnitude to genetic influences on personality and have a far greater influence than shared environmental influences (Bouchard, 1997; Plomin, Chipuer, & Neiderhiser, 1994). Several early studies of nonshared environment–personality correlations suggested that personality plays a significant role in the selection or creation of the individual's personal environment. For example, EPQ Neuroticism and Extraversion are good predictors of life events (e.g., Magnus, Diener, Fujita, & Pavot, 1993; Poulton & Andrews, 1992). Similarly, all genetic variance on controllable, desirable, and undesirable life events in women is shared with genetic influences underlying EPQ Neuroticism, Extraversion, and Openness to Experience (measured by a short version of the NEO Personality Inventory [NEO-PI]; Costa & McCrae, 1985) whereas genetic influences underlying the personality scales had little effect on uncontrollable life events simply because this variable was not heritable (Saudino, Pedersen, Lichtenstein, McClearn, & Plomin, 1997). Kendler and Karkowski-Shuman (1997) showed that the genetic risk factors for major depression increased the probability of experiencing significant life events in the interpersonal and occupational/financial domains. Clearly, individuals play an active role in creating their own environments.

More recent research does not attempt to identify the nature of these environmental effects; rather, it investigates the relative roles of genes and the environment on personality development. For example, Hopwood and colleagues (2011) examined genetic and environmental influences on personality trait stability and growth during the transition to adulthood. This study investigated the patterns and origins of personality trait changes in people ages 17–29 using three waves of twin data on the Multidimensional Personality Questionnaire (MPQ). Results suggested that both genetic and nonshared environmental factors accounted for personality changes over time. Trait changes were more significant in the first relative to the second half of the transition to adulthood, and the traits tended to become more stable during the second half of this transition, with all the traits yielding test–retest correlations between .74 and .78.

In summary, twin research has made important contributions to understanding not only the origins of personality but also the patterns of covariation among personality characteristics. Genetic influences on personality have consistently been found to be significant, and it appears that all personality traits have a substantial heritable component. This suggests that an important avenue of research is to identify the specific genes contributing to both individual differences in specific traits and the relationships among traits. However, this has not proved as successful as initially expected.

## Identifying Putative Genes

Although the classic twin study design capitalizes on common variance found within and between measures and can do much to identify realms of behavior that have a significant genetic underpinning, it is not designed to help localize the actual putative genes themselves. Given the consistency of twin research and the magnitude of genetic effects, it was once thought that it would be relatively easy to identify putative genes for personality, and that the more detailed mapping of the human genome would help to identify potential genes. The two main methods used to identify genes are the "linkage" and "association" methods, which track the inheritance of DNA segments in families and populations to localize the location of the alleles to a relatively small part of the chromosome.

"Linkage studies" use the known locations of genes as road signs or "markers" for a disease gene to obtain an approximate idea of where the disease gene is located on a chromosome. If the disease gene is proximal to the marker gene, the likelihood of the disease and marker genes being transmitted together from parent to offspring is high, and the likelihood of them being separated during meiosis is much less than if they are far apart. The likelihood that the disease and marker genes will be transmitted together given their distance apart can be computed as a likelihood odds ratio (LOD) score and tracked in families. Two genes are "linked" if they are transmitted together as expected. Linkage studies are popular but appear to work only if the disease gene has a defined mode of inheritance and is clearly defined. Given that multivariate twin research shows that genetic influences on personality are polygenic and multifactorial in nature, it comes as no surprise that linkage studies of personality and its disorders are virtually nonexistent and that research has focused on association methodologies, such as looking for specific small repeating sections of genes called "single-nucleotide polymorphisms" (SNPs) that identify a version of a specific gene.

The SNPs are usually related to the specific production or reception of neuropeptides implicated in any number of social behaviors in nonhumans. For example, the *APOE4* genetic polymorphism has been linked to increased risk for Alzheimer's disease in humans. Another example is the GG variant of the oxytocin receptor gene *rs53576*, which is associated with increased oxytocin receptors in the brain. These methods are more appropriate to investigating mental disorders because they do not require information on mode of inheritance and can be applied to quantitative or qualitative data (see Plomin & Caspi, 1998, for a detailed review). This method tests whether the gene of interest is present in more affected than in nonaffected individuals to investigate whether the disease form of the gene is more common in patients with the disease than in nonpatient controls. The trade-off for not needing to know the mode of inheritance is the requirement of having a clear idea of which gene is the actual disease gene. Unlike linkage studies, association studies do not pick road signs; rather, they require that the gene selected for analysis is actually involved with the disorder of interest. For example, if the neurotransmitter dopamine is found to be implicated in novelty-seeking behavior, it makes sense to choose genes implicated in dopamine production as "candidate" genes.

Recognizing the need to choose appropriate candidate genes, Cloninger (1986) developed the biosocial model of personality (see also Cloninger et al., 1994; Cloninger, Svrakic, & Przybeck, 1993) to provide some guidance in their selection. This model became influential in psychiatry research for a while because it made specific predictions about the neurochemical bases of both normal and disordered personality that were useful in selecting candidate genes. The model was associated with a specific measure, namely, the Tridimensional Personality Questionnaire (TPQ; Cloninger, Pryzbeck, Svrackic, & Wetzel, 1994). The biosocial model divided personality into (1) four temperament traits—labeled Novelty Seeking, Harm Avoidance, Reward Dependence, and Persistence—that resemble stable inherited differences in emotional response, each of which was postulated to be influenced by inherited variations in monoamine neurotransmitter systems: serotonin for harm avoidance, dopamine for novelty seeking, and norephinephrine for reward dependence and persistence; and (2) three character traits—Self-Directedness, Cooperativeness, and Self-Transcendence—that reflect learned, maturational variations in goals, values, and self-concepts (Cloninger et al., 1993, 1994).

Although definitive allelic associations have not been found for the personality traits studied to date, the results of the studies have clarified important issues regarding the nature of personality traits. The mixed findings regarding allelic association between the TCI temperament trait Harm Avoidance and *5-HTTLPR*, and between Novelty Seeking and *DRD4* suggest that the assumptions regarding simple relationships between serotonin and dopamine neurotransmitter systems and traits proposed by the biosocial model are incorrect. They also question the proposed distinction between temperament and character traits because of significant allelic associations with the TCI Cooperativeness and Self-Directedness character traits (characteristics that putatively reflect learned developmental aspects of personality) and the *5-HTTLPR* allele (Hamer, Greenberg, Sabol, & Murphy, 1999; see also Herbst, Zonderman, McCrae, & Costa, 2000; Ono et al., 1999).

A theory-guided approach has also been used in the search for genes for anxiety and depression. There are two major hypotheses regarding the etiology of anxiety and depression: the monoamine hypothesis and the hypothesis of an abnormal stress response acting partly via reduced neurogenesis. Hence, in these studies, candidate genes were usually chosen because of their involvement either in neurotransmission circuits or in the stress response and related processes such as neurogenesis (Belmaker & Agam, 2008). However, these studies have yielded mixed results (Middeldorp et al., 2010). In an attempt to clarify these associations, Middeldorp and colleagues (2010) conducted longitudinal studies of children and adults to investigate 45 SNPs in genes encoding for serotonin receptors 1A, 1D, 2A, catechol-*O*-methyltransferase (*COMT*), tryptophane hydroxylase type 2 (TPH2), brain-derived neurotrophic factor (BDNF), PlexinA2 and regulators of G-protein-coupled signaling (RGS) 2, 4, 16. Symptoms of anxious depression symptoms were assessed five times in 11 years in over 11,000 adults with 1,504 subjects genotyped and at ages 7, 10, 12, and during adolescence in over 20,000 twins, with 1,078 subjects genotyped. In both cohorts, no consistent association was found between SNPs for either the serotonergic system or core regulators of neurogenesis and anxious depression.

An early literature review of candidate gene studies on traits that predispose to anxiety and depression by Middeldorp, Ruigrok, Cath, and Boomsma (2002) placed the issues in the search for genes into context. At the time of the review, the literature (post-1996) had focused on genes involved in (1) the serotonin system, (2) the dopamine system, and (3) gene–gene interaction—and all of the results published were contradictory. The serotonin system was the most extensively investigated, with three negative findings considering the serotonin receptor (*5-HT2A*) and 11 positive and 11 negative findings regarding the serotonin transporter gene (*5-HTTLPR*). One noteworthy finding was that in five studies, gene–gene interaction effects were found: *DRD4* × *5-HTTLPR* × *COMT*; *5-HTTLPR* × *COMT*; $5HT_{2C}$ × *DRD2* × *DRD4*; *DRD4* × $5-HT_{2C}$; and chromosomes 8p × 18p × 20p × 2 1q (a linkage study). What is important about these interaction effects is that they often involved genes that did not appear to influence a trait when studied separately. More recent reviews and meta-analyses have found a similar pattern of nonreplication. Several of the most promising candidate genes, such as the monoamine oxidase A (*MAOA*) gene, which has been linked to antisocial behavior in past research (Caspi et al., 2003), have failed to replicate in subsequent work, according to several meta-analyses (de Moor et al., 2010).

From their review, Middeldorp and colleagues (2002) identified significant factors accounting for the contradictory findings: (1) small samples in some studies that led to the lack of statistical power to detect small gene effects; (2) use of different questionnaires; (3) population stratification; (4) ethnic and gender differences (e.g., Japanese vs. American participants; different ratio of males/females in each study); and (5) selection of subjects at the high and low ends of the distribution. The authors suggested that these problems might be overcome by (1) adopting within-family designs that prevent the influence of population stratification (but may lead to false-negative as well as false-positive results); (2) simultaneous linkage and association approaches that will strengthen evidence for association; (3) inclusion of large samples, preferably of one ethnic group, to detect small effects and gene–gene interaction; (4) use of endophenotypes in multivariate association analyses; (5) follow-up studies in young children (neonates, at 2 months, at 4 months, etc.); (6) consideration of longitudinal designs; and (7) the use of analogue animal studies to guide further studies in humans.

One of the problems in the literature noted in Middeldorp and colleagues' (2002) review was the use of different measures and their ability to assess the traits in question. Research using equivalent measures has unfortunately fared no better. For example, the human serotonin transporter gene *5-HTTLPR* has been shown to exist in long and short forms. The short form of this allele is dominant to the long version of the allele, with the long version of the *5-HTTLPR* genotype producing more serotonin transporter messenger RNA (mRNA) and protein than the short form in cultured cells, platelets, and brain tissue. Results have shown that individuals possessing the short form of the allele have significantly increased NEO-PI-R scores (e.g., Lesch et al., 1996) and related traits, such as Harm Avoidance as measured by the TPQ (e.g., Katsuragi et al., 1999). However, at least two other recent studies have found no associations between Harm Avoidance (Hamer et al., 1999) and NEO-PI-R Neuroticism (Gelernter, Kranzler, Coccaro, Siever, & New, 1998) and the serotonin transporter genes.

Perhaps the reason why it has been difficult to identify genes is because their effects are only "activated" by exposure to specific environmental triggers, an effect known as "gene–environment interaction." One of the most investigated genes is the serotonin transporter gene (*SLC6A4*, also known as *5-HTT*), which has been the focus of many personality studies. Caspi and colleagues (2003) showed that the *5-HTTLPR* polymorphism does not show a main effect on depression, but the s-allele increases the risk of depression once an individual is exposed to one or more life events. However, two meta-analyses, including five and 14, studies respectively, yielded no evidence for an effect of *5-HTTLPR* in interaction with life events on depression (Munafo, Durrant, Lewis, & Flint, 2009; Risch et al., 2009). Subsequently, these meta-analyses were critiqued for having given too much weight to the studies reporting null findings that employed poorer measurement of life events (Caspi, Hariri, Holmes, Uher, & Moffitt, 2010).

Middeldorp, Slof-Op, and colleagues (2010) tested for an interaction effect involving *5-HTTLPR* on a sample of 1,155 twins and their parents and siblings from 438 families, using a detailed measure of life events. They found a significant main effect of number of life events on anxious depression and neuroticism, especially when these were experienced in the past year. No interaction with *5-HTTLPR* was found for number of life events either experienced across the lifespan or across the past year, supporting the findings of the meta-analyses. It might be more useful to focus on the joint effect of several genes that are, for example, part of the same biological pathway in interaction with the environment.

The idea of analyzing several polymorphisms simultaneously was tested by Heck and colleagues (2009). They reasoned that previous studies that only examined one or a few polymorphisms within single genes neglected the possibility that the genetic associations might be more complex, comprising several genes or gene regions. As such, they performed an extended genetic association study analyzing 17 serotonergic (*SLC6A4, HTR1A, HTR1B, HTR2A, HTR2C, HTR3A, HTR6, MAOA, TPH1, TPH2*) and dopaminergic genes (*SLC6A3, DRD2, DRD3, DRD4, COMT, MAOA, TH, DBH*), which have been previously reported to be implicated with personality traits. One hundred ninety-five SNPs within these genes were genotyped in a sample of 366 general population participants (all European American), and they conducted a replication on an independent sample of a further 335 participants. Personality traits in both samples were assessed with the German version of Cloninger's TPQ. From 30 SNPs showing associations at a nominal level of significance, two intronic SNPs, *rs2770296* and *rs927544*, both located in the *HTR2A* gene, withstood correction for multiple testing. These SNPs were associated with Novelty Seeking. The effect of *rs927544* could be replicated for the Novelty Seeking subscale Extravagance, and the same SNP was also associated with Extravagance in the combined samples. Their results show that *HTR2A* polymorphisms modulate facets of novelty seeking behavior in healthy adults, suggesting that serotonergic neurotransmission is indeed involved in this phenotype.

Similarly, Derringer and colleagues (2010) led a consortium of researchers in an examination of a collection of SNPs associated with dopamine in prior research and subsequently examined associations between this collection of SNPs and sensation-seeking behavior. The findings were promising: Taking into account all the SNPs associated with sensation-seeking behaviors as an aggregate, dopamine genes worked in concert to explain around 6.6% of variation in sensation-seeking behavior. This approach is appealing because it involves conceiving of genes and personality not as simple one-to-one relationships, but instead as complex systems of genes that work in concert to express a personality trait.

## What Next?

The previous approaches have taken a type of "shotgun approach," in that they have relied on brute strength (e.g., large sample sizes) in the simultaneous examination of several polymorphisms to identify putative genes. Nevertheless, the proportion of the variance accounted for remains small—all under 10%. In contrast, much of the earlier twin research suggested that genes have a large influence on personality function, which raises the question of whether other approaches may be more successful. Middeldorp and colleagues (2002) suggested focusing on endophenotypes and stressed the need for more animal studies to guide human research. In essence, an "endophenotype" is a biological marker that may contain a useful link between genetic sequences and behavioral disorders. These biological markers are used to parse behavioral symptoms into more stable phenotypes with a clear genetic connection. The task ahead is to identify endophenotypes for the PDs.

Siever (2005) suggested that some clinical dimensions of PDs, such as affective instability, impulsivity, aggression, emotional information processing, cognitive disorganization, social deficits, and psychosis, particularly lend themselves to the study of corresponding endophenotypes. For example, the propensity to aggression can be evaluated by psychometric measures, interview, laboratory paradigms, neurochemical imaging, and pharmacological studies. These suggest that aggression is a measurable trait that may be related to a reduction in serotonergic activity. Hyperresponsiveness of the amygdala and other limbic structures may be related to affective instability, while structural and functional brain alterations underlie the cognitive disorganization in psychotic-like symptoms of STPD. Other investigators, such as Paris (2011), remain much less enthusiastic about the utility of endophenotypes. The identification and use of endophenotypes are associated with the assumption that mental processes can be reduced to activity at a neuronal level. Given that at present there is insufficient knowledge of the etiology and pathogenesis of the PDs to make their identification and subsequent use viable for the foreseeable future, it is unfortunate that the approach has had a strong influence on the conceptual basis of proposals for DSM-5.

Some recent research has attempted to identify potential endophenotypes for personality disorder. For example, Ruocco, Amirthavasagam, and Zakzanis (2012) evaluated whether the magnitude of volume reductions in the amygdala and hippocampus was associated with BPD. Volumetric magnetic resonance imaging results from 11 studies comprising 205 patients with BPD and 222 healthy controls were examined using meta-analytic techniques. Patients showed an average 11 and 13% decrease in the size of the hippocampus and amygdala, respectively. These volumetric differences were not attenuated in patients being treated with psychotropic medications. They also found that comorbid depression, posttraumatic stress disorder, and substance use disorders were unrelated to volumetric decreases in either structure.

The previous study represents a classic approach to finding endophenotypes for PD. However, what is emerging in the literature is the use of "intermediate endophenotypes" such as personality traits as endophenotypes for other major disorders. This trend in the research is occurring because certain personality traits seem to be overrepresented in people with specific disorders. For example, Ersche and colleagues (2012) identified anxious-impulsiveness and studied personality and cognitive dysfunction as endophenotypes for drug dependence. These types of studies are interesting in that their attempts to find the genes for another disorder as the methodology involves searching for genes underlying a related set of personality traits and functions. It is perhaps within these constellations of traits that the genes may be best identified, as opposed to the previously adopted approach examining traits individually and out of context; or arbitrary groupings that are not observed together in a clinical (i.e., real-world) setting.

Savitz, Van Der Merwe, and Ramesar (2008) used personality endophenotypes for a genetic association analysis of bipolar affective disorder (BPAD). They reasoned that various personality traits are overrepresented in people with BPAD and their unaffected relatives, and these traits may constitute genetically transmitted risk factors or endophenotypes of the illness. Seven different personality questionnaires comprising 19 subscales were administered to 31 European American families with BPAD ($n = 241$). Ten of 19 personality traits showed significant evidence of heritability and were therefore selected as candidate endophenotypes. The 3′ untranslated region repeat polymorphism of the dopamine transporter gene (*SLC6A3*) was associated with scales measuring Self-Directedness and Negative Affect. The short allele of the serotonin transporter gene (*SLC6A4*) promoter polymorphism showed a trend toward association with higher Harm Avoidance and Negative Affect. The *COMT* Val[158]Met polymorphism was weakly associated with Spirituality and Irritable Temperament.

## Conclusion

The search for the genes for personality function remains very much a methodological endeavor. The research over the past two decades has focused on fundamental issues such as the design of methods that are best suited to find genes for how personality function is measured and whether it is better to search for single or multiple genes. Other approaches have focused on the development of theoretical models to guide the search for genes and, more recently, on the identification of potential endophenotypes for personality. The results remain the same. Few genes have been found, yet the "circumstantial evidence," as demonstrated in heritability studies, for the role of genes remains high.

Where might the search for genes go next? Kraus (2013) suggests that one direction might be to delve deeper and examine cellular function: "One thing that early gene–personality work overlooked is that a lot has to happen to allow DNA to code for specific hormones/neuropeptides, that then have to act at the cellular level to subsequently influence personality. In short, genes need to be expressed at a cellular level in order to influence personality, and so one place where a genetic researcher might want to look to examine gene influences on personality is at this expression—that is, what genes are being unzipped by RNA, so that specific hormones/proteins are produced?"

Middeldorp and colleagues (2002) indicated that research on nonhuman subjects may provide some exciting leads. Research in honey bees is suggestive of the potential of examining RNA to predict behavior. In this work, mRNA abundance has been shown to be a significant predictor of behavioral transitions of honey bees from hive workers to foragers (Whitfield, Cziko, & Robinson, 2003). Human work in this domain is an exciting area of future research.

The genetics of PD remain an active area of research. As may be surmised from this chapter, this is due to the constant stream of revisions on the definition of PD. They are simultaneously considered to be distinct diagnoses much like a physical disease such as cancer or hypertension, and also are conceptualized as a broad disorder that shares common phenotypic similarities and genetic influences with normal personality. The revisions in DSM-5 add further complexity with its hybrid model of distinct diagnostic categories and measures of pathology. The answer to the question "What is the genetics of PD?" is entirely dependent on how one measures it—and can only be discussed in the context of that definition or measure. The value of genetic studies at this time is not so much in terms of what genes are associated with PD, the way in which one would look for the genes that cause cancer, but rather how one can use estimates of genetic influence to help create better definitions and measures of PD. Multivariate genetic analyses hold that key to refining diagnostic definitions by, for example, using the degree to which they share a common genetic basis to create internally consistent diagnostic definitions, much as factor analysis is used to create the main dimensions of personality. The true value of genetic studies is that they offer the promise of better diagnostic definitions, as opposed to finding putative genes, which is the goal of so much of the recent research.

## REFERENCES

American Psychiatric Association. (1987). *Diagnostic and statistical manual of mental disorders* (3rd ed., rev.). Washington, DC: Author.

American Psychiatric Association. (1994). *Diagnostic*

*and statistical manual of mental disorders* (4th ed.). Washington, DC: Author.

American Psychiatric Association. (2013). *Diagnostic and statistical manual of mental disorders* (5th ed.). Arlington, VA: Author.

Belmaker, R. H., & Agam, G. (2008). Major depressive disorder. *New England Journal of Medicine, 358,* 55–68.

Bouchard, T. J., Jr. (1997). The genetics of personality. In K. Blum & E. P. Noble (Eds.), *Handbook of psychiatric genetics* (pp. 273–296). Boca Raton, FL: CRC Press.

Caspi, A., Hariri, A. R., Holmes, A., Uher, R., & Moffitt, T. E. (2010). Genetic sensitivity to the environment: The case of the serotonin transporter gene and its implications for studying complex diseases and traits. *American Journal of Psychiatry, 167,* 509–527.

Caspi, A., Sugden, K., Moffitt, T. E., Taylor, A., Craig, I. W., Harrington, H., et al. (2003). Influence of life stress on depression: Moderation by a polymorphism in the 5-HTT gene. *Science, 301,* 386–389.

Cloninger, C. R. (1986). A unified biosocial theory of personality and its role in the development of anxiety states. *Psychiatric Developments, 3,* 167–226.

Cloninger, C. R., Przybeck, T., Svrakic, D., & Wetzel, R. D. (1994). *The Temperament and Character Inventory (TCI): A guide to its development and use.* St. Louis, MO: Center for Psychobiology and Personality, Washington University.

Cloninger, C. R., Svrakic, D., & Przybeck, T. R. (1993). A psychobiological model of temperament and character. *Archives of General Psychiatry, 50,* 975–990.

Costa, P. T., & McCrae, R. R. (1985). *Manual for the NEO Personality Inventory.* Odessa, FL: Psychological Assessment Resources.

Costa, P. T., & McCrae, R. R. (1992). *Revised NEO Personality Inventory and NEO Five-Factor Inventory.* Odessa, FL: Psychological Assessment Resources.

Crawford, C. B., & DeFries, J. C. (1978). Factor analysis of genetic and environmental correlation matrices. *Multivariate Behavioral Research, 13,* 297–318.

de Moor, M., Costa, P., Terracciano, A., Krueger, R., de Geus, E., Toshiko, T., et al. (2010). Meta-analysis of genome-wide association studies for personality. *Molecular Psychiatry, 17*(3), 337–349.

Derks, E. M., Dolan, C. V., & Boomsma, D. I. (2006). A test of the equal environment assumption (EEA) in multivariate twin studies. *Twin Research and Human Genetics, 9*(3), 403–411.

Derringer, J., Krueger, R., Dick, D., Saccone, S., Grucza, R., Agrawal, A., et al. (2010). Predicting sensation seeking from dopamine genes: A candidate-system approach. *Psychological Science, 21*(9), 1282–1290.

DiLalla, D. L., Carey, G., Gottesman, I. I., & Bouchard, T. J., Jr. (1996). Heritability of MMPI personality indicators of psychopathology in twins reared apart. *Journal of Abnormal Psychology, 105,* 491–499.

Eaves, L. J., Heath, A., Martin, N., Maes, H., Neale, M., Kendler, K., et al. (1999). Comparing the biological and cultural inheritance of personality and social attitudes in the Virginia 30,000 study of twins and their relatives. *Twin Research, 2,* 62–80.

Ersche, K. D., Turton, A. J., Chamberlain, S. R., Müller, U., Bullmore, E. T., & Robbins, T. W. (2012). Cognitive dysfunction and anxious–impulsive personality traits are endophenotypes for drug dependence. *American Journal of Psychiatry, 169,* 926–936.

Faraone, S. V., Tsuang, M. T., & Tsuang, D. W. (1999). *Genetics of mental disorders: A guide for students, clinicians, and researchers.* New York: Guilford Press.

Gelernter, J., Kranzler, H., Coccaro, E. F., Siever, L. J., & New, A. S. (1998). Serotonin transporter protein gene polymorphism and personality measures in African American and European American subjects. *American Journal of Psychiatry, 155,* 1332–1338.

Greene, R. L. (1991). *The MMPI-2/MMPI: An interpretive manual.* Boston: Allyn & Bacon.

Hamer, D. H., Greenberg, B. D., Sabol, S. Z., & Murphy, D. L. (1999). Role of serotonin transporter gene in temperament and character. *Journal of Personality Disorders, 13,* 312–328.

Heck, A., Lieb, R., Ellgas, A., Pfister, H., Lucae, S., Roeske, D., et al. (2009). Investigation of 17 candidate genes for personality traits confirms effects of the *HTR2A* gene on novelty seeking. *Genes, Brain and Behavior, 8,* 464–472.

Herbst, J. H., Zonderman, A. B., McCrae, R. R., & Costa, P. T. (2000). Do the dimensions of the Temperament and Character Inventory map a simple genetic architecture?: Evidence from modelcular genetics and factor analysis. *American Journal of Psychiatry, 157,* 1285–1290.

Hettema, J. M., Neale, M. C., Myers, J. M., Prescott, C. A., & Kendler, K. S. (2006). A population-based twin study of the relationship between neuroticism and internalizing disorders. *American Journal of Psychiatry, 163,* 857–864.

Hopwood, C. J., Donnellan, M. B., Blonigen, D. M., Krueger, R. F., McGue, M., Iacono, W. G., et al. (2011). Genetic and environmental influences on personality trait stability and growth during the transition to adulthood: A three wave longitudinal study. *Journal of Personality and Social Psychology, 100*(3), 545–556.

Hur, Y. M., & Craig, J. M. (2013). Twin registries worldwide: An important resource for scientific research. *Twin Research and Human Genetics, 16*(1), 1–12.

Jackson, D. N., & Messnick, S. (1962). Response styles on the MMPI: Comparison of clinical and normal samples. *Journal of Abnormal and Social Psychology, 65,* 285–299.

Jang, K. L. (2005). *The behavioral genetics of psychopathology: A clinical guide.* Mahwah, NJ: Erlbaum.

Jang, K. L., Livesley, W. J., & Vernon, P. A. (1996). Heritability of the big five personality dimensions and their facets: A twin study. *Journal of Personality, 64,* 577–591.

Jang, K. L., Livesley, W. J., & Vernon, P. A. (1999). The relationship between Eysenck's P-E-N model of personality and traits delineating personality disorder. *Personality and Individual Differences, 26*, 121–128.

Jang, K. L., Livesley, W. J., Vernon, P. A., & Jackson, D. N. (1996). Heritability of personality disorder traits: A twin study. *Acta Psychiatrica Scandinavica, 94*, 438–444.

Jang, K. L., Vernon, P. A., & Livesley W. J. (2000). Personality disorder traits, family environment, and alcohol misuse: A multivariate behavioural genetic analysis. *Addiction, 95*, 873–888.

Johnson, A. M., Vernon, P. A., & Feiler, A. R. (2008). Behavioral genetic studies of personality: An introduction and review of the results of 50+ years of research. In G. J. Boyle, G. Matthews, & D. H. Saklofske (Eds.), *The Sage handbook of personality theory and assessment* (Vol. 1, pp. 145–173). Los Angeles: SAGE.

Katsuragi, S., Kunugi, A. S., Sano, A., Tsutsumi, T., Isogawa, K., Nanko, S., et al. (1999). Association between serotonin transporter gene polymorphism and anxiety-related traits. *Biological Psychiatry, 45*, 368–370.

Kendler, K. S., Aggen, S. H., Czajkowski, N., Røysamb, E., Tambs, K., Torgersen, S., et al. (2008). The structure of genetic and environmental risk factors for DSM-IV personality disorders: A multivariate twin study. *Archives of General Psychiatry, 65*(12), 1438–1446.

Kendler, K. S., Aggen, S. H., & Patrick, C. J. (2012). A multivariate twin study of the DSM-IV criteria for antisocial personality disorder. *Biological Psychiatry, 71*(3), 247–253.

Kendler, K. S., & Karkowski-Shuman, L. (1997). Stressful life events and genetic liability to major depression: Genetic control of exposure to the environment? *Psychological Medicine, 27*, 539–547.

Kraus, M. W. (2013). Do genes influence personality?: A summary of recent advances in the nature vs. nurture debate. Retrieved July 11, 2013, from *www.psychologytoday.com/blog/under-the-influence/201307/do-genes-influence-personality*.

Larsson, H., Andershed, H., & Lichtenstein, P. (2006). A genetic factor explains most of the variation in the psychopathic personality. *Journal of Abnormal Psychology, 115*(2), 221–230.

Lesch, K. P., Bengel, D., Heils, A., Zhang Sabol, S., Greenberg, B. D., Petri, S., et al. (1996). Association of anxiety-related traits with a polymorphism in the serotonin transporter gene regulatory region. *Science, 274*, 1527–1530.

Livesley, W. J., & Jackson, D. N. (2009). *Manual for the Dimensional Assessment of Personality Problems—Basic Questionnaire (DAPP)*. London, ON, Canada: Research Psychologists' Press.

Livesley, W. J., Jackson, D. N., & Schroeder, M. L. (1992). Factorial structure of traits delineating personality disorders in clinical and general population samples. *Journal of Abnormal Psychology, 101*, 432–440.

Livesley, W. J., Jang, K. L., & Vernon, P. A. (1998). Phenotypic and genetic structure of traits delineating personality disorder. *Archives of Gneral Psychiatry, 55*(10), 941–948.

Magnus, K., Diener, E., Fujita, F., & Pavot, W. (1993). Extraversion and neuroticism as predictors of objective life events: A longitudinal analysis. *Journal of Personality and Social Psychology, 65*, 1046–1053.

McArdle. J. J., & Goldsmith, H. H. (1990). Alternative common factor models for multivariate biometric analyses. *Behavior Genetics, 20*(5), 569–608.

Middeldorp, C. M., de Geus, E. J. C., Willemsen, G., Hottenga, J., Slagboom, P. E., & Boomsma, D. I. (2010). The serotonin transporter gene length polymorphism (5-HTTLPR) and life events: No evidence for an interaction effect on neuroticism and anxious depressive symptoms. *Twin Research and Human Genetics, 13*, 544–549.

Middeldorp, C. M., Ruigrok, P., Cath, D. C., & Boomsma, D. I. (2002). Candidate genes for mood disorders in humans: A literature review [Abstract]. *American Journal of Medical Genetics, 114*, 39.

Middeldorp, C. M., Slof-Op, M. C. T., Landt, S. O., Medland, S. E., van Beijsterveldt, C. E. M., Bartels, M., et al. (2010). Anxiety and depression in children and adults: Influence of serotonergic and neurotrophic genes? *Genes, Brain and Behavior, 9*, 808–816.

Munafo, M. R., Durrant, C., Lewis, G., & Flint, J. (2009). Gene–environment interactions at the serotonin transporter locus. *Biological Psychiatry, 65*, 211–219.

Neale, M. C., & Cardon, L. R. (1992). *Methodology for genetic studies of twins and families*. London: Kluwer.

Neale, M. C., Eaves, L. J., & Kendler, K. S. (1994). The power of the classical twin study to resolve variation in threshold traits. *Behavior Genetics, 24*(3), 239–258.

Ono, Y., Yoshimura, K., Mizushima, H., Manki, H., Yagi, G., Kanba, S., et al. (1999). Environmental and possible genetic contributions to character dimensions of personality. *Psychological Report, 84*, 689–696.

Paris, J. (2011). Endophenotypes and the diagnosis of personality disorders. *Journal of Personality Disorders, 25*, 260–268.

Pedersen, N. L., McClearn, G. E., Plomin, R., & Nesselroade, J. R. (1991). The Swedish Adoption/Twin Study of Aging: An update. *Acta Geneticae Medicae et Gemellologiae, 40*, 7–20.

Plomin, R., & Caspi, A. (1998). DNA and personality. *European Journal of Personality, 12*, 387–407.

Plomin, R., Chipuer, H. M., & Neiderhiser, J. M. (1994). Behavioral genetic evidence for the importance of nonshared environment. In E. M. Hetherington & D. Reiss (Eds.), *Separate social worlds of siblings: The impact of nonshared environment on development* (pp. 1–31). Hillsdale, NJ: Erlbaum.

Plomin, R., DeFries, J. C., & McClearn, G. E. (1990). *Behavioral genetics: A primer* (2nd ed.). New York: Freeman.

Poulton, R. G., & Andrews, G. (1992). Personality as a new cause of adverse life events. *Acta Psychiatrica Scandinavica, 85,* 35–38.

Risch, N., Herrell, R., Lehner, T., Liang, K. Y., Eaves, L., Hoh, J., et al. (2009). Interaction between the serotonin transporter gene (5-HTTLPR), stressful life events, and risk of depression: A meta-analysis. *Journal of the American Medical Association, 301,* 2462–2471.

Ruocco, A. C., Amirthavasagam, S., & Zakzanis, K. K. (2012) Amygdala and hippocampal volume reductions as candidate endophenotypes for borderline personality disorder: A meta-analysis of magnetic resonance imaging studies. *Psychiatry Research: Neuroimaging, 201,* 245–252.

Saudino, K. J., Pedersen, N. L., Lichtenstein, P., McClearn, G. E., & Plomin, R. (1997). Can personality explain genetic influences on life events? *Journal of Personality and Social Psychology, 72,* 196–206.

Savitz, J., Van Der Merwe, L., & Ramesar, R. (2008). Personality endophenotypes for bipolar affective disorder: A family-based genetic association analysis. *Genes, Brain and Behavior, 7,* 869–876.

Schroeder, M. L., Wormworth, J. A., & Livesley, W. J. (1992). Dimensions of personality disorder and their relationships to the Big Five dimensions of personality. *Psychological Assessment, 4,* 47–53.

Siever, L. J. (2005). Endopehnotypes in the personality disorders. *Dialogues in Clinical Neuroscience, 7*(2), 139–151.

Torgersen, S., Czajkowski, N., Jacobson, K., Reichborn-Kjennerud, T., Røysamb, E., Neale, M. C., et al. (2008). Dimensional representations of DSM-IV Cluster B personality disorders in a population-based sample of Norwegian twins: A multivariate study. *Psychological Medicine, 38,* 1617–1625.

Waller, N. G., & Shaver, P. R. (1994). The importance of nongenetic influences on romantic love styles: A twin family study. *Psychological Science, 5,* 268–274.

Whitfield, C., Cziko, A. M., & Robinson, G. E. (2003). Gene expression profiles in the brain predict behavior in individual honey bees. *Science, 302,* 296–299.

Wiggins, J. S. (1966). Substantive dimensions of self-report in the MMPI item pool. *Psychological Monographs: General and Applied, 80,* 1–42.

# CHAPTER 14

# Neurotransmitter Function in Personality Disorder

Jennifer R. Fanning and Emil F. Coccaro

Among the major developments in psychiatry research in the past decade, two of the most significant ones have been the continually expanding knowledge about biological systems underlying disordered behavior and the growing recognition of the dimensional nature of disorders that historically, from a diagnostic perspective, have been treated as categorical. While efforts to understand the biology underlying psychopathology have been under way for decades, in recent years these efforts have been advanced by the growing availability of methods, such as neuroimaging, that allow complex functional systems to be studied centrally (in the brain) in living research participants. From a diagnostic perspective, there has been a slow shift over the past two decades toward recognizing the dimensional nature of psychopathology (Trull & Durrett, 2005). In the case of personality disorders (PDs), this encompasses a growing recognition of the continuity between normal and disordered personality traits (Markon, Krueger, & Watson, 2005; Widiger & Costa, 2012), and between PDs and Axis I disorders (Krueger, 2005; Krueger & Tackett, 2003). Interestingly, the value of conceptualizing psychopathology along dimensions has been appreciated by researchers studying the biological basis of disorders (and in particular PDs) for several decades, as many of the early findings in biological psychiatry centered on relationships between biological indices and dimensions of behavior (e.g., impulsive aggression) rather than on discrete diagnostic categories. We review in this chapter the research on neurotransmitter function in PDs and present evidence of the biological bases of these disorders from both categorical and dimensional perspectives.

Several models have sought to characterize the dimensions of PD within a neurobiological framework (Paris, 2005). One of these is Cloninger's tridimensional model, linking temperament to specific neurotransmitter systems. This system describes four temperament dimensions (novelty seeking, harm avoidance, reward dependence, and persistence) and three character dimensions (self-directedness, cooperativeness, and self-transcendence) (Cloninger, Svrakic, & Przybeck, 1993). Another by Depue and Lenzenweger (2001) organizes personality along five dimensions: extraversion (positive emotionality), neuroticism (negative emotionality), fear, affiliation, and nonaffective constraint. Livesley, Jang, and Vernon (1998) found that a four-factor model of personality pathology, characterized by emotional dysregulation, dissociality, inhibition, and compulsivity, provided a good fit for the data in general population, clinical, and twin samples, and a four-factor underlying genetic structure fit the phenotypic factor solution well. Siever and Davis (1991) provide a useful heuristic model of personality psychopathology, in which core psychopathological disturbances are characterized along four dimensions: affective instability, aggression/

impulsivity, cognitive/perceptual organization, and anxiety/inhibition. Importantly, they suggest that these dimensions underlie both Axis I and Axis II psychopathology. An implication of this approach is that behavioral disturbances in Axis I and Axis II disorders share neurobiological underpinnings. Siever and Weinstein (2009) describe the relationship between these four dimensions and DSM PD. "Affective instability" (AI) reflects rapidly changing mood states that are often extreme in their intensity. In PDs, AI often occurs in response to interpersonal events. AI is particularly characteristic of Cluster B ("dramatic") PDs. The types of events that trigger AI may differ across the specific disorders. In bipolar PD (BPD), AI may manifest as intense relationships and clinging behavior in response to interpersonal stressors such as perceived abandonment. In histrionic PD (HPD), AI may lead to exaggerated behavioral responses. In anxious/inhibited individuals, AI may result in greater social avoidance. AI and negative emotionality are also features of Axis I mood disorders, although the course of these is episodic, whereas in PD it is chronic. Aggression and impulsivity can be thought of as a reduced threshold for responding motorically to stimuli, either internal or external. Aggressive and impulsive behaviors are often carried out without consideration of future consequences and are therefore often destructive and maladaptive. Aggression and impulsivity are most strongly associated with BPD and antisocial PD (ASPD). In BPD, aggression and impulsivity can manifest in both self- and other-directed harm behaviors, as well as in suicide attempts, substance use, and other self-destructive behavior. In ASPD, aggression and impulsivity are more likely to reflect a disregard for social norms and impulsive behavior in pursuit of reward, and often involves violating the rights of others. Aggression and impulsivity are features of Axis I impulse control disorders, including intermittent explosive disorder, pyromania, and kleptomania. "Cognitive and perceptual disorganization" reflects the inability to perceive, attend to, and process stimuli and make use of previous experience and information about the present context to respond appropriately. These abilities are impaired in individuals with schizotypal PD (STPD), as they are in psychotic disorders broadly, and this impairment often results in impaired social cognition, poor relatedness, and ultimately impaired social functioning. "Anxiety and inhibition" are characterized by negative anticipation of future events, anticipation of negative evaluation by others, and heightened perception of danger or threat. This negative anticipation is accompanied by negative affect (anxiety and fear) and physiological symptoms, and is characteristic of Cluster C ("anxious") PD, as well as several Axis I disorders.

Several methods are available to study neurotransmitter functioning in humans, including assessment of neurotransmitter concentrations in biological samples such as plasma or cerebrospinal fluid (CSF), assessment of biological responses to pharmacological challenges, and neuroimaging methods such as positron emission tomography (PET). In this chapter, we review the existing data specifically regarding neurotransmitter function in subjects with PDs. This review also includes a review of neuropeptides. The chapter is organized around neurotransmitter systems, and we present research using both categorical and dimensional models of PD.

## Serotonin

The most extensively studied neurotransmitter with respect to PDs has been serotonin (5-hydoxytryptamine; 5-HT). A rich literature points to the involvement of serotonin in suicidal, impulsive, aggressive, and antisocial behavior, all of which are characteristic of Cluster B PDs. Early studies on serotonin focused on the role of serotonin in suicidal behavior (Asberg, 1997; Asberg, Schalling, Traskman-Bendz, & Wagner, 1987). After work in this area revealed that individuals who had committed suicide had lower concentrations of brain 5-HT or the 5-HT metabolite 5-hydroxyindoleacetic acid (5-HIAA) in postmortem studies compared to those who died by other causes (Bourne et al., 1968; Pare, Yeung, Price, & Stacey, 1969; Shaw, Eccleston, & Camps, 1967), researchers began to look for an association between serotonin metabolites and lesser forms of self-directed aggression including suicidal ideation and history of suicide attempt. Many of these studies have focused on 5-HIAA, which is a major metabolite of serotonin. 5-HIAA is thought to reflect serotonin turnover via the degradation of serotonin following release into the synapse. 5-HIAA in CSF correlates with 5-HIAA in the brain and therefore has been utilized as a marker of central serotonergic activity (Stanley,

Traskman-Bendz, & Dorovini-Zis, 1985). In one early study, Asberg, Traskman, and Thoren (1976) studied 68 depressed inpatients and found a bimodal distribution of CSF 5-HIAA, with 29% of patients comprising the group with lower levels of the metabolite. Patients who attempted suicide during the current depressive episode and those using violent methods to attempt suicide were significantly more likely to belong to the group with low 5-HIAA. Other researchers have observed lower levels of CSF 5-HIAA in individuals who have attempted suicide compared to healthy individuals (Brown, Goodwin, Ballenger, Goyer, & Major, 1979; Brown et al., 1982; Lidberg, Tuck, Asberg, Scalia-Tomba, & Bertilsson, 1985), and a meta-analysis of studies concluded that there is strong support for the relationship between suicide and CSF levels of 5-HIAA. Specifically, individuals who had attempted suicide had lower CSF 5-HIAA on average compared to psychiatric controls. The authors found mixed support for the notion that lower 5-HIAA was associated with violent (as opposed to nonviolent) suicide attempts (Lester, 1995).

Other studies point to alterations in 5-HT receptor number and function associated with suicidal behavior. Stanley and Mann (1983) observed 44% increased $5\text{-HT}_2$ receptor sites in the frontal cortices of suicide victims over controls, which was concomitant with decreased presynaptic [$^3$H]imipramine binding sites (Stanley, Virgilio, & Gershon, 1982). Similar findings were reported in a subsequent study in which the authors again observed a 28% increase in $5\text{-HT}_2$ receptors in suicide victims compared to controls but no difference in $5\text{-HT}_1$ receptors (Mann, McBride, & Bruce, 1986). In this study there was no correlation between the number of $5\text{-HT}_1$ and $5\text{-HT}_2$ receptors in either group. Simeon and colleagues (1992) examined CSF 5-HIAA and platelet imipramine binding ($B_{max}$) and affinity ($K_d$) in patients with PD, with or without self-mutilating behavior. The authors found that $B_{max}$ correlated negatively with degree of self-mutilation and impulsivity within the self-mutilating group. However, there were no differences in 5-HT indices between the two groups. Patients with BPD comprised approximately 60% of each group. These studies implicate presynaptic serotonergic function in self-destructive and suicidal behavior.

Pharmacochallenge studies also point to a role of serotonin dysfunction in suicidal behavior. In an early study, Metzler, Perline, Tricou, Lowy, and Robertson (1984) found that depressed patients who had attempted suicide had increased cortisol response when administered the 5-HT precursor 5-hydroxytryptophan (5-HTP) compared to depressed patients with suicidal ideation only or no suicidality. This finding was interpreted as reflecting increased postsynaptic 5-HT receptor sensitivity secondary to decreased (presynaptic) serotonergic activity. However, subsequent studies have more often found blunted hormonal responses to serotonergic challenge agents. Coccaro and colleagues (1989) observed reduced prolactin (PRL) response to d,l-fenfluramine (d,l-FEN) challenge among psychiatric patients with a history of suicide attempt compared to psychiatric patients with no history and compared to controls. Fenfluramine has frequently been used as a serotonergic probe. It enhances serotonin transmission by causing 5-HT release and inhibiting 5-HT reuptake. In doing so, it stimulates receptors in the hypothalamus, which causes the pituitary gland to release PRL into plasma, where it can be assayed. New and colleagues (1997) studied the relationship between nonsuicidal self-injury (NSSI) and suicide attempt history and 5-HT functioning in a sample of 97 patients with PD. Patients with a history of suicide attempt and NSSI showed the most blunted PRL[d,l-FEN] response, followed by patients with NSSI alone, compared to those with no history of self-aggressive behavior. More than half of patients with a suicide attempt history (56%) and NSSI (78%) were diagnosed with BPD. In a later study, New and colleagues (2004) also observed decreased PRL[d,l-FEN] in men (most of whom were diagnosed with PD) with a lifetime history of suicide attempt. This was observed both in patients with a major affective disorder and patients with PD.

An extensive literature has explored the role of serotonin in aggression and violence. One of the earliest studies to explore this relationship examined CSF 5-HIAA in adult military men with aggressive or impulsive behavior (Brown et al., 1979). CSF 5-HIAA was negatively correlated ($r = -0.78$) with self-reported life history or aggression. Moreover, a subgroup of the sample diagnosed with impulsive PDs had lower 5-HIAA compared to subjects diagnosed with nonimpulsive PDs (e.g., schizoid PD [SPD], obsessive–compulsive PD [OCPD]). Those participants with a history of suicide attempt ($n = 11$) had higher aggression scores, lower 5-HIAA, and higher 3-methoxy-4-hydroxyphenylglycol

(MHPG) compared to subjects with no such history (Brown et al., 1979). The correlation between CSF 5-HIAA and life history of aggression was replicated in a subsequent sample of men with BPD ($r = -0.53$; Brown et al., 1982). Several studies have observed lower levels of CSF 5-HIAA in impulsive violent offenders compared to healthy controls (Lidberg et al., 1985; Virkkunen, Nuutila, Goodwin, & Linnoila, 1987), while others have reported correlations between the metabolite and life history of aggressive behavior (Limson et al., 1991). Not all study results have been positive (e.g., Coccaro, Kavoussi, Cooper, & Hauger, 1997; Hibbeln et al., 2000). Coccaro, Kavoussi, Hauger, Cooper, and Ferris (1998) found no relation between CSF 5-HIAA and life history of aggression in samples with various PDs. Likewise, Simeon and colleagues (1992) found no relation between several indices of 5-HT functioning and life history of aggression or impulsivity in a sample of individuals with PDs and a history of self-harm. However, in a more recent study, Coccaro, Lee, and Kavoussi (2010) found that when both CSF 5-HIAA and CSF homovanillic acid (HVA) are placed in the same statistical model, CSF 5-HIAA demonstrates a significant positive correlation with aggression. This is consistent with reduced 5-HT receptor responsiveness demonstrated in pharmacochallenge studies (see Coccaro & Lee, 2010).

Pharmacochallenge studies have also provided evidence of a relationship between central serotonin functioning and aggression. Coccaro and colleagues (1989) observed a relationship between PRL[d,l-FEN] challenge and life history of aggression ($r = -.57$) and self-reported aggressive tendency ($r = -.52$) in patients with PD. Trait antisociality (Minnesota Multiphasic Personality Inventory [MMPI] Psychopathic Deviance; $r = -.33$) and Trait Suspiciousness ($r = -.03$) did not significantly correlate with PRL[d,l-FEN]. Coccaro, Kavoussi, and Hauger (1995) found a strong inverse correlation ($r = -.85$) between the PRL response to d-FEN challenge and the Direct Assault scale of the Buss–Durkee Hostility Inventory (BDHI), although not with life history of aggressive behavior, in a mixed sample of individuals with PDs (e.g., SPD, passive–aggressive PD [PAPD]). A subsequent study did find a relationship between PRL[d-FEN] and life history of aggression in PD research subjects (Coccaro et al., 1997). Similar associations were observed in a large sample of patients by New and colleagues (2004) between PRL[d,l-FEN] and BDHI Irritability/Assaultiveness in men with PD ($r = -.21$) that was not accounted for by current depression. Other studies have also found a relationship between blunted hormonal response to serotonergic challenge in patients with BPD (Paris et al., 2004), antisocial individuals (Moss, Yao, & Panzak, 1990; O'Keane et al., 1992), and substance abusers (Moeller et al., 1994; but see Fishbein, Lozovsky, & Jaffe, 1989).

Extensive research has also investigated the relationship between serotonin and antisocial behavior, with several reports of low CSF 5-HIAA in groups with prominent antisocial behavior (Virkkunen et al., 1987). In a meta-analysis, Moore, Scarpa, and Raine (2002) examined the relationship between CSF 5-HIAA and antisocial behavior in antisocial and healthy individuals. The authors found an overall moderate size effect ($d = -0.45$) for the relationship, and the effect was larger ($d = -1.37$) in individuals under age 30. The results were not significantly moderated by gender, diagnosis of alcohol use disorder, history of suicide attempt, or target of crime (person vs. property; Moore et al., 2002). Researchers have also observed reduced endocrine responses to serotonergic probes in individuals with ASPD (e.g., PRL[d,l-FEN]; O'Keane et al., 1992). A challenge to interpreting these findings has been that criminal populations examined in these studies often have engaged in violent crimes and are therefore more aggressive than healthy control subjects, in addition to being more antisocial.

In spite of these limitations, there appears to be considerable support in the literature that 5-HT is involved in behaviors that can broadly be described as impulsive rather than premeditated. As an example, Linnoila and colleagues (1983) found lower levels of 5-HIAA among murderers and attempted murderers who had committed impulsive crimes compared to those who committed premeditated crimes. Several hypotheses have been offered to explain the role of 5-HT in modulating behavior. Spoont (1992) proposed that 5-HT stabilizes information flow by supporting phase coherence in neural activity, and thereby modulates reactivity to stimuli, both internal and external. Thus, high levels of 5-HT will be associated with behavioral rigidity, while low levels of 5-HT will be associated with impulsivity and stimulus reactivity (Spoont, 1992). Similarly, Linnoila and Virkkunen (1992) postulated that a "low serotonin syndrome" characterizes many individuals who engage in violent, impulsive, and antisocial behavior. This hypothesis was largely derived from studies of 5-HIAA. These authors conclude that 5-HT largely serves to constrain behavior, such that a deficit in 5-HT is associated with increased impulsivity. Another model, the "irritable aggression model" (Coccaro, Kavoussi, & Lesser, 1992), suggests that a net hyposerotonergic state is associated with greater irritability, which can be conceptualized as a lower threshold for responding to noxious stimuli. This is consistent with findings of an inverse correlation between self-reported irritability and PRL[d,l-FEN] (Coccaro et al., 1989) and Brown and colleagues' (1982) observation that the relationship between history of suicide attempt and PRL[d,l-FEN] became nonsignificant when they controlled for self-reported impulsivity. Furthermore, research in both animals and humans suggests that noxious, threatening, or provocative stimuli may be necessary to elicit aggressive behavior in a net hyposerotonergic state (Berman, McCloskey, Fanning, Schumacher, & Coccaro, 2009; Marks, Miller, Schulz, Newcorn, & Halperin, 2007).

While early studies on the relationship between serotonin and aggression produced large effect sizes, a recent meta-analysis has yielded a more modest estimate of this relationship. Duke, Bègue, Bell, and Eisenlohr-Moul (2013) analyzed 171 studies on the serotonin–aggression relationship that used (1) a 5-HIAA assay; (2) acute tryptophan depletion (ATD); (3) a pharmacochallenge; and (4) endocrine challenge methods. The authors found a small ($r = -.12$) significant inverse relation between measures of 5-HT functioning and aggression. Pharmacochallenge studies yielded the largest effect size (−0.21), whereas 5-HIAA yielded the smallest (−0.06, ns). Small significant average effects were found for ATD (−0.10) and endocrine challenge (−0.14), while cortisol response was not significantly related to aggression (−0.02). Of note, characteristics of the samples (e.g., gender, age, psychopathology, and history of aggression) did not moderate the relationships between indices of 5-HT functioning and aggression. Furthermore, type of drug did not moderate the relationship between pharmacological or endocrine challenge and aggression. These results, as well as null results and conflicting findings in the literature, suggest that the relationship between 5-HT and behavior is more complex than previously realized.

Serotonergic neurons project broadly throughout the brain, with particularly dense projections occurring in the cerebral cortex, limbic structures, basal ganglia, and brainstem. The 5-HT system also comprises at least 14 types of receptors. Furthermore, certain receptor subtypes ($5-HT_{1A}$ and $5-HT_{1B}$) are expressed both pre- and postsynaptically. There is evidence (much of it preclinical) that 5-HT receptor subtypes exert unique and perhaps even opposing effects on aggression. For example, aggressive individuals have been shown to have blunted response to $5-HT_{1A}$ receptor agonists (Cleare & Bond, 1997; Coccaro, Gabriel, & Siever, 1990) and suicidal subjects have demonstrated unique patterns of $5-HT_{1A}$ receptor binding, although results have been mixed (Bortolato et al., 2013). $5-HT_{1B}$ agonists may also reduce aggression via effects on impulsivity and $5-HT_{1B}$ heteroreceptors (situated postsynaptically on nonserotonergic neurons) in the hypothalamus may be involved in regulating aggression that is offensive as opposed to reactive (Olivier & van Oorschot, 2005). The relationship between the $5-HT_{2A}$ receptor and impulsive aggression has been mixed, with some studies finding inverse associations with $5-HT_{2A}$ indices (Meyer et al., 2008; Soloff, Price, Mason, Becker, & Meltzer, 2010) and others finding positive associations (Rosell et al., 2010) in areas of prefrontal cortex. Rosell and colleagues (2010) saw increased $5-HT_{2A}$ availability associated with current, but not past, impulsive aggression in subjects with PD, suggesting that dynamic changes in this index may reflect state changes in aggressive behavior. Finally, the $5-HT_{2C}$ receptor has been of interest because of its possible antiaggressive effects when stimulated (Bortolato et al., 2013).

Neuroimaging methodologies represent a significant advance in the area of psychiatry research. Methods such as PET offer the potential to examine neurotransmitter functioning centrally, which may provide a more accurate measure of 5-HT system activity and functioning. PET has been used to localize deficient serotonergic functioning in the brain. In one of the earliest PET studies in subjects with PD, Siever and colleagues (1999) imaged glucose metabolism in six impulsively aggressive patients with mixed PD and five healthy control subjects following administration of a single 60-mg dose of d,l-FEN and placebo in a within-subjects design study. In healthy individuals d,l-FEN was associated with increased glucose metabolism particularly in the left orbitofrontal (OFC) area and anterior cingulate cortex (ACC), while patients with PD showed attenuated (blunted) effects in these areas. Only the inferior parietal lobe showed increased metabolism in response to the drug in subjects with PD. PRL[d,l-FEN] (placebo-corrected) responses did not differ between patients and healthy controls. PRL[d,l-FEN] correlated ($r = .58$ and $r = .63$) with regions of interest in medial frontal cortex and right middle cingulate, respectively, although these correlations were not significant, likely due to the small sample size. A similar finding was obtained in a larger follow-up study. New and colleagues (2002) studied 13 impulsively aggressive patients with mixed PD and 13 healthy subjects using a meta-chlorophenylpiperazine (mCPP) versus placebo challenge. Healthy subjects but not subjects with PD showed increased glucose metabolism in OFC and ACC (areas involved in inhibiting aggressive behavior) following mCPP relative to placebo. In addition, a 12-week course of treatment with the selective serotonin reuptake inhibitor (SSRI) fluoxetine was shown to normalize OFC function in impulsively aggressive patients with BPD, supporting the notion that deficits in OFC function are at least partially supported by abnormalities in serotonin function (New et al., 2004).

Other studies suggest that individuals with BPD may have abnormal 5-HT synthesis. In one study, men with BPD showed lower trapping of a 5-HT precursor analogue (implicating reduced 5-HT synthesis capacity) in medial frontal gyrus, anterior cingulate gyrus (ACG), superior temporal gyrus, and corpus striatum compared to healthy controls, while women with BPD had lower trapping in right ACT and superior temporal gyrus (Leyton et al., 2001). Another study using PET radiotracer for the serotonin transporter (5-HTT) also showed reduced 5-HTT availability in ACG in impulsively aggressive subjects (Frankle et al., 2005). Finally, Koch and colleagues (2007), using single-photon emission computed tomography (SPECT), examined binding of [I-123]ADAM to the serotonin transporter and found increased binding in subjects with BPD in both the hypothalamus and brainstem. ADAM binding correlated significantly with impulsivity but not with depression.

Aggression, suicidality, impulsivity, and antisociality have all been linked to abnormal 5-HT functioning. Teasing apart these constructs to understand the role of serotonin in disordered behavior has been challenging for several reasons. One has been the tendency to interpret differences between groups as indicative of a role of 5-HT in a particular construct of interest (e.g., antisociality or self-injury; Berman, Tracy, & Coccaro, 1997; Moore et al., 2002; O'Keane et al., 1992), when in fact the groups overlap on multiple relevant constructs. In addressing this limitation, it has become common practice for studies to include separate measures of aggression and impulsivity; however, studies do not always control for covariation across these constructs to identify the unique relationship between these constructs and 5-HT functioning.

Whatever the precise role or roles of serotonin, it appears to exert its effects on broad domains of behavior rather than specific psychiatric diagnoses. Accordingly, the association between low CSF 5-HIAA and impulsive behaviors has been found in a number of patient groups, including those with depression (Asberg et al., 1976; Banki, Arató, Papp, & Kurcz, 1984; Lopez-Ibor, Saiz-Ruiz, & de los Cobos, 1985; Träskman, Asberg, Bertilsson, & Sjöstrand, 1981), substance use (Banki et al., 1984; Limson et al., 1991), and schizophrenia (Banki et al., 1984; Ninan et al., 1984; van Praag, 1983). Other studies have failed to find differences between subjects with PD and other groups, or differences have been explained by variables such as impulsivity or aggression. Gardner, Lucas, and Cowdry (1990) found no difference in CSF 5-HIAA between female patients with BPD and healthy control patients, although patients with a history of suicide attempt had lower 5-HIAA than those with parasuicidal behavior only. Coccaro and colleagues (1989) observed reduced PRL[d,l-FEN] in patients with PD compared to healthy controls; however, current patients did not differ from patients with acute or remitted affective disorders. Patients with BPD had reduced PRL[d,l-FEN] response compared to patients with other PDs and compared to controls, but no differences were found among patients with STPD, PPD, or HPD and "other" PDs. The difference between subjects with BPD and other subjects was not accounted for by differences in current depression severity. Soloff, Meltzer, Becker, Greer, and Constantine (2005) observed a blunted PRL[d,l-FEN] response in male (but not female) subjects with BPD compared to healthy control subjects. However, the effect was made nonsignificant by accounting for trait impulsivity, aggression, and antisociality. These findings support the notion that serotonergic disturbances are associated with broad dimensions of behavior rather than specific diagnostic categories.

In summary, an extensive literature supports a role for serotonin in impulsivity, antisociality, aggression, and suicidality, all of which are core features of PDs reflecting impaired inhibitory control. Evidence suggests that serotonin modulates activity in areas of prefrontal cortex, including OFC and ACC, which are implicated in "top-down" control of limbic responding to stimuli. Individuals with PD display impaired serotonergic functioning in these brain regions, which may account for some of the symptoms of these disorders. Over time, a complex picture of the serotonin system has emerged, one that involves both broad and specific functions, tonic and phasic activity, and multiple receptor subtypes, and it is clear that early models (e.g., "Low Serotonin") are no longer adequate to describe the role of 5-HT in disordered behavior. Neuroimaging methods have the potential to greatly enhance our understanding of neurotransmitter function; however, drugs with antiaggressive effects are also need to elucidate the precise mechanisms at work.

## Dopamine

Dopamine (DA) is a catecholamine neurotransmitter involved in a range of functions, including learning, memory, and movement. DA has been most strongly implicated in BPD, aggressive behavior, and STPD. In BPD, DA dysfunction has been associated with emotional dysregulation, impulsivity, and cognitive-perceptual impairment (see Friedel, 2004, for a review). Patients with BPD show increased affective and psychotic-like features in response to DA challenge using amphetamine, relative to healthy subjects (Schulz et al., 1985). In another study, two patients with BPD who were administered methylphenidate experienced increased affective symptoms (e.g., anger, fear, and dysphoria), motor agitation, and cognitive disturbance, which were similar to the patients' own previous stress-related symptom exacerbations (Wolkowitz & Cowdry, 1987). These effects did not occur with placebo. Some of the most convincing evidence that DA is involved in symptoms of BPD comes from treatment studies involving antipsychotic agents, which act primarily through blockade of dopamine ($D_2$) receptors. Several of these drugs have been shown to ameliorate affective and behavioral dimensions of BPD, including depression, anxiety, anger, paranoia, impulsivity, and interpersonal sensitivity (Friedel, 2004). However, the nonspecific effects of these drugs with regard to their receptor activity make it difficult to draw firm conclusions about the mechanisms of their effects.

Compared to serotonin, the evidence for the role of DA in human aggression has been limited. Preclinical studies have revealed hyperactivity of the DA system in the mesocorticolimbic pathway during and after a provocative aggressive encounter, possibly reflecting motivational aspects of aggressive behavior (Miczek, Fish, De Bold, & De Almeida, 2002). In humans, HVA, a major metabolite of dopamine, has been studied as an index of DA turnover. Several studies have examined the relationship between HVA and aggression, but the findings have been mixed. Some studies find no relationship between CSF HVA concentration and aggression or suicide (Brown et al., 1979, 1982; Lidberg et al., 1985; Virkkunen et al., 1987), whereas other studies demonstrate an inverse relationship. Linnoila and colleagues (1983) observed reduced CSF HVA in antisocial impulsive violent offenders, and Virkkunen, De Jong, Bartko, Goodwin, and Linnoila (1989) reported that recidivist violent offenders had lower CSF HVA concentrations than their nonrecidivist violent offender controls. Limson and colleagues (1991) observed an inverse correlation between CSF HVA and aggression in alcohol-dependent and healthy individuals, and a similar relationship was reported in a sample of healthy volunteers and subjects with PD when CSF 5-HIAA and CSF HVA were placed in the same statistical model (Coccaro et al., 2010). There is some evidence of dopaminergic involvement in psychopathy, a PD characterized by callousness and unemotionality (Factor 1 psychopathy) and antisociality (Factor 2 psychopathy). Soderstrom, Blennow, Manhem, and Forsman (2001) observed a positive correlation between CSF HVA ($r = .41$; marginally significant) and Factor 1 psychopathy and Factor 2 psychopathy ($r = .65$) in 22 violent offenders. CSF 5-HIAA and HVA intercorrelate significantly; therefore, it is possible that these effects may be partly attributable to serotonergic function. The interaction between serotonin and dopamine may have implications for aggressive behavior, with DA playing a facilitating role in aggression and serotonin a constraining role (Seo, Patrick, & Kennealy, 2008). In line with this notion, Soderstrom and colleagues observed a relationship between the ratio of 5-HT to DA (HVA:5-HIAA) and Factor 1 ($r = .53$) and Factor 2 ($r = .52$) psychopathy. The relationship between HVA and HVA:5-HIAA was replicated for Factor 2 psychopathy in a follow-up study of violent offenders (Soderstrom, Blennow, Sjodin, & Forsman, 2003). Finally, evidence for the involvement of DA in aggression comes from research showing that drugs targeting DA receptors (albeit nonspecifically) are effective in reducing aggression in humans (see Comai, Tau, Pavlovic, & Gobbi, 2012, for a review).

STPD was included in DSM after it was observed that relatives of individuals with schizophrenia often display signs of the disorder in attenuated forms (Kety, Rosenthal, Wender, Schulsinger, & Jacobsen, 1976). While schizophrenia is characterized by frank delusions or hallucinations, disorganized speech and behavior, and negative symptoms, STPD is characterized by milder manifestations of these symptoms, such as unusual beliefs, inappropriate affect, and social anxiety. Like individuals with schizophrenia, those with STPD also show evidence of nonpsychotic cognitive dysfunction, particularly in working memory, and this cognitive dysfunction is associated with impaired interpersonal functioning (Mitropoulou et al., 2002, 2005). DA has long been thought to play a role in the pathophysiology of schizophrenia; however, models of DA functioning in schizophrenia have changed significantly over time. Currently it is thought that schizophrenia is characterized by increased dopaminergic activity at $D_2$ receptors in the associative striatum (giving rise to psychotic symptomatology), normal or decreased activity at DA receptors in the ventral striatum (linked to negative symptoms), and *decreased* dopaminergic activity at $D_1$ receptors in prefrontal cortex (accounting for cognitive symptoms; see Laruelle, 2014, for a recent review).

Given the close relationship between schizophrenia and STPD, dopamine has been of interest to researchers seeking to better understand STPD. Dopamine agonist (e.g., amphetamine) administered as a pharmacological challenge has been shown to increase psychotic symptoms in some individuals with BPD (Schulz et al., 1985). Amphetamine has also been associated with a greater increase in psychotic symptoms, thought disturbance, and activation in patients with BPD and STPD compared to BPD alone (Schulz, Cornelius, Schulz, & Soloff, 1988), although in another study no increase in positive symptoms was observed following the same dose of amphetamine administration in individuals with STPD (Siegal, Mitropoulou, Amin, Kirrane, & Silverman, 1996). More recently, researchers using SPECT found that individuals with STPD (relative to other PDs) show evidence of enhanced DA release in the striatum following amphetamine challenge (Abi-Dargham et al., 2004). Individuals with STPD have also been found to have increased concentration of HVA in plasma relative to healthy and other control subjects with PD, and HVA concentration has been shown to correlate significantly with psychotic-like symptoms but not deficit symptoms (Amin et al., 1997; Siever & Davis, 1991). Similar results were obtained when HVA was measured in CSF of 10 patients with STPD and patients with other PD diagnoses (Siever & Trestman, 1993). Mitropolou and colleagues (2004) induced a metabolic challenge using an infusion of 2-Deoxyglucose (2-DG) to create a hypoglycemic state to study the DA response in individuals with STPD. Previous research indicated that individuals with schizophrenia had enhanced DA response to 2-DG compared to healthy control subjects, suggestive of increased DA activity. The authors found no difference between STPD and healthy subjects in the DA response to the challenge, suggesting that, compared to patients with schizophrenia, those with STPD have more intact dopaminergic functioning. Together these results suggest that individuals with STPD may be abnormally sensitive to the effects of DA, and that basal DA functioning is related to the attenuated psychotic-like symptoms found in STPD and BPD. However, there is also evidence that individuals with STPD have relatively better intact DA functioning than their counterparts with schizophrenia, perhaps reflecting a buffer against more severe psychotic symptoms.

Decreased dopaminergic functioning may also be involved in the pathophysiology of deficit symptoms of STPD. First-degree relatives of patients with schizophrenia have been reported to have lower mean plasma HVA compared to healthy control subjects regardless of the presence of STPD, a pattern opposite to those found in patients with STPD. When examined closely, the relatives were found to primarily have deficit-type symptoms (e.g., constricted affect, lack of close friends) and plasma HVA correlated inversely with these symptoms (Amin et al., 1999). However, other studies have failed to find a correlation between plasma HVA levels and negative or deficit symptoms (Amin et al., 1997; Siever & Davis, 1991). Abi-Dargham and colleagues (2004) found that amphetamine administration improved negative symptoms in individuals with STPD, although the improvement did not correlate with DA activity in response to the challenge.

DA is also implicated in modulating cognitive functions, particularly those subserved by the frontal cortex, striatum, and associative brain areas (Cropley, Fujita, Innis, & Nathan, 2006) such as working memory (Arnsten, 1998). Amphetamine has been shown to reduce perseverative errors on the Wisconsin Card Sorting Task (WCST; Siegal et al., 1996) and to improve visual working memory performance (Kirrane et al., 2000) in patients with STPD. In one study, amphetamine-induced DA release in the striatum correlated with schizotypal personality traits in healthy volunteers, specifically, with disorganized schizotypal traits (Woodward et al., 2011). Thus, it appears that DA may play an important role in the pathophysiology of schizophrenia as well as STPD. Given the heterogeneous nature of symptoms in these disorders and the complexity of the DA system, elucidating the exact nature of this role is an area of ongoing research.

In summary, individuals with STPD display features similar to but less severe than those in individuals with schizophrenia. Although they typically do not present with the frank psychotic symptoms seen in schizophrenia, individuals with STPD may endorse subclinical, psychotic-like experiences and show similar cognitive deficits and attenuated negative and disorganized symptoms. DA is implicated in the pathophysiology of schizophrenia, and evidence suggests that abnormalities are also present in STPD, albeit in attenuated form, and may underlie key symptom domains of the disorder. Relative sparing of dopaminergic function in subcortical regions has been suggested to account for the absence of frank psychosis in STPD (Kirrane & Siever, 2000). Given the likely complex role of the dopaminergic system in schizophrenia and related disorders, there is a continued need for research into the pathways and mechanisms involved.

## Norepinephrine

Norepinephrine (NE) is involved in modulating an organism's responses to stimuli. The central NE system originates in the locus coeruleus and surrounding brain structures, and comprises both tonic and phasic activity. NE activity appears to vary with degrees of wakefulness and arousal, as well as when orienting to novel stimuli, focusing attention, and enacting behavioral responses (Berridge & Waterhouse, 2003) and is involved in the stress response as part of hypothalamic–pituitary–adrenal (HPA) axis (Dunn & Swiergiel, 2009). A role of NE in behavioral domains such as affective instability, suicidal behavior, and aggression has been suggested (Siever & Davis, 1991); however, empirical support for these hypotheses has so far been both limited and mixed (Oquendo & Mann, 2000).

Preclinical studies suggest that NE plays a "permissive" role in aggression by facilitating "fight-or-flight" responses to threat (Miczek & Fish, 2005). Findings in humans have been inconsistent. MHPG, a metabolite of NE, has been studied as a marker of NE activity. One early study reported a positive correlation between MHPG in CSF ($r = .64$; Brown et al., 1979); however, other studies have reported no relation between MHPG and aggression/antisociality (Brown et al., 1982; Lidberg et al., 1985; Virkkunen et al., 1989, 1994), and some have found an inverse relationship between plasma MHPG and aggression (Coccaro, Lee, & McCloskey, 2003). Virkunnen and colleagues (1987) observed a positive correlation between criminal behavior (but not violent crime) and MHPG in arsonists, but also higher concentrations of NE in healthy participants compared to violent criminals and arsonists. Coccaro, Lawrence, Klar, and Siever (1991) used clonidine, an alpha-2-NE receptor agonist, to assess the sensitivity of alpha-2-NE receptor sensitivity in patients with PD, remitted mood affective disorder (MAD), and healthy subjects via growth hormone (GH) response in plasma. The authors found that GH response differed only between the group with MAD and the other two groups, with PD and healthy subjects showing greater GH response and a positive correlation between GH response and irritability but not assaultiveness (Coccaro et al., 1991). This finding, however, was not replicated in a separate study in a larger group of subjects (Coccaro et al., 2010). In contrast, Gerra and colleagues (1994) found that among siblings of heroin abusers, those with antisocial personality traits showed blunted growth hormone response to clonidine challenge (indicative of subsensitive alpha-2-NE receptors) and beta-endorphin response to clonidine challenge (indicative of subsensitive alpha-1-NE receptors) compared to healthy siblings of heroin abusers and healthy control subjects. Differences in these reports may be due to the high correlation between irritability and depression in this sample of heroin-abusing subjects.

HPA axis dysfunction is implicated in BPD; however, basal NE function has generally not been distinguishable between individuals with and without BPD. Researchers in one study found no difference between BPD and healthy subjects in urine NE (Simeon, Knutelska, Smith, Baker, & Hollander, 2007), while those in another found no difference in urine NE or MHPG between bulimic women with borderline personality features and healthy women (Vaz-Leal, Rodríguez-Santos, García-Herráiz, & Ramos-Fuentes, 2011). Nater and colleagues (2010) found that patients with BPD did not differ from healthy subjects in plasma NE response to a stress challenge paradigm (the Trier Social Stress Test). Studies have also used pharmacochallenge methods to assess NE functioning in BPD. Paris and colleagues (2004) found no difference between patients with BPD and healthy subjects in GH response to clonidine (GH[CLON]). Later time to peak GH[CLON] response was positively associated with self-reported assaultiveness ($r = .47$) but the GH response was unrelated to mood symptoms and impulsivity (Paris et al., 2004). Cortisol is a product of HPA axis reactivity in response to stress. Abnormalities in basal and acute cortisol levels have been associated with various psychiatric disorders, and are likely to reflect long-term changes in HPA axis functioning, perhaps in combination with predisposing individual variation. However, understanding of this complex system and its links to disorders and symptoms remains incomplete. Zimmerman and Choi-Kain (2009) reviewed more than a dozen studies of HPA axis functioning in BPD, including studies that examined basal cortisol levels, cortisol response to dexamethasone challenge (an index of negative feedback inhibition of HPA axis activity), and cortisol response to psychosocial stress challenge. Results of these studies were mixed with respect to both basal cortisol and cortisol response to challenge, with some studies showing no difference between patients with BPD and controls, and others showing conflicting findings. History of childhood trauma and comorbid depression and posttraumatic stress disorder (PTSD) are likely to significantly predict cortisol functioning (Zimmerman & Choi-Kain, 2009). Furthermore, acute symptom profiles may also be particularly relevant to HPA functioning in BPD. In line with this notion, Simeon and colleagues (2007) found that participants with BPD and dissociative symptoms showed greater cortisol reactivity to a stress paradigm compared to healthy subjects and subjects with BPD without dissociation.

Abnormal NE and HPA axis functioning are implicated in other psychiatric disorders, including PTSD and anxiety disorders. Specifically, increased activation of the NE system, particularly under conditions of stress, may reflect sensitization to stimuli associated with the original stressor or feared stimulus (Southwick et al., 1999; Sullivan, Coplan, Kent, & Gorman, 1999). Anxiety disorders are also associated with enhanced cortical arousal and cortical reactivity to threat-stimuli (see Clark et al., 2009, for a review), both of which have been linked to the activity of the NE system (Nieuwenhuis, Aston-Jones, & Cohen, 2005). To date, however, very little work has focused specifically on NE in the anxious cluster (Cluster C) PDs.

## Glutamate

Glutamate, the primary excitatory neurotransmitter in the central nervous system, is involved in neurodevelopment, learning, and memory. Recent years have seen a growing interest in the role that glutamate plays in psychiatric disorder, including in schizophrenia (Laruelle, 2014), depression (Duman, 2014), and anxiety disorders (Bermudo-Soriano, Perez-Rodriguez, Vaquero-Lorenzo, & Baca-Garcia, 2012). Accordingly, a small but developing literature has examined the role of glutamate in personality psychopathology.

In general, it is thought that glutamate plays a facilitory role in aggressive behavior. Studies in cats and rodents show that stimulation of the hypothalamus (e.g., the "hypothalamic attack area") induces defensive aggressive behavior, and that aggression is induced by glutamate and inhibited by gamma-aminobutyric acid (GABA) and serotonin in this region (Haller, 2013). While limited data are available in humans, glutamate concentrations assessed in CSF have been shown to correlate with both aggression and impulsivity in subjects with PD and healthy subjects, although glutamate levels did not differ between healthy subjects and those with PD. Glutamate concentration did not differ as a function of PD cluster (A, B, or C;

Coccaro, Lee, & Vezina, 2013). Higher levels of glutamic acid have been observed in CSF of pathological gamblers compared to healthy research participants (Nordin, Gupta, & Sjödin, 2007). Furthermore, there is preclinical evidence that interfering with glutamate by administration of N-methyl-D-aspartate (NMDA) receptor antagonists or by inhibiting glutamate synthesis can reduce aggression in mice. In humans, treatment with memantine (an NMDA receptor antagonist) has been shown to reduce agitation and aggression in individuals with Alzheimer's disease (Wilcock, Ballard, Cooper, & Loft, 2008).

Preliminary studies suggest a possible role of glutamate in BPD, in particular the affective instability, impulsivity, and self-harm behaviors. Using proton magnetic resonance spectroscopy (MRS), Rüsch and colleagues (2010) found higher glutamate levels in the left ACC (an area involved in emotional and behavioral regulation) but not in the cerebellum in women with BPD and attention-deficit/hyperactivity disorder (ADHD), compared to healthy women. In a larger follow-up study, Hoerst and colleagues (2010) observed greater glutamate concentration in the ACC of women with BPD without ADHD, and glutamate concentration correlated with BPD symptom dimensions, including impulsivity, affect regulation, and dissociation. Other researchers found higher levels of glutamate in the ACC in youth with elevated emotional dysregulation (Wozniak et al., 2012). There has been growing interest in the use of drugs that target glutamate as a treatment for BPD and BPD symptoms. A case study of two patients with BPD and chronic self-harming behavior indicated that these patients reduced their self-harming behavior and desire to engage in self-harming when riluzole, a glutamate antagonist, was used to augment existing pharmacotherapy (Pittenger & Coric, 2005). Although a detailed review is beyond the scope of this chapter, Grosjean and Tsai (2007) proposed a detailed hypothesis of how disrupted NMDA transmission may contribute to symptoms of BPD, suggesting that this effect is heavily influenced by exposure early in life to abuse, neglect, and other adversity.

In summary, there is evidence that glutamate mediates behaviors such as aggression and impulsivity, and that abnormal glutamate activity may contribute to the pathophysiology of PDs and Axis I disorders. In schizophrenia, there is growing evidence that glutamate is an important component of the pathophysiology of the disorder, contributing to positive, negative, and cognitive symptoms (Coyle, 2006). Accordingly, it is very likely that over the next several years, attention to the role of this neurotransmitter in psychopathology will continue to increase.

## Gamma-Aminobutyric Acid

While glutamate is the primary excitatory neurotransmitter in the central nervous system, GABA is the primary *inhibitory* neurotransmitter. GABA receptors are expressed heavily in areas of frontal and limbic cortex and are found at both inhibitory–inhibitory and inhibitory–excitatory synapses. Studies of the relationship between GABA and impulsivity and aggression have been mixed. Preclinical studies have shown that aggressive animals show reduced brain levels of GABA and glutamic acid decarboxylase (GAD), an enzyme that catalyzes glutamate into GABA. In humans, GABA levels in plasma have been shown to correlate negatively with trait aggressiveness in psychiatrically healthy individuals. Lee, Petty, and Coccaro (2009) found an inverse relationship between trait impulsivity (but not aggression) and CSF GABA levels in individuals with PD and healthy control subjects. However, GABA levels were also found to be higher in individuals with a history of suicide attempt (Lee et al., 2009). Drugs that enhance GABAergic effects (including the antipsychotic clozapine, the anticonvulsants topiramate and valproate, and the mood stabilizer lithium) have been shown to reduce aggression (see Comai et al., 2012, for a review), suicide and suicide attempts (lithium; Baldessarini, Tondo, & Hennen, 2003), and behavioral dysregulation (carbamazepine; Cowdry & Gardner, 1988). High levels of state aggression and impulsivity (but not affective instability) have been associated with better treatment response (i.e., greater reduction in aggression) to valproate in patients with BPD (Hollander, Swann, Coccaro, Jiang, & Smith, 2005). These studies suggest that GABA functions in an inhibitory manner in relation to aggression. Other studies, however, suggest a more complex relationship. Certain allosteric modulators of $GABA_A$ receptors show a biphasic, bidirectional relationship with GABA. Specifically, these substances, which include some benzodiazapines, barbiturates, and alcohol, enhance aggression at low doses and reduce aggression at high doses. This "paradoxical" effect is likely to be influenced by the particular subunit composition of the benzodiazepine receptor at GABA$_A$ receptor sites, which may explain why some benzodiazepines show no such aggression-heightening effect. Furthermore, in the case of alcohol, alcohol-heightened aggressive behavior in mice is enhanced by repeated early exposure to alcohol (Miczek & Fish, 2005). Individuals with BPD may be particularly prone to paradoxical reactions to benzodiazepines. Cowdry and Gardner (1988) observed that patients with BPD engaged in more severe acts of aggression and self-aggression while taking alprazolam compared to placebo in a 6-week double-blind crossover trial.

## Vasopressin

Arginine vasopressin (AVP) and oxytocin (OXT) are neuropeptides that play a key role in the regulation of social cognition and behavior. Chronic interpersonal dysfunction is a hallmark of PD in general, and interpersonal stressors are common precipitants of mood and behavioral dysregulation in PDs; however, the function of AVP in human social cognition is just beginning to be understood. For example, intranasal AVP has been shown not only to reduce recognition of negative facial expressions in men (Uzefovsky, Shalev, Israel, Knafo, & Ebstein, 2012) but also to enhance recognition of both happy and angry faces (Guastella, Kenyon, Alvares, Carson, & Hickie, 2010).

Stress activates the HPA axis, setting into motion a hormonal cascade that includes the secretion of corticotropin-releasing hormone (CRH), adrenocorticotropic hormone (ACTH), and cortisol. AVP is involved in this system, interacting with CRF to increase the release of ACTH from the anterior pituitary. AVP is anxiogenic, and may play a role in mediating the development of depression and anxiety following stress (Beurel & Nemeroff, 2014). Preclinical research suggests that vasopressin plays a facilitory role in aggressive behavior. AVP microinjections into the hypothalamus of hamsters increase offensive aggression (Ferris et al., 1997), while vasopressin V1A receptor antagonists injected in anterior hypothalamus in hamsters inhibit intermale aggressive behavior in hamsters (Ferris et al., 2006; Ferris & Potegal, 1988). Serotonin has been shown to block AVP-facilitated aggression (Delville, Mansour, & Ferris, 1996). An early study on basal AVP levels in humans found no difference between clinical groups (ASPD, intermittent explosive disorder, and alcohol dependence disorder) and healthy individuals in CSF AVP concentrations (Virkkunen et al., 1994). However, CSF AVP has been found to correlate ($r = .41$) with life history of aggressive behavior. While AVP was found to inversely correlate with PRL[d-FEN] response, it was also an independent predictor of aggressive behavior in hierarchical regression analysis (Coccaro et al., 1998). In the latter study, AVP did not correlate with a measure of trait impulsivity, state depression, or state anxiety, and AVP levels did not vary as a function of any subtype of PD. Research suggests that AVP modulates an organism's response to stress, but possibly in a sex-specific manner (Taylor et al., 2000). Thompson, Gupta, Miller, Mills, and Orr (2004) found that AVP (but not placebo) led male participants to display similarly agonistic facial responses (corrugator electromyogram [EMG]) to both angry and neutral faces. In women, AVP was associated with decreased agonistic facial responses to same-sex happy and angry faces and increased affiliative facial responses to neutral and happy faces (Thompson, George, Walton, Orr, & Benson, 2006). Functional magnetic resonance imaging (fMRI) studies show that vasopressin activates neural structures involved in fear regulation and mentalizing (Zink et al., 2011; Zink, Stein, Kempf, Hakimi, & Meyer-Lindenberg, 2010). In one fMRI study designed to assess the role of AVP in cooperative versus agonistic behavior, male participants engaged in a prisoner's dilemma game with a confederate. Those who received intranasal AVP showed increased cooperative behavior, and cooperation was associated with increased activation in stria terminalis and lateral septum, which are part of vasopressinergic circuitry (Rilling et al., 2012). In another study (Brunnlieb, Münte, Krämer, Tempelmann, & Heldmann, 2013), male participants engaged in a laboratory aggression paradigm with a research confederate, during which the pair set noise levels of blasts of varying intensity for each other. Intranasal AVP administration showed no effects on aggressive behavior; however, it was associated with activation in the amygdala when participants were deciding the level of noise to set for the other person, an effect that was not observed with the placebo. Given its role in social-cognitive and emotional processes and the stress response, AVP dysregulation may contribute to the behavioral and emotional disturbances seen in PDs. It is not surprising then that a rapidly growing body of research is investigating the role of AVP in personality and other psychiatric disorders.

## Oxytocin

Like vasopressin, OXT plays a role in regulating social behavior, although often the nature of these relationships is in the opposite direction. For example, with regard to aggression, while CSF vasopressin levels display a positive correlation with aggression, CSF OXT correlates inversely with aggression (Lee et al., 2009). Intranasal OXT administration has been linked to improved emotional recognition, empathy (Hurlemann et al., 2010), and attachment (Buchheim et al., 2009). OXT administration has also been shown to enhance positive communication between couples during a disagreement and to decrease cortisol response during the interaction (Ditzen et al., 2013). OXT may also increase trust (Kosfeld, Heinrichs, Zak, Fischbacher, & Fehr, 2005). However, the effects of OXT on mood and behavior may not all be positive. OXT (compared to placebo) has been shown to increase negative emotions such as envy and *schadenfreude* (Shamay-Tsoory et al., 2009) and to increase noncooperation toward members of outgroups (see De Dreu, 2012, for a review). Like vasopressin, OXT is involved in the stress response; however, OXT has anxiolytic properties and is thought to serve an important role in buffering stress (Neumann & Landgraf, 2012). In one study, healthy men who received a dose of intranasal OXT and social support prior to engaging in a stressful social task (giving a public speech) showed lower cortisol response and decreased anxiety.

Individuals with BPD have difficulty forming stable relationships and regulating mood and aggressive impulses. It is therefore of interest whether dysregulation of OXT may contribute to the symptoms of BPD, and whether enhancing OXT function may lead to a reduction in symptoms (Stanley & Siever, 2010). Women with BPD have been reported to have reduced OXT concentrations in plasma (Bertsch, Schmidinger, Neumann, & Herpertz, 2013). Furthermore, trauma exposure early in life (which is common among individuals with BPD) has been found to inversely predict CSF OXT levels in women (Bertsch, Schmidinger, et al., 2013; Heim et al., 2009). The strongest relationships have been found for emotional abuse and neglect; smaller effects have been found for physical abuse and emotional neglect. CSF OXT also showed a strong negative correlation with state anxiety. The results suggest that adverse experiences early in life may decrease OXT functioning, which is associated with mood disturbance. However, it is not clear that higher levels of endogenous OXT are necessarily predictive of better functioning. Another study indicated that higher levels of OXT in plasma correlate inversely with relationship quality in women (Taylor et al., 2006). Studies employing OXT challenge have similarly yielded mixed results. In individuals with BPD, augmenting OXT through intranasal administration has been shown to reduce both dysphoria and plasma cortisol levels following a stress challenge (Simeon et al., 2011). In a modified prisoner's dilemma task, participants with BPD who received intranasal OXT were less trusting of their partner and less likely to cooperate even when they anticipated cooperation on the part of their partner (Bartz et al., 2011). Whether OXT enhanced or decreased cooperation (relative to placebo) was moderated by attachment style. Whereas OXT had no effect on cooperation among low-anxiety participants, it decreased cooperation among highly anxious and avoidant participants, and *increased* cooperation among highly anxious nonavoidant participants. These results would suggest that OXT is acting to enhance predispositions to approach or avoid cooperation among highly anxious individuals. In another study, women with BPD showed enhanced amygdala activation when viewing angry and fearful faces, but OXT reduced the effect of angry faces on amygdala activation, suggesting reduced sensitivity to threat in women in BPD (Bertsch, Gamer, et al., 2013).

In summary, research on OXT in BPD is both preliminary and mixed. There is some evidence that OXT may be anxiolytic in patients with BPD; however, it may also exacerbate preexisting behavioral tendencies. Further research is needed to better understand whether and how OXT may be involved in the pathogenesis of BPD. Currently, the potential therapeutic role of OXT in BPD remains unclear.

## Other Neurochemical Systems

Besides the major neurotransmitter and neuropeptide systems reviewed here, the roles of other neurotransmitter and neuropeptide systems have been investigated as to their roles in behavior and psychopathology. Although a thorough review of this research is beyond the scope of this chapter, these systems include testosterone (aggression, psychopathy; Carré, McCormick, & Hariri, 2011; Yildirim & Derksen, 2012); endogenous opioids (BPD; Stanley & Siever, 2010); acetylcholine (BPD; Gurvits, Koenigsberg, & Siever, 2000); neuropeptide Y (aggression; Coccaro, Lee, Liu, & Mathe, 2012); substance P (aggression; Coccaro, Lee, Owens, Kinead, & Nemeroff, 2012); and inflammatory cytokines (aggression; Coccaro, Lee, & Coussons-Read, 2014, 2015; Serafini et al., 2013). In addition, it has become increasingly apparent that behavior is subserved by complex interactions between neurotransmitter systems, and there have been some preliminary investigations into the way that neurotransmitter systems interact to influence behavior. Some hypotheses account for these interactions, for example, serotonin and DA (aggression; Seo et al., 2008) and, more recently testosterone–cortisol ratio (aggression; Terburg, Morgan, & van Honk, 2009) and others. Our understanding of these relationships will no doubt continue to grow over the coming years.

## Conclusions

While diagnostic systems have been slow to shift from categorical to dimensional models, it is apparent that the dimensional approach has a rich history in the neurobiological literature, particularly with regard to PDs. While the literature on neurotransmitter (NT) functioning in PDs has grown large over the years, a number of challenges continue to confront researchers attempting to understand their role in disordered behavior. The first concerns the most appropriate model for characterizing psychopathology (e.g., which dimensions of behavior provide the best model in relation to biological functioning). A second issue is the complexity of NT function, which depends not only on central NT levels but also tonic and phasic activity of NTs; on the function of NT receptors, including distribution, number, density, sensitivity, and changes over time; and finally on the interaction among NT systems. The effect of environmental variables (e.g., early life adversity) on NT function and the effect of the latter on gene expression add to the complexity of the NT–psychopathology relationship. A related issue concerns the way in which NTs are assessed. More advanced methodologies (including fMRI, PET, and SPECT) are able to localize NT function in specific brain areas and are increasingly being applied to research on PDs. However, due to the costs entailed in using these methods, less specific assessment methods (e.g., assays of saliva and plasma) continue to be widely utilized. In spite of these challenges, a growing literature points to the involvement of NTs and neuropeptides in behavior and psychopathology. Psychometric advances in understanding the structure of psychopathology and technological advances in assessing NT function will no doubt aid in understanding better the role these chemicals play in disordered behavior.

## REFERENCES

Abi-Dargham, A., Kegeles, L. S., Zea-Ponce, Y., Mawlawi, O., Martinez, D., Mitropoulou, V., et al. (2004). Striatal amphetamine-induced dopamine release in patients with schizotypal personality disorder studied with single photon emission computed tomography and [123I]iodobenzamide. *Biological Psychiatry, 55,* 1001–1006.

Amin, F., Siever, L., Silverman, J. M., Coccaro, E., Mitropoulou, V., Trestman, R. L., et al. (1997). Plasma HVA in schizotypal personality disorder. In A. J. Friedhoff & F. Amin (Eds.), *Plasma homovanillic acid studies in schizophrenia, implications for presynaptic dopamine dysfunction* (pp. 133–149). Washington, DC: American Psychiatric Press.

Amin, F., Silverman, J. M., Siever, L. J., Smith, C. J., Knott, P. J., & Davis, K. L. (1999). Genetic antecedents of dopamine dysfunction in schizophrenia. *Biological Psychiatry, 45,* 1143–1150.

Arnsten, A. F. T. (1998). Catecholamine modulation of prefrontal cortical cognitive function. *Trends in Cognitive Sciences, 1,* 436–447.

Asberg, M. (1997). Neurotransmitters and suicidal behavior: The evidence from cerebrospinal fluid studies. *Annals of the New York Academy of Sciences, 836,* 158–181.

Asberg, M., Schalling, D., Traskman-Bendz, L., & Wagner, A. (1987). Psychobiology of suicide, impulsivity, and related phenomena. In Herbert Y. Meltzer (Ed.), *Psychopharmacology: The third generation of progress* (pp. 665–668). New York: Raven Press.

Asberg, M., Traskman, L., & Thoren, P. (1976).

5-HIAA in the cerebrospinal fluid: A biochemical suicide predictor? *Archives of General Psychiatry, 33,* 1193–1197.

Baldessarini, R. J., Tondo, L., & Hennen, J. (2003). Lithium treatment and suicide risk in major affective disorders: Update and new findings. *Journal of Clinical Psychiatry, 64*(Suppl. 5), 44–52.

Banki, C. M., Arató, M., Papp, Z., & Kurcz, M. (1984). Biochemical markers in suicidal patients: Investigations with cerebrospinal fluid amine metabolites and neuroendocrine tests. *Journal of Affective Disorders, 6,* 341–350.

Bartz, J., Simeon, D., Hamilton, H., Kim, S., Crystal, S., Braun, A., et al. (2011). Oxytocin can hinder trust and cooperation in borderline personality disorder. *Social Cognitive and Affective Neuroscience, 6,* 556–563.

Berman, M. E., McCloskey, M. S., Fanning, J. R., Schumacher, J. A., & Coccaro, E. F. (2009). Serotonin augmentation reduces response to attack in aggressive individuals. *Psychological Science, 20,* 714–720.

Berman, M. E., Tracy, J., & Coccaro, E. F. (1997). The serotonin hypothesis of aggression revisited. *Clinical Psychology Review, 17,* 651–665.

Bermudo-Soriano, C. R., Perez-Rodriguez, M. M., Vaquero-Lorenzo, C., & Baca-Garcia, E. (2012). New perspectives in glutamate and anxiety. *Pharmacology, Biochemistry, and Behavior, 100,* 752–774.

Berridge, C. W., & Waterhouse, B. D. (2003). The locus coeruleus–noradrenergic system: Modulation of behavioral state and state-dependent cognitive processes. *Brain Research Reviews, 42,* 33–84.

Bertsch, K., Gamer, M., Schmidt, B., Schmidinger, I., Walther, S., Kästel, T., et al. (2013). Oxytocin and reduction of social threat hypersensitivity in women with borderline personality disorder. *American Journal of Psychiatry, 170,* 1169–1177.

Bertsch, K., Schmidinger, I., Neumann, I. D., & Herpertz, S. C. (2013). Reduced plasma oxytocin levels in female patients with borderline personality disorder. *Hormones and Behavior, 63,* 424–429.

Beurel, E., & Nemeroff, C. B. (2014). Interaction of stress, corticotropin-releasing factor, arginine vasopressin and behaviour. *Current Topics in Behavioral Neuroscience, 18,* 67–80.

Bortolato, M., Pivac, N., Muck Seler, D., Nikolac Perkovic, M., Pessia, M., & Di Giovanni, G. (2013). The role of the serotonergic system at the interface of aggression and suicide. *Neuroscience, 236,* 160–185.

Bourne, H. R., Bunney, W. E., Colburn, R. W., Davis, J. M., Davis, J. N., Shaw, D. M., et al. (1968). Noradrenaline, 5-hydroxytryptamine, and 5-hydroxyindoleacetic acid in hindbrains of suicidal patients. *Lancet, 292,* 805–808.

Brown, G. L., Goodwin, F. K., Ballenger, J. C., Goyer, P. F., & Major, L. F. (1979). Aggression in humans correlates with cerebrospinal fluid amine metabolites. *Psychiatry Research, 1,* 131–139.

Brown, L., Ebert, H., Goyer, F., Jimerson, D. C., Klein, J., Bunney, W., et al. (1982). Aggression, suicide, and serotonin: Relationships to CSF amine metabolites. *American Journal of Psychiatry, 139,* 741–746.

Brunnlieb, C., Münte, T. F., Krämer, U., Tempelmann, C., & Heldmann, M. (2013). Vasopressin modulates neural responses during human reactive aggression. *Social Neuroscience, 8,* 148–164.

Buchheim, A., Heinrichs, M., George, C., Pokorny, D., Koops, E., Henningsen, P., et al. (2009). Oxytocin enhances the experience of attachment security. *Psychoneuroendocrinology, 34,* 1417–1422.

Carré, J. M., McCormick, C. M., & Hariri, A. R. (2011). The social neuroendocrinology of human aggression. *Psychoneuroendocrinology, 36,* 935–944.

Clark, C. R., Galletly, C. A., Ash, D. J., Moores, K. A., Penrose, R. A., & McFarlane, A. C. (2009). Evidence-based medicine evaluation of electrophysiological studies of the anxiety disorders. *Clinical EEG and Neuroscience, 40,* 84–112.

Cleare, A. J., & Bond, A. J. (1997). Does central serotonergic function correlate inversely with aggression?: A study using D-fenfluramine in healthy subjects. *Psychiatry Research, 69,* 89–95.

Cloninger, C. R., Svrakic, D. M., & Przybeck, T. R. (1993). A psychobiological model of temperament and character. *Archives of General Psychiatry, 50,* 975–990.

Coccaro, E., Kavoussi, R., & Hauger, R. (1995). Physiological responses to D-fenfluramine and ipsapirone challenge correlate with indices of aggression in males with personality disorder. *International Clinical Psychopharmacology, 10,* 177–179.

Coccaro, E., Lee, R., Liu, T., & Mathe, A. (2012). Cerebrospinal fluid neuropeptide Y-like immunoreactivity correlates with impulsive aggression in human subjects. *Biological Psychiatry, 72,* 997–1003.

Coccaro, E., Lee, R., & McCloskey, M. S. (2003). Norepinephrine function in personality disorder: Plasma free MHPG correlates inversely with life history of aggression. *CNS Spectrums, 8,* 731–736.

Coccaro, E., Lee, R., Owens, M. J., Kinead, B., & Nemeroff, C. B. (2012). Cerebrospinal fluid substance P-like immunoreactivity correlates with aggression in personality disordered subjects. *Biological Psychiatry, 72,* 243–283.

Coccaro, E. F., Gabriel, S., & Siever, L. J. (1990). Buspirone challenge: Preliminary evidence for a role for central 5-HT$_{1a}$ receptor function in impulsive aggressive behavior in humans. *Psychopharmacology Bulletin, 26,* 393–405.

Coccaro, E. F., Kavoussi, R. J., Cooper, T. B., & Hauger, R. L. (1997). Central serotonin activity and aggression: Inverse relationship with prolactin response to D-fenfluramine, but not CSF 5-HIAA concentration, in human subjects. *American Journal of Psychiatry, 154,* 1430–1435.

Coccaro, E. F., Kavoussi, R. J., Hauger, R. L., Cooper, T. B., & Ferris, C. F. (1998). Cerebrospinal fluid vasopressin levels: Correlates with aggression and serotonin function in personality-disordered subjects. *Archives of General Psychiatry, 55,* 708–714.

Coccaro, E. F., Kavoussi, R. J., & Lesser, J. C. (1992). Self- and other-directed human aggression: The role of the central serotonergic system. *International Clinical Psychopharmacology, 6,* 70–83.

Coccaro, E. F., Lawrence, T., Klar, H. M., & Siever, L. J. (1991). Growth hormone responses to intravenous clonidine challenge correlate with behavioral irritability in psychiatric patients and healthy volunteers. *Psychiatric Research, 39*(2), 129–139.

Coccaro, E. F., & Lee, R. (2010). Cerebrospinal fluid 5-hydroxyindolacetic acid and homovanillic acid: Reciprocal relationships with impulsive aggression in human subjects. *Journal of Neural Transmission, 117,* 241–248.

Coccaro, E. F., Lee, R., & Coussons-Read, M. (2014). Elevated plasma inflammatory markers in individuals with intermittent explosive disorder and correlation with aggression in humans. *JAMA Psychiatry, 71*(2), 158–165.

Coccaro, E. F., Lee, R., & Coussons-Read, M. (2015). Cerebrospinal fluid and plasma C-reactive protein and aggression in personality-disordered subjects: A pilot study. *Journal of Neural Transmission, 122*(2), 321–326.

Coccaro, E. F., Lee, R., & Kavoussi, R. J. (2010). Aggression, suicidality, and intermittent explosive disorder: Serotonergic correlates in personality disorder and healthy control subjects. *Neuropsychopharmacology, 35*(2), 435–444.

Coccaro, E. F., Lee, R., & Vezina, P. (2013). Cerebrospinal fluid glutamate concentration correlates with impulsive aggression in human subjects. *Journal of Psychiatric Research, 47,* 1247–1253.

Coccaro, E. F., Siever, L. J., Klar, H. M., Maurer, G., Cochrane, K., Cooper, T. B., et al. (1989). Serotonergic studies in patients with affective and personality disorders. *Archives of General Psychiatry, 46,* 587–599.

Comai, S., Tau, M., Pavlovic, Z., & Gobbi, G. (2012). The psychopharmacology of aggressive behavior: A translational approach: Part 2. Clinical studies using atypical antipsychotics, anticonvulsants, and lithium. *Journal of Clinical Psychopharmacology, 32,* 237–260.

Cowdry, R. W., & Gardner, D. L. (1988). Pharmacotherapy of borderline personality disorder. *Archives of General Psychiatry, 45,* 111–119.

Coyle, J. T. (2006). Glutamate and schizophrenia: Beyond the dopamine hypothesis. *Cellular and Molecular Neurobiology, 26,* 365–384.

Cropley, V. L., Fujita, M., Innis, R. B., & Nathan, P. J. (2006). Molecular imaging of the dopaminergic system and its association with human cognitive function. *Biological Psychiatry, 59,* 898–907.

De Dreu, C. K. (2012). Oxytocin modulates cooperation within and competition between groups: An integrative review and research agenda. *Hormones and Behavior, 61,* 419–428.

Delville, Y., Mansour, K. M., & Ferris, C. F. (1996). Serotonin blocks vasopressin-facilitated offensive aggression: Interactions within the ventrolateral hypothalamus of golden hamsters. *Physiology and Behavior, 59,* 813–816.

Depue, R. A., & Lenzenweger, M. F. (2001). A neurobehavioral dimensional model. In W. J. Livesley (Ed.), *Handbook of personality disorders: Theory, research, and treatment* (pp. 136–176). New York: Guilford Press.

Ditzen, B., Nater, U. M., Schaer, M., La Marca, R., Bodenmann, G., Ehlert, U., et al. (2013). Sex-specific effects of intranasal oxytocin on autonomic nervous system and emotional responses to couple conflict. *Social Cognitive and Affective Neuroscience, 8,* 897–902.

Duke, A. A., Bègue, L., Bell, R., & Eisenlohr-Moul, T. (2013). Revisiting the serotonin–aggression relation in humans: A meta-analysis. *Psychological Bulletin, 139,* 1148–1172.

Duman, R. S. (2014). Pathophysiology of depression and innovative treatments: Remodeling glutamatergic synaptic connections. *Dialogues in Clinical Neuroscience, 16*(1), 11–27.

Dunn, A. J., & Swiergiel, A. H. (2009). The role of corticotropin-releasing factor and noradrenaline in stress-related resposnes, and the inter-relationships between the two systems. *European Journal of Pharmacology, 583,* 186–193.

Ferris, C. F., Lu, S.-F., Messenger, T., Guillon, C. D., Heindel, N., Miller, M., et al. (2006). Orally active vasopressin V1a receptor antagonist, SRX251, selectively blocks aggressive behavior. *Pharmacology, Biochemistry, and Behavior, 83,* 169–174.

Ferris, C. F., Melloni, R. H., Koppel, G., Perry, K. W., Fuller, R. W., & Delville, Y. (1997). Vasopressin/serotonin interactions in the anterior hypothalamus control aggressive behavior in golden hamsters. *Journal of Neuroscience 17,* 4331–4340.

Ferris, C. F., & Potegal, M. (1988). Vasopressin receptor blockade in the anterior hypothalamus suppresses aggression in hamsters. *Physiology and Behavior, 44,* 235–239.

Fishbein, D. H., Lozovsky, D., & Jaffe, J. H. (1989). Impulsivity, aggression, and neuroendocrine responses to serotonergic stimulation in substance abusers. *Biological Psychiatry, 25,* 1049–1066.

Frankle, W. G., Lombardo, I., New, A. S., Goodman, M., Talbot, P. S., Huang, Y., et al. (2005). Brain serotonin transporter distribution in subjects with impulsive aggressivity: A positron emission study with [$^{11}$C]McN 5652. *American Journal of Psychiatry, 162,* 915–923.

Friedel, R. O. (2004). Dopamine dysfunction in borderline personality disorder: A hypothesis. *Neuropsychopharmacology, 29,* 1029–1039.

Gardner, D. L., Lucas, P. B., & Cowdry, R. W. (1990). CSF metabolites in borderline personality disorder compared with normal controls. *Biological Psychiatry, 28,* 247–254.

Gerra, G., Caccavari, R., Marcato, A., Zaimovic, A., Avanzini, P., Monica, C., et al. (1994). Alpha-1- and 2-adrenoceptor subsensitivity in siblings of opioid addicts with personality disorders and depression. *Acta Psychiatrica Scandinavica, 90,* 269–273.

Grosjean, B., & Tsai, G. E. (2007). NMDA neurotransmission as a critical mediator of borderline personality disorder. *Journal of Psychiatry and Neuroscience, 32,* 103–116.

Guastella, A. J., Kenyon, A. R., Alvares, G. A., Carson, D. S., & Hickie, I. B. (2010). Intranasal arginine vasopressin enhances the encoding of happy and angry faces in humans. *Biological Psychiatry, 67,* 1220–1222.

Gurvits, I. G., Koenigsberg, H. W., & Siever, L. J. (2000). Neurotransmitter dysfunction in patients with borderline personality disorder. *Psychiatric Clinics of North America, 23,* 27–40.

Haller, J. (2013). The neurobiology of abnormal manifestations of aggression—a review of hypothalamic mechanisms in cats, rodents, and humans. *Brain Research Bulletin, 93,* 97–109.

Heim, C., Young, L. J., Newport, D. J., Mletzko, T., Miller, A. H., & Nemeroff, C. B. (2009). Lower CSF oxytocin concentrations in women with a history of childhood abuse. *Molecular Psychiatry, 14,* 954–958.

Hibbeln, J. R., Umhau, J. C., George, D. T., Shoaf, S. E., Linnoila, M., & Salem, N. (2000). Plasma total cholesterol concentrations do not predict cerebrospinal fluid neurotransmitter metabolites: Implications for the biophysical role of highly unsaturated fatty acids. *American Journal of Clinical Nutrition, 71,* 331S–338S.

Hoerst, M., Weber-Fahr, W., Tunc-Skarka, N., Ruf, M., Bohus, M., Schmahl, C., et al. (2010). Correlation of glutamate levels in the anterior cingulate cortex with self-reported impulsivity in patients with borderline personality disorder and healthy controls. *Archives of General Psychiatry, 67,* 946–954.

Hollander, E., Swann, A. C., Coccaro, E. F., Jiang, P., & Smith, T. B. (2005). Impact of trait impulsivity and state aggression on divalproex versus placebo response in borderline personality disorder. *American Journal of Psychiatry, 162,* 621–624.

Hurlemann, R., Patin, A., Onur, O. A., Cohen, M. X., Baumgartner, T., Metzler, S., et al. (2010). Oxytocin enhances amygdala-dependent, socially reinforced learning and emotional empathy in humans. *Journal of Neuroscience, 30,* 4999–5007.

Kety, S. S., Rosenthal, D., Wender, P. H., Schulsinger, F., & Jacobsen, B. (1976). Mental illness in the biological and adoptive families of adopted individuals who have become schizophrenic. *Behavior Genetics, 6,* 219–225.

Kirrane, R. M., Mitropoulou, V., Nunn, M., New, A. S., Harvey, P. D., Schopick, F., et al. (2000). Effects of amphetamine on visuospatial working memory performance in schizophrenia spectrum personality disorder. *Neuropsychopharmacology 22,* 14–18.

Kirrane, R. M., & Siever, L. J. (2000). New perspectives on schizotypal personality disorder. *Current Psychiatry Reports, 2,* 62–66.

Koch, W., Schaaff, N., Pöpperl, G., Mulert, C., Juckel, G., Reicherzer, M., et al. (2007). [I-123] ADAM and SPECT in patients with borderline personality disorder and healthy control subjects. *Journal of Psychiatry and Neuroscience, 32,* 234–240.

Kosfeld, M., Heinrichs, M., Zak, P. J., Fischbacher, U., & Fehr, E. (2005). Oxytocin increases trust in humans. *Nature, 435,* 673–676.

Krueger, R. F. (2005). Continuity of Axes I and II: Toward a unified model of personality, personality disorders, and clinical disorders. *Journal of Personality Disorders, 19,* 233–261.

Krueger, R. F., & Tackett, J. L. (2003). Personality and psychopathology: Working toward the bigger picture. *Journal of Personality Disorders, 17,* 109–128.

Laruelle, M. (2014). Schizophrenia: From dopaminergic to glutamatergic interventions. *Current Opinion in Pharmacology, 14,* 97–102.

Lee, R., Petty, F., & Coccaro, E. F. (2009). Cerebrospinal fluid GABA concentration: Relationship with impulsivity and history of suicidal behavior, but not aggression, in human subjects. *Journal of Psychiatric Research, 43,* 353–359.

Lester, D. (1995). The concentration of neurotransmitter metabolites in cerebrospinal fluid of suicidal individuals: A meta-analysis. *Pharmacopsychiatry, 28,* 45–50.

Leyton, M., Okazawa, H., Diksic, M., Paris, J., Rosa, P., Mzengeza, S., et al. (2001). Brain regional alpha-[$^{11}$C]methyl-L-tryptophan trapping in impulsive subjects with borderline personality disorder. *American Journal of Psychiatry, 158,* 775–782.

Lidberg, L., Tuck, J. R., Asberg, M., Scalia-Tomba, G. P., & Bertilsson, L. (1985). Homicide, suicide, and CSF 5-HIAA. *Acta Psychiatrica Scandinavica, 71,* 230–236.

Limson, R., Goldman, D., Roy, A., Lamparski, D., Ravitz, B., Adinoff, B., et al. (1991). Personality and cerebrospinal fluid monoamine metabolites in alcoholics and controls. *Archives of General Psychiatry, 48,* 437–441.

Linnoila, M., Virkkunen, M., Scheinin, M., Nuutila, A., Rimon, R., & Goodwin, F. (1983). Low cerebrospinal fluid 5-hydroxyindoleacetic acid concentration differentiates impulsive from nonimpulsive violent behavior. *Life Sciences, 33,* 2609–2614.

Linnoila, V. M., & Virkkunen, M. (1992). Aggression, suicidality, and serotonin. *Journal of Clinical Psychiatry, 53,* 46–51.

Livesley, W. J., Jang, K. L., & Vernon, P. A. (1998). Phenotypic and genetic structure of traits delineating personality disorder. *Archives of General Psychiatry, 55,* 941–948.

Lopez-Ibor, J. J., Saiz-Ruiz, J., & de los Cobos, J. C. P. (1985). Biological correlations of suicide and aggressivity in major depression (with melancholia): 5-hydroxyindoleacetic acid and cortisol in cerebral spinal fluid, dexamethasone suppression test and therapeutic response to 5-hydroxytroptophan. *Neuropsychobiology, 14,* 67–74.

Mann, J. J., McBride, P. A., & Bruce, S. (1986). Increased serotonin2 and beta-adrenergic receptor binding in the frontal cortices of suicide victims. *Archives of General Psychiatry, 43,* 954–959.

Markon, K. E., Krueger, R. F., & Watson, D. (2005). Delineating the structure of normal and abnormal personality: An integrative hierarchical approach. *Journal of Personality and Social Psychology, 88,* 139–157.

Marks, D. J., Miller, S. R., Schulz, K. P., Newcorn, J. H., & Halperin, J. M. (2007). The interaction of psychosocial adversity and biological risk in childhood aggression. *Psychiatry Research, 151,* 221–230.

Meltzer, H. Y., Perline, R., Tricou, B. J., Lowy, M., & Robertson, A. (1984). Effect of 5-hydroxytryptophan on serum cortisol levels in major affective disorders: II. Relation to suicide, psychosis, and depressive symptoms. *Archives of General Psychiatry, 41,* 379–387.

Meyer, J. H., Wilson, A. A., Rusjan, P., Clark, M., Houle, S., Woodside, S., et al. (2008). Serotonin 2A receptor binding potential in people with aggressive and violent behaviour. *Journal of Psychiatry and Neuroscience, 33,* 499–508.

Miczek, K. A., & Fish, E. W. (2005). Monoamines, GABA, glutamate, and aggression. In R. J. Nelson (Ed.), *Biology of aggression* (pp. 114–150). New York: Oxford University Press.

Miczek, K. A., Fish, E. W., De Bold, J. F., & De Almeida, R. M. M. (2002). Social and neural determinants of aggressive behavior: Pharmacotherapeutic targets at serotonin, dopamine and gamma-aminobutyric acid systems. *Psychopharmacology, 163,* 434–458.

Mitropoulou, V., Goodman, M., Sevy, S., Elman, I., New, A. S., Iskander, E. G., et al. (2004). Effects of acute metabolic stress on the dopaminergic and pituitary–adrenal axis activity in patients with schizotypal personality disorder. *Schizophrenia Research, 70,* 27–31.

Mitropoulou, V., Harvey, P. D., Maldari, L. A., Moriarty, P. J., New, A. S., Silverman, J. M., et al. (2002). Neuropsychological performance in schizotypal personality disorder: Evidence regarding diagnostic specificity. *Biological Psychiatry, 52,* 1175–1182.

Mitropoulou, V., Harvey, P. D., Zegarelli, G., New, A. S., Silverman, J. M., & Siever, L. J. (2005). Neuropsychological performance in schizotypal personality disorder: Importance of working memory. *American Journal of Psychiatry, 162,* 1896–1903.

Moeller, F. G., Steinberg, J. L., Petty, F., Fulton, M., Cherek, D. R., Kramer, G., et al. (1994). Serotonin and impulsive/aggressive behavior in cocaine dependent subjects. *Progress in Neuro-Psychopharmacology and Biological Psychiatry, 18,* 1027–1035.

Moore, T. M., Scarpa, A., & Raine, A. (2002). A meta-analysis of serotonin metabolite 5-HIAA and antisocial behavior. *Aggressive Behavior, 28,* 299–316.

Moss, H. B., Yao, J. K., & Panzak, G. L. (1990). Serotonergic responsivity and behavioral dimensions in antisocial personality disorder with substance abuse. *Biological Psychiatry, 28,* 325–338.

Nater, U. M., Bohus, M., Abbruzzese, E., Ditzen, B., Gaab, J., Kleindienst, N., et al. (2010). Increased psychological and attenuated cortisol and alpha-amylase responses to acute psychosocial stress in female patients with borderline personality disorder. *Psychoneuroendocrinology, 35,* 1565–1572.

Neumann, I. D., & Landgraf, R. (2012). Balance of brain oxytocin and vasopressin: Implications for anxiety, depression, and social behaviors. *Trends in Neurosciences, 35,* 649–659.

New, A. S., Hazlett, E. A., Buchsbaum, M. S., Goodman, M., Reynolds, D., Mitropoulou, V. S., et al. (2002). Blunted prefrontal cortical 18 fluorodeoxyglucose positron emission tomography response to meta-chlorophenylpiperazine in impulsive aggression. *Archives of General Psychiatry, 59,* 621–629.

New, A. S., Trestman, R. L., Mitropoulou, V., Benishay, D. S., Coccaro, E., Silverman, J., et al. (1997). Serotonergic function and self-injurious behavior in personality disorder patients. *Psychiatry Research, 69,* 17–26.

New, A. S., Trestman, R. F., Mitropoulou, V., Goodman, M., Koenigsberg, H. H., Silverman, J., et al. (2004). Low prolactin response to fenfluramine in impulsive aggression. *Journal of Psychiatric Research, 38,* 223–230.

Nieuwenhuis, S., Aston-Jones, G., & Cohen, J. D. (2005). Decision making, the P3, and the locus coeruleus-norepinephrine system. *Psychological Bulletin, 131,* 510–532.

Ninan, T., van Kammen, D. P. V., Scheinin, M., Linnoila, M., Bunney, W., & Goodwin, K. (1984). CSF 5-hydroxyindoleacetic acid levels in suicidal schizophrenic patients. *American Journal of Psychiatry, 141,* 566–569.

Nordin, C., Gupta, R. C., & Sjödin, I. (2007). Cerebrospinal fluid amino acids in pathological gamblers and healthy controls. *Neuropsychobiology, 56,* 152–158.

O'Keane, V., Moloney, E., O'Neill, H., O'Connor, A., Smith, C., & Dinan, T. G. (1992). Blunted prolactin responses to D-fenfluramine in sociopathy: Evidence for subsensitivity of central serotonergic function. *British Journal of Psychiatry, 160,* 643–646.

Olivier, B., & van Oorschot, R. (2005). 5-HT$_{1B}$ receptors and aggression: A review. *European Journal of Pharmacology, 526,* 207–217.

Oquendo, M. A., & Mann, J. J. (2000). The biology of impulsivity and suicidality. *Psychiatric Clinics of North America, 23,* 11–25.

Pare, C. M. B., Yeung, D. P. H., Price, K., & Stacey, R. S. (1969). 5-hydroxytryptamine, noradrenaline, and dopamine in brainstem, hypothalamus, and caudate nucleus of controls and of patients committing suicide by coal-gas poisoning. *Lancet, 2,* 133–135.

Paris, J. (2005). Neurobiological dimensional models

of personality: A review of the models of Cloninger, Depue, and Siever. *Journal of Personality Disorders, 19,* 156–170.

Paris, J., Zweig-Frank, H., Ng Ying Kin, N. M. K., Schwartz, G., Steiger, H., & Nair, N. P. V. (2004). Neurobiological correlates of diagnosis and underlying traits in patients with borderline personality disorder compared with normal controls. *Psychiatry Research, 121,* 239–252.

Pittenger, C. K., & Coric, V. (2005). Initial evidence of the beneficial effects of glutamate modulating agents in the treatment of self-injurious behavior associated with borderline personality disorder. *Journal of Clinical Psychiatry, 66,* 1492–1493.

Rilling, J. K., DeMarco, A. C., Hackett, P. D., Thompson, R., Ditzen, B., Patel, R., et al. (2012). Effects of intranasal oxytocin and vasopressin on cooperative behavior and associated brain activity in men. *Psychoneuroendocrinology, 37,* 4461–4474.

Rosell, D. R., Thompson, J. L., Slifstein, M., Xu, X., Frankle, W. G., New, A. S., et al. (2010). Increased serotonin 2A receptor availability in the orbitofrontal cortex of physically aggressive personality disordered patients. *Biological Psychiatry, 67,* 1154–1162.

Rüsch, N., Boeker, M., Büchert, M., Glauche, V., Bohrmann, C., Ebert, D., et al. (2010). Neurochemical alterations in women with borderline personality disorder and comorbid attention-deficit hyperactivity disorder. *World Journal of Biological Psychiatry, 11,* 372–381.

Schulz, S. C., Cornelius, J., Schulz, P. M., & Soloff, P. H. (1988). The amphetamine challenge test in patients with borderline disorder. *American Journal of Psychiatry, 145,* 809–814.

Schulz, S. C., Schulz, P. M., Dommisse, C., Hamer, R. M., Blackard, W. G., Narasimhachari, N., et al. (1985). Amphetamine response in borderline patients. *Psychiatry Research, 15,* 97–108.

Seo, D., Patrick, C. J., & Kennealy, P. J. (2008). Role of serotonin and dopamine system interactions in the neurobiology of impulsive aggression and its comorbidity with other clinical disorders. *Aggression and Violent Behavior, 13,* 383–395.

Serafini, G., Pompili, M., Elena Seretti, M., Stefani, H., Palermo, M., Coryell, W., et al. (2013). The role of inflammatory cytokines in suicidal behavior: A systematic review. *European Neuropsychopharmacology, 23,* 1672–1686.

Shamay-Tsoory, S. G., Fischer, M., Dvash, J., Harari, H., Perach-Bloom, N., & Levkovitz, Y. (2009). Intranasal administration of oxytocin increases envy and schadenfreude (gloating). *Biological Psychiatry, 66,* 864–870.

Shaw, D. M., Eccleston, E. G., & Camps, F. E. (1967). 5-Hydroxytryptamine in the hind-brain of depressive suicides. *British Journal of Psychiatry, 113,* 1407–1411.

Siegal, B. V., Mitropoulou, V., Amin, F., Kirrane, R., & Silverman, J. (1996). D-amphetamine challenge effects on Wisconsin Card Sort Test performance in schizotypal personality disorder. *Schizophrenia Research, 20,* 29–32.

Siever, L. J., Buchsbaum, M. S., New, A. S., Spiegel-Cohen, J., Wei, T., Hazlett, E. A., et al. (1999). D,L-fenfluramine response in impulsive personality disorder assessed with [18F]fluorodeoxyglucose positron emission tomography. *Neuropsychopharmacology, 20,* 413–423.

Siever, L. J., & Davis, K. L. (1991). A psychobiological perspective on the personality disorders. *American Journal of Psychiatry, 148,* 1647–1658.

Siever, L., & Trestman, R. L. (1993). The serotonin system and aggressive personality disorder. *International Clinical Psychopharmacology, 8,* 33–39.

Siever, L. J., & Weinstein, L. N. (2009). The neurobiology of personality disorders: Implications for psychoanalysis. *Journal of the American Psychoanalytic Association, 57,* 361–398.

Simeon, D., Bartz, J., Hamilton, H., Crystal, S., Braun, A., Ketay, S., et al. (2011). Oxytocin administration attenuates stress reactivity in borderline personality disorder: A pilot study. *Psychoneuroendocrinology, 36,* 1418–1421.

Simeon, D., Knutelska, M., Smith, L., Baker, B. R., & Hollander, E. (2007). A preliminary study of cortisol and norepinephrine reactivity to psychosocial stress in borderline personality disorder with high and low dissociation. *Psychiatry Research, 149,* 177–184.

Simeon, D., Stanley, B., Frances, A., Mann, J., Winchel, R., & Stanley, M. (1992). Self-mutilation in personality disorders: Psychological and biological correlates. *American Journal of Psychiatry, 149,* 221–226.

Soderstrom, H., Blennow, K., Manhem, A., & Forsman, A. (2001). CSF studies in violent offenders: I. 5-HIAA as a negative and HVA as a positive predictor of psychopathy. *Journal of Neural Transmission, 108,* 869–878.

Soderstrom, H., Blennow, K., Sjodin, A.-K., & Forsman, A. (2003). New evidence for an association between the CSF HVA:5-HIAA ratio and psychopathic traits. *Journal of Neurology, Neurosurgery, and Psychiatry, 74,* 918–921.

Soloff, P. H., Meltzer, C. C., Becker, C., Greer, P. J., & Constantine, D. (2005). Gender differences in a fenfluramine-activated FDG PET study of borderline personality disorder. *Psychiatry Research: Neuroimaging, 138,* 183–195.

Soloff, P. H., Price, J. C., Mason, N. S., Becker, C., & Meltzer, C. C. (2010). Gender, personality, and serotonin-2A receptor binding in healthy subjects. *Psychiatry Research, 181,* 77–84.

Southwick, S. M., Bremner, J. D., Rasmusson, A., Morgan, C. A., Arnsten, A., & Charney, D. S. (1999). Role of norepinephrine in the pathophysiology and treatment of posttraumatic stress disorder. *Biological Psychiatry, 46,* 1192–1204.

Spoont, M. R. (1992). Modulatory role of serotonin in neural information processing: Implications for human psychopathology. *Psychological Bulletin, 112,* 330–350.

Stanley, B., & Siever, L. J. (2010). The interpersonal dimension of borderline personality disorder: Toward a neuropeptide model. *American Journal of Psychiatry, 167,* 24–39.

Stanley, M., & Mann, J. J. (1983). Increased serotonin-2 binding sites in frontal cortex of suicide victims. *Lancet, 1,* 214–216.

Stanley, M., Traskman-Bendz, L., & Dorovini-Zis, K. (1985). Correlations between aminergic metabolites simultaneously obtained from human CSF and brain. *Life Sciences, 37,* 1279–1286.

Stanley, M., Virgilio, J., & Gershon, S. (1982). Tritiated imipramine binding sites are decreased in the frontal cortex of suicides. *Science, 216,* 1337–1339.

Sullivan, G. M., Coplan, J. D., Kent, J. M., & Gorman, J. M. (1999). The noradrenergic system in pathological anxiety: A focus on panic with relevance to generalized anxiety and phobias. *Biological Psychiatry, 46,* 1205–1218.

Taylor, S. E., Gonzaga, G. C., Klein, L. C., Hu, P., Greendale, G. A., & Seeman, T. E. (2006). Relation of oxytocin to psychological stress responses and hypothalamic–pituitary–adrenocortical axis activity in older women. *Psychosomatic Medicine, 68,* 238–245.

Taylor, S. E., Klein, L. C., Lewis, B. P., Gruenewald, T. L., Gurung, R. A. R., & Updegraff, J. A. (2000). Biobehavioral responses to stress in females: Tend-and-befriend, not fight-or-flight. *Psychological Review, 107,* 411–429.

Terburg, D., Morgan, B., & van Honk, J. (2009). The testosterone–cortisol ratio: A hormonal marker for proneness to social aggression. *International Journal of Law and Psychiatry, 32,* 216–223.

Thompson, R. R., George, K., Walton, J. C., Orr, S. P., & Benson, J. (2006). Sex-specific influences of vasopressin on human social communication. *Proceedings of the National Academy of Sciences USA, 16,* 7889–7894.

Thompson, R., Gupta, S., Miller, K., Mills, S., & Orr, S. (2004). The effects of vasopressin on human facial responses related to social communication. *Psychoneuroendocrinology, 29,* 35–48.

Träskman, L., Asberg, M., Bertilsson, L., & Sjöstrand, L. (1981). Monoamine metabolites in CSF and suicidal behavior. *Archives of General Psychiatry, 38,* 631–636.

Trull, T. J., & Durrett, C. A. (2005). Categorical and dimensional models of personality disorder. *Annual Review of Clinical Psychology, 1,* 355–380.

Uzefovsky, F., Shalev, I., Israel, S., Knafo, A., & Ebstein, R. P. (2012). Vasopressin selectively impairs emotion recognition in men. *Psychoneuroendocrinology, 37,* 576–580.

van Praag, H. M. (1983). CSF 5-HIAA and suicide in non-depressed schizophrenics. *Lancet, 2,* 977–978.

Vaz-Leal, F. J., Rodríguez-Santos, L., García-Herráiz, M. A., & Ramos-Fuentes, M. I. (2011). Neurobiological and psychopathological variables related to emotional instability: A study of their capability to discriminate patients with bulimia nervosa from healthy controls. *Neuropsychobiology, 63,* 242–251.

Virkkunen, M., De Jong, J., Bartko, J., Goodwin, F. K., & Linnoila, M. (1989). Relationship of psychobiological variables to recidivism in violent offenders and impulsive fire setters: A follow-up study. *Archives of General Psychiatry, 46*(7), 600–603.

Virkkunen, M., Nuutila, A., Goodwin, F. K., & Linnoila, M. (1987). Cerebrospinal fluid monoamine metabolite levels in male arsonists. *Archives of General Psychiatry, 44,* 241–247.

Virrkunen, M., Rawlings, R., Tokola, R., Poland, R. E., Guidotti, A., Nemeroff, C., et al. (1994). CSF biochemistries, glucose metabolism, and diurnal activity rythms in alcoholic, violent offenders, fire setters, and healthy volunteers. *Archives of General Psychiatry, 51,* 20–27.

Widiger, T. A., & Costa, P. T. (2012). Integrating normal and abnormal personality structure: The Five-Factor Model. *Journal of Personality, 80,* 1471–1506.

Wilcock, G. K., Ballard, C. G., Cooper, J. A., & Loft, H. (2008). Memantine for agitation/aggression and psychosis in moderately severe to severe Alzheimer's disease: A pooled analysis of 3 studies. *Journal of Clinical Psychiatry, 69,* 341–348.

Wolkowitz, O. M., & Cowdry, R. W. (1987). Dysphoria associated with methylphenidate infusion in borderline personality disorder. *American Journal of Psychiatry, 144,* 1577–1579.

Woodward, N. D., Cowan, R. L., Park, S., Ansari, M. S., Baldwin, R. M., Li, R., et al. (2011). Correlation of individual differences in schizotypal personality traits with amphetamine-induced dopamine release in striatal and extrastriatal brain regions. *American Journal of Psychiatry, 168,* 418–426.

Wozniak, J., Gonenc, A., Biederman, J., Moore, C., Joshi, G., Georgiopoulos, A., et al. (2012). A magnetic resonance spectroscopy study of the anterior cingulate cortex in youth with emotional dysregulation. *Israel Journal of Psychiatry and Related Sciences, 49,* 62–69.

Yildirim, B. O., & Derksen, J. J. (2012). A review on the relationship between testosterone and the interpersonal/affective facet of psychopathy. *Psychiatry Research, 197,* 181–198.

Zimmerman, D. J., & Choi-Kain, L. W. (2009). The hypothalamic–pituitary–adrenal axis in borderline personality disorder: A review. *Harvard Review of Psychiatry, 17,* 167–183.

Zink, C. F., Kempf, L., Hakimi, S., Rainey, C. A., Stein, J. L., & Meyer-Lindenberg, A. (2011). Vasopressin modulates social recognition-related activity in the left temporoparietal junction in humans. *Translational Psychiatry, 1,* e3.

Zink, C. F., Stein, J. L., Kempf, L., Hakimi, S., & Meyer-Lindenberg, A. (2010). Vasopressin modulates medial prefrontal cortex–amygdala circuitry during emotion processing in humans. *Journal of Neuroscience, 30,* 7017–7022.

# CHAPTER 15

# Emotional Regulation and Emotional Processing

Paul H. Soloff

> We shall define an emotion as that which leads one's condition to become so transformed that his judgment is affected, and which is accompanied by pleasure and pain.
> —ARISTOTLE

## Definitions

What is emotion? The nature of emotion has intrigued philosophers and scientists across time, giving rise to a bewildering array of competing perspectives. Theories of emotion include cognitive, cultural, and evolutionary perspectives, which deal with the awareness and meaning of emotion, as well as physiological and neurological models, which address the biological substrate (Plutchik, 2001; Solomon, 2003). For this review, I focus narrowly on contributions of recent neuroimaging studies to advance our understanding of emotion and its regulation. Defining the neurobiology of emotion and disorders of emotion regulation will inform our clinical understanding of patients with severe personality disorders (PDs) (Putnam & Silk, 2005).

Following in the footsteps of William James and Walter Cannon, a contemporary neurobiologist, Antonio Damasio, defines emotion as a neurological response to stimuli that originate generally, but not exclusively, in the external world, and are experienced through our senses. These perceptions find mental representation as "neural maps" in regions of the brain dedicated to that purpose (e.g., sight to the visual association area). Changes in these mental representations trigger innate physiological responses in the body ("action programs"), which give rise to emotions or drives. Bodily changes produced by the physiology of emotion are experienced as "feelings" once they also attain mental representation. In this theory, emotions include disgust, fear, anger, sadness, joy, shame, contempt, pride, compassion, and admiration. Drives address more basic instinctual needs such as hunger and thirst (Damasio & Carvalho, 2013). This neurobiological model provides a useful framework for interpreting the results of modern neuroimaging studies, especially functional magnetic resonance imaging (fMRI) protocols that illuminate the neural response to cognitive and sensory inputs. However, to study emotion in the clinical setting, a more interactive, psychosocial perspective is needed.

Gross and Thompson (2006, p. 5) define emotion as a state arising from a "person–situation transaction" that compels *attention*, has particular *meaning* to an individual, and gives rise to a coordinated yet flexible multisystem *response* to the ongoing person–situation transaction. The response can be adaptive and organizing, or maladaptive and deviant. (This psychosocial definition usefully extends the neural theory of emotion into the realm of social interaction.) Writers from Aristotle to Freud have emphasized the disruptive potential of emotion to affect cognition and behavior, and the importance of mature emotion regulation for the healthy personality. "Emotion regulation" includes any process that amplifies, attenuates, or maintains an emotion (Davidson, Putnam, & Larson, 2000). "Emotion *dys*regulation" is a term applied to emotional responses that are poorly controlled, disorganizing, and impair functioning. As part of a behavioral pattern, these emotional responses give rise to symptoms of psychopathology (Cole, Michel, & Teti, 1994).

Emotion regulation is a neuropsychological process that involves both voluntary and automatic regulation of emotion in the brain. Voluntary regulation of emotion includes conscious cognitive processes, such as refocusing attention, reframing, reappraisal, distancing, and suppression. These cognitive techniques facilitate response modification (e.g., selecting alternative behaviors such as exercise or relaxation techniques to reduce the impact of negative emotion). Automatic regulation of emotion involves the rapid and unconscious interaction of cortical and limbic neural networks in the appraisal of the emotional properties of stimuli, facilitation (or inhibition) of responses, and appraisal of outcomes. Automatic appraisal of outcomes can result in conditioning of future behavioral responses or extinction learning (Putnam & Silk, 2005).

## Emotion Regulation in Healthy Subjects

Neurobiological models of emotion regulation have been developed using fMRI paradigms that require cognitive task performance in the presence of affectively valenced stimuli (e.g., aversive faces or pictures). These protocols model affective interference with cognitive processing and identify brain networks activated in emotion generation and its regulation. Although this research is still in a developmental stage, there is emerging consensus among fMRI researchers that emotion generation and regulation in healthy subjects involve "bottom-up" appraisal and arousal originating in the limbic system and basal ganglia, and "top-down" cognitive control processes originating in the ventral, dorsal, and medial regions of the prefrontal cortex (PFC) and the anterior cingulate cortex (ACC). The PFC exercises tonic control over limbic arousal, such that emotion regulation occurs simultaneously with emotion generation. As a result, emotion in healthy adults is almost always modified (Davidson et al., 2000; Gross & Thompson, 2006; Ochsner & Gross, 2006; Phillips, Ladouceur, & Drevets, 2008).

Major components of the "bottom-up" neural network include the amygdala, the insula, the hippocampus, the basal ganglia, the ventral striatum, the nucleus accumbens, and paralimbic structures. The amygdala (AMY) appraises and responds to the affective salience of stimuli, especially facial expressions. (In fMRI studies, the AMY is activated by negatively valenced faces and aversive pictures. It is involved in fearful and angry responding.) The insula processes negative emotional states (e.g., disgust), and conveys subjective awareness of internal bodily states to higher cortical centers. In fMRI studies, the insula is also activated by tasks involving trust and cooperation (King-Casas et al., 2008). The hippocampus (HIP) processes declarative, episodic, and working memory, and facilitates decision making through connections to regulatory centers in PFC. The basal ganglia, ventral striatum, and nucleus accumbens are involved in reward-based decisions, especially those involving immediate versus delayed gratification. Finally, paralimbic structures such as the fusiform, parahippocampal, and lingual gyrii contribute associative memory data on familiarity of faces and scenes (Augustine, 1996; Belin, Jonkman, Dickinson, Robbins, & Everitt, 2009; Dombrovski et al., 2012; New, Goodman, Triebwasser, & Siever, 2008; Peters & Buchel, 2010; Radua et al., 2010; Ruocco, Amirthavasagam, & Zakzanis, 2012; Wall & Messier, 2001).

The "top-down" PFC areas process mental representations of emotional states, assess the properties of stimuli, direct responses, and assess outcomes (Ochsner & Gross, 2006). Major components of the "top-down" neural system include the orbitofrontal cortex (OFC), the ACC, and the dorsolateral prefrontal cortex (DLPFC). The OFC is important for response inhibition and executive decision making. In concert with the ACC, the OFC appraises external stimuli for response, focuses attention, regulates expression of affect and impulse, and motivates adaptive responses. The OFC exerts tonic control over limbic arousal through extensive connections to the AMY. The ACC is involved in focused attention, conflict resolution, error detection, emotion regulation, and reappraisal. The DLPFC is notable for emotion-regulating cognitive strategies such as suppression and reappraisal, and for working memory (Barbas, 2007; Bledowski, Rahm, & Rowe, 2009; Bonelli & Cummings, 2007; Bush, Luu, & Posner, 2000; Carter et al., 2000; Fletcher & Henson, 2001; Tekin & Cummings, 2002). Additional areas are engaged according to the cognitive demands of the specific task (e.g., visual recognition tasks engage the superior parietal cortex/precuneus, episodic memory tasks engage the HIP, etc.).

Voluntary regulation of emotion includes suppression of emotional expression, inhibition, and reappraisal (Phillips, Ladouceur, et al., 2008). fMRI studies of healthy subjects suggest that voluntary suppression of emotion most consistently activates areas of the right DLPFC and the left ventrolateral prefrontal cortex (VLPFC), though other areas may be engaged depending on the cognitive demands of the task. Voluntary inhibition activates the bilateral DLPFC, the right dorsal ACC, and the right parietal cortex, with some variations in laterality dependent on emotional valence of the test stimulus. Voluntary cognitive change through reappraisal (re-interpreting the meaning of a stimulus to down-regulate emotional response) is associated with activation of bilateral DLPFC, dorsomedial PFC, and dorsal ACC. Suppression, inhibition, and reappraisal may share a common mediation through the OFC and its extensive connections to the limbic system (Phillips, Ladouceur, et al., 2008). Distancing is a form of cognitive reappraisal in which the subject consciously down-regulates emotional responses to aversive social situations. In an fMRI paradigm in which subjects are asked to "distance" themselves from emotional responses to aversive pictures, the neural response includes increased activation in dorsal ACC, medial and lateral PFC, precuneus and posterior cingulate, intraparietal sulci, and middle-superior temporal gyrus. As these cortical structures are engaged, activation in the amygdala is decreased (Koenigsberg et al., 2010).

Automatic behavior control includes extinction learning of previously acquired behavior and aversive conditioning. Bilateral ACC and OFC play a prominent role in these functions. Automatic attention control (e.g., disengagement of attention away from an emotional stimulus) engages the function of the rostral ACC. Automatic cognitive change, such as covert error monitoring or risk learning, implicit appraisal or reappraisal, behavior monitoring, and rule learning, engage the functions of bilateral OFC and dorsomedial PFC, dorsal ACC, bilateral HIP, and parahippocampal gyrus.

A comprehensive neural model of emotion regulation proposed by Phillips, Travis, Fagiolini, and Kupfer (2008) suggests that a lateral PFC system (i.e., DLPFC and VLPFC) processes voluntary emotion regulation, while automatic emotion regulation is processed by a medial PFC system, including dorsomedial PFC, OFC, and ACC.

## Emotion Dysregulation in Patients with PDs

The capacity to experience and regulate a wide range of emotions is a hallmark of a healthy personality (American Psychiatric Association, 2013a, Section III, p. 672). Emotion dysregulation is a core clinical symptom of PDs, though it is most closely associated with the "dramatic, emotional, erratic" patients of Cluster B. Emotion dysregulation is explicitly represented in diagnostic criteria for borderline PD (BPD; as "a marked reactivity of mood," "inappropriate, intense anger or difficulty controlling anger" [p. 663]), and histrionic PD (HPD; as "a pervasive pattern of excessive emotionality," "rapid shifting and shallow expression of emotions," and "exaggerated expression of emotion" [p. 667]), and indirectly represented in the criteria for antisocial PD (ASPD; as "irritability and aggressiveness" [p. 659]) (American Psychiatric Association, 2013b). Most empirical studies of emotion dysregulation in subjects with PD have been conducted in the context of BPD. (The clinical literature uses the terms "affective instability," "affective dysregulation" and "emotion dysregulation" interchangeably to describe the brief but extreme mood shifts that characterize response to emotional stress.) The research focus on affective instability in BPD may be related, in part, to its clinical importance as core feature of the disorder, and, importantly, as a risk factor for the suicidal threats, gestures, and acts that characterize this disorder (Koenigsberg et al., 2001). In the Collaborative Longitudinal Personality Disorders Study (CLPDS), affective instability was the only diagnostic criterion for BPD that predicted suicide attempts at the 2-year follow-up (Yen et al., 2004).

## Neuropsychological Studies in BPD

Patients with BPD report being "more sensitive" to emotional cues than their peers. In experimental studies, they experience emotions more strongly than do healthy controls, especially in response to negative affect, and are slower to return to baseline once aroused (Jacob et al., 2008; Levine, Marziali, & Hood, 1997). Studies using 24-hour ambulatory monitoring of subjects with BPD revealed heightened affective instability compared to control subjects, manifested by more sudden, large decreases from positive to negative mood states, more negative emotions, and frequent switches from anxiety to sadness and anger. Subjects with BPD were more likely to have conflicting emotions and greater inability identifying specific emotions in themselves compared to controls (Ebner-Priemer, Kuo, et al., 2007; Ebner-Priemer et al., 2008; Ebner-Priemer, Welch, et al., 2007; Reisch, Ebner-Priemer, Tschacher, Bohus, & Linehan, 2008). In experimental studies, subjects with BPD are hypersensitive to facial expressions of emotions in others compared to controls (Schulze, Domes, Köppen, & Herpertz, 2013). While especially sensitive to angry faces, they also tend to see neutral faces as fearful. Heightened detection of emotion (in others), but relative impairment in labeling of emotions (in self and others) may contribute to emotional instability and suggests an impairment in cognitive processing of emotional data (Schulze et al., 2013).

Neuropsychological studies among subjects with BPD have long demonstrated deficits in executive cognitive functions, though no single pattern is diagnostic. Deficits have been described in planning, attention, cognitive flexibility, processing speed, learning and memory, and visuospatial ability (Ruocco, 2005). These impairments are documented in baseline testing and are not attributable to comorbid major depression, alcohol abuse, or low IQ (O'Leary, 2000). In the presence of negatively valenced stimuli, subjects with BPD perform more poorly than controls on standardized tests of executive cognitive function (Fertuck, Lenzenweger, Clarkin, Hoermann, & Stanley, 2006; Silbersweig et al., 2007). This "affective interference" with cognitive processing is an exaggeration of the process found in healthy subjects. In fMRI studies, emotional distractors diminish the neural response associated with task performance. Conversely, increased concentration on task performance diminishes the neural response to emotional stimuli. Emotion modulates cognition, and cognition modulates emotion (Blair et al., 2007). Neuroimaging studies in subjects with BPD report structural (MRI) and metabolic (positron emission tomography [PET]) abnormalities in brain networks involved in control of emotion, impulse, and behavior. Taken together, these abnormalities suggest a neurobiological vulnerability to cognitive, emotional, and behavioral dysregulation in BPD.

## Neuroimaging Studies in BPD
### MRI Studies

Structural studies in subjects with BPD compared to healthy controls indicate volume loss and diminished grey-matter concentrations in areas of the frontal cortex and PFC, including OFC, DLPFC, and ACC (Hazlett et al., 2005; Sala et al., 2011; Tebartz van Elst et al., 2003). Diminished grey matter in OFC (Brodmann area [BA] 10) and ACC (BA 24), and increased white-matter volumes in VLPFC (orbital inferior frontal gyrus, BA 47), correlate with increased impulsivity, irritability, and assaultiveness (Hazlett et al., 2005). Volume loss is also reported in insular and temporal cortex. Diminished volume in the insula discriminates between suicide attempters with BPD and non-attempters with BPD (Soloff et al., 2012). The most widely replicated findings in morphometric MRI studies of BPD involve loss of volume in HIP (with and without diminished volume in AMY) (Hazlett et al., 2005; Lyoo, Han, & Cho, 1998; Rüsch et al., 2003; Sala et al., 2011; Schmahl & Bremner, 2006; Soloff, Nutche, Goradia, & Diwadkar, 2008; Soloff et al., 2012; Tebartz van Elst et al., 2003; Zetzsche et al., 2007). In some studies, diminished HIP volumes in BPD have been associated with childhood histories of trauma and abuse, which are developmental factors in the etiology of BPD and risk factors for adult suicidal behavior (Brambilla et al., 2004; Driessen et al., 2000; Irle, Lange, & Sachsse, 2005; Schmahl, Vermetten, Elzinga, & Bremner, 2003)

### PET Studies

PET studies in subjects with BPD report decreased metabolic function in areas that overlap regions of reported structural abnormality in MRI studies. These include areas of PFC, including OFC and ventromedial cortex, cingulate gyrus, and temporal cortex (Schmahl & Bremner, 2006). These structures are part of the neural network involved in emotion regulation and behavioral inhibition.

Among subjects with BPD (and other impulsive subjects with PDs) diminished glucose utilization (hypometabolism) in areas of OFC, anterior medial frontal cortex, and right temporal cortex is associated with impulsive aggression (Goyer et al., 1994). Bilateral hypometabolism in the medial OFC (BA 9, BA 10, BA 11), is reported among female subjects with BPD and is related to measures of impulsivity and aggression (Soloff, Kelly, Strotmeyer, Malone, & Mann, 2003). Impulsive aggression may be viewed as a behavioral subset of emotion dysregulation. These two PD traits may share a common neural mediation. Negative emotion triggers aggressive behavior (Davidson et al., 2000; Putnam & Silk, 2005; Siever, 2008).

Impulsive aggression is a core characteristic of patients with BPD, intermittent explosive disorder (IED), and other impulsive PDs, and is related to diminished central serotonergic function (Oquendo & Mann, 2000). Subjects with BPD (and other impulsive PDs) have diminished metabolic responses to d,l fenfluramine (FEN), or meta-chlorophenylpiperazine (mCPP), serotonergic challenge agents used in PET studies (New et al., 2002; Siever et al., 1999; Soloff, Meltzer, et al., 2003; Soloff, Meltzer, Greer, Constantine, & Kelly, 2000). Following challenge with FEN or mCPP, relative to healthy controls, subjects with BPD (and other impulsive PDs) demonstrate blunted cortical metabolic responses in the OFC, adjacent ventromedial PFC, and cingulate cortex, *areas overlapping those with structural abnormalities in BPD* (New et al., 2002; Siever et al., 1999; Soloff, Kelly, et al., 2003; Soloff et al., 2000). In an mCPP-augmented PET study, New and colleagues (2007) reported diminished connectivity between the OFC and AMY among subjects with BPD and IED compared to healthy controls. Tight coupling of metabolic activity between right OFC and ventral AMY, which is normally present in healthy control subjects, was not present in the BPD–IED group, suggesting a loss of tonic inhibitory control over impulsive aggression and emotion in the subjects with PD.

It is important to note that these structural and metabolic abnormalities in frontolimbic networks in subjects with BPD subjects *do not prove* functional impairment. However, they may adversely affect network connectivity, contributing a chronic vulnerability to emotion dysregulation and impulsive aggression under emotional stress. The vulnerability to emotion dysregulation is best studied using fMRI or functional PET techniques that examine neural responses to affectively valenced stimuli (e.g., happy, sad, angry, fearful, or neutral Ekman faces; positive, negative, or neutral International Affective Picture System [IAPS] pictures; emotional words; or painful personal scripts) (Ekman & Friesen, 1976; Lang & Cuthbert, 2001). When paired with cognitive tasks, the affective context may impair cognitive processing ("affective interference"), revealing neural pathways of emotion dysregulation. A shortcoming of these methods is that faces and pictures may not elicit actual emotion, which can only be inferred through self-report or physiological measures (Davidson & Irwin, 1999).

## Functional MRI

Viewing emotional faces or aversive pictures results in "bottom-up" hyperarousal of the AMY in subjects with BPD compared to controls (Donegan et al., 2003; Herpertz et al., 2001). In the Herpertz and colleagues (2001) study, subjects with BPD, selected for affective instability, also demonstrated increased activation in the fusiform gyrus (a limbic area involved in facial recognition), and in the left medial PFC (BA 10) and right VLPFC (BA 47), (involved in "top-down" cortical regulation of emotion). Koenigsberg and colleagues (2009) also reported increased activation in the AMY and fusiform gyrus in subjects with BPD compared to healthy controls when viewing negative pictures from the IAPS.

The balance between limbic hyperarousal and cortical regulation in subjects with BPD has been studied with fMRI using behavioral tasks that incorporate affectively valenced stimuli to interfere with cognitive processing of task performance. In an "emotional" linguistic go/no-go task, a task demand (go/no-go) is coupled with emotional words (Goldstein et al., 2007). In subjects with BPD, compared to healthy controls, Silbersweig and colleagues (2007) found relatively decreased activity levels in the medial OFC and subgenual ACC (i.e., structures mediating inhibition), and increased activity in the AMY bilaterally during the condition pairing negative emotion (negative words) with an inhibitory command (no-go). In an "emotional" Stroop task, in which subjects have to name colors in which affectively valenced words are written, healthy controls activated the ACC bilaterally, the right OFC, the right pre- and postcentral gyrus, the left middle temporal gyrus, the HIP, and the cuneus in response to negative versus neutral words. Subjects with BPD showed no differences in activation between conditions. They *failed* to show the expected pattern of activation found in healthy control subjects (Wingenfeld et al., 2009). Minzenberg, Fan, New, Tang, and Siever (2007) found significantly larger *deactivation* in subjects with BPD (relative to normal controls) in the rostral/subgenual ACC bilaterally in response to fearful Ekman faces, and in the left ACC in response to fearful versus neutral faces. Koenigsberg and colleagues (2009) used a cognitive reappraisal task in which subjects with BPD were asked to psychically distance themselves and suppress negative emotional experience while viewing aversive IAPS pictures. They were *less efficient* than control subjects in activating the ACC during the suppression task. The ACC is prominently involved in error detection, conflict resolution, and emotion regulation. In the negative affective context, activation of the ACC in subjects with BPD is diminished in these tasks relative to healthy controls.

### Imaging Borderline Psychopathology

Some PET and fMRI studies have incorporated stimuli related to borderline psychopathology in their functional paradigms in order to assess the neural processing of negative emotion in this disorder. In an [$O^{15}$] PET study, Schmahl and colleagues (2003) used autobiographical accounts of abandonment experiences ("abandonment scripts") to measure cerebral blood flow (CBF) in abused female subjects with BPD (compared to non-BPD abused females). CBF was *decreased* in these subjects in an extensive frontolimbic network that included areas of the medial and inferior frontal gyrus, ACC, superior and middle temporal gyrus, HIP–AMY complex, fusiform gyrus, and thalamus. In their "emotional linguistic go/no-go" task (described earlier), Silbersweig and colleagues (2007) paired an inhibitory task and negative emotional words having special salience for subjects with BPD. Beblo and colleagues (2006) used personalized cue words to stimulate recall of actual adverse life events ("unresolved vs. resolved negative events") defined in advance by interview. Increased activation was noted in the ACC and left posterior cingulate (involved in emotion regulation), as well as the AMY (also in the right occipital cortex, bilateral cerebellum, and midbrain). However, patients with BPD reported higher levels of anxiety and helplessness during recall of unresolved negative life experiences, suggesting a relative failure of cortical inhibition in the face of limbic hyperarousal.

Self-injurious behavior (SIB) is often a behavioral response to emotion dysregulation in patients with BPD. Subjects with BPD and histories of SIB showed significantly *less activation* in the OFC compared with controls after listening to a standardized script describing emotions leading up to an act of self-injury. They had increased activation in DLPFC while imagining the circumstances triggering the SIB, and decreased activation in the posterior ACC while imagining the act itself (Kraus et al., 2010). The DLPFC is involved in working memory, and evaluation and selection of behavioral responses, while the ACC evaluates the need for cognitive controls. Deactivation of both the OFC and ACC suggests decreased inhibition. With OFC and ACC relatively "offline," impulsive SIB is more likely to occur.

Intolerance of being alone is a core characteristic of BPD, related to attachment trauma in early life. Buchheim and colleagues (2008) studied the emotional response to recall of attachment trauma by scanning subjects with BPD while they viewed pictures illustrating attachment threats experienced alone ("monadic" pictures), or in the company of others ("dyadic" pictures). Patients with BPD were more fearful viewing attachment threats experienced alone than control subjects, and had stronger activation of the anterior mid-cingulate cortex. Buchheim and colleagues suggest that this activation is an effort to inhibit emotional pain. In viewing dyadic pictures, subjects with BPD had greater activation of the right superior temporal sulcus (STS) and less activation of the right parahippocampal gyrus compared to controls. The STS is involved in "thinking about others" and in this setting may reflect "fear-based hypervigilence in attachment relationships," suggestive of rejection sensitivity. The parahippocampus is activated by memory tasks, especially memories encoded in a positive emotional context (in healthy subjects).

## Effects of Negative Emotion on Cognitive Processing in BPD

In subjects with BPD, emotion dysregulation, impulsive aggression, and impaired executive cognitive function may be related to the effects of negative emotion on chronically vulnerable neural networks. To test this hypothesis, Soloff, White, and Diwadkar (2014) created fMRI paradigms that specifically targeted brain regions reported to be abnormal in BPD, and investigated the neural effects of negative affect on cognitive processing in each of those areas. An affective go/no-go task and an affective continuous performance task (X-CPT) used Ekman faces and targeted the OFC and ACC, respectively. An affective episodic memory task used affectively valenced IAPS pictures and targeted the HIP. The negative affective context in the go/no-go task (i.e., Negative > Positive faces), resulted in *decreased* activation in the OFC of subjects with BPD relative to controls, and increased activation in AMY. In the X-CPT protocol, subjects with BPD had *increased* activation in the ACC in the negative affective context. In memory encoding and retrieval of Negative > Positive pictures, subjects with BPD had *decreased* HIP activation compared to controls. Negative affective interference with cognitive processing was associated with functional impairment in the OFC, ACC, HIP, and AMY and associated structures of subjects with BPD compared to control subjects. Disordered function in frontolimbic networks that include these structures compromises adaptive responding, especially in social situations involving strong negative emotion. Functional impairment in these networks contributes a chronic neural vulnerability to the emotional dysregulation, impulsive aggression, and executive cognitive deficits of patients with BPD.

## Emotion Regulation in Psychotherapy and Pharmacotherapy

Functional neuroimaging techniques, such as PET and fMRI, demonstrate neural changes in patients responding to psychotherapy in psychiatric disorders as diverse as obsessive–compulsive disorder (OCD), major depressive disorder (MDD), and anxiety disorders (panic disorder, social phobia, spider phobia), using treatment modalities including exposure therapy, cognitive-behavioral therapy (CBT), and interpersonal psychotherapy (IPT) (Beauregard, 2007; Beutel, Stern, & Silbersweig, 2003; Roffman, Marci, Glick, Dougherty, & Rauch, 2005). The number of neuroimaging studies documenting neural changes with pharmacotherapy far exceeds those in psychotherapy. Among treatment responders, neural changes are related to the pathophysiology of the psychiatric disorder (demonstrated in pretreatment imaging studies) and involve "normalization" of neural structure and function in patients compared to healthy controls (e.g., normalization of HIP volume in PTSD following selective serotonin reuptake inhibitor [SSRI] treatment; Thomaes et al., 2014). Psychotherapy and pharmacotherapy may achieve similar clinical efficacy but differ in the specific neural mechanisms of change. While there may be areas of overlap, brain changes in structure and function may not be identical for the two modalities. Effects of psychotherapy on brain function vary with treatment modality. Cognitive techniques such as shifting attention, suppression, reappraisal, exposure, and extinction learning engage different neural networks. For example, extinction learning engages the ventromedial PFC to regulate AMY responses; suppression and reappraisal activate the DLPFC (Goldin, McRae, Ramel, & Gross, 2008; Ochsner, Bunge, Gross, & Gabrieli, 2002). Similarly, neural effects of medication differ depending on targeted neurotransmitter systems. A general theoretical model suggests that pharmacotherapies target emotion dysregulation in frontolimbic networks (e.g., primarily modulating "bottom-up" hyperarousal), while psychotherapies, such as CBT, target frontal lobe processing abnormalities (e.g., modulating "top-down" cognitive functions) (Beauregard, 2007).

Successful treatment with psychotherapy or pharmacotherapy decreases biases in responding to emotion associated with psychiatric symptoms such as depression or anxiety (Thomaes et al., 2014). For example, SSRI treatment in depressed patients decreases AMY reactivity to emotional processing paradigms, while increasing activation in the DLPFC and ACC. Successful treatment of depression with SSRI antidepressants is associated with increased functional connectivity between these prefrontal cortical regions and limbic structures (Murphy, 2010). Among healthy volunteers, SSRI antidepressants also reduce activation in emotion processing paradigms in the AMY, middle insula, and posterior insula compared to placebo. Decreases in activation are also noted in medial PFC and ventral ACC, which are felt to be secondary to the decrease in AMY activity (Murphy, 2010). Depressed patients who are placebo responders to antidepressant treatment demonstrate neural changes similar to active medication responders, raising the possibility that these neural changes may be a *consequence* of improvement rather than a cause. Neuroimaging studies of the placebo response to medication for nonpsychiatric indications (e.g., Parkinson's disease, analgesia) suggest that neural responses, identical to those with active medication, may occur as a result of strong expectation of symptom relief (Beauregard, 2007; Rutherford, Wager, & Roose, 2010).

There is a paucity of imaging studies of psychotherapy in patients with PDs. Schnell and Herpertz (2007) studied the treatment response to 12 weeks of Dialectical Behavior Therapy (DBT) in six female in-patients with BPD (compared to six healthy controls). fMRI protocols involved passive viewing of aversive pictures in five scanning sessions (before, during, and after treatment). Viewing aversive IAPS pictures reliably induced activations in AMY in prior studies among BPD subjects (Herpertz et al., 2001). Over the course of treatment, BPD patients as a group showed diminished reactivity to negative pictures. Among the four DBT responders, there was continuous reduction in hemodynamic modulation in lt. AMY and bilateral HIP, corresponding to diminished subjective reactivity to the negative aversive stimuli. The effects of DBT on decreasing AMY activation would enhance emotion regulation.

Dialectical behavior therapy (DBT) was developed as a treatment for suicidal behavior in patients with BPD, with an important focus on improving emotion regulation through cognitive skills training (Linehan, 1993). DBT uses cognitive strategies to teach four core principles: (1) "mindfulness" (concentrating attention on the present experience in a nonjudgmental way), (2) "distress tolerance" (dealing with emotional pain), (3) "emotion regulation" (reducing the disruptive impact of emotion), and (4) "interpersonal effectiveness" (communicating needs effectively). Cognitive-behavioral techniques, such as focused attention ("one-mind"), distraction, suppression, reappraisal, and distancing are widely used in DBT, CBT, and other cognitive-behavioral psychotherapies to regulate emotional responses. Psychodynamic therapies, while less directive, also address self-regulation of emotion and behavior as they arise in the context of interpersonal relationships (IPT) or the transference relationship with the therapist (e.g., transference-focused psychotherapy, psychoanalytic psychotherapies). Clarification and interpretation, the traditional tools of insight-oriented therapies, help patients acknowledge, bear, and put into perspective painful emotional experience.

Beauregard (2007) has proposed a general neural model for self-regulation (and change) in psychotherapy built on imaging studies of emotion regulation in healthy subjects (reviewed earlier). The process of change begins in the lateral PFC (BA 9, BA 10), which selects an appropriate cognitive strategy for down-regulating disruptive emotions. This is followed by activation of the OFC (BA 11), which modulates emotion directly through its connectivity to the AMY. The AMY reappraises the emotional significance of the stimulus, down-regulating fearful or angry emotional responses. Simultaneously, the OFC acts through connections to the rostral ventral ACC to modulate the physiology of response, and through the medial PFC (BA 10) to mediate self-conscious awareness of the process, which facilitates learning.

All psychotherapy involves emotional self-regulation and learning, which are mediated through changes in neural networks. Future neuroimaging studies may identify the treatment interventions that are most effective in regulating emotion, impulsivity, and aggression in patients with PDs.

## REFERENCES

American Psychiatric Association. (2013a). Alternative DSM-5 model for personality disorders. In *Diagnostic and statistical manual of mental disorders* (5th ed., pp. 761–781). Arlington, VA: Author.

American Psychiatric Association. (2013b). Antisocial personality disorder. In *Diagnostic and statistical manual of mental disorders* (5th ed., pp. 659–663). Arlington, VA: Author.

American Psychiatric Association. (2013c). Borderline personality disorder. In *Diagnostic and statistical manual of mental disorders* (5th ed., pp. 663–666). Arlington, VA: Author.

American Psychiatric Association. (2013d). Histrionic personality disorder. In *Diagnostic and statistical manual of mental disorders* (5th ed., pp. 667–669). Arlington, VA: Author.

Augustine, J. R. (1996). Circuitry and functional aspects of the insular lobe in primates including humans. *Brain Research: Brain Research Reviews, 22*(3), 229–244.

Barbas, H. (2007). Flow of information for emotions through temporal and orbitofrontal pathways. *Journal of Anatomy, 211*(2), 237–249.

Beauregard, M. (2007). Mind does really matter: Evidence from neuroimaging studies of emotional self-regulation, psychotherapy, and placebo effect. *Progress in Neurobiology, 81*(4), 218–236.

Beblo, T., Driessen, M., Mertens, M., Wingenfeld, K., Piefke, M., Rullkoetter, N., et al. (2006). Functional MRI correlates of the recall of unresolved life events in borderline personality disorder. *Psychological Medicine, 36*(6), 845–856.

Belin, D., Jonkman, S., Dickinson, A., Robbins, T. W., & Everitt, B. J. (2009). Parallel and interactive learning processes within the basal ganglia: Relevance for the understanding of addiction. *Behavioural Brain Research, 199*(1), 89–102.

Beutel, M. E., Stern, E., & Silbersweig, D. A. (2003). The emerging dialogue between psychoanalysis and neuroscience: Neuroimaging perspectives. *Journal of the American Psychoanalytic Association, 51*(3), 773–801.

Blair, K. S., Smith, B. W., Mitchell, D. G., Morton, J., Vythilingam, M., Pessoa, L., et al. (2007). Modulation of emotion by cognition and cognition by emotion. *NeuroImage, 35*(1), 430–440.

Bledowski, C., Rahm, B., & Rowe, J. B. (2009). What "works" in working memory?: Separate systems for selection and updating of critical information. *Journal of Neuroscience, 29*, 13735–13741.

Bonelli, R. M., & Cummings, J. L. (2007). Frontal–subcortical circuitry and behavior. *Dialogues in Clinical Neuroscience, 9*(2), 141–151.

Brambilla, P., Soloff, P. H., Sala, M., Nicoletti, M. A., Keshavan, M. S., & Soares, J. C. (2004). Anatomical MRI study of borderline personality disorder patients. *Psychiatry Research: Neuroimaging, 131*(2), 125–133.

Buchheim, A., Erk, S., George, C., Kachele, H., Kircher, T., Martius, P., et al. (2008). Neural correlates of attachment trauma in borderline personality disorder: A functional magnetic resonance imaging study. *Psychiatry Research, 163*(3), 223–235.

Bush, G., Luu, P., & Posner, M. I. (2000). Cognitive and emotional influences in anterior cingulate cortex. *Trends in Cognitive Sciences, 4*(6), 215–222.

Carter, C. S., Macdonald, A. M., Botvinick, M., Ross, L. L., Stenger, V. A., Noll, D., et al. (2000). Parsing executive processes: Strategic vs. evaluative functions of the anterior cingulate cortex. *Proceedings of the National Academy of Sciences USA, 97*(4), 1944–1948.

Cole, P. M., Michel, M. K., & Teti, L. O. (1994). The development of emotion regulation and dysregulation: A clinical perspective. *Monographs of the Society for Research in Child Development, 59*(2–3), 73–100.

Damasio, A., & Carvalho, G. B. (2013). The nature of feelings: Evolutionary and neurobiological origins. *Nature Reviews Neuroscience, 14*(2), 143–152.

Davidson, R. J., & Irwin, W. (1999). The functional neuroanatomy of emotion and affective style. *Trends in Cognitive Sciences, 3*(1), 11–21.

Davidson, R. J., Putnam, K. M., & Larson, C. L. (2000). Dysfunction in the neural circuitry of emotion regulation—a possible prelude to violence. *Science, 289*, 591–594.

Dombrovski, A. Y., Siegle, G. J., Szanto, K., Clark, L., Reynolds, C. F., & Aizenstein, H. (2012). The temptation of suicide: Striatal gray matter, discounting of delayed rewards, and suicide attempts in late-life depression. *Psychological Medicine, 42*(6), 1203–1215.

Donegan, N. H., Sanislow, C. A., Blumberg, H. P., Fulbright, R. K., Lacadie, C., Skudlarski, P., et al. (2003). Amygdala hyperreactivity in borderline personality disorder: Implications for emotional dysregulation. *Biological Psychiatry, 54*(11), 1284–1293.

Driessen, M., Herrmann, J., Stahl, K., Zwaan, M., Meier, S., Hill, A., et al. (2000). Magnetic resonance imaging volumes of the hippocampus and the amygdala in women with borderline personality disorder and early traumatization. *Archives of General Psychiatry, 57*(12), 1115–1122.

Ebner-Priemer, U. W., Kuo, J., Kleindienst, N., Welch, S. S., Reisch, T., Reinhard, I., et al. (2007). State affective instability in borderline personality disorder assessed by ambulatory monitoring. *Psychological Medicine, 37*(7), 961–970.

Ebner-Priemer, U. W., Kuo, J., Schlotz, W., Kleindienst, N., Rosenthal, M. Z., Detterer, L., et al. (2008). Distress and affective dysregulation in patients with borderline personality disorder: A psychophysiological ambulatory monitoring study. *Journal of Nervous and Mental Disease, 196*(4), 314–320.

Ebner-Priemer, U. W., Welch, S. S., Grossman, P., Reisch, T., Linehan, M. M., & Bohus, M. (2007). Psychophysiological ambulatory assessment of affective dysregulation in borderline personality disorder. *Psychiatry Research, 150*(3), 265–275.

Ekman, P., & Friesen, W. V. (1976). *Pictures of facial affect.* Palo Alto, CA: Consulting Psychologists Press.

Fertuck, E. A., Lenzenweger, M. F., Clarkin, J. F., Hoermann, S., & Stanley, B. (2006). Executive neurocognition, memory systems, and borderline personality disorder. *Clinical Psychology Review, 26*(3), 346–375.

Fletcher, P. C., & Henson, R. N. (2001). Frontal lobes and human memory: Insights from functional neuroimaging. *Brain, 124*(Pt. 5), 849–881.

Goldin, P. R., McRae, K., Ramel, W., & Gross, J. J. (2008). The neural bases of emotion regulation: Reappraisal and suppression of negative emotion. *Biological Psychiatry, 63*(6), 577–586.

Goldstein, M., Brendel, G., Tuescher, O., Pan, H., Epstein, J., Beutel, M., et al. (2007). Neural substrates of the interaction of emotional stimulus processing and motor inhibitory control: An emotional linguistic go/no-go fMRI study. *NeuroImage, 36*(3), 1026–1040.

Goyer, P. F., Andreason, P. J., Semple, W. E., Clayton, A. H., King, A. C., Compton-Toth, B. A., et al. (1994). Positron-emission tomography and personality disorders. *Neuropsychopharmacology, 10*(1), 21–28.

Gross, J. J., & Thompson, R. A. (2006). Conceptual foundations. In J. J. Gross (Ed.), *Handbook of emotion regulation* (pp. 5–18). New York: Guilford Press.

Hazlett, E. A., New, A. S., Newmark, R., Haznedar, M. M., Lo, J. N., Speiser, L. J., et al. (2005). Reduced anterior and posterior cingulate gray matter in borderline personality disorder. *Biological Psychiatry, 58*(8), 614–623.

Herpertz, S. C., Dietrich, T. M., Wenning, B., Krings, T., Erberich, S. C., Willmes, K., et al. (2001). Evidence of abnormal amygdala functioning in borderline personality disorder: A functional MRI study. *Biological Psychiatry, 50*(4), 292–298.

Irle, E., Lange, C., & Sachsse, U. (2005). Reduced size and abnormal asymmetry of parietal cortex in women with borderline personality disorder. *Biological Psychiatry, 57*(2), 173–182.

Jacob, G. A., Guenzler, C., Zimmermann, S., Scheel, C. N., Rusch, N., Leonhart, R., et al. (2008). Time course of anger and other emotions in women with borderline personality disorder: A preliminary study. *Journal of Behavior Therapy and Experimental Psychiatry, 39*(3), 391–402.

King-Casas, B., Sharp, C., Lomax-Bream, L., Lohrenz, T., Fonagy, P., & Montague, P. R. (2008). The rupture and repair of cooperation in borderline personality disorder. *Science, 321,* 806–810.

Koenigsberg, H. W., Fan, J., Ochsner, K. N., Liu, X., Guise, K., Pizzarello, S., et al. (2010). Neural correlates of using distancing to regulate emotional responses to social situations. *Neuropsychologia, 48*(6), 1813–1822.

Koenigsberg, H. W., Harvey, P. D., Mitropoulou, V., New, A. S., Goodman, M., Silverman, J., et al. (2001). Are the interpersonal and identity disturbances in the borderline personality disorder criteria linked to the traits of affective instability and impulsivity? *Journal of Personality Disorders, 15*(4), 358–370.

Koenigsberg, H. W., Siever, L. J., Lee, H., Pizzarello, S., New, A. S., Goodman, M., et al. (2009). Neural correlates of emotion processing in borderline personality disorder. *Psychiatry Research, 172*(3), 192–199.

Kraus, A., Valerius, G., Seifritz, E., Ruf, M., Bremner, J. D., Bohus, M., et al. (2010). Script-driven imagery of self-injurious behavior in patients with borderline personality disorder: A pilot FMRI study. *Acta Psychiatrica Scandinavica, 121*(1), 41–51.

Lang, P. J., & Cuthbert, B. N. (2001). *International affect pictures system (IAPS): Technical manual and affective ratings.* Gainesville: University of Florida.

Levine, D., Marziali, E., & Hood, J. (1997). Emotion processing in borderline personality disorders. *Journal of Nervous and Mental Disease, 185*(4), 240–246.

Linehan, M. M. (1993). *Cognitive-behavioral treatment of borderline personality disorder.* New York: Guilford Press.

Lyoo, I. K., Han, M. H., & Cho, D. Y. (1998). A brain MRI study in subjects with borderline personality disorder. *Journal of Affective Disorders, 50*(2–3), 235–243.

Minzenberg, M. J., Fan, J., New, A. S., Tang, C. Y., & Siever, L. J. (2007). Fronto-limbic dysfunction in response to facial emotion in borderline personality disorder: An event-related fMRI study. *Psychiatry Research, 155*(3), 231–243.

Murphy, S. E. (2010). Using functional neuroimaging to investigate the mechanisms of action of selective serotonin reuptake inhibitors (SSRIs). *Current Pharmaceutical Design, 16*(18), 1990–1997.

New, A. S., Goodman, M., Triebwasser, J., & Siever, L. J. (2008). Recent advances in the biological study of personality disorders. *Psychiatric Clinics of North America, 31*(3), 441–461.

New, A. S., Hazlett, E. A., Buchsbaum, M. S., Goodman, M., Mitelman, S. A., Newmark, R., et al. (2007). Amygdala–prefrontal disconnection in borderline personality disorder. *Neuropsychopharmacology, 32*(7), 1629–1640.

New, A. S., Hazlett, E. A., Buchsbaum, M. S., Goodman, M., Reynolds, D., Mitropoulou, V., et al. (2002). Blunted prefrontal cortical 18fluorodeoxyglucose positron emission tomography response to meta-chlorophenylpiperazine in impulsive aggression. *Archives of General Psychiatry, 59*(7), 621–629.

Ochsner, K. N., Bunge, S. A., Gross, J. J., & Gabrieli, J. D. (2002). Rethinking feelings: An fMRI study of the cognitive regulation of emotion. *Journal of Cognitive Neuroscience, 14*(8), 1215–1229.

Ochsner, K. N., & Gross, J. J. (2006). The neural architecture of emotion regulation. In J. J. Gross (Ed.), *Handbook of emotion regulation* (pp. 87–89). New York: Guilford Press.

O'Leary, K. M. (2000). Borderline personality disorder: Neuropsychological testing results. *Psychiatric Clinics of North America, 23*(1), 41–60.

Oquendo, M. A., & Mann, J. J. (2000). The biology of impulsivity and suicidality. *Psychiatric Clinics of North America, 23*(1), 11–25.

Peters, J., & Buchel, C. (2010). Episodic future thinking reduces reward delay discounting through an enhancement of prefrontal–mediotemporal interactions. *Neuron, 66*(1), 138–148.

Phillips, M. L., Ladouceur, C. D., & Drevets, W. C. (2008). A neural model of voluntary and automatic emotion regulation: Implications for understanding the pathophysiology and neurodevelopment of bipolar disorder. *Molecular Psychiatry, 13*(9), 829, 833–857.

Phillips, M. L., Travis, M. J., Fagiolini, A., & Kupfer, D. J. (2008). Medication effects in neuroimaging studies of bipolar disorder. *American Journal of Psychiatry, 165*(3), 313–320.

Plutchik, R. (2001). The nature of emotions. *American Scientist, 89*(4), 344.

Putnam, K. M., & Silk, K. R. (2005). Emotion dysregulation and the development of borderline personality disorder. *Development and Psychopathology, 17*(4), 899–925.

Radua, J., Phillips, M. L., Russell, T., Lawrence, N., Marshall, N., Kalidindi, S., et al. (2010). Neural response to specific components of fearful faces in healthy and schizophrenic adults. *NeuroImage, 49*(1), 939–946.

Reisch, T., Ebner-Priemer, U., Tschacher, W., Bohus, M., & Linehan, M. (2008). Sequences of emotions in patients with borderline personality disorder. *Acta Psychiatrica Scandinavica, 118*(1), 42–48.

Roffman, J. L., Marci, C. D., Glick, D. M., Dougherty, D. D., & Rauch, S. L. (2005). Neuroimaging and the functional neuroanatomy of psychotherapy. *Psychological Medicine, 35*(10), 1385–1398.

Ruocco, A. C. (2005). The neuropsychology of borderline personality disorder: A meta-analysis and review. *Psychiatry Research, 137*(3), 191–202.

Ruocco, A. C., Amirthavasagam, S., & Zakzanis, K. K. (2012). Amygdala and hippocampal volume reductions as candidate endophenotypes for borderline personality disorder: A meta-analysis of magnetic resonance imaging studies. *Psychiatry Research: Neuroimaging, 201*(3), 245–252.

Rüsch, N., van Elst, L. T., Ludaescher, P., Wilke, M., Huppertz, H. J., Thiel, T., et al. (2003). A voxel-based morphometric MRI study in female patients with borderline personality disorder. *NeuroImage, 20*(1), 385–392.

Rutherford, B. R., Wager, T. D., & Roose, S. P. (2010). Expectancy and the treatment of depression: A review of experimental methodology and effects on patient outcome. *Current Psychiatry Reviews, 6*(1), 1–10.

Sala, M., Caverzasi, E., Lazzaretti, M., Morandotti, N., De Vidovich, G., Marraffini, E., et al. (2011). Dorsolateral prefrontal cortex and hippocampus sustain impulsivity and aggressiveness in borderline personality disorder. *Journal of Affective Disorders, 131*(1–3), 417–421.

Schmahl, C. G., & Bremner, J. D. (2006). Neuroimaging in borderline personality disorder. *Journal of Psychiatric Research, 40*(5), 419–427.

Schmahl, C. G., Vermetten, E., Elzinga, B. M., & Bremner, J. D. (2003). Magnetic resonance imaging of hippocampal and amygdala volume in women with childhood abuse and borderline personality disorder. *Psychiatry Research: Neuroimaging, 122*(3), 193–198.

Schnell, K., & Herpertz, S. C. (2007). Effects of dialectic-behavioral-therapy on the neural correlates of affective hyperarousal in borderline personality disorder. *Journal of Psychiatric Research, 41*(10), 837–847.

Schulze, L., Domes, G., Köppen, D., & Herpertz, S. C. (2013). Enhanced detection of emotional facial expressions in borderline personality disorder. *Psychopathology, 46*(4), 217–224.

Siever, L. J. (2008). Neurobiology of aggression and violence. *American Journal of Psychiatry, 165*(4), 429–442.

Siever, L. J., Buchsbaum, M. S., New, A. S., Spiegel-Cohen, J., Wei, T., Hazlett, E. A., et al. (1999). D,L-fenfluramine response in impulsive personality disorder assessed with [$^{18}$F]fluorodeoxyglucose positron emission tomography. *Neuropsychopharmacology, 20*(5), 413–423.

Silbersweig, D., Clarkin, J. F., Goldstein, M., Kernberg, O. F., Tuescher, O., Levy, K. N., et al. (2007). Failure of frontolimbic inhibitory function in the context of negative emotion in borderline personality disorder. *American Journal of Psychiatry, 164*(12), 1832–1841.

Soloff, P. H., Kelly, T. M., Strotmeyer, S. J., Malone, K. M., & Mann, J. J. (2003). Impulsivity, gender, and response to fenfluramine challenge in borderline personality disorder. *Psychiatry Research, 119*(1–2), 11–24.

Soloff, P. H., Meltzer, C. C., Becker, C., Greer, P. J., Kelly, T. M., & Constantine, D. (2003). Impulsivity and prefrontal hypometabolism in borderline personality disorder. *Psychiatry Research: Neuroimaging, 123*(3), 153–163.

Soloff, P. H., Meltzer, C. C., Greer, P. J., Constantine, D., & Kelly, T. M. (2000). A fenfluramine-activated FDG-PET study of borderline personality disorder. *Biological Psychiatry, 47*(6), 540–547.

Soloff, P. H., Nutche, J., Goradia, D., & Diwadkar, V. (2008). Structural brain abnormalities in borderline personality disorder: A voxel-based morphometry study. *Psychiatry Research: Neuroimaging, 164*(3), 223–236.

Soloff, P. H., Pruitt, P., Sharma, M., Radwan, J., White, R., & Diwadkar, V. A. (2012). Structural brain abnormalities and suicidal behavior in borderline personality disorder. *Journal of Psychiatric Research, 46*(4), 516–525.

Soloff, P. H., White, R., & Diwadkar, V. (2014). *An fMRI study of affective interference with cognitive function in borderline personality disorder.* Paper presented at the 167th annual meeting of the American Psychiatric Association, New York.

Solomon, R. C. (2003). *What is an emotion?: Classic and contemporary readings* (2nd ed.). New York: Oxford University Press.

Tebartz van Elst, L., Hesslinger, B., Thiel, T., Geiger, E., Haegele, K., Lemieux, L., et al. (2003). Fronto-limbic brain abnormalities in patients with borderline personality disorder: A volumetric magnetic resonance imaging study. *Biological Psychiatry, 54*(2), 163–171.

Tekin, S., & Cummings, J. L. (2002). Frontal–subcortical neuronal circuits and clinical neuropsychiatry: An update. *Journal of Psychosomatic Research, 53*(2), 647–654.

Thomaes, K., Dorrepaal, E., Draijer, N., Jansma, E. P., Veltman, D. J., & van Balkom, A. J. (2014). Can pharmacological and psychological treatment change brain structure and function in PTSD?: A systematic review. *Journal of Psychiatric Research, 50*, 1–15.

Wall, P. M., & Messier, C. (2001). The hippocampal formation–orbitomedial prefrontal cortex circuit in the attentional control of active memory. *Behavioural Brain Research, 127*(1–2), 99–117.

Wingenfeld, K., Rullkoetter, N., Mensebach, C., Beblo, T., Mertens, M., Kreisel, S., et al. (2009). Neural correlates of the individual emotional Stroop in borderline personality disorder. *Psychoneuroendocrinology, 34*(4), 571–586.

Yen, S., Shea, M. T., Sanislow, C. A., Grilo, C. M., Skodol, A. E., Gunderson, J. G., et al. (2004). Borderline personality disorder criteria associated with prospectively observed suicidal behavior. *American Journal of Psychiatry, 161*(7), 1296–1298.

Zetzsche, T., Preuss, U. W., Frodl, T., Schmitt, G., Seifert, D., Munchhausen, E., et al. (2007). Hippocampal volume reduction and history of aggressive behaviour in patients with borderline personality disorder. *Psychiatry Research, 154*(2), 157–170.

# CHAPTER 16

# Neuropsychological Perspectives

Marianne Skovgaard Thomsen, Anthony C. Ruocco,
Birgit Bork Mathiesen, and Erik Simonsen

Over the years, neuropsychological research has contributed significantly to the development of theories about changes in brain structure and function in patients with various psychiatric disorders (Keefe, 1995; Lezak, 2004; Silbersweig et al., 2007). Neuropsychological assessment is useful in evaluating patients' cognitive and behavioral resources and vulnerabilities, thereby providing "a window into the daily mental processes of the psychiatric patient" (Keefe, 1995, p.7). The idea that the development of borderline personality disorder (BPD) may involve neuropsychological impairments arose in large part from anecdotal clinical evidence of cognitive limitations and findings that many patients have a history of childhood physical and psychological trauma. This chapter reviews the literature on neuropsychological research on BPD published since 1980, when the diagnosis was first included in the DSM.

## Initial Forays into Cognitive Function in BPD Using Intellectual Testing

Neuropsychological deficits were not initially suspected in BPD for several reasons. First, as O'Leary and Cowdry (1994) suggested, the psychodynamic framework originally used to describe BPD attributed the cognitive style of BPD (i.e., memory irregularities, lack of precise judgment) to defensive ego mechanisms used to ward off intolerable emotions, memories, and intrapsychic conflicts (Murray, 1993; O'Leary & Cowdry, 1994). Second, DSM-III (American Psychiatric Association, 1980) assigned cognitive features such as disorganized thinking and perceptual distortions to schizotypal personality disorder (STPD) rather than BPD to differentiate these disorders (Kroll, 1988). Third, patients with BPD appeared to fall within the normal range on intellectual tests, leading researchers to assess intrapsychic structure using less structured projective methods, such as the Rorschach test (Exner, 1986; Lerner & Lerner, 1980; Rorschach, 1975; Singer & Larson, 1981) and Thematic Apperception Test (Murray, 1943; Westen, Lohr, Silk, Gold, & Kerber, 1990). However, in the early 1990s, several exploratory studies demonstrated subtle deficits on more structured cognitive tests (O'Leary & Cowdry, 1994). Nevertheless, initial studies (e.g., Cornelius et al., 1989) failed to show clear deficits even when a comprehensive neurocognitive battery was used. This was probably because patients' performances were compared to normative data rather than a comparison group recruited specifically for the study.

Several subsequent studies, comparing patients to matched control participants on the Wechsler Adult Intelligence Test—Revised (WAIS-R; Wechsler, 1981), were designed to assess whether patients showed deficits in global intellectual functioning or discrete neurocognitive deficits on specific subtests. Burgess (1990) found no differences on the Digit Span subtest (a measure of brief auditory attention) from the WAIS-R when comparing 18 patients with BPD to 14 nonpsychiatric controls. However, O'Leary, Brouwers, Gardner, and Cowdry (1991) observed significantly lower Performance IQ scores for 16 medication-free patients with BPD as compared to 16 nonpsychiatric controls when using the WAIS-R, with especially poor performance on the Digit Symbol Coding subtest, a measure of attention and visuomotor speed. This finding was reproduced in two subsequent studies in which significant differences between patients and controls were limited to either the Digit Symbol subtest (Judd & Ruff, 1993) or the Digit Symbol and Block Design subtest (a measure of visuospatial construction) (Carpenter, Gold, & Fenton, 1993). Monarch, Saykin, and Flashman (2004), who obtained mainly similar results in a study of 10 patients with BPD and 10 controls, found significantly lower scores on a single verbal measure, the Vocabulary subtest (an oral test of vocabulary), as well as the Digit Span, Block Design, and Picture Arrangement (perceptual reasoning) subtests. Swirsky-Sacchetti and colleagues (1993) reported similar results on the Picture Arrangement Test in 10 female patients with BPD and 10 controls. However, Irle, Lange, and Sachsse (2005) reported more general impairment, with significantly reduced intellectual functioning on both the WAIS-R Verbal and Performance subscales in 30 patients with BPD (of which 19 were medicated) compared to 25 controls. Minzeberg, Poole, and Vinogradov (2008) also reported that 43 patients with BPD had significantly lower Verbal, Performance, and Full-Scale IQ scores than 26 controls on the Wechsler Abbreviated Scale of Intelligence (WASI; Wechsler, 1999). Finally, a recent study by Thomsen, Ruocco, Carcone, Mathiesen, and Simonsen (2016) reported significantly lower performance in a group of 45 women with BPD compared to 56 nonpsychiatric controls on the WAIS-IV (Wechsler, 2008) indices of verbal comprehension, working memory, and processing speed, but not in the domain of perceptual reasoning.

Three other studies have reported significantly lower Full Scale IQ scores in patients with BPD compared to nonpsychiatric controls (Irle et al., 2005; Swirsky-Sacchetti et al., 1993; Thomsen, Ruocco, Carcone, et al., 2016). It is important to note, however, that in all three studies, performances of both patients with BPD and controls fell within a normatively average range. Several studies have also revealed no statistically significant differences on global IQ measures for patients with BPD (Bazanis et al., 2002; Dowson et al., 2004; Driessen et al., 2000; Kunert, Druecke, Sass, & Herpertz, 2003; Paris, Zelkowitz, Cuzder, Joseph, & Feldman, 1999; Sprock, Rader, Kendall, & Yoder, 2000), which may reflect lower statistical power to detect potentially subtle differences in intellectual functioning in any individual study.

## Summary

The most consistent findings for patients with BPD on individual subtests of the WAIS indicate lower scores on measures of Brief Auditory Attention, Processing Speed, and Visuospatial Construction. This raises the possibility of deficits in higher-order cognitive abilities (i.e., executive functions) that are not necessarily adequately captured by global indices of intellectual functioning (Carpenter et al., 1993; Judd & Ruff, 1993; Monarch et al., 2004). However, the overall results of studies examining performance on intellectual testing in patients with BPD suggest possibly slightly lower overall intellectual function, although some investigations show lower scores and others do not. Indices of Verbal and Performance IQ have generally been found to fall within the average range, suggesting that patients may have more discrete deficits in cognitive functioning that appear to be better captured by performance on specific IQ subtests.

## Comprehensive Neuropsychological Testing Using Conventional Test Batteries

This section reviews the results of studies using more comprehensive neuropsychological batteries to assess a wide range of domains, including language, episodic memory (verbal and visual), and executive functions, such as cognitive flexibility, response inhibition, and motor coordination.

### Language

Deficits in language processing are not generally associated with BPD. An early study by

Burgess (1990) found no significant differences between patients with BPD and nonpsychiatric controls on tests assessing verbal repetition and object naming. Similarly, Judd and Ruff (1993) found no significant differences between patients with BPD and controls on the Vocabulary subtest of the WAIS-R and on a measure of verbal fluency. However, Stevens, Burkhardt, Hautzinger, Schwarz, and Unckel (2004) showed that patients with BPD performed more poorly than controls on the Vocabulary and Information (general knowledge) subtests of a German adaption of the WAIS-R (Tewes, 1991).

Monarch and colleagues (2004) examined patients with BPD ($n = 10$) and a normative comparison group ($n = 131$), and found that patients performed significantly lower on a reading measure from the Wide Range Achievement Test, as well as a verbal fluency task, and an object naming test (see also Saykin et al., 1995). Irle and colleagues (2005) replicated these findings in a comparison of 30 female patients with BPD and a history of severe childhood sexual and physical abuse with a nonpsychiatric control group. However, we should state that the sample sizes of the patient groups in these studies have generally been too small to produce reliable findings. Nevertheless, elaborating on these initial findings, Travers and King (2005) compared a group of 50 "nonorganic" patients with BPD to a group of 30 "organic" patients with BPD (i.e., those with a history of neurological problems or head injury) and found significantly poorer performance on a test of verbal fluency in the organic group than in the nonorganic group. Mathiesen, Simonsen, Soegaard, and Kvist (2014) examined 20 patients with BPD to 24 patients who had an injury to the prefrontal cortex and a diagnosis of organic personality disorder (OPD), and were thought to have a personality structure close to a borderline personality organization (Kernberg, 1967), and compared the groups on measures of language using the Danish Adult Reading Test (DART) and the Vocabulary subtest from the WAIS. Surprisingly, even when the authors controlled for a higher premorbid educational level for the OPD group, the BPD group performed significantly poorer than the OPD group on the DART. The speculation was that perhaps the emotional states of patients in the BPD group may have affected performance on the language test.

Thomsen, Ruocco, Carcone, and colleagues (2016) found significant differences across all four subscales on the Verbal Comprehension Index of the WAIS-IV in 45 patients with BPD compared to 56 nonpsychiatric controls. The Verbal Comprehension Index includes subtests that measure a variety of cognitive functions, including understanding social rules, applying verbal knowledge in specific contexts, and conceptualizing information at a higher level of abstraction. Lower performance on these tests could reflect limitations in higher-order cognitive functions that require the coordination of complex information, especially on measures that integrate social information (e.g., Picture Arrangement subtest). Additionally, deficits in accumulated verbal knowledge may have downstream influences on patients' ability to express themselves and to use knowledge appropriately, possibly contributing to the social and interpersonal problems that characterize BPD.

## Episodic Memory

While memory dysfunction is not typically considered a prominent feature of BPD, researchers have theorized that specific visual and verbal memory deficits may occur due to transient dissociations, distractibility, and attentional biases when dealing with emotional stimuli. However, there is evidence suggesting that these memory difficulties may occur even outside of the context of apparently stressful or emotional situations.

### Verbal Episodic Memory

Findings of verbal memory deficits in BPD are heterogeneous. Burgess (1990) reported significant deficits on a simple verbal memory task requiring the recall of three word-pairs after 10 minutes. A subsequent study showed that patients with BPD recalled fewer items than depressed patients (Burgess, 1991). O'Leary and colleagues (1991) found no significant differences in verbal memory in their BPD sample on the Associate Learning subtest from the Wechsler Memory Scale (WMS; Wechsler, 1945). However, Swirsky-Sacchetti and colleagues (1993) did not replicate this finding.

The WMS Logical Memory Test requires participants to listen to two stories read aloud to them, then recall the information immediately after presentation and following a 45-minute delay. Five studies found significant deficits for patients with BPD on this task (Dinn et al.,

2004; Judd & Ruff, 1993; Kirkpatrick et al., 2007; O'Leary et al., 1991; Swirsky-Sacchetti et al., 1993; Travers & King, 2005), but three studies did not (Beblo et al., 2006; Carpenter et al., 1993; Driessen et al., 2000). Interestingly, in studies where deficits were found, patients improved their memory for the stories when they were provided with recognition cues, performing at a level commensurate to controls. These findings suggest that memory problems associated with BPD may arise from difficulties in retrieving learned material rather than encoding new information (O'Leary et al., 1991).

However, Swirsky-Sacchetti and colleagues (1993) also showed that patients with BPD showed significant deficits compared to controls on measures of acquisition (i.e., learning), immediate recall, delayed recall, cued recall, and recognition, assessed with the California Verbal Learning Test (Delis, Kramer, Kaplan, & Ober, 1987). Similarly, Seres, Unoka, Bódi, Aspán, and Kéri (2009) used the Repeatable Battery for the Assessment of Neuropsychological Status (RBANS; Gold, Queern, Iannone, & Buchanan, 1999) and found that patients with BPD showed deficits on indices of immediate and delayed memory for verbal information (i.e., a word list and a short story) compared to controls, but they did not differ from patients with other mental disorders. On the other hand, other studies have not detected differences between patients with BPD and nonpsychiatric controls on verbal memory tasks (Mensebach, Beblo, et al., 2009; Thomsen, Ruocco, Carcone, et al., 2016).

*Visual Episodic Memory*

Visual memory is usually assessed using tests that instruct participants to copy a design or a series of designs, then recall the information immediately after presentation and/or following a delay. Research using the Rey–Osterrieth Complex Figure Test, which includes one large design with multiple constituent design elements, indicates that patients with BPD recall fewer details of the design immediately after copying it and after a delay (Beblo, Saavedra, et al., 2006; Carpenter et al., 1993; Dinn et al., 2004; Judd & Ruff, 1993; Kirkpatrick et al., 2007; O'Leary et al., 1991; Travers & King, 2005). However, two studies did not replicate these findings (Driessen et al., 2000; Sprock et al., 2000). On the Visual Reproduction subtest from the WMS, which comprises several less complex designs, patients with BPD appear to recall fewer details of the designs than controls (Beblo, Saavedra, et al., 2006; Carpenter et al., 1993), although O'Leary and Cowdry (1994) found no significant differences between patients and controls on this test. Recent research suggests that there may be significant heterogeneity in episodic memory deficits among patients with BPD, and that substantial variability in verbal versus visual memory performance may characterize patients (Ruocco & Bahl, 2014).

*Cognitive Flexibility*

"Cognitive flexibility," or the ability to switch between mental sets, is an executive function that requires attention, memory, and reasoning. It is assessed with a range of tests, perhaps the commonest being the Wisconsin Card Sorting Test (WCST; Berg, 1948; Heaton, 1981), which asks individuals to sort cards according to specific rules, then modify their sorting approach based on changes in task contingencies. Cognitive flexibility in BPD has also been measured with the Ruff Figural Fluency Test (Ruff, Light, & Evans, 1987), a nonverbal analogue to verbal fluency tests, which provides information regarding nonverbal capacity for divergent thinking. Additionally, the Trail Making Test—Part B, which requires participants to alternate visually sequencing a series of letters and numbers in alphabetical and ascending order, respectively, has been used to measure cognitive flexibility (Lezak, 1993; Reitan, 1971) in patients with BPD.

Early studies using the WCST showed that performance errors were associated with the presence of neurological soft-signs (Gardner, Lucas, & Cowdry, 1987; Stein et al., 1993; Van Reekum, 1993), suggesting that an organic impairment may contribute to deficits in cognitive flexibility in BPD. However, these findings were not replicated by Swirsky-Sacchetti and colleagues (1993). In contrast, a comparison of 24 patients with BPD without current mood disorder to 68 nonpsychiatric controls (Lenzenweger, Clarkin, Fertuck, & Kernberg, 2004) found that patients with BPD performed significantly poorer than controls on indices of the WCST sensitive to cognitive flexibility (i.e., perseverative errors). Effect sizes for these differences were in the medium range, and results remained significant after controlling for age and education. Interestingly, lower levels of perseverative errors were associated with higher levels of inhibitory control assessed with the Multidimensional Personality Questionnaire (MPQ; Tellegen, 1982).

Black and colleagues (2009) found a significant difference between patients with BPD and nonpsychiatric controls on the number of conceptual categories completed on the WCST, which reflects poorer concept formation. Interestingly, significant differences have been found on all scales of the WCST when comparing 41 children with BPD symptoms in a psychiatric day treatment program to 53 children in day treatment with no BPD symptoms (Paris et al., 1999). Children with BPD symptoms required more trials to complete the WCST, demonstrated more perseverative errors, and had fewer conceptual-level responses compared with their peers, leading the authors to suggest that this neuropsychological deficit in children may mirror that observed among adults with BPD.

Using the Ruff Figural Fluency Test, significant differences between patients with BPD and controls were found in the number of unique designs they produced within a time limit, suggesting deficits in the patient group's ability to organize concrete nonverbal information rapidly and fluently (Judd & Ruff, 1993; O'Leary et al., 1991). Patients appeared either to get stuck on one organizational strategy or they applied random strategies in generating designs, resulting in slower performance (Judd & Ruff, 1993).

Several studies have found significantly lowered performance in BPD samples on the Trail Making Test—Part B (Beblo et al., 2006; Dinn et al., 2004; Judd & Ruff, 1993; Monarch et al., 2004; O'Leary et al., 1991; Stein et al., 1993; van Reekum, Links, Mitton, & Fedorov, 1996), which suggests that these individuals have difficulty filtering out extraneous stimuli and selecting relevant visual details from a complex field. Performance was particularly affected in patients with BPD who had a history of organic insult (Travers & King, 2005). Even though deficits on the Trail Making Test have frequently been identified in studies, in one study that reported negative results (Sprock et al., 2000), patients with BPD and neurological problems were excluded from the study. However, in a study by Mathiesen and colleagues (2014) there were also no differences in performance between a group of patients with BPD patients and a group with organic injury, displaying borderline personality organization.

## Measuring Discrete Cognitive Abilities with Greater Relevance to BPD

Following initial studies using intellectual testing and broad-range neuropsychological batteries, research has focused on specific cognitive abilities that are more relevant to the symptoms and psychopathology of BPD frequently reported by patients, such as distractibility and impulse control difficulties (Ruocco, Lam, & McMain, 2014).

### Attention

Attention is a construct that be subdivided into different components, such as "sustained attention," which is a time-limited capacity to remain vigilant (Darby & Walsh, 2005), and "selective attention," which involves focusing on relevant stimuli while ignoring irrelevant information. Using the Stroop test, Swirsky-Sacchetti and colleagues (1993) found that 10 patients with BPD had significantly poorer performances than 10 nonpsychiatric controls on the color–word trial of the test, which reflects the ability to selectively attend to specific information (i.e., ink color) while ignoring a more automatic response (i.e., reading color words). The suggestion was that this deficit could be related to the difficulties with impulse control often observed in BPD. Subsequent studies on BPD using the Stroop test have yielded mixed results. Some studies have detected mild attentional deficits in individuals while naming the ink color of incongruent color words (Sprock et al., 2000) that have also been associated with the number of lifetime suicide attempts (Legris, Links, van Reekum, Tannock, & Toplak, 2012). Other studies found significant differences between patients with BPD and nonpsychiatric controls (Kunert et al., 2003) or a group with OPD when Verbal IQ differences between groups were controlled (Mathiesen et al., 2014).

Elaborating on earlier findings of lower attentional functioning in BPD (Judd & Ruff, 1993; O'Leary et al., 1991), Posner and colleagues (2002) used the Attentional Network Test (ANT), in a sophisticated assessment of three selective attentional networks (i.e., alerting, orienting, and conflict resolution) in 39 mainly female patients with BPD compared to a group of 22 control patients high on negative emotionality (as measured by the Adult Temperament Questionnaire) and 30 controls selected for an average level of emotionality. Groups were compared on an Eriksen flanker task, which comprises a set of response inhibition tests that assess the ability to suppress responses that are inappropriate in a particular context (Eriksen & Eriksen, 1974). The BPD group was much less able to resolve conflict between competing stimulus elements than participants with average emotionality. The suggestion was that this conflict resolution–attentional dysfunction in BPD may interface with altered emotional control at the level of the anterior cingulate cortex and corticolimbic circuitry, networks that are involved in emotion regulation (Bush, Luu, & Posner, 2000; Etkin, Egner, & Kalisch, 2011).

Performances on neuropsychological tests may also show promise as candidate intermediate phenotypes for BPD (Ruocco, Laporte, Russell, Guttman, & Paris, 2012). Using the Conners' Continuous Performance Test–II (CPT; Conners & Multi-Health Systems Staff, 2000), attention and impulse control measures were examined in 39 patients with BPD, 39 first-degree sisters of patients, and 24 nonpsychiatric controls. Patients performed worse than controls in terms of their level of attentiveness on the task and the number of commission errors. The performance of relatives was almost consistently intermediate to that of patients and controls, although relatives did not significantly differ from either group. However, a cluster analysis revealed a subgroup of relatives who showed signs of inattentiveness on the CPT (as indicated by poorer discriminability between target and nontarget stimuli) and clinically elevated response inhibition deficits (as indicated by atypically fast reaction times I response to target stimuli and many commission errors). Additionally, a substantial rate of recurrence risk of response inhibition deficits was observed among siblings without BPD, suggesting that the deficits may be heritable in affected sibling pairs and could represent a potential intermediate phenotype for BPD (although the specificity of the finding to BPD as compared to other mental disorders remains to be addressed).

Building on earlier findings of lower sustained attention in patients with BPD (Gvirts et al., 2012; Monarch et al., 2004), Thomsen, Ruocco, Carone, and colleagues (2016) found that 45 patients with BPD performed significantly worse than 56 controls on a sustained attention task (the Rapid Visual Information Processing test from the Cambridge Neuropsychological Test Automated Battery [University of Cambridge, 2006]). In a follow-up study that included a subset of these participants and reassessed them after 6 months of mentalization-based therapy, patients performed similarly to controls on this sustained attention measure, and at the same time improved on a scale assessing relational symptoms on the Zanarini Rating Scale for Borderline Personality Disorder (ZAN-BPD; Zanarini et al., 2003) (Thomsen, Ruocco, Uliaszek, Mathiesen, & Simonsen, 2016). These results suggest that patients with BPD show deficits in sustained attention and that these deficits may be resolved through a psychotherapy that emphasizes increased attention to one's own subjective experiences of the self and perceptions of others.

Overall, findings of attentional functioning in BPD are mixed, with some studies indicating poorer performance in patients with BPD and others observing no differences compared to nonpsychiatric controls. Taken together, there appear to be more consistent deficits in sustained attention in BPD, and perhaps subtler limitations in selective attention; more statistically powered research is required to make firmer conclusions. Interestingly, preliminary research suggests that deficits in sustained attention may run in families and, and among patients, lowered attention may be resolved through mentalization-based treatment for BPD.

### Decision Making

Inefficient decision-making processes may contribute to the maintenance of the poorly conceived action patterns characteristic of individuals with BPD. Measuring decision making in BPD has commonly been accomplished using the Iowa Gambling Task (IGT; Bechara, Damasio, Damasio, & Anderson, 1994). The task instructs individuals to select cards from four decks, each with its own likelihood of yielding long-term gain or loss. Poor performances on the IGT (i.e., more frequently selecting cards from decks that result in long-term loss) have been associated with reversal learning difficulties, reduced ability to avoid negative feedback, and impulsive responding to certain stimuli (Bechara, Damasio, & Damasio, 2000). Poorer decision making has been detected in most studies of BPD (Bazanis et al., 2002; Dowson et al., 2004; Haaland & Landrø, 2007; Lawrence, Allen, & Chanen, 2010; Legris, Toplak, & Links, 2014; Maurex et al., 2009; Schuermann, Kathmann, Stiglmayr, Renneberg, & Endrass,

2011; Svaldi, Philipsen, & Matthies, 2012), but not in all (Kunert et al., 2003; Sprock et al., 2000). In an early study, Bazanis and colleagues (2002) compared 42 patients with BPD and 42 nonpsychiatric controls on a set of computerized decision-making and planning tasks, including the Cambridge Gambling Task (Rogers et al., 1999) and the Tower of London task (Owen et al., 1995). Patients with BPD performed worse on the gambling task based on their longer response times, less advantageous choices between competing actions, and impulsively responding when gambling on the outcome of their decisions (i.e., early responding in their choices, when placing bets on the likelihood of their decisions being correct). Deficits in decision making in BPD have also been reported by Haaland and Landrø (2007), who compared 20 patients with BPD and 15 controls on a computerized version of the IGT. In this study, patients made fewer advantageous choices on the IGT than did the controls, and patients with BPD and comorbid substance abuse performed worse than patients with BPD alone.

Maurex and colleagues (2009) also found significant differences in decision-making ability on the IGT in 48 female patients with BPD and 30 nonpsychiatric controls, with the BPD group choosing significantly more cards from the disadvantageous decks. While a majority of the patients performed within the normal range on the IGT, 20 were below the level considered "normal." Interestingly, patients performing below the normal range had a threefold greater frequency of possessing a specific allele of the tryptophan hydroxylase-1 (*TPH-1*) gene, which is related to the serotonin system and has been linked to impulsive aggression and suicidal behavior in BPD (Zaboli et al., 2006). These results support the notion that impulsive aggressive acts and self-harming behaviors may reflect deficits in decision-making abilities (Williams et al., 2015), and that these associations might be partly related to altered serotonergic neurotransmission.

Ruocco, McCloskey, Lee, and Coccaro (2009) found more limited decision-making deficits on the IGT in a comparison of 56 individuals with a Cluster B PD (71% with BPD), 19 with a Cluster C PD, and 61 nonpsychiatric controls. The Cluster B group did not significantly differ from controls on most performance measures on the IGT, with the exception of making more disadvantageous choices on the fourth-quarter portion of the task, which may reflect a more specific deficit in reversal learning (i.e., patients learned which decks were more advantageous as much as controls did, but their performance dropped off toward the end of the task). Differences between the results of this study and previous research may be due to differences in research design and the composition of the participant groups. Their results might also reflect the fact that Cluster B and Cluster C PD groups may have mild difficulties with reversal learning, reflecting a specific limitation in flexible learning, particularly when salient reward and punishment contingencies are present. Scheuerman and colleagues (2011) found that 18 patients with BPD made more risky choices than 18 matched controls and did not improve their strategies throughout their performance on a modified version of the IGT. Compared to controls, patients with BPD patients did not discriminate between positive and negative feedback information, and they showed more impulsivity and risk taking, reflected in lower mean IGT net scores. This led the authors to conclude that impaired decision making in patients with BPD may be related to dysfunctional use of feedback information, leading to decreased learning and avoidance of disadvantageous selections. These suggestions are in line with previous results linking lowered inhibition as a possible mediating process to reinforcement learning deficiencies in patients with BPD (Chapman, Leung, & Lynch, 2008; Hochhausen, Lorenz, & Newman, 2002).

In contrast to the IGT, the Game of Dice Task (Brand et al., 2005) provides information about the losses and gains associated with specific combinations of numbers on dice before and during the game, thereby allowing participants to calculate the risk of gain and loss related to each alternative dice combination. Implementing this task in a study design involving a sample of 21 patients with BPD and 29 nonpsychiatric controls, Svaldi and colleagues (2012) found that even when patients received continuous feedback regarding the consequences of their behavior, they continued to make disadvantageous decisions. Hence, these results are in line with previous findings of deficits in decision making in patients with BPD, and they provide more direct evidence that decision-making biases are evident even when the reinforcement and punishment are clear and the probability of the outcomes are defined. The underlying cognitive abilities potentially affecting decision-making ability were also examined by Legris and colleagues (2014), who administered the IGT and various measures of cognitive functioning, including overall intellectual ability (Raven's Progressive Matrices), working memory (Digit Span subtest from the WAIS-III), selective attention (Stroop test) and motor inhibition (stop-signal task) to 41 recently treated outpatients with BPD and 41 nonpsychiatric controls. The BPD group demonstrated disadvantageous decision making that continued throughout the duration of the task as compared to controls. This deficit in decision making appeared to be independent of the other cognitive functions that were measured, including global intellectual functioning, working memory, and cognitive and motor control. Moreover, poorer performance on the IGT was the only outcome that distinguished patients from controls.

## Planning and Problem Solving

The cognitive functions of planning and problem solving are commonly assumed to reflect higher-order processes of reasoning, temporal sequencing, and abstract thinking (Kramer et al., 2014; Unterrainer & Owen, 2006). Planning ability in BPD is commonly assessed using so-called "tower" tests (for a review, see Ruocco et al., 2014), including the Tower of London (Shallice, 1982) and the Tower of Hanoi (Davis & Keller, 1998; Hofstadter, 1996) tasks, as well as the Porteus Maze Test (Porteus, 1950). In an initial study, 42 patients with BPD required significantly more attempts to arrive at the correct solution to each problem on the Tower of London task than did 42 nonpsychiatric controls (Bazanis et al., 2002). Both patients and controls required more attempts for the difficult problems than for the easier ones, but this increase was significantly greater for the patients in comparison to controls. Also, patients with BPD took significantly longer than controls to make their first attempt to a solution.

In a comparison of 23 patients with BPD and 23 nonpsychiatric controls, Kunert and colleagues (2003) found no significant differences between groups on the Tower of Hanoi task. Two subsequent studies of planning ability in BPD employed the Porteus Maze Test and reported significantly poorer performances (i.e., greater response times) in patients as compared to nonpsychiatric controls (Dinn et al., 2004). Furthermore, patients with BPD and a history of "organic" brain injury performed poorer than the "nonorganic" group on this task (Travers & King, 2005).

Similarly, Beblo and colleagues (2006) reported a strong group effect within a sample of 22 patients with BPD and 22 controls using the Tower of Hanoi task. The BPD patients required more moves and took a significantly longer time to accomplish the task. In a sample of 51 patients and 34 controls, Bustamente and colleagues (2009) reproduced the pattern reported by Beblo and colleagues but used the Tower of London task, showing that patients with BPD took longer to complete each test item but did not make significantly more moves to achieve the target solutions on the task.

In an examination of planning and problem-solving abilities in patients with BPD and their biological parents, Gvirts and colleagues (2012) examined performance on the Tower of London task in four groups: 27 patients with BPD; 29 age-matched nonpsychiatric controls; 20 healthy, unaffected parents of patients with BPD; and 22 additional age-matched controls for the parent group. Significant differences were found between the BPD group and the nonpsychiatric control group at all difficulty levels (i.e., two to five move items) on the planning task. Patients had a significantly shorter initial deliberation time before beginning the task than the control group, and they solved significantly fewer problems in the most efficient manner possible (i.e., least number of moves needed to achieve the goal configuration). Additionally, both patients and their parents showed reduced latency to initiate the first move on the task (i.e., less planning time). Parents and their respective controls did not differ significantly on measurements of attention and working memory, also included in the study.

## Response Inhibition

Response inhibition, one facet of impulsivity, has been evaluated in BPD using a variety of neuropsychological tests, such as go/no-go tasks, stop-signal tasks, Stroop tests, and the CPT. The CPT (Conners, 2000; Doughterty, Bjork, Huckabee, Moeller, & Swann, 1999) is a vigilance test used to study sustained attention and rapid impulsive responding. Typically, target and nontarget stimuli are presented, and participants are then required to respond to target stimuli while withholding responses to nontarget stimuli. More BPD symptoms are robustly associated with higher levels of CPT commission errors (Swann, Bjork, Moeller, & Dougherty, 2002), and children with BPD psychopathology have higher levels of abnormal performance on the CPT in comparison with children without BPD (Paris et al., 1999). Also, in a cross-sectional survey, Rubio and colleagues (2007) divided alcohol-dependent patients (ADPs) into three subgroups: ADP's without a Cluster C PD ($n = 178$), ADP's with BPD ($n = 29$), ADP's with antisocial PD (ASPD; $n = 40$), and an additional nonpsychiatric control group ($n = 96$). Subjects with BPD had more omissions errors on the CPT in comparison than all three control groups.

Using a computerized go/no-go task, which asks individuals to withhold their response to a nontarget stimulus and subsequently receive punishment or reward, Leyton and colleagues (2001) compared 13 patients with BPD to 11 community nonpsychiatric controls. Compared to the control group, patients with BPD made significantly more punishment–reward commission errors (i.e., responding when one should not). This pattern was reproduced by Dinn and colleagues (2004) in a study that used a more conventional go/no-go task on which nine female patients with BPD exhibited longer response latencies and made significantly more errors of omission relative to controls (Lapierre, Braun, & Hodgins, 1995). Relatedly, Rentrop and colleagues (2008) found that 20 female patients with BPD performed worse on an acoustic no-go task (but not on a go task) in comparison with 18 nonpsychiatric controls, displaying faster reaction times and a greater speed–accuracy trade-off. These findings are consistent with clinical observations that patients with BPD have difficulties inhibiting behavior and delaying responses (Berlin, Rolls, & Kischka, 2004; Links, Heslegrave, & van Reekum, 1999; van Reekum, Links, Mitton, & Fedorov, 1996).

In a comparison of 15 patients with BPD, 12 patients with other Cluster C disorders, and 15 nonpsychiatric controls, both clinical groups' performance was slower than that of the nonpsychiatric controls when color-naming negative words on an emotional Stroop task with negative and neutral words (Arntz, Appels, & Sieswerda, 2000). However, performances of the clinical groups did not differ from each other, implying that attentional bias for negative stimuli was not specific for the BPD group. A subset of the applied negative words were BPD-related, but no attentional bias for these words was detected in the BPD group.

In a subsequent similar study, Sieswerda, Arntz, Mertens, and Vertommen (2007) compared 16 patients with BPD, 18 patients with other Cluster C disorders, 16 patients with an Axis I disorder, and 16 nonpsychiatric controls on an emotional word test. General negative words and neutral words were mixed with BPD-related words and presented both supra- and subliminally to participants. Patients with BPD showed hypervigilance for both negative and positive cues but were specifically biased toward BPD-related negative words, with larger effects than the other clinical groups. Additionally, the hypervigilance found in connection with BPD-related words was associated with anxiety symptoms and a history of childhood abuse. The authors suggested that patients with BPD may have an attentional bias consistent with BPD-related themes, which may have implications for monitoring hypervigilance among patients in clinical practice.

## Summary

Studies examining narrowly defined neurocognitive abilities that are more theoretically consistent with the phenotypic structure of BPD (i.e., low impulse control, poor problem solving) suggest that patients may indeed have deficits in more discrete cognitive functions. With respect to attention, deficits are most consistent in the area of sustained attention, although there are some reports of difficulties with selective attention (i.e., on the Stroop task). Decision making has been evaluated mainly using gambling tasks that also indirectly measure risk taking, and findings are mixed, although some evidence suggests that patients with BPD make less advantageous choices on decisions that have a higher risk for monetary loss. On tower tasks requiring participants to transform an initial state to match a target goal state, patients with BPD have shown both longer and shorter planning times in different studies, and they also appear to be less efficient in their problem-solving ability because they require more than the minimum attempts to reach a goal configuration. It is not yet clear what other cognitive processes may contribute to these deficits and how emotional states may influence performance on these measures.

## Interactions between Cognition and Emotion

Emotions can impact cognitive control in various ways. Emotional stimuli are potent distractors that challenge the ability to maintain focus on goal-relevant information and impact cognitive performance by capturing attention and reallocating processing resources (Dolcos & McCarthy, 2006). The prolonged and intense emotional experiences characteristic of BPD are likely to lead to cognitive disruptions, especially when individuals with the disorder are emotionally primed (e.g., focusing on sad faces when feeling depressed; Winter et al., 2014). However, these effects may not be detected because much of the research on neuropsychological function in BPD has used test batteries that do not contain emotionally laden contents. The sparse research that has explored emotion–cognition interactions in BPD has primarily focused on emotional memory biases and emotional interference with cognitive control.

### Attentional Biases for Emotional Information

Attentional biases for emotion-laden stimuli are common in many psychiatric disorders. Empirical work has shown that these factors may reflect risk and maintaining factors in emotional dysfunction (Harvey, 2004; Mathews & MacLeod, 2005). Patients with anxiety disorders show selective attention to threatening stimuli (MacLeod, Mathews, & Tata, 1986; Mogg, Philippot, & Bradley, 2004), whereas depressed patients tend to divert attention to sad themes (Gotlib, Krasnoperova, Yue, & Joormann, 2004), and selectively recall negative information (MacLeod, Rutherford, Campbell, Ebsworthy, & Holker, 2002). Accordingly, it has been suggested that individuals with BPD have difficulties controlling attention in the context of emotional dysregulation (Linehan, 1993).

Studies investigating BPD-related biases in attention have required participants to perform an attentional task as quickly as possible while ignoring emotional distractors. Results from research on the emotional Stroop task in BPD are heterogeneous, although most studies detect attentional biases in BPD in some form. A study of 15 patients with BPD, 12 patients with Cluster C disorders, and 15 nonpsychiatric controls indicated that both clinical groups performed slower than nonpsychiatric controls when color-naming negative words on an emotional Stroop with both negative and neutral words (Arntz et al., 2000). However, performances of the clinical groups did not differ from each other, implying that attentional bias for negative stimuli was not specific for the BPD group. Additionally, no attentional bias for a subset of the BPD-related negative words was detected. In a subsequent study using the same methods, Sieswerda and colleagues (2007) compared 16 patients with BPD to 18 patients with Cluster C disorders, 16 patients with an Axis I disorder, and 16 nonpsychiatric controls. Patients with BPD showed hypervigilance for both negative and positive cues (cues or words) but were specifically biased toward BPD-related negative words, with larger effects than those found in the other clinical groups. Additionally, the hypervigilance for BPD-related words was associated with anxiety symptoms and a history of childhood abuse.

Studies by Zanarini and colleagues (2003, 2006) have shown that 80% of patients with BPD achieve remission, which suggests that it is likely that biological and cognitive correlates of BPD symptoms may change over time. It must be noted though, that what is referred to as "remission" by Zanarini and colleagues refers to the fact that individuals with BPD who previously met five or more BPD criteria meet less than five after some years. However, these individuals may still have serious and severe symptoms and be far from remission in the medical sense, since patients with BPD often suffers from serious impairments in social functioning in later life. Still, the decrease in BPD criteria met over time possibly reflects some biological change in relation to remission of symptoms. Reflecting this possibility is a study showing that Stroop performance in a group of patients with BPD appeared to change after successful psychotherapy (Sieswerda et al., 2007). This study also reported that patients who showed attentional biases for the BPD-related words prior to therapy and showed symptomatic improvement following 3 years of cognitive-behavioral therapy also demonstrated a significant reduction in attentional bias, and their performance did not differ from the control group. The Stroop scores of patients who did not recover after treatment did not apparently change.

A different approach to investigate attentional biases is visual probe tasks. These computerized tasks present participants with supra- or subliminal visual primers in the form of emotional words or images. Individuals with no attentional bias are expected to show similar response times for all types of stimuli, independent of location, whereas individuals with a significant attentional bias are expected to be quicker in detecting stimuli appearing in the space just occupied by an emotional cue.

von Ceumern-Lindenstjerna and colleagues (2010) compared female adolescents with BPD, females with mixed psychiatric diagnoses, and nonpsychiatric controls, and did not find general group differences in attentional biases when mood at the time of the experiment was not taken into account. This led the authors to suggest that initial orienting to negative emotional stimuli may be more an indicator of severity of psychopathology in adolescents than being specifically related to BPD. However, there was a strong correlation between current negative mood and attentional bias toward negative faces, suggesting a difficulty for patients with BPD in disengaging attention from negative facial expressions when in a negative mood. The authors speculated that heightened attentional processing of negative emotional stimuli might exacerbate an already negative mood in patients with BPD, and they recommended that therapeutic interventions modulate attentional processes as a possible clinical implication of these findings.

Overall, although findings on attentional biases in BPD are mixed, a majority of studies suggest that BPD is associated with hypervigilance for emotion-laden material, especially when the material is specific to BPD. Higher levels of hypervigilance for, and difficulties disengaging from, emotional materials appear to be associated with higher levels of childhood abuse, negative mood, and severity of BPD symptoms, suggesting that attentional biases may play a key role in the development and maintenance of BPD.

## Memory Biases

Research on memory biases in BPD has focused on two different types of memory: selective memory for specific negative information and overgeneral autobiographical memory (i.e., remembering life events in very general terms, as opposed to more detailed, specific memories). Selective memory biases have been assessed using a directed forgetting paradigm in which participants are given a list of words with instructions about which words to remember and which to forget. Individuals who remember emotional words when instructed to forget them are assumed to have a memory bias for emotional information, whereas individuals who tend to forget emotional words are assumed to have an "avoidant retrieval style" (Gordon & Connolly, 2010).

Korfine and Hooley (2000) presented a community sample of individuals with BPD and nonpsychiatric community controls with a directed-forgetting task adapted from McNally, Metzger, Lasko, Clancy, and Pitman (1998) that included words salient to BPD. Participants were presented with either BPD-specific positive or neutral words, then instructed to either remember or forget each word. While there were no group differences in their recall of positive and neutral words, patients with BPD recalled more BPD-specific words that they were asked to forget. Domes and colleagues (2006) reported similar results using a directed forgetting task but only on negative stimuli (BPD-specific themes were not included). These results suggest that the presence of affectively valenced stimuli may decrease inhibitory ability in individuals with BPD. This implies that cognitive control functions may be impacted by emotional arousal, and that there are deficits in the intentional inhibition of aversive words, especially those with BPD-specific themes.

Mensebach and colleagues (2009) used a different approach to investigate memory biases that asked individuals to remember a list of words with and without distractions, which were either negative or neutral words. A tendency to forget more words in the context of negative compared to neutral distractors was assumed to reflect heightened sensitivity to negative stimuli. Compared to controls, patients with BPD showed lower recall of target words, but only when negative words were used as distractors. This finding can be considered consistent with research using the directed forgetting task because it suggests that negatively valenced emotional materials might disproportionately interfere with the encoding and/or subsequent recall of information in BPD.

"Autobiographical memory" (AM) is knowledge about one's own life, including knowledge of specific events, and recall of general events periods of life (Conway & Pleydell-Pearce, 2000). An important outcome variable used to evaluate AM is the number of specific versus general memories reported by an individual.

"Overgeneral memory" may be studied using the Autobiographical Memory Test (AMT; Williams & Broadbent, 1986), which requires individuals to recall specific events from their own lives based on positive, negative, or neutral cue words. The tendency to produce overgeneral memories is associated with depression, posttraumatic stress disorder (PTSD), suicidal behavior, and poor problem solving (Williams et al., 2007). Since these features are prevalent in BPD, the occurrence of overgeneral memories may expected to be associated with the disorder. However, this has not always been the case. In one study, patients with BPD retrieved significantly more overgeneral memories than did nonpsychiatric controls (Jones et al., 1999). Interestingly, the number of retrieved general memories correlated significantly with scores on a dissociation measure but not with mood, depression, anxiety, or anger symptoms. This suggests that dissociation may function as a coping mechanism for avoiding negative episodic memories. Subsequent studies failed to replicate the finding (Arntz, Meeren, & Wessel, 2002) except in subgroups with comorbid depression (Spinhoven, Van der Does, Van Dyck, & Kremers, 2006) or suicidal behavior (Maurex et al., 2009). Even this finding was not replicated by Reid and Startup (2010), although they did report that patients with BPD were less specific in their recollection of autobiographical memories than nonpsychiatric controls, but this difference was largely mediated by differences in education and intellectual function.

Overgeneral memory is commonly thought to be associated with less efficient executive functioning (Dalgleish et al., 2007) and poorer memory, source memory, and attention in individuals with major depression (Raes et al., 2006). Although results from Reid and Startup (2010) suggest that lower intellectual ability may play a role in overgeneralized memories, the authors concluded that this factor is unlikely to provide a complete explanation of the association between clinical states and overgeneral memories given that several studies have found the same effect over and above intelligence and cognitive ability (de Decker, Hermans, Raes, & Eelen, 2003; Park, Goodyer, & Teasdale, 2002; Wessel, Meeren, Peeters, Arntz, & Merckelbach, 2001; Williams et al., 1996). Supporting these findings, Kremers, Spinhoven, Van der Does, and Van Dyck (2006) found no association between overgeneral memories and social problem solving in BPD.

Comparing women with BPD to women with unipolar major depression and nonpsychiatric controls, Renneberg, Theobald, Nobs, and Weisbrod (2005) found that individuals in the BPD group had a negative tone to their autobiographical memories that was similar to those in the depressed group. However, the patients with BPD showed both greater specificity in their memories and shorter latency when recalling their memories than the control groups, suggesting that they had more rapid and easier access to specific negative memories. The authors speculated that this memory style might be related to emotional dysregulation. This association was also noted by Jørgensen and colleagues (2012), who compared patients with BPD to patients with obsessive–compulsive disorder and to nonpsychiatric controls. The BPD group recalled substantially more negative autobiographical memories than both control groups. The authors ascribed this negativity memory bias in BPD to a possible overload of negative life events that led to their self-concept and identity being dominated by memories of negative experiences and possibly to dysfunctional emotion regulation, memory disturbances, and a negative self-image (see also Bech, Elkit, & Simonsen, 2015).

## Summary and Conclusions

Neuropsychological research on BPD has yielded various results, with some findings more consistent than others, and in many instances, the number of positive findings seem to be counterbalanced by an equal number of negative ones, so that it is difficult to draw substantive conclusions. This is perhaps not surprising given the heterogeneous nature of the disorder. Initial studies showed that patients did not show decrements in global intellectual functioning but fell within the average range compared to age-based normative data. These studies, however, highlighted potential areas of deficit on subtests of intellectual tests that mainly involved attention, visuospatial construction, verbal comprehension, and perhaps higher-order executive functions. However, as with other mental disorders, no specific pattern of neurocognitive deficits has yet to be ascribed to BPD. Investigations of more narrowly defined cognitive abilities showed subtle inefficiencies in sustained attention, episodic memory, response control (i.e., motor response inhibition), decision making, problem solving, and planning. These findings are supported by meta-analytic results demonstrating deficits in several cognitive domains, including attention, cognitive flexibility, learning and memory, planning, processing speed, and visuospatial abilities (Ruocco, 2005). Subsequent neuropsychological research incorporating affectively valenced materials suggests that emotions may play a pivotal role in these deficits, and that interactions between emotion and cognition should be incorporated into neurocognitive models of BPD.

This review has identified issues that future research should address to characterize the nature and extent of neuropsychological deficits in BPD. First, it may be informative to study neurocognitive functions in adolescents with BPD, which might identify deficits that are present early in the development of the disorder and are not associated with factors that may arise during the course of illness (e.g., treatment with multiple medications). Second, given the heterogeneous nature of BPD, it may be more productive to explore neuropsychological deficits associated with specific dimensions of BPD psychopathology, such as impulsivity, affective instability, and identity disturbance. Third, research needs to clarify what cognitive deficits are specific to BPD as compared to other frequently comorbid clinical disorders (e.g., posttraumatic stress disorder). Fourth, it is important to investigate whether neuropsychological deficits persist in groups of patients that have never been treated with psychotropic medications (Kunert et al., 2003). Fifth, given that several cognitive deficits may underlie BPD, it may be important to consider the role of these deficits as potential predictors or moderators of outcomes for psychological and biological interventions for the disorder. Sixth, performance validity tests should be incorporated into the assessment of neuropsychological functioning in BPD given emerging research that indicates a small but significant proportion of patients who participate in research may not be fully compliant with cognitive testing (Ruocco, 2016). Seventh, there is a need for studies to explore the relationships between neuropsychological deficits and differences in brain structure and function to provide a better understanding of the neurobiological mechanisms that may be involved. Finally, greater attention should be given to potential sex differences in cognitive functioning in patients with BPD, especially given that most neuropsychological research on the disorder has been carried out with females.

# REFERENCES

American Psychiatric Association. (1980). *Diagnostic and statistical manual of mental disorders* (3rd ed.). Washington, DC: Author.

Arntz, A., Appels, C., & Sieswerda, S. (2000). Hypervigilance in borderline disorder: A test with the emotional Stroop paradigm. *Journal of Personality Disorders, 14*(4), 366–373.

Arntz, A., Meeren, M., & Wessel, I. (2002). No evidence for overgeneral memories in borderline personality disorder. *Behaviour Research and Therapy, 40*(9), 1063–1068.

Bazanis, E., Rogers, R. D., Dowson, J. H., Taylor, P., Meux, C., Staley, C., et al. (2002). Neurocognitive deficits in decision-making and planning of patients with DSM-III-R borderline personality disorder. *Psychological Medicine, 32*(8), 1395–1405.

Beblo, T., Saavedra, A. S., Mensebach, C., Lange, W., Markowitsch, H.-J., Rau, H., et al. (2006). Deficits in visual functions and neuropsychological inconsistency in borderline personality disorder. *Psychiatry Research, 145*(2), 127–135.

Bech, M., Elklit, A., & Simonsen, E. (2015). Autobiographical memory in borderline personality disorder—a review. *Personality and Mental Health, 9*(2), 162–171.

Bechara, A., Damasio, A., & Damasio, H. (2000). Emotion, decision making and the orbitofrontal cortex. *Cerebral Cortex, 10*(3), 295–307.

Bechara, A., Damasio, A., Damasio, H., & Anderson, S. (1994). Insensitivity to future consequences following damage to human prefrontal cortex. *Cognition, 50*(1), 7–15.

Berg, E. A. (1948). A simple objective technique for measuring flexibility in thinking. *Journal of General Psychology, 39*(1), 15–22.

Berlin, H., Rolls, E., & Kischka, U. (2004). Impulsivity, time perception, emotion and reinforcement sensitivity in patients with orbitofrontal cortex lesions. *Brain, 127*(5), 1108–1126.

Black, D. W., Forbush, K. T., Langer, A., Shaw, M., Graeber, M. A., Moser, D. J., et al. (2009). The neuropsychology of borderline personality disorder: A preliminary study on the predictive variance of neuropsychological tests vs. personality trait dimensions. *Personality and Mental Health, 3*(2), 128–141.

Brand, M., Fujiwara, E., Borsutzky, S., Kalbe, E., Kessler, J., & Markowitsch, H. J. (2005). Decision-making deficits of Korsakoff patients in a new gambling task with explicit rules: Associations with executive functions. *Neuropsychology, 19*(3), 267–277.

Burgess, J. W. (1990). Cognitive information processing in borderline personality disorder: A neuropsychiatric hypothesis. *Jefferson Journal of Psychiatry, 8*(2), Article 7.

Burgess, J. W. (1991). Relationship of depression and cognitive impairment to self-injury in borderline personality disorder, major depression, and schizophrenia. *Psychiatry Research, 38*(1), 77–87.

Bush, G., Luu, P., & Posner, M. I. (2000). Cognitive and emotional influences in anterior cingulate cortex. *Trends in Cognitive Sciences, 4*(6), 215–222.

Bustamante, M. L., Villarroel, J., Francesetti, V., Ríos, M., Arcos-Burgos, M., Jerez, S., et al. (2009). Planning in borderline personality disorder: Evidence for distinct subpopulations. *World Journal of Biological Psychiatry, 10*(4–2), 512–517.

Carpenter, C., Gold, J., & Fenton, W. (1993, May 22–27). *Neuropsychological testing results in borderline inpatients.* Paper presented at the 146th annual meeting of the American Psychiatric Association., San Fransisco, CA.

Chapman, A. L., Leung, D. W., & Lynch, T. R. (2008). Impulsivity and emotion dysregulation in borderline personality disorder. *Journal of Personality Disorders, 22*(2), 148–164.

Conners, C. K. (2004). *Conner's Continuous Performance Test II: Technical guide.* Toronto, ON, Canada: Multi-Health Systems.

Conners, C. K., & Multi-Health Systems Staff. (2000). *Conners' Continuous Performance Test II (CPT II V. 5).* North Tonawanda, NY: Multi-Health Systems.

Conway, M. A., & Pleydell-Pearce, C. W. (2000). The construction of autobiographical memories in the self-memory system. *Psychological Review, 107*(2), 261–288.

Cornelius, J. R., Soloff, P. H., George, A. V. A., Schulz, S. C., Tarter, R., Brenner, R. P., et al. (1989). An evaluation of the significance of selected neuropsychiatric abnormalities in the etiology of borderline personality disorder. *Journal of Personality Disorders, 3*(1), 19–25.

Dalgleish, T., Williams, J. M. G., Golden, A.-M. J., Perkins, N., Barrett, L. F., Barnard, P. J., et al. (2007). Reduced specificity of autobiographical memory and depression: The role of executive control. *Journal of Experimental Psychology: General, 136*(1), 23–42.

Darby, D., & Walsh, K. W. (2005). *Neuropsychology: A clinical approach.* New York: Churchill Livingstone.

Davis, H., & Keller, F. (1998). *Colorado Assessment Test manual.* Colorado Springs: Colorado Assessment Tests.

de Decker, A., Hermans, D., Raes, F., & Eelen, P. (2003). Autobiographical memory specificity and trauma in inpatient adolescents. *Journal of Clinical Child and Adolescent Psychology, 32*(1), 22–31.

Delis, D. C., Kramer, J. H., Kaplan, E., & Ober, B. A. (1987). *CVLT, California Verbal Learning Test: Adult Version: Manual.* San Antonio, TX: Psychological Corporation.

Dinn, W. M., Harris, C., Aycicegi, A., Greene, P., Kirkley, S., & Reilly, C. (2004). Neurocognitive function in borderline personality disorder. *Progress in Neuro-Psychopharmacology and Biological Psychiatry, 28*(2), 329–341.

Dolcos, F., & McCarthy, G. (2006). Brain systems mediating cognitive interference by emotional distraction. *Journal of Neuroscience, 26*(7), 2072–2079.

Domes, G., Winter, B., Schnell, K., Vohs, K., Fast, K., & Herpertz, S. C. (2006). The influence of emotions on inhibitory functioning in borderline personality disorder. *Psychological Medicine, 36*(8), 1163–1172.

Dougherty, D., Bjork, J., Huckabee, H., Moeller, F., & Swann, A. (1999). Laboratory measures of aggression and impulsivity in women with borderline personality disorder. *Psychiatry Research, 85*(3), 315–326.

Dowson, J. H., McLean, A., Bazanis, E., Toone, B., Young, S., Robbins, T. E., et al. (2004). Impaired spatial working memory in adults with attention-deficit/hyperactivity disorder: Comparisons with performance in adults with borderline personality disorder and in control subjects. *Acta Psychiatrica Scandinavica, 110*(1), 45–54.

Driessen, M., Herrmann, J., Stahl, K., Zwaan, M., Meier, S., Hill, A., et al. (2000). Magnetic resonance imaging volumes of the hippocampus and the amygdala in women with borderline personality disorder and early traumatization. *Archives of General Psychiatry, 57*(12), 1115–1122.

Eriksen, B. A., & Eriksen, C. W. (1974). Effects of noise letters upon the identification of a target letter in a nonsearch task. *Perception and Psychophysics, 16*(1), 143–149.

Etkin, A., Egner, T., & Kalisch, R. (2011). Emotional processing in anterior cingulate and medial prefrontal cortex. *Trends in Cognitive Sciences, 15*(2), 85–93.

Exner, J. E. (1986). Some Rorschach data comparing schizophrenics with borderline and schizotypal personality disorders. *Journal of Personality Assessment, 50*(3), 455–471.

Gardner, D., Lucas, P. B., & Cowdry, R. W. (1987). Soft sign neurological abnormalities in borderline personality disorder and normal control subjects. *Journal of Nervous and Mental Disease, 175*(3), 177–180.

Gold, J. M., Queern, C., Iannone, V. N., & Buchanan, R. W. (1999). Repeatable battery for the assessment of neuropsychological status as a screening test in schizophrenia: I. Sensitivity, reliability, and validity. *American Journal of Psychiatry, 156*(12), 1944–1950.

Gordon, H. M., & Connolly, D. A. (2010). Failing to report details of an event: A review of the directed forgetting procedure and applications to reports of childhood sexual abuse. *Memory, 18*(2), 115–128.

Gotlib, I. H., Krasnoperova, E., Yue, D. N., & Joormann, J. (2004). Attentional biases for negative interpersonal stimuli in clinical depression. *Journal of Abnormal Psychology, 113*(1), 121–135.

Gvirts, H. Z., Harari, H., Braw, Y., Shefet, D., Shamay-Tsoory, S., & Levkovitz, Y. (2012). Executive functioning among patients with borderline personality disorder (BPD) and their relatives. *Journal of Affective Disorders, 143*(1), 261–264.

Haaland, V. Ø., & Landrø, N. I. (2007). Decision making as measured with the Iowa Gambling Task in patients with borderline personality disorder. *Journal of the International Neuropsychological Society, 13*(4), 699–703.

Harvey, A. G. (2004). *Cognitive behavioural processes across psychological disorders: A transdiagnostic approach to research and treatment.* Oxford, UK: Oxford University Press.

Heaton, R. K. (1981). *A manual for the Wisconsin Card Sorting Test.* Odessa, FL: Psychological Assessment Resources.

Hochhausen, N. M., Lorenz, A. R., & Newman, J. P. (2002). Specifying the impulsivity of female inmates with borderline personality disorder. *Journal of Abnormal Psychology, 111*(3), 495–501.

Hofstadter, D. R. (1996). *Metamagical themas: Questing for the essence of mind and pattern.* New York: Basic Books.

Irle, E., Lange, C., & Sachsse, U. (2005). Reduced size and abnormal asymmetry of parietal cortex in women with borderline personality disorder. *Biological Psychiatry, 57*(2), 173–182.

Jones, B., Heard, H., Startup, M., Swales, M., Williams, J., & Jones, R. (1999). Autobiographical memory and dissociation in borderline personality disorder. *Psychological Medicine, 29*(6), 1397–1404.

Jørgensen, C. R., Berntsen, D., Bech, M., Kjølbye, M., Bennedsen, B. E., & Ramsgaard, S. B. (2012). Identity-related autobiographical memories and cultural life scripts in patients with borderline personality disorder. *Consciousness and Cognition, 21*(2), 788–798.

Judd, P. H., & Ruff, R. (1993). Neuropsychological dysfunction in borderline personality disorder. *Journal of Personality Disorders, 7*(4), 275–284.

Keefe, R. S. (1995). The contribution of neuropsychology to psychiatry. *American Journal of Psychiatry, 152*(1), 6–15.

Kernberg, O. F. (1967). Borderline personality organization. *Journal of the American Psychoanalytic Association, 15*(3), 641–685.

Kirkpatrick, T., Joyce, E., Milton, J., Duggan, C., Tyrer, P., & Rogers, R. D. (2007). Altered memory and affective instability in prisoners assessed for dangerous and severe personality disorder. *British Journal of Psychiatry, 190,*, S20–S26.

Korfine, L., & Hooley, J. M. (2000). Directed forgetting of emotional stimuli in borderline personality disorder. *Journal of Abnormal Psychology, 109*(2), 214–221.

Kramer, J. H., Mungas, D., Possin, K. L., Rankin, K. P., Boxer, A. L., Rosen, H. J., et al. (2014). NIH EXAMINER: Conceptualization and development of an executive function battery. *Journal of the International Neuropsychological Society, 20*(1), 11–19.

Kremers, I., Spinhoven, P., Van der Does, A., & Van Dyck, R. (2006). Social problem solving, autobiographical memory and future specificity in outpatients with borderline personality disorder. *Clinical Psychology and Psychotherapy, 13*(2), 131–137.

Kroll, J. (1988). *The challenge of the borderline patient.* New York: Norton.

Kunert, H. J., Druecke, H. W., Sass, H., & Herpertz, S. (2003). Frontal lobe dysfunctions in borderline personality disorder?: Neuropsychological findings. *Journal of Personality Disorders, 17*(6), 497–509.

Lapierre, D., Braun, C. M., & Hodgins, S. (1995). Ventral frontal deficits in psychopathy: Neuropsychological test findings. *Neuropsychologia, 33*(2), 139–151.

Lawrence, K. A., Allen, J. S., & Chanen, A. M. (2010). Impulsivity in borderline personality disorder: Reward-based decision-making and its relationship to emotional distress. *Journal of Personality Disorders, 24*(6), 785–799.

Legris, J., Links, P. S., van Reekum, R., Tannock, R., & Toplak, M. (2012). Executive function and suicidal risk in women with borderline personality disorder. *Psychiatry Research, 196*(1), 101–108.

Legris, J., Toplak, M., & Links, P. S. (2014). Affective decision making in women with borderline personality disorder. *Journal of Personality Disorders, 28*(5), 698–719.

Lenzenweger, M., Clarkin, J., Fertuck, E. A., & Kernberg, O. F. (2004). Executive neurocognitive functioning and neurobehavioral systems indicators in borderline personality disorder: A preliminary study. *Journal of Personality Disorders, 18*(5), 421–438.

Lerner, P., & Lerner, H. (1980). Rorschach assessment of primitive defenses in borderline personality structure. In J. S. Kwawer (Ed.), *Borderline phenomena and the Rorschach test* (pp. 257–274). New York: International Universities Press.

Leyton, M., Okazawa, H., Diksic, M., Paris, J., Rosa, P., Mzengeza, S., et al. (2001). Brain regional $\alpha$-[$^{11}$C] methyl-L-tryptophan trapping in impulsive subjects with borderline personality disorder. *American Journal of Psychiatry, 158*(5), 775–782.

Lezak, M. (1993). Newer contributions to the neuropsychological assessment of executive functions. *Journal of Head Trauma Rehabilitation, 8,* 24–31.

Lezak, M. D. (2004). *Neuropsychological assessment* (4th ed.). New York: Oxford University Press.

Linehan, M. M. (1993). *Cognitive-behavioral treatment of borderline personality disorder.* New York: Guilford Press.

Links, P. S., Heslegrave, R., & van Reekum, R. (1999). Impulsivity: Core aspect of borderline personality disorder. *Journal of Personality Disorders, 13*(1), 1–9.

MacLeod, C., Mathews, A., & Tata, P. (1986). Attentional bias in emotional disorders. *Journal of Abnormal Psychology, 95*(1), 15–20.

MacLeod, C., Rutherford, E., Campbell, L., Ebsworthy, G., & Holker, L. (2002). Selective attention and emotional vulnerability: Assessing the causal basis of their association through the experimental manipulation of attentional bias. *Journal of Abnormal Psychology, 111*(1), 107–123.

Mathews, A., & MacLeod, C. (2005). Cognitive vulnerability to emotional disorders. *Annual Review of Clinical Psychology, 1,* 167–195.

Mathiesen, B. B., Simonsen, E., Soegaard, U., & Kvist, K. (2014). Similarities and differences in borderline and organic personality disorder. *Cognitive Neuropsychiatry, 19*(1), 1–16.

Maurex, L., Zaboli, G., Wiens, S., Åsberg, M., Leopardi, R., & Öhman, A. (2009). Emotionally controlled decision-making and a gene variant related to serotonin synthesis in women with borderline personality disorder. *Scandinavian Journal of Psychology, 50*(1), 5–10.

McNally, R. J., Metzger, L. J., Lasko, N. B., Clancy, S. A., & Pitman, R. K. (1998). Directed forgetting of trauma cues in adult survivors of childhood sexual abuse with and without posttraumatic stress disorder. *Journal of Abnormal Psychology, 107*(4), 596–601.

Mensebach, C., Beblo, T., Driessen, M., Wingenfeld, K., Mertens, M., Rullkoetter, N., et al. (2009). Neural correlates of episodic and semantic memory retrieval in borderline personality disorder: An fMRI study. *Psychiatry Research: Neuroimaging, 171*(2), 94–105.

Mensebach, C., Wingenfeld, K., Driessen, M., Rullkoetter, N., Schlosser, N., Steil, C., et al. (2009). Emotion-induced memory dysfunction in borderline personality disorder. *Cognitive Neuropsychiatry, 14*(6), 524–541.

Minzenberg, M. J., Poole, J. H., & Vinogradov, S. (2008). A neurocognitive model of borderline personality disorder: Effects of childhood sexual abuse and relationship to adult social attachment disturbance. *Development and Psychopathology, 20*(1), 341–368.

Mogg, K., Philippot, P., & Bradley, B. P. (2004). Selective attention to angry faces in clinical social phobia. *Journal of Abnormal Psychology, 113*(1), 160–165.

Monarch, E. S., Saykin, A. S., & Flashman, L. A. (2004). Neuropsychological impairment in borderline personality disorder. *Psychiatric Clinics of North America, 27*(1), 67–82.

Murray, H. A. (1943). *Thematic Appercention Test manual.* Cambridge, MA: Harvard University Press.

Murray, J. B. (1993). Relationship of childhood sexual abuse to borderline personality disorder, posttraumatic stress disorder, and multiple personality disorder. *Journal of Psychology, 127*(6), 657–676.

O'Leary, K. M., Brouwers, P., Gardner, D., & Cowdry, M. (1991). Neuropsychological testing of patients with borderline personality disorder. *American Journal of Psychiatry, 148*(1), 106–111.

O'Leary, K. M., & Cowdry, R. W. (1994). Neuropsychological testing results in borderline personality disorder. In K. R. Silk (Ed.), *Biological and neurobehavioral studies of borderline personality disorder* (pp. 127–159). Washington DC: American Psychiatric Press.

Owen, A. M., Sahakian, B. J., Hodges, J. R., Summers, B. A., Polkey, C. E., & Robbins, T. W. (1995). Dopamine-dependent frontostriatal planning deficits in early Parkinson's disease. *Neuropsychology, 9*(1), 126–140.

Paris, J., Zelkowitz, P., Cuzder, J., Joseph, S., & Feldman, R. (1999). Neuropsychological factors associated with borderline pathology in children. *Journal of the American Academy of Child and Adolescent Psychiatry, 38*(6), 770–774.

Park, R. J., Goodyer, I., & Teasdale, J. (2002). Categoric overgeneral autobiographical memory in adolescents with major depressive disorder. *Psychological Medicine, 32*(2), 267–276.

Porteus, S. D. (1950). *The Porteus Maze Test and intelligence.* Palo Alto, CA: Pacific Books.

Posner, M., Rothbart, M., Vizueta, N., Levy, K., Evans, D., Thomas, K., et al. (2002). Attentional mechanisms of borderline personality disorder. *Proceedings of the National Academy of Sciences USA, 99,* 16366–16370.

Raes, F., Hermans, D., Williams, J. M. G., Demyttenaere, K., Sabbe, B., Pieters, G., et al. (2006). Is overgeneral autobiographical memory an isolated memory phenomenon in major depression? *Memory, 14*(5), 584–594.

Reid, T., & Startup, M. (2010). Autobiographical memory specificity in borderline personality disorder: Associations with co-morbid depression and intellectual ability. *British Journal of Clinical Psychology, 49*(3), 413–420.

Reitan, R. M. (1971). Trail making test results for normal and brain-damaged children. *Perceptual and Motor Skills, 33*(2), 575–581.

Renneberg, B., Theobald, E., Nobs, M., & Weisbrod, M. (2005). Autobiographical memory in borderline personality disorder and depression. *Cognitive Therapy and Research, 29*(3), 343–358.

Rentrop, M., Backenstrass, M., Jaentch, B., Kaiser, S., Roth, A., Unger, J., et al. (2008). Response inhibition in borderline personality disorder: Performance in a go/nogo task. *Psychopathology, 41,* 50–57.

Rogers, R. D., Owen, A. M., Middleton, H. C., Williams, E. J., Pickard, J. D., Sahakian, B. J., et al. (1999). Choosing between small, likely rewards and large, unlikely rewards activates inferior and orbital prefrontal cortex. *Journal of Neuroscience, 19*(20), 9029–9038.

Rorschach, H. (1975). *Psychodiagnostik.* New York: Grune & Stratton.

Rubio, G., Jimenez, M., Rodriguez-Jimenez, R., Martinez, I., Iribarren, M. M., Jimenez-Arriero, M. A., et al. (2007). Varieties of impulsivity in males with alcohol dependence: The role of Cluster-B personality disorder. *Alcoholism: Clinical and Experiemntal Research, 31*(11), 1826–1832.

Ruff, R. M., Light, R. H., & Evans, R. W. (1987). The Ruff Figural Fluency Test: A normative study with adults. *Developmental Neuropsychology, 3*(1), 37–51.

Ruocco, A. C. (2005). The neuropsychology of borderline personality disorder: A meta-analysis and review. *Psychiatry Research, 137*(3), 191–202.

Ruocco, A. C. (2016). Compliance on neuropsychological performance validity testing in patients with borderline personality disorder. *Psychological Assessment, 28,* 345–350.

Ruocco, A. C., & Bahl, N. (2014). Material-specific discrepancies in verbal and visual episodic memory in borderline personality disorder. *Psychiatry Research, 220,* 694–697.

Ruocco, A. C., Lam, J., & McMain, S. F. (2014). Subjective cognitive complaints and functional disability in patients with borderline personality disorder and their nonaffected first-degree relatives. *Canadian Journal of Psychiatry, 59*(6), 335–344.

Ruocco, A. C., Laporte, L., Russell, J., Guttman, H., & Paris, J. (2012). Response inhibition deficits in unaffected first-degree relatives of patients with borderline personality disorder. *Neuropsychology, 26*(4), 473–482.

Ruocco, A. C., McCloskey, M. S., Lee, R., & Coccaro, E. F. (2009). Indices of orbitofrontal and prefrontal function in Cluster B and Cluster C personality disorders. *Psychiatry Research, 170*(2), 282–285.

Ruocco, A. C., Rodrigo, A. H., Lam, J., Di Domenico, S. I., Graves, B., & Ayaz, H. (2014). A problem-solving task specialized for functional neuroimaging: Validation of the Scarborough adaptation of the Tower of London (S-TOL) using near-infrared spectroscopy. *Frontiers in Human Neuroscience, 8,* 185.

Ruocco, A. C., Swirsky-Sacchetti, T., Chute, C. L., Mandel, S., Platek, S. M., & Zillmer, E. A. (2008). Distinguishing between neuropsychological malingering and exaggerated psychiatric symptoms in a neuropsychological setting. *The Clinical Neuropsychologist, 22*(3), 547–564.

Saykin, A. J., Gur, R. C., Gur, R. E., Shtasel, D. L., Flannery, K. A., Mozley, L. H., et al. (1995). Normative neuropsychological test performance effects of age, education, gender and ethnicity. *Applied Neuropsychology, 2,* 79–88.

Schuermann, B., Kathmann, N., Stiglmayr, C., Renneberg, B., & Endrass, T. (2011). Impaired decision making and feedback evaluation in borderline personality disorder. *Psychological Medicine, 41*(9), 1917–1927.

Seres, I., Unoka, Z., Bódi, N., Aspán, N., & Kéri, S. (2009). The neuropsychology of borderline personality disorder: Relationship with clinical dimensions and comparison with other personality disorders. *Journal of Personality Disorders, 23*(6), 555–562.

Shallice, T. (1982). Specific impairments of planning. *Philosophical Transactions of the Royal Society B: Biological Sciences, 298,* 199–209.

Sieswerda, S., Arntz, A., Mertens, I., & Vertommen, S. (2007). Hypervigilance in patients with borderline personality disorder: Specificity, automaticity, and predictors. *Behaviour Research and Therapy, 45*(5), 1011–1024.

Silbersweig, D., Clarkin, J. F., Goldstein, M., Kernberg, O. F., Tuescher, O., Levy, K. N., et al. (2007). Failure of frontolimbic inhibitory function in the context of negative emotion in borderline personality disorder. *American Journal of Psychiatry, 164*(12), 1832–1841.

Singer, M. T., & Larson, D. G. (1981). Borderline personality and the Rorschach test. *Archives of General Psychiatry, 38*(6), 693–698.

Spinhoven, P., Van der Does, A. J. W., Van Dyck, R., & Kremers, I. P. (2006). Autobiographical memory in depressed and nondepressed patients with borderline personality disorder after long-term psychotherapy. *Cognition and Emotion, 20*(3–4), 448–465.

Sprock, J., Rader, T. J., Kendall, J. P., & Yoder, C. Y. (2000). Neuropsychological functioning in patients with borderline personality disorder. *Journal of Clinical Psychology, 56*(12), 1587–1600.

Stein, D. J., Hollander, E., Cohen, L., Frenkel, M., Saoud, J. B., DeCaria, C., et al. (1993). Neuropsychiatric impairment in impulsive personality disorders. *Psychiatry Research, 48*(3), 257–266.

Stevens, A., Burkhardt, M., Hautzinger, M., Schwarz, J., & Unckel, C. (2004). Borderline personality disorder: Impaired visual perception and working memory. *Psychiatry Research, 125*(3), 257–267.

Svaldi, J., Philipsen, A., & Matthies, S. (2012). Risky decision-making in borderline personality disorder. *Psychiatry Research, 197*(1), 112–118.

Swann, A. C., Bjork, J. M., Moeller, G., & Doughterty, D. M. (2002). Two models of impulsivity: Relationship to personality traits and psychopathology. *Biological Psychiatry, 51,* 988–994.

Swirsky-Sacchetti, T., Gorton, G. G., Samuel, S., Sobel, R., Genetta-Wadly, A., & Burleigh, B. (1993). Neuropsychological function in borderline personality disorder. *Journal of Clinical Psychology, 49*(3), 385–396.

Tellegen, A. (1982). *Brief manual for the Multidimensional Personality Questionnaire.* Unpublished manuscript, University of Minnesota, Minneapolis.

Tewes, U. (1991). *Hamburg–Wechsler Intelligentztest für Erwachsene (HAWIE-R) (Revision 1991): Handbuch und testanweisund.* Bern, Switzerland: Huber.

Thomsen, M. S., Ruocco, A. C., Carcone, D., Mathiesen, B. B., & Simonsen, E. (2016). Neurocognitive deficits in borderline personality disorder: Associations with dimensions of childhood trauma and personality psychopathology. *Journal of Personality Disorders.* [Epub ahead of print]

Thomsen, M. S., Ruocco, A. C., Uliaszek, A. A., Mathiesen, B. B., & Simonsen, E. (2016). Changes in neurocognitive functioning after six months of mentalization based treatment for borderline personality disorder. *Journal of Personality Disorders, 31*(3), 1–19.

Travers, C., & King, R. (2005). An investigation of organic factors in the neuropsychological functioning of patients with borderline personality disorder. *Journal of Personality Disorders, 19*(1), 1–18.

University of Cambridge. (2006). *The Cambridge Neuropsychological Test Automated Battery.* Cambridge, UK: Author.

Unterrainer, J. M., & Owen, A. M. (2006). Planning and problem solving: From neuropsychology to functional neuroimaging. *Journal of Physiology (Paris), 99*(4), 308–317.

van Reekum, R. (1993). Acquired and developmental brain dysfunction in borderline personality disorder. *Canadian Journal of Psychiatry, 38,* 4–10.

van Reekum, R., Links, P. S., Mitton, M. J. E., & Fedorov, C. (1996). Impulsivity, defensive functioning, and borderline personality disorder. *Canadian Journal of Psychiatry, 41,* 81–84.

von Ceumern-Lindenstjerna, I.-A., Brunner, R., Parzer, P., Mundt, C., Fiedler, P., & Resch, F. (2010). Attentional bias in later stages of emotional information processing in female adolescents with borderline personality disorder. *Psychopathology, 43*(1), 25–32.

Wechsler, D. (1945). *Wechsler Memory Scale manual.* New York: Psychological Corporation.

Wechsler, D. (1981). *Wechsler Adult Intelligence Scale.* New York: Psychological Corporation.

Wechsler, D. (1999). *Wechsler Abbreviated Intelligence Scale (WASI).* San Antonio, TX: Psychological Corporation.

Wechsler, D. (2008). *Wechsler Adult Intelligence Scale–Fourth Edition (WAIS-IV).* San Antonio, TX: Pearson.

Wessel, I., Meeren, M., Peeters, F., Arntz, A., & Merckelbach, H. (2001). Correlates of autobiographical memory specificity: The role of depression, anxiety and childhood trauma. *Behaviour Research and Therapy, 39*(4), 409–421.

Westen, D., Lohr, N., Silk, K. R., Gold, L., & Kerber, K. (1990). Object relations and social cognition in borderlines, major depressives, and normals: A Thematic Appercetion Test analysis. *Psychological Assessment, 2*(4), 355–364.

Williams, G., Daros, A. R., Graves, B., McMain, S. F., Links, P. S., & Ruocco, A. C. (2015). Executive functions and social cognition in highly lethal self-injuring patients with borderline personality disorder. *Personality Disorders: Theory, Research, and Treatment, 6,* 107–116.

Williams, J. M. G., Barnhofer, T., Crane, C., Herman, D., Raes, F., Watkins, E., & Dalgleish, T. (2007). Autobiographical memory specificity and emotional disorder. *Psychological Bulletin, 133*(1), 122–148.

Williams, J. M. G., & Broadbent, K. (1986) Autobiographical memories in suicide attempters. *Journal of Abnormal Psychology, 95*(2), 144–149.

Williams, J. M. G., Ellis, N. C., Tyers, C., Healy, H., Rose, G., & MacLeod, A. K. (1996). The specificity of autobiographical memory and imageability of the future. *Memory and Cognition, 24*(1), 116–125.

Winter, D., Elzinga, B., & Schmahl, C. (2014). Emotions and memory in borderline personality disorder. *Psychopathology, 47*(2), 71–85.

Zaboli, G., Gizatullin, R., Nilsonne, Å., Wilczek, A., Jönsson, E. G., Ahnemark, E., et al. (2006). Tryptophan hydroxylase-1 gene variants associate with a group of suicidal borderline women. *Neuropsychopharmacology, 31*(9), 1982–1990.

Zanarini, M. C., Frankenburg, F. R., Hennen, J., Reich, D. B., & Silk, K. R. (2006). Prediction of the 10-year course of borderline personality disorder. *American Journal of Psychiatry, 163*(5), 827–832.

Zanarini, M. C., Vujanovic, A., Parachini, E., Boulanger, J., Frankenburg, F., & Hennen, J. (2003). Zanarini Rating Scale for Borderline Personality Disorder (ZAN-BPD): A continuous measure of DSM-IV borderline psychopathology. *Journal of Personality Disorders, 17*(3), 233–242.

# CHAPTER 17

# Childhood Adversities and Personality Disorders

Joel Paris

## Adversities Associated with Mental Disorders

Mental health clinicians and researchers have long been interested in the impact of adverse events during childhood on adults. There can be little doubt that a wide variety of mental disorders are associated with childhood adversity (Perez-Fuentes et al, 2013; Rutter & Maughan, 1997). Yet most people exposed to any particular risk do not develop any disorder, while people developing the same disorder may have been exposed to entirely different risks (Cichetti, 2004). Some people with mental disorders will have had a relatively normal childhood. Clinicians need to recognize the complexity of the relationship between life stressors and psychopathology.

Risk factors are not equivalent to causes. While adversities increase the eventual risk for developing mental disorders, they only make negative outcomes more likely. A large body of research (Rutter, 2012a, 2012b) shows that resilience to adversity is not the exception, but the rule. In short, negative childhood experiences do not *necessarily* lead to psychopathological sequelae in adult life.

One reason for confusion is that studies in clinical and community populations may lead to different conclusions. In clinical populations, patients with a variety of disorders report more psychosocial adversities during childhood than do nonpatients. But in community populations, the very same adversities lead to clinically significant pathology in only a minority of those who are exposed (Cicchetti, 2004). On the other hand, patients with an underlying temperamental vulnerability may react to stressors more intensely and are much more likely to be more affected (Rutter, 2006). These individual differences in sensitivity to stressful events resolve the contradiction between the frequency of childhood adversities in patients and the fact that most people manage to overcome them. The lesson for clinicians is they should not insist on identifying past events to account for current symptoms.

A failure to distinguish between risk factors and causes has also led to the misinterpretation of research findings linking adversities to mental disorders. If one reads, for example, that a large number of patients with a personality disorder (PD) report a history of child abuse, it is tempting to assume that these early experiences account for etiology, and to search for them actively. However, correlations between risk factors and disorders do not prove causal relationships. Often, such associations are accounted for by *third-variable* effects. Long-term sequelae may be due to coexisting adversities, and to the cumulative effects of multiple risks (Rutter, 2012a). Moreover, individual vulnerabilities mediate interactions between adversity and long-term outcome. For example, children with difficult temperaments are more likely to be in conflict with peers and parents, increasing the likelihood of social rejection or maltreatment (Rutter, 2012b).

Moreover, findings that are statistically significant may mask the fact that only a minority of subjects in a study are affected. One can be impressed by effects if they are dramatic for some, even when they are either subtle or absent for others. Family breakdown provides an instructive example. Children of divorce and children from intact families show few large-scale differences in the long-term risk for developing mental disorders, but a vulnerable minority accounts for the statistically higher prevalence of sequelae in this population (Amato & Booth, 2000). Moreover, many of the negative effects of divorce for children are attributable to third variables: additional risks such as poverty, change of neighborhood, or depression in a custodial parent. Parental divorce is not the worst thing that can happen to children. It is unexpected parental separations that are most traumatic, while the dissolution of marriages marked by open conflict can actually reduce symptoms in children (Amato & Booth, 2000). The increased risk for psychopathology in the children of divorce ultimately depends on "cascades" of adversity that all too often follow family breakdown (Rutter, 2012a).

This helps to explain why even the most overtly traumatic events do not necessarily to lead to pathological sequelae. In the empirical literature on childhood sexual abuse (Fergusson & Mullen, 1999; Finkelhor, Ormrod, Turner, & Hamby, 2005) and on childhood physical abuse (Malinovsky-Rummell & Hansen, 1993), a consistent pattern emerges. While there are statistical relationships between exposure to trauma and pathological sequelae, serious negative outcomes occur in about one-fourth of those exposed (Fergusson & Mullen, 1999). Most of these children are relatively resilient to being abused. Clinical practice, where those who are most affected present for treatment, gives a misleading impression of this relationship.

The principle that *most* children are resilient to adversity is crucial. The ubiquity of protective mechanisms is both fortunate and logical. Given the adverse nature of life in the human environment of evolutionary adaptiveness (Beck, Davis, & Freeman, 2015), resilience was favored by natural selection.

A large literature elucidates the mechanisms underlying resilience (Rutter, 2012a, 2012b). Studies of children at risk (e.g., Werner & Smith, 1992) have documented how a positive temperament and life events outside the family can confer some degree of "immunity" to adversity.

On the biological side, children with positive personality traits and higher levels of intelligence are more resourceful, and better at finding ways to cope with negative experiences. There is even evidence that adversity can sometimes cause "steeling," increased resilience to future stressful events (Rutter, 2012b). In contrast, children with negative personality traits and lower levels of intelligence tend to experience adversities as more stressful than do those with a better temperament. In addition, positive relationships can buffer negative ones. Thus, problems with nuclear family members can be compensated for by attachments to extended family, or to non-family members. For example, children at risk can promote resilience by spending more time outside the home with alternative attachment figures.

A third problem in interpreting associations between early negative events and psychopathology is the use of retrospective data. It is difficult to rely on patients with serious current symptoms to provide accurate reports of childhood after the passage of decades. On the whole, being ill creates a recall bias, so that memories of the past are negatively colored by present suffering (Hardt & Rutter, 2004). The main way around the problem is to confirm the findings of retrospective studies in prospective research, as has indeed been done in community studies (Caspi & Roberts, 1999; Cohen, Crawford, Johnson, & Kasen, 2005) and in children at risk due to child abuse (Widom, Cjaza, & Paris, 2009). Since long-term follow-up studies are rare, one may also use sibling concordance data or objective data such as court records (Rutter & Maughan, 1997). Even so, few studies on adults have included collection of corroborating data. And since prospective research, following large cohorts of normal children, or children with identified risks for psychopathology, is expensive, the number of existing studies is limited.

Another issue concerns the timing of adverse events. On theoretical grounds, it has sometimes been assumed that psychosocial stressors occurring early in life should produce more sequelae than stressors occurring later on. This theoretical principle, termed "the primacy of early experience," has long been a conventional wisdom (Millon & Davis, 1996), and it remains a tenet of attachment theory (Cassidy & Shaver, 2012). Yet in spite of its ubiquity, primacy has a shaky evidence base (Paris, 2000). The problem is that the effects of timing are confounded with those of cumulative dosing. In other words, when problems start early, they are much more likely to be chronic, making it difficult to separate timing from dosing (Rutter, 2012b).

The relationship between childhood adversities and mental disorders can best be understood in light of a diathesis–stress model of mental disorders (Monroe & Simons, 1991). In this framework, disorders emerge when stressors uncover underlying vulnerabilities, and diatheses determine the type of pathology that develops. This theory accounts for the inconsistent relationship between adversity and outcome, as well as for the fact that similar risk factors are found in different mental disorders.

In summary, the existing literature on adversity and resilience justifies these preliminary conclusions:

1. A majority of children exposed to any specific adversity will not develop any mental disorder.
2. Multiple adversities have "cumulative" effects: The greater the number of negative events during childhood, the more likely are pathological sequelae.
3. Resilience mechanisms buffer adversities and can prevent long-term sequelae.
4. If adversities follow each other in a cascade, then resilience mechanisms can be overwhelmed.
5. Adversities rarely have any specific relationship to mental disorders, and the psychosocial risk factors for many categories tend to be similar.
6. There is only limited evidence that timing plays a crucial role in the effects of childhood adversities.

## Childhood Adversities Associated with PDs

A series of systematic investigations have provided documentation for clinical observations of associations between childhood adversities and PDs. Most of this research has focused on borderline PD (BPD). The main risk factors that have been identified are (1) dysfunctional families (the effects of parental psychopathology, family breakdown, or poor parenting); (2) traumatic experiences (e.g., childhood sexual abuse or physical abuse); and (3) social stressors.

### Dysfunctional Families

*Parental Psychopathology*

As is the case for most people with psychiatric diagnoses, patients with PDs tend to have parents or other close relatives who have significant psychopathology (Livesley, 2003). These disorders tend to fall in the same "spectrum" (impulsive, affective, or cognitive). Linehan (1993) suggested that emotion dysregulation may run in families. Zanarini (1993) suggested that since antisocial PD (ASPD), BPD, and substance abuse segregate together in family studies, they form a group of "impulsive spectrum disorders" associated with a common temperament. Similarly, patients with schizoid, paranoid, and schizotypal PDs tend to have relatives with schizophrenia or schizophrenia spectrum disorders, and patients with avoidant, dependent, and compulsive PDs may have relatives with anxiety disorders (Siever & Davis, 1991). These relationships reflect heritable and temperamental similarities, as well as trauma, family dysfunction, and family breakdown that tend to accompany parental psychopathology. These vulnerabilities also interact with adversity. Cloninger, Sigvardsson, and Bohman (1982) found that adopted children with an antisocial biological parent are most likely to develop the same disorder when they also experience family dysfunction.

These mechanisms have been most thoroughly investigated in impulsive PD. In a classic study, Robins (1966) examined the predictors of whether children with conduct disorder develop psychopathy (or ASPD) as adults. By far, the most important risk factor consisted of having a psychopathic parent (usually the father), which predicted antisocial personality in a child independent of other co-occurring risks. The findings concerning BPD have been similar, in that first-degree relatives of patients tend to have either "impulsive spectrum" disorders (antisocial personality, substance abuse, borderline personality), or mood disorders (White, Gunderson, Zanarini, & Hudson, 2003).

*Family Breakdown*

The long-term effects of family breakdown can be subtle, but in some cases they are all too real (Amato & Booth, 2000). Studies in community populations may not reflect the impact of separation on vulnerable children: those who are temperamentally sensitive or exposed to multiple adversities.

The rate of family breakdown in patients with PDs is greater than that in community populations. Even 20 years ago, 50% of patients with PDs, most of who were raised in the 1960s, prior to a later "epidemic" of divorce, were found to have experienced parental separation, associated with multiple psychosocial adversities (Paris, Zweig-Frank, & Guzder, 1994a, 1994b; Zanarini, 2000).

## Parenting Practices

The idea that children who develop PDs have experienced early emotional neglect derives from psychodynamic models. Attachment theory (Cassidy & Shaver, 2012) assumes that emotional security in adults is grounded in consistent empathic and supportive responses during childhood, and that abnormal personality is the result of negative and neglectful relationships with parents.

Theories of parenting describe two basic components in the task of raising children: providing love and support, and allowing them to become independent (Rowe, 1981). These two dimensions (affection vs. neglect, and autonomy vs. overprotection) emerge consistently from empirical research on effective parenting practices (Parker, 1983). The same principles have been applied to empirical studies of the dimensions of parenting. Self-report instruments such as the Parental Bonding Instrument (PBI; Parker, 1983) have been standardized in community samples. It should be kept in mind that these scales are retrospective, and they also have a heritable component, reflecting the effect of personality traits on perceptions of life experience (Plomin & Bergeman, 1991). Individuals with a greater temperamental need for affirmation and reassurance may be more likely to perceive their parenting as inadequate.

For example, empirical studies in PD using the PBI (Paris & Frank, 1989) have suggested that patients with BPD experience both neglect and overprotection from both parents. The question is whether these reports reflect historical reality, involving "biparental failure," or a discrepancy between greater needs and what "good enough" parents can reasonably offer.

A similar formulation, developed for BPD by Linehan (1993), is the concept of an "invalidating environment." In this view, children who have greater needs due to emotion dysrgegulation are exquisitely sensitive to parents who dismiss their feelings and their need for support. A self-report scale has been developed to measure this construct (Robertson, Kimbrel, & Nelson-Gray, 2013).

Very little empirical research exists on the relationship between parenting practices and PDs outside the impulsive spectrum. Overprotection would be of relevance for patients with avoidant traits. Kagan (1994), who followed a cohort of children with high levels of "behavioral inhibition," has suggested that overprotective responses by parents to children with this temperament interfere with deconditioning of anxiety, but the evidence for this hypothesis remains sketchy.

## Traumatic Experiences

### Childhood Sexual Abuse

Childhood sexual abuse is a well-established risk factor for BPD, but it does not follow that traumatic experiences must be a main etiological factor for the disorder (Paris, 2008). First, the relationship between trauma and BPD is far from specific, with similar experiences reported by patients with a range of other diagnoses. Second, only about one-third to one-half of all patients with BPD have a history of severe childhood trauma, while meta-analyses report a relatively weak relationship between exposure and outcome (Fossati, Madeddu, & Maffei, 1999). Third, community studies show that most people who experience childhood trauma never develop PDs, or any form of mental disorder (Browne & Finkelhor, 1986; Fergusson & Mullen, 1999; Rind & Tromofovitch, 1997). Fourth, long-term effects of trauma do not result from exposure alone; they but also reflect constitutional vulnerability (McNally, 2003).

Fifth, research often fails to take into account the severity of traumatic experiences, or what have been called the "parameters" of abuse and adversity (Browne & Finkelhor, 1986). For example, the impact of sexual trauma depends to a great extent on the identity of the perpetrator, the nature of the act, and the duration of the experience (Finkelhor et al., 2005). Some published reports describe experiences, such as single incidents, that very rarely produce pathological sequelae in community populations. In studies specifically examining the parameters of abuse (Paris et al., 1994a, 1994b), the range of reported trauma was similar to what is found in the community. Thus, many cases accounting for high rates of patients with BPD do not involve repeated episodes, sexual intercourse, or incest, but single events of molestation by a nonrelative or stranger, and about one-third of patients with BPD report no traumatic events whatsoever during childhood. Severe abuse experiences, such as an incestuous perpetrator, severity of sexual act, or high frequency and duration, and traumatic events are more likely to play an etiological role (Paris, 2008). But severe childhood abuse is associated with a more severe and chronic course of disorder in BPD (Soloff, Lynch, & Kelly, 2002).

Research on trauma and PDs has also failed to address the role of third-variable effects derived from family dysfunction, parenting practices, or parental psychopathology. Thus, it is difficult to determine whether sequelae are attributable to trauma alone, or to the cumulative effects of multiple adversities. Community studies show that child abuse does not occur in isolation, and that negative sequelae can often be accounted for by family dysfunction (Nash, Hulsely, Sexton, Harralson, & Lambert, 1993).

Because childhood trauma is an emotional issue, some of the research on this subject has been affected by prior beliefs. For example, some reports (e.g., Herman, Perry, & van der Kolk, 1989) have been based on studies conducted on patient populations undergoing therapies designed to "recover" repressed memories. In general, one should only accept as valid memories that have never been forgotten, and have not been elicited for the first time in psychotherapy.

Nonetheless, the most general conclusion one can make from research is that abuse is at relevant psychosocial risk factor for PD, and that it plays a greater role in certain subgroups of patients.

## Other Forms of Trauma

The relationship between physical abuse during childhood and BPD is less consistent than that for sexual abuse. But physical abuse is associated with the development of ASPD (Pollock et al., 1990). Patients with BPD also report a high frequency of exposure to witnessing violent incidents during childhood (Laporte & Guttman, 1996), which is associated with dysfunction in families. Several studies suggest that patients with BPD have been exposed to verbal and emotional abuse (Paris, 2008).

No symptoms, or set of symptoms, is a "marker" for a traumatic history. For example, dissociation and self-harm are found in BPD, whether or not patients have a history of childhood trauma (Zweig-Frank, Paris, & Guzder, 1994). Moreover, the capacity to dissociate has a heritable component (Jang, Paris, Zweig-Frank, & Livesley, 1998) that can be amplified by adverse experiences.

In summary, three conclusions seem justified by the evidence:

1. Parental psychopathology, family breakdown, and traumatic events are risk factors for personality disorders, particularly the borderline and antisocial categories.
2. Risk factors show heterogeneity within categories of disorder, as well as overlap between categories.
3. Psychological risk factors, by themselves, cannot fully account for the development of PDs.

## Social Stressors

The role of social stressors in PDs has not been well researched, but indirect evidence suggests they could play an important role (Paris, 2003).

Time cohort effects on prevalence are well established for ASPD (Robins & Regier, 1991), a diagnosis that increased in prevalence after the World War II. Since parasuicide, completed suicide, substance abuse, and criminality all increased during the same era, similar cohort effects on prevalence could apply to BPD (Millon, 1993). Possible mechanisms include the breakdown of traditional social structures, as well as a relative absence of secure attachments in contemporary society (Linehan, 1993; Paris & Lis, 2013).

The best documented difference in the cross-cultural prevalence of PDs is the rarity of the diagnosis of ASPD in Taiwan (Hwu, Yeh, & Chang, 1989), a society whose traditional and more integrated structure has had protective effects against adversity. When PDs increase in prevalence, it may not be because families are more dysfunctional than in the past, but because the social support needed to buffer trait vulnerabilities and intrafamilial stressors is less available. Although these forces affect everyone, they have a greater impact on those who are vulnerable because of biological and psychological risk factors. The modern world is also marked by rapid social change, in which young people are now expected to find an "identity" in the absence of traditional guidance and support from the community, placing those with problematical personality traits and negative family experiences at greater risk (Paris, 2013).

## Adversity in the Context of Gene–Environment Interactions

Gene–environment interactions are a key component of diathesis–stress models of psychopathology (Rutter, 2006). Childhood adversities are more likely to be pathogenic when they interact with underlying genetic vulnerability. Thus, PDs arise when temperamental and trait variants that predispose to behavioral and affective disturbances interact with psychosocial adversities (Rutter, 1987). In other words, PDs can be conceptualized as the outcome of interactions between diatheses (trait profiles) and stressors (psychosocial adversities).

Applying this model, a wide range of trait variability is compatible with normality. While trait variations are insufficient by themselves to account for PDs, they are the main determinant of which type can develop. Moreover, trait profiles influence the extent to which an individual is vulnerable to develop any disorder. Siblings have surprisingly few personality traits in common, and even when exposed to the same family environment, only one child in a family tends to develop a PD (Laporte, Paris, Russell, & Guttman, 2011).

Psychological and social factors may be crucial determinants of whether underlying traits are amplified, thereby leading to overt disorders. Individuals differ in their *exposure* to and *susceptibility* to environmental factors (Kendler & Eaves, 1986). Problematic traits can create negative feedback loops by interfering with the development of peer relationships and parental attachments, leading to amplification of these characteristics (Rutter, 1987).

## Limitations of Current Research Findings and Methods

The following future directions might shed light on the many unanswered questions in this field:

1. Long-term prospective studies of typically developing children and children at risk to document the effects of childhood adversity in adult life.
2. Multivariate studies examining both biological factors and psychosocial adversities in the same patients.
3. Twin studies with a prospective follow-up component, allowing for the separation of genetic and environmental factors.
4. Epidemiological studies examining risk factors for personality traits and disorders in the community.
5. Studies of clinical populations to examine a wider range of categories of disorder, as well as the trait dimensions underlying PDs.

## Clinical Implications

PDs are complex, multidimensional forms of psychopathology. This is particularly the case for highly symptomatic categories such as BPD (Paris, 2008). The role of childhood adversity must therefore be seen within a broad etiological model that is multidimensional, and that describes complex interactions between multiple stressors and multiple diatheses.

These conclusions have implications for the treatment of patients with PDs. If childhood adversities increase the risk for personality pathology but are not necessarily their primary cause, then clinicians should not assume that psychotherapy must always focus on uncovering childhood traumas. At present, the most effective therapies for PDs, as documented by research (Paris, 2010), are those that focus on methods of improving present levels of functioning by teaching patients to make more adaptive use of their personality traits.

### REFERENCES

Amato, P. R., & Booth, A. (2000). *A generation at risk: Growing up in an era of family upheaval.* Cambridge, MA: Harvard University Press.

Beck, A. T., Davis, D. D., & Freeman, A. (2015). *Cognitive therapy of personality disorders* (3rd ed.). New York: Guilford Press.

Browne, A., & Finkelhor, D. (1986). Impact of child sexual abuse: A review of the literature. *Psychological Bulletin, 99,* 66–77.

Caspi, A., & Roberts, B. W. (1999). Personality change and continuity across the lifetime. In L. A. Pervin & O. P. John (Eds.), *Handbook of personality: Theory and research* (2nd ed., pp. 300–326). New York: Guilford Press.

Cassidy, J., & Shaver, P. R. (Eds.). (2012). *Handbook of attachment: Theory, research and clinical aspects* (2nd ed.). New York: Guilford Press.

Cicchetti, D. (2004). An odyssey of discovery: Lessons learned through three decades of research on child maltreatment. *American Psychologist, 59,* 4–14.

Cloninger, C. R., Sigvardsson, S., & Bohman, M. (1982). Predisposition to petty criminality in Swedish adoptees II: Cross-fostering analysis of gene–environment interaction. *Archives of General Psychiatry, 39,* 1242–1253.

Cohen, P., Crawford, T. N., Johnson, J. G., & Kasen, S. (2005). The children in the community study of developmental course of personality disorder. *Journal of Personality Disorders, 19,* 466–486.

Fergusson, D. M., & Mullen, P. E. (1999). *Childhood sexual abuse: An evidence based perspective.* Thousand Oaks, CA: SAGE.

Finkelhor, D., Ormrod, R. K., Turner, H. A., & Hamby, S. L. (2005). The victimization of children and youth: A comprehensive, national survey. *Child Maltreatment, 10,* 5–25.

Fossati, A., Madeddu, F., & Maffei, C. (1999). Borderline personality disorder and childhood sexual abuse: A meta-analytic study. *Journal of Personality Disorders, 13,* 268–280.

Hardt, J., & Rutter, M. (2004). Validity of adult retrospective reports of adverse childhood experiences: Review of the evidence. *Journal of Child Psychology and Psychiatry, 45,* 260–273.

Herman, J. L., Perry, J. C., & van der Kolk, B. A. (1989). Childhood trauma in borderline personality disorder. *American Journal of Psychiatry, 146,* 490–495.

Hwu, H. G., Yeh, E. K., & Chang, L. Y. (1989). Prevalence of psychiatric disorders in Taiwan defined by the Chinese Diagnostic Interview Schedule. *Acta Psychiatrica Scandinavica, 79,* 136–147.

Jang, K., Paris, J., Zweig-Frank, H., & Livesley, W. J. (1998). A twin study of dissociative experience. *Journal of Nervous and Mental Diseases, 186,* 345–351.

Kagan, J. (1994). *Galen's prophecy: Temperament in human nature.* New York: Basic Books.

Kendler, K. S., & Eaves, L. J. (1986). Models for the joint effect of genotype and environment on liability to psychiatric illness. *American Journal of Psychiatry, 143,* 279–289.

Laporte, L., & Guttman, H. (1996). Traumatic childhood experiences as risk factors for borderline and other personality disorders. *Journal of Personality Disorders, 10,* 247–259.

Laporte, L., Paris, J., Russell, J., & Guttman, H. (2011). Psychopathology, trauma, and personality traits in patients with borderline personality disorder and their sisters. *Journal of Personality Disorders, 25*(4), 448–462.

Linehan, M. M. (1993). *Dialectical behavior therapy for borderline personality disorder.* New York: Guilford Press.

Livesley, W. J. (2003). *Practical management of personality disorder.* New York: Guilford Press.

Malinovsky-Rummell, R., & Hansen, D. J. (1993). Long-term consequences of physical abuse. *Psychological Bulletin, 114,* 68–79.

McNally, R. J. (2003). *Remembering trauma.* Cambridge, MA: Belknap Press/Harvard University Press.

Millon, T. (1993). Borderline personality disorder: A psychosocial epidemic. In J. Paris (Ed.), *Borderline personality disorder: Etiology and treatment* (pp. 197–210). Washington, DC: American Psychiatric Press.

Millon, T., & Davis, R. D. (1996) *Disorders of personality: DSM-IV and beyond* (2nd ed.). New York: Wiley.

Monroe, S. M., & Simons, A. D. (1991). Diathesis–stress theories in the context of life stress research. *Psychological Bulletin, 110,* 406–425.

Nash, M. R., Hulsey, T. L., Sexton, M. C., Harralson, T. L., & Lambert, W. (1993). Long-term sequelae of childhood sexual abuse: Perceived family environment, psychopathology, and dissociation. *Journal of Consulting and Clinical Psychology, 61*(2), 276–283.

Paris, J. (2000). *Myths of childhood.* Philadelphia: Brunner/Mazel.

Paris, J. (2003). *Personality disorders over time: Precursors, course, and outcome.* Washington, DC: American Psychiatric Press.

Paris, J. (2008). *Treatment of borderline personality disorder: A guide to evidence-based practice.* New York: Guilford Press.

Paris, J. (2010). Estimating the prevalence of personality disorders. *Journal of Personality Disorders, 24,* 405–411.

Paris, J. (2013). *Psychotherapy in an age of narcissism.* Basingstoke, UK: Palgrave Macmillan.

Paris, J., & Frank, H. (1989). Perceptions of parental bonding in borderline patients. *American Journal of Psychiatry, 146,* 1498–1499.

Paris, J., & Lis, E. (2013). Can sociocultural and historical mechanisms inluence the development of borderline personality disorder? *Transcultural Psychiatry, 50,* 140–151.

Paris, J., Zweig-Frank, H., & Guzder, J. (1994a). Psychological risk factors in recovery from borderline personality disorder in female patients. *Comprehensive Psychiatry, 34,* 410–413.

Paris, J., Zweig-Frank, H., & Guzder, J. (1994b). Risk factors for borderline personality in male outpatients. *Journal of Nervous and Mental Disease, 182,* 375–380.

Parker, G. (1983). *Parental overprotection: A risk factor in psychosocial development.* New York: Grune & Stratton.

Perez-Fuentes, G., Olfson, M., Villegas, L., Morcillo, C., Wang, S., & Blanco, C. (2013). Prevalence and correlates of child sexual abuse: A national study. *Comprehensive Psychiatry, 54,* 16–27.

Plomin, R., & Bergeman, C. (1991). Genetic influence on environmental measures. *Behavioral and Brain Sciences, 14,* 373–427.

Pollock, V. E., Briere, J., Schneider, L., Knop, J., Mednick, S. A., & Goodwin, D. W. (1990). Childhood antecedents of antisocial behavior: Parental alcoholism and physical abusiveness. *American Journal of Psychiatry, 147,* 1290–1293.

Rind, B., & Tromofovitch, P. (1997). A meta-analytic review of findings from national samples on psychological correlates of child sexual abuse. *Journal of Sexual Research, 34,* 237–255.

Robertson, C. D., Kimbrel, N. A., & Nelson-Gray, R. O. (2013). The Invalidating Childhood Environment Scale (ICES): Psychometric properties and relationship to borderline personality symptomatology. *Journal of Personality Disorders, 27,* 402–410.

Robins, L. (1966). *Deviant children grown up.* Baltimore: Williams & Wilkins.

Robins, L. N., & Regier, D. A. (Eds.). (1991). *Psychiatric disorders in America.* New York: Free Press.

Rowe, D. C. (1981). *The limits of family influence: Genes, experience, and behavior.* New York: Guilford Press.

Rutter, M. (1987). Temperament, personality, and personality disorders. *British Journal of Psychiatry, 150,* 443–448.

Rutter, M. (2006). *Genes and behavior: Nature–nurture interplay explained.* London: Blackwell.

Rutter, M. (2012a). Annual research review: Resilience—clinical implications. *Journal of Child Psychology and Psychiatry, 54,* 474–487.

Rutter, M. (2012b). Resilience as a dynamic concept. *Development and Psychopathology, 24,* 335–344.

Rutter, M., & Maughan, B. (1997). Psychosocial adversities in psychopathology. *Journal of Personality Disorders, 11,* 19–33.

Siever, L. J., & Davis, K. L. (1991). A psychobiological perspective on the personality disorders. *American Journal of Psychiatry, 148,* 1647–1658.

Soloff, P. H., Lynch, K. G., & Kelly, T. M. (2002). Childhood abuse as a risk factor for suicidal behavior in borderline personality disorder. *Journal of Personality Disorders, 16,* 201–214.

Werner, E. E., & Smith, R. S. (1992). *Overcoming the odds: High risk children from birth to adulthood.* Ithaca, NY: Cornell University Press.

White, C. N., Gunderson, J. G., Zanarini, M. C., & Hudson, J. I. (2003). Family studies of borderline personality disorder: A review. *Harvard Review of Psychiatry, 12,* 118–119.

Widom, C., Cjaza, C., & Paris, J. (2009). A prospective investigation of borderline personality disorder in abused and neglected children followed up into adulthood. *Journal of Personality Disorders, 23,* 433–446.

Zanarini, M. C. (1993). Borderline personality as an impulse spectrum disorder. In J. Paris (Ed.), *Borderline personality disorder: Etiology and treatment* (pp. 67–86). Washington, DC: American Psychiatric Press.

Zanarini, M. C. (2000). Childhood experiences associated with the development of borderline personality disorder. *Psychiatric Clinics of North America, 23,* 89–101.

Zweig-Frank, H., & Paris, J. (1991). Parents' emotional neglect and over-protection according to the recollections of patients with borderline personality disorder. *Amercan Journal of Psychiatry, 148,* 648–651.

Zweig-Frank, H., Paris, J., & Guzder, J. (1994). Psychological risk factors for dissociation in female patients with borderline and non-borderline personality disorders. *Journal of Personality Disorders, 8,* 203–209.

# CHAPTER 18

# Developmental Psychopathology

Rebecca L. Shiner and Timothy A. Allen

How do personality disorders (PDs) originate and develop over time? Much of the early clinical interest in PDs in the 20th century arose from rich, complex psychodynamic theories about the origins of such disorders. The clinicians who developed these theories looked to discussions with their patients to find the origins of PDs, and they formulated theories suggesting that PDs develop out of problematic childhood experiences. The fifth edition of the *Diagnostic and Statistical Manual of Mental Disorders* (DSM-5; American Psychiatric Association [APA], 2013) Section II, suggests possible developmental precursors to the 10 categorical PDs it covers. Despite these various claims about the childhood origins of PDs, relatively little is known empirically about the developmental pathways leading to PDs. We offer in this chapter some promising avenues for explaining the emergence and development of PDs by drawing from the existing literature on normal personality development in the first two decades of life.

We adopt a developmental psychopathology framework (Cicchetti, 1993, 2013) for PDs; developmental psychopathology focuses on the developmental mechanisms underlying the emergence, manifestation, and outcomes of psychological disorders from a life-course perspective. Three tenets of developmental psychopathology are particularly helpful in exploring the origins of PDs. First, the study of normal development is critical for understanding pathological development. The same basic biological, psychological, and contextual processes underlie both normal and abnormal development; therefore, findings from the study of normal development are relevant for explaining the development of psychological disorders. In this case, the literature on normal personality development can be tapped for its potential in explaining the development of PDs. Second, psychological disorders can best be understood by tracing the pathways leading to and following from the development of those disorders (Cicchetti, 1993, 2013). These pathways are often complex (Cicchetti & Rogosch, 1996) because different pathways and processes may lead to similar outcomes (known as "equifinality"), and similar origins may yield a broad range of outcomes (known as "multifinality"). In the case of PDs, several different processes may lead to similar pathological personality outcomes in different individuals; for example, borderline traits may arise from extreme temperaments in some people and from traumatic experiences in others. Conversely, youth with similar starting points (e.g., similarly high levels of negative emotionality in childhood) may have different adolescent or adult outcomes, with some people developing PDs and others not. Third, a complete understanding of psychological disorders can only be achieved by investigating those disorders at multiple levels of analysis, ranging from biological levels (molecular, genetic, and structural and functional brain perspectives) to individual levels (trait, social-cognitive, and narrative perspectives) to contextual levels (family, peers, school, neighborhood, socioeconomic status [SES], and cultural perspectives; Cicchetti, 2013). In the case of PDs, categorical diagnoses and pathological traits may be examined from all of these perspectives, and the interaction of various levels may be especially important for explaining the emergence of pathological personality functioning.

We offer in this chapter a developmental psychopathology perspective on the development of PDs. DSM-5 Section III, Alternative Model for PDs, argues that personality pathology consists of two important components: (1) pathological personality traits and (2) impairment in other aspects of personality functioning (e.g., identity, relationships, emotion regulation) (APA, 2013). We agree with this basic formulation for personality pathology (see Shiner, 2009, for a more detailed theoretical model); thus, we use this basic framework of personality disturbance throughout the chapter. Normal-range personality traits are relevant to understanding both aspects of personality disturbance; for the first, pathological personality traits represent extreme manifestations of normal-range personality traits, and for the second, normal-range personality traits may serve as risk factors leading to impairment in other aspects of personality functioning. Thus, we have chosen to focus the three sections of this chapter on the development of both normal-range and pathological personality traits in childhood and adolescence. First, we review what is known about the nature of normal-range personality traits in childhood, adolescence, and adulthood, then we address how these relate to pathological personality traits, particularly in childhood and adolescence. Second, we summarize current work on the development of PD-relevant traits in youth, including their continuity and change over time and the role of genes and the environment in shaping such traits. Third, we offer a model for the potential role of pathological traits in the development of PDs and discuss how early disturbed traits may lead to significant impairment in other aspects of personality functioning. Through the chapter, we use the term "PD" when we refer to studies examining PD diagnoses, "PD symptoms" when we refer to studies examining PD diagnostic criteria, and "PD traits" when we refer to studies looking at pathological personality traits. We hope that this chapter provides a useful starting point for designing future longitudinal, prospective studies on the developmental pathways leading to PDs.

## Personality Traits in Childhood, Adolescence, and Adulthood

Developmental psychopathologists have long argued that studies examining normative developmental processes offer useful information for explaining the emergence of psychological disorders, while a better understanding of pathological development can likewise shed light on normative functioning (Cicchetti, 1993, 2013; Sroufe, 1990). Adopting this approach in the current context, it is likely that research on normative personality traits may highlight specific developmental processes that contribute to the emergence, manifestation, course, and consequences of early PDs. Thus, the rich literature on normative personality and temperament differences in children and youth provides a useful starting point for investigations into personality pathology (Shiner, 2009). In this first section, we provide an overview of the research on the structure and processes underlying both normal-range and pathological personality traits in youth and adults.

### The Nature of Early Individual Differences in Personality Traits

Personality traits are relatively stable and consistent behavioral, cognitive, and affective tendencies. These traits reflect basic individual differences that have been relevant to human adaptation and are continually shaped by individuals' life experiences (Caspi & Shiner, 2006; McAdams & Pals, 2006). Emerging research has begun to link individual differences in personality traits to biological systems that have been essential for human functioning in an evolutionary context. For instance, traits have been shown to be related to neural networks responsible for reward sensitivity and processing, threat detection and sensitivity to punishment, exploration of novelty, social bonding and aggression, and the higher-order cognitive processing of goal-relevant information (DeYoung & Gray, 2009; Shiner & DeYoung, 2013). These biological systems, much like traits, display a developmental course whereby they become more specialized and differentiated as a result of both genetic and environmental influences.

Individual differences in traits are observable from the earliest days of a child's life. Traditionally, early individual differences have been studied by researchers under the rubric of "temperament"—early-emerging basic dispositions in the domains of activity, positive and negative affectivity, attention, and self-regulation that are closely linked with biological processes and partially shaped by heredity (Rothbart, 2011; Shiner et al., 2012). As development progresses, temperament traits become both broader and more differentiated as children acquire new competencies (Shiner, 2009). The development of traits is likely to involve a reciprocal process: Children's experiences influence the development of their traits, while their traits in turn influence the type of experiences they are most likely to have (Shiner & Caspi, 2012). As early as the preschool years, this interactive process yields individual differences in traits that exhibit considerable overlap with adult personality structure (De Pauw, Mervielde, & Van Leeuwen, 2009).

There is now a relative consensus among adult personality researchers for a five-factor model of personality, also known as the Big Five, which includes the traits Extraversion, Neuroticism, Conscientiousness, Agreeableness, and Openness/Intellect (Digman, 1990; John, Naumann, & Soto, 2008; McCrae & Costa, 1999). This model is increasingly being extended to describe individual differences in children and adolescents (Caspi & Shiner, 2006; Shiner & DeYoung, 2013). The five factors have been identified in developmental studies using different reporters, employing both questionnaires and *q*-sort measures (Shiner & DeYoung, 2013). Children as young as 5 years old describe their personalities along the Big Five dimensions in the context of puppet interviews (Measelle, John, Ablow, Cowan, & Cowan, 2005). Children's and adolescents' self-reports of personality increasingly conform to a Big Five structure over time (Soto, John, Gosling, & Potter, 2008). Taken together, these findings provide convincing evidence that the Big Five traits have considerable utility in describing individual differences extending across most of the life course.

### Big Five Personality Traits in Development: Underlying Processes

The Big Five personality dimensions, along with the lower-level facets with which they are associated, are presented in the first two columns of Table 18.1. In what follows, we articulate a developmental taxonomy of normative personality traits, linking each of the Big Five dimensions in childhood and adolescence with the biological systems in which they are likely to reflect variations.

*Extraversion,* or positive emotionality/surgency, as it is often referred to in temperament models (Rothbart, 2011), reflects an individual's preference to actively engage with or approach novelty in the environment. This trait appears to be linked to the behavioral approach system identified by Gray—specifically, a neurobiological system that relies heavily on dopaminergic activity and is responsible for activating approach tendencies that reflect a drive to achieve reward (DeYoung & Gray, 2009; Gray, 1982). Children scoring high on Extraversion tend to be described as dominant, outgoing, sociable, expressive, and energetic. In contrast, children scoring low on Extraversion are frequently characterized as shy, inhibited, or withdrawn. *Neuroticism,* or negative emotionality, as it is described in some temperament models (Rothbart, 2011), encompasses two separable tendencies: consistent patterns of anxiety and fearfulness on the one hand, and anger or irritability on the other. Gray and MacNaughton (2000) argue that these internalizing and externalizing aspects of Neuroticism may in part reflect the joint contribution of a behavioral inhibition system (BIS) and a fight–flight–freeze system (FFFS). The BIS is primarily responsible for passive avoidance in situations in which two goals may be in conflict, while the FFFS tends to reflect active avoidance in response to more proximate stressors (DeYoung & Gray, 2009; Shiner & DeYoung, 2013). Highly neurotic children are prone to low self-worth, feelings of guilt and shame, and insecurity. They are described as moody, vulnerable, anxious, and easily frightened. In contrast, low neuroticism, or high emotional stability, reflects a child's propensity for high frustration tolerance, low stress reactivity, and self-confidence.

*Conscientiousness/Constraint,* which is the analogue to a temperament trait called "effortful control" (Evans & Rothbart, 2007), reflects tendencies toward voluntary self-control and self-regulation. Neurobiological research has linked conscientiousness with lateral prefrontal networks that are important for planning and abstract rule-following (DeYoung et al., 2010). Moreover, temperament research has linked measures of effortful control to the development of prefrontal attention systems and, specifically, the anterior cingulate gyrus (Posner, Rothbart, Sheese, & Tang, 2007). Highly conscientious children tend to be responsible, orderly, planful, and achievement-striving, whereas children low on this dimension have been described as impulsive, disorganized,

**TABLE 18.1. Normative Big Five Traits and PD Traits in Children and Adolescents**

| Big Five trait and its PD trait counterpart | Big Five Trait: Lower-level facets[a] | PD Trait: Lower-level facets[b] |
|---|---|---|
| BF: Extraversion<br>PD: Introversion | Sociability<br>Positive emotions<br>Assertiveness<br>Approach<br>Activity level/energy[c] | Shyness<br>Paranoid traits<br>Withdrawn traits |
| BF: Neuroticism<br>PD: Emotional Instability | Fearfulness<br>Insecurity/low self-confidence<br>Anxiousness<br>Anger/irritability<br>Sadness | Dependency<br>Insecure attachment<br>Anxious traits |
| BF: Conscientiousness<br>PD: Compulsivity | Achievement striving<br>Orderliness<br>Achievement striving<br>Self-control<br>Attention | Perfectionism<br>Extreme order<br>Extreme achievement striving |
| BF: Agreeableness<br>PD: Disagreeableness | Hostility/aggression (R)<br>Empathy (vs. egocentrism)<br>Compliance<br>Prosocial behavior | Irritable–aggressive traits<br>Dominance–egocentrism<br>Hyperactive traits |
| BF: Openness/Intellect<br>PD: Not currently identified | Creativity<br>Curiosity<br>Intellect<br>Perceptual sensitivity | |

*Note.* BF, Big Five; PD, personality disorder.
[a]The Big Five trait lower-level facets are from Shiner and DeYoung (2013). Reprinted with permission from Oxford University Press.
[b]The PD trait lower-level facets are from De Clercq, De Fruyt, Van Leeuwen, and Mervielde (2006). Reprinted with permission from the American Psychological Association.
[c]There is some evidence that activity level may be an additional sixth trait in childhood (Shiner & DeYoung, 2013), but activity level/energy becomes a facet of Extraversion by adolescence.

distractible, and careless. *Agreeableness* reflects children's differences in self-regulation and tendencies to be benevolent, prosocial, empathic, cooperative with peers and family members, and polite. Conversely, disagreeable children are antagonistic, rude, and unkind to peers. While there has been limited research on the biological correlates of Agreeableness, there is some evidence suggesting that Agreeableness may be linked to the empathy and social information-processing networks that activate the mirror neuron system, the superior temporal sulcus, and the medial prefrontal cortex (DeYoung et al., 2010). Finally, children scoring high on *Openness/Intellect* are bright, quick, eager to learn, creative, imaginative, and perceptually sensitive. Historically, this trait has lacked an empirical basis in the developmental literature. In recent years, however, several studies have emerged to suggest that Openness can, in fact, be measured reliably quite early in life (De Pauw et al., 2009; Herzhoff & Tackett, 2012). As in the case of Agreeableness, there has been limited neurobiological research on Openness/Intellect; however, there is some evidence that the Intellect facet of this trait may be related to the left frontal pole and posterior middle frontal cortex, areas that are important for working memory, intelligence, and intellectual engagement (DeYoung et al., 2010).

### The Structure of Pathological Traits in Development

The current DSM-5 Section II classification model conceptualizes PDs as discrete entities, distinguishable from one another on a qualitative, as opposed to quantitative, level (APA, 2013). In recent decades, however, the DSM PD classification model has been criticized for several reasons: (1) PDs have excessively high comorbidity for supposedly distinct disorders (Clark, 2007); (2) the most prevalent PD diagnosis is PD not otherwise specified, suggesting that most patients exhibit symptoms that cut across diagnostic boundaries (Johnson et al., 2005; Verheul & Widiger, 2004); and (3) the range of symptoms relevant to PDs is inadequately covered by current PD diagnoses (Geiger & Crick, 2009). In light of these and other difficulties with the categorical model, many researchers have argued for adopting a dimensional view of personality pathology. Consistent with a developmental psychopathology framework, a dimensional model of PDs sheds the preconception that normative personality functioning is qualitatively different than personality pathology and instead adopts the perspective that both PDs and normal-range personality traits exist along a spectrum of personality functioning (Shiner & Tackett, 2014; Widiger & Costa, 2013). This spectrum model suggests that both normal and pathological personality traits rest along a continuum, and that personality pathology may represent the extreme ends of a continuously distributed personality trait or cluster of traits, rather than distinct categories of dysfunction.

Research on the Big Five model has proven to be an important avenue for researchers aiming to adopt a dimensional model of personality pathology. There is now considerable research in adults to suggest that the Big Five model captures meaningful variation in personality pathology (Markon, Krueger, & Watson, 2005; Widiger & Costa, 2013). Similar dimensions have also been identified in studies investigating PD traits (Clark, 2007; Livesley, 2007). The Alternative DSM-5 Model for PDs in Section III ("Emerging Measures and Models") requires the presence of pathological personality traits for a diagnosis of PD. This alternative dimensional model organizes pathological traits into five domains mapping onto the Big Five: negative affectivity versus emotional stability, detachment versus extraversion, antagonism versus agreeableness, disinhibition versus conscientiousness, and psychoticism versus lucidity (APA, 2013, pp. 779–781). In addition, each of the five broad dimensions is described by between three and eight more specific, narrow-band facets in an effort to enhance the model's precision in characterizing a wide range of personality dysfunction.

Consistent with the research on dimensional models of personality pathology in adults, researchers investigating pathological personality traits in children and adolescents have demonstrated that early personality dysfunction overlaps considerably with the Big Five model, though there is currently little support for the fifth dimension, Psychoticism. PD trait questionnaire measures created for adults have been adapted for use with adolescents, and findings suggest that similar higher-order pathological traits validly represent the structure of personality pathology in adolescents (Linde, Stringer, Simms, & Clark, 2013; Ro, Stringer, & Clark, 2012; Tromp & Koot, 2008, 2010). In contrast to the "top-down" evidence from adult measures adapted for adolescents, "bottom-up" data on pathological personality traits in youth come from a questionnaire designed to measure maladaptive extreme variants of normal-range personality traits in youth (Dimensional Personality Symptom Item Pool; De Clercq, De Fruyt, Van Leeuwen, & Mervielde, 2006; De Clercq, De Fruyt, & Widiger, 2009; De Fruyt & De Clercq, 2013). This measure yields four higher-order traits that are comparable to four traits found in the adult research, namely, Introversion, Disagreeableness, Compulsivity, and Emotional Instability. Although these studies in youth suggest that the basic structure of pathological traits is similar to that observed in adults, more work is needed to determine whether there are significant developmental differences in the nature of those traits (e.g., Kushner, Tackett, & De Clercq, 2013).

The pathological personality traits observed in children and adolescents are presented in Table 18.1; the traits and potential lower-order facets are placed next to the comparable Big Five traits. The *Introversion* dimension reflects excessive shyness, withdrawal, and suspiciousness. At the high end of the *Negative Affectivity* dimension, youth tend to experience anxious symptoms, dependence, low self-confidence, and interpersonal insecurity. The third PD dimension in youth, *Compulsivity,* taps perfectionism, extreme achievement striving, and extreme order. *Antagonism* includes tendencies toward hostility, aggression, manipulativeness, self-centeredness, and impulsive activity on the pathological end. The research on maladaptive traits in adults often identifies a disinhibition/low conscientiousness trait that is separate from an antagonism/disagreeableness trait (Samuel & Widiger, 2008), whereas research on youth indicates that disinhibition is an aspect of Antagonism/Disagreeableness and that Compulsivity (maladaptive high conscientiousness) forms a separate trait (De Clercq et al., 2006; Tromp & Koot, 2008). Finally, *psychoticism* or *peculiarity* (Harkness & McNulty, 1994; Tackett, Silberschmidt, Krueger, & Sponheim, 2008; Verbeke & De Clercq, 2014) has been hypothesized as the fifth and final dimension of personality pathology in adults. Though developmental research is scarce on this dimension (Tackett, Balsis, Oltmanns, & Krueger, 2009), Psychoticism is hypothesized to reflect a propensity for cognitive or perceptual aberrations, similar to those present in Cluster A PDs. This set of pathological traits observed in youth provides a useful starting point for charting the emergence of PDs in childhood and adolescence.

## The Development of Traits Relevant to Personality Disorders

As pathological personality traits are central to current models of PDs, it is important to understand the early development of such traits. In this section, we review current research on stability and change in PD symptoms traits and normal-range personality traits in childhood and adolescence, and point to some of the known genetic and environmental influences on early PD-relevant traits.

### Stability and Change in PD-Relevant Symptoms and Traits

*Rank-Order Stability*

Two different kinds of stability are especially important in research on continuity and change in personality traits (Caspi & Shiner, 2006): rank-order stability and mean-level stability. "Rank-order stability" refers to the degree to which the relative ordering of individuals on a given trait is maintained over time. If the individuals in a group maintain their same relative position on a trait over time, rank-order stability will be high, even if the group as a whole increases or decreases on that trait over time. Correlations between scores on the same trait measured across two points in time (i.e., test–retest correlations) are typically used to estimate rank-order stability.

In adolescence and early adulthood, PD symptoms and traits tend to show moderate to strong levels of rank-order stability, with the cross-time correlations often falling in the range of .40–.65 across the full range of PD symptoms and traits (reviewed in Shiner & Tackett, 2014); in other words, PD symptoms and traits do not appear to vary in their relative rank-order stability. Interestingly, PD symptoms and traits show comparable levels of stability in adulthood (Clark, 2007; Ferguson, 2010), which suggests that PD symptoms are as stable in adolescence as in adulthood. Few studies have examined the rank-order stability of PD symptoms in childhood; however, two studies found that childhood PD symptoms and pathological traits displayed moderate to strong rank-order stability over periods of 1 and 2 years (Crick, Murray-Close, & Woods, 2005; De Clercq, Van Leeuwen, van den Noortgate, De Bolle, & De Fruyt, 2009). Furthermore, one of those studies (De Clercq et al., 2009) found that the within-child stability of pathological traits was also high, which means that the absolute levels of PD traits within each child tended to remain high.

Given that the developmental psychopathology perspective emphasizes the relevance of normal functioning for explaining psychopathology, it is important to compare these findings for rank-order stability of PD symptoms and traits with those for normal-range personality traits in youth. A meta-analysis reported by Roberts and DelVecchio (2000) demonstrated that traits as measured by the five-factor model become increasingly stable over the life course. The following estimated population cross-time correlations for traits were obtained for childhood and adolescence: 0–2.9 years = .35; 3–5.9 years = .52; 6–11.9 years = .45; and 12–17.9 years = .47. These results suggest that individual differences show more modest continuity during infancy and toddlerhood, then show a rather large increase in stability during the preschool years; this moderate stability is maintained throughout childhood and adolescence. Traits continue to become more stable during adulthood. As is true in the literature on PD symptoms and traits, all normal-range traits seem to show comparable levels of stability. More recent studies using well-established Big Five trait measures in childhood and adolescence have found higher levels of rank-order trait stability than those obtained in the meta-analysis (reviewed in Shiner, 2014), perhaps because the more recent studies have used more reliable and valid trait measures. The findings for rank-order stability of PD symptoms, pathological traits, and normal-range traits suggest that moderate to strong stability is already apparent by adolescence and may even be in place by late childhood.

## Mean-Level Stability

The second type of stability, "mean-level stability," indicates whether there are increases or decreases in the average trait level of a population during different periods of life; in other words, people may tend to display higher or lower levels of particular traits during different parts of the lifespan. Research on mean-level continuity and change is important because it indicates whether there are peak periods for high levels of PD symptoms or traits during the life course. The limited existing research on mean-level stability of PD symptoms suggests that average levels of PD symptoms may peak in mid-adolescence, then decline across the years of later adolescence and early adulthood (Cohen, Crawford, Johnson, & Kasen, 2005; Johnson et al. 2000), with the greatest declines for narcissistic symptoms and the least declines for obsessive–compulsive symptoms. Likewise, average levels of borderline PD (BPD) traits have been found to decline modestly from ages 14 to 18 (Bornovalova, Hicks, Iacono, & McGue, 2013). Average PD symptom levels and pathological trait levels also continue to decline in adulthood (Clark, 2007).

Research on mean-level change in normal-range personality traits generally dovetails with the findings for PD symptoms in adolescence (Shiner, 2014). The studies on mean-level trait changes in childhood and early adolescence are not entirely consistent. However, there is some evidence that children develop better emotional self-regulation and higher levels of conscientiousness and agreeableness from earlier to later childhood, but these changes are followed by mean-level decreases in these positive traits in the transition from childhood to adolescence (Shiner, 2014; see, e.g., Soto, John, Gosling, & Potter, 2011). In other words, youth tend to become less conscientious and agreeable as they enter adolescence; in addition, girls may tend to become higher in neuroticism (Soto et al., 2011). Across the later adolescent and early adult years, there is a movement toward greater personality maturity on average, with decreases in neuroticism and increases in agreeableness and conscientious from late adolescence through middle age (Roberts, Walton, & Viechtbauer, 2006). Given that many PDs are characterized by high neuroticism and low agreeableness and conscientiousness, it is not surprising that on average, PD symptoms may peak in early or mid-adolescence and later decline. These findings suggest that the manifestations of PDs may be most intense during the adolescent years, when individuals tend to be the least conscientious and agreeable and, for females, the highest in negative emotionality.

## Influences on PD-Relevant Symptoms and Traits

Because other chapters in this volume review research on the etiology of PDs, here we provide a more limited review of influences on PD-relevant symptoms and traits in childhood and adolescence. We focus on genetic and contextual influences on PD symptoms and relevant traits in childhood and adolescence, with an emphasis on how the findings for PD symptoms and for normal-range personality traits fit together.

### Genetic Influences

Behavior genetics studies have been used to estimate the genetic and environmental influences on PD symptoms and normal-range personality traits in childhood and adolescence. A twin study was used to examine influences on parent reports of PD symptoms in children (Coolidge, Thede, & Jang, 2001); this study obtained heritability estimates ranging from .50 to .81, with no shared/family-wide environmental effects, and with moderate effects of the non-shared/child-specific environment on PD symptoms. Two twin studies that examined PD symptom counts in adults obtained similar results (reviewed in South, Reichborn-Kjennerud, Eaton, & Krueger, 2012). The average heritability of PD symptoms obtained across these three studies was .4–.5, indicating moderate heritability. There is also evidence for a genetic basis for BPD symptoms; a recent twin study of 12-year-olds obtained a heritability of .66 for BPD characteristics (Belsky et al., 2012). Likewise, a twin study obtained a heritability of BPD traits of .25 at age 14 and .48 at age 18 (Bornovalova et al., 2013).

Behavior genetics studies likewise have been used to examine influences on temperament and personality traits in youth. In general, these studies have found evidence for moderate heritability of temperament and personality traits and moderate effects of the non-shared/child-specific environment on traits, with either no effects or small effects of the shared environment (Saudino & Wang, 2012). A handful of behavior genetics studies have also addressed the question of whether genetic influences, environmental experiences, or both contribute to the stability and change in youth traits over time. By using a twin study design that measures twin pairs' standing on temperament and personality traits at two or more points in time, it is possible to parse the genetic and environmental components that contribute to the covariance and differences in those trait scores over time. Different genetic influences on the same trait may emerge at different points in development, just as different environments may lead to differences in traits over time (Saudinio & Wang, 2012). These studies suggest that, in general, genetic influences account for both stability and change in traits in childhood and adolescence, whereas non-shared/child-specific environmental factors account only for change in traits over time (Saudino & Wang, 2012; Shiner, 2014); shared/family-wide environmental factors generally have little influence over change and stability in traits. In other words, children's unique environments may cause them to shift their relative standing on traits over time, and new genetic effects on traits that are independent of earlier ones emerge at later points in development.

The behavior genetics findings have several implications for the development of PDs earlier in life. There are likely to be moderate genetic influences on pathological personality traits given that there are moderate genetic influences on both PD symptom counts in childhood and temperament and personality traits in childhood and adolescence. However, new genetic effects on PD-relevant traits may emerge at later points in childhood and adolescence. Child-specific environmental experiences (meaning those experiences that differentiate siblings from each other) influence youths' PD symptoms and temperament/personality traits, and they also contribute to change in traits over time. Thus, the family experiences likely to be most relevant to the development of PDs are those that are unique to each youth in a family, rather than those that cause siblings to become more alike. Person-specific experiences within the family could include family events that are encountered by only one child in the family (e.g., separation from parents at a specific time, a specific parent–child relationship) or family events that are experienced uniquely by each child (e.g., parental psychopathology or marital conflict that is experienced uniquely by each sibling).

*Contextual Influences*

A wide variety of contextual factors have been examined as predictors of PD symptoms and diagnoses in youth. Disturbances in the family environment predict many different PDs in childhood, adolescence, and early adulthood; these disturbances include low parental nurturing, harsh punishment, parental conflict, parent psychopathology, and maltreatment (Shiner & Allen, 2013; Shiner & Tackett, 2014). Children facing these adverse family experiences lack the socialization experiences that normally help children learn how to follow societal rules, inhibit impulses, and regulate emotions and behavior (Bradley et al., 2011; Kim, Cicchetti, Rogosch, & Manly, 2009). Beyond the family, peer relationships, SES and poverty, the school environment, and neighborhoods may also play a role in causing or worsening PDs in youth (Shiner & Allen, 2013; Shiner & Tackett, 2014). The etiological contributions of adversity to PD development are discussed in more detail by Paris (Chapter 17, this volume).

Research on contextual influences on normal-range personality traits offers helpful insights into possible environmental effects on pathological personality development. There is now convincing evidence that youths' traits interact with their environments to predict many different nontrait outcomes, including internalizing and externalizing symptoms, as well as competence and adaptation in the areas of academics, peer relationships, and emotion regulation (Bates, Schermerhorn, & Petersen, 2012; Caspi & Shiner, 2008; Lengua & Wachs, 2012; Rothbart & Bates, 2006). However, the normative studies that are more relevant to PDs are those that examine contextual influences on changes in personality traits over time, given that PDs involve pathological personality traits. The best of these studies control for earlier levels of the trait and focus on predicting changes in those traits from earlier environmental factors.

Family functioning and other contextual factors predict changes in children's neuroticism/negative emotionality and conscientiousness/self-control in childhood. Across several studies of young children, children's negative emotionality tends to decrease when caregivers respond with high sensitivity and responsiveness (Bates et al., 2012). Children's negative emotionality seems to be worsened by disorganized, chaotic, and noisy home environments (Matheny & Phillips, 2001) and by parents' punitive responses to expressions of negative emotions (Eisenberg et al., 1999). Shyness or behavioral inhibition also shows changes in response to contextual factors. Behaviorally inhibited children receiving intrusive, derisive, or overprotective parenting remain more consistently inhibited across time than inhibited children receiving other parenting (Fox, Henderson, Marshall, Nichols, & Ghera, 2005). Thus, when parents fail to provide an environment that helps children manage negative emotions—specifically, when parents create an insensitive, punitive, chaotic, and hostile environment—children's negative emotionality tends to increase over time. In contrast, behaviorally inhibited children who do not receive supportive opportunities to overcome their fears tend to remain withdrawn or become more withdrawn over time.

Children's self-control and regulation are predicted by environmental factors as well. For example, improvements in effortful control or behavioral control have been predicted by greater maternal responsiveness (Kochanska, Murray, & Harlan, 2000) and by lower levels of punitive responses (Eisenberg et al., 1999). In contrast, high levels of family risk factors (e.g., single parenting, low parental education, poverty) have been associated with declines in task persistence (Halverson & Deal, 2001) and with lower levels of executive control (Li-Grining, 2007). These findings are consistent with a broader literature that indicates that children with weaker self-control are more vulnerable to the negative effects of adverse parenting (Bates et al., 2012; Rothbart & Bates, 2006) or broader environmental disadvantages such as risky neighborhoods or dropping out of school (Caspi & Shiner, 2008; Lengua & Wachs, 2012; Meier, Slutske, Arndt, & Cadoret, 2008). Thus, youth may struggle to master self-control when they do not regularly encounter environments that provide structure and positive responsiveness, and this may be especially true for youth who are already predisposed to lower levels of self-control.

Two important caveats are needed for the existing research on contextual influences on PD development. First, it is possible that some family variables may predict the later development of PD in youth not because the family factors are causing PD in youth but because the predictors (i.e., family factors) and the outcomes (i.e., PDs) are both the result of a third variable (e.g., genes shared between parents and offspring). Genetically informative designs will be needed to determine whether there are true environmental effects on PD outcomes. For example, two recent twin studies found that the association of childhood trauma and adult PD criterion counts was best accounted for by common genetic or environmental influences (Berenz et al., 2013) and that the association of childhood abuse and adult BPD traits was best accounted for by common genetic influences (Bornovalova, Huibregtse, et al., 2013), calling into question the claim that early maltreatment or trauma causes BPD in adulthood (but for evidence for maltreatment as a true environmental contributor to childhood BPD characteristics, see Belsky et al., 2012). Second, contextual factors (e.g., adversity) may be the most important contributing factors in some instances, whereas intrapersonal factors (e.g., early personality traits) may be more salient in others. For example, youth with conduct disorder (a precursor to antisocial PD [ASPD]) include groups of youth for whom contextual adversity appears to be an important contributor and those for whom adversity appears to be less influential than genetically influenced tendencies toward callous–unemotional traits (Hyde, Shaw, & Hariri, 2013). There are likely to be other such instances of equifinality in the development of PDs—that is, cases in which youth come to develop similar PDs through different pathways.

## The Role of Personality Traits in the Development of Personality Disorders

In this section, we address the role of personality traits in the development of PDs by focusing on aspects of PDs that extend beyond pathological personality traits. We present a framework for how personality traits relate to other aspects of personality functioning, and we suggest some processes through which youths' early traits might affect the development of other aspects of PDs.

### Differentiating Personality Traits from Other Aspects of Personality Functioning

PDs include more than simply pathological personality traits; they also include impairment in other aspects of personality functioning. McAdams and colleagues (McAdams & Olson, 2010; McAdams & Pals, 2006) have developed a conceptual model for normal-range personality characteristics that is helpful in parsing the various aspects of personality that are relevant to understanding the development of PDs. This model clarifies the differences between traits and others aspects of personality by dividing personality into three aspects: (1) the dispositional signature, (2) characteristic adaptations, and (3) narrative identity. The "dispositional signature" refers to traits as the earliest emerging aspects of personality; traits account for the relatively consistent differences in the ways people tend to think, feel, and behave across situations and over time. "Characteristic adaptations," in contrast, refer to differences in "motivational, social-cognitive, and developmental adaptations contextualized in time, place, and/or social role" (McAdams & Pals, 2006, p. 208). Characteristic adaptations include constructs such as goals, plans, coping and emotion regulation strategies, mental representations, and schemas, among others. These aspects of personality tend to vary across contexts (e.g., people have different attachment relationships with different people or divergent goals in separate domains of life) and developmental periods (e.g., typical coping strategies vary in childhood, adolescence, and adulthood). Finally, this model highlights individual differences in "narrative identity"—the stories that people construct in an effort to unify events of the past, expectations for the future, and the realities of the present. Personal narratives help young people to develop and articulate a coherent, clear sense of identity that guides their actions and choices.

The new DSM-5 dimensional model of PDs likewise differentiates between pathological personality traits and other aspects of personality dysfunction (American Psychiatric Association [APA], 2013). These other aspects of personality dysfunction include problems in domains that would be defined as characteristic adaptations and narrative identity in McAdams and colleagues' model. Specifically, the new dimensional model requires moderate or greater impairment in self and interpersonal functioning in two or more of these domains: identity, self-direction, empathy, and intimacy (for more information, see APA, 2013, p. 762).

All of these areas of impairment are likely to be involved in PDs in youth, as well as in adults. Two characteristic adaptations that are likely to be especially relevant for youth are attachment and associated mental representations of close relationships and emotion regulation/coping strategies (Shiner, 2009; Shiner & Tackett, 2014). Both attachment and emotion regulation have important implications for a person's capacity to form a healthy sense of self, relate effectively to others, and cope in adaptive ways with stress and adversity. Moreover, there is extensive empirical work implicating both attachment and emotion regulation in the emergence of personality pathology (Gratz, Tull, & Gunderson, 2008; Gratz et al., 2009; Sroufe, Carlson, Levy, & Egeland, 1999; Weston & Riolo, 2007). Youth vary considerably in their capacities for empathy by middle childhood (Shiner, 2009), so this aspect of impairment is relevant for youth as well. PDs also involve difficulties with developing a clear sense of goals and identity; these aspects of personality are under construction during adolescence, and they may emerge as problems during this critical period (Shiner, 2009; Shiner & Tackett, 2014). There is some evidence that severity of dysfunction in self and interpersonal domains predicts PD outcomes in adolescents (DeFife, Goldberg, & Westen, 2013).

## Youths' Early Personality Traits and the Development of Personality Impairment

All of the previously described areas of pathological personality functioning—impairment in emotion regulation, mental representations of relationships, goals, and identity—are likely to be affected by youths' early-emerging personality traits (Shiner & Caspi, 2012). Youths' personality traits may serve as risk factors for problems in all of these areas because personality traits may set in motion processes that lead to impairment in other important aspects of personality functioning that extend far beyond traits. Children's early-emerging traits shape their experiences of the environment by influencing several tendencies (Shiner & Caspi, 2012). We describe those processes here and offer an example for each.

First, youths' personality traits shape their susceptibility to learning processes (e.g., positive and negative reinforcement; punishment). For example, children with callous and unemotional personality characteristics show, on average, lesser amygdala responses to threat (Hyde et al., 2013) and may therefore be less able to learn to avoid threatening situations. Second, early traits influence youths' likelihood of evoking particular responses from other people. Preschoolers with lower self-control evoke less positive teaching strategies in their mothers (less use of cognitive assistance and more use of directive strategies) than preschoolers with better self-control (Eisenberg et al., 2010). Third, individuals' personality traits shape their construal or interpretation of daily experiences.

For example, adolescents' BPD traits predict tendencies to avoid staying in contact with uncomfortable thoughts and emotions (Schramm, Venta, & Sharp, 2013), which suggests that such youth interpret aversive daily experiences more negatively. Fourth, and finally, youths' traits influence the selection of environments in which to spend time. Socially anxious adolescents tend to select friends who are themselves socially anxious and, over time, these friendships lead to greater social anxiety for both friends (Van Zalk, Van Zalk, Kerr, & Stattin, 2011). Over time, these processes come to influence children's personality development in more pervasive ways, and for some youth, early negative traits may set off a chain of processes leading to impairment in other aspects of their personality functioning.

There is already convincing evidence that personality pathology in the adolescent years predicts impairment in a number of areas. For adolescents, critical developmental tasks involve the development of friendships and romantic relationships, and the cultivation of skills for education and work (Roisman, Masten, Coatsworth, & Tellegen, 2004), as well as the maintenance of closeness to family members while developing increasing autonomy (Allen et al., 2006). Adolescent PDs put youth at risk for later overall impairment in adulthood (Skodol, Johnson, Cohen, Sneed, & Crawford, 2007), as well as relationship problems with family members, peers, and romantic partners, and difficulties in the areas of academic achievement and work (Shiner & Tackett, 2014). The risks for later impairment well into adulthood are as high for PDs as for other psychiatric disorders in adolescence (Crawford et al., 2008). Impairment may become an increasingly stable aspect of personality pathology as youth transition from adolescence to adulthood. There is some evidence that although the normative trend is toward greater personality maturity in early adulthood, not all youth benefit from increased personality maturity as they enter adulthood (Roberts, Wood, & Caspi, 2008). Rather, some people show maladaptive changes in their personality traits. Young people who lack normative experiences with adult roles (a group that may include youth with early personality pathology) may be particularly vulnerable to such negative changes in personality (Roberts et al., 2008).

It is important to recognize that although children's early traits may influence their tendencies toward personality impairment, these non-trait aspects of personality functioning are likely to be influenced by many other factors beyond traits (McAdams & Olson, 2010; McAdams & Pals, 2006). In other words, impairment is not simply another manifestation of pathological personality traits; is likely to have its own separate genetic, psychological, and contextual influences. These other influences on impaired identity, goals, close relationships, and emotion regulation are important areas for future research.

## Conclusions and Directions for Future Research

In this chapter, we have offered a developmental psychopathology model for the emergence of personality pathology in the first two decades of life. Like the DSM-5 Section III Alternative Model for PDs, the model articulated in this chapter is predicated on the notion that personality pathology involves two components: (1) pathological personality traits and (2) impairment in other aspects of personality functioning. As we have argued, youths' normal-range personality traits are relevant for understanding both components. In this section, we offer some ideas for how future research on PDs may profit from more thorough investigation of youths' emerging personality traits.

Like adults, children and adolescents manifest the Big Five personality traits of Extraversion, Neuroticism, Conscientiousness, Agreeableness, and Openness to Experience/Intellect, and researchers are making progress in identifying the psychological and biological processes that underlie individual differences in these traits. The existing research on pathological personality traits in youth points to the likelihood that early pathological traits take a somewhat similar form in childhood, adolescence, and adulthood. Specifically, youth exhibit differences in the pathological traits of introversion, negative affectivity, compulsivity, and antagonism. Although preliminary work on these pathological traits is promising, far more research is needed to determine the form of pathological traits in youth. There are some notable differences between the PD traits identified in research with children and adolescents and the PD traits identified in research on adults (e.g., a clear disinhibition trait is seen in adults but not in youth; De Clercq et al., 2006; Tromp & Koot, 2008). Future work should focus on exploring possible developmental differences in the structure of pathological traits in youth. Furthermore, in an effort to better serve younger populations struggling with PDs, researchers should examine the validity of the DSM-5 dimensional model in populations of children and adolescents.

Current research on stability and change in PD symptoms and PD-relevant traits indicates that these individual differences seem to manifest moderate to strong rank-order stability by childhood. Research on mean-level stability of PD symptoms and PD-relevant traits suggests that personality pathology may peak at some point during adolescence, then decline during later adolescence and adulthood. These findings call into question the common assumption that PD symptoms are ephemeral or trivial in childhood and adolescence. For both rank-order and mean-level stability, however, more research on continuity and change in PD symptoms and pathological traits is needed to reach firm conclusions.

Behavior genetics research on normal-range traits in childhood indicates that youths' traits are moderately heritable and influenced by child-specific environments; the single behavior genetics study of PD symptoms in childhood reached the same conclusions (Coolidge et al., 2001). Change in normal-range traits in childhood and adolescence is influenced by both genetic factors and child-specific environments. A wide variety of contextual factors (e.g., parenting, schools, peer relationships, neighborhoods) predict changes in normal-range traits in childhood, and such factors are likely to play a causal role in the development of PDs as well. Longitudinal, prospective studies of the development of personality pathology in childhood and adolescence are needed to better understand the pathways leading to PDs. Such studies would benefit from the use of genetically informative designs to determine true genetic and environmental influences on personality pathology. It will be important for these studies to address the emergence of the two components of PDs—pathological personality traits and impairment in other aspects of personality functioning—in order to determine whether these two components mutually influence each other over time, and whether they have shared and/or distinctive causes. PDs are important enough and emerge early enough in the life course that they warrant more intensive, longitudinal study during childhood and adolescence. Only by better understanding the developmental pathways leading to PDs will we be able to more effectively prevent and treat them.

# REFERENCES

Allen, J. P., Insabella, G., Porter, M. R., Smith, F. D., Land, D., & Phillips, N. (2006). A social-interactional model of the development of depressive symptoms in adolescence. *Journal of Consulting and Clinical Psychology, 74,* 55–65.

American Psychiatric Association. (2013). *Diagnostic and statistical manual of mental disorders* (5th ed.). Arlington, VA: Author.

Bates, J. E., Schermerhorn, A. C., & Petersen, I. T. (2012). Temperament and parenting in developmental perspective. In M. Zentner & R. L. Shiner (Eds.), *Handbook of temperament* (pp. 425–441). New York: Guilford Press.

Belsky, D. W., Caspi, A., Arseneault, L., Bleidorn, W., Fonagy, P., Goodman, M., et al. (2012). Etiological features of borderline personality related characteristics in a birth cohort of 12-year-old children. *Development and Psychopathology, 24,* 251–265.

Berenz, E. C., Amstadter, A. B., Aggen, S. H., Knudsen, G. P., Reichborn-Kjennerud, T., Gardner, C. O., et al. (2013). Childhood trauma and personality disorder criterion counts: A co-twin control analysis. *Journal of Abnormal Psychology, 122,* 1070–1076.

Bornovalova, M. A., Hicks, B. M., Iacono, W. G., & McGue, M. (2013). Longitudinal twin study of borderline personality disorder traits and substance use in adolescence: Developmental change, reciprocal effects, and genetic and environmental influences. *Personality Disorders: Theory, Research, and Treatment, 4,* 23–32.

Bornovalova, M. A., Huibregtse, B. M., Hicks, B., M., Keyes, M., McGue, M., & Iacono, W. (2013). Tests of a direct effect of childhood abuse on adult borderline personality disorder traits: A longitudinal discordant twin design. *Journal of Abnormal Psychology, 122,* 180–194.

Bradley, B., Westen, D., Mercer, K. B., Binder, E. B., Jovanovic, T., Crain, D., et al. (2011). Association between childhood maltreatment and adult emotional dysregulation in a low-income, urban, African American sample: Moderation by oxytocin receptor gene. *Development and Psychopathology, 23,* 439–452.

Caspi, A., & Shiner, R. L. (2006). Personality development. In W. Damon & R. Lerner (Series Eds.) & N. Eisenberg (Vol. Ed.), *Handbook of child psychology: Vol. 3. Social, emotional, and personality development* (6th ed., pp. 300–365). New York: Wiley.

Caspi, A., & Shiner, R. L. (2008). Temperament and personality. In M. Rutter, D. Bishop, D. Pine, S. Scott, J. Stevenson, E. Taylor, & A. Thapar (Eds.), *Rutter's child and adolescent psychiatry* (5th ed., pp. 182–199). London: Blackwell.

Cicchetti, D. (1993). Developmental psychopathology: Reactions, reflections, projections. *Developmental Review, 13,* 471–502.

Cicchetti, D. (2013). An overview of developmental psychopathology. In P. Zelazo (Ed.), *Oxford handbook of developmental psychology* (pp. 455–480). New York: Oxford University Press.

Cicchetti, D., & Rogosch, F. A. (1996). Equifinality and multifinality in development. *Development and Psychopathology, 8,* 597–600.

Clark, L. A. (2007). Assessment and diagnosis of PD: Perennial issues and emerging conceptualization. *Annual Review of Psychology, 58,* 227–257.

Cohen, P., Crawford, T. N., Johnson, J. G., & Kasen, S. (2005). The Children in the Community study of developmental course of PD. *Journal of Personality Disorders, 19,* 466–486.

Coolidge, F. L., Thede, L. L., & Jang, K. L. (2001). Heritability of personality disorders in childhood: A preliminary investigation. *Journal of Personality Disorders, 15,* 33–40.

Crawford, T. N., Cohen, P., First, M. B., Skodol, A. E., Johnson, J. G., & Kasen, S. (2008). Comorbid Axis I and Axis II disorders in early adolescence: Outcomes 20 years later. *Archives of General Psychiatry, 65,* 641–648.

Crick, N. R., Murray-Close, D., & Woods, K. (2005). Borderline personality features in childhood: A short-term longitudinal study. *Development and Psychopathology, 17,* 1051–1070.

De Clercq, B., De Fruyt, F., Van Leeuwen, K., & Mervielde, I. (2006). The structure of maladaptive personality traits in childhood: A step toward an integrative developmental perspective for DSM-V. *Journal of Abnormal Psychology, 115,* 639–657.

De Clercq, B., De Fruyt, F., & Widiger, T. A. (2009). Integrating a developmental perspective in dimensional models of personality disorders. *Clinical Psychology Review, 29,* 154–162.

De Clercq, B., Van Leeuwen, K., van den Noortgate, W., De Bolle, M., & De Fruyt, F. (2009). Childhood personality pathology: Dimensional stability and change. *Development and Psychopathology, 21,* 853–869.

DeFife, J. A., Goldberg, M. G., & Westen, D. (2015). Dimensional assessment of self and interpersonal functioning in adolescents: Implications for DSM-5's general definition of personality disorder. *Journal of Personality Disorders, 29*(2), 248–260.

De Fruyt, F., & De Clercq, B. (2013). Childhood antecedents of personality disorder: A five-factor model perspective. In T. A. Widiger & P. T. Costa, Jr. (Eds.), *Personality disorders and the five-factor model of personality* (3rd ed., pp. 43–60). Washington, DC: American Psychological Association.

De Pauw, S. S. W., Mervielde, I., & Van Leeuwen, K. G. (2009). How are traits related to problem behavior in preschool children?: Similarities and contrasts between temperament and personality. *Journal of Abnormal Child Psychology, 37,* 309–325.

DeYoung, C. G., & Gray, J. R. (2009). Personality neuroscience: Explaining individual differences in affect, behavior, and cognition. In P. J. Corr & G. Matthews (Eds.), *The Cambridge handbook of personality psychology* (pp. 323–346). Cambridge, UK: Cambridge University Press.

DeYoung, C. G., Hirsh, J. B., Shane, M. S., Papademetris, X., Rajeevan, N., & Gray, J. R. (2010). Testing predictions from personality neuroscience: Brain structure and the big five. *Psychological Science, 21*(6), 820–828.

Digman, J. M. (1990). Personality structure: Emergence of the five-factor model. *Annual Review of Psychology, 41,* 417–440.

Eisenberg, N., Fabes, R. A., Shepard, S. A., Guthrie, I. K., Murphy, B. C., & Reiser, M. (1999). Parental reactions to children's negative emotions: Longitudinal relations to quality of children's social functioning. *Child Development, 70,* 513–534.

Eisenberg, N., Vidmar, M., Spinrad, T. L., Eggum, N. D., Edwards, A., Gaertner, B., et al. (2010). Mothers' teaching strategies and children's effortful control: A longitudinal study. *Developmental Psychology, 46*(5), 1294–1308.

Evans, D. E., & Rothbart, M. K. (2007). Developing a model for adult temperament. *Journal of Research in Personality, 41*(4), 868–888.

Ferguson, C. J. (2010). A meta-analysis of normal and disordered personality across the life span. *Journal of Personality and Social Psychology, 98,* 659–667.

Fox, N. A., Henderson, H. A., Marshall, P. J., Nichols, K. E., & Ghera, M. M. (2005). Behavioral inhibition: Linking biology and behavior within a developmental framework. *Annual Review of Psychology, 56,* 235–262.

Geiger, T. C., & Crick, N. R. (2009). Developmental pathways to personality disorders. In R. E. Ingram & J. M. Price (Eds.), *Vulnerability to psychopathology: Risk across the lifespan* (2nd ed., pp. 57–112). New York: Guilford Press.

Gratz, K. L., Tull, M. T., & Gunderson, J. G. (2008). Preliminary data on the relationship between anxiety sensitivity and BPD: The role of experiential avoidance. *Journal of Psychiatric Research, 42,* 550–559.

Gratz, K. L., Tull, M. T., Reynolds, E. K., Bagge, C. L., Latzman, R. D., Daughters, S. B., et al. (2009). Extending extant models of the pathogenesis of BPD to childhood borderline personality symptoms: The roles of affective dysfunction, disinhibition, and self- and emotion-regulation deficits. *Development and Psychopathology, 21,* 1263–1291.

Gray, J. A. (1982). *The neuropsychology of anxiety: An enquiry into the functions of the septohippocampal system.* New York: Oxford University Press.

Gray, J. A., & McNaughton, N. (2000). *The neuropsychology of anxiety: An enquiry into the functions of the septo-hippocampal system* (2nd ed.). New York: Oxford University Press.

Halverson, C. F., & Deal, J. E. (2001). Temperamental change, parenting, and the family context. In T. D. Wachs & G. A. Kohnstamm (Eds.), *Temperament in context* (pp. 61–79). Mahwah, NJ: Erlbaum.

Harkness, A. R., & McNulty, J. L. (1994). The Personality Psychopathology Five (PSY-5): Issue from the pages of a diagnostic manual instead of a dictionary. In S. Strack & M. Lorr (Eds.), *Differentiating normal and abnormal personality* (pp. 291–315). New York: Springer.

Herzhoff, K., & Tackett, J. L. (2012). Establishing construct validity for Openness-to-Experience in middle childhood: Contributions from personality and temperament. *Journal of Research in Personality, 46*(3), 286–294.

Hyde, L. W., Shaw, D. S., & Hariri, A. R. (2013). Understanding youth antisocial behavior using neuroscience through a developmental psychopathology lens: Review, integration, and directions for research. *Developmental Review, 33,* 168–223.

John, O. P., Naumann, L. P., & Soto, C. J. (2008). Paradigm shift to the integrative Big Five trait taxonomy. In O. P. John, R. W. Robins, & L. A. Pervin (Eds.), *Handbook of personality: Theory and research* (3rd ed., pp. 114–158). New York: Guilford Press.

Johnson, J. G., Cohen, P., Kasen, S., Skodol, A. E., Hamagami, F., & Brook, J. S. (2000). Age-related change in personality disorder trait levels between early adolescence and adulthood: A community-based longitudinal investigation. *Acta Psychiatrica Scandinavica, 102,* 265–275.

Johnson, J. G., First, M. B., Cohen, P., Skodol, A. E., Kasen, S., & Brook, J. S. (2005). Adverse outcomes associated with personality disorder not otherwise specified in a community sample. *American Journal of Psychiatry, 162,* 1926–1932.

Kim, J., Cicchetti, D., Rogosch, F. A., & Manly, J. T. (2009). Child maltreatment and trajectories of personality and behavioral functioning: Implications for the development of personality disorders. *Development and Psychopathology, 21,* 889–912.

Kochanska, G., Murray, K. T., & Harlan, E. T. (2000). Effortful control in early childhood: Continuity and change, antecedents, and implications for social development. *Developmental Psychology, 36*(2), 220–232.

Kushner, S. C., Tackett, J. L., & De Clercq, B. (2013). The joint hierarchical structure of adolescent personality pathology: Converging evidence from two approaches to measurement. *Journal of the Canadian Academy of Child and Adolescent Psychiatry, 22*(3), 199–205.

Lengua, L. J., & Wachs, T. D. (2012). Temperament and risk: Resilient and vulnerable responses to adversity. In M. Zentner & R. L. Shiner (Eds.), *Handbook of temperament* (pp. 519–540). New York: Guilford Press.

Li-Grining, C. P. (2007). Effortful control among low-income preschoolers in three cities: Stability, change, and individual differences. *Developmental Psychology, 53*(1), 208–221.

Linde, J. A., Stringer, D. M., Simms, L. J., & Clark, L. A. (2013). The Schedule for Nonadaptive and Adaptive Personality for Youth (SNAP-Y): A new measure for assessing adolescent personality and personality pathology. *Assessment, 20,* 387–404.

Livesley, W. J. (2007). A framework for integrating dimensional and categorical classifications of personality disorder. *Journal of Personality Disorders, 21,* 199–224.

Markon, K. E., Krueger, R. F., & Watson, D. (2005). Delineating the structure of normal and abnormal personality: An integrative hierarchical approach. *Journal of Personality and Social Psychology, 88,* 139–157.

Matheny, A. P., & Phillips, K. (2001). Temperament and context: Correlates of home environment with temperament continuity and change, newborn to 30 months. In T. D. Wachs & G. A. Kohnstamm (Eds.), *Temperament in context* (pp. 81–101). Mahwah, NJ: Erlbaum.

McAdams, D. P., & Olson, B. D. (2010). Personality development: Continuity and change over the life course. *Annual Review of Psychology, 61,* 517–542.

McAdams, D. P., & Pals, J. L. (2006). A new Big Five: Fundamental principles for an integrative science of personality. *American Psychologist, 61,* 204–217.

McCrae, R. R., & Costa, P. T. (1999). A five-factor theory of personality. In L. A. Pervin & O. P. John (Eds.), *Handbook of personality: Theory and research* (2nd ed., pp. 139–153). New York: Guilford Press.

Measelle, J. R., John, O. P., Ablow, J. C., Cowan, P. A., & Cowan, C. P. (2005). Can children provide coherent, stable, and valid self-reports on the big five dimensions?: A longitudinal study from ages 5 to 7. *Journal of Personality and Social Psychology, 89*(1), 90–106.

Meier, M. H., Slutske, W. S., Arndt, S., & Cadoret, R. J. (2008). Impulsive and callous traits are more strongly associated with delinquent behavior in higher risk neighborhoods among boys and girls. *Journal of Abnormal Psychology, 117*(2), 377–385.

Posner, M. I., Rothbart, M. K., Sheese, B. E., & Tang, Y. (2007). The anterior cingulate gyrus and the mechanism of self-regulation. *Cognitive, Affective, and Behavioral Neuroscience, 7*(4), 391–395.

Ro, E., Stringer, D., & Clark, L. A. (2012). The Schedule for Nonadaptive and Adaptive Personality: A useful tool for diagnosis and classification of personality disorder. In T. A. Widiger (Ed.), *Oxford handbook of personality disorders* (pp. 58–81). New York: Oxford University Press.

Roberts, B. W., & DelVecchio, W. F. (2000). The rank-order consistency of personality traits from childhood to old age: A quantitative review of longitudinal studies. *Psychological Bulletin, 126,* 3–25.

Roberts, B. W., Walton, K. E., & Viechtbauer, W. (2006). Patterns of mean-level change in personality traits across the life course: A meta-analysis of longitudinal studies. *Psychological Bulletin, 132,* 1–25.

Roberts, B. W., Wood, D., & Caspi, A. (2008). The development of personality traits in adulthood. In O. P. John, R. W. Robins, & L. A. Pervin (Eds.), *Handbook of personality: Theory and research* (3rd ed., pp. 375–398). New York: Guilford Press.

Roisman, G. I., Masten, A. S., Coatsworth, J. D., & Tellegen, A. (2004). Salient and emerging developmental tasks in the transition to adulthood. *Child Development, 75,* 123–133.

Rothbart, M. K. (2011). *Becoming who we are: Temperament and personality in development.* New York: Guilford Press.

Rothbart, M. K., & Bates, J. E. (2006). Temperament. In

W. Damon & R. Lerner (Series Eds.) & N. Eisenberg (Vol. Ed.), *Handbook of child psychology: Vol. 3. Social, emotional, and personality development* (6th ed., pp. 99–166). New York: Wiley.

Samuel, D. B., & Widiger, T. A. (2008). A meta-analytic review of the relationships between the five-factor model and DSM-IV-TR personality disorders: A facet level analysis. *Clinical Psychology Review, 28*(8), 1326–1342.

Saudino, K. J., & Wang, M. (2012). Quantitative and molecular genetic studies of temperament. In M. Zentner & R. L. Shiner (Eds.), *Handbook of temperament* (pp. 315–346). New York: Guilford Press.

Schramm, A. T., Venta, A., & Sharp, C. (2013). The role of experiential avoidance in the association between borderline personality features and emotion regulation in adolescents. *Personality Disorders: Theory, Research, and Treatment, 4*, 138–144.

Shiner, R. L. (2009). The development of personality disorders: Perspectives from normal personality development in childhood and adolescence. *Development and Psychopathology, 21*, 715–734.

Shiner, R. L. (2014). The development of temperament and personality traits in childhood and adolescence. In M. Mikulincer & P. Shaver (Eds.), M. L. Cooper & R. Larsen (Assoc. Eds.), *APA handbook of personality and social psychology: Vol. 3. Personality processes and individual differences* (pp. 85–105). Washington, DC: American Psychological Association.

Shiner, R. L., & Allen, T. A. (2013). Assessing personality disorders in adolescents: Seven guiding principles. *Clinical Psychology: Science and Practice, 20*, 361–377.

Shiner, R. L., Buss, K. A., McClowry, S. G., Putnam, S. P., Saudino, K. J., & Zentner, M. (2012). What is temperament *now*? Assessing progress in temperament research on the twenty-fifth anniversary of Goldsmith et al. (1987). *Child Development Perspectives, 6*(4), 436–444.

Shiner, R. L., & Caspi, A. (2012). Temperament and the development of personality traits, adaptations, and narratives. In M. Zentner & R. L. Shiner (Eds.), *Handbook of temperament* (pp. 497–516). New York: Guilford Press.

Shiner, R. L., & DeYoung, C. G. (2013). The structure of temperament and personality traits: A developmental perspective. In P. D. Zelazo (Ed.) *The Oxford handbook of developmental psychology: Vol. 2. Self and other* (pp. 113–141). Oxford, UK: Oxford University Press.

Shiner, R. L., & Tackett, J. L. (2014). Personality disorders in children and adolescents. In E. J. Mash & R. A. Barkley (Eds.), *Child psychopathology* (3rd ed., pp. 848–896). New York: Guilford Press.

Skodol, A. W., Johnson, J. G., Cohen, P., Sneed, J. R., & Crawford, T. N. (2007). Personality disorder and impaired functioning from adolescence to adulthood. *British Journal of Psychiatry, 190*, 415–420.

Soto, C. J., John, O. P., Gosling, S. D., & Potter, J. (2008). The developmental psychometrics of big five self-reports: Acquiescence, factor structure, coherence, and differentiation from ages 10 to 20. *Journal of Personality and Social Psychology, 94*(4), 718–737.

Soto, C. J., John, O. P., Gosling, S. M., & Potter, J. (2011). Age differences in personality traits from 10 to 65: Big Five domains and facets in a large cross-sectional sample. *Journal of Personality and Social Psychology, 100*, 330–348.

South, S. C., Reichborn-Kjennerud, T., Eaton, N. R., & Krueger, R. F. (2012). Behavior and molecular genetics of personality disorders. In T. A. Widiger (Ed.), *The Oxford handbook of personality disorders* (pp. 143–165). New York: Oxford University Press.

Sroufe, L. A. (1990). Considering normal and abnormal together: The essence of developmental psychopathology. *Development and Psychopathology, 2*, 335–347.

Sroufe, L. A., Carlson, E. A., Levy, A. K., & Egeland, B. (1999). Implications of attachment theory for developmental psychopathology. *Development and Psychopathology, 11*, 1–13.

Tackett, J. L., Balsis, S., Oltmanns, T. F., & Krueger, R. F. (2009). A unifying perspective on personality pathology across the life span: Developmental considerations for the fifth edition of the *Diagnostic and Statistical Manual of Mental Disorders*. *Development and Psychopathology, 21*, 687–713.

Tackett, J. L., Silberschmidt, A. L., Krueger, R. F., & Sponheim, S. R. (2008). A dimensional model of personality disorder: Incorporating DSM Cluster A characteristics. *Journal of Abnormal Psychology, 117*, 454–459.

Tromp, N. B., & Koot, H. M. (2008). Dimensions of personality pathology in adolescents: Psychometric properties of the DAPP-BQ-A. *Journal of Personality Disorders, 22*, 623–638.

Tromp, N. B., & Koot, H. M. (2010). Dimensions of normal and abnormal personality: Elucidating DSM-IV personality disorder symptoms in adolescents. *Journal of Personality, 78*, 839–864.

Van Zalk, N., Van Zalk, M., Kerr, M., & Stattin, H. (2011). Social anxiety as a basis for friendship selection and socialization in adolescents' social networks. *Journal of Personality, 79*, 499–525.

Verbeke, L., & De Clercq, B. (2014). Integrating oddity traits in a dimensional model for personality pathology precursors. *Journal of Abnormal Psychology, 123*(3), 598–612.

Verheul, R., & Widiger, T. A. (2004). A meta-analysis of the prevalence and usage of the personality disorder not otherwise specified (PD-NOS) diagnosis. *Journal of Personality Disorders, 18*, 309–319.

Weston, C. G., & Riolo, S. A. (2007). Childhood and adolescent precursors to adult personality disorders. *Psychiatric Annals, 37*, 114–120.

Widiger, T. A., & Costa, P. T., Jr. (Eds.). (2013). *Personality disorders and the Five-Factor model of personality* (3rd ed.). Washington, DC: American Psychological Association.

# CHAPTER 19

# An Attachment Perspective on Callous and Unemotional Characteristics across Development

Roseann M. Larstone, Stephanie G. Craig, and Marlene M. Moretti

There is an extensive history of research on the etiology and course of serious conduct problems and treatment outcomes among antisocial and violent youth (e.g., Moffitt et al., 2008). A consistent finding from this work is that children and adolescents with conduct problems display considerable heterogeneity in the type and severity of their behavior problems, social and interpersonal functioning (e.g., quality of interpersonal relationships; school dropout, incarceration), and response to treatment. This heterogeneity suggests that there are meaningful subgroups (e.g., child vs. adolescent onset; see Moffitt, 2006) and multiple pathways to serious and persistent conduct problems and aggression (e.g., Frick & Viding, 2009; Moffitt, 1993, 2006). The identification of heterogeneous clusters in the etiology and developmental course of severe conduct problems has become a pressing research priority (Frick & Marsee, 2006; Frick & White, 2008) with important implications for intervention.

One well-developed line of research that has shed light on heterogeneity among children with serious behavior problems focuses on callous–unemotional (CU) traits (Frick & White, 2008; Waller et al., 2012). Historically, CU traits (e.g., lack of empathy and guilt; shallow affect; uncaring attitudes) (Cleckley, 1941; Hare, Hart, & Harpur, 1991) have been thought to represent a core deficit that is associated with early-onset and persistent antisocial and aggressive behavior. Children and teens who have high levels of CU traits have been shown to demonstrate more severe, chronic and aggressive patterns of behavior than do children who show conduct problems in the absence of CU traits (e.g., Frick & White, 2008; Kimonis, Bagner, Linares, Blake, & Rodriguez, 2014). Conduct problems in conjunction with high levels of CU traits are associated with low punishment sensitivity and lack of responsiveness to others' emotions (particularly fear; see Blair, Leibenluft, & Pine, 2014; Dadds & Rhodes, 2008). CU traits are predominant in current conceptualizations of psychopathy, suggesting a link between the developmental literature on CU traits and aggression in youth on the one hand, and the clinical literature on psychopathy on the other (Hare, 1993; Kimonis, Frick, Cauffman, Goldweber, & Skeem, 2012). Apart from CU traits, the affective component of psychopathy, there are two additional defining features of psychopathy: the interpersonal (e.g., arrogant and deceitful; narcissistic view of self and manipulative behavior) and the behavioral features (e.g., impulsive/irresponsible; see Frick & White, 2008).

Youth with high levels of CU traits show low levels of fearfulness and a preference for thrill-seeking, novel, and dangerous activities in both nonreferred (Frick, Cornell, et al., 2003) and referred samples (Pardini, 2006). Compared to youth with low levels of CU traits, those with high levels of such traits are less sensitive to punishment cues, show lower levels of empathy, express less emotion, and show less reactivity to threatening and emotionally distressing stimuli from a young age. This may reflect a genetic basis to their CU traits and aggressive/antisocial behavior (Dadds & Rhodes, 2008). Given these findings, it is unsurprising that CU traits are described as dispositional and have been shown to be relatively stable from late childhood to early adolescence, particularly according to parent report (Frick & White, 2008). Importantly, however, at least two studies have reported decreases over longitudinal follow up in nonreferred youth with initially high levels of CU traits (e.g., Frick, Kimonis, Dandreaux, & Farell, 2003; Pardini, Lochman, & Powell, 2007).

There is no question that CU traits are central to the development of serious conduct disorder and a core component of psychopathology, particularly antisocial personality disorder (ASPD) and psychopathy, but are there multiple pathways to CU traits? The current chapter presents two contemporary and sometimes competing views regarding the etiological and developmental trajectory of CU traits in relation to aggression and related empirical findings. The first model, which is dominant in the literature, adopts a developmental genetic and neurobiological perspective. This etiological perspective of CU traits in childhood and adolescence is congruent with, but not identical to, the construct of primary psychopathy in adults. Primary psychopathy is characterized by trait fearlessness, impulsivity, high social dominance, high self-esteem, and low anxiety, a constellation of features that are generally viewed as an expression of underlying genetic influences (e.g., Blair, Peschardt, Budhani, Mitchell, & Pine, 2006).

Of particular interest relative to this discussion is a second developmental model, originally proposed by Karpman (1941, 1948) and based on an emerging literature that conceptualizes CU features or characteristics as an "acquired adaptation" to environmental influences, particularly exposure to chronic trauma and adverse social contexts (Bennett & Kerig, 2014; Kerig & Becker, 2010; Porter, 1996). This variant of CU traits is commonly conceptualized as being analogous to secondary psychopathy.

Secondary psychopathy in adults is linked with trauma exposure and occurs in conjunction with posttraumatic stress disorder (PTSD) symptoms (Hicks, Vaidyanathan, & Patrick, 2010). Based on the field of developmental traumatology, the central premise of this view is that children exposed to severe maltreatment, especially when perpetrated within their primary relationships with caregivers (i.e., betrayal trauma), cope through avoidance, emotional detachment, and the development of callousness (see also Ford, Chapman, Mack, & Pearson, 2006; Karpman, 1941; Kerig, Bennett, Thompson & Becker, 2012; Porter, 1996).

Respectively, these two etiological models can be referred to as describing the development of "primary" versus "acquired" CU traits. In this chapter, we selectively review newly emerging research focused on the heterogeneity in developmental pathways to CU traits. Where the literature specific to CU traits is sparse, we supplement our discussion with research on the etiological factors that distinguish primary and secondary psychopathy in adolescence, which encompasses interpersonal, behavioral, and affective features. We discuss what we term "broad" CU traits, in which the literature does not distinguish between the two variants and specify primary and acquired CU, where appropriate, to reflect the available evidence. Using a developmental traumatology framework, we examine the shared and unique clinical features, etiological factors, including attachment-related processes and treatment response associated with primary versus acquired CU. We argue that these two pathways are not mutually exclusive; however, understanding distinctive features will undoubtedly improve the quality and effectiveness of our prevention and treatment efforts. We also discuss limitations in the current state of the literature and future directions for research.

## Clinical Features

A considerable body of research demonstrates that antisocial youth with CU traits differ developmentally on behavioral, emotional, and neural indices from antisocial and aggressive individuals who do not show CU traits (Frick, Ray, Thornton, & Kahn, 2014; Frick & White, 2008). Below we review the available evidence that has furthered our understanding of how primary versus acquired CU traits are expressed from studies investigating these constructs in samples of youth diagnosed with conduct disorder and those involved in the juvenile justice system. Conduct disorder describes a heterogeneous group of children and adolescents, only a small minority of whom develops severe and chronic forms of antisocial behavior (e.g., Frick et al., 2014). The inclusion of CU traits as a modifier in DSM-5 (American Psychiatric Association [APA], 2013) was to identify a clinically meaningful subtype of conduct disorder (i.e., limited prosocial emotions specifier; APA, 2013), although the diagnostic criteria do not distinguish between primary and acquired CU variants.

Primary CU is defined by shallow affect; deficient empathy, guilt, and remorse; callousness toward the feelings of others; and deficits in emotion processing that give rise to low emotional arousal—characteristics that are evident at a young age (e.g., Blair et al., 2006, 2014). In studies specifically examining primary CU traits in relation to psychopathology, these features are associated with less severe conduct problems, lower levels of physical aggression, and less emotional and behavioral dysregulation compared to the acquired variant (Kahn et al., 2013). Compared to the acquired CU variant, primary CU has been found to be associated with lower anxiety, greater self-esteem and lower behavioral inhibition in community-based and clinic-referred youth (Fanti, Demetriou, & Kimonis, 2013; Kahn et al., 2013). There is evidence of the emergence of punishment insensitivity in early childhood, particularly in contexts where perpetrating antisocial or aggressive behavior may lead to a reward or achievement of a social goal (Dadds & Salmon, 2003).

Individuals with acquired CU features also show shallow affect and low empathy; however, such youth often report greater previous exposure to trauma than do youth showing the primary CU variant (Bennett & Kerig, 2014; Kahn et al., 2013; Kimonis et al., 2012). Compared to the primary variant, acquired CU has been found to be associated with greater levels of anxiety, impulsivity, negative affect (depression), and reactive aggression (Gill & Stickle, 2016; Kimonis et al., 2012). In a community sample, youth with acquired CU were found to have lower self-esteem, higher anxiety, and greater narcissism (Fanti et al., 2013).

Porter (1996) proposed that salient clinical features associated with callousness–unemotionality emerge differently in children with acquired CU, with low empathy appearing first, eventually followed by the emergence of overt behavior problems; whereas in the case of primary CU, the core personality characteristics associated with the CU construct and related behavior problems (e.g., lying) theoretically emerge concurrently. The onset of acquired CU features in children who have been chronically exposed to early adverse events including victimization is now thought to represent an adaptive response to overwhelming interpersonal trauma. For example, symptoms such as affective numbing are associated with reductions in distress associated with trauma exposure. However, at the same time, emotional numbing increases risk for perpetrating aggression because, over time, children and youth become impervious to recognizing others' distress, thus reducing the interpersonal signaling functions of affective cues (e.g., facial expressions) that would inhibit aggression. This pathway to CU traits differs from that presumed to underlie primary CU traits in several ways, as we discuss in later sections. Importantly, trauma exposure is not a typical hallmark in children with primary CU traits, and the onset of behavior problems typically occurs in close conjunction with the emergence of CU features (Kahn et al., 2013).

Despite limited evidence, taken together, research suggests that there may be overlapping and distinctive clinical features in individuals showing primary versus acquired CU traits. These differences in clinical presentation suggest that there may be diverse etiological factors that give rise to both variants. Specifically, primary CU traits may represent the early expression of genetic and neurodevelopmental factors, and acquired CU features may in greater measure reflect the influence of environmental factors. We review in the next section the available evidence on established and newly identified etiological factors across both variants.

## Etiology

There is a long history of research on the etiology of psychopathy (see Patrick & Brislin, Chapter 24, this volume). Some perspectives emphasize biological (e.g., Blair et al., 2006, 2014; Blair, 2007) and others environmental or social origins (e.g., Karpman, 1941; Porter, 1996) of the disorder and related personality characteristics (i.e., psychopathic traits including novelty seeking, low affective empathy, impulsivity, and fearlessness). The last decade has seen the emergence and refinement of developmental theories and models that have pointed to underlying affective and cognitive deficits that precede the manifestation of CU traits in youth. This is a rich area of investigation, as recent research has just begun to distinguish between the developmental origins of primary and acquired CU traits. Below we review recent studies from genetic, emotional and moral development, and social-relational (i.e., parenting and trauma) perspectives that describe the emergence of CU traits generally, then across the two subtypes, where evidence is available.

## Environmental and Genetic Influences

Studies examining genetic contributions to broad CU traits in adolescents and young adults suggest that genetic influences on developmental trajectories (e.g., stable high; increasing; decreasing; stable low) and stability of such traits may be high (Fontaine, Rijsdijk, McCrory, & Viding, 2010). For example, a recent population-based longitudinal study of twin pairs in middle childhood (i.e., ages 7–12 years) reported a high degree of heritability in male twins showing stable high levels of CU traits as assessed by teacher report (Fontaine et al., 2010). Studies examining CU traits in samples of identical and fraternal twins using different informants (i.e., self-, parent-, and teacher-report) and assessing heritability in childhood and adolescence, show that approximately 40–67% of the variance may be attributable to genetic effects (e.g., Larsson, Andershed, & Lichtenstein, 2006; Viding, Frick, & Plomin, 2007).

Although research on the role of genetic factors in the etiology of primary versus acquired CU is limited, emerging research in the field of epigenetics suggests there may be different pathways leading to the emergence of CU traits (e.g., Cecil et al., 2014). Epigenetics refers to the study of heritable changes in gene expression (i.e., which genes are active vs. inactive); that is, how genetic material is expressed in different contexts (Moore, 2015; p. 10). One line of epigenetic research in the study of CU traits has focused on changes in the oxytocin (OXT) system. OXT is a neuropeptide that has a role in promoting affiliative and prosocial behavior (e.g., trust, empathy, and attachment) (Cecil et al., 2014). OXT can be examined via circulating blood levels through polymorphisms in the OXT receptor gene ($OXTR$) and assessing its relationship with the perception of emotion and trust (Dadds et al., 2014; Meyer-Lindenberg, Domes, Kirsch, & Heinrichs, 2011). Recent research has shown that higher levels of DNA methylation (i.e., an epigenetic signaling mechanism that cells use to keep genes in the "off" position) in $OXTR$ is related to lower levels of circulating OXT in the context of high CU in older children (Dadds et al., 2014). In a recent study that examined possible differences in developmental pathways to CU traits, Cecil and colleagues (2014) investigated a sample of youth with conduct problems, grouped according to high versus low internalizing problems (i.e., anxiety and depression) to prospectively examine associations between early environmental risk exposure and $OXTR$ methylation in the prediction of CU traits at age 13. Pre- and postnatal environmental risks (e.g., parental psychopathology; adverse life events) were assessed. Epigenetic changes (i.e., DNA methylation) to the $OXTR$ were assessed at birth and ages 7 and 9. In youth with low levels of internalizing problems, CU traits at age 13 were associated with DNA methylation at the $OXTR$ gene at birth. $OXTR$ methylation at birth was also associated with lower levels of victimization during childhood in youth with low internalizing problems. In youth with high levels of anxiety and depression, $OXTR$ methylation was not associated with CU traits at age 13. Instead, prenatal environmental risks such as family conflict were associated with higher CU traits. This suggests that adolescents with low internalizing problems had higher levels of DNA methylation in the $OXTR$ gene at birth, which may contribute to CU characteristics. In contrast, in youth with high levels of internalizing problems, CU traits were found to be independently associated with prenatal environmental adversity. These findings lend support to the idea there are two distinct pathways to the development of CU traits. However, it is unclear to what extent such effects differentially influence the two variants.

## Emotional Processing

To better understand the heterogeneity of CU features, researchers have examined differences in emotion regulation processes, including emotion recognition (Bennett & Kerig, 2014; Kimonis, Frick, Cauffman, Goldweber, & Skeem, 2012; Kimonis, Frick, Fazekas, & Loney, 2006; Kimonis, Frick, Muñoz & Aucoin, 2008). As noted earlier, CU traits are associated with fundamental deficits in emotional arousal in response to others' expressions of fear and distress. In a recent review of the CU literature in children and youth, impairments in emotion recognition were noted across 26 studies, with samples of children varying in age and across studies using different measurements and methodologies (Frick et al., 2014b).

Although few studies have examined emotion regulation in cases of primary versus acquired CU, the results of those that have done so are consistent with the dual pathway notion of development. More specifically, different types of emotion regulation deficits have been associated with primary versus acquired CU characteristics (Bennett & Kerig, 2014; Kimonis et al., 2006, 2008, 2012). In a sample of adjudicated adolescents (26% female, $M_{age}$ = 16.15 years) Bennett and Kerig (2014) found that compared to youth identified as having primary CU, youth with acquired CU (i.e., high CU features, trauma exposure and elevated posttraumatic stress symptoms) showed significantly less acceptance of emotions, less ability to identify and differentiate their own emotions, and greater emotional numbing. Acquired CU was also associated with greater sensitization to detecting the expression of negative affect in others' facial expression, specifically, disgust. In other words, compared to youth with primary CU, those with the acquired variant were more likely to detect negative affect in others and were more distressed by it. CU features in these youth may be evoked to buffer or protect them from distress. In contrast, youth with primary CU are less likely to detect negative affect in others and are less distressed as a function of this deficit. For example, Kimonis and colleagues (2012) found that in a sample of male juvenile offenders ($M_{age}$ = 16 years) boys with secondary psychopathy were more likely to report negative emotionality (e.g., depression, anxiety, anger, attention problems) than those identified as having primary psychopathy. They were also more likely to attend to negative emotional stimuli than their counterparts with primary psychopathy (e.g., a picture of a crying child) in laboratory-based tasks. These findings are consistent with the adult psychopathy literature indicating that those with secondary psychopathic traits demonstrate less severe emotion recognition deficits as compared to individuals with primary psychopathy (e.g., Prado, Treeby, & Crowe, 2015). These studies support the idea that those with primary CU have a deficit in emotion recognition and emotion deficits (e.g., less sensitivity to negative stimuli), which is believed to be at the core of psychopathic personality. On the other hand, a person with the acquired variant may be overly sensitive or overwhelmed by emotional stimuli and may therefore have difficulty processing emotions (e.g., show less acceptance of emotions and more emotional numbing).

## Moral Development

The specific emotion recognition and emotion regulation deficits noted in primary versus secondary CU have important implications for understanding developmental trajectories in aggressive and antisocial behavior from childhood to early adulthood. As noted by Blair, Colledge, Murray, and Mitchell (2001), normative processing of emotions is a prerequisite for adaptive social and moral development. According to Kimonis and colleagues (2008), developmental theories of moral socialization posit that during early normative development, a child's transgression (e.g., acts of aggression toward peers) is typically met with distress cues from the victim (e.g., crying) or with a parent's response (e.g., anger or disapproval) that signals a threat of punishment. Both responses typically result in increased anxiety or discomfort in the child that is coded as a moral emotion. The child is therefore conditioned or learns over time to avoid negative behaviors. As a result of this process, strong emotions of fear and guilt are typically elicited in the child at even the thought of a future transgression, which acts as a socializing agent even in the absence of a parent or caregiver (Kimonis et al., 2008). However, children who show a reduced negative emotional response to the distress of others (i.e., primary variant) do not experience this conditioning in the same way and therefore do not develop the associated empathic concern (Blair et al., 2006). On the other hand, children who are hyperresponsive and highly reactive (i.e., acquired variant) may have impairments in conscience development (Kochanska, 1993). This model of moral development has been important in framing and understanding the development of CU traits, as it emphasizes an essential developmental process that is disrupted in the development of empathy.

In the context of etiological theories of psychopathy, Blair (2001) proposed a Violence Inhibition Mechanism (VIM), a biologically based system that has been implicated in the development of primary psychopathy and CU traits (Frick et al., 2014b). This theory suggests that a neurocognitive deficit plays an important role in the development of emotional processing and moral development:

> "At its simplest, the VIM is thought to be a system that when activated by distress cues, the sad and fearful expressions of others, results in increased autonomic activity, attention and activation of the brain stem threat response system (usually resulting in freezing). According to the model, moral socialisation occurs through the pairing of the activation of the mechanism by distress cues with representations of the acts which caused the distress cues (moral transgressions—for example, one person hitting another)." (Blair, 2001, p. 730)

The primary neurocognitive mechanism in relation to deficits in affective empathy in the context of broad CU traits involves reduced amygdala and ventromedial prefrontal cortex responsiveness to others' distress cues (Blair, 2007). Dysfunction in the ventromedial prefrontal cortex and striatum is associated with impairments in decision making (Blair, 2013). Due to this biological deficit, Blair suggests that individuals with primary psychopathy have a developmental disorder that results in a breakdown of social moralization.

In relation to acquired CU, youth who have experienced trauma, particularly in relation to caregivers, might also go on to show dysregulated affect (i.e., hyperarousal) and may go on to experience disruptions in moral development due to an active attempt to avoid interpersonal cues as they become emotionally overwhelmed (Kerig & Becker, 2010). Recent research with adjudicated youth identified as having secondary psychopathy were shown to have higher levels of past PTSD symptoms including hyperarousal versus youth identified as having the primary variant (Tatar, Cauffman, Kimonis, & Skeem, 2012). Affective hyperarousal may have a deleterious effect on children's and youths' ability to effectively attend to and process socialization cues from caregivers (Frick & Morris, 2004). This process may impact the typical development of social-cognitive skills and moral socialization. In other words, children and youth with primary CU traits (i.e., emotional deficits) may be insufficiently aroused by emotional cues, while those with acquired CU traits may learn to avoid attending to emotional cues because they are emotionally overwhelming (e.g., parental anger; Frick & Morris, 2004).

## Trauma

Trauma and child maltreatment have been shown to disrupt normative processes of emotional recognition and processing (Young & Widom, 2014). The presence of ongoing and chronic trauma or maltreatment may interrupt the normal socialization process of moral development by emotionally overwhelming a youth with negative interpersonal stimuli. The importance of trauma in the definition of acquired CU traits is demonstrated by the presence of anxiety and higher rates of trauma (e.g., physical abuse, sexual abuse, neglect) as differentiating factors (e.g., Bennett & Kerig, 2014; Kahn et al., 2013).

There is emerging support for distinguishing between primary and acquired CU traits on the basis of maltreatment histories. For example, a study with 227 incarcerated adolescent boys with secondary psychopathy showed greater incidence of sexual abuse compared to the primary variant, whereas those individuals identified as having the primary variant reported higher rates of parental neglect compared to the secondary variant (Kimonis, Fanti, Isoma, & Donoghue, 2013). Youth classified in this study as having primary CU were differentiated from individuals in the secondary group on the basis of lower anxiety and showed higher scores on the unemotional subscale of the Inventory of Callous and Unemotional Traits (ICU). In studies we discussed previously (Bennett & Kerig, 2014; Kahn et al., 2013; Kimonis et al., 2012), researchers also found higher rates of trauma in those with acquired versus primary CU. Likewise, there is evidence from the adult literature that incarcerated individuals with secondary psychopathy have more extensive trauma histories, including child abuse (Blagov et al., 2011) than those with primary psychopathy (Tatar et al., 2012). Although some studies indicate that individuals with primary CU traits or psychopathy have experienced trauma (e.g., Hicks et al., 2010), trauma has not been found to be a robust predictor of primary CU traits.

Although much of this research focuses on general traumatic experiences or negative life events (e.g., Sharf, Kimonis, & Howard, 2014), other studies indicate that interpersonal trauma, particularly actions perpetrated by someone close to the individual (i.e., betrayal trauma), may have a more profound effect on emotional development. Kerig and colleagues (2012) found that numbing of fear and sadness mediated the relationship between betrayal trauma and CU features in an adjudicated sample of youth ($M_{age}$ = 16.16, 25% female). Coping with trauma through emotional numbing and inhibition of empathy for others is reinforced because this strategy effectively lowers distress (e.g., reduced psychological distress and somatic symptoms) and may be especially adaptive in contexts where children cannot escape trauma. By extension, reexperiencing trauma via memory is also minimized through children's use of avoidance and emotional numbing of their own negative emotions (Porter, 1996). Porter's developmental model suggests that when youth effectively inhibit their capacity to feel, they experience a deactivation or dissociation from processes involved with emotional development and moral reasoning, and as a result do not develop age-appropriate skills in these domains.

## Parenting

The quality of the parent–child relationship remains a necessary factor in the development of emotional regulation and moral development, and it has been implicated in the development of broad CU traits. Retrospective studies have shown that adolescents with high levels of broad CU traits tend to recall early family environments characterized by parental rejection; poor parental bonding, neglect, or separation; and inconsistent or severe punishment (e.g., Gao, Raine, Chan, Venables, & Mednick, 2010). Some longitudinal research indicates that exposure to harsh and inconsistent parenting practices is associated with higher levels of broad CU traits over time (e.g., Barker, Oliver, Viding, Salekin, & Maughan, 2011). However, some recent findings suggest that parenting factors such as harshness, coerciveness, and inconsistency may be more associated with conduct problems without CU traits (Barker & Maughan, 2009), whereas low warmth specifically has been found to be consistently associated with chronically elevated levels of broad CU traits (e.g., Pardini et al., 2007; Waller et al., 2014).

Parental warmth has emerged as a particularly salient correlate for youth high on broad CU traits and is associated with the development of both primary and acquired CU traits. The relationship between low parental warmth and broad CU traits has been demonstrated in preschool-age children (Waller et al., 2012), school-age children (ages 4–12; Larsson, Viding, & Plomin, 2008; Pasalich, Dadds, Hawes, & Brennan, 2011), and adolescents (Kimonis, Cross, Howard, & Donoghue, 2013). In a sample of toddlers (age 2 at baseline), parental warmth was related to CU behavior at age 3, over and above associations with behavior problems (Waller et al., 2014). Kimonis, Cross, and colleagues (2013) found that adolescent male offenders with high levels of CU traits retrospectively reported lower levels of maternal warmth and involvement. Specifically, low maternal warmth and involvement were related to the uncaring dimension (i.e., low psychophysiological responding to others' distress), which is the core of the CU construct. This relationship remained significant after the researchers accounted for other important environmental influences, such as maltreatment. Although there is a scarcity of findings on specific parenting practices and acquired CU traits, it has been suggested that unemotional or harsh parenting, or parental deficits in emotion communication and regulation, negatively impact the development of emotion recognition and sensitivity in children, placing children at greater risk for developing CU traits (Daversa, 2010). The evidence suggests that maternal warmth is an important protective factor in both primary and acquired variants; however, this hypothesis has yet to be tested.

## Attachment Processes

Kochanska, Aksan, Knaack, and Rhines (2004) suggested that normal socialization (e.g., emotional and moral development) requires a two-step process. The first process involves attachment. According to Bowlby (1944), "attachment" is a biologically based regulatory system that promotes survival by ensuring that children effectively communicate distress to their caregivers, who in turn provide protection. When children experience their parents as sensitive and responsive, they trust that their caregivers will provide reliable care, and they derive security from the relationship that allows them to explore the world. Over time, transactions within the parent–child relationship form a regulatory system that modulates the child's behavior and affect. Disruptions to the attachment system may occur as a function of parents' responsiveness to their child. Bowlby also recognized the impact of disrupted attachment on moral development and child aggression. He argued that early experiences of extended parental rejection or separation could disrupt the attachment system and give rise to "affectionless" offending, a pattern of aggression that stemmed from the inability to detect or respond to pain and suffering in victims. There are many similarities between Bowlby's descriptions of youth who engaged in affectionless offending and youth now described as possessing CU features.

Primary and acquired CU features are associated with different types of disruptions to the attachment system. One possibility is that deficits in the detection and identification of emotional cues place children at risk for insecure attachment because of a fundamental disruption in communication between the parent and child. Compared to other children, those with primary CU may experience less intense emotions related to fear and distress and/or be less effective in communicating these emotions to their parent. In turn, the parent may be less responsive to the child, or their response may not be synchronous with the child's affective states and needs. Over time, this primary deficit in emotion detection and communication disrupts the pattern of communication between parent and child. At the same time, the child is less inclined to turn to the parent for support and comfort and does not perceive the parent as a secure base from which to explore the world. It is therefore possible that children with primary CU traits will show deficits in reciprocal eye gazing, disrupting the development of shared partnership and derailing the development of attachment security. Consistent with this view, Dadds, Jambrak, Pasalich, Hawes, and Brennan (2011) found that boys ($N = 92$, $M_{age} = 8.9$ years) with high CU traits showed impaired reciprocal eye gazing with both maternal and paternal attachment figures. Although this study did not differentiate between primary and acquired CU traits, the theoretical rationale proposed by the authors is most consistent with problems most distinctive in cases of primary CU.

Attachment disruption may arise quite differently in children with acquired CU traits. In such cases, children show typical emotion detection or communication; however, their caregivers are likely respond in ways that discourage or punish the direct expression of bids for safety and security. Children who experience parental rejection or maltreatment in response to their bids for safety and security are less likely to develop an organized and secure attachment strategy. Exposure to profound maltreatment is associated with the child's lack of an organized attachment strategy, which may be expressed in features that resemble affective numbing and emotion avoidance. Repeated exposure to trauma in the absence of safe haven with a caregiver provokes intense fear in the child, who has little recourse other than to inhibit feelings through emotional numbing and to curb the direct expression of need for parental comfort and support. Over time, such experiences effectively deactivate the attachment system, reducing a child's motivation to seek proximity to and to derive comfort and security from attachment figures. If an organized attachment strategy emerges, it is likely to be anxious/avoidant (i.e., fearful attachment) and characterized by indirect or masked expressions of emotion. Without the presence of a secure attachment system, there is likely to be disruption to the emotion regulation system, specifically in the form of emotion dysregulation, which has been implicated in the development of both externalizing (Moretti & Obsuth, 2009) and internalizing symptoms (Moretti & Craig, 2013). For example, in a treatment study examining an attachment-based parenting intervention, changes in emotion dysregulation were found to mediate the relationship between both attachment avoidance and attachment anxiety in adolescents with behavioral concerns (Moretti, Osbuth, Craig, & Bartolo, 2015). However, there is currently a lack of available studies specifically investigating the relationship between CU traits and attachment (Frick et al., 2014b) to support these speculations.

## Treatment

The presence of CU traits may designate a group of children or adolescents who are particularly resistant to treatment and intervention. Much of the available evidence suggests that CU traits, particularly in combination with oppositional defiant disorder (ODD) features, predict poorer treatment outcomes for children when compared to those with conduct problems and low levels of CU traits. For example, based on a large-scale review of the available literature, Frick and colleagues noted that youth with CU traits are more resistant to and less likely to participate in treatment (Frick et al., 2014b). Hawes and Dadds (2005) examined a 10-week parenting intervention (Integrated Family Intervention for Child Conduct Problems) for boys between the ages 4 and 8 with ODD or CD and found that CU traits predicted poor treatment outcomes. Recently developed treatments have shifted the focus from managing behavior to addressing specific etiological factors that have been found to be associated with primary versus acquired CU. Although no treatment studies to date have examined primary versus acquired CU, different treatments may be more effective depending on the variant of CU under investigation.

The quality of parent–child interactions is implicated as one of the core etiological factors in youth with acquired CU traits (e.g., Kerig et al., 2012). In concordance with findings we discussed earlier in relation to parental warmth, treatment studies show that interventions that promote improvements in harsh and inconsistent parenting, and parental warmth and involvement, are associated with reductions in symptoms of psychopathy and CU traits in children (e.g., McDonald, Dodson, Rosenfield, & Jouriles, 2011; Pasalich, Witkiewitz, McMahon, Pinderhughes, & the Conduct Problems Prevention Research Group, 2016). Given the differences in emotional processing and related trauma history (particularly betrayal trauma; see Kerig et al., 2012), children and youth may respond well to treatments that target the rebuilding of secure attachment relationships. Although treatment studies have improved with the increased understanding of the etiology of CU traits, few studies have examined the differential treatment effects of primary and acquired CU traits; therefore, there is little we can conclude based on the available evidence.

## Future Directions

This chapter has provided an overview of the literature and newly emerging theoretical perspectives that further our understanding of the development of CU traits, both generally and across primary and acquired variants. There is some evidence to support a two-step process in the case of acquired CU traits that begins with the attachment relationship, which in turn affects socialization processes (e.g., emotional regulation and moral development) through the parent–child relationship. There is evidence that exposure to chronic trauma or maltreatment may impact and alter the attachment relationship and/or the socialization processes that are salient in normal development. Despite emerging evidence of two distinct developmental pathways to CU traits, there are a number of limitations in the literature that require careful attention before we are able to draw more definitive conclusions.

Foremost among these, there is considerable behavioral, developmental, and trait heterogeneity within the construct of conduct problems including the presence of CU traits (Frick et al., 2014a; Klahr & Burt, 2014). Such heterogeneity makes it difficult to draw conclusions regarding PD-related outcomes, including ASPD and psychopathy. In addition to this, although the construct of secondary psychopathy is well established in the literature, the notion of "acquired" CU traits is a relatively new concept. Hence, we may expect that CU traits will for some time be conceptualized as a unitary construct in the literature. Furthermore, research on CU traits has been typified by inconsistencies in the measurement and conceptualization of the construct. As discussed elsewhere (see Patrick & Brislin, Chapter 24, this volume), CU traits in children and youth have been assessed with psychopathy measures (e.g., Psychopathy Checklist—Revised [PCL-R]; Hare, 1991), measures assessing empathy, and more recently, the ICU (Frick, 2004). Limitations regarding measurement using such instruments include, in the case of the PCL-R, conflating affective (e.g., CU traits), interpersonal (e.g., arrogance), and behavioural components (e.g., aggression and delinquency) of psychopathy, which could have theoretical and practical implications.

With respect to terminology, in using the PCL-R as an accepted measure in developmental studies of CU traits and the term "psychopathy" interchangeably with "CU traits," it is possible that researchers are failing to identify a subsample of youth who do not show interpersonal and behavioral components of the same kind and severity as youth with clinically elevated levels of psychopathic features. There is a growing interest in the emergence of CU traits in the absence of aggression and conduct problems. Porter (1996) theorized that those with acquired CU or secondary psychopathy may show a delay in the development of conduct problems and severe patterns of aggression as they learn to dampen their emotional expression and experience during childhood. Unfortunately, there is no empirical evidence to support this theory, and this remains an open question. Future research needs to address the issue of conflating the components of psychopathy and to parse the components to better understand the emergence and development of CU traits independent of conduct problems. Future research should adopt consistent terminology and avoid using the terms "psychopathy" and "CU traits" interchangeably.

In order to address many of these concerns, there are a number of methodological considerations that need to be addressed. There have been several cross-sectional studies examining varied associations among parenting, antisocial behavior, and CU traits in children (see Waller, Gardner, & Hyde, 2013), and identifying high- versus low-anxiety CU subtypes in adolescents (e.g., Kimonis et al., 2012); however, a smaller but growing body of longitudinal research has examined CU traits and possible pathways across development. Longitudinal research that examines risk factors (e.g., trauma), and protective factors (e.g., parental warmth) will help researchers understand the differential and shared environmental risk factors for both primary and acquired CU traits. Another growing concern in the research field is the lack of diversity in the populations being examined. The majority of research on CU traits, and indeed on psychopathy, has been primarily with males involved with the justice system. Although it is likely that this population is selected for the increased likelihood of sampling youth high on CU traits, selecting youth samples involved with the justice department conflates aggressive and antisocial behavior with CU traits. In addition, the scarcity of females in sampling does not allow many opportunities for examining gender differences; it is possible that there are significant gender differences in the development and expression of primary and acquired CU traits.

## Conclusion

It may appear from our discussion that there are two distinct and nonoverlapping pathways to CU traits—one that is more biologically driven and another that is more environmentally based.

However, as we described earlier, individuals showing primary CU traits do indeed report exposure to negative/harsh parenting and trauma; similarly, it is unclear as to whether youth with acquired CU features are significantly impacted by more biologically based mechanisms. Clearly, both biological and environmental influences shape developmental pathways. Even models that hold to the idea that the magnitude of genetic effects remain latently stable over development but the expression of genetic influences varies from one age versus another may be in question. The field of epigenetics points to the need for more transactional models whereby the potential for genetic expression is shaped and reshaped through environmental influences. The next few decades will usher in new innovative frameworks, each with its own challenges, but with the cumulative impact of pushing the field further. Perhaps the most exciting ripple effect of these new frameworks will be the revision of our understanding of what interventions, for whom, and most importantly *at what points in development,* exert the most powerful and lasting therapeutic benefits. Revisiting these key questions about the impact of psychological interventions with a new understanding of the dynamic transactions of genetic and environmental influences will offer immense opportunities to develop, refine, and reinvent effective treatments.

## REFERENCES

American Psychiatric Association. (2013). *Diagnostic and statistical manual of mental disorders* (5th ed.). Arlington, VA: Author.

Barker, E. D., & Maughan, B. (2009). Differentiating early-onset persistent versus childhood-limited conduct problem youth. *Amercian Journal of Psychiatry, 166,* 900–908.

Barker, E. D., Oliver, B. R., Viding, E., Salekin, R. T., & Maughan, B. (2011). The impact of prenatal maternal risk, fearless temperament and early parenting on adolescent callous-unemotional traits: A 14-year longitudinal investigation. *Journal of Child Psychology and Psychiatry, 52,* 878–888.

Bennett, D. C., & Kerig, P. K. (2014). Investigating the construct of trauma-related acquired callousness among delinquent youth: Differences in emotion processing. *Journal of Traumatic Stress, 27*(4), 415–422.

Blagov, P. S., Patrick, C. J., Lilienfeld, S. O., Powers, A. D., Phifer, J. E., Venables, N., et al. (2011). Personality constellations in incarcerated psychopathic men. *Personality Disorders: Theory, Research, and Treatment, 2*(4), 293–315.

Blair, R. J. R. (2001). Neurocognitive models of aggression, the antisocial personality disorders, and psychopathy. *Journal of Neurology, Neurosurgery and Psychiatry, 71,* 727–731.

Blair, R. J. R. (2007). The amygdala and ventromedial prefrontal cortex in morality and psychopathy. *Trends in Cognitive Sciences, 11*(9), 387–392.

Blair, R. J. R. (2013). The neurobiology of psychopathic traits in youths. *Nature Review Neuroscience, 14,* 786–799.

Blair, R. J., Colledge, E., Murray, L., & Mitchell, D. G. V. (2001). A selective impairment in the processing of sad and fearful expressions in children with psychopathic tendencies. *Journal of Abnormal Child Psychology, 29*(6), 491–498.

Blair, R. J. R., Leibenluft, E., & Pine, D. S. (2014). Conduct disorder and callous–unemotional traits in youth. *New England Journal of Medicine, 371*(23), 2207–2216.

Blair, R. J. R., Peschardt, K. S., Budhani, S., Mitchell, D. G., & Pine, D. S. (2006). The development of psychopathy. *Journal of Child Psychology and Psychiatry, 47*(3–4), 262–276.

Bowlby, J. (1944). Forty-four juvenile thieves: Their characters and home life. *International Journal of Psychoanalysis, 25,* 19–52, 107–127.

Cecil, C. A., Lysensko, L. J., Jaffee, S. R., Pingault, J.-B., Smith, R. G., Relton, C. L., et al. (2014). Environmental risk, Oxytocin Receptor Gene (OXTR) methylation and youth callous–unemotional traits: A 13-year longitudinal study. *Molecular Psychiatry, 19,* 1071–1077.

Cleckley, H. (1941). *The mask of sanity.* St. Louis, MO: Mosby.

Dadds, M. R., Cauchi, A. J., Wimalaweera, S., Hawes, D. J., & Brennan, J. (2012). Outcomes, moderators, and mediators of empathic-emotion recognition training for complex conduct problems in childhood. *Psychiatry Research, 199*(3), 201–207.

Dadds, M. R., Jambrak, J., Pasalich, D., Hawes, D. J., & Brennan, J. (2011). Impaired attention to the eyes of attachment figures and the developmental origins of psychopathy. *Journal of Child Psychology and Psychiatry, 52*(3), 238–245.

Dadds, M. R., Moul, C., Cauchi, A., Dobson-Stone, C., Hawes, D. J., Brennan, J., et al. (2014). Methylation of the oxytocin receptor gene and oxytocin blood levels in the development of psychopathy. *Development and Psychopathology, 26,* 33–40.

Dadds, M. R., & Rhodes, T. (2008). Aggression in young children with concurrent callous–unemotional traits: Can the neurosciences inform progress and innovation in treatment approaches? *Philosophical Transactions of the Royal Society B: Biological Sciences, 363,* 2567–2576.

Dadds, M. R., & Salmon, K. (2003). Punishment insensitivity and parenting: Temperament and learning as interacting risks for antisocial behavior. *Clinical Child and Family Psychology Review, 6*(2), 69–86.

Daversa, M. T. (2010). Early environmental predictors of the affective and interpersonal constructs of psychopathy. *International Journal of Offender Therapy and Comparative Criminology, 54*(1), 6–21.

Fanti, K. A., Demetriou, C. A., & Kimonis, E. R. (2013). Variants of callous–unemotional conduct problems in a community sample of adolescents. *Journal of Youth and Adolescence, 42,* 964–979.

Fontaine, N. M., Rijsdijk, F. V., McCrory, E. J., & Viding, E. (2010). Etiology of different developmental trajectories of callous–unemotional traits. *Journal of the American Academy of Child and Adolescent Psychiatry, 49*(7), 656–664.

Ford, J. D., Chapman, J., Mack, J. M., & Pearson, G. (2006). Pathways from traumatic child victimization to delinquency: Implications for juvenile and permanency court proceedings and decisions. *Juvenile and Family Court Journal, 57,* 13–26.

Frick, P. J. (2004). *The Inventory of Callous–Unemotional Traits.* Unpublished rating scale, University of New Orleans, New Orleans, LA.

Frick, P. J., Cornell, A. H., Bodin, S. D., Dane, H. A., Barry, C. T., & Loney, B. R. (2003). Callous–unemotional traits and developmental pathways to severe conduct problems. *Developmental Psychology, 39,* 246–260.

Frick, P. J., Kimonis, E. R., Dandreaux, D. M., & Farell, J. M. (2003). The 4 year stability of psychopathic traits in non-referred youth. *Behavioral Sciences and the Law, 21*(6), 713–736.

Frick, P. J., & Marsee, M. A. (2006). Psychopathy and developmental pathways to antisocial behavior in youth. In C. J. Patrick (Ed.), *Handbook of psychopathy* (pp. 353–375). New York: Guilford Press.

Frick, P. J., & Morris, A. S. (2004). Temperament and developmental pathways to conduct problems. *Journal of Clinical Child and Adolescent Psychology, 33*(1), 54–68.

Frick, P. J., Ray, J., Thornton, L. C., & Kahn, R. E. (2014a). Annual research review: A developmental psychopathology approach to understanding callous–unemotional traits in children and adolescents with serious conduct problems. *Journal of Child Psychology and Psychiatry, 55*(6), 532–548.

Frick, P. J., Ray, J., Thornton, L. C., & Kahn, R. E. (2014b). Can callous–unemotional traits enhance the understanding, diagnosis, and treatment of serious conduct problems in children and adolescents?: A comprehensive review. *Psychological Bulletin, 140,* 1–57.

Frick, P. J., & Viding, E. (2009). Antisocial behavior from a developmental psychopathology perspective. *Development and Psychopathology, 21*(4), 1111–1131.

Frick, P. J., & White, S. F. (2008). Research review: The importance of callous–unemotional traits for developmental models of aggressive and antisocial behavior. *Journal of Child Psychology and Psychiatry, 49*(4), 359–375.

Gao, Y., Raine, A., Chan, F., Venables, P. H., & Mednick, S. A. (2010). Early maternal and paternal bonding, childhood physical abuse and adult psychopathic personality. *Psychological Medicine, 40,* 1007–1016.

Gill, A. D., & Stickle, T. R. (2016). Affective differences between psychopathy variants and genders in adjudicated youth. *Journal of Abnormal Child Psychology, 44,* 295–307.

Hare, R. D. (1991). *The Hare Psychopathy Checklist—Revised.* Toronto, ON, Canada: Multi Health Systems.

Hare, R. D. (1993). *Without conscience: The disturbing world of the psychopaths among us.* New York: Guilford Press.

Hare, R. D., Hart, S. D., & Harpur, T. J. (1991). Psychopathy and the DSM-IV criteria for antisocial personality disorder. *Journal of Abnormal Psychology, 100*(3), 391–398.

Hawes, D. J., & Dadds, M. R. (2005). The treatment of conduct problems in children with callous–unemotional traits. *Journal of Consulting and Clinical Psychology, 73*(4), 737–741.

Hicks, B. M., Vaidyanathan, U., & Patrick, C. J. (2010). Validating female psychopathy subtypes: Differences in personality, antisocial and violent behavior, substance abuse, trauma, and mental health. *Personality Disorders, 1*(1), 38–57.

Kahn, R. E., Frick, P. J., Youngstrom, E. A., Kogos Youngstrom, J., Feeny, N. C., & Findling, R. L. (2013). Distinguishing primary and secondary variants of callous–unemotional traits among adolescents in a clinic-referred sample. *Psychological Assessment, 25*(3), 966–978.

Karpman, B. (1941). On the need of separating psychopathy into two distinct clinical types: The symptomatic and the idiopathic. *Journal of Criminal Psychopathology, 3,* 112–137.

Karpman, B. (1948). Conscience in the psychopath: Another version. *American Journal of Orthopsychiatry, 18*(3), 455–491.

Kerig, P. K., & Becker, S. P. (2010). From internalizing to externalizing: Theoretical models of the processes linking PTSD to juvenile delinquency. In S. J. Egan (Ed.), *Posttraumatic stress disorder (PTSD): Causes, symptoms and treatment* (pp. 33–78). Hauppauge, NY: Nova Science.

Kerig, P. K., Bennett, D. C., Thompson, M., & Becker, S. P. (2012). "Nothing really matters": Emotional numbing as a link between trauma exposure and callousness in delinquent youth. *Journal of Traumatic Stress, 25*(3), 272–279.

Kimonis, E. R., Bagner, D. M., Linares, D., Blake, C. A., & Rodriguez, G. (2014). Parent training outcomes among young children with callous–unemotional conduct problems with or at-risk for developmental delay. *Journal of Child and Family Studies, 23*(2), 437–448.

Kimonis, E. R., Cross, B., Howard, A., & Donoghue, K. (2013). Maternal care, maltreatment and callous–unemotional traits among urban male juvenile offenders. *Journal of Youth and Adolescence, 42,* 165–177.

Kimonis, E. R., Fanti, K. A., Isoma, Z., & Donoghue, K. (2013). Maltreatment profiles among incarcerated boys with callous–unemotional traits. *Child Maltreatment, 18*(2), 108–121.

Kimonis, E. R., Frick, P. J., Cauffman, E., Goldweber, A., & Skeem, J. (2012). Primary and secondary variants of juvenile psychopathy differ in emotional processing. *Developmental Psychopathology, 24*(3), 1091–1103.

Kimonis, E. R., Frick, P. J., Fazekas, H., & Loney, B. R. (2006). Psychopathy, aggression, and the processing of emotional stimuli in non-referred girls and boys. *Behavioral Sciences and the Law, 24*(1), 21–37.

Kimonis, E. R., Frick, P. J., Muñoz, L. C., & Aucoin, K. J. (2008). Callous–unemotional traits and the emotional processing of distress cues in detained boys: Testing the moderating role of aggression, exposure to community violence, and histories of abuse. *Developmental Psychopathology, 20*(2), 569–589.

Klahr, A. M., & Burt, S. A. (2014). Evaluation of the known behavioral heterogeneity in conduct disorder to improve its assessment and treatment. *Journal of Child Psychology and Psychiatry, 55,* 1300–1310.

Kochanska, G. (1993). Toward a synthesis of parental socialization and child temperament in early development of conscience. *Child Development, 64*(2), 325–347.

Kochanska, G., Aksan, N., Knaack, A., & Rhines, H. M. (2004). Maternal parenting and children's conscience: Early security as moderator. *Child Development, 75*(4), 1229–1242.

Larsson, H., Andershed, H., & Lichtenstein, P. (2006). A genetic factor explains most of the variation in the psychopathic personality. *Journal of Abnormal Psychology, 115*(2), 221–230.

Larsson, H., Viding, E., & Plomin, R. (2008). Callous–unemotional traits and antisocial behavior genetic, environmental, and early parenting characteristics. *Criminal Justice and Behavior, 35*(2), 197–211.

McDonald, R., Dodson, M. C., Rosenfield, D., & Jouriles, E. N. (2011). Effects of a parenting intervention on features of psychopathy in children. *Journal of Abnormal Child Psychology, 39*(7), 1013–1023.

Meyer-Lindenberg, A., Domes, G., Kirsch, P., & Heinrichs, M. (2011). Oxytocin and vasopressin in the human brain: Social neuropeptides for translational medicine. *Nature Reviews Neuroscience, 12*(9), 524–538.

Moffitt, T. E. (1993). Adolescence-limited and life-course-persistent antisocial behavior: A developmental taxonomy. *Psychological Review, 100*(4), 674–701.

Moffitt, T. E. (2006). Life-course-persistent versus adolescence-limited antisocial behavior. In D. Cicchetti & D. J. Cohen (Eds.), *Developmental psychopathology: Vol 3. Risk, disorder, and adaptation* (2nd ed., pp. 570–598). Hoboken, NJ: Wiley.

Moffitt, T. E., Arseneault, L., Jaffee, S. R., Kim-Cohen, J., Koenen, K. C., Odgers, C. L., et al. (2008). Research review: DSM-V conduct disorder: Research needs for an evidence base. *Journalf of Child Psychology and Psychiatry, 49*(1), 3–33.

Moore, D. S. (2015). *The developing genome: An introduction to behavioral epigenetics.* New York: Oxford University Press.

Moretti, M. M., & Craig, S. G. (2013). Maternal versus paternal physical and emotional abuse, affect regulation and risk for depression from adolescence to early adulthood. *Child Abuse and Neglect, 37*(1), 4–13.

Moretti, M. M., & Obsuth, I. (2009). Effectiveness of an attachment-focused manualized intervention for parents of teens at risk for aggressive behaviour: The Connect Program. *Journal of Adolescence, 32,* 1347–1357.

Moretti, M. M., Obsuth, I., Craig, S. G., & Bartolo, T. (2015). An attachment-based intervention for parents of adolescents at risk: Mechanisms of change. *Attachment and Human Development, 17*(2), 119–135.

Pardini, D. A. (2006). The callousness pathway to severe violent delinquency. *Aggressive Behavior, 32,* 590–598.

Pardini, D. A., Lochman, J. E., & Powell, N. (2007). The development of callous–unemotional traits and antisocial behavior in children: Are there shared and/or unique predictors? *Journal of Clinical Child and Adolescent Psychology, 36,* 319–333.

Pasalich, D. S., Dadds, M. R., Hawes, D. J., & Brennan, J. (2011). Do callous–unemotional traits moderate the relative importance of parental coercion versus warmth in child conduct problems?: An observational study. *Journal of Child Psychology and Psychiatry, 52,* 1308–1315.

Pasalich, D. S., Witkiewitz, K., McMahon, R. J., Pinderhughes, E. E., & Conduct Problems Prevention Research Group. (2016). Indirect effects of the fast track intervention on conduct disorder symptoms and callous–unemotional traits: Distinct pathways involving discipline and warmth. *Journal of Abnormal Child Psychology, 44*(3), 587–597.

Porter, S. (1996). Without conscience or without active conscience?: The etiology of psychopathy revisited. *Aggression and Violent Behavior, 1*(2), 179–189.

Prado, C. E., Treeby, M. S., & Crowe, S. F. (2015). Examining relationships between facial emotion recognition, self-control, and psychopathic traits in a non-clinical sample. *Personality and Individual Differences, 80,* 22–27.

Sharf, A., Kimonis, E. R., & Howard, A. (2014). Negative life events and posttraumatic stress disorder among incarcerated boys with callous–unemotional traits. *Journal of Psychopathology and Behavioral Assessment, 36*(3), 401–414.

Tatar, J. R., Cauffman, E., Kimonis, E. R., & Skeem, J. L. (2012). Victimization history and posttraumatic stress: An analysis of psychopathy variants in male juvenile offenders. *Journal of Child and Adolescent Trauma, 5*(2), 102–113.

Viding, E., Frick, P. J., & Plomin, R. (2007). Aetiology of the relationship between callous–unemotional traits and conduct problems in childhood problems in childhood. *British Journal of Psychiatry, 190*(Suppl. 49), S33–S38.

Waller, R., Gardner, F., & Hyde, L. W. (2013). What are the associations between parenting, callous–unemotional traits, and antisocial behavior in youth?: A systematic review of evidence. *Clinical Psychology Review, 33,* 593–608.

Waller, R., Gardner, F., Hyde, L. W., Shaw, D. S., Dishion, T. J., & Wilson, M. N. (2012). Do harsh and positive parenting predict parent reports of deceitful–callous behavior in early childhood? *Journal of Child Psychology and Psychiatry, 53*(9), 946–953.

Waller, R., Gardner, F., Viding, E., Shaw, D. S., Dishion, T. J., Wilson, M. N., et al. (2014). Bidirectional associations between parental warmth, callous unemotional behavior, and behavior problems in high-risk preschoolers. *Journal of Abnormal Child Psychology, 42*(8), 1275–1285.

Young, J. C., & Widom, C. S. (2014). Long-term effects of child abuse and neglect on emotion processing in adulthood. *Child Abuse and Neglect, 38,* 1369–1381.

# PART V

# DIAGNOSIS AND ASSESSMENT

## INTRODUCTION

The three chapters in Part V cover different aspects of assessment for both clinical and research purposes. They share the assumption that effective treatment requires a more detailed assessment than has generally been assumed. Accumulating evidence suggests that diagnostic evaluation confined to confirmation of a DSM or ICD categorical diagnosis is not sufficient for treatment purposes, that categorical diagnoses have limited prognostic value, and that an assessment of severity of personality disorder (PD) is more useful in predicting outcome than specific diagnoses (Crawford, Koldobsky, Mulder, & Tyrer, 2011). Also, global diagnoses are not particularly helpful for treatment planning or when selecting interventions because both medication and psychotherapeutic interventions are usually selected to treat specific symptoms or impairments. This means that most clinicians effectively decompose a global diagnosis into its components such as symptom clusters or specific problems, then identify the best way to treat each component. Although clinicians seem to do this intuitively and implicitly as treatment proceeds, there are advantages to making this process more explicit and systematic, so as to ensure that all problems are addressed.

Besides these problems with traditional diagnoses, there is also emerging recognition of the value of assessing functional impairment and the dynamics of personality pathology as opposed to the more structural features emphasized by official classifications and trait-based assessment. Structural features are important, but they need to be supplemented with an evaluation of how the different features of PD interact to create the complex processes underlying substantive impairments. These requirements suggest that a more comprehensive strategy is needed to address interrelationships among diagnosis, assessment, and treatment planning. These issues are addressed by the chapters in this section.

Chapter 20, by Lee Anna Clark, Jaime L. Shapiro, Elizabeth Daly, Emily N. Vanderbleek, Morgan R. Negrón, and Julie Harrison, reviews empirically validated diagnostic and assessment methods, and updates the equivalent chapter in the first edition by reviewing measures that have been extensively revised or are new since the publication of the original chapter (2001). It then proceeds to discuss the DSM-5 alternative model in terms of measures of personality functioning and the trait model. The chapter offers an alternative perspective on the DSM-5 trait model to the perspectives discussed in other chapters (see Livesley, Chapter 1; Davis Samaco-Zamora, & Millon, Chapter 2; Benjamin, Critchfield, Karpiak, Smith, & Mestel, Chapter 22). The chapter concludes with consideration of some important issues that need to be addressed for further progress in assessing PD. Here, the authors raise the important issue of construct clarity. Although they are primarily concerned with clarifying the nature of personality dysfunction and differentiating it from trait dimensions, they have put their finger on a problem with wider currency. Some years ago, Block (1995) drew attention to this problem with personality generally by referring to what he called the "jingle-jangle effect," which refers to the problems created by using multiple terms to refer to the same construct (the jingle effect) and by using the same term to refer to multiple constructs. Lack of construct clarity and the attendant need for critical conceptual analysis are probably the biggest obstacles to establishing a coherent body of knowledge about PD. It is difficult to see how progress can be made until a valid nomenclature replaces the current mishmash of poorly defined constructs that are often little more than folk concepts masquerading as scientific constructs. "Impulsivity" is an obvious example. The term is applied to behaviors as typologically and functionally diverse as trichotillomania, recklessness, acting with a sense of urgency when distressed, as well as what is probably nearer the mark—the tendency to act on the spur of the moment without cognitive processing or regard for the consequences. There is also the tendency to coin new terms or combination of terms to refer to old constructs, creating uncertainty about the relationship between new findings and previous research and whether the new terms represent progress or merely fashion.

Clark and colleagues note the need for valid measures and greater clarity regarding the definition of PD. Although as they note there is some consensus that PD has two main components—"self" and "interpersonal" pathology—it is important to begin to specify what each entails. This definition was originally advanced as a preliminary way to assess the personality disorganization that characterizes disordered personality, with the assumption that the impairments associated with both components would subsequently be specified in detail. An unfortunate consequence of the DSM is that constructs and definitions tend to become ossified as opposed to being viewed as works in progress. It would be unfortunate if this occurred with the DSM-5 definition of PD, first because it would be helpful for treatment purposes to develop greater clarity about the impairments associated with self pathology in particular and, second, because as Clark and colleagues have noted, the DSM-5 definition is problematic. The underlying message of this chapter is an important one: that the assessment, and, we would add, the study of PD generally, needs to advance on a solid empirical basis, and that we need to give more attention to using a wider range of assessment methods than has been the case thus far.

In Chapter 21, John F. Clarkin, W. John Livesley, and Kevin B. Meehan discuss a systematic approach to clinical assessment. After reviewing the different methods described in the literature and used by different therapeutic models, they outline a comprehensive strategy with three components. First, the presence of general PD and severity are determined. The proposed approach assumes that PD involves a profound impairment in the organization and coherence of the personality system, and proposes that self pathology and chronic impairment in the capacity for effective interpersonal relationships are indicators of impaired personality organization. The approach draws on the same conceptual approach adopted by DSM-5 but seeks to remedy conceptual limitations and inconsistencies in DSM-5 criteria. Severity is then conceptualized in terms of self and interpersonal pathology. The value of this approach is that it attempts to separate the assessment of PD and severity from the assessment of trait dimensions. This is a requirement for dimensional assessment because an extreme position on a dimension does not necessarily imply pathology (Livesley, 2001; Livesley & Jang, 2005; Parker & Barrett, 2000; Wakefield, 1992, 2008). The second component is an evaluation of individual differences in clinical presentation based on clinically significant personality traits. Trait assessment is proposed as an evidence-based way to represent individual differences. Third, Clarkin and colleagues argue that effective treatment also requires an evaluation of personality dysfunction. This is achieved by decomposing disorder into functional domains. Although the impairments characterizing the disorder may be parsed in multiple ways, they suggest that four broad domains are sufficient to accommodate the impairments that clinicians typically consider in treatment: (1) symptoms, (2) impairments in the mechanisms regulating and modulating behavior and experience, (3) interpersonal problems, and (4) self/identity pathology. The value to domain-focused assessment is that it helps to ensure attention to all aspects of personality—both strengths and limitations—during diagnostic assessment. It also begins to link assessment with treatment planning and selection of interventions, since most interventions are selected to address specific impairments, and different forms of intervention are generally required to treat the different domains.

In Chapter 22, on using interpersonal reconstructive therapy (IRT) to select interventions for treating comorbid and treatment-resistant PD, Lorna Smith Benjamin, Kenneth L. Critchfield, Christie Pugh Karpiak, Tracey Leone Smith, and Robert Mestel describe an approach to case formulation that uses the structural analysis of social behavior (SASB) to focus on personality patterns. The approach nicely complements the previous chapters in the section by offering an additional perspective on assessment that focuses on not only the structure of PD but also the processes underlying clinical manifestations of the disorder. This combined focus on both the personality structures and processes extends the contributions of other chapters that focused more on personality structures. However, it is personality processes and their effects that are the primary focus of intervention. The chapter illustrates the value of this framework with several case illustrations.

The three chapters in Part V provide a good illustration of the value of adopting pluralism as part of the conceptual foundation for studying PDs. The different chapters do not describe competing approaches to diagnostic assessment; rather, they are complementary approaches designed to serve different purposes. There will also be some comprehensive assessment circumstances that require some combination of all methods.

## REFERENCES

Block, J. (1995). A contrarian view of the five-factor approach to personality description. *Psychological Bulletin, 117,* 187–215.

Crawford, M. J., Koldobsky, N., Mulder, R., & Tyrer, P. (2011). Classifying personality disorder according to severity. *Journal of Personality Disorders, 25,* 321–330.

Livesley, W. J. (2001). Commentary on reconceptualising personality disorder categories using trait dimensions. *Journal of Personality, 69,* 277–286.

Livesley, W. J., & Jang, K. L. (2005). Differentiating normal, abnormal, and disordered personality. *European Journal of Personality, 19,* 257–268.

Parker, G., & Barrett, E. (2000). Personality and personality disorder: Current issues and directions. *Psychological Medicine, 30,* 1–9.

Wakefield, J. C. (1992). Disorder as harmful dysfunction: A conceptual critique of DSM-III-R's definition of mental disorder. *Psychological Review, 99,* 232–247.

Wakefield, J. C. (2008). The perils of dimensionalization: Challenges in distinguishing negative traits from personality disorders. *Psychiatric Clinics of North America, 31,* 379–393.

# CHAPTER 20

# Empirically Validated Diagnostic and Assessment Methods

Lee Anna Clark, Jaime L. Shapiro, Elizabeth Daly,
Emily N. Vanderbleek, Morgan R. Negrón, and Julie Harrison

*Plus ça change, plus c'est la même chose.*
[The more things change, the more they stay the same.]
—Jean-Baptiste Alphonse Karr (1849)

There is no more fitting phrase than the opening quotation to describe what has happened in the personality disorder (PD) field in the 15 years since the publication of the first edition of this handbook. An alternative PD model composed of personality (self and interpersonal) impairment and pathological traits appears in Section III of the fifth edition of the *Diagnostic and Statistical Manual of Mental Disorders* (DSM-5; American Psychiatric Association [APA], 2013). In the main Section II are reproduced the familiar-but-much-maligned 10 PD categories, which first appeared in more or less their current form 38 years ago in DSM-III, and in exactly their current form 23 years ago in DSM-IV (hereafter, DSM-IV/5-II). The ultimate goal of much of the new research in PD assessment during the last 23 years has been to replace the problematic categorical system with a trait-dimensional model, but the work itself primarily has demonstrated that trait-dimensional systems are able to capture and reflect the current categories well. As such, ironically, the work may have served to "validate" and thereby perpetuate the current system—complete with its problematic comorbidity and within-PD heterogeneity—rather than to eliminate the system and implement a superior one.

The version of this chapter in the previous edition focused on assessment instruments, detailing the properties (e.g., number of items, administration time), psychometrics (e.g., internal consistency, temporal stability), and convergent and discriminant validity evidence of various measures available for assessing PD categories and relevant trait dimensions. For the most part, an update of that chapter would not differ radically from the original. Additional research with the various measures has changed what we know about them very little. We describe a few exceptions later in the chapter but, for the most part, rather than re-reviewing these measures, we simply list them in Table 20.1, along with any key recent references, and refer interested readers to the earlier version of this chapter, to recent reviews of PD measures (e.g., McDermut & Zimmerman, 2008; Widiger & Boyd, 2009), and to the literature for new details about these measures. A few measures are no longer widely used; we list these also in Table 20.1 and do not mention them further.

**TABLE 20.1. Measures Assessing Personality and Personality Pathology with Few or No Changes Since 2000**

| Measures (alphabetical order) | Abbreviation | References (original or, if available, key update[s]) |
|---|---|---|
| | | Diagnostically based measures |
| *Interviews* | | |
| Diagnostic Interview for DSM-IV Personality Disorders | DIPD | Morey et al. (2012)[a]; Zanarini et al. (2000) |
| International Personality Disorder Examination | IPDE | Loranger, Janca, & Sartorius (1997)[b] |
| Personality Disorder Interview–IV | PDI-IV | Samuel, Edmundson, & Widiger (2011) |
| Structured Clinical Interview for DSM-IV Axis II PD | SCID-II | First & Gibbon (2004) |
| Structured Interview for DSM Personality–IV | SIDP-IV | Jane, Pagan, Turkheimer, Fiedler, & Oltmanns (2006); Zimmerman, Rothschild, & Chelminski (2005) |
| *Questionnaires* | | |
| Coolidge Axis II Inventory | CATI | Coolidge (2000)[b] |
| Coolidge Personality and Neuropsychological Inventory for Children | CPNI | Coolidge, Thede, Stewart, & Segal (2002) |
| Coolidge Correctional Inventory | CCI | Coolidge, Segal, Klebe, Cahill, & Whitcomb (2009) |
| Short Form of the Coolidge Axis II Inventory | SCATI | Coolidge, Segal, Cahill, & Simenson (2010) |
| Millon Clinical Multiaxial Inventory–III | MCMI-III | Millon & Bloom (2008); Rossi, Elklit, & Simonsen (2010) |
| Minnesota Multiphasic Personality Inventory PD scales | MMPI-PD | Jones (2005) |
| Personality Assessment Inventory[c] | PAI | Morey (2014) |
| Personality Disorder Questionnaire–IV | PDQ-IV | de Reus, van den Berg, & Emmelkamp (2013); Okada & Oltmanns (2009) |
| Schedule for Nonadaptive and Adaptive Personality–2 | SNAP-2 | Clark, Simms, Wu, & Casillas (2014) |
| Wisconsin Personality Inventory | WISPI | Klein et al. (1993)[b]; Smith, Klein, & Benjamin (2003) |

Trait-based measures

*Interviews*

| | | |
|---|---|---|
| Diagnostic Interview for Borderline Patients—Revised | DIB-R | Tragresser et al. (2010); Zanarini, Frankenburg, & Vujanovic (2002) |
| Diagnostic Interview for Narcissism | DIN | Gunderson et al. (1990)[b] |
| Personality Assessment Schedule | PAS | Tyrer (1988)[d] |
| Structured Interview for the Five-Factor Model | SI-FFM | Trull & Widiger (1997); Trull et al. (1998)[b] |

*Questionnaires*

| | | |
|---|---|---|
| Dimensional Assessment of Personality Pathology | DAPP | Livesley & Jackson (2010) |
| Extended Interpersonal Adjective Scales | EIAS | Wright, Pincus, & Lenzenweger (2012) |
| Inventory of Interpersonal Problems—PD scales | IIP-PD | Pilkonis, Kim, Proietti, & Barkham (1996)[d] |
| NEO-Personality Inventory—Revised | NEO PI-R | Costa & McCrae (1992)[d] |
| Personality Adjective Check List | PACL | Strack (2008) |
| Personality Psychopathology Five | PSY-5 | Harkness et al. (2014); Harkness, Finn, McNulty, & Shields (2012); Harkness, Reynolds, & Lilienfeld (2014) |
| Schedule for Nonadaptive and Adaptive Personality–2 | SNAP-2 | Clark et al. (2014); Ro, Stringer, & Clark (2012); Simms & Clark (2006) |
| Schizotypal Personality Questionnaire | SPQ | Raine (1991)[d] |
| Schizotypy Questionnaire | STA | Claridge & Broks (1984)[b] |
| Structural Analysis of Social Behavior Intrex Questionnaire[e] | SASB-IQ | Benjamin (1996)[b] |
| Temperament-Character Inventory—Revised | TCI-R | Farmer & Goldberg (2008) |

*Note.* Only the last of multiple versions of instruments are included, unless substantively different.
[a]One of many studies reporting on the Collaborative Longitudinal of Personality Disorders Study, which used the DIPD–IV as a core measure of DSM-IV PDs.
[b]Not widely used since 2000.
[c]Assesses "major clinical constructs" (i.e., not diagnoses per se).
[d]Continues to be used, but no key update available.
[e]Assesses interpersonal dimensions (i.e., not traits per se).

The bulk of this chapter, therefore, is devoted to assessment measures and issues that have changed or developed since the first edition:

1. We first describe measures that have been revised or are new since 2000, dividing this section into (a) measures with revisions or new developments, (b) new measures of DSM PDs and (c) new measures that offer alternative approaches to assessing personality and PD trait dimensions.
2. We then turn to the DSM-5 alternative model and (a) discuss measures of personality functioning, a largely new domain in the PD field, especially with regard to its assessment, and (b) describe new trait-dimension-focused measures that are directly associated with the alternative model.
3. We touch on issues that need to be considered to move PD assessment forward on a solid empirical basis, including (a) clarifying both the nature of personality functioning and traits, and their relations to disability (i.e., impairment in functioning other than personality functioning per se), and also ongoing issues surrounding PD dimensions, categories, and hybrid models, and (b) methodological (e.g., self-report vs. interview), reliability (interrater agreement and temporal stability) and validity issues, such as using diverse information sources (e.g., self vs. informants), and the nature of change in personality and PD.

## New or Revised Assessment Instruments

### Revisions to or Developments Regarding Existing Measures

#### Psychopathy Checklist—Revised, 2nd Edition

The Psychopathy Checklist—Revised, 2nd Edition (PCL-R; Hare, 2003), based, like its predecessor, the PCL, on Hare's (1970) modification of Cleckley's (1976) concept of psychopathy, assesses 20 psychopathic characteristics. Early factor analyses (e.g., Hare et al., 1990) indicated that these characteristics formed two correlated factors: emotional–interpersonal aspects and antisocial behavioral aspects of psychopathy. Cooke and Michie (2001) proposed a three-factor hierarchical model, with an overarching psychopathy factor, composed of deficient affective experience, arrogant and deceitful interpersonal style, and impulsive and irresponsible behavioral style, thus splitting the original Factor 1 into two components and maintaining Factor 2 intact. Hare and colleagues (e.g., Hare & Neumann, 2008) then argued that the data better supported a four-factor model—affective, interpersonal, lifestyle, and antisocial behavior—which subdivides each of the original factors into two components. It appears that the two-, three-, and four-factor models form a systematic hierarchy from one through four factors. However, the three- and four-factor models both have strong adherents who persist in advocating for one model over the other. Williams, Paulhus, and Hare (2007) also developed the 64-item Self-Report Psychopathy Scale: Version III, which provides both a total score and subscale scores corresponding to the factors of the four-factor model. In any case, the PCL-R remains the dominant psychopathy assessment instrument.

#### Psychopathic Personality Inventory—Revised

Much of the new research on the Psychopathic Personality Inventory—Revised (PPI-R; Lilienfeld & Widows, 2005) also concerns its higher order structure, although the nature of the controversy is different from that surrounding the PCL-R. All generally agree that (1) the PPI-R has two factors, which have come to be called Fearless Dominance (FD) and Impulsive Antisociality (IA; Benning, Patrick, Hicks, Blonigen, & Krueger, 2003), and (2) IA corresponds primarily to the original PCL-R Factor 2 (Hare, 2003). However, there is considerable debate about whether FD corresponds to PCL-R Factor 1 and, more broadly, assesses an aspect of psychopathy at all. In a meta-analytic review of PPI construct validity, Miller and Lynam (2012) reported that (1) the two PPI-R factors were largely uncorrelated (whereas the PCL-R factors are moderately strongly correlated), (2) FD related weakly both to various Factor 1 indices and to psychopathy total scores, and (3) FD largely indexed adaptive features, such that these authors interpreted it as reflecting stable extraversion (E). Lilienfeld and colleagues (2012), however, countered that (1) the fact that FD correlated with adaptive characteristics was not evidence per se against it as an aspect of psychopathy, noting the concept of the successful psychopath, and (2) FD correlated both with measures of psychopathy not reviewed by Miller and Lynam (2012), and other theoretically relevant correlates of psychopathy such as narcissism, sensation seeking, functional impulsivity, low fear-potentiated startle, and skin conductance in response to aversive stimuli. Resolution of these issues awaits further research.

## Interpersonal Dependency Inventory

The Interpersonal Dependency Inventory (IDI; Hirschfeld et al., 1977) was developed to assess dependency broadly, by incorporating conceptions of this construct from object relations, attachment, and social learning theories. Although DSM dependent PD (DPD) has not received a great deal of research attention (Blashfield & Intoccia, 2000), we include a measure of the construct because there is clinical interest in DPD (see Bornstein, 2012) and research interest in the personality trait of dependency. A review of the dependency assessment literature (Morgan & Clark, 2010) found support for a two-factor model of Passive–Submissive and Active–Emotional dependency, plus a third, unrelated factor: Detachment/Autonomy. The IDI's three subscales—Emotional Reliance on Another Person, Lack of Social Self-Confidence, and Assertion of Autonomy—are strong markers of these factors, respectively. The IDI's authors suggested various alternatives for deriving a total dependency score, but most researchers simply have summed the three subscale scores. Loas and colleagues (2002) compared five formulas for scoring the IDI, recommending one that included all three subscales as having the best sensitivity/specificity ratio, but we know of no cross-validation attempts. Because Morgan and Clark's (2010) review indicated that assertion of autonomy is an independent dimension and therefore should not be included in an overall dependency score, summing the scores on only the Emotional Reliance on Another Person and Lack of Social Self-Confidence scales would appear to provide the best assessment of dependency; however, this requires further research consideration.

## Narcissistic Personality Inventory

The Narcissistic Personality Inventory (NPI; Raskin & Hall, 1979, 1981) was based on the DSM-III criteria for narcissistic PD (NPD), but was intended as a measure of trait narcissism, not of the PD per se and, as such, has been used most widely in the social-psychological literature (see review by Cain, Pincus, & Ansell, 2008). The NPI continues to be cited frequently, garnering more citations in 2015 than in any previous year, according to the Web of Science. Emmons (1984) proposed a four-factor structure for the NPI that has been widely used, but recent research suggests that a three-factor solution, consisting of Entitlement/Exploitativeness, Grandiose Exhibitionism, and Leadership/Authority, is more robust (Ackerman et al., 2011). The NPI total score is correlated with high levels of Extraversion (E) and low levels of Agreeableness (A) (Miller, Gaughan, Pryor, Kamen, & Campbell, 2009), but Ackerman and colleagues (2011) reported differential relations for the three factors. Specifically, all three factors were related to low A, but only the Leadership/Authority and Grandiose Exhibitionism factors correlated with E, whereas the Entitlement/Exploitativeness factor was positively related to Neuroticism (N). These results suggest that the NPI contains both adaptive and maladaptive content, some of which may be obscured when the total score is used. This, together with recent developments in the assessment of pathological narcissism, discussed in a subsequent section, indicate that narcissism is a complex, multidimensional construct that may not be well captured by a single score, except for very high or very low scorers.

## New Measures of DSM PDs

### Multisource Assessment of Personality Pathology

The Multisource Assessment of Personality Pathology (MAPP; Oltmanns & Turkheimer, 2006) was designed for both self- and peer-informant assessment of the DSM-IV/5-II PD criteria. The items are lay "translations" of the criteria into nontechnical language (e.g., avoidant criterion 6, "Views self as socially inept, personally unappealing, or inferior to others," is rendered as "I'm [or "S/he thinks s/he is] not as much fun or as attractive as other people"), plus 24 buffer items that assess positive qualities. Respondents are asked to indicate what percent of the time the target individual (self or peer) is "like this" on either a 0- to 3-point or 0- to 4-point scale, depending on the study. Internal consistency reliability coefficients are moderate to very high (range = .57–.96), with average levels higher in a large sample of young-adult military recruits (Oltmanns, Gleason, Klonsky, & Turkheimer, 2005) than in a sample of adults ages 55–65 (Carlson, Vazire, & Oltmanns, 2013).

Average convergent validity of the self-report MAPP with the Personality Disorder Questionnaire–4 (PDQ-4; Hyler, 1994) and the Structured Clinical Interview for DSM-IV Axis II PD (SCID-II; First & Gibbon, 2004) in a sample of college students was moderately strong ($r = .74$) using dimensional scores, whereas categorized scores yielded lower agreement ($r = .40$; Okada & Oltmanns, 2009). Had kappas been reported, they likely would have been lower still, commensurate with previous findings (Clark, Livesley, & Morey, 1997). Mean convergent validity with the Schedule for Nonadaptive and Adaptive Personality (SNAP; Clark, 1993) PD diagnostic scores in two large samples of young adults (college students and military recruits) was more modest ($r = .46$; Oltmanns & Turkheimer, 2006), perhaps because the SNAP scales assess DSM-III-R and/or because its items were written to assess personality traits, not specific PD diagnostic criteria.

Oltmanns and Turkheimer (2006) report extensive information about the MAPP including, for example, that the predictive validity of peer- and self-report MAPP scores are stronger, respectively, for indices of externalizing versus internalizing psychopathology, and that "meta-perception" scores (how individuals think others would rate them) provide significantly more information about how peers actually rate them than do self-reports. In summary, the MAPP appears to be a promising new instrument for gathering peer-report data on the DSM-IV/5-II PD criteria. Of course, as such, it has all the liabilities of those PD categories (e.g., comorbidity).

### NEO Personality Inventory—Revised DSM PD Prototype Profiles

The NEO Personality Inventory (Costa & McCrae, 1992), a 240-item inventory of the dominant five-factor model (FFM) of personality, assesses six facets for each trait. It was designed to assess normal-range personality traits, but meta-analyses have shown that the scales relate systematically to DSM PDs (Samuel & Widiger, 2008; Saulsman & Page, 2004). Individual scale–PD correlations are modest (~.20–.50), but profile-level relations are considerably stronger. Using all 30 facets, Lynam and Widiger (2001) and Samuel and Widiger (2004) derived consensus prototype NEO PI-R profiles for the 10 specific DSM-IV/5-II PDs plus psychopathy based on, respectively, PD researchers' and clinicians' ratings of prototypical cases. The average intraclass correlations (ICCs) between these profiles and Samuel and Widiger's (2008) meta-analytic results were .50 and .55, respectively.

In a series of studies, Miller, Bagby, Pilkonis, Reynolds, and Lynam (2005; Miller et al., 2010) correlated Lynam and Widiger's (2001) DSM NEO profiles with various PD scores, and consistently found convergent/discriminant patterns averaging ~.40 and ~.20, respectively. Including informant reports added an average 8% of explanatory variance for half the PDs (Miller, Pilkonis, & Morse, 2004). Decuyper, De Clercq, De Bolle, and De Fruyt (2009) corroborated these results in a Belgium adolescent sample. Thus, NEO profiles reflect considerable overlapping variance with the DSM PDs and have the advantage of providing a complete trait-dimensional profile rather than categorical diagnostic labels, thereby providing more specific clinical information about each individual (Clark et al., 2015). Nonetheless, they also reflect all DSM PDs' weaknesses.

### "Pathological NEO PI-R" Facet-Based Measures of DSM-IV/5-II PDs and Psychopathy

Recently, Lynam, Miller, Widiger, and colleagues began developing a set of scales to assess the DSM-IV/5-II PD diagnoses plus psychopathy, comprising pathological versions of the NEO PI-R trait facets to strengthen convergent correlations (Edmundson, Lynam, Miller, Gore, & Widiger, 2011; Glover, Miller, Lynam, Crego, & Widiger, 2012; Gore, Presnall, Miller, Lynam, & Widiger, 2012; Lynam et al., 2011; Lynam, Loehr, Miller, & Widiger, 2012; Mullins-Sweatt et al., 2012; Samuel, Riddell, Lynam, Miller, & Widiger, 2012). Facets were selected rationally for each PD based on reported empirical correlations, expert ratings, and a description of the DSM PDs using the FFM (Widiger, Trull, Clarkin, Sanderson, & Costa, 2002); then, items were written to assess PD-specific maladaptive variants of each relevant facet. For example, for schizotypal PD (STPD), the NEO PI-R Anxiousness facet was recast as Social Anxiousness, and STPD-specific items (e.g., "Social situations tend to make me very anxious") were written to replace the NEO PI-R's more generic items (e.g., "I often feel tense and jittery"; Edmundson et al., 2011, p. 323). The item pools were refined using internal consistency criteria, yielding maladaptive-FFM measures with nine to 18 subscales (mode = 12). For each measure, the resulting subscales generally showed good convergent and discriminant validity with the NEO PI-R and other measures of the target PD and its related traits.

However, at least two aspects of this enterprise are concerning. First, the large number of items limits its clinical utility. Altogether, the measures contain 845 items, comprising 86 scales, with an average of three scales for most NEO PI-R facets (range = 0–7), each tailored for a putatively distinct PD. Moreover, measures for three DSM-IV/5-II PDs have not (yet) been developed![1] Second, given the well-established problems with the DSM PDs, developing a new set of FFM scales to assess them, including as many as seven presumably highly correlated variations of the same trait facet, would seem to undermine two major advantages of a trait-dimensional approach to PD assessment: (1) It provides an alternative method for assessing and diagnosing the entire PD domain parsimoniously using a single comprehensive structure, which would allow the field (2) to transition from the problematic DSM PD constructs toward a more valid system. The creation of multiple subscales for the same personality trait construct allows assessment of fine-grain colorations of each facet, but at the cost of parsimony and the risk of maintaining constructs that, it seems to us, the field should be allowing to fade away.

### Alternative Approaches to Assessing Normal–Abnormal Range Personality Traits

At the same time that consensus has built around the FFM as the structure of normal–abnormal range personality traits, measures of alternative approaches have been developed that typically are similar, but not identical, to the FFM. In this section, we briefly describe these measures, one of which—Zuckerman's Alternative Five (Zuckerman, Kuhlman, Joireman, Teta, & Kraft, 1993)—existed prior to the original version of this chapter. It was not reviewed therein owing to its primary focus on normal-range personality traits but, because the close relation of personality and psychopathology has become established, we now include it. We also review a non-FFM measure of narcissism.

### A New Approach to Narcissism: The Pathological Narcissism Inventory

Lay conceptions of narcissism focus on its grandiose, self-centered, entitled, exploitative aspects, whereas clinical–theoretical approaches to narcissism also include vulnerable aspects: hypersensitivity, defensiveness, and shame when the ideal self-view is threatened. Until recently, narcissism measures were described as assessing either grandiosity (GN) or vulnerability (VN), and such measures have been shown to be largely uncorrelated (e.g., Daly & Clark, 2014; Wink, 1991). Together with the recent NPI research discussed earlier, this lack of correlation challenges a conceptualization of narcissism as a single construct with two aspects. Pincus and colleagues (2009) opined that two problems in the literature are that (1) the NPI assesses normal-range, not pathological, narcissism, and (2) existing narcissism measures are insufficiently multidimensional. They developed the Pathological Narcissism Inventory (PNI; Pincus et al., 2009)—a 52-item self-report inventory with seven subscales, four purportedly tapping VN and three tapping GN[2]—to be a multifaceted measure of pathological narcissism based on clinical–theoretical conceptualizations.

If narcissism is a single construct, then its VN and GN aspects should be moderately to strongly intercorrelated and should correlate at least moderately with existing measures of VN and GN. However, it is not clear that these actually were goals in developing the PNI, as the authors seem to be asserting that normal-range and pathological narcissism are distinct constructs rather than different ranges of the same construct. Moreover, accruing data suggest the PNI does not have these properties (e.g., Daly & Clark, 2014; Maxwell, Donnellan, Hopwood, & Ackerman, 2011; Pincus et al., 2009). Specifically, (1) the PNI-GN Exploitative scale correlates notably more weakly with the remaining six scales (~.15) than they do with each other (~.40); (2) the PNI-VN scales correlate (~.50) with other VN scales, but only the PNI-Exploit-

---

[1] Four, if one considers antisocial PD to be distinct from psychopathy.

[2] Pincus et al. (2009) initially presented the Entitlement Rage subscale as measuring GN, but recently recategorized it as a VN measure (Pincus, 2013).

ative scale correlates at all strongly with other measures of GN (~.40); (3) the other PNI-GN scales relate similarly weakly to other GN and VN scales (~.25 vs. .20, respectively); and (4) the PNI-VN scales correlate at the same moderate level with neuroticism (~.40) as they do with each other. Thus, whereas it is arguable that the PNI scales (except for Exploitative) meet the requirement of moderate intercorrelation for a multidimensional construct, and that the PNI-VN scales assess the VN construct, it does not appear that the PNI-GN scales assess a pathological version of GN as it typically is conceptualized. As suggested earlier, this may be because its authors did not intend the PNI to assess simply a pathological version of existing GN concepts and scales, but instead targeted a rather different conceptualization of GN, and perhaps even of VN. Thus, it remains unknown whether it is possible to develop a narcissism measure with VN and GN components that are both moderately to strongly intercorrelated, and that correlate at least moderately with existing measures of VN and GN. Moreover, how well the PNI assesses its authors' revised conceptualization of narcissism and how that revised conceptualization relates to narcissism's traditional conceptualization clearly needs further explication.

### Alternative FFM

In contrast to the standard FFM, which was developed largely atheoretically, based initially on the English personality-descriptive lexicon (see Goldberg, 1993, for a history of the FFM), the alternative FFM (A-FFM) was developed as a biologically based model of personality, operationalized with the Zuckerman–Kuhlman Personality Questionnaire (Zuckerman, 2008; Zuckerman et al., 1993). Nonetheless, it shows generally good convergent and discriminant validity with other higher-order measures of personality (e.g., Zuckerman & Cloninger, 1996; Zuckerman et al., 1993), and is used widely cross-culturally, having been translated into multiple languages in both its 99-item full form (e.g., Rossier et al., 2007) and a 50-item short form (Aluja et al., 2006).

The measure has undergone a recent major revision, and now has four 10-item facet scales for each domain (Aluja, Kuhlman, & Zuckerman, 2010). The facet scales are generally internally consistent (mean = .78; range = .56–.90), and the domain scales have high alpha values (mean = .91; range = .88–.93). At the FFM domain level, N and E align well across models, with $r$'s in the .60–.75; Activity and Aggressiveness align moderately ($r$'s ~ .50) with C and low A; and FFM Openness (O) and A-FFM Impulsive Sensation Seeking (ISS) each have no clear counterpart in the other model, although ISS facet Experience Seeking correlated .39 with O, and the ISS facet Impulsivity/Boredom Susceptibility correlated –.45 with C. (See also Aluja et al., 2013, for its relations with Eysenck's and Gray's structural models in a Spanish version.) More research is needed to evaluate the construct validity of the revised version, especially its facets.

### Five Dimensional Personality Test

The Five Dimensional Personality Test (5DPT; van Kampen, 2012) is a 100-item measure developed over a number of years as a theory-based extension of Eysenck's three-factor model (Eysenck & Eysenck, 1985), retaining N and E, and dividing Psychoticism into three factors: Insensitivity (cf. FFM low A), Orderliness (cf. FFM Conscientiousness [C]), and Absorption (cf. FFM O; Tellegen & Atkinson, 1974); see van Kampen (2009) for the history of its development. van Kampen (2006) reported that four dimensions of the 5DPT mapped onto the higher-order factors of the Dimensional Assessment of Personality Pathology (DAPP; Livesley & Jackson, 2010): Emotional Dysregulation (N), Inhibition (low E), Dissocial (Insensitivity, low A) and Compulsivity (Orderliness, "pathological C"), and van Kampen (2012) demonstrated the measure's clear convergent/discriminant correlational pattern with both the NEO-Five-Factor Inventory (Costa & McCrae, 1992) and the HEXACO (Honesty–Humility, Emotionality, Extraversion, Agreeableness, Conscientiousness, Openness to Experience; Ashton & Lee, 2007), discussed in a later section. Although it appears not to be have been studied in relation to the DSM PDs, there is no reason to believe it would behave any differently from other FFM measures. Thus, the 5DPT provides a theoretical basis for the lexically based FFM, which will be important in helping the PD field move from a purely descriptive to an explanatory model.

## Dimensional Personality Symptom Item Pool

The Dimensional Personality Symptom Item Pool (DIPSI; De Clercq, De Fruyt, Van Leeuwen, & Mervielde, 2006) was constructed using a "bottom-up" approach by writing maladaptively extreme variants of items in the FFM normal-range Hierarchical Personality Inventory for Childen (Mervielde & De Fruyt, 1999, 2002) in an effort to establish a taxonomy of personality pathology in childhood and adolescence. The DIPSI has 27 facets comprising its four higher-order dimensions of Emotional Instability, Disagreeableness, Compulsivity, and Introversion. The first three factors show a clean convergent/discriminant pattern against the DAPP's higher-order structure in adolescents, with Introversion relating to DAPP Emotional instability, as well as Inhibition (De Clercq, De Fruyt, & Widiger, 2009). Notably absent from the DIPSI are traits related to psychosis.

The DIPSI's developers have been active in developing its construct validity (we found almost two dozen articles despite the relatively newness of the measure), and other research groups are beginning to find support for the instrument's construct validity as well. For example, Tackett and colleagues (2014) found that all four of the DIPSI's factors related to the total problems score on the Childhood Behavior Checklist (Achenbach, 2001), with Disagreeableness and Emotional Instability particularly strongly correlated ($r \sim .75-.80$). Furthermore, following a laboratory-based stress induction task, significant interactions were found between PD traits and cortisol recovery, such that early recovery (usually considered adaptive) was associated with *more* behavior problems when PD traits were elevated, suggesting that adolescents with personality pathology may not fully process negative environmental stimuli, leading to deficient learning from negative consequences. Thus, the DIPSI is a promising measure for extending knowledge about personality pathology into adolescence and childhood.

## HEXACO (Honesty–Humility, Emotionality, Extraversion, Agreeableness, Conscientiousness, Openness to Experience)

Based on a review of lexical studies in multiple languages, Ashton and Lee have argued that a six-factor solution better reflects natural-language personality structure, is more grounded theoretically, and better accommodates a broader range of traits than the FFM (Ashton & Lee, 2001, 2007). Ashton and colleagues (2004) provide an excellent summary description of the HEXACO's six scales and how they overlap and contrast with the FFM. We have bolded the letters used to form the HEXACO acronym:

(a) A variant of E**X**traversion, defined by sociability and liveliness (though not by bravery and toughness); (b) a variant of **A**greeableness, defined by gentleness, patience, and agreeableness (but also including anger and ill temper at its negative pole); (c) **C**onscientiousness (emphasizing organization and discipline rather than moral conscience); (d) **E**motionality (containing anxiety, vulnerability, sentimentality, lack of bravery, and lack of toughness, but not anger or ill temper); (e) **H**onesty–Humility; (f) Intellect/Imagination/Unconventionality (**O**penness to Experience). (p. 356)

Their theoretical arguments are that H, A, and E can be interpreted in terms of prosociality versus antisociality, specifically "fairness/nonexploitation, forgiveness/nonretaliation, and empathy/attachment," whereas EX, C, and O involve active engagement in "social, task-related, and idea-related endeavours" (Ashton & Lee, 2001, p. 327). Moreover, they claim that the model "predicts several personality phenomena that are not explained within the B5/FFM, including the relations of personality factors with theoretical biologists' constructs of reciprocal and kin altruism and the patterns of sex differences in personality traits" (Ashton & Lee, 2007, p. 150). From a PD perspective, support for the model (vs. the FFM) has been reported primarily in predicting indices of psychopathy (e.g., Ashton & Lee, 2008; de Vries & van Kampen, 2010; Gaughan, Miller, & Lynam, 2012; Lee & Ashton, 2005). To accommodate schizotypy, however, a seventh dimension is needed (Ashton, Lee, de Vries, Hendrickse, & Born, 2012). Ashton and Lee have been prolific in documenting support for the model (a search for Ashton, Lee, and HEXACO returned almost 50 articles), and it has been picked up by the field as well: A search for "HEXACO NOT Ashton NOT Lee" returned 164 hits. Although only 15 of those concerned PD, they all were dated 2009 or later, so it appears the PD researchers have "discovered" HEXACO, making it a promising new domain of inquiry in the PD literature.

## Computerized Adaptive Test of Personality Disorder

The Computerized Adaptive Test of Personality Disorder (CAT-PD; Simms et al., 2011) is a measure developed using item response theory to assess pathological personality traits efficiently (see Simms et al., 2011, regarding its development). Its 33 traits comprise five domains—Negative Emotionality, Positive Emotionality, Antagonism, (Dis)Constraint, and Psychoticism—that largely correspond to the domains of the DSM-5 Section III model (Wright & Simms, 2014). The full item pool is 1,366 items, but only 188 are administered adaptively because the computer program selects items iteratively (i.e., one at a time) to maximize information for each individual's trait levels (Weiss, 1985). The CAT version is not yet available, but a 216-item static form has been developed, with mean alphas of .83 and .85 in patient and community samples, respectively (Wright & Simms, 2014). The adaptive and full scales correlate > .90, whereas the static–full form correlations average around .85; median test–retest reliability over an average of 2 weeks was .77 (Simms, 2014). CAT-PD scales mapped conceptually and empirically onto 24 of the 25 scales of the Personality Inventory for DSM-5 (PID-5; Krueger, Derringer, Markon, Watson, & Skodol, 2012), with a mean correlation of .77 (range = .58–.90); conversely, nine CAT-PD scales mapped onto no PID-5 scale (Simms, 2014). Thus, although clearly more research is needed, given its comprehensiveness, sophisticated development process, relative brevity, and that it is a public-domain instrument, the CAT-PD is a strong addition to the set of measures assessing personality pathology.

## The DSM-5 Section III Alternative Model for PD

### Personality Functioning

#### Theoretical Background

In recent years, interest has emerged in assessing personality functioning, a theoretically fundamental component of personality pathology that distinguishes mere statistically abnormal personality from disordered personality (e.g., Bender, Morey, & Skodol, 2011). In contemporary PD theories, maladaptive personality functioning is common to all PDs, and is consistently conceptualized as impairment in the self and/or interpersonal domains in both evolutionary theory on the adaptive function of personality (e.g., Livesley & Jang, 2005) and object relations (OR) theory (Huprich & Greenberg, 2003), with parallels to social cognition theory (see Bender et al., 2011), which is based on the idea that personality psychopathology emanates from disturbances in thinking about oneself and others, as well as the inability to interact adaptively with others.

#### Prior Reviews

Assessment instruments developed to measure OR have been reviewed in detail previously, so we offer only a brief summary of their content, referring interested readers to the reviews themselves. Fishler, Sperling, and Carr (1990) reviewed both projective and objective measures of interpersonal relatedness from both OR (particularly separation–individuation) and attachment theory (early bonding experiences shape later attachments). Stricker and Healey (1990) discussed the reliability and validity of OR projective measures, whereas Smith (1993) identified the most widely used OR measures across various methods, noting concerns with interrater reliability for projective measures.

Three relatively recent reviews collectively include most, if not all, interview-based OR measures. Huprich and Greenberg (2003) evaluated 12 widely used OR measures and concluded that, contrary to common belief among psychodynamic researchers, OR could be measured through self-report. As part of a broader review, Koelen and colleagues (2012) highlighted measures that had been used in treatment research and, finally, Bender and colleagues (2011) described in some detail five measures pertaining to mental representations of self and other. A major limitation of the OR assessment literature is that there are multiple conceptualizations of OR, which lead to different emphases and thus difficulty integrating concepts across measures (Huprich & Greenberg, 2003). For example, some measures emphasize quality of OR, whereas others assess the ability to form distinct representations of self and other.

## Level of Personality Functioning Scale

The DSM-5-III PD model includes a clinician rating form, the Level of Personality Functioning Scale (LPFS; APA, 2013), which operationalizes self-domain impairment as problems with identity and self-direction, whereas problems with empathy and intimacy comprise interpersonal dysfunction. Detailed descriptions are provided for each of five levels (0 = *no impairment* to 4 = *extreme impairment*). Because of the newness of the measure, very little research on it has been published to date. Few and colleagues (2013) reported interrater reliability coefficients ranging from .47 to .49 for the four domains, which they appropriately called "fair" agreement (p. 1057), noting that the ratings were complicated by the fact that each level was described with multiple phrases that may not fit a patient equally well. They found that both self- and interpersonal LPFS scores correlated significantly with several measures of emotional distress, DSM-IV/5-II PD diagnoses, number of PD symptoms, and DSM-5 (PID-5) self-report traits, and reported that the LPFS did not account for significant additional variance in predicting DSM-IV/5-II PDs above clinician-rated DSM-5 traits.

Somewhat in contrast, Zimmermann and colleagues (2014) reported an interrater reliability coefficient of .51 using untrained undergraduates which, interestingly, they labeled "acceptable" (p. 397). They reported that raters also agreed well with the judgments of two clinicians who used an expert-rater measure of personality dysfunction severity. Notably, Zimmermann and colleagues addressed the issues of complex descriptors by having the raters rate each of the dimensions' three facets (e.g., for the identity dimension: identity definition [awareness of self; role-appropriate boundaries], self-appraisal [positivity and accuracy], and emotional tolerance and regulation)—which then were aggregated across facets and dimensions to yield a single score.

Finally, Morey, Krueger, and Skodol (2013) asked 337 clinicians to rate a patient with whom they had had 5 or more contact hours on all the DSM-IV/5-II and DSM-5-III criteria, including the LPFS. They reported validity correlations in the .35–.50 range, with the clinicians' ratings of occupational, social, and leisure functioning (alpha = .72); level of risk for self-harm, violence, or criminality (alpha = .67), level of treatment needed (self-help to hospitalization), and prognosis; moreover, the LPFS had greater incremental predictive power than the number of PD criteria met for three of these four variables (the exception being risk). Thus, to date, the LPFS is yielding mixed results and, not surprisingly, more research is needed to understand better the nature of this new measure and what it assesses.

## Self-Report Assessment of Personality Functioning

MEASURE OF DISORDERED PERSONALITY FUNCTIONING[3]

Development of the Measure of Disordered Personality Functioning (MDPF; Parker et al., 2004) was based on Parker and colleagues' (2002) hypothesis that measuring disordered functioning might be a better screen for PD than diagnostic criteria, which combine descriptions of personality traits (style) and disordered functioning that, in turn, may contribute to high PD comorbidity; that is, if multiple PDs describe similar disordered functioning, comorbidity may occur even if the associated personality traits are distinct (Parker et al., 2002, 2004). Thus, separate assessment of personality functioning and traits/style could make PD diagnoses more precise and clarify the nature of individuals' disorders.

The 65-item MDPF assesses two higher-order factors of personality dysfunction, Non-Coping (self) and Non-Cooperativeness (interpersonal), composed of 11 dysfunctional domains. Discriminant analyses between PD and no-PD groups indicated that traits and functioning were virtually equally capable of discriminating the two groups (Parker et al., 2004). Two 10-item scales, Non-Cooperativeness and Non-Coping correlated an average of .57 and .27 with self- and clinician-rated PD, respectively, indicating considerable overlap between these domains, at least in self-report. Although the MDPF has not been used widely, that may change with the introduction of the construct of personality functioning in DSM-5-III, in part because of its

---

[3] Parker et al. (2004) did not name the scale, but refer to it simply as "Disordered Functioning (DF)"; we have taken the liberty of giving it a name to clarify that it is a measure, not just a construct, and that it specifically measures personality functioning.

## GENERAL ASSESSMENT OF PERSONALITY DISORDER

The General Assessment of Personality Disorder (GAPD; Livesley, 2010) is based on Livesley's evolutionary-based theory that disordered personality functioning represents a failure to achieve adaptive solutions to universal life tasks (Livesley & Jang, 2005).

The GAPD was designed to have two higher-order dimensions, Self Pathology and Interpersonal Pathology, with 19 subscales measuring various dysfunctional aspects, including OR content (e.g., poorly differentiated representations of others). Berghuis, Kamphuis, Verheul, Larstone, and Livesley (2013) found this structure in the original 144-item version, but using an eight-facet, 85-item version, Hentschel and Livesley (2013b) found a one-factor model (median loading = .83). Nevertheless, Self Pathology subscales had significant incremental validity in predicting PD severity over interpersonal pathology. The GAPD discriminated patients with and without PD and also differentiated personality pathology severity based on number of PDs (Berghuis et al., 2013). Similarly, the GAPD correctly classified 81.9% of patients into those with and without PD, with good sensitivity, specificity, and positive and negative predictive power (Hentschel & Livesley, 2013a). Mean Cronbach's alpha coefficient for the eight facet scales was .84 (range = .67–.95) and average correlations with DSM-IV/5-II PDs ranged from ≤ .15 (histrionic, obsessive–compulsive, and antisocial PD) to >.45 (avoidant, depressive, paranoid, schizotypal, and borderline PD); mean = .33 (Hentschel & Livesley, 2013b), suggesting the GAPD-assessed constructs are distinct though not unrelated to PD diagnoses. However, when examined in relation to the DAPP, a number of correlations were ≥ .75 between traits and self pathology, and three correlations were ~.60 with interpersonal dysfunction, suggesting that discriminant validity may be a challenge for the GAPD, at least in self-report.

## SEVERITY INDICES OF PERSONALITY PROBLEMS

Development of the Severity Indices of Personality Problems (SIPP; Verheul et al., 2008) was based on a premise similar to that of the GAPD: Maladaptive personality functioning—the core of personality pathology—reflects a developmental deficiency in adaptive capacities. It is intended to evaluate the changeable core components of maladaptive personality functioning as opposed to the more stable personality style (traits). This 118-item measure contains five higher-order domains (Self-Control, Identity Integration, Relational Capacities, Responsibility, and Social Concordance) and 16 lower-order facets. The authors reported a median alpha coefficient of .77 (range = .69–.84), and median within- versus across-domain correlations of .56 and .39, respectively. Temporal stability averaged .93 (range = .87–.95) over 2- to 3-week intervals in a student sample. However, every SIPP facet correlated at least .52 (up to .65) with one or more personality traits, indicating considerable overlap in domains. In an adolescent sample, the SIPP yielded a similar factor structure and alpha coefficients, discriminated community and patient (with and without PD) subsamples, and displayed sensitivity to change after treatment (Feenstra, Hutsebaut, Verheul, & Busschbach, 2011). The SIPP is gaining in recognition and use, which likely will accelerate with the introduction of personality functioning in DSM-5-III.

In developing the LPFS, Morey and colleagues (2011) rated the level of personality functioning for each GAPD and SIPP item, then used item response theory (IRT) analysis to develop empirically a combined scale. The resulting 93-item measure (alpha = .96; average inter-item $r$ = .21) correlated .51 with the number of PD criteria in two large, mostly patient samples. This measure's greatest promise is that it can be adapted for computer administration. Given that it is intended to assess a single, general, personality dysfunction construct, it is likely that administration would be quite brief.

## SUMMARY

A general concern with the three existing self-report personality functioning measures is that although they are intended to assess personality functioning independently from traits, they all have been found to correlate moderately to strongly with traits, and have been shown to co-load with traits onto the same factors when jointly factor-analyzed (Clark & Ro, 2014b; Ro & Clark, 2013). This overlap is no doubt partly due to similar item content that confounds traits and functioning in all three measures. For example, MDPF Disagreeableness and Impulsivity subscales' content is routinely found in similarly named trait measures. It is an interesting question as to whether the problem is that these personality-functioning measures inappropriately contain trait variance and/or that trait measures inappropriately assess personality functioning, or simply that the constructs themselves are inherently empirically overlapping, so that there simply are true limits on the degree to which they are distinguishable.

## DSM-5-III Trait Measures

### Personality Inventory for DSM-5

The Personality Inventory for DSM-5 (PID-5; Krueger et al., 2012) is a 220-item self-report instrument that measures the maladaptive personality traits included in DSM-5-III. Each item is rated on a 4-point scale—0 = *very false or often false,* 1 = *sometimes or somewhat false,* 2 = *sometimes or somewhat true,* and 3 = *very true or often true.* The PID-5 assesses 25 personality trait facets, with each trait facet consisting of four to 14 items, which can be combined into the five broader trait domains of Negative Affect, Detachment, Antagonism, Disinhibition, and Psychoticism. The PID-5 has demonstrated acceptable to good psychometric properties. Alphas for each of the facets ranged from .72 to .96 in a normative sample, with a median of .86, and ranged from .72 to .96 in an outpatient sample, with all facet scales demonstrating alphas greater than .70 (Krueger et al., 2012; Quilty, Ayearst, Chmielewski, Pollock, & Bagby, 2013). The five trait domains demonstrate good convergence with other measures, including the MMPI-2 Personality Psychopathology Five domains (Anderson et al., 2013). Initial research also suggests that the PID-5 domains reflect the domains of the Five-Factor model of normative personality (Quilty et al., 2013; Thomas et al., 2013). For a more detailed description of the PID-5, please refer to Ofrat, Krueger, and Clark (Chapter 4, this volume).

### PID-5 Brief Form

The PID-5 Brief Form (PID-5-BF; Krueger, Derringer, Markon, Watson, & Skodol, 2014) is a 25-item self-report measure with five PID-5 items per domain to assess the five DSM-5-III trait domains. The items use the same 4-point response format as the PID-5. As far as we could determine, no data have been published to date on this measure, but our laboratory is preparing a manuscript on the measure, scored from the full 220-item form in both patient and community samples (for details regarding the samples and data collection procedures, see Clark et al., 2015; Watson, Stasik, Ro, & Clark, 2013). Scale means are significantly higher ($p < .05$) in the patient sample, coefficient alphas are moderately high (median ~.75), with all average interitem correlations (AICs) in the recommended range (.15 to .50; Clark & Watson, 1995), so the fact that the coefficient alpha levels are only moderately high is due to the short scale length. The pattern of convergent (mean $r$ ~.90) and discriminant (mean $r$ ~.45) correlations with the corresponding domain scales in the full 220-item PID-5 is excellent (the moderately high discriminant correlations reflect those of the full PID-5). Finally, 1- to 2-year retest correlations were moderately high (~.60–.70). In summary, although replication is needed that is based on administering the PID-5-BF per se, the measure shows promising psychometric properties, such that it may be useful as a screening instrument to determine whether more in-depth assessment of personality pathology is needed.

### PID-5 Informant Rating Form

The PID-5 Informant Rating Form (PID-5-IRF; Markon, Quilty, Bagby, & Krueger, 2013) is a 218-item measure developed by rewording the PID-5 self-report items in the third person and removing two items with unacceptably low discrimination. Rating scale and scoring are the same as the self-report form; informants rate how well each item describes the individual generally. Initial development and validation used two normative samples and a high-risk community sample. Alphas were in the acceptable range (.72–.95) in both cross-validation samples. Self-informant agreement range was .38–.62 and .18–.40, in the normative and cross-validation samples, respectively, with the strongest agreement in the Disinhibition and Antagonism domains, the weakest in Psychoticism, and a convergent/discriminant pattern comparable to those found in the general psychopathology literature (Achenbach, Krukowski, Dumenci, & Ivanova, 2005). Moreover, the PID-5-IRF replicated the original PID-5 structure. The PID-5-IRF can be used either in tandem with or independent of PID-5 self-report data. Together with the PID-5, it provides useful personality trait information from a second perspective; however, its greatest utility may be when the validity of self-report is a concern due to the inability or unwillingness of the individual to provide veridical personality trait information (e.g., in legal settings).

### DSM-5 Clinicians' Personality Trait Rating Form

The DSM-5 Clinicians' Personality Trait Rating Form (DSM-5 CPTRF; American Psychiatric Association, 2013) also assesses the 25 pathological personality trait facets and five domains of the DSM-5-III PD model, with each item consisting simply of the brief description of the facet that is in the DSM-5-III. Clinicians base their ratings on personality-relevant information gathered using structured or other interviews, or on their interactions with patients in therapy. Rating scale and domain scoring are the same as the self-report form. Few and colleagues (2013) reported variable interrater reliability in a sample of 109 patients interviewed with the SCID-II (First & Gibbon, 2004)) by trained graduate students. Intraclass correlations for the trait facet ratings ranged from .12 (Perseveration) to .83 (Impulsivity), with a mean of .57. For the domain scores, generated by summing relevant trait facets, mean ICC was .66, ranging from .58 (Negative Affectivity) to .84 (Disinhibition). Convergence with patients' PID-5 domain and facet scores was strong: mean domain $r = .63$ (range = .50 for Psychoticism to .68 for Negative Affectivity) and facet mean $r = .52$ (range = .32 for Perseveration to .68 for Withdrawal).

In our laboratory, graduate student through PhD-level interviewers made DSM-5-III ratings after administering a Structured Interview for DSM-IV (SIDP-IV; Pfohl, Blum, & Zimmerman, 1997) to a mixed sample of 299 outpatients and community adults screened for high-risk for PD (Clark & Ro, 2014a). We found mean domain and facet ICCs of .67 and .69, respectively (range = .44 for Distractibility to .91 for Separation insecurity; domain ICC were all between .61 and .69), and mean domain and facet convergence with the PID-5 of .44 and .40, respectively (range = .25 for Perseveration to .59 for Intimacy Avoidance; domain range was .29 for Psychoticism to .53 for Detachment). These early data are promising regarding the DSM-5 CRF's interrater reliability and convergence with self-report data, especially for the domains.

### DSM-5-III Informant Personality Trait Rating Form

The DSM-5-III Informant Personality Trait Rating Form (DSM-5 IPTRF; Clark, Watson, & Krueger, 2014) assesses the same 25 pathological personality trait facets and five domains of the DSM-5-III PD model as the other measures in this series. Each of the 25 items consists of a brief description of the facet, revised from the DSM-5 CPTRF so as to be understood easily by lay informants. Rating scale and domain scoring are the same as the other DSM-5-III forms. In our laboratory, up to two informants were contacted when participants gave permission to do so. Consenting informants for 326 participants (138 of whom had two informants) completed several self-report measures online. Based on their personal knowledge of the person, informants rated what the primary participant generally was like. When two informants provided data, their scores were averaged.

Coefficient alphas for the domains were excellent (mean = .81, range = .79–.85). Between informants, ICCs for the domains and facets, respectively, were moderate, averaging .32 for domains and .25 for facets, with ranges of .27/.28 (Detachment, Psychoticism/Negative Affectivity) to .42 (Disinhibition) for the domains and .05 (Restricted Affectivity) to .43 (Irresponsibility) for the facets. Agreement with the primary participants' PID-5 domain scores was comparable to other self-informant personality data: *mean* $r = .29$ (range = .18 for Antagonism to .39 for Disinhibition). Facet score agreement was poor to good (mean = .25, range = .08 for Manipulativeness and Grandiosity to .37 for Depressivity and Attention Seeking). Thus, preliminary data are promising for using the DSM-5-III IPTRF to obtain personality trait information from a second perspective. Moreover, its brief 25-item format may make it more useful than the full 220-item PID-5-IRF in some settings.

## Assessment Issues for Future Research

The focus of this chapter is diagnostic and assessment methods, but in that context we first consider briefly theoretical and empirical issues that need resolution going forward. Perhaps most important is clarifying the nature of the relatively new construct of personality functioning and its relations to personality traits, plus the relations of both these constructs to disability (i.e., impairment in functioning *other than* personality functioning per se). Second, with the appearance of the DSM-5-III alternative PD model, the issue of categorical–dimensional hybrid models joins the long-standing debate regarding PD dimensions and categories. Third, data increasingly have indicated that personality is not "set like plaster," but changes at a moderate, though decreasing, rate throughout adulthood (Clark, 2007). We discuss PD assessment issues related to these findings. In closing, we discuss briefly the (NIMH) of Mental Health's Research Domain Criteria (RDoC), which has reemphasized multimethod assessment and may serve as a framework both for organizing research on the myriad assessment issues raised here, as well as moving the field into new assessment frontiers.

## Construct Clarity

### Personality Functioning

Personality dysfunction is a relatively new concept in the PD domain, and much work remains before it is fully conceptualized and reliably, validly measured. There is good conceptual agreement that the higher-order components of personality dysfunction are "self" and "interpersonal" pathology, but research is just beginning on the topology of lower-order components and how best to assess both higher and lower levels of personality-functioning structure. Moreover, whether both self and interpersonal pathology are needed for PD diagnosis is still widely debated. For example, DSM-5-III Criterion A is *described* consistently in terms of both self and interpersonal pathology, but the formal requirement for diagnosis allows for *either* self *or* interpersonal pathology. Relatedly, the *International Classification of Diseases* (ICD-11) PD proposal (Tyrer et al., 2011) defines PD only by interpersonal and trait psychology, though adding self-pathology is being considered.

It may be that self- and interpersonal dysfunction are so interrelated that their distinction is purely conceptual (e.g., Bender et al., 2011); that is, interpersonal relationships necessarily involve both the self and others, so interpersonal pathology intrinsically refers to how one views the self in relation to others; conversely, a strong sense of identity necessarily involves clear differentiation of self from others, such that self pathology naturally includes poor self–other boundaries. The constructs are interrelated empirically as well, establishing that using current assessment instruments, self and interpersonal pathology are components of a single, broad dimension of personality functioning (e.g., Clark & Ro, 2014b; Hentschel & Livesley, 2013b).

### Personality Traits

A less obvious but nonetheless important challenge is the extent to which personality functioning and traits can be measured distinctly. Clark and Ro (2014b) found that when personality traits and functioning were factor-analyzed together, self pathology subscales loaded with both internalizing personality traits (e.g., N) and measures from the broader functioning literature assessing well-being and life satisfaction. In turn, interpersonal personality pathology subscales loaded with interpersonal and externalizing personality traits, such as intimacy problems and low cooperativeness. Thus, the distinction between self/internalizing and interpersonal/externalizing dimensions was stronger and clearer than that between personality traits and functioning. Similarly, recall that the LPFS did not contribute additional variance in predicting DSM-IV PDs beyond clinician-rated DSM-5 personality traits (Few et al., 2013). One possible explanation of these results is that our purportedly well-established trait measures actually are "contaminated" with personality functioning variance; in developing personality trait scales over the past 7 decades or so, researchers may have included personality functioning variance "naturally," that is, without consideration of a possible distinction between personality traits and functioning. If so, this fact suggests that, at the very least, the constructs are highly intertwined, and distinguishing them empirically is difficult. At most, the distinction is artificial and impossible to make empirically. In either case, it may be that personality dysfunction and trait pathology are both inherent components of PD, but that *assessing* them separately is not only unnecessary but also impossible. Further research is needed to clarify these fundamental questions.

## Disability

A third conceptual challenge in PD (indeed, in all psychopathology) assessment concerns the role of social/occupational disability, that is, the functional consequences of disorder. The DSM-5 Task Force struggled with distinguishing disorder from disability and decided that, to date, "it has not been possible to completely separate normal and pathological symptoms expressions," so they retained a clinical significance criterion (CSC), a generic criterion of distress or disability to establish disorder thresholds, typically phrased as "the disturbance causes clinically significant distress or impairment in social, occupational, or other important areas of functioning" (APA, 2013, p. 21). However, the Personality and Personality Disorders Work Group decided to define PD without a CSC, so the alternative PD model has no separate reference to disability or to distress, except as inherent in certain personality traits (e.g., negative affectivity) and functioning (e.g., impaired emotional regulation).

Thus, whether to assess social/occupational disability associated with PD separately is representative of a larger debate on the definition of mental disorder. Wakefield (1992) conceptualized mental disorder as "harmful dysfunction," a failure in the evolutionarily designed natural function of a mental mechanism (e.g., cognition or, in this case, personality) that results in harm to the individual, as judged by social norms. This evolutionarily-based conceptualization of mental disorder is consistent with prominent theories of personality functioning as adaptive failure (e.g., Livesley & Jang, 2005). In contrast, the World Health Organization's International Classification of Functioning, Disability, and Health (ICF; WHO, 2001) distinguishes dysfunction from its associated harm, and considers only the former to be the basis for diagnosis. The ICF uses "disability" as an umbrella term encompassing both *impairments* in body (including psychological) functions and *activity limitations and participation restrictions,* which are the consequences of impairment in psychological functioning. To those familiar with DSM terminology, these ICD terms are confusing and/or cumbersome, so we label them "intrinsic" and "extrinsic" disability, respectively. Thus, personality dysfunction and pathological trait levels represent intrinsic disability (the impairment in psychological functioning that characterizes PD), whereas the social/occupational consequences of these dysfunctions constitute extrinsic disability which, consistent with ICD-11, is not part of DSM-5-III PD diagnosis.

In the DSM-5-III PD model, extrinsic disability can and should be assessed separately from personality functioning for clinical decision-making purposes. Again, however, the distinction is difficult to sustain, both conceptually and empirically, as personality dysfunction includes concepts that could be considered extrinsic disability. For example, the definition of extreme impairment in intimacy includes "engagement with others is detached, disorganized, or consistently negative" (APA, 2013, p. 778) which, to use the ICD-11 term, seems like an "activity limitation" in close relationships, a consequence of the impairment in the capacity for intimacy, and thus an extrinsic disability. Moreover, it seems both indistinguishable from DSM-5 CSC's "impairment in social functioning" and, arguably, a judgment based on social norms, fulfilling the harm component of Wakefield's definition (indeed, Wakefield [2013] made this point) and thus, again, an extrinsic disability. Accordingly, although the *intent* was to exclude extrinsic disability in defining the alternative PD model, it is not clear that this was accomplished completely, and an important question for future research is whether it even can be accomplished or whether the concepts are inseparably intertwined.

Furthermore, current trait assessments also often include extrinsic disability. For example, measures of detachment often include items assessing participation in social activities (e.g., "I avoid social events") or involvement in interpersonal relationships (e.g., "I have trouble opening up to people"), both of which could be considered ICF activity limitations and participation restrictions. When Clark and Ro (2014b) factor-analyzed an extensive set of personality trait, personality functioning and psychosocial functioning/extrinsic disability measures, an extrinsic disability factor emerged, but not all scales intended to assess disability loaded on it. Rather, some disability scales loaded more strongly on a factor that primarily was marked by traits related to negative affectivity and self-functioning measures. Thus, going forward, we need research that will help to clarify the overlap and distinctiveness of all three construct areas involved in PD assessment: personality dysfunction, trait pathology, and extrinsic disability.

## Dimensions, Categories, or a Hybrid Model?

Decades of debate have not ended disagreement on whether PD is better characterized by dimensions or categories, nor has considerable comparative research, which almost universally supports dimensional approaches. In DSM-5-III, a hybrid dimensional–categorical model was introduced, in which personality–dysfunction and specified pathological–trait dimensions comprise specific PD types, with cutoff scores to determine caseness. The model rests on a firmer conceptual base than that of DSM-IV/5-II because it distinguishes personality dysfunction and pathological traits although, as discussed, both theoretical and empirical problems with this formulation need to be resolved in future research. A survey of 400 members of two PD-focused organizations found that the majority of respondents ($N = 96$) endorsed a hybrid model over a pure dimensional or categorical one (Bernstein, Iscan, Maser, Boards of Directors of the Association for Research in Personality Disorders, & International Society for the Study of Personality Disorders, 2007), and the DSM-5 Task Force thought that a hybrid model would ease the transition to a purely dimensional model. Thus, there is some support in the field for a hybrid model, although there also has been considerable negative reaction to the particular DSM-5-III formulation (e.g., Gunderson, 2013; Livesley, 2012; Paris, 2013).

Due to its hybrid nature, the DSM-5-III model retains several major flaws of categorical diagnoses:

1. It does not address the issue that PD categories are not natural kinds (Haslam, 2002); that is, there are no points of rarity among the PD types, or between the presence and absence of PD. This claim has not been tested specifically with the DSM-5-III model traits, but research with highly similar trait dimensions is clear on this point (Eaton, Krueger, South, Simms, & Clark, 2011).
2. It does not solve the problem of within-diagnosis heterogeneity. Except for narcissistic PD, the hybrid model permits diagnosis via various trait combinations Moreover, Clark and colleagues (2015) found that individuals meeting criteria for any specific PD averaged five *additional* pathological traits.
3. It does not decrease comorbidity. Clark and colleagues' (2015) research also indicated that, as with the DSM-IV/5-II PD types, the majority of individuals diagnosed with any specific DSM-5-III PD type met criteria for two or more PD types.

Furthermore, the hybrid model introduces considerable complexity due to having versions of the personality–dysfunction subdomains that are specific to each PD type; in a few cases, even the pathological traits are defined differently across the specific PD types. Rating the level of personality dysfunction is aided by the $4 \times 4$ (levels by subdomains) matrix that the DSM-5 provides (see APA, 2013, pp. 775–778), but the degree of abstraction needed to consider how each PD-specific formulation would be manifest across the four levels of personality dysfunction is so formidable as to virtually assure that neither clinicians nor researchers will use them except perhaps in an impressionistic manner. In summary, although the DSM-5-III hybrid model may offer some comfort via the familiar DSM PD categories, it is a specious refuge, and should be only a temporary stopping point on the way to a PD formulation built on a solid dimensional foundation.

## Stability versus Change

### Self-Reports and Interviews, Dimensions and Categories

Data from the Collaborative Longitudinal Personality Study (CLPS; e.g., McGlashan et al., 2005), the McLean Study of Adult Development (Zanarini, Frankenburg, Hennen, & Silk, 2003), and the Longitudinal Study of Personality Disorders (Lenzenweger, Johnson, & Willett, 2004) have all highlighted that DSM PDs are not as stable over time as originally conceptualized, and that most change in PD is toward remission. One reason for this is that PD criteria vary in the extent to which they assess stable traits (e.g., "impulsivity or failure to plan ahead"; APA, 2013, p. 659) versus specific behaviors that are likely to occur less frequently, in part because they are dependent on situational circumstances (e.g., "transient, stress-related paranoid ideation or severe dissociative symptoms"; APA, 2013; p. 663). Thus, without thorough assessment of an individual's long-term patterns, it may appear that a diagnostic criterion is met, whereas the observed behavior actually depends on circumstances that may change over relatively short time periods, leading to diagnostic instability. Accordingly, because the major findings of PD change have relied on criterion-based diagnoses made via structured interviews (a different one in each case), they may not represent new findings but simply may reflect the qualitative variation in PD criteria and poor test–retest reliability of interview-based PD diagnoses that were well documented 20 years ago (Clark et al., 1997; Loranger et al., 1991; Shea, 1992; Zimmerman, 1994).

Durbin and Klein (2006) compared the 10-year stability of interview-based PD/PD traits and self-reported, normal-range personality traits, and Samuel, Hopwood, and colleagues (2011) used the CLPS data to compare PD/PD traits' 2-year stability using both self-report and interviews, each scored both categorically and dimensionally. In both studies, as always, dimensional scores were more stable than categorical scores. However, when *dimensional* scores were compared across assessment method, the results were remarkably similar, despite the different time intervals: PD–interview stabilities were .60 and .59, respectively, whereas self-reported trait stability was .69 in both studies. In contrast, categorical diagnoses had comparable, low (kappas ~ .38) 2-year stability across assessment methods. The take-home message of these studies is not new: More stable results will be obtained using dimensions than categories, especially when assessed via self-report. However, it also has become clearer that not all observed instability represents unreliability: Some of it does represent true change.

Finally, Morey and colleagues (2012) reported on the 6-, 8-, and 10-year *predictive* power of interview-based PD categories and dimensions, self-reported PD traits, and normal-range traits for a range of "important clinical outcomes" (p. 1705) in the CLPS data. At virtually all time points, self-reported PD traits evinced the greatest predictive power and interview-based categorical diagnoses the least. Interview-based PD dimensions and self-reported normal-range traits *combined* roughly equaled the predictive power of self-reported PD traits. Together with the stability data, these results suggest that although, indeed, PD can and does change, dimensional self-report scores provide more reliable assessment of change than interview-based diagnoses. Thus, these results run counter to the common belief that clinician-based scores are more valid than self-reports, insofar as reliability is a limiting factor for validity. Instead, they indicate that the more economical assessment method is also the more reliable and, thereby, likely the more valid.

## Normal-Range and Pathological Trait Change

Increased knowledge of change in normal-range personality is contributing to our understanding of change in PD. First, stability is comparable across normal- and abnormal-range personality traits (Roberts & DelVecchio, 2000). Second, nomothetically, normal-range traits become more adaptive with age (Roberts, Walton, & Viechtbauer, 2006). Specifically, N decreases, whereas A and C increase. These normative changes are consistent with the observed decrease in PD/PD traits discussed earlier. Second, normal-range personality traits become more stable with age (Roberts & DelVecchio, 2000). It is likely that this trend also applies to individuals with PD, such that pathological trait levels in older (vs. younger) individuals are less likely to decline because they are more likely to have stabilized. However, corroborative research is needed, as is research into the mechanisms of stability and change.

One hypothesized mechanism, called the "corresponsive principle" (Roberts, Wood, & Caspi, 2008) has some empirical support: Individuals, particularly in late adolescence and early adulthood, seek out environments that support—and experiences that serve to reinforce—their personality traits (Lüdtke, Roberts, Trautwein, & Nagy, 2011). Over time, people settle into these niches, which serves to stabilize personality. Thus, assessment of current life circumstances may reveal possible points of intervention to support personality change, especially in younger individuals. Other mechanisms hypothesized by Roberts and colleagues (2008) include the "role continuity" principle (that having consistent life roles stabilizes personality), the "identity development" principle (that developing, committing to, and maintaining an identity serves to stabilize personality), and the "social investment" principle (that social roles carry expectations of increasingly mature traits). However, the latter two principles either have not been tested or counterevidence has accrued (Roberts, 2014). Much research remains to be done, which necessarily will require reliable, valid assessment.

## Conclusions

As mentioned previously, the NIMH has embarked on a new approach to psychopathology research using the RDoC matrix that emphasizes synthesis across (1) multiple dimensional domains (e.g., effortful control, self-knowledge), many of which are highly relevant to personality and its pathology, and (2) multiple units of analysis (e.g., from self-reports to brain circuitry). To date, other than by obtaining verbal responses to items or questions from the individuals themselves, either via self-report or interview, virtually every other potential method of personality assessment (e.g., informant reports, laboratory tasks, coded observations of natural behavior, coding from written records or documents) is underused, and our ability to link these assessments and the personality dimensions they represent with neurobiological processes is in its infancy.

It is outside the scope of this chapter to discuss even the relatively small amount of alternative-method research that exists, so we simply assert that these methods need to be used more frequently, and new paradigms need to be developed and tested rigorously if we hope to expand our knowledge of normal and pathological personality development–change and maintenance–stability by more than small increments.

Because of the relevance of personality for a broad range of psychopathology, PD research, which already has made great progress toward implementing a dimensional model, is well positioned to lead the field in developing new approaches to understanding personality and PD via innovative assessment methods. Given that the bedrock of scientific progress is reliable and valid quantification of empirical phenomena, our success at this endeavor truly rises and falls with the quality of our assessments, so we urge the field to take advantage of the all-too-rare opportunity to focus on assessment, represented by the NIMH's RDoC approach to move toward a broader and deeper understanding of personality and its pathology.

## REFERENCES

Achenbach, T. M. (2001). *Child Behavior Checklist for Ages 6–18*. Burlington: University of Vermont, Department of Psychiatry.

Achenbach, T. M., Krukowski, R. A., Dumenci, L., & Ivanova, M. Y. (2005). Assessment of adult psychopathology: Meta-analyses and implications of cross-informant correlations. *Psychological Bulletin, 131*, 361–382.

Ackerman, R. A., Witt, E. A., Donnellan, M. B., Trzesniewski, K. H., Robins, R. W., & Kashy, D. A. (2011). What does the Narcissistic Personality Inventory really measure? *Assessment, 18*, 67–87.

Aluja, A., Escorial, S., García, L. F., García, Ó., Blanch, A., & Zuckerman, M. (2013). Reanalysis of Eysenck's, Gray's, and Zuckerman's structural trait models based on a new measure: The Zuckerman–Kuhlman–Aluja Personality Questionnaire (ZKA-PQ). *Personality and Individual Differences, 54*(2), 192–196.

Aluja, A., Kuhlman, M., & Zuckerman, M. (2010). Development of the Zuckerman–Kuhlman–Aluja Personality Questionnaire (ZKA-PQ): A factor/facet version of the Zuckerman–Kuhlman Personality Questionnaire (ZKPQ). *Journal of Personality Assessment, 92*(5), 416–431.

Aluja, A., Rossier, J., García, L. F., Angleitner, A., Kuhlman, M., & Zuckerman, M. (2006). A cross-cultural shortened form of the ZKPQ (ZKPQ-50-cc) adapted to English, French, German, and Spanish languages. *Personality and Individual Differences, 41*(4), 619–628.

American Psychiatric Association. (2013). *Diagnostic and statistical manual of mental disorders* (5th ed.). Arlington, VA: Author.

Anderson, J. L., Sellbom, M., Bagby, R. M., Quilty, L. C., Veltri, C. O, Markon, K. E., et al. (2013). On the convergence between PSY-5 domains and PID-5 domains and facets: Implications for assessment of DSM-5 personality traits. *Assessment, 20*, 286–294.

Ashton, M. C., & Lee, K. (2001). A theoretical basis for the major dimensions of personality. *European Journal of Personality, 15*(5), 327–353.

Ashton, M. C., & Lee, K. (2007). Empirical, theoretical, and practical advantages of the HEXACO model of personality structure. *Personality and Social Psychology Review, 11*(2), 150–166.

Ashton, M. C., & Lee, K. (2008). The HEXACO model of personality structure and the importance of the H factor. *Personality and Social Psychology Compass, 2*(5), 1952–1962.

Ashton, M. C., Lee, K., de Vries, R. E., Hendrickse, J., & Born, M. P. (2012). The maladaptive personality traits of the Personality Inventory for DSM-5 (PID-5) in relation to the HEXACO personality factors and schizotypy/dissociation. *Journal of Personality Disorders, 26*(5), 641–659.

Ashton, M. C., Lee, K., Perugini, M., Szarota, P., de

Vries, R. E., Blas, L. D., et al. (2004). A six-factor structure of personality-descriptive adjectives: Solutions from psycholexical studies in seven languages. *Journal of Personality and Social Psychology, 86*(2), 356–366.

Bender, D. S., Morey, L. C., & Skodol, A. E. (2011). Toward a model for assessing level of personality functioning in DSM-5, part I: A review of theory and methods. *Journal of Personality Assessment, 93*(4), 332–346.

Benjamin, L. S. (1996). *Interpersonal diagnosis and treatment of personality disorders* (2nd ed.). New York: Guilford Press.

Benning, S. D., Patrick, C. J., Hicks, B. M., Blonigen, D. M., & Krueger, R. F. (2003). Factor structure of the Psychopathic Personality Inventory: Validity and implications for clinical assessment. *Psychological Assessment, 15,* 340–350.

Berghuis, H., Kamphuis, J. H., Verheul, R., Larstone, R., & Livesley, J. (2013). The General Assessment of Personality Disorder (GAPD) as an instrument for assessing the core features of personality disorders. *Clinical Psychology and Psychotherapy, 20*(6), 544–557.

Bernstein, D. P., Iscan, C., Maser, J., Boards of Directors of the Association for Research in Personality Disorders, & International Society for the Study of Personality Disorders. (2007). Opinions of personality disorder experts regarding the DSM-IV personality disorders classification system. *Journal of Personality Disorders, 21*(5), 536–551.

Blashfield, R. K., & Intoccia, V. (2000). Growth of the literature on the topic of personality disorders. *American Journal of Psychiatry, 157*(3), 472–473.

Bornstein, R. F. (2012). From dysfunction to adaption: An interactionist model of dependency. *Annual Review of Clinical Psychology, 8,* 291–316.

Cain, N. M., Pincus, A. L., & Ansell, E. B. (2008). Narcissism at the crossroads: Phenotypic description of pathological narcissism across clinical theory, social/personality psychology, and psychiatric diagnosis. *Clinical Psychology Review, 28*(4), 638–656.

Carlson, E. N., Vazire, S., & Oltmanns, T. F. (2013). Self-other knowledge asymmetries in personality pathology. *Journal of Personality, 81,* 155–170.

Claridge, G., & Broks, P. (1984). Schizotypy and hemisphere function: I. Theoretical considerations and the measurement of schizotypy. *Personality and Individual Differences, 5,* 633–648.

Clark, L. A. (1993). *Manual for the Schedule for Nonadaptive and Adaptive Personality.* Minneapolis: University of Minnesota Press.

Clark, L. A. (2007). Assessment and diagnosis of personality disorder: Perennial issues and emerging conceptualization. *Annual Review of Psychology, 58,* 227–258.

Clark, L. A., Livesley, W. J., & Morey, L. (1997). Personality disorder assessment: The challenge of construct validity. *Journal of Personality Disorders, 11,* 205–231.

Clark, L. A., & Ro, E. (2014a). *Interview-rated DSM-5-III alternative-model traits reflect DSM-IV/5, Section II personality disorder diagnoses with high fidelity.* Paper presented at the second annual conference of the North American Society for the Study of Personality Disorder, Boston.

Clark, L. A., & Ro, E. (2014b). Three-pronged assessment and diagnosis of personality disorder and its consequences: Personality functioning, pathological traits, and psychosocial disability. *Personality Disorders: Theory, Research, and Treatment, 5*(1), 55–69.

Clark, L. A., Simms, L. J., Wu, K. D., & Casillas, A. (2014). *Schedule for Nonadaptive and Adaptive Personality.* Notre Dame, IN: University of Notre Dame.

Clark, L. A., Vanderbleek, E., Shapiro, J., Nuzum, H., Allen, X., Daly, E. J., et al. (2015). The brave new world of personality disorder-trait specified: Effects of additional definitions on coverage, prevalence, and comorbidity. *Psychopathology Review, 2*(1), 52–82.

Clark, L. A., & Watson, D. B. (1995). Constructing validity: Basic issues in objective scale development. *Psychological Assessment, 7,* 309–319.

Clark, L. A., Watson, D., & Krueger, R. F. (2014). *DSM-5 Informant Personality Trait Rating Form (DSM-5-IRF).* Unpublished manuscript available from L. A. Clark, University of Notre Dame, Notre Dame, IN.

Cleckley, H. (1976). *The mask of sanity* (5th ed.). St. Louis, MO: Mosby.

Cooke, D. J., & Michie, C. (2001). Refining the construct of psychopathy: Towards a hierarchical model. *Psychological Assessment, 13,* 171–188.

Coolidge, F. L. (2000). *Coolidge Axis II Inventory: Manual.* Colorado Springs, CO: Author.

Coolidge, F. L., Segal, D. L., Cahill, B. S., & Simenson, J. T. (2010). Psychometric properties of a brief inventory for the screening of personality disorders: The SCATI. *Psychology and Psychotherapy: Theory, Research, and Practice, 83*(4), 395–405.

Coolidge, F. L., Segal, D. L., Klebe, K. J., Cahill, B. S., & Whitcomb, J. M. (2009). Psychometric properties of the coolidge correctional inventory in a sample of 3,962 prison inmates. *Behavioral Sciences and the Law, 27*(5), 713–726.

Coolidge, F. L., Thede, L. L., Stewart, S. E., & Segal, D. L. (2002). The Coolidge Personality and Neuropsychological Inventory for Children (CPNI): Preliminary psychometric characteristics. *Behavior Modification, 26*(4), 550–566.

Costa, P. T., Jr., & McCrae, R. R. (1992). *Revised NEO Personality Inventory (NEO-PI-R) and NEO Five-Factor Inventory (NEO-FFI) professional manual.* Odessa, FL: Psychological Assessment Resources.

Daly, E. J., & Clark, L. A. (2014). *Trait narcissism in the personality hierarchy.* Poster presented at the 28th annual meeting of the Society for Research in Psychopathology, Evanston, IL.

De Clercq, B., De Fruyt, F., Van Leeuwen, K., & Mervielde, I. (2006). The structure of maladaptive personality traits in childhood: A step toward an integrative developmental perspective for DSM-V. *Journal of Abnormal Psychology, 115*(4), 639–657.

De Clercq, B., De Fruyt, F., & Widiger, T. A. (2009). Integrating a developmental perspective in dimensional models of personality disorders. *Clinical Psychology Review, 29*(2), 154–162.

Decuyper, M., De Clercq, B., De Bolle, M., & De Fruyt, F. D. (2009). Validation of FFM PD counts for screen personality pathology and psychopathy in adolescence. *Journal of Personality Disorders, 23*(6), 587–605.

de Reus, R. J. M., van den Berg, J. F., & Emmelkamp, P. M. G. (2013). Personality diagnostic questionnaire 4+ is not useful as a screener in clinical practice. *Clinical Psychology and Psychotherapy, 20*(1), 49–54.

de Vries, R. E., & van Kampen, D. (2010). The HEXACO and 5DPT models of personality: A comparison and their relationships with psychopathy, egoism, pretentiousness, immorality, and Machiavellianism. *Journal of Personality Disorders, 24*(2), 244–257.

Durbin, C. E., & Klein, D. N. (2006). Ten-year stability of personality disorders among outpatients with mood disorders. *Journal of Abnormal Psychology, 115*(1), 75–84.

Eaton, N. R., Krueger, R. F., South, S. C., Simms, L. J., & Clark, L. A. (2011). Contrasting prototypes and dimensions in the classification of personality pathology: Evidence that dimensions, but not prototypes, are robust. *Psychological Medicine, 41*(6), 1151–1163.

Edmundson, M., Lynam, D. R., Miller, J. D., Gore, W. L., & Widiger, T. A. (2011). A five-factor measure of schizotypal personality traits. *Assessment, 18*, 321–334.

Emmons, R. A. (1984). Factor analysis and construct validity of the Narcissistic Personality Inventory. *Journal of Personality Assessment, 48*, 291–300.

Eysenck, H. J., & Eysenck, M. W. (1985). *Personality and individual differences.* New York: Plenum Press.

Farmer, R. F., & Goldberg, L. R. (2008). A psychometric evaluation of the revised temperament and character inventory (TCI-R) and the TCI-140. *Psychological Assessment, 20*(3), 281–291.

Feenstra, D. J., Hutsebaut, J., Verheul, R., & Busschbach, J. J. V. (2011). Severity Indices of Personality Problems (SIPP–118) in adolescents: Reliability and validity. *Psychological Assessment, 23*(3), 646–655.

Few, L. R., Miller, J. D., Rothbaum, A. O., Meller, S., Maples, J., Terry, D. P., Collins, B., et al. (2013). Examination of the Section III DSM-5 diagnostic system for personality disorders in an outpatient clinical sample. *Journal of Abnormal Psychology, 122,* 1057–1069.

First, M. B., & Gibbon, M. (2004). *The Structured Clinical Interview for DSM-IV Axis I Disorders (SCID-I) and the Structured Clinical Interview for DSM-IV Axis II disorders (SCID-II).* Hoboken, NJ: Wiley.

Fishler, P. H., Sperling, M. B., & Carr, A. C. (1990). Assessment of adult relatedness: A review of empirical findings from object relations and attachment theories. *Journal of Personality Assessment, 55*(3–4), 499–520.

Gaughan, E. T., Miller, J. D., & Lynam, D. R. (2012). Examining the utility of general models of personality in the study of psychopathy: A comparison of the HEXACO-PI-R and NEO PI-R. *Journal of Personality Disorders, 26*(4), 513–523.

Glover, N., Miller, J. D., Lynam, D. R., Crego, C., & Widiger, T. A. (2012). The five-factor narcissism inventory: A five-factor measure of narcissistic personality traits. *Journal of Personality Assessment, 94,* 500–512.

Goldberg, L. R. (1993). The structure of phenotypic personality traits. *American Psychologist, 48*(1), 26–34.

Gore, W. L., Presnall, J. R., Miller, J. D., Lynam, D. R., & Widiger, T. A. (2012). A five-factor measure of dependent personality traits. *Journal of Personality Assessment, 94,* 488–499.

Gunderson, J. G. (2013). Seeking clarity for future revisions of the personality disorders in DSM-5. *Personality Disorders: Theory, Research, and Treatment, 4*(4), 368–376.

Gunderson, J. G., Ronningstam, E., & Bodkin, A. (1990). The diagnostic interview for narcissistic patients. *Archives of General Psychiatry, 47,* 676–680.

Hare, R. D. (1970). *Psychopathy: Theory and research.* New York: Wiley.

Hare, R. D. (2003). *Manual for the Revised Psychopathy Checklist* (2nd ed.). Toronto: Multi-Health Systems.

Hare, R. D., Harpur, T. J., Hakstian, A. R., Forth, A. E., Hart, S. D., & Newman, J. P. (1990). The Revised Psychopathy Checklist: Reliability and factor structure. *Psychological Assessment, 2*(3), 338–341.

Hare, R. D., & Neumann, C. S. (2008). Psychopathy as a clinical and empirical construct. *Annual Review of Clinical Psychology, 4,* 217–246.

Harkness, A. R., Finn, J. A., McNulty, J. L., & Shields, S. M. (2012). The Personality Psychopathology–Five (PSY-5): Recent constructive replication and assessment literature review. *Psychological Assessment, 24*(2), 432–443.

Harkness, A. R., McNulty, J. L., Finn, J. A., Reynolds, S. M., Shields, S. M., & Arbisi, P. (2014). The MMPI-2-RF Personality Psychopathology Five (PSY-5-RF) scales: Development and validity research. *Journal of Personality Assessment, 96*(2), 140–150.

Harkness, A. R., Reynolds, S. M., & Lilienfeld, S. O. (2014). A review of systems for psychology and psychiatry: Adaptive systems, Personality Psychopathology Five (PSY-5), and the DSM-5. *Journal of Personality Assessment, 96*(2), 121–139.

Haslam, N. (2002). Kinds of kinds: A conceptual taxonomy of psychiatric categories. *Philosophy, Psychiatry, and Psychology, 9*(3), 203–217.

Hentschel, A. G., & Livesley, W. J. (2013a). Differentiating normal and disordered personality using the General Assessment of Personality Disorder (GAPD). *Personality and Mental Health, 7*(2), 133–142.

Hentschel, A. G., & Livesley, W. J. (2013b). The General Assessment of Personality Disorder (GAPD): Factor structure, incremental validity of self-pathology, and relations to DSM-IV personality disorders. *Journal of Personality Assessment, 95*(5), 479–485.

Hirschfeld, R. M. A., Klerman, G. L., Gough, H. G., Barrett, J., Korchin, S. J., & Chodoff, P. (1977). A measure of interpersonal dependency. *Journal of Personality Assessment, 41,* 610–618.

Huprich, S. K., & Greenberg, R. P. (2003). Advances in the assessment of object relations in the 1990s. *Clinical Psychology Review, 23*(5), 665–698.

Hyler, S. E. (1994). *Personality Diagnostic Questionnaire–4 (PDQ-4).* New York: New York State Psychiatric Institute.

Jane, J. S., Pagan, J. L., Turkheimer, E., Fiedler, E. R., & Oltmanns, T. F. (2006). The interrater reliability of the Structured Interview for DSM-IV Personality. *Comprehensive Psychiatry, 47*(5), 368–375.

Jones, A. (2005). An examination of three sets of MMPI-2 personality disorder scales. *Journal of Personality Disorders, 19*(4), 370–385.

Klein, M. H., Benjamin, L. S., Rosenfeld, R., Treece, C., Husted, J., & Greist, J. H. (1993). The Wisconsin Personality Disorders Inventory: Development, reliability, and validity. *Journal of Personality Disorders, 7*(4), 285–303.

Koelen, J. A., Luyten, P., Eurelings-Bontekoe, L., Diguer, L., Vermote, R., Lowyck, B., et al. (2012). The impact of level of personality organization on treatment response: A systematic review. *Psychiatry: Interpersonal and Biological Processes, 75*(4), 355–374.

Krueger, R. F., Derringer, J., Markon, K. E., Watson, D., & Skodol, A. E. (2012). Initial construction of a maladaptive personality trait model and inventory for DSM-5. *Psychological Medicine, 42,* 1879–1890.

Krueger, R. F., Derringer, J., Markon, K. E., Watson D., & Skodol, A. E. (2014). *Personality Inventory for DSM-5, Brief Form.* Washington, DC: American Psychiatric Press. Retrieved from *www.psychiatry.org/psychiatrists/practice/dsm/educational-resources/assessment-measures.*

Lee, K., & Ashton, M. C. (2005). Psychopathy, Machiavellianism, and narcissism in the Five-Factor Model and the HEXACO model of personality structure. *Personality and Individual Differences, 38,* 1571–1582.

Lenzenweger, M. F., Johnson, M. D., & Willett, J. B. (2004). Individual growth curve analysis illuminates stability and change in personality disorder features: The longitudinal study of personality disorders. *Archives of General Psychiatry, 61*(10), 1015–1024.

Lilienfeld, S. O., Patrick, C. J., Benning, S. D., Berg, J., Sellbom, M., & Edens, J. F. (2012). The role of fearless dominance in psychopathy: Confusions, controversies, and clarifications. *Personality Disorders: Theory, Research, and Treatment, 3*(3), 327–340.

Lilienfeld, S. O., & Widows, M. R. (2005). *Psychopathic Personality Inventory—Revised: Professional manual.* Lutz, FL: Psychological Assessment Resources.

Livesley, W. J. (2010). *General Assessment of Personality Disorder.* Port Huron, MI: Sigma Assessments Systems.

Livesley, W. J. (2012). Tradition versus empiricism in the current DSM-5 proposal for revising the classification of personality disorders. *Criminal Behavior and Mental Health, 22,* 81–90.

Livesley, W. J., & Jackson, D. N. (2010). *Manual for the Dimensional Assessment of Personality Pathology—Basic Questionnaire.* Port Huron, MI: Sigma Press.

Livesley, W. J., & Jang, K. L. (2005). Differentiating normal, abnormal, and disordered personality [Special issue]. *European Journal of Personality, 19*(4), 257–268.

Loas, G., Corcos, M., Perez-Diaz, F., Verrier, A., Guelfi, J. D., Halfon, O., et al. (2002). Criterion validity of the Interpersonal Dependency Inventory: A preliminary study on 621 addictive subjects. *European Psychiatry, 17,* 477–478.

Loranger, A. W., Janca, A., & Sartorius, N. (1997). *Assessment and diagnosis of personality disorders: The ICD-10 International Personality Disorder Examination (IPDE).* Cambridge, UK: Cambridge University Press.

Loranger, A. W., Lenzenweger, M. F., Gartner, A. F., Susman, V. L., Herzig, J., Zammit, G. K., et al. (1991). Trait–state artifacts and the diagnosis of personality disorders. *Archives of General Psychiatry, 48*(8), 720–728.

Lüdtke, O., Roberts, B. W., Trautwein, U., & Nagy, G. (2011). A random walk down university avenue: Life paths, life events, and personality trait change at the transition to university life. *Journal of Personality and Social Psychology, 101,* 620–637.

Lynam, D. R., Gaughan, E. T., Miller, J. D., Miller, D. J., Mullins-Sweatt, S., & Widiger, T. A. (2011). Assessing the basic traits associated with psychopathy: Development and validation of the elemental psychopathy assessment. *Psychological Assessment, 23,* 108–124.

Lynam, D. R., Loehr, A., Miller, J. D., & Widiger, T. A. (2012). A five-factor measure of avoidant personality: The FFAvA. *Journal of Personality Assessment, 94,* 466–474.

Lynam, D. R., & Widiger, T. A. (2001). Using the five-factor model to represent DSM-IV personality disorders: An expert consensus approach. *Journal of Abnormal Psychology, 110,* 401–412.

Markon, K. E., Quilty, L. C., Bagby, R. M., & Krueger,

R. F. (2013). The development and psychometric properties of an informant-report form of the PID-5. *Assessment, 20,* 370–383.

Maxwell, K., Donnellan, M. B., Hopwood, C. J., & Ackerman, R. A. (2011). The two faces of Narcissus?: An empirical comparison of the Narcissistic Personality Inventory and the Pathological Narcissism Inventory. *Personality and Individual Differences, 50*(5), 577–582.

McDermut, W., & Zimmerman, M. (2008). Personality disorders, personality traits, and defense mechanisms measures. In A. J. Rush, M. B. First, & D. Blacker (Eds.) *Handbook of psychiatric measures* (2nd ed., pp. 687–729). Arlington, VA: American Psychiatric Publishing.

McGlashan, T. H., Grilo, C. M., Sanislow, C. A., Ralevski, E., Morey, L. C., Gunderson, J. G., et al. (2005). Two-year prevalence and stability of individual DSM-IV criteria for schizotypal, borderline, avoidant, and obsessive–compulsive personality disorders: Toward a hybrid model of Axis II disorders. *American Journal of Psychiatry, 162*(5), 883–889.

Mervielde, I., & De Fruyt, F. (1999). Construction of the Hierarchical Personality Inventory for Children (HiPIC). In I. Mervielde, I. Deary, F. De Fruyt, & F. Ostendorf (Eds.), *Personality psychology in Europe* (Vol. 7, pp. 107–127). Tilburg, The Netherlands: Tilburg University Press.

Mervielde, I., & De Fruyt, F. (2002). Assessing children's traits with the Hierarchical Personality Inventory for Children. In B. De Raad & M. Perugini (Eds.), *Big Five assessment* (pp. 129–146). Seattle: Hogrefe & Huber.

Miller, J. D., Bagby, R. M., Pilkonis, P. A., Reynolds, S. K., & Lynam, D. R. (2005). A simplified technique for scoring DSM-IV personality disorders with the Five-Factor Model. *Assessment, 12,* 404–415.

Miller, J. D., Gaughan, E. T., Pryor, L. R., Kamen, C., & Campbell, W. K. (2009). Is research using the Narcissistic Personality Inventory relevant for understanding narcissistic personality disorder? *Journal of Research in Personality, 43,* 482–488.

Miller, J. D., & Lynam, D. R. (2012). An examination of the psychopathic personality inventory's nomological network: A meta-analytic review. *Personality Disorders: Theory, Research, and Treatment, 3*(3), 305–326.

Miller, J. D., Maple, J., Few, L. R., Morse, J. Q., Yaggi, K. E., & Pilkonis, P. A. (2010). Using clinician-rated Five-Factor Model data to score the DSM-IV personality disorders. *Journal of Personality Assessment, 92,* 296–305.

Miller, J. D., Pilkonis, P. A., & Morse, J. Q. (2004). Five-factor model prototypes for personality disorders: The utility of self-report and observer ratings. *Assessment, 11,* 127–138.

Millon, T., & Bloom, C. (2008). *The Millon Inventories: A practitioner's guide to personalized clinical assessment* (2nd ed.). New York: Guilford Press.

Morey, L. C. (2014). The Personality Assessment Inventory. In R. P. Archer & S. R. Smith (Eds.), *Personality assessment* (2nd ed., pp. 181–228). New York: Routledge/Taylor & Francis Group.

Morey, L. C., Berghuis, H., Bender, D. S., Verheul, R., Krueger, R. F., & Skodol, A. E. (2011). Toward a model for assessing level of personality functioning in DSM-5, part II: Empirical articulation of a core dimension of personality pathology. *Journal of Personality Assessment, 93*(4), 347–353.

Morey, L. C., Hopwood, C. J., Markowitz, J. C., Gunderson, J. G., Grilo, C. M., McGlashan, T. H., et al. (2012). Comparison of alternative models for personality disorders, II: 6-, 8- and 10-year follow-up. *Psychological Medicine, 42*(8), 1705–1713.

Morey, L. C., Krueger, R. F., & Skodol, A. E. (2013). The hierarchical structure of clinician ratings of proposed DSM-5 pathological personality traits. *Journal of Abnormal Psychology, 122*(3), 836–841.

Morgan, T. A., & Clark, L. A. (2010). Passive–submissive and active–emotional trait dependency: Evidence for a two-factor model. *Journal of Personality, 78*(4), 1325–1352.

Mullins-Sweatt, S., Edmundson, M., Sauer-Zavala, S., Lynam, D. R., Miller, J. D., & Widiger, T. A. (2012). Five-factor measure of borderline personality traits. *Journal of Personality Assessment, 94*(5), 475–487.

Okada, M., & Oltmanns, T. F. (2009). Comparison of three self-report measures of personality pathology. *Journal of Psychopathology and Behavioral Assessment, 31,* 358–367.

Oltmanns, T. F., Gleason, M. E. J., Klonsky, E. D., & Turkheimer, E. (2005). Meta-perception for pathological personality traits: Do we know when others think that we are difficult? *Consciousness and Cognition, 14,* 739–751.

Oltmanns, T. F., & Turkheimer, E. (2006). Perceptions of self and others regarding pathological personality traits. In R. F. Krueger & J. Tackett (Eds.), *Personality and psychopathology: Building bridges* (pp. 71–111). New York: Guilford Press.

Paris, J. (2013). Anatomy of a debacle: Commentary on "Seeking clarity for future revisions of the personality disorders in DSM-5." *Personality Disorders: Theory, Research, and Treatment, 4*(4), 377–378.

Parker, G., Both, L., Olley, A., Hadzi-Pavlovic, D., Irvine, P., & Jacobs, G. (2002). Defining disordered personality functioning. *Journal of Personality Disorders, 16*(6), 503–522.

Parker, G., Hadzi-Pavlovic, D., Both, L., Kumar, S., Wilhelm, K., & Olley, A. (2004). Measuring disordered personality functioning: To love and to work reprised. *Acta Psychiatrica Scandinavica, 110*(3), 230–239.

Pfohl, B., Blum, N., & Zimmerman, M. (1997). *Structured Interview for DSM-IV Personality: SIDP-IV.* Washington, DC: American Psychiatric Press.

Pilkonis, P. A., Kim, Y., Proietti, J. M., & Barkham, M. (1996). Scales for personality disorders developed from the Inventory of Interpersonal Problems. *Journal of Personality Disorders, 10,* 355–369.

Pincus, A. L. (2013). The Pathological Narcissism Inventory. In J. S. Ogrodniczuk (Ed.), *Understanding and treating pathological narcissism* (pp. 93–110). Washington, DC: American Psychological Association.

Pincus, A. L., Ansell, E. B., Pimentel, C. A., Cain, N. M., Wright, A. G. C., & Levy, K. N. (2009). Initial construction and validation of the Pathological Narcissism Inventory. *Psychological Assessment, 21,* 365–379.

Quilty, L. C., Ayearst, L., Chmielewski, M., Pollock, B. G., & Bagby, R. M. (2013). The psychometric properties of the Personality Inventory for DSM-5 in an APA DSM-5 field trial sample. *Assessment, 20,* 362–369.

Raine, A. (1991). The SPQ: A scale for the assessment of schizotypal personality based on DSM-III-R criteria. *Schizophrenia Bulletin, 17,* 555–564.

Raskin, R. N., & Hall, C. S. (1979). Narcissistic Personality Inventory. *Psychological Reports, 45*(2), 590.

Raskin, R. N., & Hall, C. S. (1981). The Narcissistic Personality Inventory: Alternate form reliability and further evidence of construct validity. *Journal of Personality Assessment, 45,* 159–162.

Ro, E., & Clark, L. A. (2013). Interrelations between psychosocial functioning and adaptive- and maladaptive-range personality traits. *Journal of Abnormal Psychology, 122*(3), 822–835.

Ro, E., Stringer, D., & Clark, L. A. (2012). The Schedule for Nonadaptive and Adaptive Personality: A useful tool for diagnosis and classification of personality disorder. In T. A. Widiger (Ed.), *Oxford handbook of personality disorders* (pp. 58–81). New York: Oxford University Press.

Roberts, B. W. (2014). *Personality trait development in adulthood*. Paper presented at the 4th Purdue Symposium on Psychological Sciences, West Lafayette, IN.

Roberts, B. W., & DelVecchio, W. F. (2000). The rank-order consistency of personality traits from childhood to old age: A quantitative review of longitudinal studies. *Psychological Bulletin, 126,* 3–25.

Roberts, B. W., Walton, K. E., & Viechtbauer, W. (2006). Patterns of mean-level change in personality traits across the life course: A meta-analysis of longitudinal studies. *Psychological Bulletin, 132,* 1–25.

Roberts, B. W., Wood, D., & Caspi, A. (2008). The development of personality traits in adulthood. In O. P. John, R. W. Robins, & L. A. Pervin (Eds.), *Handbook of personality psychology: Theory and research* (3rd ed., pp. 375–398). New York: Guilford Press.

Rossi, G., Elklit, A., & Simonsen, E. (2010). Empirical evidence for a four-factor framework of personality disorder organization: Multigroup confirmatory factor analysis of the Millon Clinical Multiaxial Inventory–III personality disorder scales across Belgian and Danish data samples. *Journal of Personality Disorders, 24*(1), 128–150.

Rossier, J., Aluja, A., García, L. F., Angleitner, A., De Pascalis, V., Wang, W., et al. (2007). The cross-cultural generalizability of Zuckerman's alternative five-factor model of personality. *Journal of Personality Assessment, 89*(2), 188–196.

Samuel, D. B., Edmundson, M., & Widiger, T. A. (2011). Five factor model prototype matching scores: Convergence within alternative methods. *Journal of Personality Disorders, 25*(5), 571–585.

Samuel, D. B., Hopwood, C. J., Ansell, E. B., Morey, L. C., Sanislow, C. A., Markowitz, J. C., et al. (2011). Comparing the temporal stability of self-report and interview assessed personality disorder. *Journal of Abnormal Psychology, 120*(3), 670–680.

Samuel, D. B., Riddell, A. D. B., Lynam, D. R., Miller, J. D., & Widiger, T. A. (2012). A five-factor measure of obsessive–compulsive personality traits. *Journal of Personality Assessment, 94,* 456–465.

Samuel, D. B., & Widiger, T. A. (2004). Clinicians' personality descriptions of prototypic personality disorders. *Journal of Personality Disorders, 18*(3), 286–308.

Samuel, D. B., & Widiger, T. A. (2008). A meta-analytic review of the relationships between the five-factor model and DSM-IV-TR personality disorders: A facet level analysis. *Clinical Psychology Review, 28*(8), 1326–1342.

Saulsman, L. M., & Page, A. C. (2004). The five-factor model and personality disorder empirical literature: A meta-analytic review. *Clinical Psychology Review, 23*(8), 1055–1085.

Shea, M. T. (1992). Some characteristics of the Axis II criteria sets and their implications for assessment of personality disorders. *Journal of Personality Disorders, 6,* 377–381.

Simms, L. J. (2014, March). *The CAT-PD Project: Introducing an integrative model and efficient measure of personality disorder traits*. Symposium presented at the annual meeting of the Society for Personality Assessment, Arlington, VA.

Simms, L. J., & Clark, L. A. (2006). The Schedule for Nonadaptive and Adaptive Personality (SNAP): A dimensional measure of traits relevant to personality and personality pathology. In S. Strack (Ed.), *Differentiating normal and abnormal personality* (pp. 431–450). New York: Springer.

Simms, L. J., Goldberg, L. R., Roberts, J. E., Watson, D., Welte, J., & Rotterman, J. H. (2011). Computerized adaptive assessment of personality disorder: Introducing the CAT–PD Project. *Journal of Personality Assesment, 93,* 380–389.

Smith, T. E. (1993). Measurement of object relations: A review. *Journal of Psychotherapy Practice and Research, 2*(1), 19–37.

Smith, T. L., Klein, M. H., & Benjamin, L. S. (2003). Validation of the Wisconsin Personality Disorders

Inventory-IV with the SCID-II. *Journal of Personality Disorders, 17*(3), 173–187.

Strack, S. (2008). *Essentials of Millon™ Inventories assessment* (3rd ed.). Hoboken, NJ: Wiley.

Stricker, G., & Healey, B. J. (1990). Projective assessment of object relations: A review of the empirical literature. *Psychological Assessment, 2*(3), 219–230.

Tackett, J. L., Kushner, S. C., Josephs, R. A., Harden, K. P., Page-Gould, E., & Tucker-Drob, E. (2014). Hormones: Empirical contribution: Cortisol reactivity and recovery in the context of adolescent personality disorder. *Journal of Personality Disorders, 28*(1), 25–39.

Tellegen, A., & Atkinson, G. (1974). Openness to absorbing and self-altering experiences ("absorption"), a trait related to hypnotic susceptibility. *Journal of Abnormal Psychology, 83*(3), 268–277.

Thomas, K. M., Yalch, M. M., Krueger, R. F., Wright, A. G., Markon, K. E., & Hopwood, C. J. (2013). The convergent structure of DSM-5 personality trait facets and five-factor model trait domains. *Assessment, 20*, 308–311.

Tragesser, S. L., Solhan, M., Brown, W. C., Tomko, R. L., Bagge, C., & Trull, T. J. (2010). Longitudinal associations in borderline personality disorder features: Diagnostic Interview for Borderlines—Revised (DIB-R) scores over time. *Journal of Personality Disorders, 24*(3), 377–391.

Trull, T., & Widiger, T. A. (1997). *Structured Interview for the Five-Factor Model*. Odessa, FL: Psychological Assessment Resources.

Trull, T., Widiger, T. A., Useda, J. D., Holcomb, J., Doan, B.-T., Axelrod, S. R., et al. (1998). A structured interview for the assessment of the five-factor model of personality. *Psychological Assessment, 10*, 229–240.

Tyrer, P. (1988). *Personality disorders: Diagnosis, management and course*. London: Wright.

Tyrer, P., Crawford, M., Mulder, R., Blashfield, R., Farnam, A., Fossati, A., et al. (2011). The rationale for the reclassification of personality disorder in the 11th revision of the *International Classification of Diseases* (ICD-11). *Personality and Mental Health, 5*(4), 246–259.

van Kampen, D. (2006). The Dutch DAPP-BQ: Improvements, lower- and higher-order dimensions, and relationship with the 5DPT. *Journal of Personality Disorders, 20*(1), 81–101.

van Kampen, D. (2009). Personality and psychopathology: A theory-based revision of Eysenck's PEN model. *Clinical Practice and Epidemiology in Mental Health, 5*, 9–21.

van Kampen, D. (2012). The 5-dimensional personality test (5DPT): Relationships with two lexically based instruments and the validation of the absorption scale. Journal of *Personality Assessment, 94*(1), 92–101.

Verheul, R., Andrea, H., Berghout, C. C., Dolan, C., Busschbach, J. J. V., van der Kroft, P. J. A., et al. (2008). Severity Indices of Personality Problems (SIPP-118): Development, factor structure, reliability, and validity. *Psychological Assessment, 20*(1), 23–34.

Wakefield, J. C. (1992). The concept of mental disorder: On the boundary between biological facts and social values. *American Psychologist, 47*, 373–388.

Wakefield, J. C. (2013). DSM-5 and the general definition of personality disorder. *Clinical Social Work Journal, 41*(2), 168–183.

Watson, D., Stasik, S., Ro, E., & Clark, L. A. (2013). Integrating normal and pathological personality: Relating the DSM-5 trait dimensional model to general traits of personality. *Assessment, 20*(3), 312–326.

Weiss, D. J. (1985). Adaptive testing by computer. *Journal of Consulting and Clinical Psychology, 53*, 774–789.

Widiger, T. A., & Boyd, S. E. (2009). *Personality disorders assessment instruments*. In James N., Butcher (Ed.) *Oxford handbook of personality assessment* (pp. 336–363). New York: Oxford University Press.

Widiger, T. A., Trull, T. J., Clarkin, J. F., Sanderson, C., & Costa, P. T., Jr. (2002). A description of the DSM-IV personality disorders with the five-factor model of personality. In P. T. Costa, Jr., & T. A. Widiger (Eds.), *Personality disorders and the five-factor model of personality* (2nd ed., pp. 89–99). Washington DC: American Psychological Association.

Williams, K. M., Paulhus, D. L., & Hare, R. D. (2007). Capturing the four-factor structure of psychopathy in college students via self-report. *Journal of Personality Assessment, 88*(2), 205–219.

Wink, P. (1991). Two faces of narcissism. *Journal of Personality and Social Psychology, 61*, 590–597.

World Health Organization. (2001). *ICF: International classification of functioning, disability, and health*. Geneva, Switzerland: Author.

Wright, A. G. C., Pincus, A. L., & Lenzenweger, M. F. (2012). Interpersonal development, stability, and change in early adulthood. *Journal of Personality, 80*(5), 1339–1372.

Wright, A. G. C., & Simms, L. J. (2014). On the structure of personality disorder traits: Conjoint analyses of the CAT-PD, PID-5, and NEO-PI-3 trait models. *Personality Disorders: Theory, Research, and Treatment, 5*(1), 43–54.

Zanarini, M. C., Frankenburg, F. R., Hennen, J., & Silk, K. R. (2003). The longitudinal course of borderline psychopathology: 6-year prospective follow-up of the phenomenology of borderline personality disorder. *American Journal of Psychiatry, 160*(2), 274–283.

Zanarini, M., Frankenburg, F. R., & Vujanovic, A. A. (2002). Inter-rater and test–retest reliability of the Revised Diagnostic Interview for Borderlines. *Journal of Personality Disorders, 16*, 270–276.

Zanarini, M. C., Skodol, A. E., Bender, D., Dolan, R., Sanislow, C., Schaefer, E., et al. (2000). The collaborative longitudinal personality disorders study: Reliability of Axis I and II diagnoses. *Journal of Personality Disorders, 14*(4), 291–299.

Zimmerman, M. (1994). Diagnosing personality disorders: A review of issues and research methods. *Archives of General Psychiatry, 51,* 225–245.

Zimmerman, M., Rothschild, L., & Chelminski, I. (2005). The prevalence of DSM-IV personality disorders in psychiatric outpatients. *American Journal of Psychiatry, 162*(10), 1911–1918.

Zimmermann, J., Benecke, C., Bender, D. S., Skodol, A. E., Schauenburg, H., Cierpka, M., et al. (2014). Assessing DSM-5 level of personality functioning from videotaped clinical interviews: A pilot study with untrained and clinically inexperienced students. *Journal of Personality Assessment, 96*(4), 397–409.

Zuckerman, M. (2008). Zuckerman–Kuhlman Personality Questionnaire (ZKPQ): An operational definition of the Alternative Five Factorial Model of Personality. In G. J. Boyle, G. Matthews, & D. H. Saklofski (Eds.), *The Sage handbook of personality theory and assessment: Vol. 2. Personality* (pp. 219–238). Thousand Oaks, CA: SAGE.

Zuckerman, M., & Cloninger, C. R. (1996). Relationships between Cloninger's, Zuckerman's, and Eysenck's dimensions of personality. *Personality and Individual Differences, 21,* 283–285.

Zuckerman, M., Kuhlman, D. M., Joireman, J., Teta, P., & Kraft, M. (1993). A comparison of three structural models for personality: The Big Three, the Big Five, and the Alternative Five. *Journal of Personality and Social Psychology, 65*(4), 757–768.

# CHAPTER 21

# Clinical Assessment

John F. Clarkin, W. John Livesley, and Kevin B. Meehan

> I suppose it is tempting, if the only tool you have is a hammer, to treat everything as if it were a nail.
> —Maslow (1966)

As the conception of personality dysfunction has become more differentiated and complex, and the treatment options have grown, the need for more precise assessment strategies has become evident. For maximum efficiency and treatment effectiveness, differentiated assessment and treatment tailored to the individual are intimately related. Initial clinical assessment provides not only the information needed to construct a formulation and plan treatment but also an opportunity to begin shaping the treatment alliance, building a commitment to change, and encouraging the patients' self-appraisal and self-reflection.

There are a limited number of ways the clinician may approach the clinical assessment of personality disorders (PDs) (Beutler, Someah, Kimpara, & Miller, 2016). First, many clinicians traditionally utilize specific categorical diagnoses, such as borderline or antisocial PD, as articulated by DSM-5 (American Psychiatric Association [APA], 2013). Second, clinicians often use their own personal approach to assessment, related to their training, theoretical orientation, and experience. PD diagnoses are often established by a clinical interview, guided by the diagnostic criteria, though in some cases a self-report measure or a structured diagnostic interview is utilized as well. Third, clinicians then often institute one of the empirically supported treatments (ESTs) recommended for that categorical diagnosis. Most clinicians label themselves as "eclectic" in orientation, so the assessment guides their choice of treatment strategies.

Our goal is to question the assumptions underlying each step in this assessment process, and to offer guidelines for an integrated set of options from which a clinician can draw for the assessment of personality dysfunction. To set the stage for our review of assessment recommendations, we first consider the limitations of assessment based on diagnostic categories, the need to assess severity of dysfunction, the growing focus on domains of dysfunction rather than categorical classification, and, finally, the nature of PD. These considerations are important in shaping current approaches to assessment of individuals with suspected personality pathology. We then discuss various assessment strategies that attempt to link a coherent and planned assessment to case formulation and subsequent treatment strategies. Most of these assessment methods eschew a categorical diagnostic approach to personality dysfunction, and opt instead for dimensional assessment of crucial domains of function–dysfunction. Finally, we discuss the importance of integrating assessment into the ongoing treatment process. In doing so, we seek to outline an approach to evaluating personality dysfunction that integrates a conceptualization of the psychopathology with diagnosis and treatment planning.

## Characterizing Personality Dysfunction

There is growing recognition that diagnostic assessment as guided by DSM-5 (APA, 2013) is inadequate for assessment and its relationship to case formulation and treatment planning. We review the reasons for this conclusion and point to other useful articulations.

### Categorical Approaches to PD Diagnosis

Diagnostic practice and contemporary treatments implicitly consider all individuals meeting a diagnostic threshold to be the same. Unfortunately, this clearly is not the case. The multiple shortcomings of categorical diagnoses include extensive diagnostic overlap, limited structural validity, and poor coverage. Since nearly 40% of patients with PDs cannot be adequately diagnosed using DSM-IV (Westen & Arkowitz-Westen, 1998), PD not otherwise specified is often the most common diagnosis in clinical practice (Verheul & Widiger, 2004). This poses significant limitations for treatment. In fact, personality pathology encompasses most aspects of personality, creating enormous heterogeneity, even among those with the same categorical diagnosis. Responding to this heterogeneity with appropriate levels of treatment intensity and interventions requires a thorough evaluation of all aspects of personality dysfunction.

Patients with the same categorical diagnosis may evidence dissimilar symptom features that have significant implications for treatment planning. For example, for those meeting criteria for borderline personality disorder (BPD), it is not uncommon to present with high levels of affective dysregulation that disorganize cognitive control when distress is elevated. For such patients, treatment planning would therefore emphasize regulating emotional arousal to prevent distress that overwhelms cognitive control. However, for other patients with BPD who seek to overcontrol emotional experiences and become avoidant of contexts that have the potential for distress, treatment planning may instead emphasize reducing efforts to avoid and overcontrol affects, and instead increase activity and social engagement. Neither of these disparate treatment paths would be indicated by a diagnosis of BPD alone.

Patients with the same diagnosis may also evidence dissimilar trait features that have implications for adaptive functioning. For example, some patients with BPD have elevated trait features of sensation seeking and recklessness. These particular traits are more commonly associated with antisocial personality disorder (ASPD). The need for stimulation and excitement associated with these traits contributes to the crises and maladaptive lifestyles often associated with borderline pathology. The management of such patients is likely to differ from that of other patients with BPD who are more socially avoidant. This suggests the need to assess all traits, not just the narrow range described by each DSM-IV/DSM-5 diagnosis.

Last, patients with the same diagnosis may also evidence *within-individual heterogeneity* of like-symptom and trait features. Research utilizing experience sampling methods is being increasingly utilized to evaluate the intraindividual variability of PD features in daily social interactions, and findings have important implications for how we conceptualize the ebb and flow of personality pathology over time. For example, while patients with BPD have been found to evidence higher overall mean levels of negative affect as compared to controls, greater affective variability was observed with regard to positive affect (Russell, Moskowitz, Zuroff, Sookman, & Paris, 2007); however, at a trait level, a given patient with BPD may present with heightened negative affect but overall normative levels of positive affect. The flux of positive emotion may be empirically distinctive and clinically disruptive, such that the continual experience of having and then losing a good feeling may itself be a contributor to heightened distress. However, neither DSM-5 PD symptoms nor trait domains capture the specific nature of oscillations within pathological dispositions; therefore, this kind of heterogeneity is not well characterized by categorical diagnoses.

Personality pathology involves all aspects of personality that lead to diverse problems, including symptoms, dysregulation of emotions and impulses, interpersonal problems, and self-identity pathology. Evaluation of these domains is important because the evidence suggests that treatment outcome is domain-specific (Piper & Joyce, 2001): interventions that lead to change for one set of problems do not necessarily work for another. This suggests that interventions need to be selected according to the domain being treated rather than a global categorical diagnosis.

## Dimensional Approaches to PD Diagnosis

In response to the growing concerns about categorical approaches to PD diagnosis, a number of dimensions of pathology have been clinically articulated and empirically evaluated to better capture the complexity of the psychopathology. Dimensional models are more consistent with data characterizing personality pathology than category models (Trull & Durrett, 2006). Also, as noted earlier, the extensive heterogeneity among patients with the same categorical diagnosis severely limits the value of a diagnosis in treatment planning. Dimensional models account for heterogeneity better, and provide a comprehensive assessment of both adaptive and maladaptive features. The comprehensiveness of dimensional models also means that they can accommodate important forms of personality pathology not recognized by the DSM system, such as sadistic and oppositional traits. A number of dimensions are discussed, many of which are not mutually exclusive. However, as can be seen in the DSM-5 Section III Model (APA, 2013), efforts to integrate these disparate dimensions into a comprehensive system have proved challenging.

## Dimensions of Severity

For personality pathology, severity has been found to predict outcome better than diagnostic category (Crawford, Koldobsky, Mulder, & Tyrer, 2011). Despite growing recognition that severity is central to treatment planning, the assessment of severity remains a subject of confusion. Several proposals have been advanced, and we review a few here. However, it is useful to keep in mind that while researchers are looking for the optimal way to arrive at a summary score for severity, such a rating may not be particularly useful to the clinician. It may be more useful to identify areas of deficit indicative of severity that are likely to be modifiers of treatment response.

Parker was among the first to highlight the significance of severity and the problem of confounding severity and personality category (see Parker & Barrett 2000). Parker and colleagues (2004) recommended a general rating based on failures in cooperating and coping with the interpersonal world. Bornstein (1998) also recommended a severity rating of global personality pathology but focused on the dysfunction suffered by the individual patient. He noted areas of dysfunction, such as distorted cognition, inappropriate affectivity, impaired interpersonal functioning, and impulse control problems. Widiger, Costa, and McCrae (2002) recommended using the Global Assessment of Functioning (GAF) score. Tyrer and Johnson (1996) viewed severity as the extent of comorbidity—the sum of all criteria observed across all PD. In a reanalysis of a longitudinal study, Hopwood and colleagues (2011) found that generalized severity was most predictive of current and future dysfunction, but personality style indicated specific areas of difficulty. Based on their findings, this group recommended a three-part assessment: (1) global rating of severity (sum of all PD criteria as proposed by Tyrer & Johnson, 1996), (2) ratings of stylistic elements of PD (captured as factors representing peculiarity, withdrawal, fearfulness, instability, and deliberateness), and (3) a rating of normative traits.

Although there is little agreement, a common approach is to base a rating of severity on the amount of personality pathology present as indexed by either the number of DSM-5 PDs or total number of diagnostic criteria. Thus, a case meeting criteria for a single disorder is considered less severe than a case meeting criteria for two or more disorders, and a case manifesting 15 diagnostic criteria is considered more severe than one showing 10 criteria. Although there is evidence supporting this assumption (Dimaggio et al., 2013), the method equates severity with breadth of pathology (the number of criteria present) and not with degree of impairment. Thus, it is conceivable for a patient to manifest a wide range of criteria that are all relatively mild.

## Trait Dimensions

Trait assessment is closely linked to intervention strategies because most interventions target specific traits in their environmental context, symptom clusters, or domains of dysfunction rather than global diagnoses (Leising & Zimmermann, 2011; Livesley, 2003; Sanderson & Clarkin, 2013). This is relevant not only to psychotherapy but also to the use of medication with BPD to target specific symptom clusters, such as cognitive dysregulation, emotional lability, and impulsivity (Soloff, 2000). Likewise, psychotherapeutic interventions focus on specific behaviors such as deliberate self-harm, and specific traits such as emotional dysregulation, aggression, and abandonment anxiety. Overall, the typical level of clinical intervention is at the level of specific primary traits or their component behaviors (Leising & Zimmermann, 2011).

However, clinicians and researchers alike often face the challenge of deciding which trait model to use. Although this appears to be a difficult problem due to multiple competing models, there are only two main choices: whether to use a model of normal personality or a specific model of PD. Alternative ways to classify PDs based on models of normal personality include Eysenck's three-dimensional model (1987; Eysenck & Eysenck, 1985), the five-factor approach (Costa & Widiger, 1994), Cloninger's biologically based model (1987; Svrakic, Whitehead, Przybeck, & Cloninger, 1993), and the interpersonal circumplex (Kiesler, 1986; Wiggins, 1982).

Dimensional assessment of traits can be accomplished by two questionnaires that were specifically designed to evaluate PD: the Schedule for Nonadaptive and Adaptive Personality (SNAP; Clark, 1993) and the Dimensional Assessment of Personality Pathology—Basic Questionnaire (DAPP-BQ; Livesley & Jackson, 2009). Both were developed using a "bottom-up" strategy that began with a representative pool of descriptive terms, then gradually built a final structure based on the empirical structure identified in the original pool. With the SNAP, the original descriptors were personality terms used in DSM-III, whereas the DAPP-BQ relied on terms identified through a broad literature search. Nevertheless, the final structure of the two measures is remarkably similar (Clark & Livesley, 1994; Harkness, 1992).

However, our preference is to use a clinically based model of assessment that incorporates traditional clinical concepts (Clark, 1990; Livesley, Jackson, & Schroeder, 1992; Livesley & Jang, 2000). There is a reasonable consensus that four broad factors provide an adequate representation of the trait structure of PD (Widiger & Simonsen, 2005). Table 21.1 lists the primary traits associated with each higher-order factor, and Table 21.2 defines each primary trait.

## Dimensionally Derived Types

There is a growing consensus that traits, as assessed by self-report questionnaires, must be transformed in some manner to provide more direct treatment relevant information. Even Krueger, who was so instrumental in inserting traits into DSM-5, Section III, notes that traits are abstract in terms of conceptualizing the specific patient (Krueger, Eaton, South, Clark, & Simms, 2010). A more "person-centered" approach recommended by these authors is to use statistical procedures such as finite mixture modeling to delineate groups of similar individuals based on a trait instrument, such as the SNAP. The emerging seven clusters of individuals reflect both normal and problematic adjustment. Clusters labeled "normal personality" (low on mistrust, aggression, self-harm, and eccentric perceptions), "worker bees" (high levels of positive temperament, propriety, and workaholism, and low aggression), and "repressors"

**TABLE 21.1. Traits Constellations and Primary Traits**

| Secondary domain | Primary trait |
|---|---|
| Emotional dysregulation | **Anxiousness** |
| | **Emotional lability:** |
| |     **Emotional reactivity** |
| |     **Emotional intensity** |
| | Pessimistic anhedonia |
| | **Submissiveness** |
| | **Insecure attachment** |
| | Cognitive dysregulation |
| | Need for approval |
| | Social apprehensiveness |
| | Oppositional |
| | Self-harming acts |
| | Self-harming ideas |
| Dissocial | **Callousness:** |
| |     **Lack of empathy/remorselessness** |
| |     **Exploitativeness** |
| |     **Egocentrism** |
| |     **Sadism** |
| |     **Hostile-dominance** |
| | Conduct problems |
| | Impulsivity |
| | Sensation seeking |
| | Narcissism |
| | Suspiciousness |
| Social avoidance | **Low affiliation** |
| | **Restricted emotional expression** |
| | Avoidant attachment |
| | Self containment |
| | Inhibited sexuality |
| | Attachment need |
| Compulsivity | **Orderliness** |
| | Conscientiousness |

*Note.* The most salient traits for each factor as shown in **bold**.

## TABLE 21.2. Primary Traits of PD

| Primary trait | Definition |
|---|---|
| Anxiousness | Readily feels fearful, worried, tense, and threatened; lifelong sense of tension and feeling "on the edge"; broods about unpleasant experiences, unable to divert attention from painful thoughts; unable to make decisions due to fear of making a mistake; pervasive sense of guilt |
| Attachment need | Strong need for attachment relationships; distressed by lack of intimacy |
| Avoidant attachment | Avoids attachment relationships; fearful of attachments; does not seek out others when stressed or distressed; shows little reaction to separations or reunions |
| Cognitive dysregulation | Thoughts tend to become disorganized when stressed; may experience brief stress psychosis; tends to experience feelings of depersonalization or derealization and show dissociative behavior; often manifests schizotypal cognition (e.g., mild paranoid thoughts, illusions, and pseudohallucinations) |
| Conduct problems | Violates social norms and laws; violent; resorts to threats and intimidation; often has a history of juvenile antisocial behavior; tends to engage in substance misuse; routinely prevaricates and rationalizes actions; deliberately flouts authority |
| Conscientiousness | Strong sense of duty and obligation; completes all tasks thoroughly and meticulously |
| Egocentrism | Preoccupied with self; perceptions dominated by own point of view, interests, and concerns; defines and pursues own needs without regard for those of others; believes he or she knows what is best for others |
| Emotional intensity | Feels and expresses emotions intensely; overreacts emotionally; exaggerates emotional significance of events |
| Emotional reactivity | Experiences frequent and unpredictable emotional changes; moody; irritable with low threshold for annoyance, impatient; intense, frequently and easily aroused to anger; poor anger control |
| Exploitativeness | Takes advantage of others for personal gain; charming and ingratiating when suites his or her own purpose; believes that others are easily manipulated or conned; considers self to be adroit at taking advantage of others |
| Hostile dominance | Antagonistic and unfriendly to others; verbally abusive; enjoys taking charge, assumes leadership roles, likes to influence others, frustrated when not in charge |
| Impulsivity | Does things on the spur of the moment; many actions unplanned or without much thought about the consequences; fails to follow established plans; impulsivity overrules previous experiences; hence, he or she appears not to learn from experience |
| Inhibited sexuality | Lacks interest in sexuality; derives little pleasure from sexual experiences; fearful of sexual relationships |
| Insecure attachment | Fears losing attachments; coping depends on presence of attachment figure; urgently seeks proximity with attachment figure when stressed; strongly protests separations; intolerant of aloneness; avoids being alone and plans adequate activities to avoid being alone |
| Lack of empathy | Does not notice or respond to others feelings or problems; has difficulty understanding others feelings; lacks guilt about the effects of own actions; unable to express remorse |
| Low affiliation | Seeks out situations that do not include other people; declines opportunities to socialize; does not initiate social contact |

*(continued)*

**TABLE 21.2.** *(continued)*

| Primary trait | Definition |
|---|---|
| Narcissism | Grandiose, exaggerates achievements and abilities, craves admiration; preoccupied with fantasies of unlimited success, power, brilliance, or beauty; feels and acts as if entitled; acts to be noticed; strong need for acceptance and approval |
| Need for approval | Strong need for demonstrations of acceptance and approval; constantly seeks reassurance that he or she is a worthy person |
| Oppositionality | Resists satisfactory performance of routine tasks, hence failing to meet others' requests and expectations; resents authority figures; lacks ambition, rarely takes the initiative; shows low levels of activity and fails to take control of own life; fails to get things done on time, "forgets" to do things; does not plan or organize ahead; passively resists cooperating with others |
| Orderliness | Methodical and organized; concerned with cleanliness; concerned with details, time, punctuality, schedules, and rules |
| Pessimistic anhedonia | Derives little pleasure for experiences or relationships; no sense of fun; pervasive feelings of hopelessness; negative expectations for the future; accentuates the negative; strongly adheres to negative beliefs |
| Restricted emotional expression | Does not express emotions; appears unemotional; avoids emotional situations; shows little reaction to emotionally arousing situations |
| Sadism | Cruel; humiliates and demeans others; fascinated by violence and torture; amused by/enjoys the suffering of others; considers others to be worthless; despises others; cynical |
| Self-containment | Reluctant to share personal information; avoids inadvertent self-disclosure; fears personal information may be used against self; self-reliant and self-sufficient; prefers to cope independently, does not to seek help from others; fears having to rely on others |
| Self-harming acts | Deliberate self-damaging acts (e.g., self-mutilation, drug overdoses) |
| Self-harming ideas | Frequent thoughts about suicide and hurting self; stress or distress readily activates thoughts of self-harm |
| Sensation seeking | Craves excitement; needs variety; has difficulty tolerating the normal or routine; reckless, enjoys taking unnecessary risks and does not heed his or her own limitations; denies the reality of personal danger |
| Social apprehensiveness | Fears hurt and rejection; poor social skills; uncertain about appropriate social behavior, awkward in social settings |
| Submissiveness | Subservient and unassertive; subordinates self and his or her own needs to those of others; passively follows the interests and desires of others; submits to abuse and intimidation to maintain relationships; seeks advice and reassurance about all courses of action; readily accepts others suggestions and often appears gullible |
| Suspiciousness | Mistrusts other people; hyperalert to signs of trickery or harm; searches for hidden meanings in events, questions others' loyalty, and often feels persecuted |

*Note.* Adapted from Livesley and Clarkin (2015) with permission from The Guilford Press.

(high levels of positive temperament and low levels of most other scales, including negative temperament, mistrust, and aggression) suggest various forms of adjustment. Other clusters manifested various combinations of traits suggesting personality dysfunction: "distressed–dependent" (high levels of negative temperament, self-harm, dependency, and detachment), "wild-oat spreaders" (high levels of positive temperament, exhibitionism, and entitlement), "severe PD" (elevated negative temperament, mistrust, manipulativeness, aggression, self-harm, eccentric perceptions, dependency, detachment, disinhibition, and impulsivity), and "rebels" (high aggression and low dependency). The appeal of this approach is that it transforms abstract trait dimensions into empirically based yet clinically recognizable types.

### DSM-5 Section III Model of Diagnosis and Assessment

The DSM-5 Section III model of diagnosis and related assessment is described by the study group as a "hybrid" approach, combining dimensional ratings of self and other functioning and dimensional assessment of traits. These dimensional ratings are combined with a categorical diagnosis of one of six PD categories. The DSM-5 proposal defined "self pathology" in terms of identity and self-directedness and "interpersonal pathology" as problems with intimacy and empathy.

Unfortunately, the proposed descriptions of both self and interpersonal pathology are too ambiguous for reliable clinical assessment. Also, the proposal fails to capture the basic idea that identity defines one's sense of self and place in the social contexts in which one lives. The suggestion that identity involves "experience of oneself as unique" may lead to identity being equated with narcissistic tendencies. It is also culturally bound, in that it seems to be more applicable to Western cultures than to cultures that emphasize connectedness to other persons (Mulder, 2012). Equally problematic is the description of self-directedness that confuses the motivational aspect of the self with the conceptually unrelated concept of prosocial behavior and the metacognitive process of self-reflection. Given these problems, we suggest an alternative scheme later in this chapter.

A major goal of the DSM-5 PD work group was to insert the dimensional trait approach to personality assessment and diagnosis into the official diagnostic system (Krueger & Markon, 2014). The empirical process of constructing self-report questionnaires using factor analysis to define homogeneous traits or domains of functioning/behavior has a long tradition in psychology (Clark, 2007). Most recently, Krueger and colleagues constructed the Personality Inventory for DSM-5 (PID-5; Krueger, Derringer, Markon, Watson, & Skodol, 2012) to assess personality traits highlighted in the DSM-5 Section III model. This 220-item assessment instrument reliably measures 25 specific traits of maladaptive personality functioning. The development of this instrument is in its infancy, and most psychometric assessments to date have been limited to nonclinical samples (Meehan & Clarkin, 2015). Krueger and Markon (2014) are quite enthusiastic about the inclusion of the empirically based trait assessment method in DSM-5 Section III. However, there are a number of difficulties with the use of the traits assessed by self-report for guiding treatment (see Meehan & Clarkin, 2015). For example, Hopwood, Wright, Ansell, and Pincus (2013) point out that conceptions of traits have emphasized stability and generality across situations, prioritizing between-person differences, whereas clinical practice often focuses on dynamic within-person processes. Clinical intervention is often focused on the interaction between the patient and the situational context experienced in a subjective way within which symptoms emerge. We describe later in this chapter how trait information can inform the clinical interview, or how the clinical interview can provide information to make ratings of patient traits.

### An Integrated Approach to Characterizing Personality Dysfunction

Although there is currently little consensus on how to define a PD, some trends are emerging that provide the outline of a practical clinical definition. The DSM-III (APA, 1980) definition of PD as maladaptive traits initially led to simple definitions based on having an extreme level of traits that are expressed rigidly or in maladaptive ways (Cloninger, 2000; Eysenck, 1987; Kiesler, 1986; Leary, 1957, Wiggins & Pincus, 1989). The idea has not proved useful because an extreme level of a trait does not necessarily imply disordered functioning (Parker &

Barrett, 2000; Verheul et al., 2008). Moreover, terms such as "maladaptive" and "inflexible" are too vague and poorly defined (Wakefield, 2008) for reliable assessment.

Definitions based solely on traits also fail to recognize that personality includes other features besides traits, such as motives, roles, goals, strategies, values, representations of self and others, and life narratives (McAdams, 1994; McAdams & Pals, 2006). Equally important, they neglect the integrating and organizing aspects of personality (Allport, 1961; Cervone & Shoda, 1999; McAdams, 1994; Rutter, 1987). As Millon (1996) noted, personality "is not a potpourri of unrelated traits and miscellaneous behaviors but a tightly knit organization of stable structures (e.g., internalized memories and self-images) and coordinated functions (e.g., unconscious mechanisms and cognitive processes)" (p. 13). Similarly, Mischel and Shoda (1995) noted that the "personality system functions literally as a whole—a unique network of organized interconnections among cognitions and affects, not a set of separate, independent discrete variables, forces, factors, or tendencies. The challenge becomes to understand the psychological meaning of the organization of the relationships within the person" (pp. 258–259). This aspect of personality is directly applicable to defining PD because the essential feature of disorder is an enduring disturbance of the organizational and integrative aspects of personality (Kernberg & Caligor, 2005; Livesley, 2003; Livesley & Jang, 2000; Rutter, 1987; Wakefield, 2008).

As background to this issue, we note the unfortunate divide between the study of normal and disordered personality. This divide has hindered the development of a definition of PD from benefiting from the evolution of an understanding of the self and advances in social-cognitive approaches. These approaches have emphasized the functional and adaptive aspects of the self (self-regulation, self-direction, and self-defense), as well as concepts of identity and object relations, leading to the recognition of the self as a causal agent, with growing emphasis on emotion as a motivating force (Carver, 2011; Carver & Scheier, 1998; Kernberg & Caligor, 2005; Mischel & Morf, 2003; Sheldon & Elliot, 1999). These are ideas that have obvious implications for conceptualizing the functional disturbances in self and interpersonal relationships. In the next section, we draw on ideas about the organizational component of personality, and the cognitive and motivational aspects of the self, to formulate a working definition of PD to guide assessment.

## PD as Adaptive Impairment

Defining PD as impairment in the organization and integration of personality immediately raises the question of what indicators are clinically useful in evaluating such a generalized impairment. Clinicians have traditionally focused on two general indicators: chronic interpersonal problems and an impaired sense of self or identity. General and interpersonal psychiatry consider impaired interpersonal functioning to be the core feature of PD (Hopwood et al., 2013; Pincus & Hopwood, 2012; Rutter, 1987; Vaillant & Perry, 1980). Rutter (1987), for example, defined PD as "characterized by a persistent, pervasive abnormality in social relationships and social functioning generally" (p. 454). In contrast, the psychoanalytic literature has focused on self pathology as illustrated by Kohut's (1971) description of the lack of a cohesive self-structure in narcissistic conditions and Kernberg's (1984) concept of identity diffusion (disorganized representations of self and others) in borderline personality organization. Interestingly, this clinical tradition predates and is consistent with more recent cognitive models of the self as a cohesive structure of self-schemas.

The conception of PD emerging from clinical practice is also consistent with ideas about the adaptive origins of personality. Personality structures presumably evolved because they fostered fitness in our remote ancestors. The gradual emergence of community living over the last 2 million years created the need for mechanisms to manage the problems created by social living. To function effectively in the small social groups that were the context in which many personality structures and mechanisms evolved, required the development of a sense of self or identity that defined one's place in the group, the capacity for attachment and intimacy, and the ability to function in an altruistic and prosocial manner. Combining this understanding of the adaptive functions of personality with clinical conceptions of PD suggests that the working definition of disorder involves at least one of the following: (1) an impaired sense of self and identity; (2) a seriously impaired capacity for intimacy and attachment; and/or (3) a poorly developed capacity for prosocial, altruistic, and cooperative behavior

(Livesley, 1998, 2003). The definition of PD in the proposed revisions for DSM-5 Section III drew on this conceptualization.

## Clinical Definition of PD

We propose an alternative approach that defines self pathology in terms of cognitive and motivational impairments (Livesley, 2003). The cognitive component is described as problems with the *differentiation* and *integration* of the person's knowledge of the self. Knowledge about the self accumulates during development through interaction with the social environment. As self-knowledge accumulates, the self takes structure. Poor differentiation of the self is manifested as an impoverished set of self-schemas or mental representations, lack of clarity or certainty about personal attributes, a sense of inner emptiness, and defective interpersonal boundaries. In parallel with the process of differentiation is an integrative process that combines items of self-knowledge or self-schemas into different images of the self, resulting ultimately in an autobiographical sense of self that organizes diverse aspects of self-knowledge into an overarching self-narrative. The interconnections created within self-knowledge form the basis for a subjective sense of personal unity, continuity, and coherence that characterizes an adaptive self-system (Harter, 2012; Toulmin, 1978). Problems of integration include lack of a sense of historicity or continuity in one's experience of the self, fragmentary self-representations, and disconnected self-states (Kernberg, 1984; Livesley, 2003).

The second component of the self is motivational: Meaningful goals contribute to the coherence of the self. Goals integrate by drawing together different aspects of personality, linking needs and wishes with the abilities and skills needed to attain them. It is this striving toward a goal that integrates, not its attainment (Allport, 1961). As Read, Jones, and Miller (1990) noted, "Behavioral organization becomes understandable in terms of the individuals goals, plans, resources, and beliefs" (p. 1060). Striving to attain goals contributes to a sense of personal autonomy and agency that gives meaning, direction, and purpose to life (Carver, 2011; Carver & Scheier, 1998; Shapiro, 1981).

The interpersonal component of PD is more straightforward. It involves impaired capacity for (1) intimacy, attachment, and affiliative relationships and (2) prosocial and cooperative behavior. In evolutionary terms, these may be considered impaired functioning in kinship and societal relationships, respectively. We describe later in this chapter how the clinical interview can provide information to assess these dimensions of personality.

## Methods for Assessing Personality Pathology

One can distinguish between the process and the content of clinical assessment. The process of assessment depends a great deal on the treatment context within which the clinician is working. Assessment by clinical interview is the time-honored and most easily used method in private practice and individual practitioners' offices. Clinic settings may combine the clinical interview with a limited number of self-report questionnaires. Research settings often replace the clinical interview with semistructured interviews to enhance reliability of diagnosis.

The content of the assessment is composed of problem areas or domains of dysfunction that are prominent in the current functioning of the patient, and are causing distress and dysfunction in relating to the environment. Reviews of psychotherapy research models of personality functioning and trait research have all guided the clinical focus to specific domains of dysfunction. Given the heterogeneity of patients who meet a particular PD diagnosis and the almost universal occurrence of "comorbidity" of the PDs, the transdiagnostic approach to treatment focused on specific domains of dysfunction is gaining in popularity. However, given the complexity of the human organism and its functioning, it is not surprising that there are differences in the domains of dysfunction emphasized by various clinical leaders and researchers.

### Considerations in Assessing Personality Pathology

The clinician who conducts the initial clinical assessment of an individual suspected of personality dysfunction or PD either explicitly or implicitly makes a number of decisions on the process and content of the assessment. We suggest that the clinician keep an eye on the following aspects of each model to be examined: the domains of dysfunction highlighted in the model, the approach to discrepancies between patient self-report and observed behavior (either by clinician assessor or significant others), the combination of clinical interview with other procedures, and the relative emphasis on categorical diagnosis and dimensional description of the pathology.

Undertaking to assess a patient, the clinician must first decide what aspects of dysfunction on which to focus. This is precisely where choices must be made because the advocates of the various treatments for the PDs emphasize different impairments. Unfortunately, while the empirically supported treatments focus on different domains of dysfunction, there is little evidence that the treatments are specific to the domains of dysfunction they emphasize. Hence, they offer limited guidance in identifying critical assessment variables.

A second clinical decision is whether the patient crosses the threshold into PD. Although this decision is usually considered categorical, it is essentially dimensional: To what extent and to what degree does a patient show stigmata of personality pathology? There is a wide range of personality difficulties to consider here. Does a successful man with narcissistic traits whose spouse experiences him as distant and not interested in her meet criteria for PD, or not? One could sensibly ask: Does it really matter? There are marital conflicts that have brought the couple to treatment, and whether the husband's traits suffice for a diagnosis is likely immaterial. In contrast, consider the patient who has multiple symptoms (anxiety, depression, angry outbursts, wrist cutting, and creation of conflict in relationships) and meets the severity criteria for self and other relations and severe trait disturbances that clearly place her in the realm of PD. These examples illustrate the distinction between personality dysfunction and PD. Although this distinction may not be important in initiating treatment, it has implications for how treatment is conducted—severity is the main factor determining treatment intensity and intervention strategy.

A major decision for the clinical assessor is whether to use a clinically guided interview or a semistructured interview with predetermined areas of inquiry. The former is the time-honored approach (MacKinnon, Michels, & Buckley, 2009) that has the advantage of favoring the freedom of a talented and experienced clinician. The latter provides an assurance of standard coverage of crucial areas and allows clinicians to compare their assessments with those of others. On balance, we recommend using the clinical interview as the primary assessment tool for routine clinical practice because it allows the clinician to elicit information in ways that foster the alliance and engage patients in treatment. This is important because many patients drop out either during assessment or between assessment and therapy, even under the carefully constructed conditions of a randomized clinical trial (Giessen-Bloo et al., 2006). Assessors should not lose sight of the process of the interview and rapport in the quest for information.

In collecting assessment information, a pertinent decision required of the assessor is the balance between extensive evaluation of present functioning and a focus on the past through obtaining a developmental history. Within the dictates of time, we recommend a thorough evaluation of present functioning, with relatively less attention to the past, except where it has direct implications for present functioning. Yet information about past difficulties in development, traumatic experiences, and the history of current ways of relating to others is most relevant. Thus, when time constraints are not a problem, it is always valuable to have detailed developmental and life-history information.

Yet another issue for the clinical assessor is the potential discrepancy between what the patient reports about his or her symptoms and interpersonal functioning, and how others may describe the patient. As the severity of personality pathology increases, it is more likely that the patient will have a view that is discrepant from that of other observers in terms of perceptions of self and others. There is a growing empirical basis to documenting the discrepancy between self-perception and other perception in individuals with PD (Bornstein, 2015). The astute clinical assessor is keenly aware of this potential discrepancy and takes measures to correct it. Both reports from significant others and close observation of patient behavior in interaction with the assessor serve as avenues to correct the discrepancy.

A final decision is whether to supplement the interview with ancillary measures such as questionnaires and more extensive assessment instruments. Whereas self-report questionnaires and, in fact, a whole battery of psychological and neurocognitive tests can be used to evaluate the patient (Clarkin, McClough, & Mattis, 2014), efficiency and limited resources in many mental health systems lead clinicians to use the interview as the most efficient way to approach diagnostic assessment and treatment planning.

## Treatment-Specific Clinical Assessment Recommendations

Perhaps surprisingly, the clinical literature contains few systematic recommendations for assessing individuals with a potential personality disorder. Recommendations also vary widely, though many recommend a broad assessment strategy. Widiger and Lowe (2012), for example, provided a comprehensive review of the instruments and empirical research on assessment related to treatment planning. They acknowledge that clinicians do not typically use structured interviews (e.g., Structured Clinical Interview for DSM-IV Axis II [SCID-II], International Personality Disorder Examination [IPDE]) and recommend a combination of patient self-report measures, clinical interview, and selected components of semistructured interviews based on the patient's individual domains of difficulty.

Our review of assessment procedures that follows (see Table 21.3) is not intended to be exhaustive. Rather, we have selected a range of assessment orientations to provide the reader with representative alternatives based on both theory (Linehan, 2015; Luyten, Fonagy, Lowyck, & Vermote, 2011) and empirical tailoring of patient characteristics and treatment factors (Beutler & Clarkin, 2014).

## Assessment Related to Cognitive and Dialectical Behavior Interventions

Beck and colleagues (Beck, Davis, & Freeman, 2015; Pretzer & Beck, 2005) were pioneers in modifying cognitive therapy for the PDs. Assessment is utilized to arrive at a case formulation that will guide intervention. This cognitive therapy approach conceptualizes each PD as involving a set of schemas, assumptions, and interpersonal strategies. Treatment is focused on the role of dysfunctional beliefs and assumptions of the patient. In their manual for schema-focused therapy, Young, Klosko, and Weishaar (2003), emphasize a case formulation approach

**TABLE 21.3. Prominent Assessment Approaches**

| | Assessment procedure | Attitude toward diagnosis | Targets of assessment |
|---|---|---|---|
| DSM-5, Section III | Interview PID-5 | Dimensional plus categorical diagnosis | Self- and other functioning; traits; categorical diagnoses |
| Dialectical behavior therapy (Linehan, 1993, 2015) | Interview | Diagnosis plus domains of emotion dysregulation, impulsivity, and self-concept | Problem behaviors and use of skills |
| Mentalization-based treatment | Interview Ancillary measures | Transdiagnostic | Four modes of mentalizing: internal–external; self–others; cognitive–affective; automatic–controlled |
| Transference-focused psychotherapy (Yeomans, Clarkin, & Kernberg, 2015) | Structural interview | Levels of personality organization | Identity, defenses, object relations, coping, aggression, moral values |
| Interpersonal theory | Interview Questionnaires EMA | Transdiagnostic | Interpersonal problems; interpersonal complementarity; agentic and communal needs |
| Systematic treatment selection (Beutler & Clarkin, 2014) | Interview Instruments | Transdiagnostic | Functional impairment; level of social support; problem complexity; ways of coping; resistance to outside influence |
| Integrated modular treatment (Livesley & Clarkin, 2015) | Interview | Transdiagnostic | Symptoms; regulation and modulation; interpersonal; self and identity |

based on a broad assessment strategy covering dysfunctional life patterns, early maladaptive schemas and their origins, coping styles and responses, and temperament that makes little reference to formal diagnosis. Davidson (2007) recommends a similar approach in her account of cognitive therapy for PDs. With these purely cognitive therapies, assessment is designed to provide the information needed to construct a road map that allows treatment to be tailored to the individual within the parameters of the cognitive model.

Originally designed to treat patients with suicidal behavior and BPD, dialectical behavior therapy (DBT; Linehan, 1993) and its skills training modules have been utilized to treat patients with a range of emotion dysregulation conditions. The target patient populations are loosely related to specific diagnostic disorders, and more related to trait-like difficulties such as emotion dyscontrol (over- or under-) and related issues of impulsivity, interpersonal dysfunctions, and self-image (Linehan, 2015). The goals of initial assessment are crisply described as five in number: (1) assessment of patient difficulties, (2) determination of treatment intensity and type, (3) orienting the patient to skills training, (4) developing a collaborative commitment, and (5) developing the treatment alliance. The most distinctive aspect of assessment for DBT is the emphasis on ongoing assessment throughout the treatment for both emotion regulation difficulties and use of skills taught in the treatment itself.

### Assessment by Systematic Treatment Selection

In an extensive stepwise approach to matching the individual patient with a tailored treatment for that individual, Beutler and colleagues (2016; see the recent summary) have developed what is called Systematic Treatment Selection (STS). This integrative model of assessment and treatment delivery highlights not patient diagnosis but rather participant factors, interventions, and relationship qualities.

The first step in this empirically driven process was to identify patient factors that predict change in psychotherapy, using reviews of the outcome literature (Beutler, Clarkin, & Bongar, 2000; Castonguay & Beutler, 2006). Four major clusters of patient variables were correlated with change: (1) functional impairment (comorbidity, chronicity, social support, symptom intensity), (2) coping style and response to stress (externalizing and internalizing patterns), (3) trait-like resistance ranging from avoidance to reactance, and (4) subjective distress. The second step was to identify common and specific characteristics of psychotherapy whose effects are moderated by patient qualities. Reviews of the psychotherapy literature (Malik, Beutler, Alimohamed, Gallagher-Thompson, & Thompson, 2003) resulted in the identification of six major dimensions of treatment: (1) intensity (duration and frequency), (2) format (multiperson and individual), (3) treatment mode (pharmacology, psychosocial, community), (4) focus (insight/awareness vs. symptom focus), (5) therapist directiveness (directive vs. evocative), and (6) means of affective regulation (affect control vs. affect discharge/cathartic). A final step was to validate the optimal "fit" between patient characteristics and treatment dimensions for optimal treatment effectiveness.

By utilizing five data sets, Beutler and Forrester (2014) found that the fit between patient impairment and mode of treatment, resistance traits and directiveness of the intervention, and coping style by symptom change/insight objectives contributed strongly both to the development of the therapeutic relationship and to change. STS/innerlife (Beutler, Williams & Norcross, 2008) is an online treatment assessment and planning system that uses a self-report format to identify patient status on symptom scales and a variety of moderating and mediating variables of change. The instrument assesses patient–treatment fit, as well as the patients' readiness for change.

### Assessment of Personality Organization

Many clinical theorists recognize the crucial role of the organized and integrated manner in which the normal personality functions. This is precisely what is missing in trait assessment. Kernberg's (1984) structural interview is an attempt to assess the levels of organization of the personality. Instead of beginning the clinical assessment with a standard psychiatric history, the structural interview focuses on the patients' current symptoms, interpersonal relations, conceptions of self and others, and motivation for treatment.

The initial phase of the structural interview is an inquiry about the patient's reason for appearing for assessment, the nature of current difficulties, and what is expected from treatment. This opening provides the patient an opportunity to disclose current symptoms and difficulties, and attitudes toward the need for treatment. The patient's ability to remember and respond to the questions in coherent and/or confused ways begins to reveal the nature of the patient's personality organization. In listening to the patient's response, the interviewer can evaluate the patient's awareness of pathology and need for treatment, and the expectations (realistic or unrealistic) of treatment. The patient's manner of listening to and responding to the interviewer's questions also provides indirect evidence of sensorium, memory, and some evaluation of intelligence.

The middle phase of the structural interview focuses on potential pathological character traits. The interviewer asks the patient to describe in his or her own words, and in detail, a significant other in the patient's life, and to describe him- or herself. With these descriptions of self and significant other, the interviewer can begin to evaluate the presence of various degrees of integrated or contradictory representations of self and others. Individuals with neurotic organization reveal integrated, albeit sometimes conflicted, representations of self and others. Those with borderline personality organization present with identity diffusion. The termination phase of the interview provides an opportunity to evaluate the patient's motivation for treatment, to manage any acute dangers that have been revealed, and to assess the ability and extent to which the patient can tolerate and respond to the interviewer's statements about his or her perceptions of the patient's problems and difficulties. In each phase of the interview, the interviewer is interested in not just the content of the patient's answers (e.g., patient is depressed, describes self as without intimate relations), but most importantly the coherence and/or incoherence and discrepancies of the answers, and any difficulties in responding that the patient demonstrates.

Caligor and Clarkin (2013) provide clinical illustrations of patients at the various levels of personality organization and how these levels influence behavior. As the level of organization decreases and becomes more diffuse, there is a need for the treatment intervention to be more structured by treatment contract in order to protect the patient–therapist relationship and provide controls for destructive acting out. In addition, as the personality organization is in the borderline range, there is more need for the therapist to address here-and-now distortions of patient interactions with the therapist and significant others.

As an aide to those who have not been trained in administering the Structural Interview and/or for those interested in doing clinical research, this clinical-research group has constructed the Structured Interview for Personality Organization (STIPO) (Clarkin, Caligor, Stern, & Kernberg, 2004; Stern et al., 2010), and the shorter and revised Structured Interview for Personality Organization—Revised (STIPO-R). Both semistructured interviews are available to interested clinicians (see *www.istfp.org*). With its structured questions and probes, the STIPO provides the clinician with a needed guide to the assessment of key domains of functioning for a psychodynamic diagnosis distinguishing patients with borderline personality organization from those with neurotic personality organization. Whereas the STIPO lacks the clinical intuitiveness and subtlety of the structural interview, this semistructured interview provides a standardized way to gather information and score it objectively, which is very helpful for research purposes. The goal of the STIPO is to arrive at a structural diagnosis (neurotic organization, high- and low-level borderline organization) through assessment of six essential constructs: identity (including capacity to invest in work/profession, sense of self, mental representations of others), object relations (interpersonal relations, intimate relations, and sexuality), defensive functioning, aggression (self- and other-directed), coping styles, and moral values. The individual with neurotic organization manifests a consolidated identity, relatively stable and enduring object relations, and an absence of primitive defenses, with varying degrees of rigidity in coping. Moral values may be overly harsh and rigid, and reality testing is intact. The high-level borderline patient has mild to moderate identity diffusion; split and superficial object relations, with some degree of stability; and impaired empathy. There are not only primitive defenses and maladaptive coping, with aggression directed against self and others, but also a desire for love and intimacy. Moral values are variable, and there are moderate difficulties in reality testing. The low-level borderline is somewhat more severe than the high-level borderline on all six dimensions, most prominently in the poor object relations (no empathy, no capacity to maintain consistent object relations), aggression (dangerous aggression toward self and others), and absence of an organized value system (antisocial features, behavior). The STIPO can distinguish among pathological groups, with treatment planning implications (Di Pierro, Preti, Vurro, & Madeddu, 2014).

## Assessment of Mentalization

A major treatment approach to personality pathology with empirical support for treatment of BPD is the mentalization-based treatment of Bateman and Fonagy (2006). This approach to assessment and treatment is grounded in attachment theory that posits the characteristic interactional patterns of those with secure and insecure attachment styles. The intersection of attachment systems, stress, and mentalization are crucial to understanding the individual. Activation and deactivation of the attachment systems are related to arousal and stress regulation. Insecurely attached individuals are prone to either hyperactivation or deactivation strategies that tend to interfere with more productive resilience, affiliation, and building of lasting relations with others.

The clinical assessor can use a number of interviews, scales, and questionnaires to evaluate the patients' various dimensions of mentalizing (Luyten, Fonagy, Lowyck, & Vermote, 2012). However, a more practical form of assessment can be accomplished in several detailed clinical interviews in which the assessor probes for mentalization in current and past relationships, and in the way the patient experiences his or her symptoms and difficulties. It is recommended that the clinical assessor probe in detail in order to form a mentalizing profile on the four polarities involved in mentalizing: (1) ability to perceive and self-correct initial impressions based on external appearances, (2) ability to integrate knowledge about self and others without undue focus on self, (3) ability to integrate both cognitive and affective knowledge of self and others, and (4) ability to mentalize in both stressful and nonstressful conditions.

It should not be assumed that these authors are suggesting assessment of mentalization in isolation. The manual for mentalization-based therapy (Bateman & Fonagy, 2004) indicates that structured diagnostic interviews are used to establish diagnosis prior to treatment. In a subsequent volume, however, Bateman and Fonagy (2006) discuss assessment of mentalizing and the interpersonal relationships largely using clinical methods and indicators such as chaotic life style, unstable housing, suicide risk, substance abuse, and problems with impulse control—features that we refer to as severity indicators.

## Assessment Guided by Interpersonal Theory

With its core assumption that the most important expressions of personality and psychopathology occur in phenomena involving more than one person, contemporary interpersonal theory of personality (Cain & Ansell, 2015; Pincus, 2005; Pincus & Ansell, 2013) is uniquely positioned to provide a framework for clinical assessment of personality functioning and disorder. Contemporary interpersonal theory incorporates aspects of object relations theory and the cognitive-affective model of personality functioning (Mischel & Shoda, 2008). Interpersonal functioning is assumed to involve not only interactions between people but also mental representations of self and others in the present and the past.

Interpersonal complementarity is present when the agentic and communal needs of both persons are met in the interpersonal interaction, typically in interpersonal situations in which dominance from one calls for submission from the other, and friendliness pulls for friendliness, and hostility pulls for hostility. Deviations from this complementarity are likely to disrupt interpersonal relations, and chronic deviations may indicate personality pathology. Dysregulation (failure to achieve security and self-esteem) in the interpersonal field and distortions (inaccurate mental representations of interpersonal situations) are characteristic of personality pathology.

Hopwood and colleagues (2013) outline clinical assessment of personality pathology using a combination of a battery of self-report instruments, such as the Personality Assessment Inventory (Morey, 1991), patient and clinician ratings of their interactions, daily diary reports of interactions, and informant information, along with the clinical interview. The central task of the assessor is to construct a formulation of when and how maladaptive patterns emerge, and to relate this information to transdiagnostic treatment goals and strategies. Similar to the approach to assessment in object relations orientations, interpersonal theory emphasizes the interaction between clinical assessor and patient as a major source of information on the interpersonal behavior of the patient.

The empirical basis of the interpersonal theory and its approach to assessment of interpersonal behavior has been dramatically enhanced by the recent utilization of ecological momentary assessment (EMA) strategies to rate interpersonal perceptions of self and others over time, utilizing the interpersonal circumplex (Roche, Pincus, Conroy, Hyde, & Ram, 2013; Roche, Pincus, Rebar, Conroy, & Ram, 2014). Instead of relying on generalized self-report information over an extended period of time or trait instruments subject to memory recall, EMA capitalizes on immediate report of interactions with others in the daily environment surrounding the subject.

### Assessment for an Integrated Treatment Approach

Livesley and Clarkin (2015) recommend an assessment strategy based on an analysis of heterogeneity of personality and the match of patients to the most appropriate level of treatment intensity and selective use of treatment strategies from all treatment orientations. This has been referred to as an "integrated modular treatment" approach. Besides obtaining a thorough personal history and evaluation of mental state, including any comorbid symptom constellations (e.g., depression, anxiety), this orientation describes a need to evaluate three sets of personality variables: (1) severity of the disorder; (2) clinically relevant individual differences in personality traits; and (3) impairments in four domains of personality functioning (i.e., symptoms, regulation and modulation mechanisms, interpersonal domain, and self or identity domain).

This information is used to construct a case formulation and treatment plan derived logically from the formulation that (1) links evaluation of severity and domains of impairment to treatment intensity, therapeutic pathways, and intervention strategies and (2) includes practical decisions about frequency of treatment, treatment setting, likelihood of crises, and so forth. Although it appears quite complex, this type of assessment occurs implicitly with all treatments because clinicians need to isolate specific features in order to identify effective interventions. We advocate decomposing global diagnoses such as ASPD and BPD into four domains of functionally related impairments: symptoms, regulation and modulation, interpersonal, and self or identity. The value of this approach is that it systematically links assessment to treatment goals and methods, something that is not possible with a categorical diagnosis.

Thorough and accurate assessment of PD requires that we look not only at traits but also at domains linked to specific intervention modules. Because personality pathology can be parsed into domains in various ways, we sought to base domains on descriptive concepts closely tied to the traditional subdivisions of personality, clinical descriptions of PD, and the problem clinicians typically address in therapy. Four functional domains are specified:

1. *Symptoms:* A wide variety of symptoms are associated with personality disorders, including dysphoria, anxiety, deliberate self-harm, dissociative features, quasi-psychotic symptoms, aggression, rage, and violent behavior.
2. *Regulation and modulation:* Problems arising from impaired regulatory structures that inhibit behavioral responses and mediate action and metacognitive processes involved in modulating personality processes:
   a. Undercontrol of emotions and impulses, resulting in unstable emotions, frequent mood changes, impulsive behaviors, violence, and impulsive aggression.
   b. Overcontrol of emotions and impulses, resulting in constricted emotions and inhibited behavior.
3. *Interpersonal:* Problems range from inability to establish social relationships, problems with intimacy and attachment, conflicted interpersonal behaviors, unstable relationships, callousness, and disregard for the well-being and welfare of others.
4. *Self or Identity:* Problems with the contents and structure of self and identity, including difficulties with the regulation of self-esteem, maladaptive self-schemas, unstable sense of self or identity, poorly developed self-system, and dysfunctional and biased perceptions of self in relation to others.

Every clinician develops his or her own preferred approach to the initial assessment interview, and it is not our intent to discuss in detail how the initial evaluation should be structured. However, our assumption is that the interview will cover (1) current symptoms and problems, and reasons for seeking help, including a recent history of symptoms and problems and their onset; (2) personal history, including information about the nuclear family and early development, reactions to major developmental transitions (e.g., early school experiences, adolescence, sexuality, peer relationships, experiences of abuse, trauma, and other forms of adversity), and important memories; and (3) examination of mental state.

### Assessing PD and Severity

Evaluation of self and interpersonal pathology based on the previously discussed conceptualization is not as daunting and subjective a task as it may appear. The definitions of self and interpersonal pathology shown in Table 21.4 are sufficiently precise to construct reliable self-report scales that differentiate PD from other mental disorders (Berghuis, Kamphuis, Verheul, Larstone, & Livesley, 2012; Hentschel & Livesley, 2013a, 2013b), and these definitions are easily applied in clinical assessment. Establishing the presence or absence of disorder need not be a lengthy process that requires assessing all facets of self pathology. Rather, we suggest that clinicians become familiar with the concepts and use the definitions as a prototype to evaluate the degree to which the patient matches the description. Most clinical interviews provide sufficient information to make a reliable evaluation. For example, patients may mention uncertainty about who they are or what they think or feel, or that they lose themselves in other people or do not know what they want from life. Such statements, respectively, hint at poor differentiation of the self, uncertainty about personal qualities, boundary problems, and low self-directedness that can readily be pursued to establish a diagnosis of PD. This information can then be supplemented with a few specific questions to explore different facets of the definition.

In the absence of an agreed measure of severity (noted earlier in this chapter), we propose using a clinical evaluation based on the degree of impairment in the core features of PD, thereby combining the diagnosis of PD with assessment of severity. Although severity is a graded construct, we suggest that until a generally accepted rating scale is available, it is sufficient for most clinical purposes to recognize two levels of severity: PD and severe PD. This approach is reminiscent of Kernberg's (1984) delineation of levels of personality organization (i.e., neurotic, high-level borderline, and low-level borderline organization). Table 21.4 describes differences in severity for each defining feature of PD. We recommend using these descriptions to make a global determination of severity.

When making this assessment, it is important to distinguish severity of pathology from intensity of distress. Some forms of PD may show little distress even though there is severe impairment in personality functioning, for example, patients with high levels of social avoidance (DSM-IV/DSM-5 schizoid PD). In contrast, extreme levels of distress may occur with relatively low severity.

### Clinical Assessment of Self Pathology

We find it helpful to begin assessing these problems by eliciting a self-description: "Perhaps we could now talk about how you see yourself. What sort of person do you think you are? How would you describe yourself?" This question usually produces important diagnostic information relatively quickly. Having posed the question, the interviewer observes how the patient responds.

Those with a poorly differentiated self often struggle with the task and comment about being unsure about who they are. Others provide a brief description that consists of a few general or concrete attributes—for example, "I am not sure what to say. I am a nice person, I like dancing, and I am very attached to my dog. . . . I do not know what else to say." A few probing questions to elicit more information usually reveal the extent of differentiation problems. Poor differentiation is often accompanied by feelings of "inner emptiness" that is easily assessed by asking: "Do you feel as if there is nothing inside, as if you are empty and hollow inside?" Information on interpersonal boundaries is especially important because the distinction between self and others is a prerequisite for the emergence of the self. Useful questions to explore boundary problems include "Do you ever feel very vulnerable and exposed because it feels as if nothing separates you from other people?"; "Do you ever confuse other people's ideas with your own?"; and "Do ever worry that you will lose the sense of who you really are or lose yourself in others?"

The differences between mild to moderate PD and severe PD are reflected in the degree of differentiation. Lower severity typically produces a self-description limited to a few concrete qualities, and there is some uncertainty about personal qualities. With severe disorder, the self-concept is severely impoverished, lead-

**TABLE 21.4. Definition of PD and Levels of Severity**

PD is characterized by an impaired self/identity and/or chronic interpersonal dysfunction that differ markedly from the expectations of the individual's culture.

Self pathology

Impaired self/identity as manifested by at least one of the following: (1) poor differentiation, (2) fragmented self-concept, and (3) low self-directedness.

1. Differentiation: Poorly developed self structure with limited development of self-schemas and impaired interpersonal boundaries
   - *Personality disorder:* self-description is limited to a few relatively concrete qualities with a lack of clarity and certainty about personal qualities, feelings, and wants, leading to a poorly developed sense of identity; wants and emotions do not feel real or authentic (e.g., questions whether emotions are real or genuine); relies extensively on others to confirm the appropriateness of thoughts and experiences and to help decide how they feel; interpersonal boundaries are present but poorly developed; feels empty or "hollow"
   - *Severe personality disorder:* severely impoverished self-concept—has difficulty describing personal qualities and attributes; lacks a sense of identity; minimal interpersonal boundaries leading to enmeshed relationships and the "sense of losing oneself" when with others, which may lead to dissociation; assumes that personal experiences and those of others are identical

2. Integration: Self-structure is poorly integrated, leading to a fragmented and unstable sense of self and a limited sense of personal unity and continuity
   - *Personality disorder:* experiences shifting and poorly integrated or unrelated self-states but is able to recall experiences in other self-states than the current state; sense of self varies substantially across situations; feels a sense of discontinuity between the self presented to the world and the "real" self
   - *Severe personality disorder:* integration is minimal—self-experience consists of a series of discrete disconnected experiences and distinct self-state, with little recall experiences across different self-states

3. Self-directedness: Difficulty setting and attaining satisfying personal goals
   - *Personality disorder:* low motivation leading to difficulty establishing realistic goals; unable to sustain work on achieving long-term goals; limited sense of personal autonomy and agency
   - *Severe personality disorder:* lacks the ability to establish lasting long-term goals; lacks direction and purpose; passive and lacks motivation; lacks a sense of agency and autonomy and shows

Interpersonal pathology

Chronically impaired interpersonal functioning as manifested either by impaired capacity for intimacy and attachment and/or socialization.

Intimacy and attachment: Impaired capacity for close relationships
   - *Personality disorder:* Exhibits one or more to the following difficulties: (a) impaired capacity for intimacy due to personality traits (e.g., narcissism, insecure attachment, compulsivity), although he or she may be able to tolerate more distant social relationships; (b) unstable and conflicted relationships; (c) difficulty tolerating the autonomy and individuality of others; (d) attachment problems involving either difficulty establishing adult patterns of attachment or inability to function as a responsible attachment figure
   - *Severe personality disorder:* Severely impaired capacity to relate to others involving either difficulty differentiating self and other (symbiotic relationships) or avoidance of relationships

Prosocial behavior: Impaired socialization as evidenced by severely impaired prosocial behavior and/or moral development
   - *Personality disorder:* Impaired respect for culturally typical moral behavior; impairment in altruistic behavior
   - *Severe personality disorder:* Lacks the capacity for culturally typical moral behavior; devoid of altruism

*Note.* Adapted from Livesley and Clarkin (2015) with permission from The Guilford Press.

ing to difficulty describing personal qualities and attributes. Instead, the self is defined very much by the moment and the expectations of others. There are also differences in boundaries: With increasing severity, interpersonal boundaries become almost nonexistent, leading to enmeshed relationships and a sense of losing oneself by merging with others.

Patients with integration problems may respond to the request for a self-description by commenting that it is difficult to describe themselves because their ideas about themselves change frequently. For example, patients may note, "It is hard to say. . . . My feelings about myself change all the time" or "Sometimes it feels as if there are lots of different me's." Such statements suggest discontinuity in experiences of the self that can be assessed further by asking questions such as "Does your sense of who you are change a lot from day to day?"; "Do you have contradictory feelings about yourself and who you are?"; and "Do you ever get the feeling that you are several different people?"

The previous responses are typical of patients with emotional dysregulation problems as associated with DSM-IV/DSM-5 BPD. In more schizoid or socially withdrawn individuals, problems with integration may take the form of feeling that the self presented to the world is a façade, and that the "real" self is hidden inside and never exposed to others. Differences in severity are less marked than in the case of differentiation problems. A major differentiating feature is that with severe pathology, there is greater disjunction between self-states, such that experiences when in one state are poorly recalled in another state. For example, one patient with severe disorder showed several self-states, including a more settled optimistic state and a state of intense agitation associated with almost painful feelings of inner emptiness that he found terrifying, a state that was largely characterized by a combination of intense anger and neediness. When experiencing the state of inner emptiness, he found it difficult to recall or even imagine that he ever felt any different, even when he had been in a more settled state only a few hours previously. This inability to recall that he had felt different increased his distress because the despair felt timeless, as if it had always existed and always would.

Low self-directedness, the motivational component of the self, has several components: low self-efficacy—a sense of being unable to control oneself and one's destiny; a lack of meaning and purpose to life; and difficulty setting and attaining long-term goals. All components can usually be evaluated when taking a personal history because it often becomes apparent whether the individual has lived a life imbued with purpose, with clearly defined goals, or whether life has been less purposeful. This initial assessment can then be followed up with a few questions: "Do you feel as if you are not in control of your own life, as if there is nothing that you can do to change your life?"; "Does it feel as if your life has meaning? Does it seem as if nothing that you do has much purpose?"; and "Do you have difficulty deciding what you want to achieve in life and in setting goals?" Patients with less severe pathology often set goals, but their goals often change rapidly, due to uncertainty about self-attributes, including goals, and they have difficulty sustaining the effort to achieve longer term objectives. With increasing pathology, there is an almost total lack of goal setting that is associated with low motivation and a pervasive sense of passivity.

### Clinical Assessment of Interpersonal Pathology

Information on interpersonal functioning is readily elicited in a clinical interview. Standard questions about relationships with significant others, childhood peer relationships, and adult relationships, including romantic relationships, usually provide sufficient information to evaluate the ability to establish meaningful relationships and the capacity to sustain attachment and intimacy. Exploration of current circumstances adds additional information about the extent and quality of relationships, number of friends, and the stability of relationships, which is readily translated into a clinical evaluation of the intimacy and affiliative component of interpersonal pathology. Just as the assessor asks the patient to describe his or her self, one can also ask the patient to describe a significant other, to evaluate the depth (differentiation) and degree of integration of the representation of that person. Patients with less severe disorder often form relationships but have difficulty with sustained intimacy and attachment, which may or may not be associated with unstable and conflicted relationships. Greater severity is associated with a substantially impaired capacity to relate to others, involving either difficulty differentiating self and other, which in turn leads to symbiotic relationships, or almost total avoidance of relationships.

A comprehensive clinical interview also reveals information about impaired socialization, leading to problems with prosocial and moral behavior, which can usually be clarified with a few questions. These questions include whether the patient likes working with others or has problems with cooperation, whether he or she would ever "sacrifice him- or herself to help others," or whether "the patient would make sure to get what he or she wants, regardless of the consequences for others." Greater severity is associated with an absence of concern for others, disregard for culturally typical moral behavior, and an absence of altruism.

## ASSESSING TRAIT CONSTELLATIONS AND PRIMARY TRAITS

The second part of the assessment of PD is to evaluate individual differences in clinically important personality characteristics. An understanding of the individual's salient personality characteristics is needed to establish treatment pathways and identify suitable intervention strategies. Although categorical diagnoses have traditionally been used prior to treatment, we advocate dimensional classification because of the well-established limitations of categorical diagnoses, extensive evidence supporting dimensional diagnosis, and direct links between traits such as emotional lability and impulsivity and treatment methods. Despite the evidence, however, there is considerable resistance to using dimensional assessment.

A practical alternative to a questionnaire is to assess traits during the clinical interview. The most comprehensive way is to assess all primary traits shown in Table 21.1 using information obtained from an interview, supplemented as needed with questions based on the definitions of each trait, to establish whether the trait is present to a clinically significant degree. Table 21.2 provides detailed definitions of each trait based in part on Livesley and Jackson (2009). A more parsimonious approach is to assess only the most salient traits in each cluster using interview information and clarifying questions (Livesley, 1998). These traits are shown in bold in Table 21.1. The most salient traits are those with the highest loadings in the analyses used to establish the structure (Livesley & Jackson, 2009; Livesley, Jang, & Vernon, 1998). If these screening traits are considered clinically significant (i.e., they are associated with impaired social and/or occupational functioning), the remaining traits defining the cluster can be assessed to provide a detailed picture of the constellation. With this strategy, traits can be assessed relatively quickly, at least for clinical purposes. For example, the emotional dependency cluster can be assessed based on four traits—emotional lability, anxiousness, insecure attachment, and submissive dependency—and the underlying conflict between neediness and fear of rejection can be assessed at the same time by inquiring about attachment needs. The diagnostic process would extend to the salient traits of the dissocial (antisocial/psychopathic), social avoidance (schizoid/avoidant), and compulsivity constellations. In many cases, this information is sufficient for planning and initiating treatment. More detailed assessment may subsequently be incorporated into treatment.

The trait system is not independent of functional domains; rather, it cuts across domains. For example, traits such as anxiousness and emotional lability predispose to mood symptoms, interpersonal problems, and self pathology, and cognitive dysregulation predisposes to impaired thinking when stressed and the development of quasi-psychotic symptoms, such as illusions and pseudohallucinations. Interpersonal traits such as callousness, insecure attachment, and social avoidance play an important role in the development of interpersonal problems.

Because domain assessment identifies impairments that form treatment targets, it helps to map the broad directions of therapy. It also helps to structure discussions with patients about the personal concerns that they want to address in treatment, which is part of working with the patient to establish the collaborative goals that will be the focus of therapeutic work. Table 21.5 describes the relationships among domains, goals, and assessment, and illustrates typical problems associated with each domain. This list is not intended to provide an exhaustive account of each problem domain; rather, it illustrates the range of issues to consider in each domain. We suggest that these guidelines form the basis for a systematic assessment of each domain. At some point toward the end of the assessment process, it is useful to conduct a systematic evaluation of each domain, rather like the systematic review that is part of a mental state examination. This information obtained during the clinical interview will include details of impairments across domains, so that completion of a domain assessment need not be time-consuming. It is a useful way to conclude

**TABLE 21.5. Relationships between Domains, Goals, and Assessment**

| Domain | Treatment goals | Assessment |
|---|---|---|
| Symptoms | Reduce symptoms | Nature and severity of symptoms |
| Emotion/impulse control: | | |
| • Undercontrol | Control suicidal, parasuicidal, and other self-harming behavior | Frequency and intensity of suicidal ideation; frequency and nature of self-harm |
| | Improve emotion/impulse regulation | Emotional lability; anxiousness; impulse control |
| | Improve self-reflection | Self-reflection abilities |
| | Enhance ability to understand mental states | Capacity to understand mental states of self and others |
| | Increase effortful control | Capacity for attention control |
| • Overcontrol | Reduce emotional constriction; improve self-reflection; enhance ability to understand mental states | Restricted emotional expression; self-reflection abilities; capacity to understand mental states of self and others |
| | More contextually adaptive application of effortful control | Capacity for attention control |
| Interpersonal | Improve interpersonal relationships and behavior | Interpersonal traits; capacity for relationships; interpersonal patterns; interpersonal conflicts; moral development; capacity for cooperation; capacity for empathy |
| Self and identity | Increase self-esteem | Level and stability of self-esteem |
| | Modulate maladaptive self-schema | Core self-schemas |
| | Promote more adaptive sense of self and identity | Sense of self and identify |
| | Develop a personal niche | Assessment compatibility of personality and environment |

*Note.* Adapted from Livesley and Clarkin (2015) with permission from The Guilford Press.

the assessment because it paves the way for a discussion of the formulation and treatment options.

The structured approach to assessment that we present as an alternative to the usual determination of categorical diagnoses is designed to be more clinically useful by focusing on functional impairments. It is not our intention to imply that the detailed methods we have discussed should be followed slavishly or that all aspects of the assessment should be completed prior to therapy. Instead, we seek to offer a scheme for thinking systematically about assessment in the context of therapy, and about the relationship among assessment, treatment planning, and the interventions that are likely to be useful at different phases of treatment. Our goal was to outline the kinds of variables therapists should consider, while recognizing that much of this information will be fleshed out during therapy. However, we think that it is helpful for the therapist to have a broad understanding of level of severity, salient personality traits and constellations, and critical impairments within each domain prior to starting therapy because this information is required to construct the formulation needed to negotiate the treatment contract.

Although our recommendations differ from traditional diagnostic assessment prior to therapy, the approach is consistent with emerging trends in the taxonomy of PD, and the emphasis being placed on understanding the functional impairments associated with these disorders. Like other recommendations, some of which we reviewed earlier, we advocate for a broad but flexible assessment of all aspects of personality, including assets and liabilities, and sources of both resilience and vulnerability. We have also proposed a combination of functional and structural impairments. As indicated in the discussion of self pathology, it is important to assess structural aspects of personality that have higher-order integrative functions. Our approach shows parallels to Kernberg's (1984) structural interview that combines aspects of a traditional assessment, including chief complaint, current difficulties, and mental status information, with exploration of the individual's active and current representations of self in relationship to others. This approach enables the clinician to have a vivid picture of the patient's current functioning, a major focus of intervention, with less attention to personal history.

## Assessement and Treatment Process

The product of a thoughtful integrative assessment is a mutually created understanding of the patient at many levels of experience. While such understanding is essential for making diagnostic decisions and treatment recommendations in the early phases of treatment, it is important to note that the assessment provides the foundation of the subsequent treatment process. We briefly discuss the assessment process as an alliance-building activity, as well as the need for ongoing assessment as part of any treatment process with patients with PDs.

### Enhancing Treatment Alliance through Assessment

The assessment process should be used to foster engagement because of the association between the quality of the alliance and early dropout. This means that alliance-building techniques should be used throughout the assessment (Hilsenroth & Cromer, 2007) even if this means a somewhat longer assessment process. The alliance is fostered when the clinician conducts the assessment in a way that conveys respect and demonstrates competence in assessing and treating PD. The patient's perception of the relationship is also enhanced when the therapist is nurturing, collaborative, and understanding (Bachelor, 1995). Nurturance is conveyed by attentive, nonjudgmental listening and empathic attunement to the patient's feelings, problems, and situation.

Hilsenroth and Cromer (2007) identified three clinician behaviors that promote a positive alliance during assessment. First, the alliance is fostered by a longer and collaborative in-depth assessment that allows ample opportunity for the patient to voice concerns and discuss the cognitive and emotional aspects of these concerns. Rapport is increased by using clear, concrete, and "experience-near" language and avoiding jargon. Second, detailed exploration of patients' immediate concerns fosters the alliance and helps patients to commit to therapy. A key feature is to help patients to discuss not only factual details about their concerns but also sources of distress, while taking steps to ensure that patients are not overwhelmed by their distress. Third, it is important to seek constant feedback from patients about how they think the assessment is going and how they feel about discussing their problems. It also helps to incorporate a psychoeducational element by explaining features of the disorder as they are discussed during assessment, and by helping patients to develop new insights into the problems they present.

After completing the assessment process, dominated by many assessment questions, the patient deserves a summary feedback statement from the assessor, who can then make a link to possible treatment alternatives. This feedback process is in some ways less complex when the major difficulty is a mood state, such as anxiety and/or depression. In the case of a PD, does one give feedback related to the current difficulties, or does one indicate the complex nature of a specific PD ("You meet the criteria for narcissistic personality disorder") or a generic personality disorder? Our own clinical experience, and that of teaching developing clinicians, is that the general diagnosis of PD, with some indication of the severity, sets the stage for recommending a treatment of appropriate length and intensity.

### Integrating Assessment into the Ongoing Treatment Process

Initial clinical assessment is necessary to focus the intervention, but as the relationship between patient and therapist evolves, the initial assessment picture becomes amplified with additional information. The use of the daily diary card to facilitate the communication between patient and therapist about ongoing difficulties in DBT (Linehan, 1993), is an excellent example of continual assessment of patient progress during treatment that keeps both patient and therapist focused on progressive goals. Others have used patient reports of treatment progress (Lambert,

2007). We have indicated elsewhere (Livesley & Clarkin, 2015) that the need in treatment of patients with PDs is essentially the need to continuously monitor the therapeutic alliance and patient motivation for change. In fact, one of the many indicators of a deepening therapeutic process may be the unfolding of previously inaccessible representations of self, others, and adjoining affect states (Clarkin, Yeomans, & Kernberg, 2006), which then need further elaboration and evaluation. Thus assessment is an essential component of the ongoing treatment process.

## Concluding Comments

Although our review of disparate approaches to conceptualizing and assessing personality pathology reveals little consensus, several convergent themes emerge. The strength of most of these approaches is their primary dependence on the clinical interview and their attention to a direct link to case formulation and selection of treatment strategies and techniques. With the pressures of insurance companies, managed care, and the insistence of treatments of the briefest duration, most clinicians depend on the clinical interview, supplementing additional questionnaire assessment only as necessitated by the particulars of a given patient. It is difficult to imagine that this situation will change.

Most of these treatment assessment systems favor dimensional assessment of key domains of functioning over any form of categorical diagnosis. This consensus on the limited value of categorical diagnosis is striking. Instead of a focus on categorical diagnosis, the domains of dysfunction highlighted across systems vary as related to the background conception of the latent structure of the personality dysfunction. Even among these differences, there is an emerging consensus on the centrality of the core of personality pathology, that is, the deficits in self- and other-representations, and their manifestation in disturbed interpersonal connections and interactions. Consistent with the dominant cognitive–affective processing system analysis of personality functioning (Mischel & Shoda, 2008), many of these diagnostic systems favor an assessment interview that focuses on patients' articulation of representations of self and other (Bateman & Fonagy, 2006; Kernberg & Caligor, 2005), distortions in the rhythm of interpersonal interaction (Hopwood et al., 2013), and the need to translate trait information into the specifics of patients' specific environment (Livesley & Clarkin, 2015). This approach is also consistent with the way therapy is conducted: Interventions tend to focus on relatively specific features of personality pathology, such as emotional lability and aggressivity, rather than global diagnoses (Leising & Zimmermann, 2011; Sanderson & Clarkin, 2013).

This having been said, some assessment systems have a tendency to focus on a single domain of dysfunction. There is little doubt that emotion dysregulation (Linehan, 1993) and mentalization (Bateman & Fonagy, 2006) are key domains of human functioning that may lead to personality dysfunction. Treatments based on a central notion, such as DBT's targeting of emotion dysregulation, may have been initially focused on BPD but have now been translated to neighboring disorders for whom emotion dysregulation is also a core feature (i.e., substance use disorders). However, given the complexity of human organization and functioning, and interaction with the vagaries of the environment, it is unlikely that one domain of pathology can explain the variance in human function and dysfunction.

It is a positive development that many of the systems reviewed point to the need to assess the coherent organization of personality and deviations from coherent organization. This organizing principle is captured in concepts such as cognitive–affective units (Mischel & Shoda, 2008); internal representations of self and others (Kernberg, 1984); mentalization capacities to articulate complex, coherent, and realistic conceptions of self and others (Bateman & Fonagy, 2006); and dominant personality traits (Livesley & Clarkin, 2015), with ways to capture these organizing aspects in the clinical interview. Experts in psychotherapy research, Beutler, Someah, Kimpora, and Miller (2016) have exposed the futility of developing an empirically supported treatment approach based on the narrow basis of single diagnoses. Beutler's STS approach is unique in its focus on a range of patient characteristics that have little to do with specific diagnoses, and that call for flexibility and adaptation from the therapist. This explicit attention to the two-way interaction and match between patient characteristics and therapist approach is unique, but it is inferred by the other approaches.

Finally, most of the approaches highlight the need for the clinician assessor to evaluate the content of the patient's description of symptoms and interpersonal functioning in comparison to how the patient actually relates to the assessor. Discrepancies between the patient's verbal reports and the experience of the clinical interviewer are important sources of information. By definition, patients with personality dysfunction manifest distortions in the way they experience and relate to others, and this includes the nature of their attitudes and behavior toward the clinical assessor.

In the spirit of integration that is applied to treatment approaches, we suggest the following principles of clinical assessment of patients with suspected personality dysfunction:

- A primary goal of assessment is to intimately link the assessment with subsequent clinical intervention.
- None of the assessment systems define themselves by the categorical diagnoses of DSM-5.
- The specific domains of assessment focus vary according to theoretical orientation and treatment strategies, but there are common overlapping areas of concern, including behaviors that are dangerous to the patient and disrupt interpersonal interchange, emotion regulation, and representations of self and others.
- In addition to assessment of the problems prominent for the specific patient (e.g., suicidal behavior, interpersonal dysfunction), an integrated assessment evaluates the multiple levels of human functioning related to each problem area (i.e., specific behaviors in specific environmental contexts, related cognitive affective units or mental representations of the events).
- Much more important than PD category, the severity of the personality dysfunction is a major variable related to treatment intensity and setting.
- The clinical interview is the most efficient method of clinical assessment. While the use of impersonal self-report questionnaires and semistructured interviews may usefully augment the assessment process, the clinical interview provides a mechanism for enhancing the unique relationship between patient and therapist.
- Assessment is an ongoing process, not a single event at the beginning of treatment. This ongoing process is a major factor in monitoring not only patient improvement but also the relationship quality between therapist and patient.

## ACKNOWLEDGMENT

Portions of this chapter are based on Livesley and Clarkin (2015). Adapted with permission from The Guilford Press.

## REFERENCES

Allport, G. W. (1961). *Pattern and growth in personality: A psychological interpretation.* New York: Holt, Rinehart & Winston.

American Psychiatric Association. (1980). *Diagnostic and statistical manual of mental disorders* (3rd ed.). Washington, DC: Author.

American Psychiatric Association. (2000). *Diagnostic and statistical manual of mental disorders* (4th ed., text rev.). Washington, DC: Author.

American Psychiatric Association. (2013). *Diagnostic and statistical manual of mental disorders* (5th ed.). Arlington, VA: Author.

Bachelor, A. (1995). Clients' perception of the therapeutic alliance: A qualitative analysis. *Journal of Consulting Psychology, 42,* 323–337.

Bateman, A., & Fonagy, P. (2004). *Psychotherapy for borderline personality disorder: Mentalization-based treatment.* Oxford, UK: Oxford University Press.

Bateman, A., & Fonagy, P. (2006). *Mentalization-based treatment for borderline personality disorder.* Oxford, UK: Oxford University Press.

Beck, A. T., Davis, D., & Freeman, A. (2015). *Cognitive therapy of personality disorders* (3rd ed.). New York: Guilford Press.

Berghuis, H., Kamphuis, J. H., Verheul, R., Larstone, R., & Livesley, W. J. (2012). The General Assessment of Personality Disorder (GAPD) as an instrument for assessing the core features of personality disorders. *Clinical Psychology and Psychotherapy, 20*(6), 544–557.

Beutler, L. E., & Clarkin, J. F. (2014). *Systematic treatment selection: Toward targeted therapeutic interventions.* New York: Routledge.

Beutler, L. E., Clarkin, J. F., & Bongar, B. (2000). *Guidelines for the systematic treatment of the depressed patient.* New York: Oxford University Press.

Beutler, L. E., & Forrester, B. (2014). What needs to change: Moving from "research informed" practice to "empirically effective" practice. *Journal of Psychotherapy Integration, 24*(3), 168–177.

Beutler, L. E., Someah, K., Kimpara, S., & Miller, K. (2016). Selecting the most appropriate treatment for each patient. *International Journal of Clinical and Health Psychology, 16*(1), 99–108.

Beutler, L. E., Williams, O. B., & Norcross, J. N. (2008). Innerlife.com.: A copyrighted software package for treatment planning. Retrieved from www.webpsychcorp.com.

Bornstein, R. F. (1998). Reconceptualizing personality disorder diagnosis in DSM-5: The discriminant validity challenge. *Clinical Psychology: Science and Practice, 5*(3), 333–343.

Bornstein, R. F. (2015). Process-focused assessment of personality pathology. In S. K. Huprich (Ed.), *Personality disorders: Toward theoretical and empirical integration in diagnosis and assessment* (pp. 271–290). Washington, DC: American Psychological Association.

Cain, N. M., & Ansell, E. B. (2015). An integrative interpersonal framework for understanding personality pathology. In S. K. Huprich (Ed.), *Personality disorders: Toward theoretical and empirical integration in diagnosis and assessment* (pp. 345–365). Washington, DC: American Psychological Association.

Caligor, E., & Clarkin, J. F. (2010). An object relations model of personality and personality pathology. In J. F. Clarkin, P. Fonagy, & G. Gabbard (Eds.), *Psychodynamic psychotherapy for personality disorders: A clinical handbook* (pp. 3–36). Washington, DC: American Psychiatric Publishing.

Carver, C. S. (2011). Self-awareness. In M. R. Leary & J. P. Tangney (Eds.), *Handbook of self and identity* (pp. 50–68). New York: Guilford Press.

Carver, C. S., & Scheier, M. F. (1998). *On the self-regulation of behavior*. Cambridge, UK: Cambridge University Press.

Castonguay, L. G., & Beutler, L. E. (2006). *Principles of therapeutic change that work*. New York: Oxford University Press.

Cervone, D., & Shoda, Y. (1999). Social-cognitive theories and the coherence of personality. In D. Cervone & Y. Shoda (Eds.), *The coherence of personality* (pp. 3–33). New York: Guilford Press.

Clark, L. A. (1990). Toward a consensual set of symptom clusters for assessment of personality disorder. In J. Butcher & C. Spielberger (Eds.), *Advances in personality assessment* (Vol. 8, pp. 243–266). Hillsdale, NJ: Erlbaum.

Clark, L. A. (1993). *Manual for the Schedule for Nonadaptive and Adaptive Personality (SNAP)*. Minneapolis: University of Minnesota Press.

Clark, L. A. (2007). Assessment and diagnosis of personality disorder: Perennial issues and an emerging reconceptualization. *Annual Review of Psychology, 58,* 227–257.

Clark, L. A., & Livesley, W. J. (1994). Two approaches to identifying the dimensions of personality disorder. In P. T. Costa, Jr., & T. A. Widiger (Eds.), *Personality disorders and the five-factor model of personality* (pp. 261–277). Washington, DC: American Psychological Association Press.

Clarkin, J. F., Caligor, E., Stern, B., & Kernberg, O. F. (2004). *Structured Interview of Personality Organization (STIPO)*. Unpublished manuscript, Personality Disorders Institute, Weill Cornell Medical College, New York, NY.

Clarkin, J. F., McClough, J., & Mattis, S. (2014). Psychological assessment. In R. E. Hales, S. C. Yudofsky, & L. W. Roberts (Eds.), *The American Psychiatric Publishing textbook of psychiatry* (6th ed., pp. 61–88). Washington, DC: American Psychiatric Publishing.

Clarkin, J. F., Yeomans, F. E., & Kernberg, O. F. (2006). *Psychotherapy for borderline personality: Focusing on object relations*. Washington, DC: American Psychiatric Publishing.

Cloninger, C. R. (1987). A systematic method for the clinical description and classification of personality variants. *Archives of General Psychiatry, 44,* 573–588.

Cloninger, C. R. (2000). A practical way to diagnose personality disorder: A proposal. *Journal of Personality Disorders, 14,* 99–106.

Costa, P. T., Jr., & Widiger, T. A., (Eds.). (1994). *Personality disorders and the five factor model of personality*. Washington, DC: American Psychological Association.

Crawford, M. J., Koldobsky, N., Mulder, R., & Tyrer, P. (2011). Classifying personality disorder according to severity. *Journal of Personality Disorders, 25,* 321–330.

Davidson, K. (2007). *Cognitive therapy for personality disorders: A guide for clinicians*. New York: Routledge.

Di Pierro, R., Preti, E., Vurro, N., & Madeddu, F. (2014). Dimensions of personality structure among patients with substance use disorders and co-occurring personality disorders: A comparison with psychiatric outpatients and healthy controls. *Comprehensive Psychiatry, 55,* 1398–1404.

Dimaggio, G., Carcione, A., Nicolò, G., Lysaker, P. H., d'Angerio, S., Conti, M. L., et al. (2013). Differences between axes depend on where you set the bar: Associations among symptoms, interpersonal relationship and alexithymia with number of personality disorder criteria. *Journal of Personality Disorders, 27,* 371–382.

Eysenck, H. J. (1987). The definition of personality disorders and the criteria appropriate to their definition. *Journal of Personality Disorders, 1,* 211–219.

Eysenck, H. J., & Eysenck, M. W. (1985). *Personality and individual differences: A natural science approach*. New York: Plenum Press.

Giesen-Bloo, J., van Dyck, R., Spinhoven, P., van Tilberg, W., Dirksen, C., van Asselt, T., et al. (2006). Outpatient psychotherapy for borderline personality disorder: Randomized trial of schema-focused therapy vs transference-focused therapy. *Archives of General Psychiatry, 63,* 649–658.

Harkness, A. R. (1992). Fundamental topics in the personality disorders: Candidate trait dimensions from the lower regions of the hierarchy. *Psychological Assessment, 4,* 251–259.

Harter, S. (2012). *The construction of the self*. New York: Guilford Press.

Hentschel, A. G., & Livesley, W. J. (2013a). Differentiating normal and disordered personality using the General Assessment of Personality Disorder (GAPD). *Personality and Mental Health, 7,* 133–142.

Hentschel, A. G., & Livesley, W. J. (2013b). The General Assessment of Personality Disorder (GAPD): Factor structure, incremental validity of self pathology, and relations to DSM-IV personality disorders. *Journal of Personality Assessment, 95,* 479–485.

Hilsenroth, M. J., & Cromer, T. D. (2007). Clinical interventions related to alliance during the initial interview and psychological assessment. *Psychotherapy: Research, Theory, and Practice, 44,* 205–208.

Hopwood, C. J., Malone, J. C., Ansell, E. B., Sanislow, C. A., Grilo, C. M., McGlashan, T. H., et al. (2011). Personality assessment in DSM-5: Empirical support for rating severity, style, and traits. *Journal of Personality Disorders, 25,* 305–320.

Hopwood, C. J., Wright, A. G., Ansell, E. B., & Pincus, A. L. (2013). The interpersonal core of personality pathology. *Journal of Personality Disorders, 27*(3), 270–295.

Kernberg, O. F. (1984). *Severe personality disorders: Psychotherapeutic strategies*. New Haven, CT: Yale University Press.

Kernberg, O. F., & Caligor, E. (2005). A psychoanalytic theory of personality disorders. In M. E. Lenzenweger & J. F. Clarkin (Eds.), *Major theories of personality disorder* (2nd ed., pp. 114–156). New York: Guilford Press.

Kiesler, D. J. (1986). The 1982 interpersonal circle: An analysis of DSM-III personality disorders. In T. Millon & G. L. Klerman (Eds.), *Contemporary directions in psychopathology: Toward the DSM-IV* (pp. 571–597). New York: Guilford Press.

Kohut, H. (1971). *The analysis of the self*. New York: International Universities Press.

Krueger, R. F., Derringer, J., Markon, K. E., Watson, D., & Skodol, A. E. (2012). Initial construction of a maladaptive personality trait model and inventory for DSM-5. *Psychological Medicine, 42,* 1879–1890.

Krueger, R. F., Eaton, N. R., South, S. C., Clark, L. A., & Simms, L. J. (2010). Empirically derived personality disorder prototypes: Bridging dimensions and categories in DSM-5. In D. A. Regier, W. E. Narrow, E. A. Kuhl, D. J. Kupfer, & the American Psychiatric Association (Eds.), *The conceptual evolution of DSM-5* (pp. 97–118). Washington, DC: American Psychiatric Publishing.

Krueger, R. F., & Markon, K. E. (2014). The role of the DSM-5 personality trait model in moving toward a quantitative and empirically based approach to classifying personality and psychopathology. *Annual Review of Clinical Psychology, 10,* 477–501.

Lambert, M. (2007). Presidential address: What we have learned from a decade of research aimed at improving psychotherapy outcome in routine care. *Psychotherapy Research, 17*(1), 1–14.

Leary, T. (1957). *Interpersonal diagnosis of personality: A functional theory and methodology for personality evaluation*. New York: Ronald Press.

Leising, D., & Zimmermann, J. (2011). An integrative conceptual framework for assessing personality and personality pathology. *Review of General Psychology, 15,* 317–330.

Linehan, M. M. (1993). *Cognitive-behavioral treatment of borderline personality disorder*. New York: Guilford Press.

Linehan, M. M. (2015). *DBT skills training manual* (2nd ed.). New York: Guilford Press.

Livesley, W. J. (1998). Suggestions for a framework for an empirically based classification of personality disorder. *Canadian Journal of Psychiatry, 43,* 137–147.

Livesley, W. J. (2003). Diagnostic dilemmas in the classification of personality disorder. In K. Phillips, M. First, & H. A. Pincus (Eds.), *Advancing DSM: Dilemmas in psychiatric diagnosis* (pp. 153–189). Washington, DC: American Psychiatric Publishing.

Livesley, W. J., & Clarkin, J. F. (2015). Diagnosis and assessment. In W. J. Livesley, G. DiMaggio, & J. F. Clarkin (Eds.), *Integrated treatment for personality disorder: A modular approach* (pp. 51–79). New York: Guilford Press.

Livesley, W. J., & Jackson, D. N. (2009). *Dimensional Assessment of Personality Pathology—Basic Questionnaire technical manual*. Port Huron, MI: Sigma Press.

Livesley, W. J., Jackson, D. N., & Schroeder, M. L. (1992). Factorial structure of personality disorders in clinical and general population samples. *Journal of Abnormal Psychology, 101,* 432–440.

Livesley, W. J., & Jang, K. L. (2000). Toward an empirically based classification of personality disorder. *Journal of Personality Disorders, 14,* 137–151.

Livesley, W. J., Jang, K. L., & Vernon, P. A. (1998). The phenotypic and genetic architecture of traits delineating personality disorder. *Archives of General Psychiatry, 55,* 941–948.

Luyten, P., Fonagy, P., Lowyck, B., & Vermote, R. (2011). Assessment of mentalization. In A. Bateman & P. Fonagy (Eds.), *Handbook of mentalizing in mental health practice* (pp. 43–66). Washington, DC: American Psychiatric Publishing.

MacKinnon, R. A., Michels, R., & Buckley, P. J. (2009). *The psychiatric interview in clinical practice* (2nd ed.). Washington, DC: American Psychiatric Publishing.

Malik, M. L., Beutler, L. E., Alimohamed, S., Gallagher-Thompson, D., & Thompson, L. (2003). Are all cognitive therapies alike?: A comparison of cognitive and noncognitive therapy process and implications for the application of empirically supported treatments. *Journal of Consulting and Clinical Psychology, 71*(1), 150–158.

Maslow, A. H. (1966). *The psychology of science.* New York: Harper.

McAdams, D. P. (1994). Can personality change?: Levels of stability and growth in personality across the life span. In T. F. Heatherton & J. L. Weinberger (Eds.), *Can personality change?* (pp. 299–313). Washington, DC: American Psychological Association Press.

McAdams, D. P., Pals, J. L. (2006). A new Big Five: Fundamental principles for an integrative science of personality. *American Psychologist, 61,* 204–217.

Meehan, K. B., & Clarkin, J. F. (2015). A critical evaluation of moving toward a trait system for personality disorder assessment. In S. K. Huprich (Ed.), *Personality disorders: Toward theoretical and empirical integration in diagnosis and assessment* (pp. 85–106). Washington, DC: American Psychological Association.

Millon, T. (1996). *Personality and psychopathology.* New York: Wiley.

Mischel, W., & Morf, C. C. (2003). The self as a psychosocial dynamic processing system: A meta-perspective on a century of the self in psychology. In M. R. Leary & J. P. Tangney (Eds.), *Handbook of self and identity* (pp. 15–43). New York: Guilford Press.

Mischel, W., & Shoda, Y. (1995). A cognitive-affective system theory of personality: Reconceptualizing situations, dispositions, dynamics, and invariance in personality structure. *Psychological Review, 102,* 246–268.

Mischel, W., & Shoda, Y. (2008). Toward a unified theory of personality: Integrating dispositions and processing dynamics within the cognitive-affective processing system. In O. P. John, R. W. Robins, & L. A. Pervin (Eds.), *Handbook of personality: Theory and Research* (3rd ed., pp. 208–241). New York: Guilford Press.

Morey, L. C. (1991). *Personality Assessment Inventory professional manual.* Odessa, FL: Psychological Assessment Resources.

Mulder, R. T. (2012). Cultural aspects of personality disorder. In T. A. Widiger, (Ed.,) *Oxford handbook of personality disorders* (pp. 260–274). Oxford, UK: Oxford University Press.

Parker, G., & Barrett, E. (2000). Personality and personality disorder: Current issues and directions. *Psychological Medicine, 30,* 1–9.

Parker, G., Hadzi-Pavlovic, D., Both, L., Kumar, S. Wilhelm, K., & Olley, A. (2004). Measuring disordered personality functioning: To love and to work reprised. *Acta Psychiatrica Scandinavica, 110,* 230–239.

Pincus, A. L. (2005). A contemporary integrative interpersonal theory of personality disorders. In M. Lenzenweger & J. F. Clarkin (Eds.), *Major theories of personality disorder* (2nd ed., pp. 282–331). New York: Guilford Press.

Pincus, A. L., & Ansell, E. B. (2013). Interpersonal theory of personality. In J. Suls & H. Tennen (Eds.), *Handbook of psychology: Vol. 5. Personality and social psychology* (2nd ed., pp. 141–159). Hoboken, NJ: Wiley.

Pincus, A. L., & Hopwood, C. J. (2012). A contemporary interpersonal model of personality pathology and personality disorder. In T. A. Widiger (Ed.), *Oxford handbook of personality disorders* (pp. 372–398). New York: Oxford University Press.

Piper, W. E., & Joyce, A. S. (2001). Psychosocial treatment outcome. In W. J. Livesley (Ed.), *Handbook of personality disorders* (pp. 323–343). New York: Guilford Press.

Pretzer, J. L., & Beck, A. T. (2005). A cognitive theory of personality disorders. In M. F. Lenzenweger & J. F. Clarkin (Eds.), *Major theories of personality disorder* (2nd ed., pp. 43–113). New York: Guilford Press.

Read, S. J., Jones, D. K., & Miller, L. C. (1990). Traits as goal-based categories: The importance of goals in the coherence of dispositional categories. *Journal of Personality and Social Psychology, 56,* 1048–1061.

Roche, M. J., Pincus, A. L., Conroy, D. E., Hyde, A. L., & Ram, N. (2013). Pathological narcissism and interpersonal behavior in daily life. *Personality Disorders: Theory, Research, and Treatment, 4,* 315–323.

Roche, M. J., Pincus, A. L., Rebar, A. L., Conroy, D., & Ram, N. (2014). Enriching psychological assessment using a person-specific analysis of interpersonal processes in daily life. *Assessment, 21*(5), 515–528.

Russell, J. J., Moskowitz, D. S., Zuroff, D. C., Sookman, D., & Paris, J. (2007). Stability and variability of affective experience and interpersonal behavior in borderline personality disorder. *Journal of Abnormal Psychology, 116*(3), 578–588.

Rutter, M. (1987). Temperament, personality and personality disorder. *British Journal of Psychiatry, 150,* 443–458.

Sanderson, C., & Clarkin, J. F. (2013). Further use of the NEO-PI-R personality dimensions in differential treatment planning. In T. A. Widiger & P. T. Costa (Eds.), *Personality disorders and the five factor model of personality* (3rd ed., pp. 325–348). Washington, DC: American Psychological Association.

Shapiro, D. (1981). *Autonomy and rigid character.* New York: Basic Books.

Sheldon, K. M., & Elliot, A. J. (1999). Goal striving, need satisfaction, and longitudinal well-being: The self-concordance model. *Journal of Personality and Social Psychology, 76,* 482–497.

Soloff, P. H. (2000). Psychopharmacology of borderline personality disorder. *Psychiatric Clinics of North America, 23,* 169–190.

Stern, B., Caligor, E., Clarkin, J. F., Critchfield, K. L., MacCornack, V., Lenzenweger, M. F., et al. (2010). The Structured Interview of Personality Organization (STIPO): Preliminary psychometrics in a clinical sample. *Journal of Psychological Assessment, 91,* 35–44.

Svrakic, D. M., Whitehead, C., Przybeck, T. R., & Cloninger, C. R. (1993). Differential diagnosis of personality disorders by the seven factor model of temperament and character. *Archives of General Psychiatry, 50,* 991–999.

Toulmin, S. (1978). Self-knowledge and knowledge of the "self." In T. Mischel (Ed.), *The self: Psychological and philosophical issues* (pp. 291–317). Oxford, UK: Oxford University Press.

Trull, T., & Durrett, C. (2005). Categorical and dimensional models of personality disorder. *Annual Review of Clinical Psychology, 1,* 355–380.

Tyrer, P., & Johnson, T. (1996). Establishing the severity of personality disorder. *American Journal of Psychiatry, 153,* 1593–1597.

Vaillant, G. E., & Perry, J. C. (1980). Personality disorders. In H. Kaplan, A. M. Freedman, & B. Sadock (Eds.), *Comprehensive textbook of psychiatry* (3rd ed., pp. 1562–1590). Baltimore: Williams & Wilkins.

Verheul, R., Andrea, H., Berghout, C. C., Dolan, C., Busschback, J., van der Kroft, P., Bateman, A., et al. (2008). Severity indices of personality problems (SIPP-118): Development, factor structure, reliability, and validity. *Psychological Assessment, 20,* 23–34.

Verheul, R., & Widiger, T. A. (2004). A meta-analysis of the prevalence and usage of the personality disorder not otherwise specified (PDNOS) diagnosis. *Journal of Personality Disorders, 18,* 309–319.

Wakefield, J. C. (2008). The perils of dimensionalization: Challenges in distinguishing negative traits from personality disorders. *Psychiatric Clinics of North America, 31,* 379–393.

Westen, D., & Arkowitz-Westen, L. (1998). Limitations of Axis II in diagnosing personality pathology in clinical practice. *American Journal of Psychiatry, 155,* 1767–1771.

Widiger, T. A., Costa, P. T., Jr., & McCrea, R. R. (2002). A proposal for Axis II: Diagnosing personality disorders using the five-factor model. In P. T. Costa, Jr. & T. A. Widiger (Eds.), *Personality disorders and the five-factor model of personality* (2nd ed., pp. 431–456). Washington, DC: American Psychological Association.

Widiger, T. A., & Lowe, J. R. (2012). Personality disorders. In M. M. Anthony & D. H. Barlow (Eds.), *Handbook of assessment and treatment planning for psychological disorders* (2nd ed., pp. 571–605). New York: Guilford Press.

Widiger, T. A., & Simonsen, E. (2005). Alternative dimensional models of personality disorder. *Journal of Personality Disorders, 19,* 110–130.

Wiggins, J. S. (1982). Circumplex models of interpersonal behaviour. In J. P. Kendall & J. N. Butcher (Eds.), *Handbook of research methods in clinical psychology* (pp. 183–221). New York: Wiley.

Wiggins, J. S., & Pincus, A. L. (1989). Conceptions of personality disorder and dimensions of personality. *Psychological Assessment, 1,* 305–316.

Yeomans, F. E., Clarkin, J. F., & Kernberg, O. F. (2015). *Transference-focused psychotherapy for borderline personality disorder: A clinical guide.* Washington, DC: American Psychiatric Publishing.

Young, J. E., Klosko, J. S., & Weishaar, M. E. (2003). *Schema therapy: A practitioner's guide.* New York: Guilford Press.

CHAPTER 22

# Using Interpersonal Reconstructive Therapy to Select Effective Interventions for Comorbid, Treatment-Resistant, Personality-Disordered Individuals[1]

Lorna Smith Benjamin, Kenneth L. Critchfield, Christie Pugh Karpiak,
Tracey Leone Smith, and Robert Mestel

Personality disorder (PD) has been the stepchild of psychiatric diagnosis ever since the diagnostic "revolution" of 1982, with publication of DSM-III. The intent was to identify diagnoses that were reliable, specific, and sensitive, which means that clinicians should agree about a diagnosis, it should not be applied indiscriminately, and it should be detectable if present. In the early stages of planning DSM-5 (Kupfer, First, & Regier, 2002), PDs (and affective disorders) were targeted as a continuing diagnostic challenge because of robust findings of comorbidity. On average, it appeared that if a person has one PD, he or she may have several more. Worse yet, it became clear that comorbidity is associated with treatment resistance or severity (Merikangas & Weissman, 1986, p. 274).

By the time of DSM-5 was published, comorbidity among affective and other disorders (e.g., anxiety, depression) was addressed by supplementary "dimensional" measures (PROMIS), while comorbidity among PDs was addressed by a very complex new model placed in a separate section (III). When using that system, patients are to be assessed for (1) levels of personality functioning, which involve ratings of Self ("Identity" and "Self-Direction") and of Interpersonal Functioning (Empathy and Intimacy); in addition, there is an assessment of (2) Pathological personality traits, which involves ratings on five "dimensions" based on factor analysis (Negative Affectivity, Detachment, Antagonism, Disinhibition, and Psychoticism). Within each of those trait domains, 25 trait facets are used to characterize five specific PDs (antisocial [ASPD], avoidant [AVPD], borderline [BPD], narcissistic [NPD], obsessive–compulsive [OCPD], and schizotypal [STPD]). For example, ASPD is defined by manipulativeness, callousness, deceitfulness, hostility, risk taking, impulsivity plus ratings of identity, self-di-

---

[1] The first edition's version of this chapter described the well-validated structural analysis of social behavior (SASB) model and the newer interpersonal reconstructive therapy (IRT) models. There was an emphasis on the supporting literature for IRT, much of it collected by Karpiak. This version includes natural biology featured in Benjamin (2018); new databases, including Critchfield's research about the reliability and validity of the case formulation method and change in IRT clinic patients; Smith's (2002) database from her study of Benjamin's predictions for antecedents of personality disorder; and Mestel's large German patient database. Karpiak and Smith also created independent databases that establish reliability of the SASB medium form.

rection, and empathy and intimacy. The *raison d'être* of this alternative system for personality diagnosis is that it can address comorbidity by creating profiles for individual on various basic dimensions identified by factor analysis. The factor loadings are used to determine each individual's position on the underlying dimensions defined by the factors. Presumably, the factors represent the underlying nature of personality; no independent evidence is offered to support that assumption. Interestingly, the comorbidity among affective and other disorders is not seen to be so problematic as to require construction of an equally complex route to diagnose anxiety or depression, for example. Perhaps that is because the "neurobiology" of some of them is known, and treatments with medication can successfully address them. For example, symptoms of depression are associated with a deficit of serotonin and (some) antidepressants address that by blocking serotonin reuptake mechanisms. There is no comparable neurobiological analysis of or related interventions for PD per se.

For tests of the validity of diagnosis and treatment models, the need for integrative theory is clear (*Psychotherapy Research,* 25th Anniversary Issue, 2012). Ideally, such theory would include descriptions of mechanisms of pathology that can be activated during treatment and favorably affect outcome. Studies of mechanisms would significantly enhance understanding of effectiveness. Emphasis on mechanisms has been recommended by Insel (2013), director of NIMH, who noted that randomized controlled trials (RCTs) can only account for a percentage of the people in the trial. In contrast, the procedure of relating mechanisms of change to outcome potentially can account for every subject. The idea would be that those who did not show improvement would have a demonstrated deficiency in the functioning of mechanisms.

Our purpose in this chapter is to describe a reliable, specific, and sensitive-case formulation method (IRT; Benjamin, 2003) that focuses on personality patterns and accommodates comorbidity among and between PDs and affective disorders by invoking a natural biological analysis (Benjamin, 2018). The natural biology offers an attachment-based description of mechanisms of pathology and of change. It is wholly compatible with treatment by medication and by psychotherapy.

An early version of this approach was applied to DSM-III/DSM-IV definitions of personality (Benjamin, 1996a). It included a description of likely developmental antecedents for each PD and clearly argued ways of making differential diagnoses. In Benjamin (2003, 2018), methods to identify developmental antecedents for affective disorders and PDs at the individual level (regardless of diagnosis) are emphasized along with individualized treatment recommendations. Early results of IRT treatments with a population called CORDS (Comorbid, Often Rehospitalized, Dysfunctional, and Suicidal) are summarized in this chapter.

## IRT Case Formulations

IRT case formulations begin with a list of symptoms and identification of related current stresses. Then affective symptoms (e.g., anger, anxiety and depression) are linked to attempts to cope with threat and find safety. This is accomplished by exploring the interpersonal contexts in which the affective symptoms appear, using free association to link perceived stresses and responses to antecedent interactions with attachment figures, and learn how and why the symptoms, maladaptive though they may be in reality, are experienced as adaptive.

### *Example of an IRT Case Formulation*

Roger, 42-year-old man, was depressed and recently had lost his job because of disagreements with coworkers. He believed that his boss had conspired to get rid of him, and he was consulting a lawyer to see whether he had legal recourse. The issue at the time of hospitalization was his uncontrolled rage, which had included attacks on one particular child and uncontrolled anger on the job. He was fond of alcohol, and when on a binge, often became suicidal. During one of these episodes, the police were called, and he was taken to the hospital. His worst stress at the time of the interview was the recent death of his mother. Much against his will and hers, she had been placed in a nursing home, where she failed to thrive and died shortly thereafter. His response to his unenviable situation was to drink, rage, and be depressed. His self-descriptions included the following: "I have rage attacks; It feels normal when I am crazy; I do drink sometimes but I do not remember what I do. I can dissociate from reality. But mostly, I am very logical and kind. I love my family." His current diagnosis was major depressive disorder and alcohol dependence. He was referred for assessment of Axis II complications. There was strong evidence of brain damage and associated dysfunction (e.g., Performance IQ was far below his relatively high Verbal IQ). A stroke had been ruled out by medical tests. Roger's in-hospital medication was Paxil.

The case formulation interview quickly centered on Roger's father, whom he described in the same terms he used to describe himself: His father also "felt regular when crazy." This man would rage unpredictably, and the specific targets of his rage were Roger's mother (for alleged infidelity) and Roger. Father's attacks on him usually included full-strength fisticuffs to the head. But there were other forms of threat, too. For example, the father shot Roger's pet cat and threw it in the trash, allegedly because the cat might scratch the boy. The father also frequently called Roger stupid.

## Copy Processes

The links between past and present happen by one or more of three copy processes (and their exact opposites, defined later in the section on SASB). For Roger, identification with his father was reflected in the fact that, like his father, his rage attacks earned him the title of "ogre" in his own marital family. Like his father, he targeted one particular child for abuse and accused his wife of infidelity. And as noted earlier, Roger offered the same unusual description for his father and himself: "I feel normal when crazy." Roger recapitulated his relationship with his father by being paranoid in relation to male authorities (the boss at work). He introjected his father's attacks as suicidal ideation and also thoughts of himself as stupid. Staff members agreed that, given the history, it was likely that the brain damage was the consequence of chronic blows to the head.

Roger also was identified with his mother, whom he described as "kind and logical." She had often been knocked out by the father's beatings. When the father had an affair, she divorced him and then was severely depressed and neglected the children. Like his mother, Roger was nonfunctional because of severe depression and alcoholism. Feeling he had failed to protect his mother and having lost his job, he despaired. The situation recapitulated earlier experiences of unbearable helplessness and loss, and Roger turned his rage against himself.

An IRT case formulation includes a functional analysis of threat affects (e.g., anger, anxiety, and depression). In general, anger has the function of creating distance or control as a way of coping with threat. Anxiety has the function of mobilizing the individual to find a way to cope with threat, and it is not resolved until there is success in that. Depression is a defensive adaptation of last resort: It reduces threat value by facilitating hiding via psychological walling off and inhibition of self-expression, sometimes to the point of surrender. Anger prevailed as Roger tried to control his wife, coworkers, and son. Roger likely was vulnerable to anxiety, too, but he did not speak of it, probably because his efforts to cope were so dominated by his reflexive access to anger. His depression reflected defeat in his efforts to control family and coworkers and was made worse as he introjected his father's message that he was stupid, as well as criticism and rejection from the men at work. In addition, Roger qualified for the label paranoid PD because of his frequent suspicions of harm and deception, sensitivity to threat, inappropriate responses of counterattack, and recurrent suspicious about his wife's fidelity. In summary, Roger's presenting suicidality, his anger, depression, alcoholism, paranoia, and alienation from his wife and his fellow workers all had copy process connections to his interactions with others.

## Gifts of Love

Copy processes, whether they support adaptive (Green) or maladaptive (Red) patterns, are sustained by loyalty to and love for internalized representations of attachment figures called "family in the head" in IRT.[2] The process of copying is a Gift of Love (GOL) to family in the head, a demonstration of loyalty to and love for the internal working models of attachment figures. For example, as Roger beat his son, he was showing loyalty to and love for (GOL) the father in his head. As he lost himself in alcoholism, he showed loyalty to and love for his mother. The term GOL reflects the fact that copying attachment figures during early development is supported by a primitive brain (subcortical) sense of well-being. Nature provides it, along with a powerful preference to maintain proxim-

---

[2]This replaces the term IPIR (important persons and their internalized representations) from Benjamin (2003). The reason is that many readers objected to so many acronyms. Any attachment figure, biologically related or not, belongs to "family in the head."

ity to the attachment figure, to support survival. There is a sense of safety and well-being when in proximity to, obeying, and pleasing attachment figures when under threat (which includes separation from the attachment figure when the mammal is young). The patterns set by this process (i.e., maintain proximity, copy their ways, and all will be well) are meant by nature to last a lifetime. The mechanism is that throughout the lifetime, the individual maintains a relationship with family in the head (internalized representations with mechanisms discussed in the section on natural biology). This means that Roger's copy processes represent GOLs to internalizations of his father and mother, and that by copying their ways, he could feel safe and, as he said, "normal."

If GOLs support maladaptive copy processes, then it follows they are the primary treatment target. If Roger could give up loyalty to destructive versions of parental rules and values modeled for him, he could become free to be his Birthright Self, the person he would have become if he had been provided Secure Base conditions as a child. The idea that Secure Base conditions offered by the parent are internalized as secure base is Bowlby's. Secure Base has been shown to relate powerfully to all forms of good health and function by many hundreds of research studies (Cassidy & Shaver, 2008). Research with Bowlby's concept typically involves classifying parental and child attachment types in categories that include Secure Base conditions (offered; received). Parental offering of Secure Base conditions is described here (and later in the SASB section) as friendly, sensitive protectiveness, gradually accompanied by support for age-appropriate amounts of autonomy. The result of secure-base parenting is a well attached child with a well-defined sense of separate self, able to show balance between focus on self and others. In IRT, internalized secure base and secure-base patterns of personality define normality, and it is the reconstructive therapy goal.

## Reliability, Specificity, and Sensitivity of Case Formulations

Evidence that the case formulation method is reliable, specific, and sensitive was provided in Critchfield, Benjamin, and Levenick (2015), based on a subsample of case formulations from over 270 inpatients referred to LSB (the interviewer) for consultation, usually for "suspected Axis II involvement." This applied research was on individuals who had not responded to treatment as usual; not surprisingly the cases were complex, comorbid, and reliably included PD. Tallies of diagnoses in the medical records, results of Structured Clinical Interview for DSM-IV Axis II and Axis II (SCID-I and SCID-II) and of Beck's rating scales for depression and anxiety lead to the label CORDS: Comorbid, Often Rehospitalized (average prior lifetime hospitalizations = 4, median = 2), Dysfunctional (average Global Assessment of Functioning [GAF] at admission = 25) and Suicidal (average of 2.1 lifetime suicide attempts, median = 2.0). Roger was qualified for the CORDS label; he presented with a suicide attempt (not his first); was dysfunctional, depressed, and anxious; abused alcohol; and had symptoms of attenuated psychosis and paranoid PD.

Reliability of the case formulations was established by kappas between two independent sets of judges at different sites. Of the many comparisons involved, the most complex and directly relevant is whether independent judges could link specific symptoms to a current relationship (e.g., Roger was angry with his boss, his coworkers for unfairness, and his wife for infidelity) that is connected to a specific attachment figure (Roger's father) by a specific process (e.g., identification with his father in his relationship with his boss, his wife, and his son.) The kappa for these links among judgments made by graduate trainees was .75 and between site consensus with a team of professionals was .77. According to Fleiss (1981), a kappa > .75 marks excellent agreement.

Specificity of the case formulation method was established by asking 38 judges to view five case formulation videos and accurately match each of the five patients to his or her actual case formulation by drawing from a list of seven possibilities. Thirty-five of the 38 judges made significantly more correct matches than was expected by chance.

Sensitivity was established in two ways. First, there was an SASB coded profile for each symptom-relevant relationship; this was based on the patients' descriptions of relationships as documented in the case reports. SASB is described later in this chapter. Sensitivity was also assessed using Spearman's rho to compare 8-point profiles from patients' self-ratings on the SASB Intrex to SASB-coded profiles generated from descriptions in the case reports.

The many significant rho results demonstrated that patients' self-ratings matched the patterns reported in the case reports. That concordance between interview data and patient ratings is important because it affirms that the interviewer elicited rather than forced the observed links.

## Natural Biology of a Case Formulation

The natural biology in IRT, explained in detail in Benjamin (2018), grounds the IRT case formulation and treatment models in basic biological science. If attachment figures provide secure base conditions, the nervous system functions in adaptive ways. Normal function is apparent if safety and threat are managed by adaptively cued sequences of affects, behaviors, and cognitions in the primitive brain. The sequences are called C1AB chains in IRT, and they are cued by lessons from attachment figures. A chain begins with apprehension of threat or safety (C1) accompanied by specific affects (A) that predispose behaviors (B) that are adaptive in the perceived context. An example of an adaptive sequence, C1AB is "See the bear (C1), fear it (A), run away (B)." By contrast, here is an astonishing example of a maladaptive instruction about safety. Living near a highway, John's upper-class mother, who overtly envied the attention her husband gave their son, took him to a "lesson in safety." At dusk, they arrived at the interstate highway far from an intersection; the lesson was to run across when she told him it was safe even though he could see an oncoming truck (C1). He was terrified (A) and ran as fast as he could, barely escaping the truck (B). Not surprisingly, as an adult he showed the copy process of recapitulation as he repeatedly engaged in self-sabotaging behaviors that courted disaster while implementing the "lesson" as GOLs to his mother.

Natural biology records copy processes, whether adaptive or maladaptive, with mirror neurons and complex brain circuits that include, among other things, affect regulating the hypothalamic–pituitary–adrenal (HPA) axis and Family in the Head. C1AB chains can be identified during an interview simply by asking for the components of a critical event. For example, Roger could be asked, "Can you recall a recent time when you lost it with your son?" If the answer is "yes," then follow with "What was going on (C1)? What did you feel (A)? What did you do (B)." Next, ask, "What does that remind you of?" The associative result likely yields "raw data" about a C1AB. Roger's responses revealed the identification with his father. His statement that it "felt normal" to abuse his son was evidence of a GOL to his father.

Mechanisms that direct C1AB threat chains involve connections to natural stress chemistry (e.g., epinephrine, cortisol) to mobilize for "fight or flight." Copying is followed by safety system chemistry because doing as the caregiver did or said (verbally or nonverbally) is as calming as hugging an attachment figure. Calming and pleasant affects are managed largely by the parasympathetic nervous system, which calls for release of serotonin, dopamine, oxytocin, and opioids.[3] Those processes explain why Roger experienced aggressing against a son was a normal thing to do when he copied his father and was calmed by doing what father his did. Adaptive function and rationality, called C2 to represent higher (cortical) brain function, have little to do with it. The primitive brain follows primitive rules: Just copy what attachment figures perceived (C1), felt (A) and did (B), and all will be well. It is as if nature says, "What they did is right and good; your safety depends on believing that and complying with their instructions."

Natural biology supports the psychoanalytic idea of developmental stages. In IRT, the stages are simple: First, there is attachment that is vital for protection, nurturance, and training. There is no attempt in IRT theory to detail the cortical and subcortical circuits that put it all together. That challenge is being addressed by many others. Porges's (1994) polyvagal theory is an excellent example of credible description of circuitry; he focuses on mechanisms regarding safety and threat in terms of complex interactions between respiratory and cardiac function. Second, there is differentiation that is vital if the offspring is to function as a distinct member of the troop (community). Third, there is a time of peer play and continued instruction for developing social and cognitive skills. Then there is bonding that facilitates the creation of and support and education of the next generation. Failure at any of these stages can result in dysfunction. With CORDS, the most common developmental problem is differentiation failure.

---

[3] IRT offers diagnostic descriptions for distortion of safety related affects (e.g. substance abuse, eating disorders, mania), but they are not discussed here.

While considering the impact of attachment relationships on the development of the nervous system and consequent behavior, it is important to reiterate that IRT interviews are characterized by (1) specificity of the narrative that helps activate the primitive brain memory and (2) focus on interactions as is characteristic in the basic sciences. Try to imagine chemistry, physics, or astronomy without being very specific about interactive "behaviors" of chemicals, particles, moving objects, the heart and lungs, or the planets and stars. It follows that clinical psychology and psychiatry also should be well attuned to contexts and interactions if basic science is the desired methodology. Theory that explains interactions might then replace discussions of fixed traits and of independent human entities moving through the world imposing their will or getting their needs met.

Inheritance, of course, also affects definitions of threat and safety. The startle response is a good example of an inherited response to threat. Instructions for these inherited dispositions are embedded in sequences in the DNA. But genes also are affected by environment. Its effect is recorded by well-known processes of expressing and silencing genes and by newly discovered epigenetic processes. An early investigator of epigenetic process (Meaney, 2010, p. 41), after 20 years of careful experimentation on anxiety in rats, reported that "environmental conditions in early life structurally alter DNA, providing a physical basis for the influence of the perinatal environmental signals on phenotype over the life of the individual." Similarly, at the National Institute of Mental Health (NIMH) laboratory of ethology directed by S. Suomi, epigenetic process in chimpanzees has shown (Spinelli et al., 2010, p. 1153) that "adverse early-life environment during infancy is associated with long-term alterations in the serotonin system." In summary, genes are very much involved in symptoms of mental disorder, but they are shaped by interactions with the environment, as well as by sequences in DNA present at birth.

## Structural Analysis of Social Behavior

Since the 1970s (Benjamin, 1974), SASB-based assessments of clinical and research material have contributed to the development of IRT case formulations and treatment models (Benjamin, 2003). Reviews of a variety of uses of SASB by others are in Benjamin (1996b), Benjamin, Rotweiler, and Critchfield (2006), and Constantino (2000). The most influential precursors to SASB were Harry Stack Sullivan, Henry Murray, Timothy Leary, Earl Schaefer, and Harry Harlow. Details appeared in Benjamin (1974) and have been summarized repeatedly (e.g., Benjamin, 2010). Combined with natural biology, the SASB model is particularly useful in providing parsimonious descriptions of a normal developmental sequences and affects, behaviors and cognitions. This is essential in setting therapy goals and making decisions about interventions.

A simplified version of the full SASB model (Benjamin, 1974, 1979) appears in Figure 22.1 (from Benjamin 2003). Like many of other models for describing social behavior (e.g., single circumplex models; see Leary, 1957; Schaefer, 1965; Wiggins, 1982), the horizontal axis in Figure 22.1 ranges from hostility to love and is called the "affiliation axis." The description of the vertical axis in SASB, called the "interdependence axis," is different from interpersonal models that stay closer to Leary's original version. They appear in a single plane and their vertical dimension holds that Submit is the opposite of Control. The SASB model appears in three planes, and the vertical dimension on each plane is different. The three planes represent three types of focus: transitive focus on other (**bold** print in Figure 22.1), intransitive focus on self (underlined print) and transitive focus turned inward (*italicized* print). As shown in Figure 22.1, rather than describing Submit as the "opposite" of Control, on the SASB model, Emancipation is the opposite of Control, while Submit is the complement of Control. Each of the eight positions in Figure 22.1 is defined in terms of location on the affiliation and interdependence axes. Think of the extremes as + or –2 units from the center of the figure. By rules of plane geometry, Attack is at –2 units of affiliation and 0 units of interdependence. Emancipate is +2 units of independence (the upper half of the vertical axis) and 0 units of affiliation. That means that Blame is at (–1, –1) while its opposite, Affirm, is at (+1, +1). Each of the eight positions in Figure 22.1 is defined in terms of location on the affiliation and interdependence axes. The extremes are + or –2 units from the center of the figure.) By rules of plan geometry, Attack is at –2 units of affiliation and 0 units of interdependence. Emancipate is +2 units of independence (the upper half of the vertical

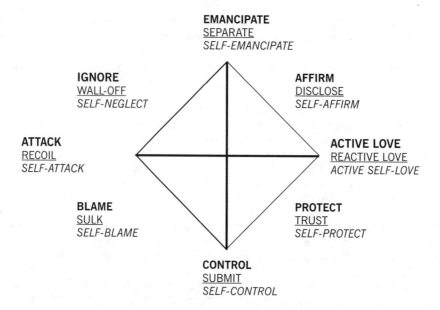

**FIGURE 22.1.** The SASB one-word cluster model. **Bold** print indicates transitive focus on other. Underlined print indicates intransitive focus on self. *Italicized* print indicates transitive focus introjected inward on the self. From Benjamin (1996a, p. 55). Copyright © 1996 The Guilford Press. Reprinted by permission.

axis) and 0 units of affiliation. So, for example, Blame is at (−1, −1) while its opposite, Affirm, is at (+1, +1).

Interpersonal and intrapsychic relationships with self and others can reliably be described in terms of combinations of the underlying primitive basics either by self-ratings on the SASB Intrex questionnaires (Benjamin, 2000) or by an objective observer coding system. Summaries of self-ratings on the Intrex questionnaires and/or of objective observer codes are available by SASB software (*intrex@psych.utah.edu*). Self-ratings are made on a 100-point scale to indicate aptness of the description and the frequency that it happens. The number 50 is the marker between "true" and "false." Objective observer codes of video made by judgments of underlying dimensions, as described earlier, yield SASB profiles comparable to those from self-ratings. Observer codes of video also may be analyzed for sequences, which can be taken to higher powers using Markov chain logic to yield estimates of transition states, identify steady states, and more (Benjamin, 1986; Benjamin & Cushing, 2000; Knobloch-Fedders et al., 2014).

The SASB medium and short form questionnaires assess relationships in terms of the simple SASB model in Figure 22.1. Items reflect great intensity at the poles of the axes, and this is consistent with natural biology. For example, Attack (Figure 22.1) is described as "Without thought about what might happen, $X$ wildly, hatefully, destructively attacks $Y$." This is opposed by Active Love, "$X$ happily, gently, very lovingly approaches $Y$, and warmly invites $Y$ to be as close as he or she would like." This language is noticeably more intense and primitive than the words "Cold-Hearted and Warm-Agreeable," used to define extremes on the single-surface interpersonal circle.

### SASB Defines Secure Base

To the extent possible, all definitions and concepts in SASB and IRT are as detailed and concrete as possible. For example, Bowlby's secure base is described by SASB codes of video of secure interactions between mothers and toddlers (Teti, Heaton, Benjamin, & Gelfand, 1995): Affirm/Disclose; Self-Affirm; Active Love/Reactive Love/Self-Love; and Protect/Trust/Self-Protect. In summary, secure base is characterized as consistently friendly with moderate enmeshment (interdependence) and moderate autonomy (independence). Secure Base is normal behavior, and it is the reconstructive goal in

IRT. This position was powerfully supported by a study that used SASB coding to a short video of mother–toddler interactions of 100 maltreating mothers and 100 matched controls (Skowron, Cipriano-Essel, Benjamin, Pincus, & Van Ryzin, 2013). They used a special version of SASB software to track physiological threat and safety responses in parallel with SASB codes of mother–child interactions. The physiology of maltreating mothers showed that they were distressed when the child was autonomous and felt safer when the child was submissive. The opposite was true for the nonmaltreating moms, who were most comfortable when the child was completing the task on his or her own. This is consistent with the definition of "secure base" as attached, yet clearly defined as separate (differentiated); it also reconfirms secure base as characteristic of normal populations.

### Validations of the Structure of the SASB Model

The structure of the model has been confirmed by naive raters' dimensional ratings of the questionnaire items written to describe points of the SASB models (Benjamin, 2000, 2010) and by factor-analytic reconstructions of the model using data generated when raters apply the Intrex items to themselves and their relationships (as distinct from rating the dimensions of the items per se; Benjamin, 1974, 2000). See reviews of publications using SASB (Benjamin, 1996b; Benjamin et al., 2006).

### Predictive Principles: Similarity, Complementarity, Introjection, and Antithesis

In addition to describing patterns in a valid and reliable way, the SASB model provides predictions about what is likely to follow a given position. The predictive principle of similarity defines identification. As Roger blamed his wife for infidelity, his behavior and the SASB codes (e.g., Blame, which is a hostile, transitive action) were the same as codes for his father in relation to his mother. In research studies, if the profiles for one relationship share more than half the variance with profiles of another, they are said to be similar. Complementarity is shown in Figure 22.1 by the pairing of **bold** print points with underlined points. For example, Sulk is the complement of Blame. Its coordinates are the same as Blame (–1, –1). The only difference is the focus. Sulk is intransitive and Blame is transitive. Complementary pairings each are focused on the same individual (transitive person focuses on intransitive person, and intransitive person focuses on self), and both are at comparable points on the horizontal and vertical coordinates of interpersonal space. Complementarity is the most frequently observed predictive principle (Benjamin, 2018).

The third predictive principle is Introjection, and it is marked by pairing of **bold** and *italicized* points in Figure 22.1. As Roger turns his father's Blame inward, he feels Self-Blame, a feature that dominated his suicidal thoughts. Introjection also is very common. An Antithesis is the complement of the opposite. Everything is reversed: interpersonal focus, value of attachment, and value of interdependence. For example, the antithesis of Blame is Disclose. This means there is a shift from Transitive (–1, –1) to Intransitive (+1, +1). The principle is useful for providing corrective interventions. A good response to Blame often is to Disclose (about the impact): "Roger, I would like it if you could trust me. It bothers me a lot as you keep accusing me of something that is just not true." An adolescent characterized by Separate in response to parental Control is a common example of antithesis.

### Examples of Clinical Uses of SASB-Based Descriptions

Mean ratings by 133 normal subjects of their mothers' perceived transitive actions (diamonds) and the raters' intransitive responses (squares) when they were ages 5–10 are presented in Figure 22.2. It is clear that their highest scores, well above the true marker of 50, are in the secure base region of interpersonal space: Affirm/Disclose, ActiveLove/PassiveLove, and Protect/Trust. Hostile patterns received very low average ratings from this group. The rho between the profile for normal mother transitive and rater intransitive is 1.00, $p > .005$, and that is evidence of complementarity. Given that SASB questionnaire items are presented in a randomly determined order, it is remarkable that these group profiles are so similar. Yet this same form of complementarity can be seen at the individual level by correlating the 8-point within-subject profiles for [Mother transitive] with [Rater intransitive]. If such a "within-$r$" is .71 or more, over half the variance between pro-

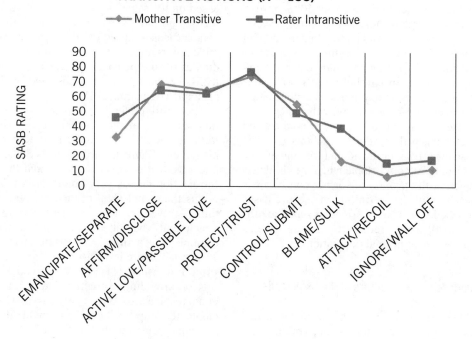
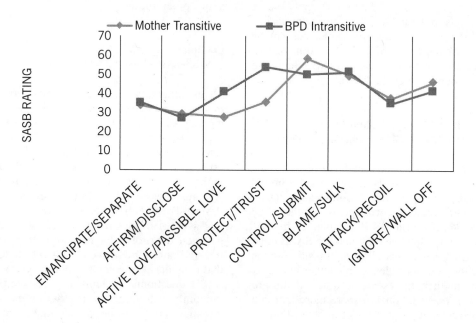

**FIGURE 22.2.** Comparison of mothers' transitive (top) and raters' intransitive (bottom) interpersonal patterns in normal, BPD, anakastic PD, and NPD samples. Normal data are from University students in Wisconsin, 1980, and PD data are from patients at the HELIOS Klinik in Bad Gronenbach, Germany, courtesy of Robert Mestel, Director of Research.

files is correlated, and the connection is taken to be noteworthy. Within-$r$'s of this magnitude are very common, no matter where the complementary pairs peak in their profiles. For the mother–child pairs shown in top part of Figure 22.2, within-$r$ average .81, with $SD = .25$. The validity of complementarity defined by SASB was affirmed by Gurtman (2000), using a different between-subjects method of testing complementarity in normal and patient populations. Complementarity has served as an independent variable in therapy studies in which Svartberg and Stiles (1992) predicted therapy outcome from therapist competence and patient complementarity.

The profiles for normal raters (top of Figure 22.2) are very different from profiles generated by patients for 1,980 patients with BPD (bottom) at Helios Klinik (Bad Gronenbach, Germany). Patient ratings of mother transitive and self-intransitive are markedly more hostile and less friendly. In addition, rho (.524) testing group profiles for complementarity between patients with BPD and their mothers were not significant. Inspection of bottom part of Figure 22.2 shows that the average patient profiles for intransitive patterns with mother were rotated 45 degrees in the friendly direction. The patient's peak was at Trust rather than Submit, which directly would complement the mother's peak at Control. That particular deviation from complementarity is seen (not shown here) for NPD and anakastic PD as well. In general, patient raters' self-described intransitive profiles in relation to early attachment figures peak on Trust rather than Submit even as the parent is elevated on Control and Hostility. The same patterns are observed with fathers.

This rotation in the direction of Trust is explained by natural biology, which notes that young primates are predisposed to attach (trust, maintain proximity) to caregivers, no matter how the caregivers treat them 10. Harlow (1958) argued that critical variables for attachment in the baby primate is frequent proximity early in life and reliable offering of contact comfort. It is enhanced greatly, of course, if the parent also is responsive to the child's needs (Bretherton, 1992), which Harlow's artificial laboratory "mothers" of baby monkeys could not do. Still, Harlow's argument that vital components of attachment during early development are proximity and contact comfort is supported by observations of clinicians who work with abused children. They love their caregivers and usually want to return to them no matter how they badly they have been treated by them. This evidence of positive attachment even to a hostile caregiver further supports the GOL concept.

The predictive principle of Similarity is shown in Figure 22.3 by normal raters' observations of marital modeling by mother and father. Their relationships received highest ratings in the secure base region except that for intransitive states (bottom), mothers Submit ($p < .05$) and Sulk ($p < .05$) more in relation father, while fathers take more autonomy from mothers ($p < .05$). Data support the other predictive principles, too, but the most common ones are complementarity, similarity, and introjection (Benjamin, 2018). Use of SASB predictive principles to identify copy processes in IRT case formulations was discussed earlier. SASB is more complex relative to other models (Carson, 1969) but offers substantial clinical advantages, including the ability to connect perceived patterns with attachment figures in childhood to perceived relationships with self and others in adulthood, as in the case formulation. In treatment, use of SASB keeps the dialogue interactive and specific enough for recognition of patterns and links among them to be accurate.

## Using SASB to Describe PD and Make Differential Diagnoses

In Benjamin (1996a), SASB codes of DSM-IV descriptions of PD provided interpersonal descriptions of each disorder and were accompanied by recommendations for differential diagnoses and treatment. Recommendations for differential diagnosis are of great interest in this discussion of comorbidity among PDs because that comorbidity, as noted earlier, is taken to be devastating to the present DSM diagnostic system for PD.

The SASB-based theoretical recommendations for making differential PD diagnoses were applied in the diagnostic reports of PD provided by the Wisconsin Personality Disorders Inventory (WISPI; Klein et al., 1993). Here, the comorbidity problem for PD is addressed on an empirical rather than a theoretical basis. Starting with canonical $R$, the $T$ for Beta scores is used to assess links between specific PDs to specific SASB codes. The rationale for using $T$ in this way is specified in Appendix 22.1. The comorbid diagnostic population in this analysis is Cluster B personality disorders (HPD = his-

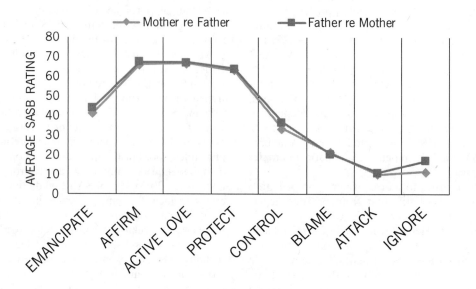

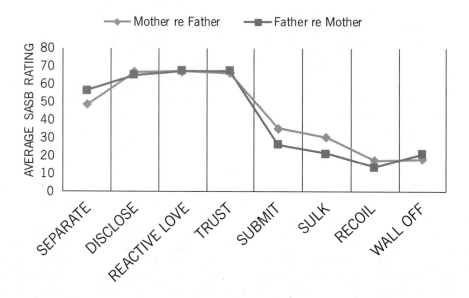

**FIGURE 22.3.** Normal parents' transitive (top) and intransitive (bottom) interpersonal patterns with each other. In this and other normal samples, the friendly behaviors are rated well above the "true" marker (= 50) and hostile behaviors are rated well below. This figure shows that the parents' transitive actions with each other are nearly identical. Their intransitive responses are similar in friendliness, but mothers Submit ($p < .05$) and Sulk ($p < .05$) more, while fathers are more autonomous ($p < .05$).

trionic; NPD = narcissistic; ASPD = antisocial; and BPD = borderline). Exploration of the method within Clusters A and C, and also in relation to the total set of PDs plus normal subjects is deferred for elsewhere.

Results of canonical $R$ that appear in Table 22.1 drew on a database collected by Smith (2002), who obtained diagnostic information by interviewing 76 psychiatric inpatients using the SCID-II (First, Spitzer, Gibbon, Williams, & Benjamin, 1997) and by administering the WISPI (Klein et al., 1993), a self-rating assessment method. Diagnoses using WISPI correlated significantly with diagnoses made by SCID-II (Smith, Klein, & Benjamin, 2003) in this same dataset. In addition to gathering diagnostic information by WISPI and SCID-II, Smith and colleagues (2003) assessed patients' views of self and others using the SASB Intrex medium form questionnaires.

In the canonical analyses that follow here, the WISPI diagnoses are primary. A brief report on results using SCID-II follows the discussion of Table 22.1, which presents results of canonical $R$'s between the mean PD scale scores on the WISPI for each of the four Cluster B disorders and the 8-point SASB profile scores for a given aspect of an attachment relationship (e.g., Me with my SO at worst). Canonical $R$ weights SASB scores, so that differences are minimized between the DSM diagnostic scores and the weighted SASB psychosocial scores. If Rao's $F$ was associated with a "noteworthy" $p$, its level is listed in the table. As we indicate below, results are highly consistent with clinical observation. Table 22.1 includes only the aspects of relationships (e.g., My introject at worst; or My transitive behaviors with mother) that had canonical $R$ with Rao's $F$ with $p \leq .10$ (with one exception at $p$ for Rao's $F < .11$). Nine of 18 = 50% of the possible aspects of relationship assessed in the SASB Intrex standard series met this criterion. The many instances of Rao's $F$ with $p < .05$ establish that, in general, interpersonal and intrapsychic descriptions of patterns with loved ones link directly to PD diagnoses.

In addition to noticing which aspects are related to PD, it is important to know specifically which interactive patterns relate to which disorders. That question is addressed here by $T$, which is a standardized beta score. $T$ identifies SASB codes that have large beta weights connecting them to a given Cluster B PD. For example, in Table 22.1 the $T$ for Self-Attack (introject worst) is 4.079 for BPD and (minus) 2.180 for HPD. So the clinician who struggles with whether to diagnose BPD or HPD should consider (among other things) primitive brain perceptions, affects, and behaviors (C1AB) related to Self-Attack. It is expected the clinician will find BPD predicts Self-Attack at worst (e.g., GOL "says" it is right and safe as is alienation from SO). For HPD, Self-Attack is negatively weighted, and even in the worst state, while intransitive behaviors in relation to SO suggest a secure base for HPD. The two disorders have dramatically different social and intrapsychic descriptors.

NPD can be confused with HPD but they too have very different "centers of gravity." HPD shows complex transitive patterns toward SO at Best (Emancipate Affirm, Love, Blame and Neglect), but even at Worst, is averse to Self-Blame and Self-Attack and reliant on SO (Discloses, Loves, Trusts). By contrast, the distinguishing markers for NPD do not suggest warm connectedness at all. There is Self-Emancipating and Control of SO at Best and Self-Protect at Worst. Interestingly, mothers of persons with NPD submitted to the NPD and were averse to having the person with NPD separate from them. This could predispose the person with NPD to manage other attachment figures in service of self-protection, with no concern about loss.

BPD and ASPD are similar in some ways but different in others. Persons with ASPD have experienced, and they deliver, hostility and neglect. The mother was remarkably unavailable and unresponsive (i.e, she was walled off, separate, and averse to submission). The person with ASPD had nothing in his or her history to suggest a secure base and only knew about punishment (from father) and separation (from mother). Reflecting on such a barren history, devoid of markers for attachment, makes one think that punishing these people compares to abusing a neglected and abused animal and expecting it to become friendly. Persons with BPD also have serious hostility in their history (Paternal Attack) but they appear to have selected a corrective SO (negative Blame). Nonetheless, persons with BPD do give SO a hard time, as they Attack SO at worst with negative weights to Protection, Affirmation and Emancipation of SO, possibly reflecting identification with father. The BPD negative $T$ for Neglect of and Emancipating SO also suggests an investment in staying connected, distinguishes BPD from ASPD and NPD, and is consistent with the DSM item for BPD regarding fear of abandonment.

TABLE 22.1. Relationships and Self-Concept Help Differentiate Cluster C Disorders

| | Rao's F | Self-Emancipate | Self-Affirm | Self-Love | Self-Protect | Self-Control | Self-Blame | Self-Attack | Self-Neglect |
|---|---|---|---|---|---|---|---|---|---|
| **1. Introject best** | | | | | | | | | |
| **Significant prediction PD to SASB** | p <.000 | .000 | | .009 | .002 | | .004 | .014 | .001 |
| Histrionic | | | | 2.666 | 2.114 | | −2.180 | | |
| Narcissistic | | (1.57) | | | | | | | |
| Antisocial | | 2.426 | −4.293 | −4.293 | | | | 1.648 | 1.994 |
| Borderline | | | −2.206 | −3.583 | −4.293 | | 3.916 | 2.621 | 2.302 |
| **2. Introject worst** | | | | | | | | | |
| **Significant prediction PD to SASB** | p <.000 | .001 | | | | | .017 | .000 | .003 |
| Histrionic | | 2.622 | | | | | −1.676 | −2.598 | |
| Narcissistic | | | | | 1.801 | | | | |
| Antisocial | | 2.380 | | | | −2.042 | | | |
| Borderline | | | (−1.60) | −2.232 | −2.270 | 1.60 | 3.286 | 4.079 | 2.873 |
| | Rao's F | Emancipate | Affirm | Active Love | Protect | Control | Blame | Attack | Neglect |
| **3. SO at best transitive** | | | | | | | | | |
| **Significant prediction PD to SASB** | p <.047 | | | | | | .035 | .036 | 1.58 (1.513) |
| Histrionic | | | 1.699 | 1.713 | | 1.872 | | | |
| Narcissistic | | | | | | | | | |
| Antisocial | | | | | | | 2.740 | 2.198 | |
| Borderline | | | | | | | (−1.539) | | |
| **5. Rater transitive with SO best** | | | | | | | | | |
| **Significant prediction PD to SASB** | p <.004 | | | | | .078 | (1.539) | .000 | .000 |
| Histrionic | | 1.747 | 1.748 | 1.772 | (1.601) | | | | |
| Narcissistic | | | | | | 1.913 | | | |
| Antisocial | | | | | | | | | |
| Borderline | | −2.163 | | | | | | 2.572 −1.962 | 2.282 |
| **9. Rater transitive with SO worst** | | | | | | | | | |
| **Significant prediction PD to SASB** | p <.075 | | | | .10 | | .014 | .008 | .005 |
| Histrionic | | | | | 1.984 | | | | |
| Narcissistic | | | | | | | | | |

| | Separate | Disclose | Reactive Love | Trust | Submit | Sulk | Recoil | Wall Off |
|---|---|---|---|---|---|---|---|---|
| Antisocial | 1.817 | (-1.621) | | -1.863 | | | 1.770 | 2.427 |
| Borderline | (-1.488) | (-1.503) | | -1.752 | | | | |

**10. Rater intransitive with SO worst**
**Significant prediction PD to SASB**

Rao's F p < .046

| | Separate | Disclose | Reactive Love | Trust | Submit | Sulk | Recoil | Wall Off |
|---|---|---|---|---|---|---|---|---|
| | .097 | .002 | | | | | .038 | .075 |
| Histrionic | | 3.668 | 1.935 | 1.795 | | | | |
| Narcissistic | | | | | | | | |
| Antisocial | | -2.148 | (-1.565) | | | | 1.787 | 2.681 |
| Borderline | | -2.874 | | | | | | |

**12. Mother intransitive**
**Significant prediction PD to SASB**

Rao's F p < .119

| | Separate | Disclose | Reactive Love | Trust | Submit | Sulk | Recoil | Wall Off |
|---|---|---|---|---|---|---|---|---|
| | | | | | .019 | .010 | | |
| Histrionic | | | | | | | | |
| Narcissistic | (-1.503) | | | | 2.063 | | | |
| Antisocial | | | | | | | | |
| Borderline | | | | | | | | |

**13. Rater transitive with mother (ages 5–10)**
**Significant prediction PD to SASB**

Rao's F p < .085

| | Emancipate | Affirm | Active Love | Protect | Control | Blame | Attack | Neglect |
|---|---|---|---|---|---|---|---|---|
| | | | | | .000 | .002 | | .105 |
| | | | | | (1.471) | | | |
| Histrionic | | | | | | | | |
| Narcissistic | | | | | 3.493 | 2.108 | | 1.763 |
| Antisocial | | | | | -2.005 | | | |
| Borderline | | | | | | | | |

**15. Father transitive with rater**
**Significant prediction PD to SASB**

Rao's F p < .066

| | Emancipate | Affirm | Active Love | Protect | Control | Blame | Attack | Neglect |
|---|---|---|---|---|---|---|---|---|
| | | | | .021 | .000 | | | |
| Histrionic | | | | | | | | |
| Narcissistic | | | | | | | -1.724 | 1.419 |
| Antisocial | | -1.946 | -2.580 | -2.711 | | | | |
| Borderline | | | | | | | | |

*Note.* Relationship aspects shown here differentiated Cluster C disorders by Rao's $F$ with $p \leq .10$, except facet 12, where $p < .119$. SASB codes with $T$ for beta indicating $p \leq .10$ are shown in roman. $T$ for beta associated with $p > .10$ and $p < .15$ appear in *italics* within parentheses. The rationale for using $T$ and for the unusual levels of $p$ appears in Appendix 22.1. SO, significant other person in adulthood.

There is much more information in Table 22.1, but perhaps these examples illustrate the value of weighting SASB profiles to help make differential diagnoses by using Canonical R to compare self descriptions of interpersonal patterns to individual scores based on standard DSM PD diagnoses. The fact that, most significantly, Rao's $F$ involved Introject and relationship with Significant Other at Best and Worst suggests those markers should be highlighted in making differential diagnoses within Cluster B.

These data make it difficult to claim accuracy when using trait descriptions that do not vary by relationship or context to describe personality patterns. In addition to recognizing that people behave differently in different social contexts, use of SASB-based detail circumvents the problems by asking clinicians to make attributions such as "She is manipulative; he is aggressive." Natural biology explains why it is important to consider the patient's perspective to understand symptoms.[4] Still another advantage is that conspicuous absence (i.e., negative beta weights) is as powerful a diagnostic marker as is conspicuous presence. That is a feature that, if incorporated in the diagnostic system for PD, could sharpen boundaries among disorders considerably, and make diagnosis of PD more like diagnoses in medicine that both "rule out" and "rule in" when making diagnoses.

Finally, it should be noted, that a parallel version of Table 22.1 based on SCID-II mean scores yielded significant Rao's $F$ for only five aspects (= 31% of possibilities) of relationship compared to nine aspects (= 56%) for WISPI. Significant trends using mean SCID-II scores were consistent with those discussed earlier, but there were fewer descriptions of differential markers. For example, BPD was marked by negative self-affirmation at Best, Blaming of SO at Worst. The mother was blamed but also was denied differentiation (negative $T$ for emancipate). There were no significant markers for NPD. As this promising approach is pursued, still other methods of diagnosing PD will be used, including Mestel's very large outpatient database that provides *International Classification of Diseases* (ICD-10) clinical diagnoses of PD.

---

[4]The C1 part of the C1AB chain emphasizes the centrality of patient perception is activating specific affects and specific behaviors linked to C1A by lessons in safety and threat.

## Parallel Models for Affect and Cognition

In Benjamin (2003), the underlying structure of SASB was extrapolated to create to two parallel models: one for affect, called SAAB, and one for cognition, called SACB. In those two names, the third letter stands for Affect and Cognition, respectively. Park (2005) tested the validity of the parallel SAAB (affect) model. Dimensional ratings of the affect words alone did yield a circumplex figure, but the vertical axis was very weak and unstable. However, a more reasonable facsimile of the theoretical SAAB model with two axes did emerge from factor analyses of subjects' ratings of applicability of affect words if they were embedded in a randomly ordered collection of words from the SASB model (Figure 22.1) that assessed social interactions with a significant other person at worst. That suggests that raters' primitive brain (C1AB brain chains) needed to be activated for them to note and rate accurately the primitive functions of the affect words.

## Revisiting Comorbidity

Comorbidity illustrated by Roger is not unusual among patients, and each symptom has its natural biological reason. Comorbidity among affective disorders is as common as comorbidity among PDs and between affective and PDs. This is illustrated in the large sample of outpatients at the HELIOS Klinik. Most of the diagnoses were gathered by routine clinical practice within an organization that requires clinicians to make a good faith effort to record all relevant diagnoses. The diagnoses may not be up to research standards (personal communication, R. Mestel, 2012). Nonetheless, diagnoses in this clinic are unusually complete and likely resulted in information that reflects the best of everyday practices. There were 14,829 individuals in the sample and 76.4% = 11,329 had no PD diagnosis, while 3,500 did. Rows in Table 22.2 list ICD-10 personality diagnoses, which total 3,597, with 97 having more than one PD (2.8% of those with any PD). The two comorbid affective categories, anxiety and depression, are listed in four columns that represent only anxiety, only depression, neither, and both. Of those who had one or more PDs, 17.6% had comorbid diagnoses of depression alone, while only 3.2% had anxiety alone; 6.1% had both anxiety and

TABLE 22.2. Comorbidity between and among PDs, Anxiety Disorder, and Depression

| Disorder | Total N | N for depression alone | N for anxiety disorder alone | N for neither | N for both |
|---|---|---|---|---|---|
| Borderline | 1,980 | 921 | 159 | 621 | 279 |
| Histrionic | 139 | 54 | 11 | 56 | 18 |
| Narcissistic | 785 | 426 | 53 | 223 | 83 |
| Antisocial | 57 | 16 | 3 | 29 | 9 |
| Dependent | 890 | 481 | 71 | 200 | 138 |
| Anakastic | 179 | 81 | 26 | 37 | 35 |
| Avoidant | 1,268 | 578 | 140 | 226 | 324 |
| Passive aggressive | 72 | 28 | 4 | 33 | 7 |
| Paranoid | 85 | 25 | 9 | 41 | 10 |
| N cases with no PD | 11,232 | | | | |
| N cases with PD | 3,597 | | | | |
| N anxiety/depression | | 2,610 | 476 | 1,466 | 903 |
| % of total 14,829 | | 17.60% | 3.20% | 9.90% | 6.10% |

*Note.* ICD-10 diagnoses were made in clinical practice under the supervision of Robert Mestel, PhD, Director of Research at the HELIOS Kliniken, in Bad Groenenbach, Germany. The rows for PDs are not completely independent because 1,858/3,597 (52.2%) of patients with PD had more than one disorder.

depression, and 9.9% had neither of these affective disorders. In other words, about 90% of the population with PDs had comorbid anxiety or depression, or both. And depression was more often comorbid with PD than was anxiety. From the point of view of IRT, none of this is surprising. Comorbid affects should serve patterns of adaptation in three coordinated domains represented by C1AB, or perception, affect, and behavior patterns.

For example, a person with BPD may be terrified to be alone because that is when incestual abuse occurred. For that person with BPD, abandonment anxiety is not much of a mystery if one understands the confusion involved in having a sexual relationship with a caregiver who is abusive. If someone with OCPD (which has highest level of comorbidity with anxiety in Table 22.2) has to keep perfect order or father will go into a rage when he comes home, anxiety about lack of order and mobilization to keep order makes sense. If a dependent person (highest frequencies for depression in Table 22.2) suffers from a sense of being overwhelmed and defeated, then depression is not a surprise.

In conclusion, comorbidity is the rule, not the exception, and its presence offers conceptual challenges that can be understood if, along with a survey of symptoms, the clinician inquires about what is going on in an individual's life, and about what he or she has learned about what to fear and how to be safe. The IRT case formulation model offers a way to do that.

## The IRT Treatment Model

Most CORDS in the IRT outpatient clinic qualified for a PD label. Interviewer assigned a PD diagnosis to 88% of the cases that, most often, were OCPD (47%) and passive–aggressive (PAPD; 34%). Comorbid diagnoses of PDs with one another were not made because the necessary and exclusionary rules in Benjamin (1996a) sharpened the focus and made differential diagnoses among the DSM-IV PDs possible. By contrast, of the 42 SCID-II interviews (First et al., 1997) administered to those who participated in inpatient IRT treatment, all qualified for one or more PD disorder diagnoses. Of these, 50% had more than one PD. OCPD was most common (54.8%), followed by avoidant PD (AVPD, 35.7%), PAPD (23.8%) and BPD (23.8%). IRT case formulations accommodate affective symptoms and problem personality patterns. As noted already, treatment interventions must free the patient from copy processes by the process of differentiation, which means relinquishing maladaptive GOLs to family in the head. But that is "against nature," and many patients do not even like to acknowledge GOLs, much less give them up.

So the first step in treatment is for the patient to agree to work toward a secure base, understanding that this means defying old rules for managing threat and safety and giving up loyalties to maladaptive rules and values sponsored by loved ones. The subjective problem is that differentiation feels like "betrayal" of family in the head, and that is both frightening and depressing. But until the patient, Roger, for example, can and will differentiate from symptoms relevant to family in the head, problems with rage and paranoia will persist. Insight is not "the cure." It is only the road map in IRT, not the journey. GOLs must be revisited over and over again in many different contexts before patients can let go of them and replace maladaptive guiding internalizations with more adaptive ones. As the goal of IRT treatments is to help the patient build secure base patterns, relationships that enable old patterns may need to be modified. Current attachment figures are invited to sessions if the patient wishes. If appropriate, referral of the guest to another therapist is offered, sometimes followed by a few sessions of couple or family therapy with the cotherapist. This goal of transformation as defined by natural biology means that IRT goals can go beyond symptom reduction or containment. If successfully accomplished, a new internal secure base will preclude the need for further intervention.

The interviewing style in an IRT treatment is simple and direct. Prescribed by the Core Algorithm, therapists should show accurate empathy; emphasize Green (adaptive responses, thoughts) more than Red (Maladaptive responses, thoughts); use the case formulation; address input, response, and impact on self; and address parallel C1Abs (i.e., do not focus exclusively on affect, or cognition or behavior). We try to follow the five IRT therapy steps shown in Figure 22.4: collaboration, learn about patterns, block maladaptive patterns, engage the will to change, and learn new patterns. Skillful and consistent use of the core algorithm is required to receive high IRT adherence ratings. According to IRT flow diagrams (not show here), these details should include Input (What set it off? What did you do?), Response (What did you do? How did you feel?) and Impact on Self (How did it affect you?). Not so long ago, emphasis on specificity repeatedly was shown to be related to outcome in psychotherapy studies (Garfield & Bergin, 1978). The fact that it now rarely is explicitly mentioned or practiced suggests that the half-life of evidence about effectiveness can be short.

## IRT Explicitly Integrates Techniques

The integrative nature of IRT can be seen by inspection of Figure 22.4, which describes IRT therapy steps and the five steps that unfold in sequence, with variability. For each step, there are illustrative interventions divided into two groups: Self-Discovery and Self-Management. Self-discovery activities are commonly drawn from dynamically oriented or existential therapies. They encourage curiosity about and acceptance of self and others. Self-management activities, shown on the right side of Figure 22.4, are more likely to be seen in cognitive-behavioral therapy (CBT) and its derivatives. They invoke change by willful effort based on logical choices. Every step is important, but the most challenging point is Step 4, Enable the Will to Change. It is divided into the familiar change stages described by Prochaska, DiClemente, and Norcross (1992): Precontemplation, Contemplation, Preparation, Action, and Maintenance. IRT theory and natural biology provide detail about how to progress through the most difficult stage of change, the action stage. This is in response to frequent queries by patients and therapists to this effect: "I see how copy process and GOL are operating but what can *I* do about it?" Natural biology helps explain why the action stage is so difficult to master. Giving up old rules for safety and threat is extremely difficult because such change is threatening at the deepest levels of primitive brain. The process is outlined by phases within the stage of action (Benjamin, 2018). It includes (1) resist the red voices and defy with green action; (2) face and relinquish yearning (that childhood would have been better); (3) envision the birthright (Secure self); face fear, disorganization, emptiness; (4) build birthright, celebrate success and happiness; and (5) face grief. After the Action stage is well under way, maintenance of gains demands a struggle with giving up fantasies based on GOL, which function very much like an addiction.

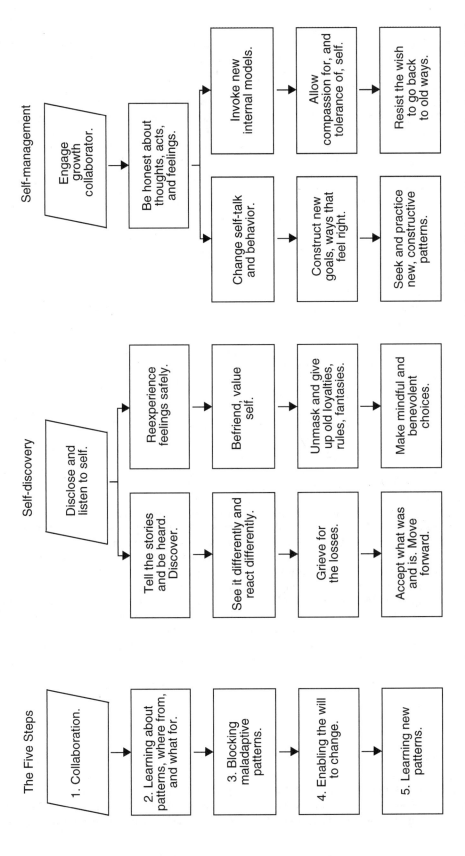

**FIGURE 22.4.** The IRT treatment model. The attachment-based IRT model explicitly integrates psychodynamic (self-discovery) and cognitive-behavioral (self-management) interventions. Step 4 is the marker between reconstruction of personality and no personality change. From Benjamin (2003, p. 88). Copyright © 2003 The Guilford Press. Reprinted by permission.

For example, if Roger tries to suppress his anger at his son (Phase 1), his father in his head likely mocks him and tells him he is a weakling and worse. This means Roger must recognize and renounce his wish for (Yearning) reconciliation with the father in his head (Phase 2) and tolerate the fear and disorientation that follows (Phase 3). If he masters all that, he might be successful in his effort to do something constructive with his son rather than berate him (Phase 1). And then he may feel disoriented, not "right," not "himself" (Phase 4). Toward the end of the Action stage, when all the losses associated with having made maladaptive choices are accepted, and when it is clear that fantasies of having had a more loving childhood are never coming true, there is lasting, nearly unbearable, unmitigated grief about these losses (Phase 5). Many patients sob for days at a time and say they have fallen into a deep, dark hole. But with much willpower, Roger can repeat the phases, use behavior technology to reprogram his sense of threat and his responses to his son (C1ABs), and begin to tolerate, then even enjoy new, more loving reactions from family. In doing so, Roger would have reconstructed his personality.

To accomplish all of this, the therapist needs considerable skill in integrative thinking and mastery of a diversity of approaches. Critchfield, Mackaronis, and Benjamin (2017) tested the claim that IRT is integrative by using the Comparative Psychotherapy Process Scale (CPPS; Hilsenroth, Blagys, Ackerman, Bonge, & Blais, 2005) to assess IRT trainees' use of the model in their sessions in the IRT clinic. IRT-naive advanced undergraduates rated nine IRT trainee session tapes on the CPPS. Results suggested the sessions included both psychodynamic–interpersonal techniques (PI) and CBT techniques at the level of "somewhat characteristic." Although in a separate task, these raters had high reliability as they rated the trainee sessions for adherence to the IRT model, their reliability for the same sessions on the CPPS scale was low. This is because item analysis suggested that trainees used both PI and CBT techniques, as required by the IRT manual, so while rating CPPS, the decision to cast an event that included both approaches in either the IP or CBT category was arbitrary. For example, there might be an IRT homework assignment that instructs the patient to note self-talk (CBT) during problem interactive patterns (I) and link them to an attachment figure (P). By giving homework focused on self-talk, the intervention resembles CBT. It also includes common interpersonal factors implicit to many effective psychotherapies of any orientation: collaboration, learning about patterns, blocking problem patterns. However, this particular homework also encourages self-study of a sort that more clearly is "psychodynamic," as it helps prepare the patient to challenge family in the head. It is uniquely characteristic of IRT in the focus on the explicit C1AB chains that link current symptoms, interpersonal stress, and copy process connections to patterns with attachment figures, and eventually to the sustaining GOLs (automatic GOL learning) so that if they keep on with the old solutions, somehow things will get "fixed."

## IRT and Evidence-Based Practice in Psychology

Evidence in support of IRT is consistent with most of the standards set forth in Evidence-Based Practice in Psychology (EBPP; Levant, 2005). These include:

1. Clinical observations. In IRT, the case formulation method was developed on the basis of clinical observations and subsequently proved to be reliable, specific to individuals, and sensitive to relevant information (Critchfield et al., 2015).
2. Each individual case formulation is an example of qualitative research as the clinician tries to learn: Why does this patient present with these symptoms now?
3. In Benjamin (1996a) there are two systematic case studies for each of the DSM-IV (and DSM-5) personality diagnoses, and the procedures for treatment later were formalized in the IRT book (Benjamin, 2003a).
4. Single-case experimental designs. Two published independent European single case studies demonstrated that Intrex ratings can reflect changes in the structure of internalizations changes during psychotherapy (Hartkamp & Schmidtz, 1999; Ulbert, Hoglend, Marble, & Sorbye, 2009).
5. Public health and ethnographic research were illustrated by Florsheim (1996), who used SASB measures of problem interpersonal patterns in different ethnic groups.
6. There are many published process–outcome studies including mechanisms of change. A scan of the APA database for full text ar-

ticles on "therapy process and SASB" recently yielded 50 studies.
7. The first year change in CORDS treated in the IRT clinic clearly represent research natural settings.
8. There are no RCTs of IRT. However, research in the IRT clinic shows that adhering to the IRT model, focusing as often as possible on mechanisms of change, enhances outcome. RCTs presumably show that one approach addresses mechanisms of change better than another. The strategy of relating activation of mechanisms of change in relation to outcome more directly addresses the key issue.
9. Meta-analysis is not possible for IRT because there are no RCTs. However, in Critchfield and Benjamin's (2006, Table 3) review of interventions shared by therapies proven effective by RCTs, there was indirect validation of IRT. All demonstrably effective strategies in that list had been mentioned in the IRT "manual" (Benjamin, 2003).

## First-Year Outcome in Treatment of CORDS in the IRT Clinic

### Pre- and Posttreatment Comparisons for the First Year of Treatment in the IRT Clinic

Treatment-resistant CORDS treated by IRT trainees for 1 year showed significant reduction in trait anger and in the number of suicide attempts compared to the preceding year. Defining "less" severely disturbed people as those with two or fewer prior hospitalizations, it also was shown that all eight less severe cases improved in depressive symptoms, while all four of the more severe cases deteriorated into depression. This interaction was significant ($p < .002$). Overall improvement in symptoms of OCPD, the most common PD among CORDS, was suggested by pre- and posttreatment comparison, $Z = -1.54$ ($-1.64$ is required for two-tailed $p < .05$). Relating activation of mechanisms of change to outcome was accomplished with nonparametric correlations between best work with GOL during the first year, and reductions in trait anger, as well as depression, were significant. There was a significant increase in symptoms of AVPD, perhaps because there were many individuals with OCPD. Treatment for that pattern begins with helping them "back off" in their attempts to control others that typically appears as withdrawal, which is a primary characteristic of AVPD. We have observed that in IRT treatments of severe disorders, things do sometimes get worse before they get better. It may be because giving up old patterns does not always directly lead to goal behaviors (secure base). Getting worse is observed when challenging family in the head; patients are overwhelmed and frightened by the task. And if that is managed, giving up old fantasies is a new reason for depression.

## Summary and Conclusions

SASB, IRT case formulation, and treatment models, and the natural biology that supports them, have been applied with supporting data to the problem of comorbidity, with emphasis on PD. A demonstration that linked SASB ratings of relationships with attachment figures to WISPI-based diagnoses of Cluster B PDs suggested that the problem of comorbidity in DSM-5 definitions of PD could be enriched and managed by using SASB-based specific descriptions of interpersonal and intrapsychic patterns to help make differential diagnoses. Moreover, a tally in a large sample of outpatients showed that comorbidity of anxiety and depression with each other and with PD is common. The IRT case formulation method, based on natural biological theory, can account for such comorbidity in reliable, specific, and sensitive ways. The case formulation guides the clinician when working with comorbid cases to change relationships with internalized representations of attachment figures that are regulating affective symptoms and associated personality patterns. What has to change is maladaptive versions of what to fear and how to be safe (i.e., primitive brain cognitions, affects, and behaviors); these need to be replaced by more secure strategies. In the IRT clinic, which now is closed, the goal was to reconstruct individuals who were suicidal, often rehospitalized, dysfunctional, and highly comorbid to achieve secure base affects and behaviors. It was documented only for four of 38 individuals who entered the research protocol. But those four did change their primitive brain rules for safety and threat and make marked progress on their reconstructive journey toward an internal secure base and have, as far as we know, remained relatively free of symptoms on a long-term basis.

## APPENDIX 22.1. Rationale for Use of Canonical T as a Marker of Contribution of SASB Measures (Y) to PD Diagnosis (X)[5]

Let an individual's four Cluster B scores be a vector $X$ and his or her eight-point SASB profile for a given facet (e.g., my introject at worst) be a vector $Y$. In SYSAT, $X$ is called an independent variable, which means it will not change and it is the variable to be predicted. $Y$ is called the dependent variable, because it will be changed to become as closely related to $X$ as possible on the basis of covariance $XY$. That is accomplished by computing beta weights for each $Y$ score (SASB) for a weighted $Y$ score vector that will maximize prediction of $X$ (diagnosis). The method uses matrix algebra with $[X]$ = PD = a 4 × 4 matrix for variance within four Cluster B scores and $[Y]$ = 8 × 8 matrix for variance within eight-point SASB profiles. Then compute:

1. Within $[Y]$ variance (SASB psychosocial)
2. Within $[X]$ variance (SCID-II PD)
3. $[X][Y]$ = covariance $X$ and $Y$
4. [$Y$ prime scores] = adjust $[Y]$ by computing weights based on $[XY]/[Y]$. Here, the shared variance $XY$ is divided by $Y$ variance alone to leave $Y$ prime representing covariance $XY$. Use $F = Y$ prime variance/within $Y$ variance to test and report $p$ for the "Significance Tests for Prediction of Each Basic Y Variable"
5. Differential calculus ensures the beta-adjusted $[Y]$ comes maximally close to $[X]$. $T$ = beta/$SD$ betas and is a "standardized" beta score associated with a $p$ based on $F$ computed by between-groups variance/within-groups variance. $T$ values are entered in Table 22.1 to indicate direction and magnitude of the association between the SASB variable (e.g., Self-Attack) and diagnostic group (e.g., BPD), where $T$ is associated with $p \leq .15$. If $p > .10$ and $< .15$, it is distinguished by parentheses and italicized print.

This analysis predicts SASB scores, given PD scores. For example, if one has BPD, then one has the SASB minima and maxima suggested by $T$ for BPD in Table 22.1. That could be useful in making differential PD diagnoses. The reverse process of using SASB scores to predict PD is declined. Rao's $F$ and its $p$ are not changed by exchanging definitions of $X$ and $Y$ variables, but betas do change: If $X$ and $Y$ were reversed, Table 22.1 should have SASB codes on rows (independent variables) and PD (dependent variables) on columns. $T$ would represent differential weighting of PD to predict SASB codes. Treatment implications are very different. One can focus in therapy on Control of SO, but not on "HPD" per se. Also, the comorbidity issue is not well addressed by that approach. It would require giving up all hope of speaking of "a" PD diagnosis.

There are two reasons for the unusually generous standards for $p$ as a measure of contributions by different tests. The first is that these results are heuristic, a demonstration of a method for making differential PD diagnoses. It does not characterize the disorders in terms of SASB codes. Means, not weights for differential prediction, would be appropriate for that. Second, the $T$ usually appears (as do means) in circumplex order and $p$ here does not capture correspondence to that underlying order. That could be done with orthogonal polynomials partialing out variance between points in a SASB profile, but the procedure is beyond the present scope.

## AUTHORS' NOTE

The University of Utah Conflict of Interest Committee requires that Lorna Smith Benjamin disclose that if ever SASB is sold to a testing company, she is entitled to an author's interest. She is an author of two published books and one in print, and receives royalties from them. She has a private practice and gives workshops for a fee about IRT and SASB. She is an author on three instruments for assessing PD but receives no royalties from them: WISPI, SCID-II, and SCID-PD.

## REFERENCES

Benjamin, L. S. (1974). Structural analysis of social behavior (SASB). *Psychological Review, 81,* 392–425.

Benjamin, L. S. (1979). Structural analysis of differentiation failure. *Psychiatry: Journal for the Study of Interpersonal Processes, 42,* 1–23.

Benjamin, L. S. (1986). Operational definition and measurement of dynamics shown in the stream of free associations. *Psychiatry: Journal for the Study of Biological and Social Processes, 49,* 104–129.

Benjamin, L. S. (1996a). *Interpersonal diagnosis and treatment of personality disorders* (2nd ed.). New York: Guilford Press.

Benjamin, L. S. (1996b). Introduction to the special section on Structural Analysis of Social Behavior (SASB). *Journal of Consulting and Clinical Psychology, 64,* 1203–1212.

Benjamin, L. S. (2000). *SASB Intrex user's manual.* Salt Lake City: University of Utah.

---

[5] Based on Cooley and Lohnes (1962, pp. 31–37).

Benjamin, L. S. (2003). *Interpersonal reconstructive therapy: An integrative personality-based treatment for complex cases.* New York: Guilford Press.

Benjamin, L. S. (2010). Structural analysis of social behavior and the nature of nature. In S. Strack & L. Horowitz (Eds.), *Handbook of interpersonal psychology: Theory, research, assessment and therapeutic interventions* (pp. 325–341). New York: Wiley.

Benjamin, L. S. (2018). *Interpersonal reconstructive therapy for anger, anxiety and depression: It's about broken hearts, not broken brains.* Washington, DC: American Psychological Association.

Benjamin, L. S., & Cushing, G. (2000) *Reference manual for coding social interactions in terms of structural analysis of social behavior.* Salt Lake City: University of Utah.

Benjamin, L. S., Rothweiler, J. R., & Critchfield, K. L. (2006). Use of structural analysis of social behavior as an assessment tool. *Annual Review of Clinical Psychology, 2,* 83–109.

Bretherton, I. (1992). The origins of attachment theory: John Bowlby and Mary Ainsworth. *Developmental Psychology, 28,* 759–775.

Carson, R. (1969). *Interaction concepts of personality.* New Brunswick, NJ: Aldine.

Cassidy, J., & Shaver, P. R. (Eds.). (2008). *Handbook of attachment: Theory, research, and clinical applications* (2nd ed.). New York: Guilford Press.

Constantino, M. J. (2000), Interpersonal process in psychotherapy through the lens of thez structural analysis of social behavior. *Applied and Preventive Psychology: Current Scientific Perspectives, 9,* 153–172.

Cooley, W. W., & Lohnes, P. R. (1962). *Multivariate procedures for the behavioral sciences.* New York: Wiley.

Critchfield, K. L., & Benjamin, L. S. (2006). Principles for psychosocial treatment of personality disorder: Summary of the APA Division 12 Task Force/NASPR review. *Journal of Clinical Psychology, 62,* 661–674.

Critchfield, K. L., Benjamin, L. S., & Levenik, K. (2015). Reliability, sensitivity, and specificity of case formulations in interpersonal reconstructive therapy: Addressing psychosocial and biological mechanisms of psychopathology. *Journal of Personality Disorders, 29,* 547–573.

Critchfield, K. L., Mackaronis, J. E., & Benjamin, L. S. (2017). Integrative use of CBT and psychodynamic techniques in interpersonal reconstructive therapy. *Journal of Psychotherapy Integration.* [Epub ahead of print]

First, M. B., Spitzer, R. L., Gibbon, M., Williams, J. B. W., & Benjamin, L. S. (1997). *Structural Clinical Interview for DMS-IV Axis II personality disorders (SCID-II).* Washington, DC: American Psychiatric Press.

Fleiss, J. L. (1981). *Statistical methods for rates and proportions* (2nd ed.). New York: Wiley.

Florsheim, P. (1996). Family processes and risk for externalizing behavior problems among African American and Hispanic boys. *Journal of Consulting and Clinical Psychology, 64,* 1222–1230.

Garfield, S. L., & Bergin, A. E. (Eds.). (1978). *Handbook of psychotherapy and behavior change: An empirical analysis* (2nd ed.). New York: Wiley.

Gurtman, M. (2000). Interpersonal complementarity: Integrating interpersonal measurement with interpersonal models. *Journal of Counseling Psychology, 48,* 97–110.

Harlow, H. (1958). The nature of love. *American Psychologist, 13,* 673–685.

Hartkamp, N., & Schmitz, N. (1999). Structures of introject and therapist patient interaction in a single case study of inpatient psychotherapy. *Psychotherapy Research, 9,* 199–215.

Hilsenroth, M. J., Blagys, M. D., Ackerman, S. J., Bonge, D. R., & Blais, M. A. (2005). Measuring psychodynamic-interpersonal and cognitive-behavioral techniques: Development of the Comparative Psychotherapy Process Scale. *Psychotherapy: Theory, Research, Practice, Training, 42*(3), 340–356.

Insel, T. R. (2013, April 29). Director's blog. Retrieved from *www.nimh.nih.gov/about/director/2013/transforming diagnosis.shtml.*

Klein, M. H., Benjamin, L. S., Rosenfeld, M. A., Treece, C., Husted, J., & Greist, J. H. (1993). The Wisconsin Personality Disorders Inventory: Development, reliability and validity. *Journal of Personality Disorders, 7,* 285–303.

Knobloch-Fedders, L. M., Critchfield, K. L., Boisson, T., Woods, N., Bitman, R., & Durbin, C. E. (2014). Depression, relationship quality, and couples' demand/withdraw and demand/submit sequential interactions. *Journal of Counseling Psychology, 61,* 264–279.

Kupfer, D. J., First, M., & Regier, D. (2002). *A research agenda for DSM-V.* Washington, DC: American Psychiatric Press.

Leary, T. (1957). *Interpersonal diagnosis of personality: A functional theory and methodology for personality evaluation.* New York: Ronald Press.

Levant, R. F. (2005). *Report of the 2005 Presidential Task Force on Evidence-Based Practice.* Washington, DC: American Psychological Association.

Meaney, M. J. (2010). Epigenetics and the biological definition of gene × environment interactions. *Child Development, 81,* 41–79.

Merikangas, K. R., & Weissman, M. M. (1986). Epidemiology of DSM-III Axis II personality disorders. In A. J. Frances & R. E. Hales (Eds.), *American Psychiatric Association annual review* (Vol. 5, pp. 258–278). Washington, DC: American Psychiatric Association.

Park, J. H. (2005). A validation study of the structural analysis of affective behavior: Further development and empirical analysis. *Dissertation Abstracts International: B: The Sciences and Engineering, 65*(10), 5418.

Porges, S. W. (1994). Orienting in a defensive world: Mammalian modifications of our evolutionary heritage: A polyvagal theory. *Psychophysiology, 32,* 301–318.

Prochaska, J. O., DiClemente, C. C., & Norcross, J. C. (1992). In search of how people change: Applications to addictive behaviors. *American Psychologist, 47,* 1102–1114.

Schaefer, E. S. (1965). Configurational analysis of children's reports of parent behavior. *Journal of Consulting Psychology, 29,* 552–557.

Skowron, E. A., Cipriano-Essel, E., Benjamin, L. S., Pincus, A. L., & Van Ryzin, M. J. (2013). Cardiac vagal tone and quality of parenting show concurrent and time-ordered associations that diverge in abusive, neglectful, and non-maltreating mothers. *Couple and Family Pychology: Research and Practice, 2,* 95–115.

Smith, T. L. (2002). Specific psychosocial perceptions and specific symptoms of personality and other psychiatric disorders. *Dissertation Abstracts International B: The Sciences and Engineering, 63*(6-B), 3026.

Smith, T. L., Klein, M. H., & Benjamin, L. S. (2003). Validation of the Wisconsin Personality Disorders Inventory–IV with the SCID-II. *Journal of Personality Disorders, 17*(3), 173–187.

Spinelli, S., Chefer, S. Carson, R. E., Jagoda, E., Lang, L., Hejlig, M., et al. (2010). Effects of early-life stress on serotonin 1a receptors in juvenile rhesus monkeys measured by positron emission tomography. *Biological Psychiatry, 67,* 1146–1153.

Svartberg, M., & Stiles, T. C. (1992). Predicting patient change from therapist competence and patient–therapists complementarity in short-term anxiety-provoking psychotherapy: A pilot study. *Journal of Consulting and Clinical Psychology, 60,* 304–307.

Teti, D. M., Heaton, N., Benjamin, L. S., & Gelfand, D. M. (1995, May 29). *Quality of attachment and caregiving among depressed mother–child dyads: Strange Situation classifications and the SASB Coding System.* Paper presented to a symposium at the annual meeting of the Society for Applied Behavioral Analysis, Washington, DC.

Ulbert, R., Hoglend, P., Marble, A., & Sorbye, O. (2009). From submission to autonomy: Approaching independent decision making: A single-case study in a randomized, controlled study of long-term effects of dynamic psychotherapy. *American Journal of Psychotherapy, 63,* 227–243.

Wiggins, J. S. (1982). Circumplex models of interpersonal behavior in clinical psychology. In P. C. Kendall & J. N. Butcher (Eds.), *Perspectives in personality* (Vol. 1, pp. 183–221). Greenwich, CT: JAI Press.

# PART VI

# SPECIFIC PATTERNS

## INTRODUCTION

Given the emphasis this volume places on an evidence-based approach to personality disorder (PD), the decision to include chapters on specific categorical diagnoses requires explanation. The first edition did not have a corresponding section because of the lack of evidence for typal diagnoses, and the situation has not changed in the intervening years, in that the evidence on this issue has become even more solid. As noted in several chapters (see Chapters 1, 4, 22), the DSM-IV/DSM-5 classification of PD lacks structural validity (see also Jacobs & Krueger, 2015). There are two main problems. First, the empirical structure of PD in clinical samples does not match the DSM proposal that these features are organized into 10 distinct diagnoses. Second, the features of PD are not organized into discrete types but rather are continuously distributed. Nevertheless, clinicians and researchers alike continue to make extensive use of these diagnoses. For this reason, we decided to include chapters on the more important conditions.

The compromise we adopted was to include categorical diagnoses showing some resemblance to the major constellations identified by empirical analyses. Factor analyses of the descriptive features of PD consistently converge on a four-factor structure (Widiger & Simonsen, 2005). The factors identified have been variously labeled emotional dysregulation/affective instability/negative affectivity/neuroticism, dissocial/antagonism/aggressiveness, social avoidance/introversion/withdrawal, and compulsivity/conscientiousness/constraint. The emotion dysregulation factor characterized by labile emotions, anxiousness, attachment insecurity, and submissive dependency bears some resemblance to borderline personality disorder. The dissocial factor resembles antisocial and psychopathic PDs. The social avoidance factor, which is defined by social withdrawal and restricted emotional expression, resembles schizoid PD and some aspects of avoidant PD. Finally, compulsivity shows some resemblance to obsessive–compulsive PD.

Based on this convergence we solicited chapters on antisocial/psychopathic, borderline, and obsessive–compulsive PDs. We would have liked to include a chapter on the schizoid/avoidant constellation of features because this is an interesting condition. Unfortunately, there is not an extensive, recent empirical literature on this condition, probably because such individuals do not seek help very often. We chose to "overweight" antisocial/psychopathic PD by including two chapters covering conceptual and clinical aspects of this condition for several reasons. The diagnosis usually receives less attention in the mental health literature than borderline personality disorder, although it is also a prevalent condition. Also, although this constellation of personality pathology has always received attention from researchers in the forensic field, research has recently become more broadly based. Hence, it seemed timely to review this work in more detail.

## REFERENCES

Jacobs, K. L., & Krueger, R. F. (2015). The importance of structural validity. In P. Zachar, D. St. Stoyanov, M. Aragona, & A. Jablensky (Eds.), *Alternative perspectives on psychiatric validation* (pp. 189–200). Oxford, UK: Oxford University Press.

Widiger, T. A., & Simonsen, E. (2005). Alternative dimensional models of personality disorder. *Journal of Personality Disorders, 19,* 110–130.

# CHAPTER 23

# Clinical Features of Borderline Personality Disorder

Joel Paris

## Historical Issues

Borderline personality disorder (BPD) was first described in 1938 by Stern, who wrote a clinical description of a group of patients who were emotionally unstable, impulsive, and sensitive to rejection in interpersonal relationships, and who often did poorly in therapy.

If read today, Stern's paper is surprisingly contemporary. But his use of the term "borderline," implying that patients were neither neurotic nor psychotic, but something in between, was misleading given the undefined the nature of the border. Yet we still use the term "borderline," mainly for lack of a better alternative. While a number of alternatives have been proposed, definitions that focus on one aspect of BPD, such as affective instability or impulsivity, fail to account for the complexity of this multidimensional disorder (Paris, 2008).

BPD is a syndrome that may be classified and described differently in the future. However, patients with this condition have a readily recognizable clinical presentation. With experience, it can usually be diagnosed in a single consultation.

The construct of BPD was ignored until the 1960s. The diagnosis did not appear in either DSM-I or DSM-II. Kernberg's (1970) concept of "borderline personality organization" was influential but overly broad, too theoretical, and lacking in empirical grounding. The turning point came when Gunderson and Singer (1975) demonstrated that patients with BPD could be identified by an observable pattern of signs and symptoms, without recourse to psychodynamic inferences. This approach was in the spirit of the contemporaneous Research Diagnostic Criteria (Feighner et al., 1972). Once the BPD diagnosis was shown to be reliable and linked to clinical features, it was accepted into DSM-III (and later, in modified form, into the *International Classification of Diseases*). An explosion of research followed, and over 3,000 papers were published over the next several decades. DSM-IV modified the definition by adding an additional criterion describing cognitive symptoms. There was no change in DSM-5, although proposals for a major redefinition that were not accepted were put in an Appendix.

## Critiques of the BPD Construct

While the BPD diagnosis suffers from heterogeneity and fuzzy boundaries, similar problems affect the classification of most mental disorders. It is neither more nor less valid than most categories in psychiatry. In the field trials associated with DSM-5, the diagnosis had good reliability at only one of two sites (Regier et al., 2013). Yet its reliability was still better than common diagnoses such as major depression.

Yet the diagnosis of BPD has long had critics. One reason is the paradigm shift within psychiatry. In the minds of many, BPD is associated with psychoanalysis, not with psychopharmacology. Over 30 years ago, Akiskal, Chen, and Davis (1985) sarcastically described borderline personality as "an adjective without a noun."

The critics of BPD would like to define it as a variant of mood disorder. As a multidimensional and highly symptomatic PD, this diagnosis has a very wide comorbidity. Most patients meet criteria for a mood disorder, an anxiety disorder, and a substance abuse disorder, and many also have eating disorders (Zanarini et al., 1998). Yet these phenomena are best seen as co-occurrence, not as "comorbidity." The DSM system of diagnosis encourages multiple diagnosis, and many of the most commonly used categories overlap with each other. The advantage of making a PD diagnosis is that most of these phenomena can be accounted for by BPD.

The idea that BPD is a mood disorder, as opposed to a PD, is based on striking symptoms of affective instability. British psychiatrist Peter Tyrer (2009, p, 87) wrote, "It is better classified as a condition of recurrent unstable mood and behaviour, or fluxithymia, which is better placed with the mood disorders." However, this conclusion begs the question as to whether affective instability is indeed a variant of mood disorders or a separate phenomenon. Past attempts to define BPD as a variant of depression to be treated with antidepressants (Akiskal et al., 1985) have been unsuccessful (Gunderson & Phillips, 1991). The more recent idea that BPD is a form of bipolar disorder (Akiskal, 2003) is also not consistent with the research literature (Paris, Gunderson, & Weinberg, 2007).

BPD does have prominent mood symptoms. But the original concept of manic–depression, developed by Kraepelin (1921), described *episodes* of depression or elation. In contrast, patients with BPD experience continually abnormal mood for years, may be in a different mood from hour to hour, are as likely to be angry as sad or elated, and have a different neurobiological profile (Koenigsberg, 2010). Moreover, mood symptoms are only one of the primary features of BPD, and do not account for impulsivity, self-harm, unstable relationships, or cognitive symptoms (Paris, 2010). Finally, patients with BPD, unlike those with classical mood disorders, respond inconsistently, or not at all, to antidepressants and mood stabilizers (Stoffers et al., 2010).

In recent years, it has been very hard to find a patient with BPD who has not been diagnosed, at one time or another, as suffering from bipolarity (Ruggero, Zimmerman, Chelminski, & Young, 2010). The attempt to reduce BPD to bipolar disorder is based on the concept that mood instability is nothing but "ultrarapid cycling" (Ghaemi, Ko, & Goodwin, 2002). This conclusion is part of a broader agenda to redefine a wide range of mental disorders as falling within a "bipolar spectrum" (Paris, 2012). There are several problems with this formulation. First and foremost, patients with BPD do not have manic or hypomanic episodes (Paris et al., 2007). And when they do, one should question the diagnosis of a PD given the distorting effects on personality of bipolar illness. Second, patients with BPD have family histories of antisocial personality, substance abuse, and depression, but not bipolarity (White et al., 2003). Third, there is little evidence that the drugs used for classical bipolar disorder are effective for mood instability in BPD (Stoffers et al., 2010).

Another critique of the BPD diagnosis has come from psychotherapists who see these patients as suffering from a form of posttraumatic stress disorder (PTSD), or what Herman (1992) called "complex PTSD." There are also problems with this proposal. First, while many patients with BPD have histories of trauma during childhood, about one-third develop symptoms without experiencing serious childhood adversity (Paris, 2008). Family studies show that BPD is unlikely to evolve without temperamental vulnerability, as measured by abnormal trait profiles (Laporte, Paris, Russell, & Guttman, 2011). Second, most patients with BPD do not meet criteria for PTSD. Redefining it as a "complex" form of the disorder is little more than hand-waving. Once again, explaining multiple clinical phenomena through a simple etiological model is bound to fail.

The most substantive critique of BPD comes from trait psychology. This approach does not attempt to redefine BPD as another disorder, but redefines it in light of its underlying trait dimensions (Costa & Widiger, 2012; Livesley, 2017). Most researchers have concluded that BPD is rooted either in emotion dysregulation (Linehan, 1993), or a combination of affective instability and impulsive behavior (Crowell, Beauchaine, & Linehan, 2009; Siever & Davis, 1991). These formulations do not, however, account for the interpersonal problems that characterize the disorder (Gunderson & Lyons-Ruth, 2008), or for its prominent cognitive abnormalities, such as hallucinations, paranoid ideas, and depersonalization (Zanarini, Frankenburg, Wedig, & Fitzmaurice, 2013) that suggest the syndrome still lies on some kind of "border" with psychosis.

BPD is a syndrome reflecting multiple trait dimensions (Paris, 2010), marked by prominent egodystonic symptoms that are not readily accounted for by trait profiles. Given the prominence of affective instability, it is not surprising that many see BPD as a variant of mood disorder. And while a dimensional approach to PD applies neatly to patients with obsessive–compulsive PD and narcissistic PD, whose problems almost entirely reflect exaggerated traits, it does not account for patients who are highly unstable and chronically suicidal.

Recognizing BPD is clinically important. To paraphrase Winston Churchill on democracy, the diagnosis, for all its problems, is a better construct than any alternatives thus far proposed. Whatever its ultimate validity, recognizing patients with BPD is important because it leads clinicians to recommend a unique pathway to treatment.

## Making the Diagnosis

In DSM-5 (American Psychiatric Association, 2013), nine criteria for BPD are listed, with five required to make a diagnosis. These criteria include affective symptoms (affective instability, anger, and emptiness), impulsive symptoms (suicidality or self-harm, and other self-damaging behaviors), interpersonal problems (unstable relationships), an unstable identity, and cognitive symptoms (paranoid and dissociative symptoms). The ICD-10 (World Health Organization, 1992) defines "emotionally unstable personality disorder, borderline type" as requiring three out of a list of five impulsive symptoms, as well as at least two symptoms from a second list of six symptoms (e.g., identity problems, unstable relationships, self-harm, and emptiness). These two definitions are similar, but their "polythetic" approach inevitably leads to heterogeneity, since no single feature is required, and there are too many ways that patients with different symptoms can receive the diagnosis. For this reason, some researchers prefer a more restrictive definition, in which symptoms are grouped by symptoms or traits.

Based on criteria developed by Gunderson and Singer (1975), the Diagnostic Interview for Borderlines—Revised (DIB-R; Zanarini, Gunderson, & Frankenburg, 1989) describes a more homogeneous group of patients than DSM-5 or ICD-10. Clinicians are asked to rate symptoms on four subscales: for affective symptoms (scored 0–2), for cognitive symptoms (scored 0–2), for impulsive symptoms (scored 0–3), and for interpersonal problems (scored 0–3). Diagnosis requires a total score of 8/10, and one cannot reach that threshold without having most of the features of BPD, and having symptoms that reflect multiple dimensions of psychopathology.

The most characteristic feature of BPD is affective instability (AI). Hypersensitivity to the environment leads to rapid changes of mood in response to interpersonal events, with slow recovery from distress (Linehan, 1993). Patients with BPD readily describe their emotions as "a roller coaster." Unlike depression or hypomania, AI is more characterized by angry outbursts than by elation or long-lasting sadness, and may have unique neurobiological characteristics (Koenigsberg, 2010). Linehan (1993) suggested that AI (or emotion dysregulation) is the key trait underlying BPD, and that it becomes amplified due to interaction with an "invalidating environment."

While self-report measures have been developed to measure AI, ecological momentary assessment (EMA; Moskowitz, 2009) offers a more precise approach. In this method, patients record emotional responses immediately after life events over the course of 2–3 weeks. Research on BPD using EMA (Ebner-Priemer et al., 2007; Russell-Archambault, Moskowitz, Sookman, & Paris, 2007; Trull, Jahng, Tomko, Wood, & Sher, 2010) confirms clinical impressions that mood shifts occur when interpersonal encounters lead to conflict and/or rejection. These observations also show how AI is different from depression, in which mood remains low even when positive events occur.

Yet AI, while central to BPD, does not fully account for the disorder. Impulsive and self-destructive behaviors are what bring patients with BPD to the emergency room or the clinic. The most characteristic behaviors are chronic and recurrent overdoses and/or self-harm (particularly cutting). BPD can be found in about 10% of patients presenting in emergency rooms with repetitive suicide attempts (Forman, Berk, Henriques, Brown, & Beck, 2004). Self-harm and overdoses are usually precipitated by interpersonal conflict. Clinicians also see a range of other impulsive behavioral patterns, such as substance abuse, bulimia, and shoplifting. These conditions need not be thought of as "comorbid" but as symptomatic expressions of a pervasive behavioral pattern.

Clinicians treating patients with BPD are usually most concerned about suicidal behaviors. Some of these features are striking and unusual. First, suicidality is chronic: Patients often describe thinking about suicide on a daily basis for years. Paradoxically, maintaining an option to die can be comforting when life is experienced as hopeless and marked by intense suffering (Paris, 2006). Second, suicidal attempts in BPD tend to be more dramatic than dangerous. Of course, some attempts are quite serious, and about 10% of patients do eventually kill themselves (Paris, 2008). But there are few other conditions in psychiatry in which patients repetitively take small overdoses, then inform other people of what they have just done. Suicidality in BPD is communicative—a way of being heard when one does not see any other way for a message to get through.

Clinicians need to understand that cutting is *not* suicidal behavior. Patients report they self-harm to relieve tension, not to die (Brown, Comtois, & Linehan, 2002). The powerful calming effect of self-harm on emotional dysregulation can make it addictive, and some patients with BPD cut on an almost daily basis (Linehan, 1993).

In addition to AI and impulsivity, patients with BPD have a pattern of unstable close relationships (Gunderson & Lyons-Ruth, 2008) that involve clinging attachment, fear of abandonment, and intense conflict with intimate partners. Problematic intimacy is a consequence of AI and impulsivity, but patients have a deficient capacity to monitor the emotional state of other people, as well as their own (Bateman & Fonagy, 2006).

The one aspect of BPD that is "borderline" is a range of cognitive symptoms (Zanarini et al., 2013). About half of patients experience transitory auditory hallucinations, usually under stress, often hearing a voice saying they are bad and should die. This contrasts with the more constant hallucinations seen in psychosis, and patients with BPD do not develop delusional elaborations of these experiences, even if they initially seem real. A very large percentage of patients with BPD also experience paranoid feelings, and depersonalization can be prolonged and painful.

## Epidemiology

The best designed surveys of the community prevalence of BPD (Coid, Yang, Tyrer, Roberts, & Ullrich, 2006; Lenzenwnweger, Lane, Loranger, & Kessler, 2007; Torgersen, Kringlen, & Cramer, 2001) have found a rate equal to or somewhat under 1%. That prevalence is the same as for schizophrenia. A widely quoted higher frequency of 4%, reported by Grant and colleagues (2004), was probably an artifact of low thresholds for diagnosis used by research assistants. A conservative reanalysis of the same data reduced the prevalence to 2% (Trull et al., 2010).

Most patients with BPD in clinical settings are female (Gunderson & Links, 2014). Yet community studies suggest an equal prevalence in men and women (Coid et al., 2006; Lenzenwenger et al., 2007). Surveys of women and men with BPD (Paris, Zweig-Frank, & Guzder, 1994a, 1994b) find few differences between male and female patients. But since females tend to be more help seeking, clinicians see more of them.

The prevalence of BPD has not been studied outside of North American and Western Europe, but the diagnosis has been shown to be recognizable in large cities in developing countries (Loranger et al., 1991). Changes associated with urbanization and globalization may have reduced the threshold for developing the disorder, and BPD may also be shaped by history (Paris & Lis, 2013). Unlike psychoses or melancholic depression, there was no clinical description of the syndrome prior to 1938, and it is possible that patients with similar psychological problems may have presented with different symptoms in the past.

## Etiology and Development

BPD, like other mental disorders, can best be understood in the light of diathesis–stress theory. Temperamental vulnerability is a necessary condition. It is well established that both BPD (Distel et al., 2008; Torgersen et al, 2001, 2012) and its underlying traits (Livesley, Jang, & Vernon, 1998) have a heritable component ranging around .40. By themselves, traits such as affective instability and impulsivity are insufficient to cause BPD. But these characteristics make people more sensitive to their environment and produce vicious cycles in which negative perceptions of other people lead to further instability (Paris, 2008).

The majority of patients with BPD report childhood adversities, and in at least one-third of cases, they describe serious traumatic events such as abuse and neglect (Paris, 2008). There are also established risk factors for sequelae in community populations (Fergusson & Mullen, 1999). But childhood adversities, by themselves, do not necessarily lead to BPD. This conclusion is supported by the resilience literature (Rutter, 2012), and by family studies documenting discordance for the disorder between siblings (Laporte et al., 2011).

BPD usually becomes clinically apparent during adolescence, and may be more frequent at this stage than in young adult populations (Chanen & McCutcheon, 2013). It is important to make the diagnosis in these patients, since dismissing problems as "adolescent turmoil" does not promote early intervention.

The childhood precursors of BPD are not well documented, but a series of studies has recently examine high-risk prepubertal populations that may have early symptoms of the disorder (Stepp, Pilkonis, Hipwell, Loeber, & Stouthamer-Loeber, 2010; Zanarini et al., 2011). Long-term follow-ups of these cohorts may shed light on whether children at risk can be identified, and whether prevention is possible.

## Outcome and Course

BPD, once believed to be a lifelong disorder, has a surprisingly good prognosis. Most patients stop meeting diagnostic criteria before middle age. Improvement over time was documented in a series of followback studies conducted in the 1980s and 1990s (McGlashan, 1986; Stone, 1990, Paris et al., 1994a, 1994b), and confirmed by large-scale prospective studies (Gunderson et al, 2011; Zanarini, Frankenburg, Reich, & Fitzmaurice, 2012). In general, impulsive symptoms remit early, while affective symptoms are slower to change. But while some patients recover completely, many continue to show residual psychosocial dysfunction. Although partially recovered patients no longer overdose or cut, they are less likely to find sustained employment, stable partners, or to bear children.

The clinical feature of BPD that most alarms clinicians is suicidality. Follow-up shows that the frequency of completed suicide is close to 5% in prospectively followed cohorts, and about 10% in followback studies (Paris, 2008). But while younger patients with BPD threaten suicide more frequently, the mean age of suicide at 27-year follow-up is 38 (Paris & Zweig-Frank, 2001). This suggests that suicide is more likely in patients who approach middle age but have failed to recover from BPD. Even so, it is encouraging that at least 90% of these patients, most of whom were chronically suicidal for years, choose to go on living.

## Clinical Implications

Patients with BPD are challenging for clinical management. The disorder is not always recognized by clinicians, and many cases called "bipolar" actually meet BPD criteria (Zimmerman et al., 2010). While it is likely that BPD will be seen in different ways in the future, it provides a frame for treatment, even in the absence of a more substantive understanding of its causes. We also know that most cases of BPD can be effectively treated (Paris, 2010). But if the diagnosis is not made, appropriate therapy will not be provided.

## REFERENCES

Akiskal, H. (2003). Demystifying borderline personality: Critique of the concept and unorthodox reflections on its natural kinship with the bipolar spectrum. *Acta Psychiatrica Scandinavica, 110,* 401–407.

Akiskal, H. S., Chen, S. E., & Davis, G. C. (1985). Borderline: An adjective in search of a noun. *Journal of Clinical Psychiatry, 46,* 41–48.

American Psychiatric Association. (2013). *Diagnostic and statistical manual of mental disorders* (5th ed.). Arlington, VA: Author.

Bateman, A., & Fonagy, P. (2006). *Mentalization-based treatment for personality disorders: A practical guide.* Oxford, UK: Oxford University Press.

Brown, M. Z., Comtois, K. A., & Linehan, M. M. (2002). Reasons for suicide attempts and nonsuicidal self-injury in women with borderline personality disorder. *Journal of Abnormal Psychology, 111,* 198–202.

Chanen, A. M., & McCutcheon, L. (2013). Prevention and early intervention for borderline personality disorder: Current status and recent evidence. *British Journal of Psychiatry, 202,* S24–S29.

Coid, J., Yang, M., Tyrer, P., Roberts, A., & Ullrich, S. (2006). Prevalence and correlates of personality disorder in Great Britain. *British Journal of Psychiatry, 188,* 423–431.

Costa, P. T., & Widiger, T. A. (Eds.). (2012). *Personality disorders and the five factor model of personality* (3rd ed.). Washington, DC: American Psychological Association.

Crowell, S., Beauchaine, T. P., & Linehan, M. M. (2009). A biosocial developmental model of borderline personality: Elaborating and extending Linehan's theory. *Psychological Bulletin, 135,* 495–510.

Distel, M. A., Trull, T. J., Derom, C. A., Thiery, E. W., Grimmer, M. A., Martin, N. G., et al. (2008). Heritability of borderline personality disorder features is similar across three countries. *Psychological Medicine, 38,* 1219–1229.

Ebner-Priemer, U. W., Kuo, J., Kleindienst, N., Welch, S. S., Reisch, T., Reinhard, I., et al. (2007). State affective instability in borderline personality disorder assessed by ambulatory monitoring. *Psychological Medicine, 37,* 961–970.

Feighner, J. P., Robins, E., Guze, S. B., Woodruff, R. A., Winokur, G., & Munoz, R. (1972). Diagnostic criteria for use in psychiatric research. *Archives of General Psychiatry, 26,* 57–63.

Fergusson, D. M., & Mullen, P. E. (1999). *Childhood sexual abuse: An evidence based perspective.* Thousand Oaks, CA: SAGE.

Forman, E. M., Berk, M. S., Henriques, G. R., Brown, G. K., & Beck, A. T. (2004). History of multiple suicide attempts as a behavioral marker of severe psychopathology. *American Journal of Psychiatry, 161,* 437–443.

Ghaemi, S. N., Ko, J. Y., & Goodwin, F. K. (2002). "Cade's disease" and beyond: Misdiagnosis, antidepressant use, and a proposed definition for bipolar spectrum disorder. *Canadian Journal of Psychiatry, 47,* 125–134.

Grant, B. F., Hasin, D. S., Stinson, F. S., Dawson, D. A., Chou, S. P., Ruan, W. J., et al. (2004). Prevalence, correlates, and disability of personality disorders in the United States: Results from the National Epidemiologic Survey on Alcohol and Related Conditions. *Journal of Clinical Psychiatry, 65,* 948–958.

Gunderson, J. G. (2009). Borderline personality disorder: Ontogeny of a diagnosis. *American Journal of Psychiatry, 166,* 530–539.

Gunderson, J. G., & Links, P. (2014). *Handbook of good psychiatric management for borderline personality disorder.* Washington, DC: American Psychiatric Publishing.

Gunderson, J. G., & Lyons-Ruth, R. (2008). BPD's interpersonal hypersensitivity phenotype: A gene–environment–developmental model. *Journal of Personality Disorders, 22,* 22–41.

Gunderson, J. G., & Phillips, K. A. (1991). A current view of the interface between borderline personality disorder and depression. *American Journal of Psychiatry, 148,* 967–975.

Gunderson, J. G., & Singer, M. T. (1975). Defining borderline patients: An overview. *American Journal of Psychiatry, 132*(1), 1–10.

Gunderson, J. G., Stout, R. L., McGlashan, T. H., Shea, M. T., Morey, L. C., Grilo, C. M., et al. (2011). Ten-year course of borderline personality disorder: Psychopathology and function from the Collaborative Longitudinal Personality Disorders Study. *Archives of General Psychiatry, 68,* 827–837.

Herman, J. L. (1992). *Trauma and recovery.* New York: Basic Books.

Kernberg, O. F. (1970). A psychoanalytic classification of character pathology. *Journal of the American Psychoanalytic Association, 18,* 800–822.

Koenigsberg, H. (2010). Affective instability: Toward an integration of neuroscience and psychological perspectives. *Journal of Personality Disorders, 24,* 60–82.

Kraepelin, E. (1921). *Manic–depressive insanity and paranoia* (R. M. Barclay, Trans.; G. M. Robertson, Ed.). Edinburgh, UK: Livingstone.

Laporte, L., Paris, J., Russell, J., & Guttman, H. (2011). Psychopathology, trauma, and personality traits in patients with borderline personality disorder and their sisters. *Journal of Personality Disorders, 25,* 448–462.

Lenzenweger, M. F., Lane, M. C., Loranger, A. W., & Kessler, R. C. (2007). DSM-IV personality disorders in the National Comorbidity Survey Replication. *Biological Psychiatry, 62,* 553–556.

Linehan, M. M. (1993). *Dialectical behavior therapy for borderline personality disorder.* New York: Guilford Press.

Livesley, W. J. (2017). *Integrated modular treatment for borderline personality disorder.* New York: Cambridge University Press.

Livesley, W. J., Jang, K. L., & Vernon, P. A. (1998). Phenotypic and genetic structure of traits delineating personality disorder. *Archives of General Psychiatry, 55,* 941–948.

Loranger, A. W., Hirschfeld, R. M. A., Sartorius, N., & Regier, D. A. (1991). The WHO/ADAMHA International Pilot Study of Personality Disorders: Background and purpose. *Journal of Personality Disorders, 5,* 296–306.

McGlashan, T. H. (1986). The Chestnut Lodge follow-up study III: Long-term outcome of borderline personalities. *Archives of General Psychiatry, 43,* 2–30.

Moskowitz, D. S. (2009). Coming full circle: Conceptualizing the study of interpersonal behaviour. *Canadian Psychology/Psychologie canadienne, 50,* 33–41.

Paris, J. (2003). *Personality disorders over time: Precursors, course, and outcome.* Washington, DC: American Psychiatric Press.

Paris, J. (2006). *Half in love with death: Managing the chronically suicidal patient.* Florence, KY: Erlbaum.

Paris, J. (2008). *Treatment of borderline personality disorder: A guide to evidence-based practice.* New York: Guilford Press.

Paris, J. (2010). Effectiveness of differing psychotherapy approaches in the treatment of borderline personality disorder. *Current Psychiatry Reports, 12,* 56–60.

Paris, J. (2012). *The bipolar spectrum*. New York: Routledge.

Paris, J., Gunderson, J. G., & Weinberg, I. (2007). The interface between borderline personality disorder and bipolar spectrum disorder. *Comprehensive Psychiatry, 48,* 145–154.

Paris, J., & Lis, E. (2013). Can sociocultural and historical mechanisms influence the development of borderline personality disorder? *Transcultural Psychiatry, 50,* 140–151.

Paris, J., Zweig-Frank, H. (2001). A 27-year follow-up of patients with borderline personality disorder. *Comprehensive Psychiatry, 42,* 482–487.

Paris, J., Zweig-Frank, H., & Guzder, J. (1994a). Psychological risk factors for borderline personality disorder in female patients. *Comprehensive Psychiatry, 35,* 301–305.

Paris, J., Zweig-Frank, H., & Guzder, J. (1994b). Risk factors for borderline personality in male outpatients. *Journal of Nervous and Mental Disease, 182,* 375–380.

Regier, D. A., Narrow, W. E., Clarke, D., Kraemer, H. C., Kuramoto, S. J., Kuhl, E. A., et al. (2013). DSM-5 field trials in the United States and Canada: Part II. Test–retest reliability of selected categorical diagnoses. *American Journal of Psychiatry, 170,* 159–170.

Ruggero, C. J., Zimmerman, M., Chelminski, I., & Young, D. (2010). Borderline personality disorder and the misdiagnosis of bipolar disorder. *Psychiatric Research, 44,* 405–408.

Russell-Archambault, J., Moskowitz, D., Sookman, D., & Paris, J. (2007). Affective instability in patients with borderline personality disorder. *Journal of Abnormal Psychology, 116,* 578–588.

Rutter, M. (2012). Resilience as a dynamic concept. *Development and Psychopathology, 24,* 335–344.

Siever, L. J., & Davis, K. L. (1991). A psychobiological perspective on the personality disorders. *American Journal of Psychiatry, 148,* 1647–1658.

Stepp, S. D., Pilkonis, P. A., Hipwell, A. E., Loeber, R., & Stouthamer-Loeber, M. (2010). Stability of borderline personality disorder features in girls. *Journal of Personality Disorders, 24,* 460–472.

Stern, A. (1938). Psychoanalytic investigation of and therapy in the borderline group of neuroses. *Psychoanalytic Quarterly, 7,* 467–489.

Stoffers, J., Völlm, B. A., Rücker, G., Timmer, A., Huband, N., & Lieb, K. (2010). Pharmacological interventions for borderline personality disorder. *Cochrane Database of Systematic Reviews, 6,* CD005653.

Stone, M. H. (1990). *The fate of borderline patients*. New York: Guilford Press.

Torgersen, S., Kringlen, E., & Cramer, V. (2001). The prevalence of personality disorders in a community sample. *Archives of General Psychiatry, 58,* 590–596.

Torgersen, S., Lygren, S., Oien, P. A., Skre, I., Onstad, S., Edvardsen, J., et al. (2000). A twin study of personality disorders. *Comprehensive Psychiatry, 41,* 416–425.

Torgersen, S., Myers, J., Reichborn-Kjenneru, T., Roysame, E., Kubarych, T. S., & Kendler, K. S. (2012). The heritability of Cluster B personality disorders assessed both by personal interview and questionnaire. *Journal of Personality Disorders, 26,* 848–866.

Trull, T. J., Jahng, S., Tomko, R. L., Wood, P. K., & Sher, K. J. (2010). Revised NESARC personality disorder diagnoses: Gender, prevalence, and comorbidity with substance dependence disorders. *Journal of Personality Disorders, 24,* 412–426.

Tyrer, P. (2009). Why borderline personality disorder is neither borderline nor a personality disorder. *Personality and Mental Health, 3,* 86–95.

White, C. N., Gunderson, J. G., Zanarini, M. C., & Hudson, J. I. (2003). Family studies of borderline personality disorder: A review. *Harvard Review of Psychiatry, 12,* 118–119.

World Health Organization. (1993). *International classification of diseases* (10th ed.). Geneva, Switzerland: Author.

Zanarini, M. C., Frankenburg, F. R., Dubo, E. D., Sickel, A. E., Trikha, A., & Levin, A. (1998). Axis I comorbidity of borderline personality disorder. *American Journal of Psychiatry, 155,* 1733–1739.

Zanarini, M. C., Frankenburg, F. R., Reich, D. B., & Fitzmaurice, G. (2012). Attainment and stability of sustained symptomatic remission and recovery among patients with borderline personality disorder and Axis II comparison subjects: A 16-year prospective follow-up study. *American Journal of Psychiatry, 169,* 476–483.

Zanarini, M. C., Frankenburg, F. R., Wedig, M., & Fitzmaurice, G. M. (2013). Cognitive experiences reported by patients with borderline personality disorder and Axis II comparison subjects: A 16-year prospective study. *American Journal of Psychiatry, 170,* 671–679.

Zanarini, M. C., Gunderson, J. G., & Frankenburg, F. R. (1989). The revised diagnostic interview for borderlines: Discriminating BPD from other Axis II disorders. *Journal of Personality Disorders, 3,* 10–18.

Zanarini, M. C., Horwood, J., Wolke, D., Waylen, A., Fitzmaurice, G., & Grant, B. F. (2011). Prevalence of DSM-IV borderline personality disorder in two community samples: 6,330 English 11-year-olds and 34,653 American adults. *Journal of Personality Disorders, 25,* 607–619.

Zimmerman, M., Galione, J. N., Ruggero, C. J., Chelminski, I., Young, D., Dalrymple, K., et al. (2010). Screening for bipolar disorder and finding borderline personality disorder. *Journal of Clinical Psychiatry, 71,* 1212–1217.

# CHAPTER 24

# Theoretical Perspectives on Psychopathy and Antisocial Personality Disorder

Christopher J. Patrick and Sarah J. Brislin

Psychopathy and antisocial personality disorder (ASPD) are related but distinguishable diagnostic conditions. Recent years have seen a shift from the view of these conditions as discrete and unitary to a conception of them as continuous and multifaceted. This shift, evident in contemporary models of personality pathology more broadly, has occurred in response to research demonstrating separable subdimensions with contrasting correlates and etiological bases. We discuss in this chapter the commonalities and distinctions between psychopathy and ASPD from the standpoint of these constituent subdimensions and what is known about their relations with criteria from differing assessment domains (self-report, clinician rating, behavioral, neurobiological). The subdimensions of alternative psychopathy inventories and those of ASPD may be viewed as partially overlapping operationalizations of core dispositional constructs, labeled boldness, meanness, and disinhibition by the triarchic model of psychopathy. These dispositional constructs have clear referents in the developmental and neurobiological literatures, and thus provide useful points of reference for organizing what is known about the causal origins and proximal mechanisms of psychopathy.

## Psychopathy and ASPD: Alternative Conceptions and Distinguishable Facets

### Historic Descriptions

The historic account of psychopathy with the strongest influence on contemporary theories and assessment approaches is Hervey Cleckley's book, *The Mask of Sanity* (1941/1976). Cleckley distinguished psychopathic individuals from others exhibiting persistent criminality or antisocial deviance through reference to core features, including shallow affect, lack of close relationships, and ostensible psychological stability in the form of low anxiety, social effectiveness, and disinclination toward suicide. Cleckley's descriptive account served as a key referent for the diagnosis of antisocial personality as described initially in the second edition of the *Diagnostic and Statistical Manual of Mental Disorders* (DSM-II; American Psychiatric Association [APA], 1968), which emphasized features of selfishness, callousness, absence of guilt, and incapacity for loyalty, along with irresponsible, unrestrained behavior.

By contrast, ASPD as defined in DSM-III (APA, 1980) focused predominantly on impulsive–antisocial tendencies—beginning in childhood and continuing into adulthood—with limited representation of affective–interpersonal features aside from deceptiveness. This change partly reflected a general shift in DSM-III toward the use of specific objective criteria, as opposed to the narrative prototype descriptions used in previous editions. Additionally, the behaviorally oriented conception of ASPD in DSM-III was strongly influenced by the work of psychiatric epidemiologist Lee Robins (1966, 1978), who demonstrated early and persistent aggressive behavior to be a key predictor of "sociopathy" in adulthood. Robins's work was in turn influenced by published writings of the time on psychopathy in criminal offender samples (Lindner, 1944; McCord & McCord, 1964), which highlighted aggression and predatory exploitativeness as salient features.

Some effort was made in DSM-III-R (APA, 1987) to improve representation of affective–interpersonal features through inclusion of a "lacks remorse" criterion in adulthood, entailing rationalization of behaviors injurious or detrimental to others. In DSM-IV (APA, 2000), this criterion was modified to cover deficient empathic tendencies by including "indifference to," as well as "rationalization of," harmful behaviors. However, the DSM-IV diagnosis of ASPD remained controversial for its neglect of characteristics such as superficial charm, grandiosity, and shallow affectivity that are considered to be central to psychopathy (Hare, Hart, & Harpur, 1991).

## Contemporary Conceptions

Notwithstanding these concerns, the DSM-IV conception of ASPD was preserved without revision in the main part (Section II) of DSM-5 (APA, 2013). However, as discussed by Olson-Ayala and Patrick (Chapter 25, this volume), DSM-5 also contains a new dimensional system for characterizing personality pathology (in Section III, "Emerging Measures and Models") that includes an alternative, trait-based definition of ASPD. Relative to the criterion-based definition of ASPD within DSM-5 Section II, the trait-based definition appears to provide more balanced coverage of affective–interpersonal and impulsive–antisocial features. As discussed further below, this impression has been confirmed by empirical analysis. Notably, ASPD, as defined in the DSM-5 dimensional system, also includes a trait-based specifier for designating a classically low-anxious, socially efficacious (i.e., "primary psychopathic") variant of ASPD.

Alternative conceptions of psychopathy are embodied in differing contemporary assessment instruments. As described by Olson-Ayala and Patrick (Chapter 25, this volume), the dominant inventory for assessment of psychopathy in adults in clinical and forensic settings is the interview-based Psychopathy Checklist—Revised (PCL-R; Hare, 2003). Adaptations of the PCL-R have been developed for use with children and adolescents, including an interview-based youth version (PCL-YV; Forth, Kosson, & Hare, 2003) and the child-oriented Antisocial Process Screening Device (APSD; Frick & Hare, 2001) and Child Psychopathy Scale (CPS; Lynam, 1997), which rely on informant ratings. Various self-report instruments also exist for assessing psychopathy. Some are patterned after the PCL-R, such as the Hare Self-Report Psychopathy Scale (SRP-III; Paulhus, Neumann, & Hare, 2016), the Levenson Self-Report Psychopathy Scale (LSRP; Levenson, Kiehl, & Fitzpatrick, 1995), and the Youth Psychopathic Traits Inventory (YPI; Andershed, Kerr, Stattin, & Levander, 2002). Others have been developed separately from the PCL-R. The most widely used of these is the Psychopathic Personality Inventory (PPI; Lilienfeld & Andrews, 1996; Lilienfeld & Widows, 2005). Newer non-PCL-R-based inventories include the Elemental Psychopathy Assessment (EPA; Lynam, Gaughan, Miller, Miller, Mullins-Sweatt, & Widiger, 2011) and the Triarchic Psychopathy Measure (TriPM; Drislane, Patrick, & Arsal, 2014; Patrick, 2010).

## Subdimensions of Psychopathy

Countering findings from an initial study (Harris, Rice, & Quinsey, 1994) suggesting that psychopathy might be typological (i.e., discrete, or "taxonic") in nature, further research has yielded compelling and consistent evidence that psychopathic tendencies are distributed continuously in the population (Edens, Marcus, Lilienfeld, & Poythress, 2006; Marcus, John, & Edens, 2004; Murrie et al., 2007). This dimensional perspective has important implications for research. It encourages investigation of both nonclinical and clinical samples, which can facilitate knowledge acquisition. Also, the dimensional perspective encourages investigation of the factors influencing severity of psychopathic tendencies as opposed to focusing on identification of a single underlying cause.

Accompanying the transition from a categorical to a dimensional perspective, a shift has also occurred from the idea of psychopathy as a unitary entity, to viewing it as a multifaceted condition encompassing distinguishable subdimensions or factors. The PCL-R, for example, contains distinct factors even though its items were selected to operate as coherent (i.e., internally consistent) indicators of a common criterion referent—namely, global ratings of resemblance to Cleckley's diagnostic description (Hare, 1980). Initial structural analyses of the PCL/PCL-R (Hare et al., 1990; Harpur, Hakstian, & Hare, 1988) suggested two factors: an affective–interpersonal factor and antisocial–deviancy factor. Subsequent work, has shown that Factor 1 can be subdivided into distinct affective and interpersonal components (Cooke & Michie, 2001), and that Factor 2 can be parsed into impulsive–irresponsible and antisocial behavior facets (Hare & Neumann, 2008).

While intercorrelated, the broad factors and narrower facets of the PCL-R show divergent relationships with external criterion variables. For example, Factor 1 shows selective associations with narcissism, instrumental aggression, and certain adaptive qualities (e.g., lack of anxiousness or depression; Hare, 2003; Hicks & Patrick, 2006), whereas Factor 2 shows preferential relations with reactive aggression, substance use problems, and suicidal behavior (Hare., 1991, 2003; Verona, Patrick, & Joiner, 2001). Factor 2 also accounts for the moderate-level relationship between the PCL-R and ASPD diagnoses or symptoms; controlling for its overlap with Factor 1, scores on PCL-R Factor 2 are unrelated to ASPD (Verona et al., 2001). Contrasting associations with clinical and personality variables have also been reported for the narrower PCL-R facets (Hall, Benning, & Patrick, 2004; Kennealy, Hicks, & Patrick, 2007; Venables & Patrick, 2012; see also Wong, Chapter 36, this volume). Moreover, the two factors of the PCL-R also show diverging relations with physiological criterion measures (e.g., Drislane, Vaidyanathan, & Patrick, 2013; Vaidyanathan, Hall, Patrick, & Bernat, 2011; Venables & Patrick, 2014; see also Patrick & Bernat, 2009). Importantly, evidence of *cooperative suppressor* effects has been reported for the two PCL-R factors (Hicks & Patrick, 2006), in which associations for each with certain criterion measures (e.g., anxiety, depression, suicidal behavior) increase after accounting for their overlap. Instances of cooperative suppression provide particularly strong evidence that psychologically distinct attributes are embedded within a putatively unitary measure.

Further evidence for the heterogeneity of psychopathy as indexed by the PCL-R is provided by findings from model-based cluster analyses of individuals obtaining high overall scores on this instrument. In an initial study, Hicks, Markon, Patrick, Krueger, and Newman (2004), using personality trait scales as cluster variates, identified two subgroups of high PCL-R scorers with markedly different trait profiles. The first, labeled the "aggressive" subtype, exhibited high scores on negative emotional traits including aggression and alienation, along with low scores on traits reflecting planfulness, conformity, and inhibitory control. The second, "stable" subtype showed low anxiousness (stress reactivity) in conjunction with high scores on traits reflecting active, agentic tendencies (i.e., social dominance, achievement, well-being). Subsequent work by other authors has corroborated this finding of distinguishable variants of high PCL-R scorers (e.g., Poythress et al., 2010; Skeem, Johansson, Andershed, Kerr, & Louden, 2007).

Clear evidence for heterogeneity has also emerged from research on psychopathic tendencies in children. Factor analyses of the PCL-R's main childhood counterpart, the APSD, have also revealed distinguishable subdimensions. Most work has focused on two factors, labeled callous–unemotional (CU) traits and impulsivity/conduct problems (I/CP). Children who score high on both of these APSD factors show diminished reactivity to distressing stimuli, failure to learn from punishment, and high levels of both reactive and proactive aggression in the context of normal or above-average intellect, whereas those scoring high on the I/CP factor alone are characteristically below average in intellect and show heightened stress reactivity and emotional lability, along with increased reactive (but not instrumental) aggression (Frick & Marsee, 2006; Frick & White, 2008). These findings for the APSD served as the major impetus for inclusion of a "low prosocial emotions" specifier for the diagnosis of conduct disorder in DSM-5—allowing for designation of a CU (i.e., "psychopathic") variant of this child behavior disorder.

Distinct subdimensions are also evident in contemporary self-report inventories for psychopathy. Like the PCL-R itself, inventories patterned after the PCL-R have correlated factors (e.g., Andershed, Hodgins, & Tengström, 2007; Levenson et al., 1995; Paulhus et al., 2016). By contrast, the PPI—which was developed to assess basic trait dispositions associated with psychopathy without specific requirements for convergence—has two higher-order factors that are largely uncorrelated (Benning, Patrick, Hicks, Blonigen, & Krueger, 2003; Benning, Patrick, Salekin, & Leistico, 2005; Ross, Benning, Patrick, Thompson, & Thurson, 2009). These factors, labeled Fearless Dominance and Impulsive Antisociality or Self-Centered Impulsivity, show divergent relations with multiple criterion variables in self-report, interview-based, and physiological domains (Benning, Patrick, Blonigen, Hicks, & Iacono, 2005; Benning, Patrick, & Iacono, 2005; Carlson, Thái, & McLaron, 2009; Lilienfeld & Widows, 2005; for a review, see Patrick & Bernat, 2009). Notably, the PPI contains one subscale, Coldheartedness, which fails to load appreciably on either of these factors—instead emerging as a separate subdimension in structural analyses (Benning et al., 2003; Benning, Patrick, Blonigen, et al., 2005). As we discussed further below, this subscale appears to index CU traits or meanness more exclusively than the other subscales of the PPI.

### Subdimensions of ASPD

The childhood criteria for ASPD in Section II of DSM-5—which mirror those for conduct disorder (CD)—include aggressive and destructive behaviors along with theft/deceptiveness and nonaggressive rule-breaking acts. Factor analyses of the CD criteria (e.g., Frick et al., 1991; Tackett, Krueger, Sawyer, & Graetz, 2003) have demonstrated that the aggressive and rule-breaking symptoms define separate, albeit correlated, factors. Tackett, Krueger, Iacono, and McGue (2005) reported evidence for overlapping as well as distinctive etiological underpinnings to these factors in a study of young male twins. In this study, additive genetic and nonshared (i.e., unique, person-specific) environmental influences contributed significantly to each, with the proportion of symptom variance attributable to genes higher for the aggressive than the rule-breaking factor (35 vs. 28%); the finding of higher heritability for the aggressive factor of CD has been corroborated by follow-up research (Burt, 2009). A contribution of shared environment (i.e., influences common to siblings reared together) was found for the rule-breaking but not the aggressive subdimension. Extending this work, Kendler, Aggen, and Patrick (2013) presented behavioral genetic evidence that (1) aggressive and rule-breaking subdimensions of CD reflect differing sources of genetic influence, and (2) the shared environmental contribution to the rule-breaking subdimension is concentrated in a subset of symptoms reflecting covert delinquent acts (e.g., stealing, telling lies).

Corresponding criteria for ASPD at the adult level include one aggression-specific criterion (irritability/aggressiveness), three clearly nonaggressive criteria (impulsivity, irresponsibility, deceitfulness), and three nonspecific criteria (failure to conform to legal norms, reckless disregard for safety, lacks remorse). Using data from an adult twin sample, Kendler, Aggen, and Patrick (2012) demonstrated two distinct factors underlying these adult symptoms as assessed by participant report—a *disinhibition* factor encompassing tendencies toward impulsivity, irresponsibility, and deceitfulness, and an *aggressive-disregard* factor reflecting irritability/aggressiveness, reckless behavior, and lack of concern for self or others. Paralleling findings for factors of CD (Kendler et al., 2013; Tackett et al., 2005), the two adult ASPD factors were found to be associated with differing sources of genetic influence.

In summary, paralleling findings of distinct factors for various inventories of psychopathy, available evidence points to separable subdimensions underlying both the child and adult symptoms of ASPD. In the next section, we consider relationships between subdimensions of psychopathy and ASPD from the standpoint of the triarchic model of psychopathy (Patrick, Fowles, & Krueger, 2009).

### Clarifying Relationships among Differing Psychopathy Measures and ASPD: The Triarchic Model

The triarchic model was advanced as a framework for integrating alternative conceptions of psychopathy, clarifying their relationships with other clinical conditions (including ASPD), and guiding research on neurobiological correlates and etiological influences. The model proposes that psychopathy as characterized in historic writings and contemporary assessment instruments encompasses three distinct but intersecting symptomatic (phenotypic) constructs: disinhibition, boldness, and meanness. "Disinhibition" entails impulsiveness, weak restraint, hostility and mistrust, and difficulties in regulating emotion. "Meanness" entails deficient empathy, lack of affiliative capacity, contempt toward others, predatory exploitativeness, and empowerment through cruelty or destructiveness. The third triarchic model construct, "boldness," encompasses tendencies toward confidence and social assertiveness, emotional resiliency, and venturesomeness.

The constructs of the model may be viewed as descriptive building blocks for differing conceptions of psychopathy. For example, Cleckley's conception, derived from observations of psychiatric inpatients, emphasizes boldness (i.e., low anxiousness, social efficacy, and insensitivity to punishment) and unrestrained–disinhibitory tendencies, whereas conceptions based on criminal samples (e.g., McCord & McCord, 1964) focus more on meanness and disinhibition. As we discuss further below, the triarchic model constructs also have behavioral referents and show replicable associations with physiological variables and, as such, may be helpful for relating psychopathy and ASPD to neurobiology (cf. Patrick, Durbin, & Moser, 2012).

The TriPM (Patrick, 2010), which consists of 58 items, was developed to assess the three constructs of boldness, meanness, and disinhibition. The Disinhibition and Meanness scales correspond to item-based factor scales from the brief form (Patrick, Kramer, et al., 2013) of the Externalizing Spectrum Inventory (ESI; Krueger et al., 2007), a measure developed to operationalize a hierarchical structural model of the externalizing spectrum of psychopathology—encompassing child and adult behavior problems, substance use problems, and disinhibitory traits. The ESI's 23 content scales load together on a general *externalizing proneness* factor, with some scales also loading on separate *callous aggression* and *substance abuse* subfactors. The ESI brief form (ESI-BF) contains shortened versions of all ESI content scales, along with item-based scales for indexing the ESI's broad factors. The general externalizing proneness and callous aggression factor scales of the ESI-BF equate with the TriPM's Disinhibition and Meanness subscales. The third subscale of the TriPM, Boldness, was developed to index fearless–dominant tendencies (cf. Benning, Patrick, Blonigen, et al., 2005) associated with the general factor of a structural model of fear and fearlessness inventories (Kramer, Patrick, Krueger, & Gasperi, 2012), including the subscales of the PPI that define its Fearless Dominance factor.

In terms of content, the TriPM Disinhibition scale assesses general externalizing proneness using items indexing irresponsibility and lack of dependability, problematic impulsivity and lack of planful control, impatient urgency, boredom proneness, alienation, theft, and fraudulence. The TriPM Meanness scale assesses callous–aggressive tendencies through items tapping lack of empathy and different forms of aggression (relational, destructive, physical), along with excitement seeking and dishonesty. The TriPM Boldness scale assesses fearless tendencies in domains of emotional experience (through items tapping resiliency, self-confidence, and optimism), interpersonal behavior (items indexing persuasiveness, social assurance, and dominance), and venturesomeness (items tapping courage, thrill seeking, and tolerance for uncertainty). Scores on the TriPM Meanness and Disinhibition scales are moderately correlated (.4–.6), with scores on Meanness and Boldness related to a more modest degree (.2–.3) and scores on Boldness and Disinhibition largely uncorrelated.

The TriPM has been used in several studies with differing populations as a referent for evaluating the content coverage of alternative psychopathy measures. Studies with undergraduate and correctional samples (Drislane et al., 2014; Sellbom & Phillips, 2013) have shown that the PPI provides balanced coverage of boldness, meanness, and disinhibition, as indexed by the TriPM, whereas other psychopathy inventories index meanness and disinhibition either more than boldness (e.g., SRP-III, YPI) or exclusively (e.g., LSRP). In turn, the subdimensions of the PPI can be understood in terms of their coverage of triarchic constructs. The PPI's Fearless Dominance factor relates strongly to TriPM Boldness and modestly to TriPM Meanness, whereas the PPI's Self-Centered Impulsivity factor relates strongly to TriPM Disinhibition and somewhat less so to Meanness—mainly due to inclusion of the PPI's Machiavellianism Egocentricity scale. The PPI Coldheartedness scale, not represented in either factor, shows a strong selective association with TriPM Meanness. These findings for the PPI suggested that its constituent items can be used to construct effective scale measures of the triarchic model constructs, and work along this line was undertaken by Hall and colleagues (2014). Parallel work has been done to construct item-based boldness, meanness, and disinhibition scales from other psychopathy measures (e.g., Drislane et al., 2015) and omnibus inventories of personality (e.g., Brislin et al., 2015; Sellbom et al., 2016).

Other recent research has used the TriPM scales or close variants to clarify similarities and differences between PCL-R psychopathy and ASPD as defined in DSM-5 Section II. One study by Venables, Hall, and Patrick (2014) showed that scores on the PCL-R as a whole contain variance associated with all three constructs of the triarchic model, whereas ASPD indexes only the meanness and disinhibition constructs—with the adult symptoms tapping disinhibition more, and the child (CD) symptoms capturing meanness more. Analyses of component scores for the PCL-R revealed Factor 1 to be associated with Boldness and Meanness scales of the TriPM but not Disinhibition, and Factor 2 to be associated with Disinhibition and Meanness but not Boldness. Scores on the PCL-R Interpersonal facet accounted mainly for the association of Factor 1 with Boldness, whereas scores on the Impulsive–Irresponsible facet accounted mainly for the association of Factor 2 with Disinhibition. Representation of meanness in Factors 1 and 2 was accounted for by the Affective and Antisocial facets of the PCL-R, respectively. Findings complementary to these were reported by Wall, Wygant, and Sellbom (2015). These investigators showed that scores on TriPM Boldness and Meanness each contributed over and above ASPD symptom scores to prediction of PCL-R Factor 1, whereas scores on TriPM Disinhibition contributed incrementally over ASPD to prediction of PCL-R Factor 2. Reciprocally, scores on TriPM Disinhibition contributed over and above total PCL-R scores to prediction of ASPD symptoms, with no incremental contribution evident for TriPM Boldness or Meanness.

Taken together, results from these studies establish that (1) PCL-R psychopathy contains greater representation of boldness and meanness than ASPD, through its Interpersonal and Affective facets, and (2) the two conditions include overlapping but somewhat distinct representation of disinhibition (i.e., as evidenced by analyses showing that disinhibition contributed over and above ASPD to the prediction of PCL-R scores and vice versa). Further research is needed to clarify in psychological terms how PCL-R psychopathy and ASPD compare in their coverage of meanness and disinhibition, and how boldness as represented in the PCL-R compares and contrasts with boldness as represented in other inventories such as the PPI.

Other studies have examined relationships between ASPD as defined in Section III of DSM-5 and constructs of the triarchic model (Anderson, Sellbom, Wygant, Salekin & Krueger, 2014; Strickland, Drislane, Lucy, Krueger, & Patrick, 2013). Results demonstrate that traits identified as diagnostic of ASPD (i.e., impulsivity, irresponsibility, and risk taking from the domain of Disinhibition, and callousness, manipulativeness, and deceitfulness from the domain of Antagonism) covary appreciably with TriPM Disinhibition and Meanness, respectively. Additionally, traits represented in the psychopathic features specifier for ASPD (i.e., anxiousness [–], attention seeking [+], and withdrawal [–]) provide effective coverage of boldness as indexed by the TriPM. These results indicate that the trait-based diagnosis of ASPD and its psychopathic features specifier provide effective coverage of core dispositional facets of psychopathy emphasized in various historic and contemporary conceptions.

## Perspectives on the Etiology of Psychopathy

Psychopathy has long been of interest to experimental psychopathologists, beginning with Lykken's (1957) experimental analysis of anxiety responding in youthful offenders classified as primary versus secondary ("neurotic") psychopaths. This focus continued with Hare's work on autonomic reactivity to stressors in adult prisoners judged to be low or high in psychopathy as described by Cleckley (see Hare, 1978) and more recently has been extended through use of human neuroscience methodologies (cf. Patrick, Venables, & Skeem, 2012). Contemporary experimental studies have focused increasingly on identifying deviations in physiological or behavioral response associated with distinct subdimensions of psychopathy (e.g., Baskin-Sommers, Zeier, & Newman, 2009; Benning, Patrick, & Iacono, 2005; Carlson et al., 2009; Dvorak-Bertsch, Curtin, Rubinstein, & Newman, 2009; López, Poy, Patrick, & Moltó, 2013; Marsh et al., 2008; Molto, Poy, Segarra, Pastor, & Montanes, 2007; Vaidyanathan et al., 2011; Venables & Patrick, 2014; for reviews, see Blair, 2013; Fowles & Dindo, 2009; Frick

& White, 2008; Patrick & Bernat, 2009). Work on subdimensions of ASPD is newer; therefore, evidence pertaining to distinct behavioral or physiological correlates of these subdimensions is more limited. As discussed below, however, knowledge of relationships between subdimensions of psychopathy and ASPD provides a basis for linking biological and behavioral findings across the two.

While findings from experimental studies of individuals scoring high in psychopathy or ASPD, or distinct facets of each, can provide insights into pathological processes underlying these conditions, there are distinct limitations to studies of this type. Experimental studies are inherently quasi-experimental, since they focus on groups that differ in preexisting characteristics rather than on groups made to differ through experimental manipulation. For this reason, studies of this type can provide information about proximal processes (e.g., affective or cognitive anomalies) relevant to observed symptoms, but not about basic causal influences. To gain understanding of causal factors contributing to psychopathy and ASPD, longitudinal–developmental and behavioral or molecular genetic studies are needed. In the sections that follow, we review what has been learned about proximal processes and causal factors in psychopathy through studies of these differing types—with reference again to the dispositional constructs of the triarchic model.

## Experimental Findings

Experimental research on psychopathy has focused most heavily on affective and cognitive processing deviations. While Cleckley (1976, p. 383) hypothesized that psychopathy entails a general deficit in affective sensitivity ("a consistent leveling of response to petty ranges and an incapacity to react with sufficient seriousness to achieve much more than pseudoexperience or quasi-experience"), evidence has emerged most consistently indicating weaknesses in reactivity to *negative* emotional stimuli. For example, following up on work by Lykken and Hare reporting deficits in electrodermal response to experimental stressors, studies over the past two decades have reliably demonstrated reduced potentiation of the defensive startle reflex during exposure to aversive cues of differing types (see review by Patrick & Bernat, 2009). Other work with youth and adults scoring high in psychopathy has yielded evidence of reduced reactivity of the amygdala, a subcortical structure implicated in fear and other emotions, to aversive visual stimuli (Birbaumer et al., 2005; Kiehl et al., 2001; Larson et al., 2013; Marsh et al., 2008; see also Gordon, Baird, & End, 2004). These findings dovetail with evidence for reduced behavioral recognition of fearful facial stimuli in high-psychopathy individuals (Marsh & Blair, 2008).

Regarding studies focusing on cognitive processing anomalies, Newman (1998; Patterson & Newman, 1993) proposed that psychopathy entails a deficit in "response modulation," defined as the ability to shift from an ongoing (dominant) action set to an alternative mode of responding when situational cues signal the need for a shift. A somewhat different but compatible perspective is that psychopathic individuals have difficulty processing peripheral cues when attention is prioritized toward more central, goal-relevant cues (Jutai & Hare, 1983; Newman & Kosson, 1986)—particularly under performance conditions that promote activation of the left hemisphere (Kosson, 1996, 1998). Recent work by Newman and colleagues (e.g., Baskin-Sommers, Curtin, & Newman, 2011; Dvorak-Bertsch et al., 2009; Larson et al., 2013) has sought to integrate affective and attentional perspectives by suggesting that negative reactivity deficits in psychopathy are most likely to arise in divided attention contexts—where aversive cues occur incidentally to targeted stimuli, and "pull" for attentional resources in a more automatic manner (cf. Lang, Bradley, & Cuthbert, 1997).

A model that relates findings pertaining to affective and cognitive–attentional anomalies to what is known about distinct subdimensions of psychopathy is the two-process (Patrick & Bernat, 2009) or dual-pathway model (Fowles & Dindo, 2009), which proposes that impairments in emotional response and cognitive–attentional processing contribute differently to affective–interpersonal and antisocial deviance components of psychopathy. This model contrasts with more traditional unitary-process perspectives, which posit that a single underlying deficit or impairment accounts for the features of psychopathy as a whole. The two processes the model focuses on are dispositional fearlessness and weak inhibitory control.

From the dual-process perspective, the "mask of sanity" that Cleckley (1976) described reflects an extreme temperament disposition arising from an underlying weakness in affective, particularly fear, reactivity. Neurobiologically, dispositional fearlessness is theorized to reflect differences in the functioning of the brain's defensive motivational system, comprising the amygdala and affiliated structures. In contrast, the major basis for the antisocial deviance component of psychopathy is hypothesized to be weak inhibitory control, or externalizing proneness—that is, the strongly heritable propensity that contributes to various impulse control problems, including child and adolescent antisocial behavior and substance use disorders (Krueger et al., 2002). In neurobiological terms, this vulnerability is presumed to reflect impairments in the functioning of higher brain systems that operate to regulate emotion and guide decision making and action.

A key point of reference for the two-process model is the finding that reduced startle potentiation during aversive cuing relates most to the affective–interpersonal component of psychopathy—whether indexed by PCL-R Factor 1 (Patrick, 1994; Vaidyanathan et al., 2011; Vanman, Mejia, Dawson, Schell, & Raine, 2003) or by PPI Fearless Dominance (Benning, Patrick, & Iacono, 2005; Dvorak-Bertsch et al., 2009). Other work with adults has shown that electrodermal response deficits in aversive cueing contexts also relate most to the affective–interpersonal features of psychopathy (Benning, Patrick, & Iacono, 2005; Dindo & Fowles, 2011; Flor, Birbaumer, Hermann, Ziegler, & Patrick, 2002; López et al., 2013). Additionally, work with child and adolescent samples has shown that participants exhibiting affective–interpersonal (CU) features along with impulsive conduct problems show deficits in laboratory behavioral measures of fear reactivity (e.g., response inhibition/withdrawal, observable distress) not shown by participants with conduct problems alone (Frick & Marsee, 2006; Frick & White, 2008).

Regarding the impulsive–antisocial component of psychopathy, Patrick, Hicks, Krueger, and Lang (2005) demonstrated a close association between this component and externalizing proneness operationalized as the common factor underlying child and adult symptoms of ASPD, substance-related problems, and disinhibitory personality traits. In turn, converging lines of evidence indicate that externalizing proneness reflects impairments in anterior brain systems that function to regulate affect and behavior in complex everyday contexts. In particular, evidence has been found for impaired performance on frontal-executive tasks (Morgan & Lilienfeld, 2000; Young et al., 2009) and reduced brain potential response in cognitive processing tasks (Patrick, Venables, et al., 2013). Well-established brain response indicators of externalizing proneness include the P300 component of the event-related potential (ERP; Iacono, Carlson, Malone, & McGue, 2002; Patrick et al., 2006) and the error-related negativity (ERN), a negative-going cortical response that follows incorrect responses in a performance task (Dikman & Allen, 2000; Hall, Bernat, & Patrick, 2007).

The two distinct mechanisms emphasized in the two-process model, dispositional fearlessness and externalizing proneness, connect most obviously and directly to the boldness and disinhibition facets, respectively, of the triarchic model of psychopathy. Direct evidence for a role of dispositional boldness in defensive reactivity deficits associated with psychopathy is provided by work demonstrating that (1) the subscales of the PPI that define its Fearless Dominance factor operate as indicators of a broad common factor when modeled together with other established scale measures of fear and fearlessness (Kramer et al., 2012), and (2) scores on this broad fear/fearlessness factor predict individual differences in aversive startle potentiation (Kramer et al., 2012; Vaidyanathan, Patrick, & Bernat, 2009).

Corresponding evidence for a role of trait disinhibition in frontal-executive task deficits (Morgan & Lilienfeld, 2000) and brain ERP deficits comes from (1) research demonstrating strong associations of both PCL-R Factor 2 and PPI Impulsive-Antisociality with disinhibitory tendencies as indexed by externalizing disorder symptoms (Blonigen, Hicks, Krueger, Patrick, & Iacono, 2005; Patrick et al., 2005) and ESI or TriPM disinhibition scores (Drislane et al., 2014; Sellbom & Phillips, 2013; Venables & Patrick, 2012; Wall et al., 2015); (2) work demonstrating a robust, genetically mediated relationship (negative in direction) between disinhibitory tendencies as indexed by externalizing symptoms and scores on a common factor reflecting covariance among task measures of executive function (Young et al., 2009); and (3) research demonstrating reduced P300 brain response in relation to PCL-R Factor 2 (Venables & Patrick, 2014) and PPI Impulsive Antisociality (Carlson et al., 2009), as well as with disinhibitory tendencies as indexed by externalizing disorder symptoms and ESI/TriPM disinhibition scores

(Patrick et al., 2006; Yancey, Venables, Hicks, & Patrick, 2013). To the extent that ASPD partly reflects disinhibitory tendencies associated with general externalizing proneness (Krueger et al., 2002)—in particular, as a function of its nonaggressive child and adult criteria—it is not surprising that it also shows parallel negative associations with executive task performance (Morgan & Lilienfeld, 2000) and P300 brain response (Bauer & Hesslebrock, 1999; Bauer, O'Connor, & Hesslebrock, 1994).

Most of what is known about experimental correlates of CU traits (meanness) comes from work with clinic-referred children and adolescents, because this subdimension of psychopathy and ASPD has been distinguished from disinhibitory tendencies only recently in the adult literature. As compared to conduct-problem youth without CU tendencies, those high in CU traits report low levels of anxiousness and neuroticism, are attracted to activities entailing novelty and risk, exhibit reduced behavioral reactivity to threatening or distressing stimuli of differing types, show impairments in passive avoidance learning (i.e., reduced ability to inhibit behavior that results in punishment), and exhibit high levels of both proactive and reactive aggression (Frick & Marsee, 2006; Frick & White, 2008). Additionally, as noted earlier, youth high in CU traits also show reduced amygdala reactivity to fearful facial stimuli (Marsh & Blair, 2008). Findings along these lines have been interpreted as indicating a role for dispositional fearlessness, or perhaps emotional insensitivity more broadly (Blair, 1995, 2001), in early-emerging CU tendencies. If this is true, the obvious question that arises is: What accounts for contrasting expressions of low dispositional fear in the form of boldness as compared to meanness? Possible explanations are considered in the next section on developmental research findings.

### Concepts and Findings from the Developmental Literature

Evidence from the developmental literature supports the idea of basic dispositions corresponding to disinhibition and boldness early in life contributing to the emergence of behavioral deviance over time. The early childhood counterpart to disinhibition is "difficult temperament" (Frick & Morris, 2004; Thomas & Chess, 1977), which entails high negative affect and irritability, overactivity, poor performance in contexts requiring sustained attention, and difficulty adapting to changes in the environment. This pattern of proclivities is associated with increased likelihood of conduct problems beginning early in childhood and continuing through adolescence into adulthood. In particular, impairments in the ability to manage unanticipated stresses and to regulate emotional reactions, reflected in low frustration tolerance and intense angry outbursts, are seen as crucial to the emergence of early, persisting conduct problems (Frick & Morris, 2004). A related concept in the developmental literature is that of effortful control, which is considered a core temperament dimension by some (e.g., Kochanska, Murray, & Harlan, 2000; Rothbart, 2007). Theorized to be dependent on the development of focused (executive) attention skills early in life, and encompassing abilities to resist distraction, regulate emotion, and inhibit prepotent responses, weak effortful control is considered central to the unrestrained aggressive behavior that commonly occurs with difficult temperament. The concept of weak effortful control also aligns closely with the construct of disinhibition in the triarchic model.

The counterpart to boldness in the developmental literature is fearless temperament, which entails tolerance for novelty or mild threat and active approach toward unfamiliar objects/situations. Kochanska (1997) and her colleagues (Kochanska & Aksan, 2006; Kochanska, Gross, Lin, & Nichols, 2002) presented evidence that variations in temperamental fear/fearlessness are important in early conscience development. In particular, these investigators found that parents' use of gentle discipline (i.e., instilling awareness of adverse effects through feedback) predicted development of internalized conscience among children with higher but not lower fear. Conscience development in children with low fear was predicted instead by degree of positive interaction and attachment with parental figures. These results indicate that reward-oriented approaches focusing on connectedness with parental figures are more likely to foster socialization in fearless children than mild punishment-based approaches. Extending this work, Fowles and Kochanska (2000) reported that gentle discipline fosters conscience development in children who exhibit strong electrodermal reactivity to laboratory stressors, whereas positive connectedness predicts conscience development in children exhibiting only weak electrodermal reactivity to stressors.

These results provide a direct point of contact with data from studies of adults showing reduced electrodermal reactivity to aversive stimuli of differing types in highly bold individuals.

Besides highlighting these developmental counterparts to disinhibition and boldness as basic liability factors for the emergence of early, persisting conduct problems, the developmental literature also emphasizes the important role of person–environment transactions across time—including coercive exchanges (i.e., parent–child interactions marked by escalation of conflict and negative reinforcement of coercion) and factors affecting parent–child bonding. Difficult temperament, entailing low frustration tolerance and weak inhibitory control, has been discussed as a specific risk factor for coercive exchanges that foster routine adversarial interactions with others and a vicious cycle of antagonism–rejection. Difficult temperament has also been discussed as a factor contributing to insecure attachment, in view of the challenges it poses to parental resources and patience. These person–environment transactions represent mechanisms whereby tendencies toward callousness and antagonism (meanness) may develop over time. In cases in which difficult temperament is coupled with dispositional fearlessness, the "push" toward meanness may be even stronger (i.e., because conscience formation is unlikely to occur in such individuals in the absence of positive connectedness with parents and others). This may help account for findings indicating a role for dispositional fearlessness in CU tendencies (Frick & Marsee, 2006; Frick & White, 2008).

However, it is conceivable that distinct neurobiological processes related to the formation of empathy, affiliation, and nurturance also contribute to the emergence of meanness. For example, Jones, Happé, Gilbert, Burnett, and Viding (2010) reported evidence that antisocial youth high in CU traits show intact cognitive perspective-taking abilities but deficient emotional empathy, as evidenced by low levels of reported sympathy for victims of aggression and low reported fear when witnessing aggressive victimization. Elsewhere, Decety and Jackson (2004), on the basis of electrophysiological and neuroimaging evidence, hypothesized that emotional empathy entails the activation of shared representations—that is, internal representations pertaining to one's own behavior in the context of witnessing (or otherwise encountering) that same behavior in another person. Extrapolating from this, it may be the case that a core heritable weakness in the ability to form shared representations of others' distress, or to activate these representations at appropriate times, contributes to the facet of psychopathy referred to as "meanness." Other work points to an important role for neuromodulatory hormones, including oxytocin and vasopressin, in the development of trust and close relationships, in humans as well as other mammals (Kosfeld, Heirichs, Zak, Fischbacher, & Fehr, 2005; Young & Wang, 2004). Deficits in the production of such hormones, or hypoactivity of their receptor sites within the brain, could also contribute to CU tendencies through detrimental effects on natural affiliative processes. It is important to explore these possibilities in future experimental and longitudinal–developmental studies.

### Genetic and Environmental Influences

Behavioral and molecular genetics studies provide a valuable complement to longitudinal studies for delineating causal factors contributing to psychopathology. Behavioral genetics studies utilize data from identical and fraternal twins to estimate contributions of additive genetic influences along with shared and nonshared environmental influences to target phenotypes. Molecular genetics studies hold promise for connecting target phenotypes to physical substrates in the form of specific gene variants.

Behavioral genetic studies over the past decade have substantially advanced our understanding of the etiological bases of psychopathy and ASPD. Research focusing on psychopathy as indexed by the PPI in adult twins indicates approximately equal (50:50) contributions of genes and nonshared environment to total scores, with shared environment contributing minimally (Blonigen, Carlson, Krueger, & Patrick, 2003). The same appears true for the two factors of the PPI (i.e., genes and nonshared environment contribute about equally to scores on Fearless Dominance and Impulsive Antisociality), with differing sets of genes contributing to each, as evidenced by a negligible genetic correlation between the two (Blonigen et al., 2005). From the standpoint of the triarchic model, the implication is that genetic influences contributing to boldness per se (reflected by scores on PPI Fearless Dominance) differ from those contributing to disinhibition when coupled with meanness (as tapped by scores on PPI Impulsive Antisociality; see Sellbom & Phillips, 2013). However, behavior genetic research using the YPI, which measures boldness in a manner that overlaps with disinhibition and meanness (through items reflecting grandiosity–manipulativeness; Drislane et al., 2015), yielded evidence of a general psychopathy factor that accounted for much of the genetic variance in scores on the inventory as a whole. The implication is that boldness can be operationalized in alternative ways through use of differing item sets, such that it overlaps either more or less with disinhibition and meanness—genotypically as well as phenotypically. Extrapolating from this, it may be possible as well to index disinhibition and meanness either as separate or correlated dimensions through use of items selected to be either maximally discriminating or interrelated. Doing so may be helpful for understanding how these constructs intersect and diverge etiologically.

Other work examining the etiology of teacher-rated CU tendencies and conduct problems, as indexed by the APSD in child-age twin pairs (Larsson, Viding, & Plomin, 2008; Viding, Blair, Moffitt, & Plomin, 2005; Viding, Jones, Frick, Moffitt, & Plomin, 2008), demonstrates that CU tendencies are moderately to highly (> 60%) heritable, and that conduct problems appear more substantially heritable when accompanied by CU tendencies (70–80%) than when not (30–50%). This finding of increased heritability for conduct problems when accompanied by CU tendencies served as one impetus for inclusion of a limited prosocial emotions ("psychopathy") specifier for the diagnosis of CD in DSM-5. From the perspective of the triarchic model, the implication is that a phenotype combining tendencies toward disinhibition and meanness is more strongly determined by genes than a "pure" disinhibitory (i.e., impulsive–irresponsible but not callous–aggressive) phenotype.

As noted earlier, behavioral genetic research on symptoms of CD itself indicates higher heritability for aggressive symptoms than for non-aggressive (rule-breaking) symptoms. Research is needed to evaluate the extent of overlap between CU tendencies as indexed by the APSD or the low prosocial emotions specifier within DSM-5 and aggressive symptoms included among the criteria for CD—particularly in view of research suggesting stronger representation of callous aggression (meanness) in aggressive versus nonaggressive symptoms of CD (e.g., Venables & Patrick, 2012). It is conceivable that CD involving aggressive symptoms of certain types (e.g., initiation of fights, physical cruelty, weapons use) overlaps substantially with CD that entails high CU tendencies and, as such, is more strongly heritable. Research is also needed to evaluate the degree of continuity of CU tendencies from childhood through to adulthood, along with the continuity of aggressive symptoms of CD with adult aggressive symptoms of ASPD (cf. Kendler et al., 2012), and the extent to which the continuity of aggressive ASPD symptoms is intertwined with that of CU tendencies.

Regarding molecular genetic research, substantial excitement was generated by findings from candidate gene studies of psychopathy and ASPD-related phenotypes during the 1990s and 2000s (cf. Raine, 2008; Waldman & Rhee, 2006). However, this excitement has been greatly tempered by findings from newer large-$N$ genomewide association (GWA) studies demonstrating exceedingly small effect sizes (in most cases, below detection thresholds for significance) for genes identified by smaller-$N$ studies as potentially relevant to target psychiatric phenotypes (Kendler, 2013). Recent research indicates that this picture applies to ASPD and psychopathy. Tielbeek and colleagues (2012) undertook GWA analyses of data from a sample of 4,816 participants assessed via questionnaire for adult symptoms of ASPD ($n = 3,167$) or history of unlawful behavior more broadly ($n = 1,649$). No genes in this study evinced a signification association with antisocial behavior as defined in these ways. Another study that employed a less conservative genomewide linkage analysis approach (Gizer et al., 2012) found evidence for only a marginal association of antisocial tendencies, as indexed by self-report, with one distinct region on a single chromosome. More recently, Viding and colleagues (2013) undertook a GWA analysis of CU tendencies in 7- to 12-year-old children ($N = 2,930$), as assessed by teacher ratings, and found no genes with effects exceeding the genomewide threshold for significance.

Findings from these recent studies provide compelling evidence that effect size estimates for single genes reported in small-$n$ studies are generally erroneous, and that the moderate or higher-level heritability estimates for psychiatric phenotypes including psychopathy and ASPD emerging from twin studies almost certainly reflect the combined influence of multiple genes synergizing in complex ways with one another and environmental influences across time. While perhaps disappointing from some points of view, these results are clear in their implications and point to a need for new conceptual and analytic approaches to understanding the role of genes and environment in psychopathy and ASPD, as well as other psychiatric conditions.

## Coda: Subdimensions of Psychopathy/ASPD and Dimensional Models of Psychopathology

The triarchic conception of psychopathy emerged from efforts to integrate differing characterizations of this condition. Because the categorical diagnosis of ASPD was included in the DSM to capture psychopathy as described historically, with DSM-III and subsequent editions focusing on the life-course-persistent criminal variant highlighted by Robins, the symptomatic features of ASPD reflect distinct thematic facets of psychopathy described by the triarchic model (i.e., the disinhibition and meanness facets that relate most to aggressive–antisocial deviance; Venables & Patrick, 2012; Venables et al., 2014; Wall et al., 2015). Furthermore, because psychopathy and ASPD are conceived of as dispositionally based ("characterological") conditions, each can be effectively represented in terms of narrower or broader trait dimensions from general inventories of personality (Benning, Patrick, Blonigen, et al., 2005; Miller, Lynam, Widiger, & Leukefeld, 2001; Poy, Segarra, Estellar, López, & Moltó, 2014; Trull, 1992) or personality pathology (Hopwood, Thomas, Markon, Wright, & Krueger, 2012; Sellbom et al., 2012; Strickland et al., 2013). Furthermore, consistent with the triarchic model formulation, recent evidence (Poy et al., 2014; Strickland et al., 2013) indicates that the coverage of psychopathy and ASPD provided by inventories of personality and personality pathology is traceable to their representation of tendencies embodied in the three constructs of the model (i.e., boldness, meanness, disinhibition).

The view of psychopathy and ASPD as overlapping conditions that intersect with normal and abnormal personality dimensions, and with externalizing proneness and callous–aggressive factors of the externalizing spectrum model (Krueger et al., 2007) and the general factor of the fear–fearlessness domain (Kramer et al., 2012), has important implications for research and clinical assessment. It suggests that clinical conditions traditionally viewed as characterological and those considered more episodic in nature (i.e., externalizing conditions entailing impulsive reward seeking and internalizing conditions marked by extreme fear, distress, and/or dysphoria) can be assessed and studied in an integrative manner—through reference to common dispositional dimensions. The new dimensional-trait system in DSM-5, which shows promise for indexing psychopathy and ASPD (Strickland et al., 2013; Wall et al., 2015), can serve as one useful framework for this. Efforts being made to operationalize this system through clinician interview (Morey, Krueger, & Skodol, 2013) and informant rating approaches (Markon, Quilty, Bagby, & Krueger, 2013) along with self-report (Krueger, Derringer, Markon, Watson, & Skodol, 2012) could provide the basis for a systematic, cross-domain analysis of the system's ability to effectively index dispositional tendencies relevant to many, if not most, forms of psychopathology.

However, as a final point, it should be emphasized that trait-dimensional frameworks such as the new DSM-5 system are best viewed as movable points of reference rather than fixed anchors. For example, the trait taxonomy formulated for DSM-5 has been criticized on grounds that it departs from empirically grounded five-factor model conceptions (e.g., Trull, 2012), and the DSM-5 revision process as a whole has been criticized for failing to consider concepts and findings from modern neuroscience in updating characterizations of mental disorders (Insel et al., 2010). From this latter perspective, the trait system for personality pathology in DSM-5 may be viewed as inadequate because it lacks direct brain referents (e.g., traits that relate clearly to dimensions of neurobiological or neurobehavioral variability).

Our view is that dispositional dimensions can be defined in alternative ways, with reference to indicators from different domains of measurement, for different purposes. For example, dimensions of variability can be identified that reflect covariation between observed clinical problems and reported dispositional tendencies (e.g., Krueger et al., 2002, 2007); these dimensions will be useful in particular for predicting criterion variables in one of these domains from indicators in the other. Alternatively, dimensions of variability can be identified that reflect covariation between measures of brain response and reported dispositional tendencies (Brislin et al., 2017; Patrick et al., 2013; Yancey, Venables, & Patrick, 2016); dimensions of this type can be valuable for predicting neurophysiological and perceived-trait domains. An important goal for future research on individual differences and psychopathology would be to establish a multidomain normative database (e.g., containing interrelated measures of clinical problems, reported traits, physiological response, and behavioral response) for delineating dimensions of covariation across differing domains, and facilitating cross-domain prediction. Constructs specified by the triarchic model, which have clear referents in neurobiology and behavior (i.e., defense system reactivity, frontal inhibitory capacity, attachment system sensitivity), could serve as effective targets for this type of cross-domain mapping effort (Patrick & Drislane, 2015).

## REFERENCES

American Psychiatric Association. (1968). *Diagnostic and statistical manual of mental disorders* (2nd ed.). Washington, DC: Author.

American Psychiatric Association. (1980). *Diagnostic and statistical manual of mental disorders* (3rd ed.). Washington, DC: Author.

American Psychiatric Association. (1987). *Diagnostic and statistical manual of mental disorders* (3rd ed., rev.). Washington, DC: Author.

American Psychiatric Association. (2000). *Diagnostic and statistical manual of mental disorders* (4th ed., text rev.). Washington, DC: Author.

American Psychiatric Association. (2013). *Diagnostic and statistical manual of mental disorders* (5th ed.). Arlington, VA: Author.

Andershed, H., Hodgins, S., & Tengström, A. (2007). Convergent validity of the Youth Psychopathic Traits Inventory (YPI): Association with the Psychopathy Checklist: Youth Version (PCL:YV). *Assessment, 14,* 144–154.

Andershed, H., Kerr, M., Stattin, H., & Levander, S. (2002). Psychopathic traits in non-referred youths: Initial test of a new assessment tool. In E. Blaauw, J. M. Philippa, K. C. M. P. Ferenschild, & B. van Lodensteijn (Eds.), *Psychopaths: Current international perspectives* (pp. 131–158). The Hague, The Netherlands: Elsevier.

Anderson, J. L., Sellbom, M., Wygant, D. B., Salekin, R. T., & Krueger, R. F. (2014). Examining the associations between DSM-5 Section III antisocial personality disorder traits and psychopathy in community and university samples. *Journal of Personality Disorders, 28,* 675–697.

Baskin-Sommers, A. R., Curtin, J. J., & Newman, J. P. (2011). Specifying the attentional selection that moderates the fearlessness of psychopathic offenders. *Psychological Science, 22,* 226–234.

Baskin-Sommers, A. R., Zeier, J. D., & Newman, J. P. (2009). Self-reported attentional control differentiates the major factors of psychopathy. *Personality and Individual Differences, 47,* 626–630.

Bauer, L. O., & Hesselbrock, V. M. (1999). P300 decrements in teenagers with conduct problems: Implications for substance abuse risk and brain development. *Biological Psychiatry, 46,* 263–272.

Bauer, L. O., O'Connor, S., & Hesselbrock, V. M. (1994). Frontal P300 decrements in antisocial personality disorder. *Alcoholism: Clinical and Experimental Research, 18,* 1300–1305.

Benning, S. D., Patrick, C. J., Blonigen, D. M., Hicks, B. M., & Iacono, W. G. (2005). Estimating facets of psychopathy from normal personality traits: A step toward community-epidemiological investigations. *Assessment, 12,* 3–18.

Benning, S. D., Patrick, C. J., Hicks, B. M., Blonigen, D. M., & Krueger, R. F. (2003). Factor structure of the psychopathic personality inventory: Validity and implications for clinical assessment. *Psychological Assessment, 15,* 340–350.

Benning, S. D., Patrick, C. J., & Iacono, W. G. (2005). Psychopathy, startle blink modulation, and electrodermal reactivity in twin men. *Psychophysiology, 42,* 753–762.

Benning, S. D., Patrick, C. J., Salekin, R. T., & Leistico, A. R. (2005). Convergent and discriminant validity of psychopathy factors assessed via self-report: A comparison of three instruments. *Assessment, 12,* 270–289.

Birbaumer, N., Veit, R., Lotze, M., Erb, M., Hermann, C., Grodd, W., et al. (2005). Deficient fear conditioning in psychopathy: A functional magnetic resonance imaging study. *Archives of General Psychiatry, 62,* 799–805.

Blair, R. J. R. (1995). A cognitive developmental approach to morality: Investigating the psychopath. *Cognition, 57,* 1–29.

Blair, R. J. R. (2001). Neurocognitive models of aggression, the antisocial personality disorders, and psychopathy. *Journal of Neurology, Neurosurgery and Psychiatry, 71,* 727–731.

Blair, R. J. R. (2013). The neurobiology of psychopathic traits in youths. *Nature Reviews Neuroscience, 14,* 786–799.

Blonigen, D. M., Carlson, S. R., Krueger, R. F., & Patrick, C. J. (2003). A twin study of self-reported psychopathic personality traits. *Personality and Individual Differences, 35,* 179–197.

Blonigen, D. M., Hicks, B. M., Krueger, R. F., Patrick, C. J., & Iacono, W. G. (2005). Psychopathic personality traits: Heritability and genetic overlap with internalizing and externalizing psychopathology. *Psychological Medicine, 35,* 637–648.

Brislin, S. J., Drislane, L. E., Smith, S. T., Edens, J. F., & Patrick, C. J. (2015). Development and validation of triarchic psychopathy scales from the Multidimensional Personality Questionnaire. *Psychological Assessment, 27,* 838–851.

Brislin, S. J., Yancey, J. R., Perkins, E. R., Palumbo, I. M., Drislane, L. E., Salekin, R. T., et al. (2017). Callous-aggression and affective face processing in adults: Behavioral and brain-potential indicators. *Personality Disorders: Theory, Research, and Treatment.* [Epub ahead of print]

Burt, S. A. (2009). Are there meaningful etiological differences within antisocial behavior?: Results of a meta-analysis. *Clinical Psychology Review, 29,* 163–178.

Carlson, S. R., Thái, S., & McLaron, M. E. (2009). Visual P3 amplitude and self-reported psychopathic personality traits: Frontal reduction is associated with self-centered impulsivity. *Psychophysiology, 46,* 100–113.

Cleckley, H. (1976). *The mask of sanity* (5th ed.). St. Louis, MO: Mosby. (Original work published 1941)

Cooke, D. J., & Michie, C. (2001). Refining the construct of psychopathy: Towards a hierarchical model. *Psychological Assessment, 13,* 171–188.

Decety, J., & Jackson, P. L. (2004). The functional architecture of human empathy. *Behavioral and Cognitive Neuroscience Reviews, 3,* 71–100.

Dikman, Z. V., & Allen, J. J. (2000). Error monitoring during reward and avoidance learning in high- and low-socialized individuals. *Psychophysiology, 37,* 43–54.

Dindo, L., & Fowles, D. C. (2011). Dual temperamental risk factors for psychopathic personality: Evidence from self-report and skin conductance. *Journal of Personality and Social Psychology, 100,* 557–566.

Drislane, L. E., Brislin, S. J., Kendler, K. S., Andershed, H., Larsson, H., & Patrick, C. J. (2015). Development and validation of triarchic construct scales from the Youth Psychopathic Traits Inventory. *Journal of Personality Disorders, 27,* 838–851.

Drislane, L. E., Patrick, C. J., & Arsal, G. (2014). Clarifying the content coverage of differing psychopathy inventories through reference to the Triarchic Psychopathy Measure. *Psychological Assessment, 26,* 350–362.

Drislane, L. E., Vaidyanathan, U., & Patrick, C. J. (2013). Reduced cortical call to arms differentiates psychopathy from antisocial personality disorder. *Psychological Medicine, 43,* 825–835.

Dvorak-Bertsch, J. D., Curtin, J. J., Rubinstein, T. J., & Newman, J. P. (2009). Psychopathic traits moderate the interaction between cognitive and affective processing. *Psychophysiology, 46,* 913–921.

Edens, J. F., Marcus, D. K., Lilienfeld, S. O., & Poythress, N. G. (2006). Psychopathic, not psychopath: Taxometric evidence for the dimensional structure of psychopathy. *Journal of Abnormal Psychology, 115*(1), 131–144.

Flor, H., Birbaumer, N., Hermann, C., Ziegler, S., & Patrick, C. J. (2002). Aversive Pavlovian conditioning in psychopaths: Peripheral and central correlates. *Psychophysiology, 39,* 505–518.

Forth, A. E., Kosson, D. S., & Hare, R. D. (2003). *The Psychopathy Checklist: Youth Version manual.* Toronto, ON, Canada: Multi-Health Systems.

Fowles, D. C., & Dindo, L. (2009). Temperament and psychopathy A dual-pathway model. *Current Directions in Psychological Science, 18,* 179–183.

Fowles, D. C., & Kochanska, G. (2000). Electrodermal activity and temperament in preschool children. *Psychophysiology, 37,* 777–787.

Frick, P. J., & Hare, R. D. (2001). *The Antisocial Process Screening Device.* Toronto, ON, Canada: Multi-Health Systems.

Frick, P. J., Lahey, B. B., Loeber, R., Stouthamer-Loeber, M., Green, S., Hart, E. L., et al. (1991). Oppositional defiant disorder and conduct disorder in boys: Patterns of behavioral covariation. *Journal of Clinical Child Psychology, 20,* 202–208.

Frick, P. J., & Marsee, M. A. (2006). Psychopathy and developmental pathways to antisocial behavior in youth. In C. J. Patrick (Ed.), *Handbook of psychopathy* (pp. 353–374). New York: Guilford Press.

Frick, P. J., & Morris, A. S. (2004). Temperament and developmental pathways to conduct problems. *Journal of Clinical Child and Adolescent Psychology, 33,* 54–68.

Frick, P. J., & White, S. F. (2008). The importance of callous–unemotional traits for developmental models of aggressive and antisocial behavior. *Journal of Child Psychology and Psychiatry, 49,* 359–375.

Gizer, I. R., Ehlers, C. L., Vieten, C., Feiler, H. S., Gilder, D. A., & Wilhelmsen, K. C. (2012). Genome-wide linkage scan of antisocial behavior, depression, and impulsive substance use in the UCSF family alcoholism study. *Psychiatric Genetics, 22,* 235–244.

Gordon, H. L., Baird, A. A., & End, A. (2004). Functional differences among those high and low on a trait measure of psychopathy. *Biological Psychiatry, 56,* 516–521.

Hall, J. R., Benning, S. D., & Patrick, C. J. (2004). Criterion-related validity of the three-factor model of psychopathy personality, behavior, and adaptive functioning. *Assessment, 11,* 4–16.

Hall, J. R., Bernat, E. M., & Patrick, C. J. (2007). Externalizing psychopathology and the error-related negativity. *Psychological Science, 18,* 326–333.

Hall, J. R., Drislane, L. E., Murano, M., Patrick, C. J., Lilienfeld, S. O., & Poythress, N. G. (2014). Development and validation of triarchic construct scales from the Psychopathic Personality Inventory. *Psychological Assessment, 26,* 447–461.

Hare, R. D. (1978). Electrodermal and cardiovascular correlates of psychopathy. In R. D. Hare & D. Schalling (Eds.), *Psychopathic behavior: Approaches to research* (pp. 107–143). Chichester, UK: Wiley.

Hare, R. D. (1980). A research scale for the assessment of psychopathy in criminal populations. *Personality and Individual Differences, 1,* 111–119.

Hare, R. D. (1991). *The Hare Psychopathy Checklist—Revised.* Toronto, ON, Canada: Multi-Health Systems.

Hare, R. D. (2003). *The Hare Psychopathy Checklist—Revised* (2nd ed.). Toronto, ON, Canada: Multi-Health Systems.

Hare, R. D., Harpur, T. J., Hakstian, A. R., Forth, A. E., Hart, S. D., & Newman, J. P. (1990). The Revised Psychopathy Checklist: Reliability and factor structure. *Psychological Assessment, 2*(3), 338–341.

Hare, R. D., Hart, S. D., & Harpur, T. J. (1991). Psychopathy and the DSM-IV criteria for antisocial personality disorder. *Journal of Abnormal Psychology, 100,* 391–398.

Hare, R. D., & Neumann, C. S. (2008). Psychopathy as a clinical and empirical construct. *Annual Review of Clinical Psychology, 4,* 217–246.

Harpur, T. J., Hakstian, A. R., & Hare, R. D. (1988). Factor structure of the Psychopathy Checklist. *Journal of Consulting and Clinical Psychology, 56,* 741–747.

Harris, G. T., Rice, M. E., & Quinsey, V. L. (1994). Psychopathy as a taxon: Evidence that psychopaths are a discrete class. *Journal of Consulting and Clinical Psychology, 62,* 387–397.

Hicks, B. M., Markon, K. E., Patrick, C. J., Krueger, R. F., & Newman, J. P. (2004). Identifying psychopathy subtypes on the basis of personality structure. *Psychological Assessment, 16,* 276–288.

Hicks, B. M., & Patrick, C. J. (2006). Psychopathy and negative emotionality: Analyses of suppressor effects reveal distinct relations with emotional distress, fearfulness, and anger-hostility. *Journal of Abnormal Psychology, 115,* 276–287.

Hopwood, C. J., Thomas, K. M., Markon, K. E., Wright, A. G. C., & Krueger, R. F. (2012). DSM-5 personality traits and DSM-IV personality disorders. *Journal of Abnormal Psychology, 121,* 424–432.

Iacono, W. G., Carlson, S. R., Malone, S. M., & McGue, M. (2002). P3 event-related potential amplitude and risk for disinhibitory disorders in adolescent boys. *Archives of General Psychiatry, 59,* 750–757.

Insel, T., Cuthbert, B., Garvey, M., Heinssen, R., Pine, D. S., Quinn, K., et al. (2010). Research domain criteria (RDoC): Toward a new classification framework for research on mental disorders. *American Journal of Psychiatry, 167,* 748–751.

Jones, A. P., Happé, F. G., Gilbert, F., Burnett, S., & Viding, E. (2010). Feeling, caring, knowing: Different types of empathy deficit in boys with psychopathic tendencies and autism spectrum disorder. *Journal of Child Psychology and Psychiatry, 51,* 1188–1197.

Jutai, J. W., & Hare, R. D. (1983). Psychopathy and selective attention during performance of a complex perceptual-motor task. *Psychophysiology, 20,* 146–151.

Kendler, K. S. (2013). What psychiatric genetics has taught us about the nature of psychiatric illness and what is left to learn. *Molecular Psychiatry, 18,* 1058–1066.

Kendler, K. S., Aggen, S. H., & Patrick, C. J. (2012). A multivariate twin study of the DSM-IV criteria for antisocial personality disorder. *Biological Psychiatry, 71,* 247–253.

Kendler, K. S., Aggen, S. H., & Patrick, C. J. (2013). Familial influences on conduct disorder criteria in males reflect two genetic factors and one shared environmental factor: A population-based twin study. *JAMA Psychiatry, 70,* 78–86.

Kennealy, P. J., Hicks, B. M., & Patrick, C. J. (2007). Validity of factors of the Psychopathy Checklist—Revised in female prisoners: Discriminant relations with antisocial behavior, substance abuse, and personality. *Assessment, 14,* 323–340.

Kiehl, K. A., Smith, A. M., Hare, R. D., Mendrek, A., Forster, B. B., Brink, J., et al. (2001). Limbic abnormalities in affective processing by criminal psychopaths as revealed by functional magnetic resonance imaging. *Biological Psychiatry, 50,* 677–684.

Kochanska, G. (1997). Multiple pathways to conscience for children with different temperaments: From toddlerhood to age 5. *Developmental Psychology, 33,* 228–240.

Kochanska, G., & Aksan, N. (2006). Children's conscience and self-regulation. *Journal of Personality, 74,* 1587–1618.

Kochanska, G., Gross, J. N., Lin, M. H., & Nichols, K. E. (2002). Guilt in young children: Development, determinants, and relations with a broader system of standards. *Child Development, 73,* 461–482.

Kochanska, G., Murray, K. T., & Harlan, E. T. (2000). Effortful control in early childhood: Continuity and change, antecedents, and implications for social development. *Developmental Psychology, 36,* 220–232.

Kosfeld, M., Heinrichs, M., Zak, P. J., Fischbacher, U., & Fehr, E. (2005). Oxytocin increases trust in humans. *Nature, 435,* 673–676.

Kosson, D. S. (1996). Psychopathy and dual-task performance under focusing conditions. *Journal of Abnormal Psychology, 105,* 391–400.

Kosson, D. S. (1998). Divided visual attention in psychopathic and nonpsychopathic offenders. *Personality and Individual Differences, 24,* 373–391.

Kramer, M. D., Patrick, C. J., Krueger, R. F., & Gasperi, M. (2012). Delineating physiologic defensive reactivity in the domain of self-report: Phenotypic and etiologic structure of dispositional fear. *Psychological Medicine, 42,* 1305–1320.

Krueger, R. F., Derringer, J., Markon, K. E., Watson, D., & Skodol, A. E. (2012). Initial construction of a maladaptive personality trait model and inventory for DSM-5. *Psychological Medicine, 42,* 1879–1890.

Krueger, R. F., Hicks, B., Patrick, C. J., Carlson, S., Iacono, W. G., & McGue, M. (2002). Etiologic connections among substance dependence, antisocial behavior, and personality: Modeling the externalizing spectrum. *Journal of Abnormal Psychology, 111,* 411–424.

Krueger, R. F., Markon, K. E., Patrick, C. J., Benning, S. D., & Kramer, M. (2007). Linking antisocial behavior, substance use, and personality: An integrative quantitative model of the adult externalizing spectrum. *Journal of Abnormal Psychology, 116,* 645–666.

Lang, P. J., Bradley, M. M., & Cuthbert, B. N. (1997). Motivated attention: Affect, activation, and action. In P. J. Lang, R. F. Simons, & M. T. Balaban (Eds.), *Attention and orienting: Sensory and motivational processes* (pp. 97–135). Hillsdale, NJ: Erlbaum.

Larson, C. L., Baskin-Sommers, A. R., Stout, D. M., Balderston, N. L., Curtin, J. J., Schultz, D. H., et al. (2013). The interplay of attention and emotion: Top-down attention modulates amygdala activation in psychopathy. *Cognitive, Affective, and Behavioral Neuroscience, 13,* 757–770.

Larsson, H., Viding, E., & Plomin, R. (2008). Callous–unemotional traits and antisocial behavior: Genetic, environmental, and early parenting characteristics. *Criminal Justice and Behavior, 35,* 197–211.

Levenson, M. R., Kiehl, K. A., & Fitzpatrick, C. M. (1995). Assessing psychopathic attributes in a non-institutionalized population. *Journal of Personality and Social Psychology, 68,* 151–158.

Lilienfeld, S. O., & Andrews, B. P. (1996). Development and preliminary validation of a self-report measure of psychopathic personality traits in noncriminal populations. *Journal of Personality Assessment, 66,* 488–524.

Lilienfeld, S. O., & Widows, M. R. (2005). *Psychopathic Personality Inventory—Revised (PPI-R) professional manual.* Odessa, FL: Psychological Assessment Resources.

Lindner, R. M. (1944). *Rebel without a cause: The story of a criminal psychopath.* New York: Grune & Stratton.

López, R., Poy, R., Patrick, C. J., & Moltó, J. (2013). Deficient fear conditioning and self-reported psychopathy: The role of fearless dominance. *Psychophysiology, 50,* 210–218.

Lykken, D. T. (1957). A study of anxiety in the sociopathic personality. *Journal of Abnormal and Social Psychology, 55,* 6–10.

Lynam, D. R. (1997). Pursuing the psychopath: Capturing the fledgling psychopath in a nomological net. *Journal of Abnormal Psychology, 106,* 425–438.

Lynam, D. R., Gaughan, E. T., Miller, J. D., Miller, D. J., Mullins-Sweatt, S., & Widiger, T. A. (2011). Assessing the basic traits associated with psychopathy: Development and validation of the Elemental Psychopathy Assessment. *Psychological Assessment, 23,* 108–124.

Marcus, D. K., John, S. L., & Edens, J. F. (2004). A taxometric analysis of psychopathic personality. *Journal of Abnormal Psychology, 113,* 626–635.

Markon, K. E., Quilty, L. C., Bagby, R. M., & Krueger, R. F. (2013). The development and psychometric properties of an informant-report form of the PID-5. *Assessment, 20,* 370–383.

Marsh, A. A., & Blair, R. J. R. (2008). Deficits in facial affect recognition among antisocial populations: A meta-analysis. *Neuroscience and Biobehavioral Reviews, 32,* 454–465.

Marsh, A., Finger, E., Mitchell, D., Reid, M., Sims, C., Kosson, D. S., et al. (2008). Reduced amygdala response to fearful expressions in children and adolescents with callous–unemotional traits and disruptive behavior disorders. *American Journal of Psychiatry, 165,* 712–720.

McCord, W., & McCord, J. (1964). *The psychopath: An essay on the criminal mind.* Princeton, NJ: Van Nostrand.

Miller, J. D., Lynam, D. R., Widiger, T. A., & Leukefeld, C. (2001). Personality disorders as extreme variants of common personality dimensions: Can the five-factor model adequately represent psychopathy? *Journal of Personality, 69,* 253–276.

Moltó, J., Poy, R., Segarra, P., Pastor, M., & Montanes, S. (2007). Response perseveration in psychopaths: Interpersonal/affective or social deviance traits? *Journal of Abnormal Psychology, 3,* 632–637.

Morey, L. C., Krueger, R. F., & Skodol, A. E. (2013). The hierarchical structure of clinician ratings of proposed DSM-5 pathological personality traits. *Journal of Abnormal Psychology, 122,* 836–841.

Morgan, A. B., & Lilienfeld, S. O. (2000). A meta-analytic review of the relation between antisocial behavior and neuropsychological measures of executive function. *Clinical Psychology Review, 20,* 113–136.

Murrie, D. C., Marcus, D. K., Douglas, K. S., Lee, Z., Salekin, R. T., & Vincent, G. (2007). Youth with psychopathy features are not a discrete class: A taxometric analysis. *Journal of Child Psychology and Psychiatry, 48,* 714–723.

Newman, J. P. (1998). Psychopathic behavior: An information processing perspective. In D. J. Cooke, A. E. Forth, & R. D. Hare (Eds.), *Psychopathy: Theory, research and implications for society* (pp. 81–104). Dordrecht, The Netherlands: Springer.

Newman, J. P., & Kosson, D. S. (1986). Passive avoidance learning in psychopathic and nonpsychopathic offenders. *Journal of Abnormal Psychology, 95,* 252–256.

Patrick, C. J. (1994). Emotion and psychopathy: Startling new insights. *Psychophysiology, 31,* 319–330.

Patrick, C. J. (2010). *Operationalizing the triarchic conceptualization of psychopathy: Preliminary description of brief scales for assessment of boldness, meanness, and disinhibition.* Unpublished test manual, Florida State University, Tallahassee, FL.

Patrick, C. J., & Bernat, E. (2009). Neurobiology of psychopathy: A two-process theory. In G. G. Berntson & J. T. Cacioppo (Eds.), *Handbook of neuroscience for the behavioral sciences* (pp. 1110–1131). New York: Wiley.

Patrick, C. J., Bernat, E., Malone, S. M., Iacono, W. G., Krueger, R. F., & McGue, M. K. (2006). P300 amplitude as an indicator of externalizing in adolescent males. *Psychophysiology, 43,* 84–92.

Patrick, C. J., & Drislane, L. E. (2015). Triarchic model of psychopathy: Origins, operationalizations, and observed linkages with personality and general psychopathology. *Journal of Personality, 23*(6), 627–643.

Patrick, C. J., Durbin, C. E., & Moser, J. S. (2012). Reconceptualizing antisocial deviance in neurobehavioral terms. *Development and Psychopathology, 24,* 1047–1071.

Patrick, C. J., Fowles, D. C., & Krueger, R. F. (2009). Triarchic conceptualization of psychopathy: Developmental origins of disinhibition, boldness, and meanness. *Development and Psychopathology, 21,* 913–938.

Patrick, C. J., Hicks, B. M., Krueger, R. F., & Lang, A. R. (2005). Relations between psychopathy facets and externalizing in a criminal offender sample. *Journal of Personality Disorders, 19,* 339–356.

Patrick, C. J., Kramer, M. D., Krueger, R. F., & Markon, K. E. (2013). Optimizing efficiency of psychopathology assessment through quantitative modeling: Development of a brief form of the Externalizing Spectrum Inventory. *Psychological Assessment, 25,* 1332–1348.

Patrick, C. J., Venables, N., & Skeem, J. (2012). Psychopathy and brain function: Empirical findings and legal implications. In H. Häkkänen-Nyholm & J. Nyholm (Eds.), *Psychopathy and law: A practitioner's guide* (pp. 39–77). New York: Wiley.

Patrick, C. J., Venables, N. C., Yancey, J. R., Hicks, B. M., Nelson, L. D., & Kramer, M. D. (2013). A construct-network approach to bridging diagnostic and physiological domains: Application to assessment of externalizing psychopathology. *Journal of Abnormal Psychology, 122,* 902–916.

Patterson, C. M., & Newman, J. P. (1993). Reflectivity and learning from aversive events: Toward a psychological mechanism for the syndromes of disinhibition. *Psychological Review, 100,* 716–736.

Paulhus, D. L., Neumann, C. S., & Hare, R. D. (2016). *Self-Report Psychopathy Scale* (4th ed.). Toronto, ON, Canada: Multi-Health Systems.

Poy, R., Segarra, P., Esteller, À., López, R., & Moltó, J. (2014). FFM description of the triarchic conceptualization of psychopathy in men and women. *Psychological Assessment, 26,* 69–76.

Poythress, N. G., Edens, J. F., Skeem, J. L., Lilienfeld, S. O., Douglas, K. S., Frick, P. J., et al. (2010). Identifying subtypes among offenders with antisocial personality disorder: A cluster-analytic study. *Journal of Abnormal Psychology, 119,* 389–400.

Raine, A. (2008). From genes to brain to antisocial behavior. *Current Directions in Psychological Science, 17,* 323–328.

Robins, L. N. (1966). *Deviant children grown up.* Baltimore: Williams & Wilkins.

Robins, L. N. (1978). Sturdy predictors of adult antisocial behaviour: Replications from longitudinal studies. *Psychological Medicine, 8,* 611–622.

Ross, S. R., Benning, S. D., Patrick, C. J., Thompson, A., & Thurston, A. (2009). Factors of the Psychopathic Personality Inventory: Criterion-related validity and relationship to the BIS/BAS and five-factor models of personality. *Assessment, 16,* 71–87.

Rothbart, M. K. (2007). Temperament, development, and personality. *Current Directions in Psychological Science, 16,* 207–212.

Sellbom, M., Ben-Porath, Y., Patrick, C. J., Wygant, D. B., Gartland, D. M., & Stafford, K. P. (2012). Development and construct validation of MMPI-2-RF indices of global psychopathy, fearless-dominance, and impulsive-antisociality. *Personality Disorders: Theory, Research, and Treatment, 3,* 17–38.

Sellbom, M., Drislane, L. E., Johnson, A. K., Goodwin, B. E., Phillips, T. R., & Patrick, C. J. (2016). Development and validation of MMPI-2-RF scales to measure the Triarchic model of psychopathy. *Assessment, 23,* 527–543.

Sellbom, M., & Phillips, T. R. (2013). An examination of the triarchic conceptualization of psychopathy in incarcerated and nonincarcerated samples. *Journal of Abnormal Psychology, 122,* 208–214.

Skeem, J. L., Johansson, P., Andershed, H., Kerr, M., & Louden, J. E. (2007). Two subtypes of psychopathic violent offenders that parallel primary and secondary variants. *Journal of Abnormal Psychology, 116,* 395–409.

Strickland, C. M., Drislane, L. E., Lucy, M., Krueger, R. F., & Patrick, C. J. (2013). Characterizing psychopathy using DSM-5 personality traits. *Assessment, 20,* 327–338.

Tackett, J. L., Krueger, R. F., Iacono, W. G., & McGue, M. (2005). Symptom-based subfactors of DSM-defined conduct disorder: Evidence for etiologic distinctions. *Journal of Abnormal Psychology, 114,* 483–487.

Tackett, J. L., Krueger, R. F., Sawyer, M. G., & Graetz, B. W. (2003). Subfactors of DSM-IV conduct disorder: Evidence and connections with syndromes from the Child Behavior Checklist. *Journal of Abnormal Child Psychology, 31,* 647–654.

Thomas, A., & Chess, S. (1977). *Temperament and development.* New York: Brunner/Mazel.

Tielbeek, J. J., Medland, S. E., Benyamin, B., Byrne, E. M., Heath, A. C., Madden, P. A., et al. (2012). Unraveling the genetic etiology of adult antisocial behavior: A genome-wide association study. *PLOS ONE, 7,* e45086.

Trull, T. J. (1992). *DSM-III-R* personality disorders and the five-factor model of personality: An empirical comparison. *Journal of Abnormal Psychology, 101,* 553–560.

Trull, T. J. (2012). The five-factor model of personality and DSM-5. *Journal of Personality, 80,* 1697–1720.

Vaidyanathan, U., Hall, J. R., Patrick, C. J., & Bernat, E. M. (2011). Clarifying the role of defensive reactivity deficits in psychopathy and antisocial personality using startle reflex methodology. *Journal of Abnormal Psychology, 120,* 253–258.

Vaidyanathan, U., Patrick, C. J., & Bernat, E. M. (2009). Startle reflex potentiation during aversive picture viewing as an indicator of trait fear. *Psychophysiology, 46,* 75–85.

Vanman, E. J., Mejia, V. Y., Dawson, M. E., Schell, A. M., & Raine, A. (2003). Modification of the startle reflex in a community sample: Do one or two dimensions of psychopathy underlie emotional processing? *Personality and Individual Differences, 35,* 2007–2021.

Venables, N. C., Hall, J. R., & Patrick, C. J. (2014). Differentiating psychopathy from antisocial personality disorder: A triarchic model perspective. *Psychological Medicine, 44,* 1005–1013.

Venables, N. C., & Patrick, C. J. (2012). Validity of the Externalizing Spectrum Inventory in a criminal offender sample: Relations with disinhibitory psychopathology, personality, and psychopathic features. *Psychological Assessment, 24,* 88–100.

Venables, N. C., & Patrick, C. J. (2014). Reconciling discrepant findings for P3 brain response in criminal psychopathy through reference to the concept of externalizing proneness. *Psychophysiology, 51,* 427–436.

Verona, E., Patrick, C. J., & Joiner, T. E. (2001). Psychopathy, antisocial personality, and suicide risk. *Journal of Abnormal Psychology, 110,* 462–470.

Viding, E., Blair, R. J. R., Moffitt, T. E., & Plomin, R. (2005). Evidence for substantial genetic risk for psychopathy in 7-year-olds. *Journal of Child Psychology and Psychiatry, 46,* 592–597.

Viding, E., Jones, A. P., Frick, P., Moffitt, T. E., & Plomin, R. (2008). Genetic and phenotypic investigation to early risk factors for conduct problems in children with and without psychopathic tendencies. *Developmental Science, 11,* 17–22.

Viding, E., Price, T. S., Jaffee, S. R., Trzaskowski, M., Davis, O. S., Meaburn, E. L., et al. (2013). Genetics of callous–unemotional behavior in children. *PlOS ONE, 8,* e65789.

Waldman, I. D., & Rhee, S. H. (2006). Genetic and environmental influences on psychopathy and antisocial behavior. In C. J. Patrick (Ed.), *Handbook of psychopathy* (pp. 205–228). New York: Guilford Press.

Wall, T. D., Wygant, D. B., & Sellbom, M. (2015). Boldness explains a key difference between psychopathy and antisocial personality disorder. *Psychiatry, Psychology, and Law, 22,* 94–105.

Yancey, J. R., Venables, N. C., Hicks, B. M., & Patrick, C. J. (2013). Evidence for a heritable brain basis to deviance-promoting deficits in self-control. *Journal of Criminal Justice, 41,* 309–317.

Yancey, J. R., Venables, N. C., & Patrick, C. J. (2016). Psychoneurometric operationalization of threat sensitivity: Relations with clinical symptom and physiological response criteria. *Psychophysiology, 53,* 393–405.

Young, L. J., & Wang, Z. (2004). The neurobiology of pair bonding. *Nature Neuroscience, 7,* 1048–1054.

Young, S. E., Friedman, N. P., Miyake, A., Willcutt, E. G., Corley, R. P., Haberstick, B. C., et al. (2009). Behavioral disinhibition: Liability for externalizing spectrum disorders and its genetic and environmental relation to response inhibition across adolescence. *Journal of Abnormal Psychology, 118,* 117–130.

# CHAPTER 25

# Clinical Aspects of Antisocial Personality Disorder and Psychopathy

Lacy A. Olson-Ayala and Christopher J. Patrick

Antisocial personality disorder (ASPD) and psychopathy (psychopathic personality) have long held the public's fascination due to the aura of dangerousness that surrounds them and the severe societal costs they impose. Sensationalized fictional examples of these conditions appear regularly in books, films, and television programs such as *American Psycho, Dexter,* and *The Silence of the Lambs,* and news sources provide coverage of ostensible, real-life prototypes such as Charles Manson, O. J. Simpson, Bernie Madoff, and Jodi Arias on a seemingly constant basis. Balancing these media portrayals is a substantial body of empirical research that demystifies these conditions through clarification of their defining features, dispositional bases, and links to problems of a more familiar nature.

Our goal in this chapter is to review what is known about ASPD and psychopathy in clinical–empirical terms. The chapter includes coverage of historical and contemporary descriptive accounts of these conditions, commonly used assessment instruments, epidemiology and course, comorbidity patterns, and approaches to treatment. The chapter also provides perspective on conceptions of ASPD and psychopathy appearing in the various editions of DSM including DSM-5 (American Psychiatric Association [APA], 2013). We begin with a historical account of observation-based clinical descriptions of psychopathy and putatively related conditions, then discuss how ASPD and psychopathy are represented in the various DSM editions. We then consider alternative trait-dimensional approaches to APSD in relation to an integrative framework for conceptualizing psychopathy and antisocial behavior, the triarchic model (Patrick, Fowles, & Krueger, 2009). We provide descriptions of the most widely used interview- and self-report-based measures for assessing ASPD and psychopathy, and issues of clinical importance, including epidemiology, course, and comorbidity, are discussed. We conclude with an overview of existing methods of treatment directed at reducing the dangerousness and recidivism risk of antisocial and psychopathic individuals, and the harm these individuals cause to society.

## Historical Background

Clinical conceptions of psychopathy and antisocial personality have evolved over time through contributions of writers from different eras. Philippe Pinel (1806/1962) was the first to formally document a clinical condition entailing impulsive and reckless/erratic behavior in otherwise rational-appearing individuals. The label Pinel used for this condition was *manie sans delire* ("insanity without delirium"). J.

C. Pritchard (1835) applied the term "moral insanity" to a broader array of chronic conditions, including addictions, sexual deviations, depressive disorders, psychoses, and mental retardation. In a similar vein, Benjamin Rush (1812) ascribed problems involving impulsive acting-out behavior to "moral weakness." Some years later, the term "psychopathy" was introduced by the German psychiatrist Koch (1888) to denote conditions he considered inborn, or "organic"—including so-called character disorders, neurotic conditions of various types, and mental retardation. Kraepelin (1915) used a similar term, "psychopathic personalities," for a somewhat narrower range of conditions, including self-defeating impulsivity, sexual deviancy, and obsessional disorders, along with "degenerative" conditions consisting of antisocial (callous–destructive) and quarrelsome (hostile–alienated) variants of personality pathology.

Modern conceptions of ASPD and psychopathy trace back to the work of American psychiatrist Hervey Cleckley. His pioneering book, *The Mask of Sanity* (1941/1976), included detailed case examples that he used to distill 16 diagnostic criteria for psychopathy. These included indicators of (1) ostensible psychological health (social charm and average or better intelligence, absence of psychotic symptoms, lack of nervousness or anxious–depressive symptoms, and low suicidality); (2) emotional insensitivity and shallow interpersonal relations (shallow affectivity, self-centeredness, lack of social reciprocity, incapacity for love, deceitfulness, absence of insight); and (3) behavioral deviance (impulsive antisocial acts, irresponsibility, promiscuity, and lack of direction in life). Thus, Cleckley's conception of psychopathy as a "mask of sanity" refers to the outward appearance of psychological stability that masks affective–interpersonal abnormalities and deviant behavioral tendencies.

Another dominant theme that emerged at about the same time, from the writings of criminologically oriented scholars (e.g., Lindner, 1942; McCord & McCord, 1964; Robins, 1966, 1978), was of psychopathy as a particularly virulent form of criminal deviancy—marked by remorselessness, callous–predatory behavior, and persistent violence. This conception served as a point of reference for the diagnosis of ASPD in the third and fourth editions of the DSM, carried forth to the main diagnostic code section (II) of DSM-5, and also for Hare's (2003) conception of adult criminal psychopathy, which in turn influenced youth-oriented conceptions.

## Clinical Features and Diagnosis

Scholars have long debated the definition of "psychopathy," and it is important to note that definitions and theories have continued to evolve as empirical findings have accumulated. The impact of both Cleckley and Robins on the various DSM editions was discussed by Patrick and Brislin (Chapter 24, this volume); they noted how attempts to increase diagnostic reliability in DSM-III led to the use of behaviorally based criteria for disorders and hence heavy reliance on work by Robins (1966, 1978). Although this substantially increased reliability, concerns were raised about the validity of the diagnosis (e.g., Frances, 1980; Hare, 1983) due to the omission of features that Cleckley considered central to psychopathy—including superficial charm, lack of anxiety, absence of remorse or empathy, and general poverty of affect. Although this prompted the addition of "lack of remorse" as a criterion for ASPD in DSM-III-R, it did little to alleviate criticisms. Nevertheless, diagnostic criteria for ASPD changed little from DSM-III-R to DSM-IV, and the DSM-IV criteria were adopted in the main diagnostic section of DSM-5 (Section II; APA, 2013, p. 659).

The fact that the criteria for the categorical diagnosis of ASPD in the current and preceding two DSM editions are "polythetic," which means that only a small subset of the criteria need to be met for the diagnosis to be applied (i.e., two of 15 childhood symptoms [as evidence of conduct disorder; First, Gibbon, Spitzer, Williams, & Benjamin, 1997] and three of seven adult symptoms [APA, 2013]) has important implications. This approach results in considerable heterogeneity among individuals assigned the diagnosis. For example, some individuals may exhibit rule-breaking tendencies in childhood such as truancy and curfew violation followed by pervasively impulsive, irresponsible, and reckless behavior in adulthood, whereas others may exhibit salient aggression in the form of bullying and physical cruelty early in life, transitioning to persistent predatory offending and remorseless acts of violence in adulthood. This heterogeneity has important implications for understanding the etiology of ASPD and establishing effective treatments (i.e., contrasting symptomatic expressions may arise from differing causes and require separate approaches to treatment), and for understanding the relationship between ASPD and psychopathy (i.e., particular symptomatic configurations may be more or less likely to intersect with psychopathy).

Dimensional models provide a framework for addressing this issue of symptomatic heterogeneity, along with other well-recognized problems with categorical diagnoses of personality disorders (PDs) such as arbitrary symptom thresholds for diagnoses and high comorbidity across categories (Clark, 2007; Trull & Durrett, 2005; Widiger & Clark, 2000). As we discuss next, DSM-5 includes a new dimensional-trait system for PDs, within Section III, titled "Emerging Measures and Models."

## Dimensional Frameworks: The DSM-5 Trait System and the Triarchic Model

Recent research on PDs has emphasized trait-based systems, and it seems likely, with continued research efforts, that models of this type will eventually supersede criterion-based systems. Unlike prior editions, DSM-5 contains an alternative trait-dimensional system for characterizing personality pathology in terms of (1) impairments in self and interpersonal functioning, and (2) profiles of specific traits within broader thematic domains.

Within the DSM-5 trait-dimensional system, the impairments in functioning regarded as characteristic of APSD include identity disturbance marked by extreme self-centeredness; problems in self-directedness based on seeking immediate gratification, lack of prosocial behavior, and disregard for social conventions and legal prohibitions; deficits in guilt and empathic concern; and shallow relations with others, marked by use of deception and force. Personality traits considered typical of APSD are ones reflecting impulsive–disinhibitory and callous–antagonistic tendencies. Additionally, a diagnostic specifier is included for indicating the presence of psychopathic features—that is, tendencies toward social assertiveness and low anxiousness that operate to "mask" (see Cleckley, 1941/1976) the impulsive–disinhibitory and callous–manipulative tendencies associated with ASPD. Along somewhat related lines, a "low prosocial emotions" specifier was added to the Section II diagnosis of conduct disorder in DSM-5, for purposes of designating a psychopathic variant of this childhood precursor to ASPD entailing the presence of salient callous–unemotional tendencies (Frick, 1995; Frick & Marsee, 2006).

The new trait-based conception of ASPD in Section III of DSM-5 can be connected in turn to a recently formulated integrative conceptual framework, the triarchic model of psychopathy (Patrick et al., 2009), which was advanced to help reconcile contrasting conceptions of psychopathy and to clarify overlap and distinctiveness among different assessment inventories for psychopathy, and between psychopathy and ASPD (see Patrick & Brislin, Chapter 24, this volume). The model proposes that psychopathy encompasses three distinguishable symptomatic (phenotypic) components or facets—*disinhibition, boldness,* and *meanness*—that can be viewed as building blocks for alternative conceptions of psychopathy and differing observed variants.

Within the triarchic model, the *disinhibition* facet encompasses proclivities toward weak behavioral restraint, irresponsibility, mistrust and hostility, and difficulties in emotion regulation. The facet combines tendencies toward impulsivity and negative emotionality. By contrast, the *meanness* facet entails deficient empathy, lack of affiliative capacity, contempt toward others, predatory exploitativeness, and empowerment through cruelty and destructiveness. Concepts related to meanness include callousness (Frick, O'Brien, Wootton, & McBurnett, 1994), cold-heartedness (Lilienfeld & Widows, 2005), and antagonism (Lynam & Derefinko, 2006). The distinction between disinhibition and meanness facets is consistent with evidence from the psychopathy literature demonstrating contrasting correlates for affective–interpersonal versus impulsive–antisocial symptoms of adult psychopathy (Hare, 2003; Skeem, Polaschek, Patrick, & Lilienfeld, 2011) and impulsive/conduct problem versus callous-unemotional symptoms of child psychopathy (Frick & Marsee, 2006). The third symptomatic facet of the triarchic model, *boldness,* includes tendencies toward persuasiveness, social assurance, emotional resiliency, and venturesomeness emphasized in historic accounts of "primary" psychopathy (Cleckley, 1941/1976; Karpman, 1946; Lykken, 1957). In personality terms, boldness combines tendencies toward social dominance, low stress reactivity, and thrill/adventure seeking (Benning, Patrick, Blonigen, Hicks, & Iacono, 2005; Benning, Patrick, Hicks, Blonigen, & Krueger, 2003). The construct of boldness most clearly captures the "mask" element of Cleckley's conception of psychopathy. The three facets of the triarchic model can be combined in different ways to represent alternative conceptions of psychopathy in past and contemporary literatures.

The triarchic model shows points of convergence and divergence with the alternative representations of ASPD in Sections II and III of DSM-5. The Section II conception does not include the dominant, emotionally resilient, and fearless tendencies associated with boldness. However, the new trait-based conception in Section III includes these features in the supplemental "psychopathic features" specifier (Strickland, Drislane, Lucy, Krueger, & Patrick, 2013). Given extensive research demonstrating psychological, behavioral, and physiological differences in antisocial individuals with and without core affective–interpersonal features of psychopathy (Blair, Mitchell, & Blair, 2005; Drislane, Vaidyanathan, & Patrick, 2013; Neumann & Hare, 2008; Newman & Lorenz, 2003; Patrick, 2007; Vaidyanathan, Hall, Patrick, & Bernat, 2011), which entail boldness and meanness (Venables, Hall, & Patrick, 2014; Wall, Wygant, & Sellbom, 2015), a diagnostic distinction needs to be made between psychopathic and nonpsychopathic variants of antisocial individuals. This distinction has important clinical/treatment implications. For example, Wong, Gordon, Gu, Lewis, and Olver (2012) have argued that affective–interpersonal features associated with psychopathy pose distinct obstacles to treatment and need to be directly addressed to allow for risk-reducing change in impulsive–antisocial tendencies. More specifically, Patrick and Nelson (2013) identified features associated with meanness (i.e., social disconnectedness, lack of empathic concern) as detrimental to formation of therapeutic alliances, and features associated with boldness (i.e., high perceived self-efficacy, low stress reactivity) as working against motivation for change.

## Assessment of Psychopathy

In this section, we review the best-established instruments for use with adult criminal and noncriminal samples, and with clinical and nonclinical youth (child, adolescent) samples. Table 25.1 provides a quick reference summary of these various instruments.

### Adult Measures

Measures for assessing psychopathy in adults include the interview-based Psychopathy Checklist—Revised, designed for use in correctional and forensic samples, and various self-report inventories developed for use with noncriminal, community-based samples.

#### The Psychopathy Checklist—Revised

The Psychopathy Checklist—Revised (PCL-R; Hare, 1991, 2003) is the best known and most commonly used assessment instrument for psychopathy in research studies and clinical settings. It was developed to assess for psychopathy among incarcerated offenders using global ratings of resemblance to Cleckley's conception as the criterion (Hare, 1980). The PCL-R contains 20 items, scored on the basis of information from two separate sources: (1) a semistructured interview with the offender, and (2) institutional file records. The test manual provides a narrative description for each item to optimize reliability of scores. Each item is rated on a 2-point scale (0 = *absent,* 1 = *equivocal,* 2 = *present*), with items scores summed to yield a total psychopathy score. A score of 30 or above is considered diagnostic of psychopathy.

It is important to note that the interpersonal–affective deficits and behavioral deviance features described by Cleckley (1941/1976) are clearly represented in the PCL-R item set. However, the positive adjustment features highlighted by Cleckley, such as social efficacy, good intelligence, lack of anxiety or internalizing symptoms, and disinclination toward suicide, are not represented. Factor analyses of the PCL-R have demonstrated that its 20 items do not index a unitary construct, but rather separate into distinct (albeit correlated) factors. Initially two factors were identified, an interpersonal–affective factor (F1) encompassing superficial charm, grandiosity, conning/deceptiveness, absence of remorse or empathy, shallow affect, and externalization of blame, and an impulsive–antisocial factor (F2) encompassing early behavior problems and juvenile delinquency, impulsivity, irresponsibility, boredom proneness, parasitic lifestyle, lack of long-term

**TABLE 25.1. Summary of Inventories Used to Assess for Psychopathy in Adults and Youth**

| Sample/inventory | Rating format | No. of items | Facets/factors assessed |
|---|---|---|---|
| *Adult* | | | |
| Criminal | | | |
| PCL-R | Interviewer | 20 | Interpersonal, affective, lifestyle, antisocial |
| SRP-III | Self-report | | Callousness, interpersonal, lifestyle, criminal behaviors |
| Noncriminal | | | |
| PPI | Self-report | 187 | Fearless dominance, impulsive antisociality |
| TriPM | Self-report | | Meanness, boldness, disinhibition |
| *Child/adolescent* | | | |
| Clinical | | | |
| APSD | Parent/teacher | 20 | Impulsive/conduct problems, callous–unemotional |
| CPS | Parent/teacher | 41 | Affective–interpersonal, behavioral deviance |
| PCL:YV | Interviewer | 20 | Interpersonal, affective, lifestyle, antisocial |
| Nonclinical | | | |
| ICU | Self-report | 24 | Callousness, uncaring, unemotional |
| YPI | Self-report | 53 | Grandiose–manipulative, callous–unemotional, impulsive–irresponsible |

*Note.* PCL-R, Psychopathy Checklist—Revised (Hare, 2003); PPI, Psychopathic Personality Inventory (Lilienfeld & Andrews, 1996); SRP-III, Self-Report Psychopathy Scale–Version III (Paulhus et al., 2009); TriPM, Triarchic Psychopathy Measure (Patrick, 2010); ASPD, Antisocial Process Screening Device (Frick & Hare, 2001); CPS, Child Psychopathy Scale (Lynam, 1997); PCL-YV, Psychopathy Checklist—Youth Version (Forth et al., 2003); ICU, Inventory of Callous–Unemotional Traits (Frick, 2004); YPI, Youth Psychopathic Traits Inventory (Andershed et al., 2002).

goals, impulsive aggressiveness, and violations of conditional release (Hare et al., 1990; Harpur, Hakstian, & Hare, 1988). However, other, subsequent work supports a three-factor model in which F1 is subdivided into "deficient affective experience" and "arrogant/deceitful" factors (Cooke & Michie, 2001), and F2 is limited to trait-oriented items, or a four-factor extension of this, in which F2 is divided into trait-oriented "Lifestyle" and behaviorally oriented "Antisocial" components (Hare & Neumann, 2006).

### The Self-Report Psychopathy Scale–III

The current, third version of the Self-Report Psychopathy Scale (SRP-III; Paulhus, Hemphill, & Hare, 2009) is a 60-item inventory that assesses psychopathy in terms of components specified by the PCL-R four-factor model (Hare & Neumann, 2006). The SRP-III yields a total psychopathy score, along with scores on four interrelated subscales: Callous Affect, Interpersonal Manipulation, Erratic Lifestyle, and Criminal Tendencies.

### The Psychopathic Personality Inventory

The Psychopathic Personality Inventory (PPI; Lilienfeld & Andrews, 1996) is a 187-item inventory designed to index psychopathy in terms of personality tendencies represented in key historic conceptions; its revised version (PPI-R; Lilienfeld & Widows, 2005) contains 154 items from the original version, some in reworded form. The PPI yields a total psychopathy score, along with scores on eight subscales: Social Potency, Stress Immunity, Fearlessness, Carefree Nonplanfulness, Rebellious Nonconformity, Blame Externalization, Machiavellian Egocentricity, and Coldheartedness. Seven of these eight subscales load onto two factors labeled Fearless Dominance and Impulsive Antisociality (Benning, Patrick, Blonigen, Hicks, & Iacono, 2005) or Self-Centered Impulsivity

(Lilienfeld & Widows, 2005). The PPI's eighth subscale, Coldheartedness, indexes tendencies distinct from these two factors.

## The Triarchic Psychopathy Measure

As described in the preceding chapter, the 58-item Triarchic Psychopathy Measure (TriPM; Patrick, 2010) assesses the three constructs of the triarchic model in a targeted manner. Items are completed using a 4-point response format (*True, Somewhat True, Somewhat False, False*). The TriPM Disinhibition and Meanness scales consist of items from the Externalizing Spectrum Inventory (ESI; Krueger, Markon, Patrick, Benning, & Kramer, 2007; Patrick, Kramer, Krueger, & Markon, 2013), designed to index the ESI's general disinhibitory and callous–aggression factors, respectively. The TriPM Boldness scale assesses tendencies toward social efficacy, emotional resiliency, and venturesomeness associated with the PPI fearless dominance construct. Despite the relative newness of this measure, substantial published evidence already exists for the validity of the inventory as a whole and the convergent and discriminant validity of its subscales (e.g., Drislane, Patrick, & Arsal, 2014; Marion, Sellbom, Salekin, Toomey, Kucharski, & Duncan, 2013; Poy, Segarra, Esteller, López, & Moltó, 2013; Sellbom & Phillips, 2013; Stanley, Wygant, & Sellbom, 2013; Strickland et al., 2013).

## Child and Adolescent Measures

Most existing inventories for assessing psychopathic tendencies in children and adolescents were developed as adaptations (or "downward extensions"; Salekin, 2006) of the PCL-R. Those designed for younger children utilize an informant-rating (parent or teacher) format. Inventories for older children and adolescents employ interview- or self-report-based formats.

## Antisocial Process Screening Device

The 20-item Antisocial Process Screening Device (APSD; Frick & Hare, 2001) assesses for psychopathic tendencies in children (ages 6–13) using items formulated as age-appropriate counterparts to those of the PCL-R. Items are rated by parents or teachers and summed to yield a total psychopathy score, along with scores on factors of Callous–Unemotional (CU) and Impulsivity/Conduct Problems (I/CP). The CU factor captures lack of empathy, restricted affectivity, insensitivity to others, lack of remorse or guilt, and unconcern about performance, whereas the I/CP factor taps proneness to boredom, rashness, hotheadedness, attention seeking, and blame externalization. An alternative three-factor model of the APSD that has received less attention in the literature includes a Narcissism factor along with the CU and I/CP factors (Frick, Bodin, & Barry, 2000). A self-report version of the APSD is also available for use with adolescents.

## The Child Psychopathy Scale

The Child Psychopathy Scale (CPS), available in informant rating (Lynam, 1997; Lynam et al., 2005) and self-report versions (Spain, Douglas, Poythress, & Epstein, 2004), is designed for use with clinic-referred children and adolescents (ages 6–17). Like the APSD, it was developed to provide a youth-oriented equivalent to the adult PCL-R. The CPS provides a total psychopathy score, along with scores on 13 subscales.

## The Psychopathy Checklist—Youth Version

The Psychopathy Checklist—Youth Version (PCL-YV; Forth, Kosson, & Hare, 2003) is an adaptation of the PCL-R designed for use with court-adjudicated adolescents. Identical to the PCL-R, it is scored using information from a semistructured interview and a review of case information from institutional records. Like the PCL-R, it contains 20 items, each rated 0–2.

## Inventory of Callous–Unemotional Traits

The 24-item Inventory of Callous–Unemotional Traits (ICU; Frick, 2004) was developed as a self-report-based assessment of CU traits related to serious antisocial and aggressive behaviors in youth. Four items associated with the CU factor of the informant-rated ASPD served as primary referents in formulating items for this self-report inventory (Frick et al., 2000). Items are scored on a 4-point Likert scale ranging from 0 (*Not at all true*) to 3 (*Definitely true*). Structural analyses of the ICU item set have revealed three lower-order factors (Callousness, Uncaring, and Unemotional) that load together on a higher-order CU dimension (Kimonis et al., 2008). Recent research indicates that this inventory as a whole indexes the meanness facet of the triarchic psychopathy model (Drislane,

Patrick, & Arsal, 2014), and as such, can serve as a self-report-based operationalization of this construct in older children, adolescents, and perhaps adults.

### The Youth Psychopathic Traits Inventory

The Youth Psychopathic Traits Inventory (YPI; Andershed, Kerr, Stattin, & Levander, 2002) is a 50-item self-report inventory designed to assess the interpersonal, affective, and behavioral components of psychopathy represented in the PCL-R three-factor model (Cooke & Michie, 2001). The YPI provides a total psychopathy score, along with scores on 10 specific content scales that are combined to form scores on three factors labeled Grandiose–Manipulative, Callous–Unemotional, and Impulsive–Irresponsible. The items of the YPI are trait-oriented and simply worded, making the inventory suitable for use in both nonclinical (community) and clinical samples of older children and adolescents.

## Prevalence, Comorbidity, Subtypes, and Course and Outcomes

### Prevalence

Prevalence rates for ASPD and psychopathy can be estimated in a variety of ways. According to DSM-5, estimated prevalence figures for ASPD across different studies range from 0.2 to 3.3%. Within the general population, the estimate prevalence is higher for men (3%) as compared to women (1%). Interestingly, rates of ASPD do not differ as a function of race or ethnicity. The prevalence of ASPD within nonforensic clinical samples is typically higher than that in community samples, and the prevalence in correctional/forensic settings is markedly elevated—with estimates ranging from 50% to as high as 80% (Hare, 2003).

Prevalence estimates for psychopathy as defined by the PCL-R in adult male prison populations are 15–25% (Hare, 2003)—much lower than aforementioned rates for ASPD (i.e., 50–80%). Prevalence rates for psychopathy in the general community are less clear because the PCL-R is not suitable for use with nonoffenders and because agreed-upon diagnostic cutoffs for more easily administrable self-report inventories designed for community samples have not been established. However, using an abbreviated screening version of the PCL-R (PCL:SV; Hart, Cox, & Hare, 1995) composed of items more applicable to nonoffender samples, Farrington (2006) estimated the prevalence of psychopathy in a population-representative sample of adults from the community to be around 2%. Estimated prevalence rates for psychopathy in incarcerated female samples vary, with some studies suggesting rates comparable to those for incarcerated men and others reporting lower prevalence rates (Verona & Vitale, 2006). Within general community and patient samples, prevalence is consistently lower in women than in men (Verona & Vitale, 2006).

In contrast with categorical diagnoses of ASPD, there seems to be some evidence of ethnic and cultural differences in rates of PCL-R-defined psychopathy within male correctional samples. Specifically, some evidence exists for higher average PCL-R scores and higher rates of psychopathy (PCL-R total > 30) in African American prisoners than in European American prisoners (Kosson, Smith, & Newman, 1990; Skeem, Edens, Camp, & Colwell, 2004). Additionally, other work has provided evidence for higher rates of PCL-R-defined psychopathy in American as compared to European prison samples (Sullivan & Kosson, 2006).

### Comorbidity

It is well known that ASPD, and its childhood precursor, conduct disorder, exhibit substantial comorbidity with other clinical conditions—in particular, disruptive behavior disorders and other PDs (e.g., oppositional defiant disorder, attention-deficit/hyperactivity disorder, borderline personality disorder) and substance use disorders (i.e., alcoholism and other drug dependence; Hare, 2003; Skeem et al., 2011). Regarding the latter, some work suggests that as many as 80–85% of individuals diagnosed with ASPD meet criteria for one or more substance use disorders (Chavez, 2010; Regier et al., 1990). It is also associated with increased rates of anxiety and mood disorders (APA, 2000), and suicidal behavior (APA, 2000; Verona & Patrick, 2002).

In contrast with ASPD, psychopathy as indexed by the PCL-R is associated only modestly with substance-related disorders and is largely unrelated to trait anxiety, negative affectivity, or occurrence of anxiety and mood disorders. Compared with ASPD, PCL-R psychopathy also relates minimally to suicidal behavior (Verona, Hicks, & Patrick, 2005; Verona, Patrick,

& Joiner, 2001) while showing higher comorbidity with narcissistic and histrionic personality disorders (Hare, 2003). These differing associations for ASPD and PCL-R psychopathy appear to be attributable to the enhanced representation of affective-interpersonal (F1) features in the latter. Indeed, associations for F2 of the PCL-R—which accounts mostly for the covariation between PCL-R scores and ASPD diagnoses or symptom scores (Patrick, Hicks, Krueger, & Lang, 2005)—closely parallel those for ASPD. Reciprocally, variance unique to F1 accounts for the PCL-R's lower associations with problems of certain types (e.g., substance use disorders, negative affectivity and anxiety/mood disorders, suicidal behavior) and its heightened associations with problems of other types (e.g., narcissistic and histrionic PDs).

These differing patterns of comorbidity for ASPD and PCL-R F2 and PCL-R F1, can be understood in terms of two intersecting dimensional models—the triarchic model of psychopathy and Krueger and colleagues' (2002, 2007) externalizing spectrum (ES) model. From the perspective of the triarchic model, PCL-R F1 indexes meanness along with some aspects of boldness (Patrick et al., 2009; Venables et al., 2014), whereas PCL-R F2 indexes disinhibition plus some elements of meanness (with the meanness portion accounting for overlap with F1). The boldness- and meanness-related variance in F1 that is nonoverlapping with F2—reflecting tendencies toward dominance, stress immunity, and callous unconcern (Patrick et al., 2009; Venables et al., 2014)—can be viewed as accounting for its differential relations with clinical problems, as noted above.

The ES model intersects with the triarchic model through its general disinhibitory and callous–aggressive factors, which correspond to the disinhibition and meanness constructs of the triarchic model. The general disinhibitory factor of the ES model provides a point of reference for understanding patterns of comorbidity for ASPD. Specifically, twin modeling research has demonstrated that the basis of the observed overlap between adult and child symptoms of ASPD, and their overlap in turn with substance use disorders and other disruptive behavior disorders, lies in a highly heritable dispositional tendency—indexed phenotypically by scores on the general disinhibitory factor of the ES (Krueger et al., 2002; Young et al., 2009). The dispositional tendency indexed by the disinhibitory factor of the ES can be viewed as a general liability to impulse-related problems of various types that is shaped in specific directions of clinical expression by other etiological influences. In turn, the observed parallels in clinical correlates of PCL-R F2 with those of ASPD become understandable in light of evidence that PCL-R F2 largely taps the general disinhibitory factor of the ES model (Patrick et al., 2005).

## Variants (Subtypes) of Psychopathy

As noted earlier, the diagnostic criteria for ASPD are polythetic, resulting in substantial heterogeneity in symptom pictures among individuals receiving this diagnosis. In an effort to characterize this heterogeneity empirically, research studies have been conducted to identify subgroups of individuals with ASPD, differentiated on the basis of dispositional or behavioral tendencies. In general, work of this kind has utilized cluster analysis—a statistical technique for assigning individuals in a sample to subgroups (clusters) based on similarities versus differences in profiles of scores on measured characteristics (cluster variates). For example, Poythress and colleagues (2010) used cluster analysis to delineate distinct variants of ASPD in a large sample of incarcerated offenders. Four subgroups (clusters) were found, the first exhibiting characteristics consistent with descriptive accounts of primary psychopathy (see below), the second resembling Karpman's (1941) description of secondary psychopathy, the third scoring high on psychopathic features and harm avoidance (i.e., aversion to danger), and the fourth scoring low in features of psychopathy (nonpsychopathic ASPD group). The results of this study highlight the distinction between ASPD and psychopathy, while providing evidence for variants of highly psychopathic individuals among offenders diagnosed as ASPD. Paralleling these results, in another cluster-analytic study of offenders diagnosed with ASPD, Swogger and Kosson (2007) found evidence of primary and secondary psychopathic subgroups, along with two other subgroups characterized as (1) high in negative affect and (2) low in general psychopathology.

Empirical evidence also points to the existence of distinct subtypes within the category of individuals defined as psychopathic according to scores on the PCL-R or other measures. A particularly salient and long-standing distinction in the literature has been between primary and secondary variants of psychopathy (Karpman,

1946; Poythress & Skeem, 2006; Lykken, 1957, 1995). The term "primary" refers to individuals who exhibit the pattern of features described by Cleckley (1941/1976)—that is, severe deficits in behavioral restraint, affective sensitivity, and interpersonal connectedness masked by a low anxious, socially efficacious demeanor. By contrast, the label "secondary" psychopathy has been used for individuals who exhibit persistent behavioral deviancy in the context of high levels of anxiety/distress and hostility. In support of this notion, studies using cluster analysis to distinguish high PCL-R- scoring offenders on the basis of dispositional characteristics provide consistent evidence for two variants differentiated in particular by high versus low anxiousness (Blackburn, Logan, Donnelly, & Renwick, 2008; Hicks, Markon, Patrick, Krueger, & Newmann, 2004; Poythress et al., 2010; Skeem, Johansson, Andershed, Kerr, & Louden, 2007; Swogger & Kosson, 2007; Swogger, Walsh, & Kosson, 2008; see also Newman, Schmitt, & Voss, 1997).

Building on this work with offenders, some newer cluster-analytic studies have tested for subtypes among participants from the community at large attaining high scores on self-report measures of psychopathy. In general, the studies have also yielded evidence for subgroups of highly psychopathic individuals differing in anxiousness along with other dispositional tendencies (Lee & Salekin, 2010; Skeem et al., 2007; Swogger & Kosson, 2007). In one recent study of this type, Drislane, Patrick, Sourander, and colleagues (2014) tested for subtypes of high psychopathy scorers within a large Finnish community male sample, using scores on the facets of the triarchic model (indexed via the TriPM), along with scores on a measure of negative affectivity (NA; i.e., anxious–depressive tendencies) as cluster variates. Consistent with prior work, two subgroups were found that differed markedly in NA in relation to one another and to a low-psychopathy comparison group. The low NA psychopathy group also scored higher in boldness than either the high NA group or the low-psychopathy group, which did not differ on boldness. Both psychopathy groups scored markedly higher on disinhibition and meanness than the low-psychopathy group, while differing from one another on disinhibition (high NA > low NA) but not meanness.

Along with cluster-analytic work focusing on dispositional characteristics, behavioral and psychophysiological studies also provide evidence for distinct variants of high psychopathy individuals. For example, laboratory behavioral studies by Newman and colleagues (Arnett, Smith, & Newman, 1997; Hiatt, Lorenz, & Newman, 2002; Lorenz & Newman, 2002; Newman & Schmitt, 1998; Newman et al., 1997) demonstrated cognitive–affective processing deficits in low-anxious (primary) psychopathic offenders—including deficits in passive avoidance learning and affective/neutral stimulus differentiation—not evident in high-anxious (secondary) psychopathic offenders or low-psychopathy controls. Similarly, psychophysiological studies by this group (Sutton, Vitale, & Newman, 2002) and others (e.g., Benning, Patrick, & Iacono, 2005; Dindo & Fowles, 2011; Lykken, 1957) provided evidence for affective response deficits—in particular, reduced reactivity to aversive stimulus cues—in low-anxious psychopathic and high fearless-dominant (bold) individuals.

## Course and Outcomes

ASPD and psychopathy are considered chronic conditions. By definition, the categorical diagnosis of ASPD requires persistence of antisocial behavior from childhood through adulthood, and the PCL-R criteria for psychopathy include indicators of early deviance (behavioral problems before age 12, juvenile delinquency) along with more adult-oriented indicators. Nonetheless, longitudinal studies indicate that ASPD symptoms and impulsive–antisocial features of psychopathy tend to decline over the life course, particularly from early adulthood through the fourth decade of life (APA, 2013). By contrast, the affective–interpersonal features of psychopathy tend to be more stable from earlier to later years (Blonigen, Hicks, Krueger, Patrick, & Iacono, 2006; see also Lynam et al., 2009).

Given the reckless, unrestrained tendencies that are characteristic of ASPD and psychopathy, these conditions tend to be associated with a variety of adverse outcomes—including violence, other criminal behavior, substance-related disorders, and sexual transgressions. Within delinquent and adult samples, the PCL-R in particular has proven effective for predicting disciplinary infractions during incarceration and reoffending following release (recidivism). Regarding prediction of general (either violent or nonviolent) recidivism, meta-analytic reviews have reported small (Gendreau, Goggin, & Smith, 2002; Walters, 2003) to moderate effect sizes (Hemphill, Hare, & Wong, 1998) for overall scores on the PCL-R across varying intervals of time (see also Douglas, Vincent, & Edens, 2006). Other recent meta-analytic work (Kennealy, Skeem, Walters, & Camp, 2010) indicates that the impulsive–antisocial (F2) component of the PCL-R accounts mainly for prediction of violent reoffending. In view of the costly toll that ASPD and psychopathy exact on society—emotionally, physically, and financially—there is a critical need to establish effective methods for treating these severe clinical conditions.

## Treatment of ASPD and Psychopathy

One of the most debated topics within the study of ASPD and psychopathy is how best to treat these costly disorders, if indeed they can be treated. In fact, the long-standing idea that these conditions are untreatable (Harris & Rice, 2006; Salekin, 2002) has been challenged by recent carefully conducted outcome research (Skeem et al., 2011). In particular, empirical findings indicate that correctional treatment programs for offenders are most effective (i.e., induce the greatest reductions in criminal behavior) when they (1) prioritize delivery of intensive services to high-risk offenders; (2) focus on modifying tendencies directly associated with reoffense risk, such as criminal attitudes, substance abuse, and impulsivity; and (3) deliver treatment in a manner that is engaging for the offenders (Skeem et al., 2011). Reductions in criminal reoffending associated with treatment programs enacting these principles are modest but robust, with effect sizes ranging from 0.15 to 0.34 (Andrews & Bonta, 2006).

Clinicians have developed a range of treatments for ASPD and psychopathy, some of which have proved more effective than others (see Wong, Chapter 36, this volume). Outcomes associated with psychodynamic approaches to the treatment of antisocial behavior have been decidedly mixed, with some studies indicating *poorer* outcomes for treated individuals as compared to nontreated controls (Andrews, Bonta, & Hoge, 1990; Antonowicz & Ross, 1994). Increased rates of recidivism have also been reported for therapeutic community programs of certain types (Rice, Harris, & Cormier, 1992), although the treatment protocols of such programs have been subjected to criticism (Skeem et al., 2011). Regarding individualized behavioral therapies, strict behavior modification approaches have generally proven less effective than treatments involving a cognitive-behavioral focus (Landenberger & Lipsey, 2005).

Many of the treatments available for ASPD and psychopathy include some form of cognitive-behavioral therapy (CBT), which focuses on teaching cognitive skills presumed to be deficient in individuals who engage repeatedly in criminal behaviors (Friendship, Blud, Erikson, Travers, & Thornton, 2003; Lipsey, Chapman, & Landenberger, 2001; Samenow, 1991; Yochelson & Samenow, 1976, 1977). Reasoning and rehabilitation (R&R) therapy is one example of a CBT-based treatment for offenders. Empirical research suggests that offenders exhibit a variety of cognitive deficits of direct relevance to their criminal behaviors, such as concrete thinking, failures to consider consequences, and disregarding others' feelings, thoughts, and behaviors (Ross, Fabiano, & Ewles, 1988). R&R therapy is a structured, multifaceted intervention that targets criminogenic beliefs and cognitions, and inculcates understanding of how these thoughts are related to criminal behavior. This treatment has specific modules focusing on amelioration of cognitive deficits and improvement of self-control, critical reasoning, and consideration of values (Robinson & Porporino, 2000; Ross et al., 1988). R&R therapy is typically administered in a 2-hour group format, with groups ranging from six to 12 individuals.

Moral reconation therapy (MRT) is another CBT-oriented treatment for offenders. The primary goal is to improve the behavior of offenders by improving their moral and social capacities (Little & Robinson, 1988; Wilson, Bouffard, & MacKenzie, 2005). Similar to R&R, MRT is administered in a group format, with sessions of 1–2 hours typically conducted twice per week. The MRT approach assists individuals in identifying goals, exploring good and more difficult times in life, realizing that behaviors that have consequences, and recognizing sources of unhappiness (Little & Robinson, 1988; Wilson et al., 2005). Other CBT-oriented treatments for antisocial behavior include "Thinking for a Change" (Golden, Gatchel, & Cahill, 2006) and "aggression replacement" therapy (Glick & Goldstein, 1987). Created for adult offenders on probation and aggressive youth, respectively, these programs focus in particular on enhancement of self-control and improvement of interpersonal relations.

In general, available research suggests that the use of CBT-based interventions is modestly effective in reducing antisocial behavior and results in stable reductions in recidivism within offending samples (e.g., Andrews et al., 1990; Antonowitz & Ross, 1994; Friendship et al., 2003; Garrett, 1985; Izzo & Ross, 1990; Landenberger & Lipsey, 2005; Lipsey et al., 2001; Whitehead & Lab, 1989; Wilson et al., 2005). More specifically, on average, offender rehabilitation program reduce recidivism by 10% (Lösel, 1996). These modest but stable results generate hope for the possibility of reducing persistent criminal offending and acts of violence by antisocial and psychopathic individuals. Given the current state of literature, it appears that R&R and other CBT-focused treatments represent the best available current methods for reducing recidivism and curtailing the harm produced by antisocial and psychopathic offenders. However, further systematic research is needed to refine current best-available treatments and to establish new and more effective methods of intervention.

## REFERENCES

American Psychiatric Association. (2000). *Diagnostic and statistical manual of mental disorders* (4th ed., text rev.). Washington, DC: Author.

American Psychiatric Association. (2013). *Diagnostic and statistical manual of mental disorders* (5th ed.). Arlington, VA: Author.

Andershed, H., Kerr, M., Stattin, H., & Levander, S. (2002). Psychopathic traits in non-referred youths: A new assessment tool. In E. Blau & L. Sheridan (Eds.), *Psychopaths: Current international perspectives* (pp. 131–158). Amsterdam, The Netherlands: Elsevier.

Andrews, D. A., & Bonta, J. (2006). *The psychology of criminal conduct* (4th ed.). Cincinnati, OH: Anderson.

Andrews, D. A., Bonta, J., & Hoge, R. D. (1990). Classification for effective rehabilitation: Rediscovering psychology. *Criminal Justice and Behavior, 17,* 19–52.

Antonowitz, D. H., & Ross, R. R. (1994). Essential components of successful rehabilitation programs for offenders. *International Journal of Offender Therapy and Comparative Criminology, 38,* 97–104.

Arnett, P. A., Smith, S. S., & Newman, J. P. (1997). Approach and avoidance motivation in psychopathic criminal offenders during passive avoidance. *Journal of Personality and Social Psychology, 72,* 1413–1428.

Benning, S. D., Patrick, C. J., Blonigen, D. M., Hicks, B. M., & Iacono, W. G. (2005). Estimating facets of psychopathy from normal personality traits: A step toward community-epidemiological investigations. *Assessment, 12,* 3–18.

Benning, S. D., Patrick, C. J., Hicks, B. M., Blonigen, D. M., & Krueger, R. F. (2003). Factor structure of the Psychopathic Personality Inventory: Validity and implications for clinical assessment. *Psychological Assessment, 15,* 340–350.

Benning, S. D., Patrick, C. J., & Iacono, W. G. (2005). Psychopathy, startle blink modulation, and electrodermal reactivity in twin men. *Psychophysiology, 42*(6), 753–762.

Blackburn, R., Logan, C., Donnelly, J., & Renwick, S. J. D. (2008). Identifying psychopathic subtypes: Combining an empirical personality classification of offenders with the Psychopathy Checklist—Revised. *Journal of Personality Disorders, 22,* 604–622.

Blair, J., Mitchell, D., & Blair, K. (2005). *The psychopath: Emotion and the brain.* Malden, MA: Blackwell.

Blonigen, D. M., Hicks, B. M., Krueger, R. F., Patrick, C. J., & Iacono, W. G. (2006). Continuity and change in psychopathic personality traits: A longitudinal–biometric study. *Journal of Abnormal Psychology, 115,* 85–95.

Chavez, J. X. (2010). Assessing the incidence rates of substance use disorders among those with antisocial and borderline personality disorders in rural settings. *International Journal of Psychology, 6,* 57–66.

Clark, L. A. (2007). Assessment and diagnosis of personality disorder: Perennial issues and an emerging reconceptualization. *Annual Review of Psychology, 58,* 227–257.

Cleckley, H. (1976). *The mask of sanity* (5th ed.). St. Louis, MO: Mosby. (Original work published 1941)

Cooke, D. J., & Michie, C. (2001). Refining the construct of psychopathy: Towards a hierarchical model. *Psychological Assessment, 13,* 171–188.

Dindo, L., & Fowles, D. (2011). Dual temperamental risk factors for psychopathic personality: Evidence from self-report and skin conductance. *Journal of Personality and Social Psychology, 100,* 557–566.

Douglas, K. S., Vincent, G. M., & Edens, J. F. (2006). Risk for criminal recidivism: The role of psychopathy. In C. J. Patrick (Ed.), *Handbook of psychopathy* (pp. 533–554). New York: Guilford Press.

Drislane, L. E., Patrick, C. J., & Arsal, G. (2014). Clarifying the content coverage of differing psychopathy inventories through reference to the Triarchic Psychopathy Measure. *Psychological Assessment, 26,* 350–362.

Drislane, L. E., Patrick, C. J., Sourander, A., Sillanmäki, L., Aggen, S. H., Elonheimo, H., et al. (2014). Distinct variants of extreme psychopathic individuals in society at large: Evidence from a population-based sample. *Personality Disorders: Theory, Research, and Treatment, 5,* 154–163.

Drislane, L. E., Vaidyanathan, U., & Patrick, C. J. (2013). Reduced cortical call to arms differentiates psychopathy from antisocial personality disorder. *Psychological Medicine, 43*(4), 825–835.

Farrington, D. (2006). Family background and psychopathy. In C. J. Patrick (Ed.), *Handbook of psychopathy* (pp. 229–250). New York: Guilford Press.

First, M. B., Gibbon, M., Spitzer, R. L., Williams, J. B. W., & Benjamin, L. S. (1997). *User's guide for the Structured Clinical Interview for DSM-IV Axis II Personality Disorders.* Washington, DC: American Psychiatric Press.

Forth, A. E., Kosson, D. S., & Hare, R. D. (2003). *The Psychopathy Checklist: Youth Version manual.* Toronto, ON, Canada: Multi-Health Systems.

Frances, A. J. (1980). The DSM-III personality disorders section: A commentary. *American Journal of Psychiatry, 137,* 1050–1054.

Frick, P. J. (1995). Callous–unemotional traits and conduct problems: A two-factor model of psychopathy in children. *Issues in Criminological and Legal Psychology, 24,* 47–51.

Frick, P. J. (2004). *The Inventory of Callous–Unemotional Traits.* Unpublished rating scale, University of New Orleans, New Orleans, LA.

Frick, P. J., Bodin, S. D., & Barry, C. T. (2000). Psychopathic traits and conduct problems in community and clinic-referred samples of children: Further development of the psychopathy screening device. *Psychological Assessment, 12*(4), 382–393.

Frick, P. J., & Hare, R. D. (2001). *The Antisocial Process Screening Device (APSD).* Toronto, ON, Canada: Multi-Health Systems.

Frick, P. J., & Marsee, M. A. (2006). Psychopathy and developmental pathways to antisocial behavior in youth. In C. J. Patrick (Ed.), *Handbook of psychopathy* (pp. 353–374). New York: Guilford Press.

Frick, P. J., O'Brien, B. S., Wootton, J. M., & McBurnett, K. (1994). Psychopathy and conduct problems in children. *Journal of Abnormal Psychology, 103,* 700–707.

Friendship, C., Blud, L., Erikson, M., Travers, R., & Thornton, D. (2003). Cognitive-behavioural treatment for imprisoned offenders: An evaluation of HM Prison Service's cognitive skills programmes. *Legal and Criminological Psychology, 8,* 103–114.

Garrett, C. J. (1985). Effects of residential treatment on adjudicated delinquents: A meta-analysis. *Journal of Research on Crime and Delinquency, 22,* 287–308.

Gendreau, P., Goggin, C., & Smith, P. (2002). Is the PCL-R really the "unparalleled" measure of offender risk?: A lesson in knowledge cumulation. *Criminal Justice and Behavior, 29,* 397–426.

Glick, B., & Goldstein, A. P. (1987). Aggression replacement training. *Journal of Counseling and Development, 65,* 356–362.

Golden, L. S., Gatchel, R. J., & Cahill, M. A. (2006). Evaluating the effectiveness of the National Institute of Corrections' "Thinking for a Change" program among probationers. *Journal of Offender Rehabilitation, 43,* 55–73.

Hare, R. D. (1980). A research scale for the assessment of psychopathy in criminal populations. *Personality and Individual Differences, 1*(2), 111–119.

Hare, R. D. (1983). Diagnosis of antisocial personality disorder in two prison populations. *American Journal of Psychiatry, 140,* 887–890.

Hare, R. D. (1991). *The Hare Psychopathy Checklist—Revised.* Toronto, ON, Canada: Multi-Health Systems.

Hare, R. D. (2003). *The Hare Psychopathy Checklist—Revised* (2nd ed.). Toronto, ON, Canada: Multi-Health Systems.

Hare, R. D., Harpur, T. J., Hakstian, A. R., Forth, A. E., Hart, S. D., & Newman, J. P. (1990). The Revised Psychopathy Checklist: Reliability and factor structure. *Psychological Assessment, 2,* 338–341.

Hare, R. D., & Neumann, C. S. (2006). The PCL-R assessment of psychopathy. In C. J. Patrick (Ed.), *Handbook of psychopathy* (pp. 55–88). New York: Guilford Press.

Harpur, T. J., Hakstian, A. R., & Hare, R. D. (1988). Factor structure of the psychopathy checklist. *Journal of Consulting and Clinical Psychology, 56,* 741–747.

Harris, G. T., & Rice, M. E. (2006). Treatment of psychopathy. In C. J. Patrick (Ed.), *Handbook of psychopathy* (pp. 555–572). New York: Guilford Press.

Hart, S., Cox, D., & Hare, R. D. (1995). *Manual for the Psychopathy Checklist: Screening Version (PCL:SV).* Toronto, ON, Canada: Multi-Health Systems.

Hemphill, J. F., Hare, R. D., & Wong, S. (1998). Psychopathy and recidivism: A review. *Legal and Criminological Psychology, 3,* 141–172.

Hiatt, K. D., Lorenz, A. R., & Newman, J. P. (2002). Assessment of emotion and language in processing psychopathic offenders: Results from a dichotic listening task. *Personality and Individual Differences, 32,* 1255–1268.

Hicks, B. M., Markon, K. E., Patrick, C. J., Krueger, R. F., & Newman, J. P. (2004). Identifying psychopathy subtypes on the basis of personality structure. *Psychological Assessment, 16,* 276–288.

Izzo, R. L., & Ross, R. R. (1990). Meta-analysis of rehabilitation programs for juvenile delinquents: A brief report. *Criminal Justice and Behavior, 17,* 134–142.

Karpman, B. (1941). On the need of separating psychopathy into two distinct clinical types: The symptomatic and the idiopathic. *Journal of Criminal Psychopathology, 3,* 112–137.

Karpman, B. (1946). Psychopathy in the scheme of human typology. *Journal of Nervous and Mental Disease, 103*(3), 276–288.

Kennealy, P. J., Skeem, J. L., Walters, G. D., & Camp, J. (2010). Do core interpersonal and affective traits of PCL-R psychopathy interact with antisocial behavior and disinhibition to predict violence? *Psychological Assessment, 22*(3), 569–580.

Kimonis, E. R., Frick, P. J., Skeem, J. L., Marsee, M. A., Cruise, K., Munoz, L. C., et al. (2008). Assessing callous–unemotional traits in adolescent offenders: Validation of the Inventory of Callous–Unemotional

Traits. *International Journal of Law and Psychiatry, 31*(3), 241–252.

Koch, J. L. (1888). *Kurzgefasster leitfaden der psychiatrie* [Short textbook of psychiatry]. Ravensburg, Germany: Maier.

Kosson, D. S., Smith, S. S., & Newman, J. P. (1990). Evaluating the construct validity of psychopathy in black and white male inmates: Three preliminary studies. *Journal of Abnormal Psychology, 99,* 250–259.

Kraepelin, E. (1915). *Psychiatrie: Ein lehrbuch [Psychiatry: A textbook]* (8th ed.). Leipzig, Germany: Barth.

Krueger, R. F., Hicks, B., Patrick, C. J., Carlson, S., Iacono, W. G., & McGue, M. (2002). Etiologic connections among substance dependence, antisocial behavior, and personality: Modeling the externalizing spectrum. *Journal of Abnormal Psychology, 111,* 411–424.

Krueger, R. F., Markon, K. E., Patrick, C. J., Benning, S. D., & Kramer, M. (2007). Linking antisocial behavior, substance use, and personality: An integrative quantitative model of the adult externalizing spectrum. *Journal of Abnormal Psychology, 116,* 645–666.

Landenberger, N. A., & Lipsey, M. W. (2005). The positive effects of cognitive-behavioral programs for offenders: A meta-analysis of factors associated with effective treatment. *Journal of Experimental Criminology, 1,* 451–476.

Lee, Z., & Salekin, R. (2010). Psychopathy in a noninstitutional sample: Differences in primary and secondary subtypes. *Personality Disorders: Theory, Research, and Treatment, 1,* 153–169.

Lilienfeld, S. O., & Andrews, B. P. (1996). Development and preliminary validation of a self report measure of psychopathic personality traits in noncriminal populations. *Journal of Personality Assessment, 66,* 488–524.

Lilienfeld, S. O., & Widows, M. R. (2005). *Psychopathic Personality Inventory—Revised (PPI-R) professional manual.* Odessa, FL: Psychological Assessment Resources.

Lindner, R. M. (1942). Experimental studies in constitutional psychopathic inferiority. *Journal of Criminal Psychopathology, 3,* 252–276.

Lipsey, M. W., Chapman, G. L., & Landenberger, N. A. (2001). Cognitive-behavioral programs for offenders. *Annals of the American Academy of Political and Social Science, 578,* 144–157.

Little, G. L., & Robinson, K. D. (1988). Moral reconation therapy: A systematic step-by-step treatment system for treatment-resistant clients. *Psychological Reports, 62,* 135–151.

Lorenz, A. R., & Newman, J. P. (2002). Deficient response modulation and emotion processing in low-anxious Caucasian psychopathic offenders: Results from a lexical decision task. *Emotion, 2,* 91–104.

Lösel, F. (1996). Effective correctional programming: What empirical research tells us and what it doesn't. *Forum on Corrections Research, 6,* 33–37.

Lykken, D. T. (1957). A study of anxiety in the sociopathic personality. *Journal of Abnormal and Social Psychology, 55*(1), 6–10.

Lykken, D. T. (1995). *The antisocial personalities.* Mahwah, NJ: Erlbaum.

Lynam, D. R. (1997). Pursuing the psychopath: Capturing the fledgling psychopath in a nomological net. *Journal of Abnormal Psychology, 106,* 425–438.

Lynam, D. R., Caspi, A., Moffitt, T. E., Raine, A., Loeber, R., & Stouthamer-Loeber, M. (2005). Adolescent psychopathy and the Big Five: Results from two samples. *Journal of Abnormal Child Psychology, 33*(4), 431–443.

Lynam, D. R., Charnigo, R., Moffitt, T. E., Raine, A., Loeber, R., & Stouthamer-Loeber, M. (2009). The stability of psychopathy across adolescence. *Development and Psychopathology, 21,* 1133–1153.

Lynam, D. R., & Derefinko, K. J. (2006). Psychopathy and personality. In C. J. Patrick (Ed.), *Handbook of psychopathy* (pp. 133–155). New York: Guilford Press.

Marion, B. E., Sellbom, M., Salekin, R. T., Toomey, J. A., Kucharski, L. T., & Duncan, S. (2013). An examination of the association between psychopathy and dissimulation using the MMPI-2-RF validity scales. *Law and Human Behavior, 37*(4), 219–230.

McCord, W., & McCord, J. (1964). *The psychopath: An essay on the criminal mind.* Princeton, NJ: Van Nostrand.

Neumann, C. S., & Hare, R. D. (2008). Psychopathic traits in a large community sample: Links to violence, alcohol use, and intelligence. *Journal of Consulting and Clinical Psychology, 76*(5), 893–899.

Newman, J. P., & Lorenz, A. R. (2003). Response modulation and emotion processing: Implications for psychopathy and other dysregulatory psychopathology. In R. J. Davidson, K. R. Scherer, & H. H. Goldsmith (Eds.), *Handbook of affective sciences* (pp. 904–929). New York: Oxford University Press.

Newman, J. P., & Schmitt, W. (1998). Passive avoidance in psychopathic offenders: A replication and extension. *Journal of Abnormal Psychology, 107,* 527–532.

Newman, J. P., Schmitt, W. A., & Voss, W. D. (1997). The impact of motivationally neutral cues on psychopathic individuals: Assessing the generality of the response modulation hypothesis. *Journal of Abnormal Psychology, 106,* 563–575.

Patrick, C. J. (2007). Antisocial personality disorder and psychopathy. In W. O'Donohue, K. A. Fowler, & S. O. Lilienfeld (Eds.), *Personality disorders: Towards the DSM-V* (pp. 109–166). New York: SAGE.

Patrick, C. J. (2010). Operationalizing the triarchic conceptualization of psychopathy: Preliminary description of brief scales for assessment of boldness, meanness, and disinhibition. Unpublished test manual, Florida State University, Tallahassee, FL. Available at *www.phenxtoolkit.org/index.php?pagelink=browse.protocoldetails&id=121601.*

Patrick, C. J., Fowles, D. C., & Krueger, R. F. (2009). Triarchic conceptualization of psychopathy: Developmental origins of disinhibition, boldness, and meanness. *Development and Psychopathology, 21,* 913–938.

Patrick, C. J., Hicks, B. M., Krueger, R. F., & Lang, A. R. (2005). Relations between psychopathy facets and externalizing in a criminal offender sample. *Journal of Personality Disorders, 19*(4), 339–356.

Patrick, C. J., Kramer, M. D., Krueger, R. F., & Markon, K. E. (2013). Optimizing efficiency of psychopathology assessment through quantitative modeling: Development of a brief form of the Externalizing Spectrum Inventory. *Psychological Assessment, 25*(4), 1332–1348.

Patrick, C. J., & Nelson, L. D. (2013). Antisocial personality disorder. In J. Smits (Ed.), *Cognitive behavioral therapy: A complete reference guide: Vol. 2. CBT for specific disorders* (pp. 1263–1298). New York: Wiley-Blackwell.

Paulhus, D. L., Hemphill, J., & Hare, R. (2009). *Manual for the Self-Report Psychopathy Scale, Version III (SRP-III).* Toronto, ON, Canada: Multi-Heath Systems.

Pinel, P. (1962). *A treatise on insanity* (D. Davis, Trans.). New York: Hafner. (Original work published 1806)

Poy, R., Segarra, P., Esteller, À., López, R., & Moltó, J. (2013). FFM description of the triarchic conceptualization of psychopathy in men and women. *Psychological Assessment, 26*(1), 69–76.

Poythress, N. G., Edens, J. F., Skeem, J. L., Lilienfeld, S. O., Douglas, K. S., Frick, P. J., et al. (2010). Identifying subtypes among offenders with antisocial personality disorder: A cluster-analytic study. *Journal of Abnormal Psychology, 119,* 389–400.

Poythress, N. G., & Skeem, J. L. (2006). Disaggregating psychopathy: Where and how to look for subtypes. In C. J. Patrick (Ed.), *Handbook of psychopathy* (pp. 172–192). New York: Guilford Press.

Pritchard, J. C. (1835). *A treatise on insanity and other disorders affecting the mind.* London: Sherwood, Gilbert & Piper.

Regier, D. A., Farmer, M. E., Rae, D. S., Locke, B. Z., Keith, S. J., Judd, L. L., et al. (1990). Comorbidity of mental disorders with alcohol and other drug abuse: Results from the Epidemiologic Catchment Area (ECA) Study. *Journal of American Medical Association, 264*(19), 2511–2518.

Rice, M. E., Harris, G. T., & Cormier, C. A. (1992). An evaluation of a maximum security therapeutic community for psychopaths and other mentally disordered offenders. *Law and Human Behavior, 16,* 399–412.

Robins, L. N. (1966). *Deviant children grown up.* Baltimore: Williams & Wilkins.

Robins, L. N. (1978). Sturdy predictors of adult antisocial behaviour: Replications from longitudinal studies. *Psychological Medicine, 8,* 611–622.

Robinson, D., & Porporino, F. J. (2000). Programming in cognitive skills: The Reasoning and Rehabilitation Programme. In C. R. Hollin (Ed.), *Handbook of offender assessment and treatment* (pp. 179–193). New York: Wiley.

Ross, R. R., Fabiano, E. A., & Ewles, C. D. (1988). Reasoning and rehabilitation. *International Journal of Offender Therapy and Comparative Criminology, 32,* 29–35.

Rush, B. (1812). *Medical inquiries and observations upon the diseases of the mind.* Philadelphia: Kimber & Richardson.

Salekin, R. T. (2002). Psychopathy and therapeutic pessimism: Clinical lore or clinical reality? *Clinical Psychology Review, 22,* 79–112.

Salekin, R. T. (2006). Psychopathy in children and adolescents. In C. J. Patrick (Ed.), *Handbook of psychopathy* (pp. 389–414). New York: Guilford Press.

Samenow, S. E. (1991). Correcting errors in thinking in the socialization of offenders. *Journal of Correctional Education, 42,* 56–58.

Sellbom, M., & Phillips, T. R. (2013). An examination of the triarchic conceptualization of psychopathy in incarcerated and non-incarcerated samples. *Journal of Abnormal Psychology, 122,* 208–214.

Skeem, J. L., Edens, J. F., Camp, J., & Colwell, L. H. (2004). Are there racial differences in levels of psychopathy?: A meta-analysis. *Law and Human Behavior, 28,* 505–527.

Skeem, J. L., Johansson, P., Andershed, H., Kerr, M., & Louden, J. E. (2007). Two subtypes of psychopathic violent offenders that parallel primary and secondary variants. *Journal of Abnormal Psychology, 116,* 395–409.

Skeem, J. L., Polaschek, D. L., Patrick, C. J., & Lilienfeld, S. O. (2011). Psychopathic personality bridging the gap between scientific evidence and public policy. *Psychological Science in the Public Interest, 12*(3), 95–162.

Spain, S. E., Douglas, K. S., Poythress, N. G., & Epstein, M. (2004). The relationship between psychopathic features, violence and treatment outcome: The comparison of three youth measures of psychopathic features. *Behavioral Sciences and the Law, 22*(1), 85–102.

Stanley, J. H., Wygant, D. B., & Sellbom, M. (2013). Elaborating on the construct validity of the triarchic psychopathy measure in a criminal offender sample. *Journal of Personality Assessment, 95*(4), 343–350.

Strickland, C. M., Drislane, L. E., Lucy, M., Krueger, R. F., & Patrick, C. J. (2013). Characterizing psychopathy using DSM-5 personality traits. *Assessment, 20*(3), 327–338.

Sullivan, E. A., & Kosson, D. S. (2006). Ethnic and cultural variations in psychopathy. In C. J. Patrick (Ed.), *Handbook of psychopathy* (pp. 437–458). New York: Guilford Press.

Sutton, S. K., Vitale, J. E., & Newman, J. P. (2002). Emotion among women with psychopathy during picture perception. *Journal of Abnormal Psychology, 111,* 610–619.

Swogger, M. T., & Kosson, D. S. (2007). Identifying subtypes of criminal psychopaths: A replication and extension. *Criminal Justice and Behavior, 34,* 953–970.

Swogger, M. T., Walsh, Z., & Kosson, D. S. (2008). Psychopathy subtypes among African American county jail inmates. *Criminal Justice and Behavior, 35,* 1484–1499.

Trull, T. J., & Durrett, C. A. (2005). Categorical and dimensional models of personality disorder. *Annual Review of Clinical Psychology, 1,* 355–380.

Vaidyanathan, U., Hall, J. R., Patrick, C. J., & Bernat, E. M. (2011). Clarifying the role of defensive reactivity deficits in psychopathy and antisocial personality using startle reflex methodology. *Journal of Abnormal Psychology, 120,* 253–258.

Venables, N. C., Hall, J. R., & Patrick, C. J. (2014). Differentiating psychopathy from antisocial personality disorder: A triarchic model perspective. *Psychological Medicine, 44,* 1005–1014.

Verona, E., Hicks, B. M., & Patrick, C. J. (2005). Psychopathy and suicidality in female offenders: Mediating influences of personality and abuse. *Journal of Consulting and Clinical Psychology, 73*(6), 1065–1073.

Verona, E., & Patrick, C. J. (2002). Suicide risk in externalizing syndromes: Temperamental and neurobiological underpinnings. In T. Joiner & M. T. Rudd (Eds.), *Suicide science: Expanding the boundaries* (pp. 137–173). Norwell, MA: Kluwer.

Verona, E., Patrick, C. J., & Joiner, T. E. (2001). Psychopathy, antisocial personality, and suicide risk. *Journal of Abnormal Psychology, 110*(3), 462–470.

Verona, E., & Vitale, J. (2006). Psychopathy in women: Assessment, manifestations, and etiology. In C. J. Patrick (Ed.), *Handbook of psychopathy* (pp. 415–436). New York: Guilford Press.

Wall, T. D., Wygant, D. B., & Sellbom, M. (2015). Boldness explains a key difference between psychopathy and antisocial personality disorder. *Psychiatry, Psychology, and Law, 22,* 94–105.

Walters, G. D. (2003). Predicting criminal justice outcomes with the Psychopathy Checklist—Revised and Lifestyle Criminality Screening Form: A meta-analytic comparison. *Behavioral Sciences and the Law, 21,* 89–102.

Whitehead, J. T., & Lab, S. P. (1989). A meta-analysis of juvenile correctional treatment. *Journal of Research on Crime and Delinquency, 26,* 276–295.

Widiger, T. A., & Clark, L. A. (2000). Toward DSM-V and the classification of psychopathology. *Psychological Bulletin, 126*(6), 946–963.

Wilson, D. B., Bouffard, L. A., & MacKenzie, D. L. (2005). A quantitative review of structured, group-oriented, cognitive-behavioral programs for offenders. *Criminal Justice and Behavior, 32,* 172–204.

Wong, S. C. P., Gordon, A., Gu, D., Lewis, K., & Olver, M. E. (2012). The effectiveness of violence reduction treatment for psychopathic offenders: Empirical evidence and a treatment model. *International Journal of Forensic Mental Health, 11,* 336–349.

Yochelson, S., & Samenow, S. E. (1976). *The criminal personality: Vol. 1. A profile for change.* New York: Jason Aronson.

Yochelson, S., & Samenow, S. E. (1977). *The criminal personality: Vol. 2. The change process.* New York: Jason Aronson.

Young, S. E., Friedman, N. P., Miyake, A., Willcutt, E. G., Corley, R. P., Haberstick, B. C., et al. (2009). Behavioral disinhibition: Liability for externalizing spectrum disorders and its genetic and environmental relation to response inhibition across adolescence. *Journal of Abnormal Psychology, 118*(1), 117–130.

# CHAPTER 26

# Obsessive–Compulsive Personality Disorder and Component Personality Traits

Anthony Pinto, Emily Ansell, Michael G. Wheaton, Robert F. Krueger,
Leslie Morey, Andrew E. Skodol, and Lee Anna Clark

Obsessive–compulsive personality disorder (OCPD) involves a chronic maladaptive pattern of excessive perfectionism, preoccupation with orderliness and detail, and need for control over one's environment that leads to significant distress or impairment, particularly in areas of interpersonal functioning (de Reus & Emmelkamp, 2012). Coworkers, friends, and family often describe individuals with OCPD as overly rigid and controlling. They may find it difficult to relax, feel obligated to plan out their activities to the minute, and find unstructured time intolerable (Pinto, Eisen, Mancebo, & Rasmussen, 2008).

This chapter consists of two sections. The first reviews research on OCPD as a diagnostic category and evidence for its validity. The validators used, symptom description, prevalence, functional impairment, course of illness, comorbidity with other disorders, treatment response, temperamental antecedents, familiality, genetic risk factors, and neural substrates are based on and extend those proposed by Robins and Guze (1970) and subsequently by others (e.g., Kendler, Gardner, & Prescott, 2002). DSM-5 Work Groups used these validators to inform their decision making about the validity of individual syndromes, as well as relatedness among disorders. The second section is a review of traits either definitionally or theoretically linked to OCPD, and how these traits relate to clinical outcomes.

## Obsessive–Compulsive Personality Disorder

### Clinical Description

#### Symptoms

DSM-5 (American Psychiatric Association [APA], 2013) defines OCPD as "a pervasive pattern of preoccupation with orderliness, perfectionism, and mental and interpersonal control, at the expense of flexibility, openness, and efficiency," as indicated by the presence of at least four of the following eight criteria: (1) preoccupation with details, rules, lists, order, organization perfectionism; (2) perfectionism that interferes with task completion; (3) excessive devotion to work and productivity to the exclusion of leisure activities and friendships; (4) inflexibility about matters of morality, ethics, or values; (5) inability to discard worn-out or worthless items; (6) reluctance to delegate tasks or work to others unless they submit to the individual's way of doing things; (7) miserliness toward both self and others; and (8) rigidity and stubbornness. While the DSM-5 maintained the DSM-IV definition of OCPD, the diagnostic criteria for OCPD have undergone substantial changes with previous DSM revisions, which have posed obstacles to studying the disorder. For example, DSM-IV dropped two DSM-III-R (American Psychiatric Association, 1987) criteria—restricted expression of affection and indecisiveness—because of their poor specificity (Pfohl, 1996), and added a criterion for reluctance to delegate.

Section III of DSM-5, which reports on emerging measures and models needing further study, proposes a radical reconceptualization of personality disorders (PDs) broadly. This revision is based on a hybrid dimensional–categorical model, designed to account for the normal variation in personality traits in the population, while retaining diagnostic categories to describe individuals with personality pathology. In order to meet criteria for a PD according to this model, an individual must have significant impairment in personality functioning, manifested as difficulties in at least two of four possible domains: identity, self-direction, empathy, and intimacy. Individuals who meet criteria for a PD can be further characterized into one of six PD types based on the presence of characteristic pathological personality traits, which the DSM conceptualizes as the extreme poles of the five-factor model of personality (FFM) and Personality Psychopathology Five (PSY-5) models (APA, 2013). For example, on the continuum that ranges between disinhibition and conscientiousness, DSM-5 identifies *rigid perfectionism* as an aspect of extreme conscientiousness. The pathological trait rigid perfectionism is a requirement for an OCPD diagnosis according to the alternative model. In addition, patients must also meet criteria for at least one other characteristic OCPD pathological personality trait: perseveration (persistence at the same behavior despite repeated failures), intimacy avoidance (difficulty with close relationships, interpersonal attachments and sexual relationships), and restricted affectivity (constricted emotional experience and expression).

The alternative model represents a significant change compared to the previous criteria, which were maintained for official diagnosis (Diedrich & Voderholzer, 2015). Specifically, whereas the official diagnosis can be made with any combination of symptoms, the alternative OCPD conceptualization is hierarchical, in that all individuals must meet the rigid perfectionism criterion in order to be diagnosed. In addition, the set of alternative diagnostic criteria drops two of the official criteria: (1) inability to discard worn out or worthless items and (2) miserliness. These two deletions are in line with previous research, as difficulty discarding is associated with hoarding, which the DSM-5 now categorizes as an independent disorder (APA, 2013), and miserliness has been found to be one of the least stable OCPD criteria over time (McGlashan et al., 2005).

The implications of the changes made in these alternative criteria are not yet clear. For example, as Starcevic and Brakoulias (2014) observe, the alternative criteria appear to be "stricter," as fewer combinations of symptoms would qualify for the diagnosis. This change aims to narrow the OCPD phenotype, but it also means that some individuals who would meet existing DSM-IV/DSM-5 criteria would no longer be diagnosed under the alternative model, which may affect OCPD prevalence estimates in the community. In addition, the alternative conceptualization introduces several new criteria: intimacy avoidance, restricted affectivity, and perseveration. Therefore, psychometric work on the validity and reliability of these additional criteria represents a pressing need. The APA Board of Trustees ultimately decided that the alternative model of PDs represented too large a change to be undertaken immediately, and instead retained the DSM-IV conceptualization for official clinical diagnoses. Research to validate the alternative model is in its nascent stages; therefore, the data reviewed in this chapter primarily utilize the official conceptualization of OCPD.

### Prevalence

DSM-5 reports that OCPD is one of the most common PDs in the general population, with an estimated prevalence ranging from 2.1 to 7.9% (APA, 2013), which is a substantial increase over DSM-IV, which reported a prevalence of about 1% in community samples (APA, 1994). The higher prevalence rate reported in DSM-5 is in line with community studies, although prevalence estimates vary considerably. OCPD had the highest median prevalence (2.1%) across 12 epidemiological studies (Torgersen, 2009) and an estimated prevalence of 2.4% in the National Comorbidity Survey Replication study (NCS-R; Lenzenweger, Lane, Loranger, & Kessler, 2007). However, the National Epidemiologic Survey on Alcohol and Related Conditions (NESARC; Grant, Mooney, & Kushner, 2012) reported a rate of 7.8%. OCPD is also one of the most frequently diagnosed PDs in clinical samples—both among outpatients (13.1%: Stuart et al., 1998; 8.7: Zimmerman, Rothschild, & Chelminski, 2005) and inpatients (28.3%: Rossi, Marinangeli, Butti, Kalyvoka, & Petruzzi, 2000). Despite its prevalence, OCPD remains an underrecognized phenomenon in the community. For example, a recent community survey found very low recognition rates for OCPD, with participants much more likely to correctly identify depression, schizophrenia and obsessive–compulsive disorder (OCD) (Koutoufa & Furnham, 2014).

Although OCPD is described by DSM-5 as occurring twice as often in men as in women, support for this contention is limited, with some studies finding significant differences (Maier, Lichtermann, Klinger, Heun, & Hallmayer, 1992; Torgersen, Kringlen, & Cramer, 2001; Zimmerman & Coryell, 1989), while others find less dramatic or no gender differences (Albert, Maina, Forner, & Bogetto, 2004; Alnaes & Torgersen, 1988; Ekselius, Bodlund, von Knorring, Lindstrom, & Kullgren, 1996; Grant, Mooney, & Kushner, 2012; Gunderson et al., 2000; Morey, Warner, & Boggs, 2002). In an analysis of individual DSM-III-R criteria, Ekselius and colleagues (1996) found that only one criterion, "lack of generosity in giving," displayed gender differences, demonstrating the stated 2:1 male:female ratio. Interestingly, this criterion underwent considerable revision in the transition to DSM-IV-TR ("adopts a miserly spending style"), and this revised criterion did not display a gender difference in more recent studies (Jane, Oltmanns, South, & Turkheimer, 2007; Morey, Warner, et al., 2002), which suggests that gender differences may be smaller under DSM-IV-TR criteria. One study did report a greater propensity for males to be diagnosed with OCPD in a sample of individuals with a history of depression (Light et al., 2006).

Studies of the prevalence of OCPD cross-culturally have produced mixed results. An early study employing DSM-III criteria reported similar prevalence rates across five culturally diverse U.S. communities (Karno, Golding, Sorenson, & Burnam, 1988). Similarly, Chavira and colleagues (2003) reported no differences in OCPD prevalence rates by ethnicity in a clinical sample. In contrast, two nationally representative surveys (Grant et al., 2004, 2012) reported that OCPD was significantly less common in Asians and Hispanics than in European Americans and African Americans. However, in a recent study that recruited participants from a community mental center in a Hispanic community, Ansell and colleagues (2010) reported an OCPD prevalence estimate of 26%, which suggests that OCPD may be common in Hispanic outpatient samples.

## Functional Impairment

Significant functional impairment is common in individuals with OCPD (de Reus & Emmelkamp, 2012). For example, in the Collaborative Longitudinal Personality Disorders Study (CLPS) intake sample, nearly 90% of individuals with OCPD were rated as having at least moderate impairment in one or more areas of functioning (e.g., occupational, interpersonal relationships, recreation) or received a global assessment of functioning rating of 60 or less (Skodol et al., 2002). Interestingly, in a 2-year follow-up study, Skodol and colleagues (2005) found that improvement in OCPD pathology, defined as the proportion decrease in the number of criteria met from baseline to follow-up, was not reflected in improvements in functional impairment. A recent study using well-validated measures of quality of life and psychosocial functioning found equivalent levels of impairment in psychosocial functioning and quality of life in patients with OCPD compared to those with OCD (Pinto, Steinglass, Greene, Weber, & Simpson, 2014).

As with other PDs, impaired interpersonal functioning is a hallmark feature of OCPD. Clinical descriptions note that interpersonal conflicts frequently occur, often triggered by impossibly high standards for the behavior of others, difficulty acknowledging differing viewpoints, and rigidity (Pollak, 1987). Millon (1981) also notes that individuals with OCPD may be uncompromising and demanding, and OCPD has been linked with outbursts of anger and hostility, both at home and at work (Villemarette-Pittman, Stanford, Greve, Houston, & Mathias, 2004). In a recent study investigating interpersonal functioning in OCPD, Cain, Ansell, Simpson, and Pinto (2015) found that individuals with OCPD reported hostile-dominant interpersonal problems and sensitivities with warm-dominant behavior by others, as well as less empathic perspective taking relative to healthy controls, which may underlie some of the interpersonal problems described earlier.

In addition, OCPD has been associated with increased suicidal risk in patients with mood disorders (Raja & Azzoni, 2007). Diaconu and Turecki (2009) found that among depressed patients, individuals with OCPD reported increased current and lifetime suicidal ideation and more lifetime suicide attempts. Of special clinical concern, depressed patients with OCPD reported fewer reasons for living and less anxiety on a fear of death questionnaire, both prognostic indicators of suicide (Diaconu & Turecki, 2009). A study of the economic burden of PDs found that, along with borderline PD (BPD), OCPD is associated with the highest total economic burden in terms of direct medical costs and productivity losses of all PDs (Soeteman, Hakkaart-van Roijen, Verheul, & Busschbach, 2008).

In contrast, studies utilizing community samples have found that OCPD is not significantly associated with reduced quality of life (Cramer, Torgersen, & Kringlen, 2007); in fact, Ullrich, Farrington, and Coid (2007) found that obsessive–compulsive (and narcissistic) traits were associated with higher levels of status and wealth. Together, these data suggest that there is a range of functioning in people with OCPD: Those who seek evaluation or treatment in a clinical setting are logically more impaired and warrant help.

## Course

PDs are usually not diagnosed in childhood, but several studies have investigated the presence of OCPD traits in children. For example, Bernstein and colleagues (1993) reported that 13.5% of children ages 9–19 endorsed criteria for OCPD, making it the most frequent disorder in a large community sample. However, another study reported a very low rate of OCPD (Lewinsohn, Rohde, Seeley, & Klein, 1997). In line with this finding, a recent epidemiological study found that OCPD was less prevalent in younger individuals (aged 20–29), than in individuals older than 30 (Grant et al., 2012). One possible explanation for these somewhat conflicting reports is that some OCPD traits may manifest in childhood, but not become full blown until later in life. In line with this possibility, a recent retrospective study revealed that individuals with OCPD tend to view their traits as beginning in childhood. Pinto, Greene, Storch, and Simpson (2015) reported that adults with DSM-IV OCPD endorsed higher rates of childhood obsessive–compulsive personality traits (including perfectionism, inflexibility, and drive for order) compared to matched healthy controls.

The DSM suggests that PDs are stable across time, yet evidence for the temporal stability of OCPD diagnoses is mixed. In a follow-up study of adolescents with PDs, only 32% of those initially diagnosed with OCPD met criteria 2 years later (Bernstein et al., 1993). Importantly however, this study employed DSM-III criteria and did not report on the temporal stability of particular OCPD symptoms (e.g., rigidity and perfectionism), so it cannot be determined precisely whether these traits changed, or whether changing situational circumstances modified how problematic these traits were. Global OCPD severity predicted continued OCPD diagnosis, as odds ratios indicated that children were four times as likely to retain the OCPD diagnosis at the 2-year follow-up if they had been diagnosed initially with moderate levels of OCPD, and 15 times more likely to continue to have the diagnosis if they initially had severe symptoms. In a subsequent longitudinal study with a much longer follow-up window (12–18 years), Nestadt and colleagues (2010) found OCPD to have appreciable stability (intraclass correlation [ICC] estimate = 0.2–0.3). However, OCPD was less stable than some other PDs (antisocial, avoidant, borderline, histrionic, and schizotypal ICC estimate = 0.4–0.8). A notable limitation of these studies is that they employed DSM-III criteria, which may be less reliable and valid (Pfohl, 1996).

In the CLPS, which employed DSM-IV criteria, 38% of the participants with OCPD at baseline remitted (using a stringent definition of 12 consecutive months with two or fewer criteria) during the initial 24-month follow-up period (Grilo et al., 2004). The presence of three of the DSM-IV OCPD criteria—preoccupation with details, rigidity, and reluctance to delegate—were the strongest predictors of a continued OCPD diagnosis after 2 years (Grilo et al., 2004). Over the 2-year follow-up, rigidity, reluctance to delegate, and perfectionism were the most prevalent and stable OCPD criteria, whereas miserliness and hypermorality were least prevalent and stable (McGlashan et al., 2005). The CLPS findings point to DSM-IV OCPD as a hybrid consisting of criteria representing more stable personality traits linked to criteria that represent less stable, or intermittently expressed, symptomatic behaviors or manifestations (McGlashan et al.,

2005). Traits are known to be dimensional in nature and expression, ranging from adaptive variants to pathological exaggerations in PDs (Clark, 2007). For OCPD, such traits seem to account for most of the predictive relationship of the disorder to functional outcomes over 10-year follow-up (Morey et al., 2012). Meanwhile, symptomatic behaviors are conceptualized as behavioral manifestations of underlying traits. The presence and severity of the problematic behaviors used to compensate for pathological traits may vary with both situational factors (life events) and intrapsychic factors (increased stress).

## Comorbidity

In the CLPS intake sample, the most common lifetime comorbid Axis I conditions for individuals with OCPD were major depression (75.8%), generalized anxiety disorder (29.4%), alcohol abuse/dependence (29.4%), substance abuse/dependence (25.7%), and OCD (20.9%) (McGlashan et al., 2000). With regard to Axis II, the most common comorbid PD by far in the OCPD sample was avoidant PD (27.5%), followed by borderline (9.2%), paranoid (7.9%), and narcissistic PDs (7.2%) (McGlashan et al., 2000).

Studies using DSM-IV criteria have consistently found elevated rates of OCPD in OCD, with estimates ranging from 23 to 34% (Albert et al., 2004; Garyfallos et al., 2010; Lochner et al., 2011; Pinto, Mancebo, Eisen, Pagano, & Rasmussen, 2006; Samuels et al., 2000; Tenney, Schotte, Denys, van Megen, & Westenberg, 2003) in comparison to rates of OCPD in community samples. In the CLPS, 21% of subjects with DSM-IV OCPD met criteria for OCD (McGlashan et al., 2000). Recent data and clinical observations suggest that the presence of comorbid OCPD increases the morbidity of OCD: Compared to those without comorbid OCPD, individuals with OCD and comorbid OCPD experience younger age at onset of first OCD symptoms, poorer psychosocial functioning despite no difference in OCD severity (Coles, Pinto, Mancebo, Rasmussen, & Eisen, 2008; Garyfallos et al., 2010), more severe cognitive inflexibility (Fineberg, Sharma, Sivakumaran, Sahakian, & Chamberlain, 2007), poorer insight (Lochner et al., 2011), more depression and alcohol abuse (Gordon, Salkovskis, Oldfield, & Carter, 2013), and lower likelihood of OCD remission after 2 years (Pinto, 2009). Cavedini, Erzegovesi, Ronchi, and Bellodi (1997) reported a worse outcome for patients with OCD and comorbid DSM-III-R OCPD, as compared to those without OCPD, after 10 weeks of selective serotonin reuptake inhibitor (SSRI) treatment (either clomipramine or fluvoxamine). The authors concluded that comorbid OCPD may identify a subtype of OCD with a different pattern of SSRI response. Only one study has examined the impact of OCPD on exposure and response prevention (EX/RP) outcome for OCD. Among outpatients with primary OCD, OCPD diagnosis and greater OCPD severity (defined as the number of clinically significant DSM-IV OCPD criteria present at baseline) predicted worse EX/RP outcome (Pinto, Liebowitz, Foa, & Simpson, 2011). Of all the OCPD criteria, the presence of perfectionism was most strongly associated with poor EX/RP outcome.

The presence of OCPD has been shown to affect the prognosis of other mental disorders adversely. The presence of childhood OCP traits is an important risk factor for the development of eating disorders, with the estimated odds ratio for eating disorders increasing by a factor of 6.9 for every additional trait present. Subjects with eating disorders who reported perfectionism and rigidity in childhood had significantly higher rates of OCPD and OCD comorbidity later in life, compared with subjects with eating disorders who did not report those traits (Anderluh, Tchanturia, Rabe-Hesketh, & Treasure, 2003). In a large epidemiological study, OCPD and paranoid PD were the only PDs associated with reduced probability of remission from early-onset chronic depression (Agosti, Hellerstein, & Stewart, 2009). In prospective studies of adolescent-onset anorexia nervosa, OCPD has been associated with longer duration of illness (Strober, Freeman, & Morrell, 1997; Wentz, Gillberg, Anckarsater, Gillberg, & Rastam, 2009). In a randomized controlled trial of adolescent anorexia nervosa, patients with high levels of OCPD traits did more poorly in short-term than in long-term family therapy (Lock, Agras, Bryson, & Kraemer, 2005). OCPD also has been associated with higher risk of relapse in both depression (Grilo et al., 2010) and generalized anxiety disorder (Ansell et al., 2011). Among patients with borderline PD in the CLPS, low global functioning and more OCPD criteria reported at baseline predicted greater borderline personality pathology at 2-year follow-up (Gunderson et al., 2006).

## Etiology

Little is known about specific and general environmental risk factors or precursors that contribute to the development of OCPD. As compared to healthy controls and other psychiatric outpatients, patients with OCPD retrospectively report receiving less parental care and greater parental overprotection (Nordahl & Stiles, 1997). As with other PDs, high rates of childhood abuse and neglect have also been reported (Battle et al., 2004). However, within the CLPS sample, a unique association emerged between diagnosis of OCPD and a reported history of sexual abuse by a non-caretaking adult (Battle et al., 2004). Maladaptive perfectionism in childhood has also been described as a risk factor for later OCPD diagnosis (Franklin, Piacentini, & D'Olio, 2007).

## Biological Studies

Though severely limited, and with much research still needed, studies in the areas of family history, genetics, brain circuitry, neurochemistry, and neuropsychology have given clues to the biological etiology of OCPD.

## Family History

In a twin study using DSM-III-R, Torgersen and colleagues (2000) found a heritability estimate of 0.8 for OCPD (and 0.6 for PDs in general), which is higher than for most Axis I disorders, yet similar to that of OCD. Relations of OCPD to anorexia nervosa and OCD have been underscored by family study data, suggesting common family-based etiological factor(s). The first-degree relatives of restricting-type anorexia probands (all of whom were female) were found to have elevated rates of OCPD (compared to the relatives of normal controls), regardless of the presence of OCPD in the probands themselves (Lilenfeld et al., 1998). Strober, Freeman, Lampert, and Diamond (2007) found that relatives of probands with anorexia nervosa had a threefold greater risk of OCPD compared with relatives of never-ill controls. This familial aggregation remained significant when regression models were adjusted for the presence of OCPD in the proband and for lifetime presence of eating disorder in the relatives. The first-degree relatives of OCD probands were twice as likely to have OCPD as compared to the relatives of control probands (Samuels et al., 2000). In addition, several studies have reported increased frequencies of OCPD traits in the parents of pediatric OCD probands versus the parents of healthy children (Calvo et al., 2009; Lenane et al., 1990; Swedo, Rapoport, Leonard, Lenane, & Cheslow, 1989).

## Genetics

As mentioned, the first twin study of OCPD heritability found the disorder to be highly heritable (Torgersen et al., 2000). A more recent Norwegian, population-based study of twins applied dimensional representations of Cluster C DSM-IV PDs, and using ordinal variables based on the number of criteria endorsed instead of categorical diagnoses, found that genetic effects (both common to the other Cluster C PDs and disorder specific) account for 27% of the variance in OCPD (Reichborn-Kjennerud et al., 2007). In this study, genetic and environmental influences on OCPD were mostly specific to this PD, differentiating the disorder from the others in Cluster C. A subsequent study revealed that of the 10 DSM-IV PDs, disorder-specific genetic effects had their strongest influence on OCPD (Kendler et al., 2008). A recent longitudinal twin study found DSM-IV diagnoses to be moderately stable over time, with genetic factors contributing more than unique environmental factors to the stability of OCPD diagnoses over a 10-year follow-up (Gjerde et al., 2015).

The only study to investigate the role of the serotonin transporter polymorphism (*5-HTTL-PR*) in OCPD found no differences in allelic frequencies between OCPD and controls (Perez, Brown, Vrshek-Schallhorn, Johnson, & Joiner, 2006). Light and colleagues (2006) reported preliminary evidence that individuals with a dopamine $D_3$ receptor gene polymorphism (Gly/Gly genotype) are 2.4 times more likely to be diagnosed with OCPD.

## Brain Circuitry

No studies have investigated imaging abnormalities in patients with a principal diagnosis of OCPD.

## Neurochemistry

A study of serotonergic function in males with DSM-III OCPD found that OCPD criteria correlate negatively with prolactin response to fenfluramine, a marker of serotonergic dysfunction (Stein et al., 1996). Those with OCPD showed significantly blunted prolactin responses to fenfluramine compared with other patients with PD and normal controls. Prolactin blunting after fenfluramine also has been reported in several studies of OCD (Hewlett, Vinogradov, Martin, Berman, & Csernansky, 1992; Lucey, O'Keane, Butcher, Clare, & Dinan, 1992).

## Neuropsychology

Few studies have examined neurocognitive functioning in relation to OCPD, and much of the extant research to date has been conducted in student samples. For example, performance deficits on a nonverbal measure of executive control and working memory were related to OCP traits in a student sample, lending support to the contention that specific OCP traits may represent, at least in part, compensatory tactics that evolve in response to executive control deficits (Aycicegi-Dinn, Dinn, & Caldwell-Harris, 2009). Consistent with descriptions of a detail-oriented attentional style in OCPD (Shapiro, 1965), OCP traits in another student sample were associated with local interference: excessive visual attention to small local aspects of stimuli ("trees") when trying to identify their global aspects ("forest") (Yovel, Revelle, & Mineka, 2005). Local interference was associated particularly with perfectionism. In a study of attentional coping style, students with high levels of OCP traits engaged in more information-seeking behaviors, demonstrating difficulty in tolerating uncertainty relative to controls (Gallagher, South, & Oltmanns, 2003). In a study of adults age 55 years or older, depressed subjects with OCPD became considerably more risk-averse as a gambling task progressed, compared with controls (Chapman et al., 2007). The severity of OCPD features, rather than depression, accounted for increased risk aversion in this group. The findings support the notion that OCPD is characterized by a conservative, cautious response style that can be counterproductive. In addition, some limited neurocognitive data in patients with OCD and comorbid OCPD suggest possible deficits in cognitive flexibility on tasks associated with dorsolateral prefrontal cortex function (Aycicegi, Dinn, & Harris, 2002; Fineberg et al., 2007).

Recently, Pinto and colleagues (2014) compared individuals with OCPD and OCD on a self-control task designed to probe individuals' capacity to delay reward. Comparing patients diagnosed with DSM-IV OCPD ($N = 25$), OCD ($N = 25$), both OCD and OCPD ($N = 25$) and healthy controls ($N = 25$), they reported group differences on an intertemporal choice task that had participants decide between a smaller amount of money immediately or a larger amount offered later in time. Relative to patients with OCD and healthy controls, patients with OCPD (including those with comorbid OCD) had a greater capacity to delay reward, suggesting that patients with OCPD may exhibit excessive self-control (overcontrol). This is consistent with the behavioral presentation of many patients who can be miserly and controlling of their environment. Another recent investigation compared the neurocognitive profile of 21 adults meeting DSM-IV OCPD criteria and found that this group demonstrated cognitive inflexibility and executive planning deficits relative to 15 healthy controls on the Cambridge Automated Neuropsychological Test Battery (Fineberg et al., 2015).

## Treatment

Studies show that individuals with OCPD have higher levels of treatment utilization even after controlling for lifetime Axis I disorders. They are three times as likely to receive individual psychotherapy than patients with major depressive disorder (Bender et al., 2001) and show high rates of primary care utilization (Sansone, Hendricks, Sellbom, & Reddington, 2003). Despite this increased use of the health care system, to date, there is no empirically validated "gold standard" treatment for OCPD. In the only randomized placebo-controlled trial of pharmacotherapy in OCPD, Ansseau (1997) tested the therapeutic utility of fluvoxamine in OCPD without associated depression. In this unpublished study, patients were randomly assigned to either fluvoxamine (50 mg during the first week, then 100 mg) ($N = 12$) or placebo ($N = 12$) in double-blind conditions. Results showed a significant effect of fluvoxamine over placebo after 3 months. Below is a review of the limited psychotherapy research literature in OCPD.

### Psychodynamic Psychotherapy

Psychodynamic treatment for OCPD involves an insight-oriented approach that attempts to reveal how the OCPD symptoms function to defend the individual against internal feelings of insecurity and uncertainty. With this insight, patients then work to change their inflexible patterns of behavior and give up their rigid demands for perfection. One uncontrolled study suggests that supportive–expressive psychodynamic therapy is effective for patients with PDs, including OCPD (Barber, Morse, Krakauer, Chittams, & Crits-Christoph, 1997). This study included 14 patients with OCPD and found significant improvement after 52 sessions, but it did not include a control group. Two subsequent trials found that mixed groups of patients with PDs (including some patients with OCPD) treated with brief psychodynamic treatments improved in terms of general functioning relative to wait-list control groups (Abbass, Sheldon, Gyra, & Kalpin, 2008; Winston et al., 1994). However, neither study specifically investigated improvement among those with OCPD, and the study outcomes did not assess for changes in OCPD symptoms specifically.

## Cognitive Therapy

The cognitive approach to treating OCPD involves identifying and restructuring the dysfunctional thoughts underlying maladaptive behaviors (Bailey, 1998; Beck & Freeman, 1990; Beck, 1997). For example, patients are taught to challenge "all-or-nothing" thinking by considering the range of acceptable possibilities and to recognize instances in which they overestimate the consequences of mistakes (catastrophizing) by examining the realistic significance of minor errors. Some approaches also incorporate behavioral elements, such as behavioral experiments (e.g., purposefully making small mistakes in order to observe the actual consequences) (Sperry, 2003). Establishing rapport can be difficult with some patients due to their rigid thinking styles and difficulty with emotional expression. In light of this difficulty, Young's (1999) schema-focused therapy aims to identify and restructure patients' maladaptive schemas as they are expressed in the therapy process.

Although several cognitive and behavioral approaches to OCPD have been described (Kyrios, 1998), little empirical research has been conducted to test them. In an uncontrolled trial conducted in Hong Kong Chinese patients, Ng (2005) recruited individuals with treatment-refractory depression who also met DSM-IV criteria for OCPD and offered cognitive therapy focusing on OCPD. Ten patients were treated, and after a mean of 22.4 sessions, all showed reductions in depression and anxiety symptoms, and nine no longer met diagnostic criteria for OCPD. However, this study did not include a control group, and the sample size was small. Strauss and colleagues (2006) conducted an open trial of cognitive therapy among outpatients with avoidant PD ($N = 24$) and OCPD ($N = 16$), who received up to 52 weekly sessions. Of the patients with OCPD, results indicated that 83% had clinically significant reductions in OCPD symptom severity, and 53% had clinically significant improvement in depression severity. However, this open trial did not include a comparison condition, such as a wait-list control group or alternative treatment, precluding a firm conclusion about the efficacy of cognitive therapy for OCPD.

The largest ever treatment study for OCPD was an open trial that involved 116 outpatients with DSM-IV OCPD, who received 10 weekly sessions of group CBT (Enero et al., 2013). The authors reported that baseline distress was a significant predictor of who responded to this treatment but, notably, they did not include a control group.

Few data exist to compare the effectiveness of cognitive therapy with psychodynamic treatment. In one study, Svartberg, Stiles, and Seltzer (2004) randomized Cluster C patients to receive 40 treatment sessions of either cognitive therapy ($N = 25$) or short-term psychodynamic treatment ($N = 25$). Avoidant PD was the most frequent diagnosis in the sample, though OCPD was also represented, with eight individuals in the cognitive therapy group (32%) and nine in the psychodynamic group (36%) meeting DSM-III criteria. The results revealed that both groups significantly improved on measures of symptom distress, interpersonal problems, and core personality pathology after treatment and at 2-year follow-up. Both treatments were equally effective. However, this study did not specifically report on the improvements seen in the patients with OCPD.

## Alternative Psychotherapies

Other treatments have been explored in single-case studies. For example, two case studies have reported using adaptations of metacognitive therapy (Dimaggio et al., 2011; Fiore, Dimaggio, Nicolo, Semerari, & Carcione, 2008). Metacognitive therapy aims to improve individuals' ability to understand mental states, enhancing awareness of their own emotions, while also improving empathy and interpersonal functioning. This form of psychotherapy would seem well suited to the interpersonal problems frequently observed in individuals with OCPD, but more testing is needed. Lynch and Cheavens (2008) described an adaption of dialectical behavioral therapy (DBT) designed to target cognitive rigidity and emotional constriction, and report on its successful implementation with one individual with OCPD. DBT and other so-called "third wave" cognitive-behavioral treatments, such as acceptance and commitment therapy (ACT), have shown promise for the treatment of PDs (Ost, 2008). However, systematic evaluation of these treatments for OCPD is needed. Pinto (2016) described a case study of an individual with OCPD successfully treated with a combination of emotion regulation skills, as well as CBT targeting perfectionism, raising the possibility that psychotherapy for OCPD might be improved by incorporating elements from both traditional and "third wave" approaches.

## Construct Validity

### Factor Structure of OCPD

Clinical observations consistently have highlighted the multifactorial nature of OCPD. Freud (1908/1963) described a triad of "anal character" traits: orderliness, parsimony, and obstinacy. Shapiro (1965) emphasized the OCPD thinking style in terms of cognitive rigidity and tense deliberateness. Millon (1981) identified three self-perpetuating processes, including pervasive rigidity, adherence to rules and regulations, and guilt and self-criticism, that serve to maintain and reinforce OCPD patterns by limiting the acquisition of new perceptions of the world and the learning of more flexible strategies for living. Pollak (1987) pointed to exaggerated attempts at control over self, others, and the environment.

Factor analyses have suggested a two- or three-factor solution of OCPD. Among patients with OCD, Baer (1994) reported a two-factor solution based on the nine DSM-III OCPD criteria. The first factor included perfectionism, preoccupation with details, indecision, restricted affection, and inability to discard, whereas the second factor included rigidity, hypermorality, work devotion, and miserliness. Using DSM-IV OCPD criteria, Grilo (2004) identified a three-factor solution in a clinical sample of individuals with binge-eating disorder (BED): "rigidity" [interpersonal control and resistance to change] (consisting of rigidity, reluctance to delegate, hypermorality), "perfectionism" [cognitive or intrapersonal control] (preoccupation with details, perfectionism, work devotion), and "miserliness" (miserliness, inability to discard). Ansell, Pinto, Edelen, and Grilo (2008) followed up with a confirmatory factor analysis in a patient sample with BED and found that the miserliness factor was problematic in fit and underidentified in the analysis. The authors concluded that a two-factor solution may best represent the core pathology of OCPD. In a large day-treatment sample, Hummelen, Wilberg, Pedersen, and Karterud (2008) applied an exploratory factor analysis to all DSM-IV PD criteria and noted that the OCPD criteria fell on two factors. The first factor (perfectionism) is consistent with prior factor-analytic studies. However, the second factor (aggressiveness) included criteria from borderline (inappropriate or excessive anger), paranoid (counterattacks) and antisocial (physical aggression) PD diagnoses. The authors were also not able to replicate Grilo's (2004) three-factor model in their data using confirmatory factor analysis. Finally, Ansell and colleagues (2010) tested multifactor models of OCPD in a Hispanic psychiatric outpatient sample and found the best fit for two factors: perfectionism and interpersonal rigidity. Validation of these factors revealed differential relationships with clinical correlates, with interpersonal rigidity being associated with aggression and anger, whereas perfectionism was associated with depression and suicidal thoughts.

Huprich, Zimmerman, and Chelminski (2006) conducted an exploratory principal components analysis of the SIDP-IV avoidant, borderline, depressive, and OCPD criteria from 1,200 psychiatric outpatients to determine the inherent clustering or associations of the symptoms of these disorders. They found that avoidant and OCPD symptoms clustered in ways that may reflect a problem in how to engage with others, suggestive of an approach–avoidance conflict.

### Psychometric Properties of DSM-IV OCPD Criteria

Farmer and Chapman (2002) noted weaknesses in the psychometric properties (e.g., sensitivity, specificity, predictive power) of the DSM-IV OCPD criteria. Findings by Cooper, Balsis, and Zimmerman (2010) suggest that the criteria are differentially related to the latent construct, with some criteria only marginally related and in need of revision. Grilo, Sanislow, and colleagues (2004; Grilo et al., 2001) and Hummelen and colleagues (2008) found diagnostic efficiencies of the OCPD criteria to be variable and questioned the utility of some criteria. Specifically, these studies found preoccupation with details/order and perfectionism to be among the criteria that performed best, whereas hoarding behavior and miserliness performed poorest. Hertler (2013) outlined problems with the sensitivity and specificity of the DSM-IV OCPD criteria, noting that the lack of hallmark criteria and use of polythetic criteria make DSM-IV OCPD an indistinct diagnostic category marked by heterogeneous presentations.

Hummelen and colleagues (2008) noted that the quality of OCPD as a PD prototype category may be improved by deleting the two weakest criteria and replacing them with criteria about interpersonal difficulties (and specifically, the need for predictability in relationships), an important aspect of OCPD that was missing in the DSM-IV conceptualization. In summary, research suggests substantial variability in how well individual criteria map onto the core OCPD construct. As such, researchers have been shifting away from the categorical presence–absence of OCPD in favor of dimensional models of particular OCP traits (Pinto & Eisen, 2012).

## Traits Theoretically Linked to OCPD

Research on the traits that have been linked to OCPD has established their utility in understanding clinical phenomena and dysfunction. Traits linked to OCPD based on theoretical models include conscientiousness, neuroticism, orderliness, perfectionism, rigidity, overcommitment, and inhibition versus disinhibition. We review each of these traits here.

### The FFM: Conscientiousness and Neuroticism

Considerable research on personality traits and OCPD has focused on overlap with the FFM (Costa & Widiger, 1994). Using the consensus of experts, Lynam and Widiger (2001) proposed a combination of traits and facets within the model that would best represent OCPD relative to other disorders: high Neuroticism-facet anxiousness; low Neuroticism-facet impulsiveness; low Extraversion-facet excitement seeking; low Openness-facets of feeling, actions, ideas, and values; and high Agreeableness-facet modesty. All facets of Conscientiousness were expected to be elevated in patients with OCPD.

Although high Conscientiousness is proposed to be a distinguishing trait feature for OCPD (Lynam & Widiger, 2001), research has been less conclusive on this association. Hypothesized associations between the FFM and OCPD appear to depend on comparison groups. In the CLPS, which contains a large cohort of OCPD patients, Conscientiousness in patients with OCPD was relatively higher when compared to other patients with PDs, but lower when compared to community norms (Morey, Gunderson, et al., 2002). Associations between OCPD scales and the NEO Personality Inventory—Revised (NEO-PI-R) revealed that the majority of OCPD scales were correlated with higher domain Neuroticism and with specific facets: lower openness to actions and trust, greater order, dutifulness, and achievement striving (Samuel & Widiger, 2010). In an examination of trait and PD stability in the CLPS sample (Warner et al., 2004), models of lagged associations between FFM traits and OCPD indicate that, unlike other PDs, OCPD did not show any significant lagged effects between FFM OCPD trait change and disorder change. They concluded that traits underlying OCPD may lie outside the realm of personality captured within the FFM (Warner et al., 2004).

An additional consideration is that Conscientiousness is a multifaceted construct, with many of the facets exhibiting divergent associations with functioning variables (Roberts, Walton, & Bogg, 2005). One study identified six facets across measures of Conscientiousness, specifically industriousness, order, self-control, responsibility, traditionalism, and virtue. It may be that associations between Conscientiousness and OCPD depend on which facets underlie the version of Conscientiousness being measured, and the relative maladaptiveness of those facets. For example, orderliness has been identified as a trait facet of Conscientiousness (DeYoung, Quilty, & Peterson, 2007; Roberts & Bogg, 2004), perfectionism (Pearson & Gleaves, 2006), and OCPD (Lazare, Klerman, & Armor, 1966), but there has been little research on the psychological and functional consequences of orderliness, which makes it difficult to ascertain its utility in understanding the pathology of OCPD.

A meta-analysis of the structure of facets of impulsivity versus those of constraint/Conscientiousness (Sharma, Markon, & Clark, 2014) sheds some light on this issue. A correlated two-factor solution emerged with the first factor representing orderliness, NEO Conscientiousness-facet deliberation, and Neuroticism (vs. dysfunctional impulsivity; e.g., lack of forethought and planning), whereas the second factor was marked most strongly on one end by NEO achievement and the perseverance subscale of the UPPS Impulsive Behavior Scale (Whiteside & Lynam, 2001) as well as all other NEO Conscientiousness facets (orderliness and deliberation cross-loaded), plus workaholism and propriety (Clark, Lelchook, & Taylor, 2010) with Neuroticism marking the other end. They considered the first factor to represent maladaptive constraint (vs. impulsivity), and the second factor "will to achieve" (Digman & Takemoto-Chock, 1981) versus resourcelessness (Tyrer, Smith, McGrother, & Taub, 2007). Although both factors may be relevant in OCPD, they do so in distinct ways that, interestingly, had opposite relations with Neuroticism.

Research on the maladaptiveness of Conscientiousness and associations with functional impairment or psychopathology have been similarly inconclusive, with some research suggesting that high Conscientiousness is associated with improved health outcomes (Kern & Friedman, 2008). However, Samuel and Widiger (2011) found that Conscientiousness items that had been altered to be more extreme were associated with personality pathology. Further research is needed to determine what facets of Conscientiousness are associated with increased maladaptivity and whether alterations in the assessment of Conscientiousness have opened the construct up to overlap in variance from other traits (e.g., perfectionism or rigidity).

## Perfectionism

Trait perfectionism is a multidimensional construct with substantial empirical support for its relevance in psychopathology and functioning (Egan, Wade, & Shafran, 2011). Although the definitions of "perfectionism" vary, the general phenomenon is described as a need for perfection in behavior and presentation for both self and others (Hewitt, Flett, Besser, Sherry, & McGee, 2003). In children, perfectionism is associated with depression, anxiety, social stress, anger suppression, expression of anger, and suicidal behaviors (Boergers, Spirito, & Donaldson, 1998; Hewitt et al., 2002; Lapointe & Emond, 2005). Trait perfectionism has significant associations with psychopathology in adults, specifically, anxiety, depression, and eating disorders (Bieling, 2004; Blatt, 1995; Enns & Cox, 2005b; Hewitt, Norton, Flett, Callander, & Cowan, 1998; Lilenfeld, Wonderlich, Riso, Crosby, & Mitchell, 2006; Rice & Aldea, 2006; Shahar, Blatt, Zuroff, & Pilkonis, 2003; Shahar, Gallagher, Blatt, Kuperminc, & Leadbeater, 2004; Sutandar-Pinnock, 2003; Zuroff et al., 2000). Greater perfectionism was found in patients with eating disorders and OCPD than in patients with eating disorders and OCD (Halmi et al., 2005).

Perfectionism has considerable detrimental impact on the course of psychotherapy, particularly for depression (Blatt, Quinlan, Pilkonis, & Shea, 1995; Blatt, Zuroff, Bondi, Sanislow, & Pilkonis, 1998; Shahar et al., 2003) and OCD (Pinto et al., 2011). There is also evidence linking perfectionism with social dysfunction and interpersonal problems such as poorer marital adjustment (for both the individual and the partner) (Habke & Flynn, 2002; Haring, Hewitt, & Flett, 2003; Slaney, Pincus, Uliaszek, & Wang, 2006). In one study, only maladaptive perfectionism was associated with interpersonal problems (hostile dominant or friendly submissive), whereas adaptive perfectionism was associated with interpersonal adjustment (Slaney et al., 2006). Consistent with this, perfectionism was associated with difficulties in establishing relationships during treatment for depression (Shahar et al., 2003). Perfectionism effects appear to moderate the experience of stressful life events resulting in maladaptive outcomes (Enns & Cox, 2005a). This response may be due to perfectionism's moderation of the neuroendocrine stress response. Research examining acute stress responses (Wirtz et al., 2007) revealed that trait perfectionism is associated with hypothalamic–pituitary–adrenal (HPA) axis activation, specifically, greater cortisol response, when men are exposed to a psychosocial stressor. This effect remained even when controlling for anxiety and neuroticism, highlighting the unique influence of perfectionism on stress responses. Perfectionism also is associated with suicide-related outcomes (Blankstein, Lumley, & Crawford, 2007; Blatt, 1995; Boergers et al., 1998; Hewitt, Flett, & Turnbull-Donovan, 1992; Hewitt, Flett, & Weber, 1994; Hewitt, Newton, Flett, & Callander, 1997; Hewitt et al.,

1998; Lombardi, Florentino, & Lombardi, 1998; O'Connor & Forgan, 2007). Perfectionism is associated with greater suicidal ideation and behavior and wishing for death, independent of other known risk factors for suicide (Boergers et al., 1998; Hewitt et al., 1992, 1994, 1998; O'Connor & Forgan, 2007). In one study, perfectionism was associated with greater suicidal threat and intent, independent from depression or feelings of hopelessness (Hewitt et al., 1992). This finding extends to conceptualizations of perfectionism within DSM-IV OCPD criteria. Ansell and colleagues (2010) found associations between the OCPD factor of perfectionism and suicidal ideation, suggesting the importance of examining trait perfectionism in patients with OCPD as a risk factor for suicide-related outcomes.

## Rigidity

The construct of "rigidity," or the tendency to be controlling, stubborn, and without flexibility in one's thoughts, behaviors, and interactions with others, has been identified as a factor dimension within existing DSM-IV OCPD criteria. However, the definition of trait rigidity has varied widely across studies, with references to cognitive, behavioral, and interpersonal manifestations. No research has examined to what extent each, or perhaps all, of these manifestations are relevant to OCPD. Nonetheless, there remains significant theoretical and empirical support for the relevance of rigidity in understanding the course of psychopathology and functioning. Trait rigidity is associated with poorer outcomes for depression and eating disorders, particularly symptoms associated with anorexia nervosa (Anderluh, Tchanturia, Rabe-Hesketh, Collier, & Treasure, 2009; Bruce & Steiger, 2005; Drieling, van Calker, & Hecht, 2006; Sakado et al., 2001).

Cognitive rigidity, or deficits in executive functioning involving mental flexibility, is associated with suicide-related outcomes, particularly suicidal ideation and attempts (Marzuk, Hartwell, Leon, & Portera, 2005; Patsiokas, Clum, & Luscomb, 1979; Upmanyu, 1995). Behavioral expressions of rigidity have primarily focused on rigidity within interpersonal interactions. In one study, rigidity within relationship patterns was significantly greater in a patient population with OCPD when compared to one with borderline PD (McCarthy, Connolly Gibbons, & Barber, 2008). Rigidity in interpersonal behaviors was associated with greater interpersonal distress via less adaptability of one's interpersonal responses (Tracey, 2005). Interpersonal rigidity also was associated inversely with measures of well-being (Tracey & Rohlfing, 2010).

The impact of rigidity may extend beyond consequences for the self. Rigidity in parent–child interactions has been associated with development of later internalizing and externalizing problems in children (Hollenstein, Granic, Stoolmiller, & Snyder, 2004). Problems in the assessment of interpersonal rigidity have left questions as to its maladaptiveness (Erickson, Newman, & Pincus, 2009; McCarthy et al., 2008). It may be that rigidity of an individual across interactants is adaptive (e.g., represents an expression of identity integrity), whereas rigidity across situations with a single interactant may represent a lack of flexibility necessary for promoting relationship cohesion and decreasing interpersonal distress (McCarthy et al., 2008; Tracey, 2005; Tracey & Rohlfing, 2010). These studies highlight the relevance of trait rigidity in understanding the interpersonal difficulties associated with OCPD mentioned earlier (Cain et al., 2015).

## Overcommitment

The concept of work addiction within the construct of OCPD is reflected in the DSM-IV/DSM-5 criteria, which describe workaholism and work devotion as related criteria. The concept of trait work devotion, or overcommitment, reflects a much broader view of the pathology associated with work devotion. "Overcommitment" is defined as a maladaptive coping pattern driven by a person's high need for control and approval, which is characterized by excessive striving and an inability to withdraw from obligations (Joksimovic et al., 1999; Siegrist et al., 2004; Wirtz, Siegrist, Rimmele, & Ehlert, 2008). This trait has been associated with maladaptive work and health outcomes (e.g., exhaustion and breakdowns, musculoskeletal and cardiovascular ailments) (Joksimovic et al., 1999; Joksimovic, Starke, von dem Knesebeck, & Siegrist, 2002). It also has been associated with blunted stress reactivity (Wirtz et al., 2008). No prior research has examined trait overcommitment in relation to OCPD, but theoretical conceptualizations and descriptions of the workaholic criteria in the DSM-IV/DSM-5 suggest that the trait is likely highly related.

## Inhibition versus Disinhibition

Individuals with OCPD have been described as exhibiting affect restriction and behavioral inhibition. However, growing research suggests that this observation is only one side of the OCPD phenomenon. Additional evidence (Ansell et al., 2010; Hummelen et al., 2008; Villemarette-Pittman et al., 2004) indicates associations between OCPD and behavioral disinhibition and aggression. The idea that compulsivity and impulsivity are distinct and coexisting dimensions is not new. The coexistence of these dimensions in samples with psychopathology has been useful in understanding individuals with addiction disorders (Fineberg et al., 2010; Potenza, 2007) and may be useful in understanding traits associated with OCPD.

In one study (Villemarette-Pittman et al., 2004), the second most common diagnosis in a sample of patients referred for aggression problems was OCPD (behind antisocial PD). The authors theorized that a subset of patients with OCPD may exhibit impulse control disorders prior to the onset of the OCPD diagnosis, and that compulsive inhibition may be an attempt at regulating a behavioral disinhibition problem. Another possibility that we present here is that the overcontrolled responses in OCPD are compensatory responses (regardless of origin) that fail when the individual is put under stress (relationship, work, etc.), resulting in sudden disinhibition and aggression (Villemarette-Pittman et al., 2004). In two other studies, OCPD criteria were associated with aggression and hostility criteria (Ansell et al., 2010; Hummelen et al., 2008). Regardless of the origins, research examining the simultaneous occurrence of impulsive and compulsive traits in patients with eating disorders supports the utility of considering both inhibition and disinhibition in other patient groups, and may generalize to enhance understanding of traits associated with OCPD (Claes, Vandereycken, & Vertommen, 2002; Engel et al., 2005).

## Conclusions

This review summarizes the current literature on OCPD, both as a diagnostic category and in terms of component traits theoretically linked to the construct. We find sufficient evidence of coherence and distinctiveness in the pattern of traits associated with OCPD to recommend that OCPD continue to be identified as a distinct PD, as it is in DSM-5. Moreover, our review provides evidence for the hybrid dimensional–categorical model proposed for Section III of DSM-5, using the proposed criteria of impairment in personality functioning and maladaptive traits. OCPD is prevalent in both community and clinical samples. With some exceptions, it has been associated with maladaptive cognitions and behavior, as well as functional impairment. OCPD as a diagnostic category is related but distinct from other disorders, and its presence influences the manifestation other disorders. When OCPD co-occurs with an Axis I condition (most commonly, depression, anorexia nervosa, generalized anxiety disorder, OCD), OCPD tends to adversely impact course and treatment outcome.

Factor-analytic studies of OCPD point to a complex, heterogeneous construct that comprises core aspects of the disorder (rigidity, perfectionism, aggressiveness). An examination of the psychometric properties of DSM-IV OCPD criteria revealed several weaknesses in the current conceptualization. The poorest performing DSM-IV criteria are hoarding and miserliness. This finding supports the alternative model for OCPD proposed in DSM-5, in which both of these criteria have been dropped from the OCPD construct. In place of these dropped criteria, the new conceptualization of OCPD introduces several new OCPD diagnostic symptoms, including intimacy avoidance, restricted affectivity, and perseveration. This literature review suggests that items pertaining to interpersonal difficulties would more fully capture problematic areas of OCPD, which is consistent with these new criteria. However, research in this area is in its infancy and will require substantial future work to validate the new criteria (Skodol, 2014).

In addition, much work has yet to be done to expand the research base of OCPD in terms of treatment and etiology, both at diagnostic and component traits levels. There is no empirically validated treatment for OCPD, so treatment development remains a priority. Besides meeting a public health need, advances in treatment of OCPD and its component traits would allow for comparisons in treatment response with related disorders and would inform the treatment of comorbid cases. New research endeavors in the area of endophenotypes, unobservable characteristics (e.g., neurophysiological, biochemical, neuropsychological, and cognitive) that mediate relations between genes and behavioral phenotypes (Gottesman & Gould, 2003), may provide insights into underlying mechanisms and potential treatment targets for OCPD and its core component traits. As the field turns away from categorical models of PDs and toward dimensional approaches, future work on transdiagnostic pathological personality traits has the potential to significantly advance our understanding of the construct validity of OCPD.

## ACKNOWLEDGMENTS

We thank Kimberly Glazier, PhD, for her assistance with the systematic literature searches.

## REFERENCES

Abbass, A., Sheldon, A., Gyra, J., & Kalpin, A. (2008). Intensive short-term dynamic psychotherapy for DSM-IV personality disorders: A randomized controlled trial. *Journal of Nervous and Mental Disease, 196*(3), 211–216.

Agosti, V., Hellerstein, D. J., & Stewart, J. W. (2009). Does personality disorder decrease the likelihood of remission in early-onset chronic depression? *Comprehensive Psychiatry, 50*(6), 491–495.

Albert, U., Maina, G., Forner, F., & Bogetto, F. (2004). DSM-IV obsessive–compulsive personality disorder: Prevalence in patients with anxiety disorders and in healthy comparison subjects. *Comprehensive Psychiatry, 45*(5), 325–332.

Alnaes, R., & Torgersen, S. (1988). DSM-III symptom disorders (Axis I) and personality disorders (Axis II) in an outpatient population. *Acta Psychiatrica Scandinavica, 78*(3), 348–355.

American Psychiatric Association. (1987). *Diagnostic and statistical manual of mental disorders* (3rd ed., rev.). Washington, DC: Author.

American Psychiatric Association. (1994). *Diagnostic and statistical manual of mental disorders* (4th ed.). Washington, DC: Author.

American Psychiatric Association. (2013). *Diagnostic and statistical manual of mental disorders* (5th ed.). Arlington, VA: Author.

Anderluh, M., Tchanturia, K., Rabe-Hesketh, S., Collier, D., & Treasure, J. (2009). Lifetime course of eating disorders: Design and validity testing of a new strategy to define the eating disorders phenotype. *Psychological Medicine, 39*(1), 105–114.

Anderluh, M. B., Tchanturia, K., Rabe-Hesketh, S., & Treasure, J. (2003). Childhood obsessive–compulsive personality traits in adult women with eating disorders: Defining a broader eating disorder phenotype. *American Journal of Psychiatry, 160*(2), 242–247.

Ansell, E. B., Pinto, A., Crosby, R. D., Becker, D. F.,

Anez, L. M., Paris, M., et al. (2010). The prevalence and structure of obsessive–compulsive personality disorder in Hispanic psychiatric outpatients. *Journal of Behavior Therapy and Experimental Psychiatry, 41*(3), 275–281.

Ansell, E. B., Pinto, A., Edelen, M. O., & Grilo, C. M. (2008). Structure of DSM-IV criteria for obsessive–compulsive personality disorder in patients with binge eating disorder. *Canadian Journal of Psychiatry, 53*(12), 863–867.

Ansell, E. B., Pinto, A., Edelen, M. O., Markowitz, J. C., Sanislow, C. A., Yen, S., et al. (2011). The association of personality disorders with the prospective 7-year course of anxiety disorders. *Psychological Medicine, 41,* 1019–1028.

Ansseau, M. (1997). The obsessive–compulsive personality: Diagnostic aspects and treatment possibilities. In J. A. denBoer & H. G. M. Westenberg (Eds.), *Obsessive–compulsive spectrum disorders* (pp. 61–73). Amsterdam, The Netherlands: Syn-Thesis.

Aycicegi, A., Dinn, W. M., & Harris, C. L. (2002). Neuropsychological function in obsessive–compulsive personality with schizotypal features. *Bulletin of Clinical Psychopharmacology, 12,* 121–125.

Aycicegi-Dinn, A., Dinn, W. M., & Caldwell-Harris, C. L. (2009). Obsessive–compulsive personality traits: Compensatory response to executive function deficit? *International Journal of Neuroscience, 119*(4), 600–608.

Baer, L. (1994). Factor analysis of symptom subtypes of obsessive compulsive disorder and their relation to personality and tic disorders. *Journal of Clinical Psychiatry, 55*(Suppl.), 18–23.

Bailey, G. R., Jr. (1998). Cognitive-behavioral treatment of obsessive–compulsive personality disorder. *Journal of Psychological Practice, 4*(1), 51–59.

Barber, J. P., Morse, J. Q., Krakauer, I., Chittams, J., & Crits-Christoph, K. (1997). Change in obsessive–compulsive and avoidant personality disorders following time-limited supportive–expressive therapy. *Psychotherapy, 34,* 133–143.

Battle, C. L., Shea, M. T., Johnson, D. M., Yen, S., Zlotnick, C., Zanarini, M. C., et al. (2004). Childhood maltreatment associated with adult personality disorders: Findings from the Collaborative Longitudinal Personality Disorders Study. *Journal of Personality Disorders, 18*(2), 193–211.

Beck, A. T., & Freeman, A. (1990). *Cognitive therapy of personality disorders.* New York: Guilford Press.

Beck, J. S. (1997). Cognitive approaches to personality disorders. In J. H. Wright & M. E. Thase (Eds.), *Cognitive therapy review of psychotherapy.* Washington, DC: American Psychiatric Press.

Bender, D. S., Dolan, R. T., Skodol, A. E., Sanislow, C. A., Dyck, I. R., McGlashan, T. H., et al. (2001). Treatment utilization by patients with personality disorders. *American Journal of Psychiatry, 158*(2), 295–302.

Bernstein, D. P., Cohen, P., Velez, C. N., Schwab-Stone, M., Siever, L. J., & Shinsato, L. (1993). Prevalence and stability of the DSM-III-R personality disorders in a community-based survey of adolescents. *American Journal of Psychiatry, 150*(8), 1237–1243.

Bieling, P. J. (2004). Perfectionism as an explanatory construct in comorbidity of Axis I disorders. *Journal of Psychopathology and Behavioral Assessment, 26*(3), 193–201.

Blankstein, K., Lumley, C., & Crawford, A. (2007). Perfectionism, hopelessness, and suicide ideation: Revisions to diathesis–stress and specific vulnerability models. *Journal of Rational-Emotive and Cognitive-Behavior Therapy, 25*(4), 279–319.

Blatt, S. J. (1995). The destructiveness of perfectionism: Implications for the treatment of depression. *American Psychologist, 50*(12), 1003–1020.

Blatt, S. J., Quinlan, D. M., Pilkonis, P. A., & Shea, M. T. (1995). Impact of perfectionism and need for approval on the brief treatment of depression: The National Institute of Mental Health Treatment of Depression Collaborative Research Program revisited. *Journal of Consulting and Clinical Psychology, 63*(1), 125–132.

Blatt, S. J., Zuroff, D. C., Bondi, C. M., Sanislow, C. A., III, & Pilkonis, P. A. (1998). When and how perfectionism impedes the brief treatment of depression: Further analyses of the National Institute of Mental Health Treatment of Depression Collaborative Research Program. *Journal of Consulting and Clinical Psychology, 66*(2), 423–428.

Boergers, J., Spirito, A., & Donaldson, D. (1998). Reasons for adolescent suicide attempts: Associations with psychological functioning. *Journal of the American Academy of Child and Adolescent Psychiatry, 37*(12), 1287–1293.

Bruce, K. R., & Steiger, H. (2005). Treatment implications of Axis-II comorbidity in eating disorders. *Eating Disorders, 13*(1), 93–108.

Cain, N. M., Ansell, E. B., Simpson, H. B., & Pinto, A. (2015). Interpersonal functioning in obsessive–compulsive personality disorder. *Journal of Personality and Assessment, 97,* 90–99.

Calvo, R., Lazaro, L., Castro-Fornieles, J., Font, E., Moreno, E., & Toro, J. (2009). Obsessive–compulsive personality disorder traits and personality dimensions in parents of children with obsessive–compulsive disorder. *European Psychiatry, 24,* 201–206.

Cavedini, P., Erzegovesi, S., Ronchi, P., & Bellodi, L. (1997). Predictive value of obsessive–compulsive personality disorder in antiobsessional pharmacological treatment. *European Neuropsychopharmacology, 7*(1), 45–49.

Chapman, A. L., Lynch, T. R., Rosenthal, M. Z., Cheavens, J. S., Smoski, M. J., & Krishnan, K. R. R. (2007). Risk aversion among depressed older adults with obsessive compulsive personality disorder. *Cognitive Therapy and Research, 31,* 161–174.

Chavira, D. A., Grilo, C. M., Shea, M. T., Yen, S., Gunderson, J. G., Morey, L. C., et al. (2003). Ethnicity and four personality disorders. *Comprehensive Psychiatry, 44*(6), 483–491.

Claes, L., Vandereycken, W., & Vertommen, H. (2002). Impulsive and compulsive traits in eating disordered patients compared with controls. *Personality and Individual Differences, 32*(4), 707–714.

Clark, L. A. (2007). Assessment and diagnosis of personality disorder: Perennial issues and an emerging reconceptualization. *Annual Review of Psychology, 58,* 227–257.

Clark, M. A., Lelchook, A. M., & Taylor, M. L. (2010). Beyond the Big Five: How narcissism, perfectionism, and dispositional affect relate to workaholism. *Personality and Individual differences, 48*(7), 786–791.

Coles, M. E., Pinto, A., Mancebo, M. C., Rasmussen, S. A., & Eisen, J. L. (2008). OCD with comorbid OCPD: A subtype of OCD? *Journal of Psychiatric Research, 42,* 289–296.

Cooper, L. D., Balsis, S., & Zimmerman, M. (2010). Challenges associated with a polythetic diagnostic system: Criteria combinations in the personality disorders. *Journal of Abnormal Psychology, 119*(4), 886–895.

Costa, P. T., & Widiger, T. A. (Eds.). (1994). *Personality disorders and the five factor model of personality.* Washington, DC: American Psychological Association.

Cramer, V., Torgersen, S., & Kringlen, E. (2007). Socio-demographic conditions, subjective somatic health, Axis I disorders and personality disorders in the common population: The relationship to quality of life. *Journal of Personality Disorders, 21*(5), 552–567.

de Reus, R. J., & Emmelkamp, P. M. (2012). Obsessive–compulsive personality disorder: A review of current empirical findings. *Personality and Mental Health, 6*(1), 1–21.

DeYoung, C. G., Quilty, L. C., & Peterson, J. B. (2007). Between facets and domains: 10 aspects of the Big Five. *Journal of Personality and Social Psycholpgy, 93*(5), 880–896.

Diaconu, G., & Turecki, G. (2009). Obsessive–compulsive personality disorder and suicidal behavior: Evidence for a positive association in a sample of depressed patients. *Journal of Clinical Psychiatry, 70*(11), 1551–1556.

Diedrich, A., & Voderholzer, U. (2015). Obsessive–compulsive personality disorder: A current review. *Current Psychiatry Reports, 17*(2), 2.

Digman, J. M., & Takemoto-Chock, N. K. (1981). Factors in the natural language of personality: Reanalysis, comparison, and interpretation of six major studies. *Multivariate Behavioral Research, 16*(2), 149–170.

Dimaggio, G., Carcione, A., Salvatore, G., Nicolo, G., Sisto, A., & Semerari, A. (2011). Progressively promoting metacognition in a case of obsessive–compulsive personality disorder treated with metacognitive interpersonal therapy. *Psychology and Psychotherapy: Theory, Research and Practice, 84*(1), 70–83, 98–110.

Drieling, T., van Calker, D., & Hecht, H. (2006). Stress,

personality and depressive symptoms in a 6.5 year follow-up of subjects at familial risk for affective disorders and controls. *Journal of Affective Disorders, 91*(2–3), 195–203.

Egan, S. J., Wade, T. D., & Shafran, R. (2011). Perfectionism as a transdiagnostic process: A clinical review. *Clinical Psychology Review, 31*(2), 203–212.

Ekselius, L., Bodlund, O., von Knorring, L., Lindstrom, E., & Kullgren, G. (1996). Sex differences in DSM-III-R, Axis II personality disorders. *Personality and Individual Differences, 20*(4), 457–461.

Enero, C., Soler, A., Ramos, I., Cardona, S., Guillamat, R., & Valles, V. (2013). 2783–Distress level and treatment outcome in obsessive–compulsive personality disorder (OCPD). *European Psychiatry, 28*(1), 1.

Engel, S. G., Corneliussen, S. J., Wonderlich, S. A., Crosby, R. D., le Grange, D., Crow, S., et al. (2005). Impulsivity and compulsivity in bulimia nervosa. *International Journal of Eating Disorders, 38*(3), 244–251.

Enns, M., & Cox, B. (2005a). Perfectionism, stressful life events, and the 1-year outcome of depression. *Cognitive Therapy and Research, 29*(5), 541–553.

Enns, M. W., & Cox, B. J. (2005b). Psychosocial and clinical predictors of symptom persistence vs remission in major depressive disorder. *Canadian Journal of Psychiatry, 50*(12), 769–777.

Erickson, T. M., Newman, M. G., & Pincus, A. L. (2009). Predicting unpredictability: Do measures of interpersonal rigidity/flexibility and distress predict intraindividual variability in social perceptions and behavior? *Journal of Personality and Social Psychology, 97*(5), 893–912.

Farmer, R. F., & Chapman, A. L. (2002). Evaluation of DSM-IV personality disorder criteria as assessed by the structured clinical interview for DSM-IV personality disorders. *Comprehensive Psychiatry, 43*(4), 285–300.

Fineberg, N. A., Day, G. A., de Koenigswarter, N., Reghunandanan, S., Kolli, S., Jefferies-Sewell, K., et al. (2015). The neuropsychology of obsessive–compulsive personality disorder: A new analysis. *CNS Spectrums, 20*(5), 490–499.

Fineberg, N. A., Potenza, M. N., Chamberlain, S. R., Berlin, H. A., Menzies, L., Bechara, A., et al. (2010). Probing compulsive and impulsive behaviors, from animal models to endophenotypes: A narrative review. *Neuropsychopharmacology, 35*(3), 591–604.

Fineberg, N. A., Sharma, P., Sivakumaran, T., Sahakian, B., & Chamberlain, S. R. (2007). Does obsessive–compulsive personality disorder belong within the obsessive–compulsive spectrum? *CNS Spectrums, 12*(6), 467–482.

Fiore, D., Dimaggio, G., Nicolo, G., Semerari, A., & Carcione, A. (2008). Metacognitive interpersonal therapy in a case of obsessive–compulsive and avoidant personality disorders. *Journal of Clinical Psychology, 64*(2), 168–180.

Franklin, M. E., Piacentini, J. C., & D'Olio, C. (2007). Obsessive–compulsive personality disorder: Developmental risk factors and clinical implications. In A. Freeman & M. A. Reinecke (Eds.), *Personality disorders in childhood and adolescence* (pp. 533–558). Hoboken, NJ: Wiley.

Freud, S. (1963). Character and anal eroticism. In P. Reiff (Ed.), *Collected papers of Sigmund Freud* (Vol. 10). New York: Collier. (Original work published 1908)

Gallagher, N. G., South, S. C., & Oltmanns, T. F. (2003). Attentional coping style in obsessive–compulsive personality disorder: A test of the intolerance of uncertainty hypothesis. *Personality and Individual Differences 34*, 41–57.

Garyfallos, G., Katsigiannopoulos, K., Adamopoulou, A., Papazisis, G., Karastergiou, A., & Bozikas, V. P. (2010). Comorbidity of obsessive–compulsive disorder with obsessive–compulsive personality disorder: Does it imply a specific subtype of obsessive–compulsive disorder? *Psychiatry Research, 177*(1–2), 156–160.

Gjerde, L. C., Czajkowski, N., Røysamb, E., Ystrom, E., Tambs, K., Aggen, S. H., et al. (2015). A longitudinal, population-based twin study of avoidant and obsessive–compulsive personality disorder traits from early to middle adulthood. *Psychological Medicine, 45*(16), 3539–3548.

Gordon, O. M., Salkovskis, P. M., Oldfield, V. B., & Carter, N. (2013). The association between obsessive compulsive disorder and obsessive compulsive personality disorder: Prevalence and clinical presentation. *British Journal of Clinical Psychology, 52*(3), 300–315.

Gottesman, I. I., & Gould, T. D. (2003). The endophenotype concept in psychiatry: Etymology and strategic intentions. *American Journal of Psychiatry, 160*(4), 636–645.

Grant, B. F., Hasin, D. S., Stinson, F. S., Dawson, D. A., Chou, S. P., Ruan, W. J., et al. (2004). Prevalence, correlates, and disability of personality disorders in the United States: Results from the National Epidemiologic Survey on Alcohol and Related Conditions. *Journal of Clinical Psychiatry, 65*(7), 948–958.

Grant, J. E., Mooney, M. E., & Kushner, M. G. (2012). Prevalence, correlates, and comorbidity of DSM-IV obsessive–compulsive personality disorder: Results from the National Epidemiologic Survey on Alcohol and Related Conditions. *Journal of Psychiatric Research, 46*(4), 469–475.

Grilo, C. M. (2004). Factor structure of DSM-IV criteria for obsessive compulsive personality disorder in patients with binge eating disorder. *Acta Psychiatrica Scandinavica, 109*(1), 64–69.

Grilo, C. M., McGlashan, T. H., Morey, L. C., Gunderson, J. G., Skodol, A. E., Shea, M. T., et al. (2001). Internal consistency, intercriterion overlap and diagnostic efficiency of criteria sets for DSM-IV schizotypal, borderline, avoidant and obsessive–compulsive personality disorders. *Acta Psychiatrica Scandinavica, 104*(4), 264–272.

Grilo, C. M., Sanislow, C. A., Gunderson, J. G., Pagano, M. E., Yen, S., Zanarini, M. C., et al. (2004). Two-year stability and change of schizotypal, borderline, avoidant, and obsessive–compulsive personality disorders. *Journal of Consulting and Clinical Psychology, 72*(5), 767–775.

Grilo, C. M., Skodol, A. E., Gunderson, J. G., Sanislow, C. A., Stout, R. L., Shea, M. T., et al. (2004). Longitudinal diagnostic efficiency of DSM-IV criteria for obsessive–compulsive personality disorder: A 2-year prospective study. *Acta Psychiatrica Scandinavica, 110,* 64–68.

Grilo, C. M., Stout, R. L., Markowitz, J. C., Sanislow, C. A., Ansell, E. B., Skodol, A. E., et al. (2010). Personality disorders predict relapse after remission from an episode of major depressive disorder: A 6-year prospective study. *Journal of Clinical Psychiatry, 71,* 1629–1635.

Gunderson, J. G., Daversa, M. T., Grilo, C. M., McGlashan, T. H., Zanarini, M. C., Shea, M. T., et al. (2006). Predictors of 2-year outcome for patients with borderline personality disorder. *American Journal of Psychiatry, 163*(5), 822–826.

Gunderson, J. G., Shea, M. T., Skodol, A. E., McGlashan, T. H., Morey, L. C., Stout, R. L., et al. (2000). The Collaborative Longitudinal Personality Disorders Study: Development, aims, design, and sample characteristics. *Journal of Personality Disorders, 14*(4), 300–315.

Habke, A. M., & Flynn, C. A. (2002). Interpersonal aspects of trait perfectionism. In G. L. Flett & P. L. Hewitt (Eds.), *Perfectionism: Theory, research, and treatment* (pp. 151–180). Washington, DC: American Psychological Association.

Halmi, K. A., Tozzi, F., Thornton, L. M., Crow, S., Fichter, M. M., Kaplan, A. S., et al. (2005). The relation among perfectionism, obsessive–compulsive personality disorder and obsessive–compulsive disorder in individuals with eating disorders. *International Journal of Eating Disorders, 38*(4), 371–374.

Haring, M., Hewitt, P. L., & Flett, G. L. (2003). Perfectionism, coping, and quality of intimate relationships. *Journal of Marriage and Family, 65,* 143–158.

Hertler, S. C. (2013). Understanding obsessive–compulsive personality disorder. *SAGE Open, 3,* 3.

Hewitt, P. L., Caelian, C. F., Flett, G. L., Sherry, S. B., Collins, L., & Flynn, C. A. (2002). Perfectionism in children: Associations with depression, anxiety, and anger. *Personality and Individual Differences, 32*(6), 1049–1061.

Hewitt, P. L., Flett, G. L., Besser, A., Sherry, S. B., & McGee, B. (2003). Perfectionism is multidimensional: A reply to Shafran, Cooper and Fairburn. *Behaviour Research and Therapy, 41*(10), 1221–1236.

Hewitt, P. L., Flett, G. L., & Turnbull-Donovan, W. (1992). Perfectionism and suicide potential. *British Journal of Clinical Psychology, 31*(Pt. 2), 181–190.

Hewitt, P. L., Flett, G. L., & Weber, C. (1994). Dimensions of perfectionism and suicide ideation. *Cognitive Therapy and Research, 18,* 439–460.

Hewitt, P. L., Newton, J., Flett, G. L., & Callander, L. (1997). Perfectionism and suicide ideation in adolescent psychiatric patients. *Journal of Abnormal Child Psychology, 25*(2), 95–101.

Hewitt, P. L., Norton, G. R., Flett, G. L., Callander, L., & Cowan, T. (1998). Dimensions of perfectionism, hopelessness, and attempted suicide in a sample of alcoholics. *Suicide and Life-Threatening Behavior, 28*(4), 395–406.

Hewlett, W. A., Vinogradov, S., Martin, K., Berman, S., & Csernansky, J. G. (1992). Fenfluramine stimulation of prolactin in obsessive–compulsive disorder. *Psychiatry Research, 42*(1), 81–92.

Hollenstein, T., Granic, I., Stoolmiller, M., & Snyder, J. (2004). Rigidity in parent–child interactions and the development of externalizing and internalizing behavior in early childhood. *Journal of Abnormal Child Psychology, 32*(6), 595–607.

Hummelen, B., Wilberg, T., Pedersen, G., & Karterud, S. (2008). The quality of the DSM-IV obsessive–compulsive personality disorder construct as a prototype category. *Journal of Nervous and Mental Disease, 196*(6), 446–455.

Huprich, S. K., Zimmerman, M., & Chelminski, I. (2006). Disentangling depressive personality disorder from avoidant, borderline, and obsessive–compulsive personality disorders. *Comprehensive Psychiatry, 47*(4), 298–306.

Jane, J. S., Oltmanns, T. F., South, S. C., & Turkheimer, E. (2007). Gender bias in diagnostic criteria for personality disorders: An item response theory analysis. *Journal of Abnormal Psychology, 116,* 166–175.

Joksimovic, L., Siegrist, J., Meyer-Hammer, M., Peter, R., Franke, B., Klimek, W. J., et al. (1999). Overcommitment predicts restenosis after coronary angioplasty in cardiac patients. *International Journal of Behavioral Medicine, 6*(4), 356–369.

Joksimovic, L., Starke, D., von dem Knesebeck, O., & Siegrist, J. (2002). Perceived work stress, overcommitment, and self-reported musculoskeletal pain: A cross-sectional investigation. *International Journal of Behavioral Medicine, 9*(2), 122–138.

Karno, M., Golding, I., Sorenson, S., & Burnam, M. (1988). The epidemiology of obsessive–compulsive disorder in five US communities. *Archives of General Psychiatry, 45,* 1094–1099.

Kendler, K. S., Aggen, S. H., Czajkowski, N., Roysamb, E., Tambs, K., Torgersen, S., et al. (2008). The structure of genetic and environmental risk factors for DSM-IV personality disorders: A multivariate twin study. *Archives of General Psychiatry, 65*(12), 1438–1446.

Kendler, K. S., Gardner, C. O., & Prescott, C. A. (2002). Toward a comprehensive developmental model for major depression in women. *American Journal of Psychiatry, 159*(7), 1133–1145.

Kern, M. L., & Friedman, H. S. (2008). Do conscientious individuals live longer?: A quantitative review. *Health Psychology, 27*(5), 505–512.

Koutoufa, I., & Furnham, A. (2014). Mental health literacy and obsessive–compulsive personality disorder. *Psychiatry Research, 215*(1), 223–228.

Kyrios, M. (1998). A cognitive-behavioural approach to the understanding and management of obsessive–compulsive personality disorder. In C. Perris

& P. D. McGorry (Eds.), *Cognitive psychotherapy of psychotic and personality disorders: Handbook of theory and practice* (pp. 351–378). New York: Wiley.

Lapointe, L., & Emond, C. (2005). *Dimensions du perfectionnisme et tendances suicidaires chez des adolescents en milieu scolaire* [Relationships between suicidal behaviors and perfectionism dimensions in a non-clinical sample of adolescents] (Vol. 26). Montreal, Canada: Universite du Quebec, Departement de Psychologie.

Lazare, A., Klerman, G. L., & Armor, D. J. (1966). Oral, obsessive, and hysterical personality patterns: An investigation of psychoanalytic concepts by means of factor analysis. *Archives of General Psychiatry, 14*(6), 624–630.

Lenane, M., Swedo, S. E., Leonard, H. L., Pauls, D. L., Sceery, W., & Rapoport, J. L. (1990). Psychiatric disorders in first degree relatives of children and adolescents with obsessive–compulsive disorder. *Journal of the American Academy of Child and Adolescent Psychiatry, 29*, 407–412.

Lenzenweger, M. F., Lane, M. C., Loranger, A. W., & Kessler, R. C. (2007). DSM-IV personality disorders in the National Comorbidity Survey Replication. *Biological Psychiatry, 62*(6), 553–564.

Lewinsohn, P. M., Rohde, P., Seeley, J. R., & Klein, D. N. (1997). Axis II psychopathology as a function of Axis I disorders in childhood and adolescence. *Journal of the American Academy of Child and Adolescent Psychiatry, 36*(12), 1752–1759.

Light, K. J., Joyce, P. R., Luty, S. E., Mulder, R. T., Frampton, C. M., Joyce, L. R., et al. (2006). Preliminary evidence for an association between a dopamine D3 receptor gene variant and obsessive–compulsive personality disorder in patients with major depression. *American Journal of Medical Genetics B: Neuropsychiatric Genetics, 141*(4), 409–413.

Lilenfeld, L. R., Kaye, W. H., Greeno, C. G., Merikangas, K. R., Plotnicov, K., Pollice, C., et al. (1998). A controlled family study of anorexia nervosa and bulimia nervosa: Psychiatric disorders in first-degree relatives and effects of proband comorbidity. *Archives of General Psychiatry, 55*(7), 603–610.

Lilenfeld, L. R., Wonderlich, S., Riso, L. P., Crosby, R., & Mitchell, J. (2006). Eating disorders and personality: A methodological and empirical review. *Clinical Psychology Review, 26*(3), 299–320.

Lochner, C., Serebro, P., der Merwe, L. V., Hemmings, S., Kinnear, C., Seedat, S., et al. (2011). Comorbid obsessive–compulsive personality disorder in obsessive–compulsive disorder (OCD): A marker of severity. *Progress in Neuropsychopharmacology and Biological Psychiatry, 35*, 1087–1092.

Lock, J., Agras, W. S., Bryson, S., & Kraemer, H. C. (2005). A comparison of short- and long-term family therapy for adolescent anorexia nervosa. *Journal of the American Academy of Child and Adolescent Psychiatry, 44*(7), 632–639.

Lombardi, D. N., Florentino, M. C., & Lombardi, A. J. (1998). Perfectionism and abnormal behavior. *Journal of Individual Psychology, 54*(1), 61–71.

Lucey, J. V., O'Keane, V., Butcher, G., Clare, A. W., & Dinan, T. G. (1992). Cortisol and prolactin responses to D-fenfluramine in non-depressed patients with obsessive–compulsive disorder: A comparison with depressed and healthy controls. *British Journal of Psychiatry, 161*, 517–521.

Lynam, D. R., & Widiger, T. A. (2001). Using the five-factor model to represent the DSM-IV personality disorders: An expert consensus approach. *Journal of Abnormal Psychology, 110*(3), 401–412.

Lynch, T. R., & Cheavens, J. S. (2008). Dialectical behavior therapy for comorbid personality disorders. *Journal of Clinical Psychology, 64*(2), 154–167.

Maier, W., Lichtermann, D., Klinger, T., Heun, R., & Hallmayer, J. (1992). Prevalences of personality disroders (DSM-III-R) in the community. *Journal of Personality Disorders, 6*, 187–196.

Marzuk, P. M., Hartwell, N., Leon, A. C., & Portera, L. (2005). Executive functioning in depressed patients with suicidal ideation. *Acta Psychiatrica Scandinavica, 112*(4), 294–301.

McCarthy, K. S., Connolly Gibbons, M. B., & Barber, J. P. (2008). The relation of rigidity across relationships with symptoms and functioning: An investigation with the Revised Central Relationship Questionnaire. *Journal of Counseling Psychology, 55*(3), 346–358.

McGlashan, T. H., Grilo, C. M., Sanislow, C. A., Ralevski, E., Morey, L. C., Gunderson, J. G., et al. (2005). Two-year prevalence and stability of individual DSM-IV criteria for schizotypal, borderline, avoidant, and obsessive–compulsive personality disorders: Toward a hybrid model of Axis II disorders. *American Journal of Psychiatry, 162*(5), 883–889.

McGlashan, T. H., Grilo, C. M., Skodol, A. E., Gunderson, J. G., Shea, M. T., Morey, L. C., et al. (2000). The Collaborative Longitudinal Personality Disorders Study: Baseline Axis I/II and II/II diagnostic co-occurrence. *Acta Psychiatrica Scandinavica, 102*(4), 256–264.

Millon, T. (1981). *Disorders of personality: DSM-III, Axis II*. New York: Wiley.

Morey, L. C., Gunderson, J. G., Quigley, B. D., Shea, M. T., Skodol, A. E., McGlashan, T. H., et al. (2002). The representation of borderline, avoidant, obsessive–compulsive, and schizotypal personality disorders by the five-factor model. *Journal of Personality Disorders, 16*(3), 215–234.

Morey, L. C., Hopwood, C. J., Markowitz, J. C., Gunderson, J. G., Grilo, C. M., McGlashan, T. H., et al. (2012). Comparison of alternative models for personality disorders, II: 6-, 8- and 10-year follow-up. *Psychological Medicine, 42*(8), 1705–1713.

Morey, L. C., Warner, M. B., & Boggs, C. D. (2002). Gender bias in the personality disorders criteria: An investigation of five bias indicators. *Journal of Psychopathology and Behavioral Assessment, 24*, 55–65.

Nestadt, G., Di, C., Samuels, J. F., Bienvenu, O. J., Reti, I. M., Costa, P., et al. (2010). The stability of DSM personality disorders over twelve to eighteen years. *Journal of Psychiatric Research, 44*(1), 1–7.

Ng, R. M. (2005). Cognitive therapy for obsessive–compulsive personality disorder—a pilot study in Hong Kong Chinese patients. *Hong Kong Journal of Psychiatry, 15*(2), 50.

Nordahl, H. M., & Stiles, T. C. (1997). Perceptions of parental bonding in patients with various personality disorders, lifetime depressive disorders, and healthy controls. *Journal of Personality Disorders, 11*(4), 391–402.

O'Connor, R., & Forgan, G. (2007). Suicidal thinking and perfectionism: The role of goal adjustment and behavioral inhibition/activation systems (BIS/BAS). *Journal of Rational-Emotive and Cognitive-Behavior Therapy, 25*(4), 321–341.

Ost, L. G. (2008). Efficacy of the third wave of behavioral therapies: A systematic review and meta-analysis. *Behaviour Research and Therapy, 46*(3), 296–321.

Patsiokas, A. T., Clum, G. A., & Luscomb, R. L. (1979). Cognitive characteristics of suicide attempters. *Journal of Consulting and Clinical Psychology, 47*(3), 478–484.

Pearson, C. A., & Gleaves, D. H. (2006). The multiple dimensions of perfectionism and their relation with eating disorder features. *Personality and Individual Differences, 41*(2), 225–235.

Perez, M., Brown, J. S., Vrshek-Schallhorn, S., Johnson, F., & Joiner, T. E., Jr. (2006). Differentiation of obsessive–compulsive-, panic-, obsessive–compulsive personality-, and non-disordered individuals by variation in the promoter region of the serotonin transporter gene. *Journal of Anxiety Disorders, 20*(6), 794–806.

Pfohl, B. (1996). Obsessive–compulsive personality disorder. In T. A. Widiger, H. A. Pincus, R. Ross, M. First, & W. Wakefield (Eds.), *DSM-IV sourcebook* (Vol. 2, pp. 777–789). Washington, DC: American Psychiatric Association.

Pinto, A. (2009). *Understanding obsessive compulsive personality disorder and its impact on obsessive compulsive disorder.* Paper presented at the 16th annual Obsessive Compulsive Foundation Conference, Minneapolis, MN.

Pinto, A. (2016). Treatment of obsessive–compulsive personality disorder. In *Clinical handbook of obsessive–compulsive and related disorders* (pp. 415–429). Cham, Switzerland: Springer International.

Pinto, A., & Eisen, J. (2012). Personality features of OCD and spectrum conditions. In G. Steketee (Ed.), *The Oxford handbook of obsessive compulsive and spectrum disorders* (pp. 189–208). New York: Oxford University Press.

Pinto, A., Eisen, J. L., Mancebo, M. C., & Rasmussen, S. A. (2008). Obsessive–compulsive personality disorder. In J. S. Abramowitz, D. McKay, & S. Taylor (Eds.), *Obsessive–compulsive disorder: Subtypes and spectrum conditions* (pp. 246–270). New York: Elsevier.

Pinto, A., Greene, A. L., Storch, E. A., & Simpson, H. B. (2015). Prevalence of childhood obsessive–compulsive personality traits in adults with obsessive–compulsive disorder versus obsessive–compulsive personality disorder. *Journal of Obsessive–Compulsive and Related Disorders, 4,* 25–29.

Pinto, A., Liebowitz, M. R., Foa, E. B., & Simpson, H. B. (2011). Obsessive compulsive personality disorder as a predictor of exposure and ritual prevention outcome for obsessive compulsive disorder. *Behaviour Research and Therapy, 49*(8), 453–458.

Pinto, A., Mancebo, M. C., Eisen, J. L., Pagano, M. E., & Rasmussen, S. A. (2006). The Brown Longitudinal Obsessive Compulsive Study: Clinical features and symptoms of the sample at intake. *Journal of Clinical Psychiatry, 67,* 703–711.

Pinto, A., Steinglass, J. E., Greene, A. L., Weber, E. U., & Simpson, H. B. (2014). Capacity to delay reward differentiates obsessive–compulsive disorder and obsessive–compulsive personality disorder. *Biological Psychiatry, 75*(8), 653–659.

Pollak, J. M. (1987). Obsessive–compulsive personality: Theoretical and clinical perspectives and recent research findings. *Journal of Personality Disorders, 1*(3), 248–262.

Potenza, M. N. (2007). Impulsivity and compulsivity in pathological gambling and obsessive–compulsive disorder. *Revista Brasileira de Psiquiatria, 29*(2), 105–106.

Raja, M., & Azzoni, A. (2007). The impact of obsessive–compulsive personality disorder on the suicidal risk of patients with mood disorders. *Psychopathology, 40*(3), 184–190.

Reichborn-Kjennerud, T., Czajkowski, N., Neale, M. C., Orstavik, R. E., Torgersen, S., Tambs, K., et al. (2007). Genetic and environmental influences on dimensional representations of DSM-IV cluster C personality disorders: A population-based multivariate twin study. *Psychological Medicine, 37*(5), 645–653.

Rice, K. G., & Aldea, M. A. (2006). State dependence and trait stability of perfectionism: A short-term longitudinal study. *Journal of Counseling Psychology, 53,* 205–212.

Roberts, B. W., & Bogg, T. (2004). A longitudinal study of the relationships between conscientiousness and the social-environmental factors and substance-use behaviors that influence health. *Journal of Personality, 72*(2), 325–354.

Roberts, B. W., Walton, K. E., & Bogg, T. (2005). Conscientiousness and health across the life course. *Review of General Psychology, 9*(2), 156–168.

Robins, E., & Guze, S. B. (1970). Establishment of diagnostic validity in psychiatric illness: Its application to schizophrenia. *American Journal of Psychiatry, 126*(7), 983–987.

Rossi, A., Marinangeli, M. G., Butti, G., Kalyvoka, A., & Petruzzi, C. (2000). Pattern of comorbidity among anxious and odd personality disorders: The case of obsessive–compulsive personality disorder. *CNS Spectrums, 5*(9), 23–26.

Sakado, K., Sakado, M., Seki, T., Kuwabara, H., Kojima, M., Sato, T., et al. (2001). Obsessional personality features in employed Japanese adults with a lifetime history of depression: Assessment by the Munich Personality Test (MPT). *European Archives of Psychiatry and Clinical Neurosciences, 251*(3), 109–113.

Samuel, D. B., & Widiger, T. A. (2010). A comparison of obsessive–compulsive personality disorder scales. *Journal of Personality Assessment, 92*(3), 232–240.

Samuel, D. B., & Widiger, T. A. (2011). Conscientiousness and obsessive–compulsive personality disorder. *Personality Disorders: Theory, Research, and Treatment, 2*(3), 161–174.

Samuels, J., Nestadt, G., Bienvenu, O. J., Costa, P. T., Jr., Riddle, M. A., Liang, K. Y., et al. (2000). Personality disorders and normal personality dimensions in obsessive–compulsive disorder. *British Journal of Psychiatry, 177,* 457–462.

Sansone, R. A., Hendricks, C. M., Sellbom, M., & Reddington, A. (2003). Anxiety symptoms and healthcare utilization among a sample of outpatients in an internal medicine clinic. *International Journal of Psychiatry in Medicine, 33*(2), 133–139.

Shahar, G., Blatt, S. J., Zuroff, D. C., & Pilkonis, P. A. (2003). Role of perfectionism and personality disorder features in response to brief treatment for depression. *Journal of Consulting and Clinical Psychology, 71*(3), 629–633.

Shahar, G., Gallagher, E. F., Blatt, S. J., Kuperminc, G. P., & Leadbeater, B. J. (2004). An interactive-synergetic approach to the assessment of personality vulnerability to depression: Illustration using the adolescent version of the Depressive Experiences Questionnaire. *Journal of Clinical Psychology, 60*(6), 605–625.

Shapiro, D. (1965). *Neurotic styles.* New York: Basic Books.

Sharma, L., Markon, K. E., & Clark, L. A. (2014). Toward a theory of distinct types of "impulsive" behaviors: A meta-analysis of self-report and behavioral measures. *Psychological Bulletin, 140*(2), 374–408.

Siegrist, J., Starke, D., Chandola, T., Godin, I., Marmot, M., Niedhammer, I., et al. (2004). The measurement of effort-reward imbalance at work: European comparisons. *Social Science and Medicine, 58*(8), 1483–1499.

Skodol, A. E. (2014). Personality disorder classification: Stuck in neutral, how to move forward? *Current Psychiatry Reports, 16*(10), 1–10.

Skodol, A. E., Gunderson, J. G., McGlashan, T. H., Dyck, I. R., Stout, R. L., Bender, D. S., et al. (2002). Functional impairment in patients with schizotypal, borderline, avoidant, or obsessive–compulsive personality disorder. *American Journal of Psychiatry, 159*(2), 276–283.

Skodol, A. E., Pagano, M. E., Bender, D. S., Shea, M. T., Gunderson, J. G., Yen, S., et al. (2005). Stability of functional impairment in patients with schizotypal, borderline, avoidant, or obsessive–compulsive personality disorder over two years. *Psychological Medicine, 35*(3), 443–451.

Slaney, R. B., Pincus, A. L., Uliaszek, A. A., & Wang, K. T. (2006). Conceptions of perfectionism and interpersonal problems: Evaluating groups using the structural summary method for circumplex data. *Assessment, 13*(2), 138–153.

Soeteman, D. I., Hakkaart-van Roijen, L., Verheul, R., & Busschbach, J. J. (2008). The economic burden of personality disorders in mental health care. *Journal of Clinical Psychiatry, 69*(2), 259–265.

Sperry, L. (2003). *Handbook of diagnosis and treatment of DSM-IV-TR personality disorders* (2nd ed.). New York: Brunner/Routledge.

Starcevic, V., & Brakoulias, V. (2014). New diagnostic perspectives on obsessive–compulsive personality disorder and its links with other conditions. *Current Opinion in Psychiatry, 27*(1), 62–67.

Stein, D. J., Trestman, R. L., Mitropoulou, V., Coccaro, E. F., Hollander, E., & Siever, L. J. (1996). Impulsivity and serotonergic function in compulsive personality disorder. *Journal of Neuropsychiatry and Clinical Neuroscience, 8*(4), 393–398.

Strauss, J. L., Hayes, A. M., Johnson, S. L., Newman, C. F., Brown, G. K., Barber, J. P., et al. (2006). Early alliance, alliance ruptures, and symptom change in a nonrandomized trial of cognitive therapy for avoidant and obsessive–compulsive personality disorders. *Journal of Consulting and Clinical Psychology, 74*(2), 337–345.

Strober, M., Freeman, R., Lampert, C., & Diamond, J. (2007). The association of anxiety disorders and obsessive compulsive personality disorder with anorexia nervosa: Evidence from a family study with discussion of nosological and neurodevelopmental implications. *International Journal of Eating Disorders, 40*(Suppl.), S46–S51.

Strober, M., Freeman, R., & Morrell, W. (1997). The long-term course of severe anorexia nervosa in adolescents: Survival analysis of recovery, relapse, and outcome predictors over 10–15 years in a prospective study. *International Journal of Eating Disorders, 22*(4), 339–360.

Stuart, S., Pfohl, B., Battaglia, M., Bellodi, L., Grove, W., & Cadoret, R. (1998). The co-occurrence of DSM-III-R personality disorders. *Journal of Personality Disorders, 12*(4), 302–315.

Sutandar-Pinnock, K. (2003). Perfectionism in anorexia nervosa: A 6–24-month follow-up study. *International Journal of Eating Disorders, 33*(2), 225–229.

Svartberg, M., Stiles, T. C., & Seltzer, M. H. (2004). Randomized, controlled trial of the effectiveness of short-term dynamic psychotherapy and cognitive therapy for cluster C personality disorders. *American Journal of Psychiatry, 161*(5), 810–817.

Swedo, S. E., Rapoport, J. L., Leonard, H. L., Lenane, M. C., & Cheslow, D. (1989). Obsessive compulsive disorder in children and adolescents: Clinical and phenomenology of 70 consecutive cases. *Archives of General Psychiatry, 46,* 335–341.

Tenney, N. H., Schotte, C. K., Denys, D. A., van Megen, H. J., & Westenberg, H. G. (2003). Assessment of

DSM-IV personality disorders in obsessive–compulsive disorder: Comparison of clinical diagnosis, self-report questionnaire, and semi-structured interview. *Journal of Personality Disorders, 17*(6), 550–561.

Torgersen, S. (2009). The nature (and nurture) of personality disorders. *Scandinavian Journal of Psychology, 50*(6), 624–632.

Torgersen, S., Kringlen, E., & Cramer, V. (2001). The prevalence of personality disorders in a community sample. *Archives of General Psychiatry, 58,* 590–596.

Torgersen, S., Lygren, S., Oien, P. A., Skre, I., Onstad, S., Edvardsen, J., et al. (2000). A twin study of personality disorders. *Comprehensive Psychiatry, 41*(6), 416–425.

Tracey, T. J. G. (2005). Interpersonal rigidity and complementarity. *Journal of Research in Personality, 39*(6), 592–614.

Tracey, T. J., & Rohlfing, J. E. (2010). Variations in the understanding of interpersonal behavior: Adherence to the interpersonal circle as a moderator of the rigidity–psychological well-being relation. *Journal of Personality, 78*(2), 711–746.

Tyrer, F., Smith, L. K., McGrother, C. W., & Taub, N. A. (2007). The impact of physical, intellectual and social impairments on survival in adults with intellectual disability: A population-based register study. *Journal of Applied Research in Intellectual Disabilities, 20*(4), 360–367.

Ullrich, S., Farrington, D. P., & Coid, J. W. (2007). Dimensions of DSM-IV personality disorders and life-success. *Journal of Personality Disorders, 21*(6), 657–663.

Upmanyu, V. V. (1995). A study of suicide ideation: The intervening role of cognitive rigidity. *Psychological Studies, 40,* 126.

Villemarette-Pittman, N. R., Stanford, M. S., Greve, K. W., Houston, R. J., & Mathias, C. W. (2004). Obsessive–compulsive personality disorder and behavioral disinhibition. *Journal of Psychology, 138*(1), 5–22.

Warner, M. B., Morey, L. C., Finch, J. F., Gunderson, J. G., Skodol, A. E., Sanislow, C. A., et al. (2004). The longitudinal relationship of personality traits and disorders. *Journal of Abnormal Psychology, 113*(2), 217–227.

Wentz, E., Gillberg, I. C., Anckarsater, H., Gillberg, C., & Rastam, M. (2009). Adolescent-onset anorexia nervosa: 18-year outcome. *British Journal of Psychiatry, 194*(2), 168–174.

Whiteside, S. P., & Lynam, D. R. (2001). The five factor model and impulsivity: Using a structural model of personality to understand impulsivity. *Personality and Individual Differences, 30*(4), 669–689.

Winston, A., Laikin, M., Pollack, J., Samstag, L. W., McCullough, L., & Muran, J. C. (1994). Short-term psychotherapy of personality disorders. *American Journal of Psychiatry, 151*(2), 190–194.

Wirtz, P. H., Elsenbruch, S., Emini, L., Rudisuli, K., Groessbauer, S., & Ehlert, U. (2007). Perfectionism and the cortisol response to psychosocial stress in men. *Psychosomatic Medicine, 69*(3), 249–255.

Wirtz, P. H., Siegrist, J., Rimmele, U., & Ehlert, U. (2008). Higher overcommitment to work is associated with lower norepinephrine secretion before and after acute psychosocial stress in men. *Psychoneuroendocrinology, 33*(1), 92–99.

Young, J. E. (1999). *Cognitive therapy for personality disorders: A schema-focused approach* (3rd ed.). Sarasota, FL: Professional Resource Press.

Yovel, I., Revelle, W., & Mineka, S. (2005). Who sees trees before forest?: The obsessive–compulsive style of visual attention. *Psychological Science, 16*(2), 123–129.

Zimmerman, M., & Coryell, W. (1989). DSM-III personality disorder diagnoses in a nonpatient sample: Demographic correlates and comorbidity. *Archives of General Psychiatry, 46*(8), 682–689.

Zimmerman, M., Rothschild, L., & Chelminski, I. (2005). The prevalence of DSM-IV personality disorders in psychiatric outpatients. *American Journal of Psychiatry, 162*(10), 1911–1918.

Zuroff, D. C., Blatt, S. J., Sotsky, S. M., Krupnick, J. L., Martin, D. J., Sanislow, C. A., III, et al. (2000). Relation of therapeutic alliance and perfectionism to outcome in brief outpatient treatment of depression. *Journal of Consulting and Clinical Psychology, 68*(1), 114–124.

# PART VII
# EMPIRICALLY BASED TREATMENTS

## INTRODUCTION

Knowledge about treatment has changed as extensively as any area of personality disorder (PD) study since the first edition of this volume was published. More treatment options are now available, and outcome studies have extended our understanding of treatment efficacy. To accommodate these developments, this section has been changed substantially. The section on treatment in the previous edition sought to cover the range of treatments available at the time and to represent all schools of therapy. Developments in the field and greater emphasis on evidence-based approaches resulted in the decision to include only treatments shown to be effective in at least one randomized controlled trial (RCT). Seven specific therapies met this modest criterion: dialectical behavior therapy (DBT; Linehan, 1993), cognitive analytic therapy (CAT; Ryle, 1997), schema-focused therapy (SFT; Young, Klosko, & Weishaar, 2003), cognitive therapy for PDs (CBTpd; Davidson, 2008), transference-focused psychotherapy (TFP; Clarkin, Yeomans, & Kernberg, 1999, 2006), mentalization-based therapy (MBT; Bateman & Fonagy, 2004, 2006), and systems training for emotion predictability and problem solving (STEPPS; Blum, Bartels, St. John, & Pfohl, 2012).

The chapters on DBT, by Clive J. Robins, Noga Zerubavel, André M. Ivanoff, and Marsha M. Linehan (Chapter 29) and on cognitive analytic therapy, by Anthony Ryle and Stephen Kellett (Chapter 27), are updates of equivalent chapters in the first edition. The chapters on TFP, by John F. Clarkin, Nicole Cain, Mark F. Lenzenweger, and Kenneth N. Levy (Chapter 32), on MBT, by Anthony W. Bateman, Peter Fonagy, and Chloe Campbell (Chapter 30), and on STEPPS, by Nancee Blum, Donald W. Black, and Don St. John (Chapter 33), are new. The TFP chapter replaces a more general chapter on psychoanalysis and psychoanalytic psychotherapy because RCTs of psychoanalytic therapy for PD have primarily been conducted on TFP. MBT and STEPPS were not published in manualized form until after the publication of the first edition. The decision to include two chapters on cognitive therapy in addition to a chapter on DBT requires explanation. The original application of cognitive therapy to PD (Beck, Freeman, and Associates, 1990) has not been systematically evaluated. However, an elaboration of the approach by Young and colleagues (2003) has been shown to be effective (Giesen-Bloo et al., 2006; Masley, Gillanders, Simpson, & Taylor, 2012); hence, a chapter on

SFT (Chapter 31) by David P. Bernstein and Maartje Clercx is included. Kate M. Davidson (Chapter 28) subsequently developed a manualized form of Beck's original model for use in evaluating the approach in treating borderline and antisocial PDs (CBTpd). The subsequent evaluation demonstrated its efficacy (Davidson, Norrie, et al., 2006; Davidson, Tyrer, et al., 2006). Since CBTpd differs from SFT in several clinically important respects, we decided to include it as a separate chapter to give the reader an opportunity to consider the differences. Although both are clearly grounded in a cognitive therapy perspective, CBTpd is more closely related to Beck and colleagues' (1990) original position and therefore does not adopt the partial parenting approach of SFT or its emphasis on conceptualizing PD in terms of schema modes. CBTpd also places substantially less emphasis on the use of the treatment relationship as a vehicle for change. Since these differences have important conceptual and clinical implications that need to be considered when treating patients and developing more effective therapies, we decided that both approaches warrant inclusion.

Authors describing specific therapies were asked to cover a specific set of issues to ensure a broad overview of their approach and its assumptions, so that readers can compare the different approaches and understand how the different therapies address key issues. The topics authors were asked to address include the origins and scope of their approach; the structure and temporal course of therapy; diagnosis, assessment, and formulation; theoretical foundations in terms of the underlying model of PD, fundamental theoretical constructs, and principles of change; major strategies and interventions; treatment relationship; process of treatment; and the evidence supporting their approach.

Most chapters describe therapies that are generally long-term, in that they typically require patients to be treated for at least a year, and often longer. The exceptions are CAT, which typically lasts 24 weeks, with 4 follow-up sessions, and STEPPS, which consists of 20 sessions. Both therapies contain interesting features that raise important questions about treatment duration. An interesting feature of CAT is its focus on restructuring and integrating the disparate self-states associated with borderline pathology. Although a fragmented and unstable self-structure is a core feature of the disorder, it is not addressed by some popular therapies. Interestingly, CAT seeks to address these problems in short-term therapy. Evidence of the effectiveness of this treatment suggests the need to reconsider both the strategies required to treat the different components of personality pathology as opposed to the current emphasis on treatments for specific DSM diagnoses, and the frequency and duration of therapy. STEPPS differs from the other therapies discussed in Part VII in that it is group treatment delivered in a classroom format. It also differs from other treatments in the refreshing sense that it is not proposed as definitive therapy for borderline PD (BPD) but rather as an addition to other treatments. This is an interesting idea that is consistent with current interest in modular treatments. However, the efficacy of STEPPS and its relative cost-effectiveness suggests that it, or a version of it, might also be used as a first-line intervention as part of a program of stepped care.

Part VII contains four additional chapters. In Chapter 34, Maria Elena Ridolfi and John G. Gunderson discuss psychoeducation, an important but neglected aspect of treatment. In Chapter 36, Stephen C. P. Wong discusses evidence-based treatment of antisocial and psychopathic personality patterns. The current treatment literature is focussed almost entirely on BPD. However, we felt it was important to include a chapter on antisocial and psychopathic personality given the social and clinical significance of this condition. The section also includes updated Chapter 35 on pharmacotherapy, by Paul Markovitz. Although the role of medication in the treatment of PDs is contentious, with reviews reaching divergent conclusions, ranging from medication being a useful treatment option to it not being recommended, it continues to be widely used, and a conservative reading of the literature suggests that medication is best considered an adjunctive form of therapy that can be useful for some patients. The section concludes as did the final section in the previous edition, with a chapter on integrated therapy. In Chapter 37, W. John Livesley outlines a proposal for combining the effective components of empirically supported treatments to provide more comprehensive coverage of personality pathology tailored to the needs of individual patients.

The psychotherapy chapters should be considered in the context of current research on treatment outcome, which has grown considerably over the last 15 years. The important question for the clinician, and for the development of improved treatments, is whether these therapies differ in effectiveness and cost-effectiveness and, if so, how these differences affect treatment decisions. In the first edition, doubts were raised about the differential effectiveness of the therapies available at the time. Subsequent research has largely validated these reservations. All therapies evaluated to date in RCTs bring about significant change, but no single therapy stands out as more effective (Bartak, Soeteman, Verheul, & Busschbach, 2007; Budge et al., 2014; Cristea et al., 2017; Leichsenring & Leibing, 2003; Leichsenring, Leibing, Kruse, New, & Leweke, 2011; Mulder & Chanen, 2013). Some possible exceptions to the conclusion of similar outcome across therapies have been noted. For example, Giesen-Bloo and colleagues (2006) suggested that in their comparison of TFP and SFT, fewer dropouts occurred among those receiving SFT and their outcomes were better. However, differences were small, the sample size was limited, and questions have been raised about whether the two therapies were delivered in comparable ways (Yeomans, 2007). Comparisons of the relative cost-effectiveness among specialized treatments or between specialized treatments and good clinical care is an important research priority. In terms of treatment costs, in an economic evaluation from their RCT, Giesen-Bloo and colleagues (2006) suggested that SFT showed greater cost-effectiveness than TFP (van Asselt et al., 2008). Such economic evaluations are also useful in informing treatment decisions in contexts of limited health care resources.

Currently, there is no clear indication that there are clinically important differences in efficacy of the specialized therapies for PD. However, they are more effective than treatment as usual or treatment by experts (Budge et al., 2014; Clarke, Thomas, & James, 2013; Doering et al., 2010; Farrell, Shaw, & Webber, 2009; Koons et al., 2001; Linehan, Armstrong, Suarez, Allmon, & Heard, 1991; Linehan et al., 2006; Verheul et al., 2003). It should be noted, however, that treatment as usual is a modest standard and in some settings may involve relatively little active therapy. However, the specialized therapies are not more effective than either well-defined, manualized general psychiatric care or supportive therapy. Moreover, a recent meta-analysis of treatments for borderline PD suggests that outcome changes are modest and unstable (Cristea et al., 2017). These are important findings with substantial implications for practice and for understanding mechanisms of change. Hence, it is important to note that the failure to demonstrate differences from good clinical care appears robust. It is supported by studies comparing different therapies with different forms of good clinical care conducted by investigators with different theoretical orientations in very different settings.

Four specialized therapies, namely, DBT, TFP, CAT, and MBT, have been compared with good clinical care. In all cases, similar outcomes were reported. Clarkin, Levy, Lenzenweger, and Kernberg (2007) found few differences across multiple outcome measures in a comparison of TFP, DBT, and supportive dynamic therapy over 1 year. McMain and colleagues (2009) confirmed these findings in the case of DBT by comparing this treatment with general psychiatric management based on American Psychiatric Association (2001) guidelines for treating BPD. Chanen and colleagues (2008) reported that CAT was not significantly better than manualized good clinical care over 24 months. Finally, Bateman and Fonagy (2009) reported similar outcomes with MBT and structured clinical management. Comparisons between specialized therapies and supportive therapy also failed to find differences in effectiveness. Jørgensen and colleagues (2013) reported that outcome for MBT did not differ from that of supportive psychotherapy across a range of measures with the exception of therapist-rated global assessment of functioning, which was not a blind rating. This finding is especially important because the MBT group received substantially more intense treatment than the supportive therapy group. Differences between the groups remained nonsignificant at 18-month follow-up (Jørgensen et al., 2014).

The results of outcome studies clearly show that treatment for PD is modestly effective, but it does not seem to matter what treatment is used: Specialized therapies, good clinical care, and supportive therapy produce comparable results. It appears that nothing is gained from using a specialized therapy. However, it does seem to be important to use a structured approach (Critchfield & Benjamin, 2006), and it is noteworthy that both good clinical care and supportive therapy were also systematized and manualized in the studies that compared them to a specialized therapy.

These findings, viewed in the context of treatment for PD, may seem surprising. A generation ago, there was widespread doubt about whether PD is treatable. The advent of a range of manualized therapies supported by RCTs changed clinical practice and has radically changed the lives of many patients. As a result, there has been a tendency to consider these therapies to be definitive approaches that probably needed to be tweaked a little, but little else. This perception has been encouraged by a partisan attitude on the part of the proponents of some of these therapies, who tend to claim that their approach is more definite, more evidence-supported, or in some way more fundamental. However, when these findings are viewed in the context of research on psychotherapy outcome generally, they are congruent with well-established findings that outcomes for the treatment of most mental disorders and psychological problems are similar across all therapies (Beutler, 1991; Castonguay & Beutler, 2006a, 2006b; Luborsky, Singer, & Luborsky, 1975).

Overall, the findings of outcome research present a substantial challenge for specialized treatments. Currently, it seems difficult to justify the use of a specialized therapy rather than a less expensive and more easily delivered treatment, especially as the initial or first-line treatment method.

They also suggest the need to rethink how PD is treated. In the final chapter in this section, W. John Livesley argues that these findings suggest that treatment should seek to optimize the effect of generic interventions and adopt an integrated approach that combines the essential components of all effective therapies. Nevertheless, a review in the first edition (Piper & Joyce, 2001) noted evidence of domain specificity. This is an important but neglected issue. Since all evaluated treatments are effective, all must contain effective interventions. In addition to interventions based on generic change mechanisms, it seems likely that these therapies also contain interventions that are specific to a given treatment model. The importance of so-called "dismantling" studies that seek to identify the change mechanisms of the different therapies is now gaining recognition (Johansson et al., 2010). However, it is perhaps more important to study the slightly different but related problem of determining the most effective interventions to treat different problems and impairments that characterize PD.

The chapters on specific therapies should also be considered in the context of the limitations of current outcome research and the conceptual limitations of these treatments. Despite the progress and consistent findings, research on PD treatments remains modest, and many studies have substantial limitations, including challenges in matching therapies in terms of intensity, frequency, goals, and duration. In addition, the specialized therapies evaluated to date were primarily developed to treat BPD, and the majority of RCTs have been conducted on patients with this disorder, raising serious questions about generalizability to other forms of PD. Generalizability of findings is also limited by the comparatively small sample sizes of almost all studies (Davidson, Norrie, et al., 2006).

Recently, some evidence indicates that at least some therapies are also effective in treating other PDs. SFT, for example, seems also to be effective with other forms of PD (Bamelis, Evers, Spinhoven, & Arntz, 2014), and CBTpd seems to be applicable to both BPD (Davidson et al., 2006a, 2006b) and antisocial PD (Davidson et al., 2009).

When reviewing the therapies and comparing and contrasting the different approaches, readers should also be mindful of the fact that the therapies described are often applied to patients who differ substantially in severity. This is important because severity is strongly related to outcome (Crawford, Koldobsky, Mulder, & Tyrer, 2011). Also, the clinical literature reveals substantial differences in the settings in which these therapies were developed and typically used. MBT, for example, was developed in a day hospital setting in the United Kingdom, which suggests that it is used to treat patients with high levels of severity. In contrast, the case material included in texts on some of the cognitive therapies seems to pertain to patients with lower severity (see above comment). For example, some of the cases described are patients who are professionals or who hold executive positions. Similarly, the literature on TFT notes that patients entering treatment should not be in a crisis, and a requirement of treatment is that they obtain some kind of employment at the outset of treatment. This suggests either that patients have less severe baseline pathology or that they have had prior treatment to stabilize their condition. It also suggests that these patients are different from those presenting to general mental health services. Therapists should be mindful of these differences because therapeutic strategies that are effective or tolerable for patients at one level of severity may be counterproductive with patients at a different level.

Finally, it should also be noted that although considerable progress has been made in improving the treatment of PD, some key impairments do not seem to improve greatly with treatment. Change seems to primarily involve symptomatic improvement, reduced self-harm, decreased hospital admissions, and modest improvement in social functioning and quality of life. Substantial functional impairments remain following treatment (Kröger, Harbeck, Armbrust, & Kliem, 2013; McMain et al., 2009) and overall functioning, social adjustment, and quality of life remain poor. Also, treatment dropout is high for most treatments (Cameron, Palm Reed, & Gaudiano, 2014). This is a serious problem that needs to be addressed because the outcome for those who drop out of therapy is poor (Karterud et al., 2003).

## REFERENCES

American Psychiatric Association. (2001). *Practice guideline for the treatment of patients with borderline personality disorder*. Washington, DC: Author.

Bamelis, L. L. M., Evers, S. M. A. A., Spinhoven, P., &, Arntz, A. (2014). The results of a multicenter randomized controlled trial on the clinical effectiveness of schema therapy for personality disorders. *American Journal of Psychiatry, 171,* 305–322.

Bartak, A., Soeteman, D. I., Verheul, R., & Busschbach, J. J. V. (2007). Strengthening the status of psychotherapy for personality disorders: An integrated perspective on effects and costs. *Canadian Journal of Psychiatry, 52,* 803–810.

Bateman, A., & Fonagy, P. (2004). *Psychotherapy for borderline personality disorder: Mentalization-based treatment*. Oxford, UK: Oxford University Press.

Bateman, A., & Fonagy, P. (2006). *Mentalization-based treatment for borderline personality disorder*. Oxford, UK: Oxford University Press.

Bateman, A., & Fonagy, P. (2009). Randomized controlled trial of outpatient mentalization-based therapy versus structured clinical management for borderline personality disorder. *American Journal of Psychiatry, 166,* 1355–1364.

Beck, A. T., Freeman, A., & Associates. (1990). *Cognitive therapy of personality disorders*. New York: Guilford Press.

Beutler, L. E. (1991). Have all won and must all have prizes?: Revisiting Luborsky et al.'s verdict. *Journal of Consulting and Clinical Psychology, 59,* 226–232.

Blum, N. S., Bartels, N. E., St. John, D., & Pfohl, B. (2012). *Systems Training for Emotional Predictability and Problem Solving (Second Edition): Group treatment program for borderline personality disorder*. Coralville, IA: Level One Publishing (Blums Books).

Budge, S. L., Moore, J. T., Del Re, A. C., Wampold, B. E., Baardseth, T. P., & Nienhaus, J. B. (2014). The effectiveness of evidence-based treatments for personality disorders when comparing treatment-as-usual and bona fide treatments. *Clinical Psychology Review, 34*(5), 451–452.

Cameron, A. Y., Palm Reed, K., & Gaudiano, B. A. (2014). Addressing treatment motivation in borderline personality disorder: Rationale for incorporating values-based exercises into dialectical behavior therapy. *Journal of Contemporary Psychotherapy, 44,* 109–116.

Castonguay, L. G., & Beutler, L. E. (2006a). Common and unique principles of therapeutic change: What do we know and what do we need to know? In L.

G. Castonguay & L. E. Beutler (Eds.), *Principles of therapeutic change that work* (pp. 353–369). New York: Oxford University Press.

Castonguay, L. G., & Beutler, L. E. (Eds.). (2006b). *Principles of therapeutic change that work.* New York: Oxford University Press.

Chanen, A. M., Jackson, H. J., McCutcheon, L. K., Jovev, M., Dudgeon, P., Yuen, H. P., et al. (2008). Early intervention for adolescents with borderline personality disorder using cognitive analytic therapy: Randomised controlled trial. *British Journal of Psychiatry, 193,* 477–484.

Clarke, S., Thomas, P., & James, K. (2013). Cognitive analytic therapy for personality disorders: A randomized controlled trial. *British Journal of Psychiatry, 202,* 129–134.

Clarkin, J. F., Levy, K. N., Lenzenweger, M. F., & Kernberg, O. F. (2007). Evaluating three treatments for borderline personality disorder: A multiwave study. *American Journal of Psychiatry, 164*(6), 922–928.

Clarkin, J. F., Yeomans, F. E., & Kernberg, O. (1999). *Psychotherapy for borderline personality disorder.* New York: Wiley.

Clarkin, J. F., Yeomans, F. E., & Kernberg, O. (2006). *Psychotherapy for borderline personality: Focusing on object relations.* Washington, DC: American Psychiatric Publishing.

Crawford, M. J., Koldobsky, N., Mulder, R., & Tyrer, P. (2011). Classifying personality disorder according to severity. *Journal of Personality Disorders, 25,* 321–330.

Cristea, I. A., Gentili, C., Cotet, C. D., Palomba, D., Barbui, C., & Cuijpers, P. (2017). Efficacy of psychotherapies for borderline personality disorder: A systematic review and meta-analysis. *JAMA Psychiatry, 74,* 319–328.

Critchfield, K. L., & Benjamin, L. S. (2006). Integration of therapeutic factors in treating personality disorders. In L. G. Castonguay & L. E. Beutler (Eds.), *Principles of therapeutic change that work* (pp. 253–271). New York: Oxford University Press.

Davidson, K. (2008). *Cognitive therapy for personality disorders* (2nd ed.). London: Routledge.

Davidson, K., Norrie, J., Tyrer, P., Gumley, A., Tata, P., Murray, H., et al. (2006). The effectiveness of cognitive behavior therapy for borderline personality disorder: Results from the BOSCOT trial. *Journal of Personality Disorders, 20,* 450–465.

Davidson, K. M., Tyrer, P., Gumley, A., Tata, P., Norrie, J., Palmer, S., et al. (2006). Rationale, description, and sample characteristics of a randomised controlled trial of cognitive therapy for borderline personality disorder: The BOSCOT study. *Journal of Personality Disorders, 20*(5), 431–449.

Davidson, K. M., Tyrer, P., Tata, P., Cooke, D., Gumley, A., Ford, I., et al. (2009). Cognitive behaviour therapy for violent men with antisocial personality disorder in the community: An exploratory randomised controlled trial. *Psychological Medicine, 39,* 569–578.

Doering, S., Hörz, S., Rentrop, M., Fischer-Kern, M., Schuster, P., Benecke, C., et al. (2010). Transference-focused psychotherapy v. treatment by community psychotherapists for borderline personality disorder: Randomized controlled trial. *British Journal of Psychiatry, 196,* 389–395.

Farrell, J. M., Shaw, I. A., & Webber, M. A. (2009). A schema-focused approach to group psychotherapy for outpatients with borderline personality disorder: A randomized controlled trial. *Journal of Behavior Therapy and Experimental Psychiatry, 40,* 317–328.

Giesen-Bloo, J., van Dyck, R., Spinhoven, P., van Tilberg, W., Dirksen, C., van Asselt, T., et al. (2006). Outpatient psychotherapy for borderline personality disorder: Randomized trial of schema-focused therapy vs. transference-focused therapy. *Archives of General Psychiatry, 63,* 649–658.

Johansson, P., Høglend, P., Ulberg, R., Amlo, S., Marble, A., Bøgwald, K.-P., et al. (2010). The mediating role of insight for long-term improvements in psychodynamic therapy. *Journal of Consulting and Clinical Psychology, 78*(3), 438–448.

Jørgensen, C. R., Bøye, R., Andersen, D., Døssing Blaabjerg, A. H., Freund, C., Jordet, H., et al. (2014). Eighteen months post-treatment naturalistic follow-up study of mentalization-based therapy and supportive group treatment of borderline personality disorder: Clinical outcomes and functioning. *Nordic Psychology, 66,* 254–273.

Jørgensen, C. R., Freund, C. Bøye, R., Jordet, H., Andersen, D., & Kjolbye, M. (2013). Mentalizing-based therapy versus psychodynamic supportive therapy. *Acta Psychiatrica Scandinavica, 127,* 305–317.

Karterud, S., Pedersen, G., Bjordal, E., Brabrand, J., Friss, S., Haaseth, O., et al. (2003). Day treatment of clients with personality disorders: Experiences from a Norwegian treatment research network. *Journal of Personality Disorders, 17,* 243–262.

Koons, C. R., Robins, C. J., Tweed, J. L., Lynch, T. R., Gonzalez, A. M., Morse, J. Q., et al. (2001). Efficacy of dialectical behavior therapy in women veterans with borderline personality disorder. *Behavior Therapy, 32,* 371–390.

Kröger, C., Harbeck, S., Armbrust, M., & Kliem, S. (2013). Effectiveness, response, and dropout of dialectical behavior therapy for borderline personality disorder in an inpatient setting. *Behaviour Research and Therapy, 51,* 411–416.

Leichsenring, F., & Leibing, E. (2003). The effectiveness of psychodynamic therapy and cognitive behavioural therapy in the treatment of personality disorders: A meta-analysis. *American Journal of Psychiatry, 160,* 1223–1232.

Leichsenring, F., Leibing, E., Kruse, J., New, A. S., & Lewke, F. (2011). Borderline personality disorder. *Lancet, 377,* 74–84.

Linehan, M. M. (1993). *Cognitive-behavioural treat-*

*ment of borderline personality disorder.* New York: Guilford Press.

Linehan, M. M., Armstrong, H. E., Suarez, A., Allmon, D., & Heard, H. L. (1991). Cognitive-behavioral treatment of chronically parasuicidal borderline patients. *Archives of General Psychiatry, 48,* 1060–1064.

Linehan, M. M., Comtois, K. A., Murray, A. M., Brown, M. Z., Gallop, R. J., Heard, H. L., et al. (2006). Two-year randomized controlled trial and follow-up of dialectical behavior therapy vs. therapy by experts for suicidal behaviors and borderline personality disorder. *Archives of General Psychiatry, 63,* 757–766.

Luborsky, L., Singer, B., & Luborsky, L. (1975). Comparative studies of psychotherapies: Is it true that "everyone has won and all must have prizes"? *Archives of General Psychiatry, 32,* 995–1008.

Masley, S. A., Gillanders, D. T., Simpson, S. G., & Taylor, M. A. (2012). A systematic review of the evidence base for schema therapy. *Cognitive Behavior Therapy, 41*(3), 185–202.

McMain, S. F., Links, P. S., Gnam, W. H., Guimond, T., Cardish, R. J., Korman, L., et al. (2009). A randomized controlled trial of dialectical behavior therapy versus general psychiatry management for borderline personality disorder. *American Journal of Psychiatry, 166,* 1365–1374.

Mulder, R., & Chanen, A. M. (2013). Effectiveness of cognitive analytic therapy for personality disorders. *British Journal of Psychiatry, 202,* 89–90.

Piper, W. E., & Joyce, A. S. (2001). Psychosocial treatment outcome. In W. J. Livesley (Ed.), *Handbook of personality disorders: Theory, research, and treatment.* New York: Guilford Press.

Ryle, A. (1997). *Cognitive analytic therapy and borderline personality disorder.* Chichester, UK: Wiley.

van Asselt, A. D., Dirksen, C. D., Arntz, A., Giesen-Bloo, J. H., van Dyck, R., Spinhoven, P., et al. (2008). Out-patient psychotherapy for borderline personality disorder: Cost-effectiveness of schema-focused therapy vs. transference-focused psychotherapy. *British Journal of Psychiatry, 192*(6), 450–457.

Verheul, R., van den Bosch, L. M. C., Koeter, M. W. J., de Ridder, M. A. J., Stijnen, T., & van den Brink, W. (2003). Dialectical behaviour therapy for women with borderline personality disorder: 12-month, randomised clinical trial in The Netherlands. *British Journal of Psychiatry, 182,* 135–140.

Yeomans, F. (2007). Questions concerning the randomized trial of schema-focused therapy vs. transference-focused psychotherapy. *Archives of General Psychiatry, 64,* 609–610.

Young, J. E., Klosko, J. S., & Weishaar, M. E. (2003). *Schema therapy: A practitioner's guide.* New York: Guilford Press.

# CHAPTER 27

# Cognitive Analytic Therapy

Anthony Ryle[1] and Stephen Kellett

## The Origins and Main Features of Cognitive Analytic Therapy

Cognitive analytic therapy (CAT) originated as an integration of psychodynamic and cognitive theory/concepts to produce an active, collaborative, time-limited, and highly relational treatment model. As an integrative therapy, there should be no conflict between the cognitive and analytic elements of model during its delivery. There were two main original sources for this integration. The first source was the use of repertory grid techniques investigating aspects of structural change in patients receiving psychodynamic psychotherapy (summarized in Ryle, 1975). Therefore, the C in CAT has little in common theoretically and clinically with "Beckian" cognitive theory. The second source was the influence of the object relations school (Fairbairn, 1952) in combination with an attempt to devise ways to describe the goals, processes, and language of psychodynamic therapy in terms consistent with methodologically sound outcome research and everyday language for use with patients. Ryle (1995) then studied the notes of completed therapies, which revealed that most therapies had concentrated on one or two key issues and, crucially, that these issues had generally become evident in the first session. Moreover, such issues could be summarized and highlighted by describing the use by patients of repeated (but ultimately unsuccessful) strategies. The reasons behind chronic nonrevision by patients enabled the naming of three general patterns; (1) *traps,* in which negative assumptions generate actions that elicit consequences that then confirm the original beliefs about self, others, or the world in general; (2) *dilemmas,* in which apparent options for action (including relating to others and self-management) present as limited, polarized either–or or if–then choices; and (3) *snags,* in which appropriate goals are sabotaged, abandoned, or dismantled due to being unacceptable to others or the self (or both).

---

[1] We are sad to say that Tony Ryle, the founder of cognitive analytic therapy (CAT), died on September 29, 2016. Tony began his career as a GP and questioned why many of his patients repeatedly brought emotional and relational problems to his surgery. During his time as Director of Student Health at Sussex University and then as Consultant Psychotherapist at Guy's and St. Thomas's Hospitals, he put forward an integration of object relations theory and cognitive theory that became CAT. Tony was deeply committed to public health care and the social and developmental understanding of ill health. In developing CAT, he wanted to make available an in-depth, accessible, client-friendly collaborative psychotherapy that could be delivered within the resources of the National Health Service (NHS) to those at most need. A tribute to his vision is the success of CAT around the world and the establishment of national associations in the United Kingdom, Finland, Greece, Ireland, Australia and New Zealand, Spain, Italy, and India. Tony's legacy is in safe hands.

## Theory and Practice Links in CAT

CAT as a short-term and transdiagnostic model has a key role to play in the treatment of a wide range of mental health conditions in public services (Calvert & Kellett, 2014). CAT does this by initially identifying, describing, and reformulating the underlying dysfunctional psychological processes that manifest in the patients daily life (and are frequently reenacted within in the therapeutic relationship). The CAT therapist and patient then co-design "exits" that enable the patient to take up new, more positive/benign roles or learn how to interrupt their previously unhelpful procedures. The basic CAT treatment model involves a predetermined time limit, usually of 8, 16, or 24 weekly sessions, according to severity, complexity, and willingness to change. Longer contracts are occasionally offered according to need and complexity. Patients seen for the 8- and 16-session versions of the model are seen for one follow-up session (normally at 3 months, but negotiated with the patient) and patients seen in 24-session CAT receive four follow-ups (three sessions, 1 month apart and the final session at 6-months post-termination). Follow-up sessions are intended and designed to revisit and reinforce the use of the recognition (self-awareness) and revision work (the individualized exits) developed during therapy, rather than simply being "add-on" therapy sessions. Patients with chronic and enduring relational problems, as indicated by the diagnosis of personality disorder (PD), are typically treated within a 24-session contract. Patients with bipolar disorder in a recent pilot randomized trial of CAT, for example, were treated with a 24-session contract (Evans, Kellett, Heywood, Hall & Majid, 2016). There is evidence from routine clinical practice that CAT therapists do allocate patients with PD to the longer 24-session contract (Marriott & Kellett, 2009). If a patient with PD wanted to work on a particular single issue and was motivated to engage in therapy and change, there is no reason why an 8-session intervention could not be offered.

Early CAT sessions are devoted to the detailed assessment of the patient and the production of two helping tools: (1) *a narrative reformulation* and (2) *a diagrammatic reformulation*. These tools enable identification of key presenting problems, name the patterns that underpin them, and recognition of the historical context (often neglect and trauma) that created the pathological reciprocal roles. Early, collaborative, compassionate, noncollusive, and descriptive reformulation that is tolerable, acceptable, and digestible by a patient with PD has therefore become a defining feature of CAT. Narrative reformulation that is presented in a draft format to patients and conceived as a shared understanding is revised and completed as necessary, via patient feedback. The construction of *sequential diagrammatic reformulations* (SDR) then mirror and pictorially reinforce the roles and patterns described in narrative reformulations, but in a briefer co-constructed map-like document. This brevity enables the patient to carry and use the map to initially recognize when he or she is involved in, about to be involved, or has just enacted unhelpful roles and procedures, with associated recognition rating sheets used in CAT sessions to track the development of reflective capacity (*www.acat.me.uk*). During therapy sessions, the SDR is also used by CAT therapists to navigate the therapeutic relationship with patients with PD, often in terms repairing the frequent ruptures to the therapeutic alliance that occur (Bennett, Parry, & Ryle, 2006; Daly, Llewellyn, & McDougall, 2010). When the patient finds something that works in terms of change, then that is always labeled on the SDR as an "exit" (i.e., a different colored arrow summarizing how the exit takes the client away from pathological roles and procedures).

Assessment is carried out collaboratively, with the active participation of the patient—in CAT, reformulation is done with, not to the patient. Such narrative and diagrammatic reformulation enables the links between the patient's history and current life to be compassionately established. Potentially dysfunctional patterns and "reenactments" of past relationships (anticipation or activation of reciprocal roles) that may manifest in the therapeutic relationship are named and analyzed. Treatment of patients with CAT is therefore based on the foundation stone of *reformulation*. The aim of this is to set the patient's presenting symptoms, behaviors, thoughts, feelings, and relationships in the context of a general sequential model of underlying processes. This is to communicate clearly and consistently to the patient with PD the structure or set of roles and patterns evident in his or her life, and how these can so often echo his or her early attempts to survive abusive or neglectful early experiences—and also that set up the patient to experience the therapist in the transference in a certain manner. The early theoretical development of CAT involved the development of a model based on the idea of the *procedural sequence* as an appropriate unit of description. In this preliminary CAT model, aim-directed action was described in terms of the following recurrent sequence:

1. The context is appraised.
2. The possibility of action and the likely efficacy and consequences of available action plans are considered.
3. The selected plan is enacted.
4. The aim and the means are evaluated in the light of perceived consequences and then confirmed or revised.

Theoretical extension and evolution then involved the fuller integration of object relations theory into CAT's *procedural sequence object relations model* (PSORM; Ryle, 1985). Procedures of concern to CAT therapists are those controlling intra- and interpersonal actions and associated management of the self in the social/relational context. In seeking a relationship, the patient aims to find or elicit an appropriate response from the other, an idea expressed in the concept of a *reciprocal role procedure* (RRP). The limited and stereotyped *repertoire* of RRPs of the patient with PD is derived from early traumatic interactions with caretakers (and often siblings) that both maintain toxic contemporary relationships with others, and organize and mobilize pathological self-management (e.g., consistent self-harm). The "building blocks" and associated relational templates of the contemporary self are therefore derived and based on original interactions with others. This model parallels the ideas proposed within psychoanalysis by Ogden (1983), but it is differentiated by its emphasis on the real/actual experiences of the infant/child, as opposed to innate unconscious fantasy. It is a model close to that proposed by Mead (1934/1972) and the ideas of Vygotsky (1978) and his followers on the social formation of mind; these ideas and those of Bakhtin have been influential in the later developments of CAT, as described in Ryle (1991) and elaborated by Leiman (1992, 1994, 1995, 1997, 2000).

The emotional implications of termination for the patient with PD are considered throughout CAT (i.e., abandonment is recognized and reformulated), and the therapy aims to provide an experience of a "good ending," particularly for patients with marked abandonment histories, such as those seen in borderline personality disorder (BPD; American Psychiatric Association [APA], 2013). In the final sessions, the achievements, residual problems, ruptures that were repaired, key insights, methods of maintaining relational awareness, key relational changes, and the future consolidation of change are considered. These are summarized by both patient and therapist in "good-bye letters" exchanged in the final session. There are prompt sheets to support patients in writing their good-bye letters (Kellett, 2016).

### Diagnostic and Assessment Issues Using CAT Tools

The person with PD most likely to present to services is one with BPD, but only a minority are referred to psychotherapy services, and many are considered too disturbed for therapy. Many patients with BPD are seen in primary care settings (Moran, Jenkins, Tylee, Blizard, & Mann, 2000), and some of them are referred to general psychiatric settings for the treatment of associated depression/anxiety/somatization. In both settings, BPD is frequently undiagnosed or consists of no more than attaching the dismissive label "difficult patient." Others are seen after self-harm by emergency departments or in substance abuse or forensic settings. While a person with severe BPD will usually provide clear evidence of the diagnosis in the form of self-destructive behaviors and numerous unhelpful encounters with agencies, less severely disturbed patients may present themselves, at least initially, in compliant, coping "modes," and the diagnosis may be missed or occluded. As described in detail below, the existence of dissociated or disavowed self-states significantly adds to the reliability of accurately identifying BPD. Often patients are misdiagnosed with bipolar disorder or cyclothymia because of the presence of marked and distinct mood shifts, which are in fact manifestations of state shifts (e.g., rapid state shifting from a depressed and suicidal state to an overactive, impulsive, and disinhibited state).

In CAT, two types of screening questionnaires have been developed to assess and describe these shifts between distinct and often extreme states for patients with PD. Such tools enable the quantitative assessment of state shifting, usefully supplementing diagnostic and formulation work from clinical opinion and other-report. The 8-item Personality Structure Questionnaire (PSQ) provides a valid and reliable measure of the degree of personality integration and state shifting (Pollock, Broadbent, Clarke, Dorrian, & Ryle, 2001), with norms available for BPD populations. High PSQ scores (> 27) are indicative of structural dissociation and point to the need to further assess, identify, and characterize the different states. A recent cross-cultural validation of the PSQ (Berrios, Kellett, Fiorani, & Poggioli, 2016) investigated the construct validity of the PSQ in large community and clinical Italian samples. Confirmatory factor analysis revealed a three-factor PSQ structure of differing self-states, mood variability, and behavioral loss of control. Global PSQ scores of 26–28 were appropriate for assisting in diagnostic procedures for PD. The *states description procedure* (Ryle, 2007) also offers a clinically systematic approach to states assessment. Patients are given a list of commonly used names and profiles of states, and for each state that they regularly experience, they identify their (1) associated subjective experiences, (2) associated relationship patterns, and (3) other features. Through this procedure, patients can start to learn to identify their states as a first step toward integration. Using the states description procedure contributes significantly to the construction of accurate SDRs and to the initial control of damaging state shifts.

## Theoretical Foundations

The original attempt to integrate cognitive and psychoanalytic approaches was followed by a process of differentiation from these extant sources and by the introduction of ideas drawn from other sources. A full account of this early evolution may be found in Leiman (1994) and in Ryle (1995). This further elaboration of the clinical model has been closely supported by many observational studies, documenting the biologically driven, high-frequency, and interpersonally intense interactions (and reciprocity) of the child with those around him or her (e.g., Boyes, Giordano, & Pool, 1997; Delgado, Strawn, & Pedapati, 2014; Oliviera, 1997; Stern, 1985; Trevarthen & Aitken, 2001).

### Personality Development and Pathology

Normal personality development and psychological deviations from it are determined by early experience. Assessment during CAT emphasizes the social and psychological areas, since these have more plasticity for change and reflect the therapy context. Biological evolution over millennia has selectively favored characteristics adapted to the parallel evolution of complex, flexible social forms, dependent on great increases in brain size and on the ability to communicate (Donald, 1991). As a result, CAT conceives of the human infant as being *biologically adapted to be socially formed*. The human genotype has flourished with negligible change through widely differing historical epochs and cultures because it allows each individual to learn from, be formed by, and contribute to the particular culture into which he or she is born.

Such formation takes place initially *in utero*, then continues as the child is born into a world of semiotic meanings. As physical maturation proceeds, the child acquires a working knowledge of physical, social, and relational reality through his or her own active curiosity in a context of, and with a commentary by, caretakers (and others). CAT theory is based on Vygotsky's understanding that the self is a social creation and rejects the "monadic" assumptions that still underpin most current theories, in which the child is seen to build up representations of self and other through separate systems of information processing concerned with knowledge and feeling. In CAT theory, the individuality of the child is created and also shaped within and by relationships with others, and knowledge about the world is internalized through the signs and meanings developed and co-created with caretakers. The child does not store representations to which a mayonnaise of meaning is applied; affects and cognitions, meanings and facts, and the definitions of self and other are acquired in the course of actively engaging with others, whose own meanings also reflect and transmit those of the wider society and culture. Patterns of relationships with others (not the "objects" of psychoanalysis) are the source of the radical "dialogic" structure of the social self in CAT (Ryle & Kerr, 2002). Kerr, Finlayson-Short, McCutcheon, Beard, and Chanen (2015) therefore define a supraordinate, functionally constituted entity of the self that ranges over multiple, interacting levels. These levels range from an unconscious, "core" self to a reflective, phenotypic, idiographic, and relational self that is constituted by both interpersonal and sociocultural experiences. This construct of the self therefore partially redefines BPD as a "self-state" and relational disorder.

This developmental perspective of CAT, with its focus on reciprocal roles, was clarified and sharpened by these Vygotskian ideas and by the work of Bakhtin, with its emphasis on the continuities between external and internal dialogue. The self is conceived of as being made of relationships or "conversations" between past and present "voices" rather than as a battleground between warring internal "objects" conveying innate and conflicted instinctual forces. The stability of self-processes is a result of the early (often preverbal) acquisition of the major procedural patterns defining self–other relationships and of individuals seeking out those who reciprocate (and hence appear to confirm) their role procedures.

These ideas mean that the CAT model does not contain a replica of the dynamic unconscious of psychoanalysis and does not consider unconscious conflict as a prerequisite to the understanding PD phenomenology. In the course of their formation, *all* role procedures are, in psychoanalytic terms, compromise formations, in which action is shaped by memory, inherited predispositions, desire, reality, and the (external or internalized) reactions of others. The main procedural patterns are laid down early and continue to operate without the individual's conscious awareness. In this view, "the unconscious" is largely shaped (before speech) by social forces rather than innate fantasies (see Burkitt, 1995). Damaging, restricting, and avoidant procedures (which are often accompanied by "psychiatric" symptoms) result from the internalization of neglecting, harsh, critical, or conditional voices. The patient with a PD may lack insight into the relational origins of such voices prior to treatment, and awareness may be additionally limited by defensive procedures that are developed as alternatives to feared or forbidden positions/roles. Another form of lack of awareness in PD reflects limited awareness of the nature of one's own enacted procedures, resulting from the absence of self-reflective procedures. This is particularly the case in relation to the unstated assumptions that determine or limit the range of day-to-day actions. Once described, these patterns become readily recognized and are therefore more open to positive change and revision.

## Key Features of CAT PD Clinical Practice

Descriptions of personality and its disorders in CAT are therefore clinically based on identifying the repertoire of reciprocal roles and associated procedural sequences. In arriving at descriptions, the aim is to create the highest-level, most general account based on the assumption of a hierarchical structure, whereby lower-order "tactical" procedures operate within the terms of higher-order "strategic" procedures. While PD may be influenced and shaped by organic or inherited processes, the aim of CAT is to identify and revise the current and "here and now" dysfunctional procedures. Due to the short-term nature of the work, CAT therapists are encouraged to "push it where it moves" during sessions and concentrate on revising those roles and procedures most liable and pliable to change (i.e., within the patient's zone of proximal development). A start to this is enabled by the patient completing during or between early sessions the *psychotherapy file* (www.acat.me.uk), which is a CAT tool that names many of the common states, snags, traps, and dilemmas, and asks the patient to rate him- or herself in relation to the descriptions. The key therapeutic functions of CAT are (1) *pattern recognition* to create an observing self, (2) *noncollusion* by the CAT therapist, and (3) the development of alternatives—the final stage of revision in CAT, in which "exits" are co-created in change work by therapist and client. The observing self is often added to the SDR as a logo that encourages the patient with a PD patient to step back frequently and notice relational (self to self, self to other, and other to self) patterns. Rather than being stuck in a fixed observational position on the map, the patient is encouraged to move his or her observing eyes around the map to facilitate better self-understanding, using a *democracy of observation*.

### Sequential Diagrammatic Reformulation

In practice, descriptions that combine *sequential* elements with developmentally derived *structural* considerations are best expressed diagrammatically. In constructing such maps with patients with PDs, the first step is to collaboratively co-create in the core of the diagram the main *reciprocal role repertoires* that reflect the patient's named self-states. This is a heuristic device. Enacted role procedures are traced on procedural loops that describe associated aims, thoughts, feelings, actions and their consequences that form the links between self-states. CAT maps therefore often function to make sense of previously confusing enactments, procedures, and also dissociative experiences of patients with PDs. For many patients there is a "blank" or "zombie" state (this is also named in the *psychotherapy file*), which is an expression of a dissociative state in which the patient is cut off from thoughts and feelings (often expressed by a cloud on the map). This is frequently facilitated by the use of street drugs and alcohol in BPD. SDRs demonstrate that the consequences of problematic procedures reinforce the core procedural pattern. Such maps make it clear how each described role may be enacted and how others may be recruited to reciprocate. The form and content of SDRs also provides guidance (and a visual prompt) to CAT therapists to resist the often intense pressures and pulls to collude with negative procedures during sessions.

### Internalization

The formation of self-structures from relationships with others is a key developmental process. In Vygotsky's account, learning takes place on two planes, the first external and the second, involving some transformation, internal. Learning takes place in the "zone of proximal development" (ZPD), which is defined as the area in which the child has the potential capacity to learn, if given appropriate assistance by a more experienced other. The internalization of such learning involves the provision and mutual development of signs. As the developing child explores the world, the parent or teacher provides the "scaffolding" that links experiences and actions with meanings and mindfully controls the rate of change. These ideas have a clear relevance to CAT in terms of specific content and timing of interventions by CAT therapists. Too little scaffolding and the therapist is leaving the patient with insufficient support to enable stabilization and change, and too much scaffolding and he or she runs the risk of getting in the way of change and/or creating unhelpful dependency. In the past, others may have been damaging, restricting, prescriptive, or unsupportive, and the task of CAT therapists is to resist pressures to repeat these patterns. The content and the terms of the "conversation" or relationship between child and others will be repeated internally, as between different voices within the self, and will also continue to shape and be shaped by continuing patterns of relating to others. In this sense the self in CAT is both dialogic and permeable. CAT's emphasis on reciprocal roles and on the scaffolding created during the reformulation process represent the application of Vygotskian understandings to the process and content of the therapy.

### Flexibility

CAT is primarily a collaborative model, but there is the risk of under- and overcollaborating. The CAT therapist and the patient with PD can work effectively shoulder to shoulder on the construction of an SDR, but the therapist needs to be careful not to overcollaborate and to consistently define what is "we," "you," and "I." The between-session tasks of CAT are collaboratively designed by therapist and patient, but they are put into action solely by the patient. Helping patients to complete between-session activities that enable them to be both the "actor" (i.e., trying out an exit) and the "observer" (via some kind of record keeping) helps both experiential and reflective learning to take place. CAT therapists needs to be comfortable in three positions in relation to the patient with PD (see Figure 27.1). The CAT therapist needs to complete the naming, describing, and linking work from the "one-up" position (providing the *linking/naming to aware/named* reciprocal role). The work of therapy in which the therapist and patient collaborate is defined by the horizontal position, providing the *connecting/containing to connected/contained* reciprocal role). Crucially, the patient is an expert in his or her own experience; therefore, the CAT therapist needs to have the humility to adopt a "one-down" position in relation the patient. From this position, the therapist can learn from the patient how the patient's roles and procedures operate (providing the *describing to understood* reciprocal role). CAT therapists should move seamlessly between these positions, according to the context of the session and appropriate responsivity to the patient.

### BPD: The CAT Model

There are several problems with the concept of BPD. The clinical features contributing to the DSM-5 BPD diagnosis (APA, 2013) refer to instability or variability, but many overlap, are not quantified, and provide no satisfactory understanding of the underlying psychological processes and structures. Explanations in terms of "ego weakness" are tautological. The psychoanalytic concept of "splitting" is more

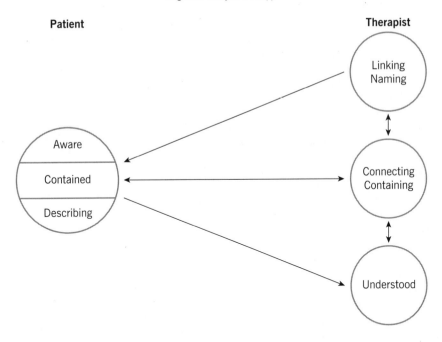

**FIGURE 27.1.** Flexibility and reciprocation in the therapeutic relationship during CAT.

explanatory, but it is frequently conceived as resulting from internal and innate rather than environmental and experiential processes. The disease model cannot be transferred crudely to personality deviations, and the evidence points to there being a common underlying set of causes of various forms of damage and distortion in individual development. Fonagy and Target (1997) viewed the inability to reflect on the psychological states of self and other as a fundamental cause of BPD, and accept that the capacity to generate inferences, predict behaviors, and form a "theory of mind" on the basis of unobservable mental states is an innate capacity. The Vygotskian account of personal formation through the internalization of external dialogue offers a more plausible and parsimonious explanation of the child's acquisition of understandings of self and others.

### The Multiple Self-States Model

In constructing SDRs in clinical practice with patients with neuroses, is usually possible to identify two or three key reciprocal role procedures that constitute the core of the map, with transitions between the roles often being smooth and appropriate. When working with patients with PDs, it is evident that reformulation can be undermined by the confusions and discontinuities of self that PD patients commonly experience (Pollock, Stowell-Smith, & Göpfert, 2006). Additionally, state shifts may also be iatrogenically induced and heightened by the interpersonal stress of the psychotherapy context itself (e.g., the threat of being abandoned by the therapist). The theoretical solution to this confusion comes with the recognition that these patients are operating discontinuously from one or another separate procedural systems, and that transitions between these are often sudden and, at times, externally unprovoked. Only when these separate "self-states" (i.e., dissociated reciprocal role patterns) are identified and described can their elicitation (i.e., appearances and disappearances) be effectively traced.

This theoretical development in clinical practice contributes to a clarification of the phenomenology of BPD, as involving structural dissociation between a number of self-states, each characterized by a distinct reciprocal role pattern (Ryle & Kerr, 2002). In BPD, state switches occur abruptly and often inappropriately, and in the absence of evident provocations; such switches reflect the inadequate development and/or the traumatic disruption of the metaprocedural system. Over time, behavior may be governed and experience may be interpreted by any of the different reciprocal role patterns in the disrupted system. Some particular roles may be perceived, sought, or provoked in the other, but are seldom, rarely, or never enacted by the self. This is a way of describing the process of projective identification, as described by Sandler (1976) and Ryle (1994); it is usually described in relation to negative roles and their affects, but it may equally apply to idealized roles. The multiple self-states model (MSSM) is consistent with the clinical evidence of partial dissociation between RRPs and with the known and evidenced associations between gross neglect and abuse in childhood and adult personality pathology (Ryle & Kerr, 2002). It offers explanations of much of the phenomenology of BPD, of the high comorbidity rates, and of patients' inadequate self-reflective capacity. The magnitude of these effects vary according to the degree of genetic predisposition/vulnerability and the degree, chronicity, and range of early abuse and neglect (Kellett, 2005). The MSSM describes three ways in which the pathology may present:

1. *Extreme roles.* The characteristic damaging patterns of self-management and relationships with others and also associated comorbid conditions (notably, depression, anxiety, and eating disorders) reflect the presence of damaging, restrictive, and often extreme repertoires of RRPs. These either repeat in some form patterns derived from the emotionally unmanageable experiences of childhood, typically *abusing/neglecting in relation to deprived/victimized,* or they represent partially dissociated patterns developed as alternatives to the (usually avoided) unmanageably intense feelings. Typical patterns range from submissive placation, perfectionist striving, or affectless coping ("joyless treadmill"), all liable to be accompanied by depression and somatization symptoms in relation to abusive demands from self and others.

2. *State shifts.* The variable and intermittent presence of many BPD features can be understood as reflecting the following phenomena: (a) *response shifts* within a given RRP (e.g., from *submissive* to *rebellious* in relation to *controlling*), (b) *role reversals* (e.g., from *victimized to abuser* to *abuser to victimized*), or (c) self-state shifts (e.g., *from ideally cared for in relation to perfect caring* to *abusive in relation to abandoning*). These state shifts frequently disrupt and sabotage apparently initially positive therapeutic relationships and may be markedly confusing for psychotherapists unless they are aware of such phenomena. State shifts account for the phenomena of each session being radically different in terms of process and content.

3. *Deficient self-reflection.* The capacity for self-reflection is impaired in BPD because the kinds of parenting (or substitute care) the patient experienced in childhood usually involved persistent inconsistency: for example, alternations between affection and abuse, or care and abandonment, combined with disinterest in the child's subjective experiences. No model of concern is internalized, and access to the language of moods, feelings, and emotions may be limited. Also, such capacity for self-reflection (as has developed) is not continuous, due to the disruption in awareness and associated learning by persistent state switches. Such switches tend to occur at the precise moment at which the established role procedure cannot accommodate either nonreciprocation from others or a new event, that is, at the moment when procedural revision would be particularly valuable (i.e., some learning would take place). The common failure of patients with BPD to take responsibility for the impact of their often abusive actions in relation to others can be attributed to such switches between states. This is particularly marked when memory or awareness of other states is either absent or considerably impaired.

## MSSM Case Example

The following is an example of the clinical use of the MSSM with a male CAT patient. During the early reformulation sessions, the following states were elicited: (1) an impulsive state in which the patient was occasionally a risk to others and more frequently a risk to himself by taking on the abusing role, (2) a lost/abandoned state in which the patient felt very desperate and lonely if relationships did not run smoothly, (3) a rescuing state in which the patient wanted to intervene to help anyone and everyone in distress, (4) a critic state in which the patient would denigrate himself for any minor perceived misdemeanor, and finally (5) a cut-off state (no thoughts or feelings) when under the influence of substances. These states also matched the patient's self-rating on the *psychotherapy file*. The patient ticked 11/22 "states" on the *psychotherapy file,* which highlighted, in particular, states related to themes of fear and mistrust. To aid with construction of an SDR reflecting the MSSM, an initial list of dominant reciprocal role procedures (described in the patient's own words) was created to represent the skeleton of interactions with self and others. Figure 27.2 provides an example of the *self-states SDRs* produced. The patient named self-states that were summaries of his reciprocal role procedures and these are described below:

- Self-state 1 "pain"
  A1 Abusive/abusing to A2   Powerless
- Self-state 2 "Robin Hood"
  B1 Idealized saver to B2   Rescued
- Self-state 3 "lost/alone"
  C1 Abandoning    to C2    Abandoned
- Self-state 4 "critic"
  D1 Ripping apart  to D1    Put down

Within the SDR, procedural patterns were added, which accounted for state shifts enabling the patient to start to make sense of the previously confusing state shifting. For example, a *state shift* the patient was able to notice was the sharp oscillation between perfect rescuing care and his dual fear of being abandoned. This was conceptualized as a state shift from idealized/saver-rescued (SS1; B2/B2) to abandoning to abandoned (SS2; C1/C2). The construction of the SDR also enabled the patient to recognize *role reversals* (Pollock et al., 2006). For example, in the critic state, he could enact an RRP toward himself of pulling himself to pieces. The patient stated that often he heard this RRP in his father's voice, and this was particularly distressing. This voice was experienced as a quiet but persistent internal dialogue for the majority of the time, but he did note that when he was extremely distressed, the voice took on the quality of an auditory hallucination. A *response shift* (Pollock et al., 2006) was apparent in reciprocation to the abusing pole, with the patient either ending up feeling terrified/powerless or mistakenly labeling his actions as abandoning. The response shift was in response to the cognition in the procedural sequence in the SDR of "I am a bad person if I don't go along."

### Research Evidence for the MSSM

The MSSM was derived in part from the elaboration of self-states SDRs, as illustrated in Figure 27.2. Bennett and Parry (1998) tested the ability of a jointly produced self-states SDRs to identify the themes emerging within early CAT sessions. Judges were required to match the self-states identified in an SDR from an individual patient using the Core Conflict Relationship Theme (CCRT; Luborsky & Crits-Christoph, 1990) and the Structural Analysis of Social Behavior—Cyclic Maladaptive Pattern (SASB-CMP; Schacht & Henry, 1994). This study showed that the self-states identified on the SDR were a valid representation of recurrent maladaptive relationship patterns. Highly accurate matching was achieved, and this finding was repeated on three subsequent cases (D. Bennett, personal communication, May 15, 1998). Golynkina and Ryle (1999), in a study of patients with BPD ($N = 20$), named the states identified by these patients and their therapists during early sessions as elements in a repertory grid (the States Grid). These were then rated against constructs concerned with sense of self and other, and describing the dominant mood and the degree of access to (and control of) core emotions. Most patients could carry out the task in relation to all their states, despite impaired access to memory in some instances. Analysis of the grids demonstrated that all the patients made meaningful discriminations between states, and that in many cases both poles of an identified RRP were described. States described by different patients shared many similarities. Thus, patients identified states derived from their early internalization of reciprocal role patterns of, for example, *abusing neglect in relation to victim or rebel,* and most showed some relating to patterns of *ideally caring to ideally cared for* and of either *soldiering on* or *affectless coping in relation to abandoning or threatening.* The States Description Procedure (Ryle, 2007), described earlier, therefore provides further support for the MSSM.

### The Practice of CAT with BPD

The dissociated self-states of BPD are unstable and, in most instances, have a single dominant RRP, often expressed in extreme behaviors—attempts to elicit confirmation (in and out of session) are correspondingly intense. This feature accounts for the range and variations in often powerful countertransference experiences elicited by patients with BPD during therapy, the often variable and chaotic content of sessions, varying interactions with clinical teams, and general life chaos. Recognizing (in the moment,

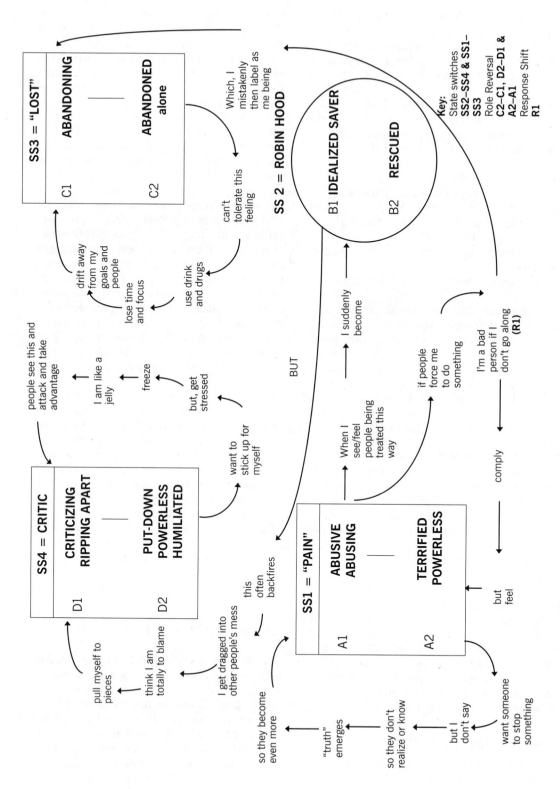

FIGURE 27.2. Sequential diagrammatic reformulation using the multiple self-states model.

via clinical supervision) and then resisting the patient's powerful "invitations" to collude with damaging procedures is the most important therapeutic function in CAT—and the scaffold for this is frequent use of the SDR within CAT sessions to analyze therapeutic interactions and also out-of-session enactments. During the reformulation phase of CAT, this work can be usefully supplemented by Leiman's "dialogic sequence analysis" (DSA; Leiman, 1997), whereby the sequences in RRP are analyzed for their reciprocity at each stage. This can be especially helpful in the case of those patients with BPD who, during tense phases evoked by therapy or difficult situations, may show marked and extremely rapid switches between states. Therefore, the chaos of the session can be halted, then usefully analyzed. DSA enables the patient to observe (often for the first time) the manner in which he or she can pinball around their SDR in response to interpersonal stress (e.g., experiencing a benevolent question by the therapist as abusive) or internal prompts (e.g., intrusive abuse memories). In such instances, each segment of the account is described in terms of the particular reciprocal roles involved; therefore, the DSA enables therapist and patient to reflect on the roles taken up. As in the previous case example, switches may be the result of response shifts, role reversals, or self-state shifts.

## Screening

Most patients referred for outpatient CAT who undergo assessment are accepted for treatment. Given that deficient self-reflection, via the operation of the MSSM, is a characteristic of BPD, patients are *not* expected to arrive with extant "psychological mindedness." Using the therapeutic relationship and the tools of CAT to develop and maintain the ability to consistently mentalize is a focus of CAT. During the early sessions, some patients prove unable to work in the CAT model, and the reasons for this might be (1) continuing substance abuse, (2) severity (e.g., manifest in massive and extreme state shifts or disruptive gross psychotic episodes), or (3) their social context is too threatening or violent to allow therapeutic work. A past history of unsuccessful interventions for PD is not usually considered a contraindication for CAT because previous interventions may have been inadequate, mistimed, or inappropriate. Attendance at screening may also signal a current willingness and ability to engage.

There are, however, some contraindications to outpatient CAT. Most patients with BPD have experienced loss of control of angry feelings and many have done physical harm to themselves and others by their aggressive and destructive actions. A patient with BPD entering a rage state will have little executive control during such state shifting due to dissociation and little memory of his or her actions during rage. Any patients with a high violence potential must be carefully screened in relation to the treatment setting in terms of patient and staff safety. Patients who might be successfully treated in secure inpatient or forensic settings may be unsuitable for treatment in primary care or outpatient clinics. Similarly, outpatient treatment may be unsafe for patients with intense suicidal preoccupations or severe and frequent self-harming behavior. Another contradiction is a high level of current substance abuse. Ideally, total withdrawal should precede CAT, for outcome is severely limited in patients continuing to abuse alcohol or street drugs, even if its use is intermittent and controlled. Combining CAT with treatment of addiction or linking it with withdrawal programs may be useful (see Leighton, 1997) and avoids the paradox of requiring recovery before treatment can start.

Some patients with BPD have accompanying life-threatening conditions that may need treatment before CAT is possible. An example would be anorexia nervosa, but even here, management and treatment within a CAT framework may be helpful (Treasure et al., 1995). In general, comorbid somatic or mood disorders would not be a contraindication to CAT—and would not be the primary focus of therapy. Determining which procedure or self-state is associated with the symptom, or which potential procedure the symptom seems to have replaced, allows CAT to then be focused on the issues of personality integration and developing or encouraging more benign, high-level interpersonal and self-management procedures. When such treatment is effective, direct treatment of the symptoms is usually unnecessary. At the time of the screening, current prescribed medication or the need for medication should be reviewed. Prescribing and management of medication are achieved best in the hands of a psychiatrist with a special interest in PD, who would be able to admit the patient for inpatient care should this become necessary. Use of minor tranquilizers is seldom indicated, due to unhelpfully inducing a "cut-off" state. In patients liable to enter states with intense paranoid or other psychotic features, antipsychotic medication may be helpful, preferably taken only when the symptoms are present. Although antidepressant medication has an uncertain impact on the depression of patients with BPD, it is sometimes of value and occasionally has marked effect on mood, which in turn may reduce borderline symptoms.

## Contracting

The basic function of the contracting is to provide a consistent and containing frame for the CAT work. When patients with PD are accepted for CAT, it is helpful to provide an overall idea of the collaborative and relational nature of CAT, the frequency and timing of sessions (weekly, 50- to 60-minute sessions), and the duration of the treatment contract itself (usually 24 weeks, with four sessions of follow-up). Clear expectations about attendance and notification of canceled sessions (by both patient and therapist) should be expressed. If the patient fails to attend a session without notification, then that session is deducted from the session total. Attitudes regarding willingness to engage in collaboratively designed between-session work should be elicited. Such therapy contracts, as well as offering a model of clarity and openness, mean that departures from the contract during CAT can also be understood as potential manifestations of the patient's procedures.

## The Reformulation Phase

At the screening session and review of the contract, the CAT therapist describes the overall nature and structure of CAT and explains the reformulation, recognition, and revision structure and stages. Naturally, there is some "bleed over" between CAT phases in most therapies. Assessment sessions leading to reformulation are explained as getting an understanding of the lived experience of the patient over the childhood, adolescent, and adult phases of life, in order to extract the core relational themes. To manage expectations, patients may be told that reformulation is based on attempting to generate a shared understanding of their problems, and the recognition phase as building relational and self-awareness, rather than striving to generate an immediate therapeutic solution. The first four to six sessions culminate in the collaborative creation of both narrative and diagrammatic reformulations. The process of reformulation starts immediately; hints of the main themes are evident in the first half of the first session, from the stories told and the patient's relational style. Prompt sheets to support patients in thinking about their past may be completed as between-session work (Strange & Kellett, 2016). The therapist leaves the agenda to the patient for much of the time, but might invite a focus from the patient at the start of each session. Competence in CAT therapy (Bennett & Parry, 2004) means connecting each detailed event to the broader pattern of which it is an example. As the main concerns are interpersonal and intrapersonal processes, individual reports or events can usually be seen as exemplifying particular reciprocal patterns of interaction (e.g., *caring–cared for, rejecting–rejected, controlling–submitting, controlling–rebelling, threatening–avoiding,* and *abusing–abused*) and in this way a *summary repertoire of RRPs* can be assembled. The CAT approach is therefore driven by a relational therapeutic approach and style.

In patients with BPD, each role is experienced as a discrete state, often initially described in terms of an extreme mood, affect or behavior. Further enquiry and between-session recognition by the patient identifies the accompanying sense of self and others, the degree to which affect is accessed or controlled, and the accompanying symptoms of each experienced self-state. Self-states are theoretical constructs describing partially dissociated reciprocal role patterns and subjective experiences associated with particular roles. The concept of the self-state also brings into focus, for both the CAT therapist and the patient, perceived or internalized reciprocals. Once the self-states have been identified in this way, careful observation and self-monitoring can identify the particular procedures generated from each role (these may be direct enactments of the role, or defensive or symptomatic replacements) and the internal and external triggers for state switches. Priority is given to recognizing states and the procedures leading to self-harm or to therapy-interfering behaviors. The final product will be a *self-states SDR,* as shown in Figure 27.2, which is actively used throughout the rest of the therapy and to manage the often strong emotions elicited by the termination phase of CAT work.

## Reformulation Letters and Reformulation Diagrams

Diagrammatic reformulation of the patient's current procedural repertoire is a paradigmatic exercise. In practice, it is typically preceded or accompanied by a letter offering a narrative reformulation. This is presented by the therapist at an early session, then refined via further discussion and review by the patient. As a between-sessions exercise, patients with PD can read and comment on the narrative reformulation (if possible) in differing self-states. This often elicits very differing reactions and responses, and provides a learning experience to the patient that he or she can experience the same "stimuli" in very different ways when in different states (e.g., comparing the achingly sad feelings in one reading with the scathing self-contempt present in another reading). These letters are the CAT therapist's gift to the patient and are an account of his or her understanding of the patient's life and problems. They should compassionately and empathically communicate a felt response from the sessions conducted, as well as an accurate account of the life history. Narrative reformulation is a model of noncollusion; the patient's ability to exist at both ends of reciprocal role poles are named (i.e., that the patient is both damaging and damaged). The letters' form involves a brief summary of key past experiences and of how the patient coped/survived, plus a description of how current patterns represent either repetitions of earlier experiences or the persistence of the alternatives developed as coping methods, which are now themselves problematic in the patient's life. These alternatives are identified as representing separate, alternating sources of experience and action. The aim of CAT is the revision of these patterns and the integration of the different self-states. The ways in which such negative patterns or roles may be manifest in the therapy relationship are outlined and speculated upon, if not already observed (e.g., experiencing an inquiry or connection by the therapist as abusive or bullying). Narrative reformulation is usually experienced as profoundly moving by the patients, and the experience of the collaborative joint work involved in forming the SDR is also a new and valued experience. The manner in which patients receive and experience narrative reformulation is often a key insight into (or provides more evidence of) chronic patterns (e.g., suppression of affect or denigration of the content). With the completion of this reformulation phase, the agenda shifts from reformulation to recognition and revision—the three R's of CAT (Ryle & Kerr, 2002). Common therapeutic errors derive from inadequately clear or incomplete SDRs and the failure to link reported events and in-session enactments to the SDR. Such linking depends heavily on the construction of a "good enough" SDR, so clinical supervision of the content and construction of self-state SDRs is important (Pickvance, 2017). During early stages of CAT, patient and therapist may collude in omitting from the SDR some area of shared difficulty (e.g., identifying that the patient can operate at both ends of reciprocal roles, or that the therapist is enjoying being put on a pedestal by the patient). Again, supervision is vital in recognizing and naming such aspects early. Generally, CAT therapists may be invited into every role described on the SDR, and only in session reflective vigilance will prevent inadvertent collusion.

### Active Phases: Recognition and Revision

Change in CAT is grounded in enlargement of the patient's capacity for accurate self-reflection, which is achieved through a combination of the formal, cognitive task of learning to recognize and exit the damaging automatic procedures, supported by the experience of a respecting and noncollusive relationship with the CAT therapist. Recognition involves self-monitoring and diary keeping; it is based on clear, accurate working diagrams that can be color-coded and used with idiosyncratic artwork to capture particular self-states (e.g., erupting volcanoes representing rage states). SDRs can operate like a transitional object for some patients. At times, the emphasis may be on particular procedures (e.g., those threatening to life or therapy), but usually the patient keeps a day-to day diary of disturbing experiences and learns to locate them on his or her SDR. Maintaining the noncollusive relationship involves the CAT therapist's frequent use of the SDR to avoid or correct acts/comments that constitute reciprocation and reinforcement of the patient's negative procedures. It is also helpful to challenge the patient's interpretation of events or ruptures in the therapeutic relationship, when they are based on the repetitive negative patterns described in the SDR—this is at the heart of the rupture repair process in CAT (Bennett et al., 2006).

These activities provide a therapeutic framework of understanding that is not only containing but also permits a sufficiently emotionally intense relationship. The intensity of this relationship is tempered by the notion of the patient's unique ZPD. Therefore, the CAT therapist will sensitively judge how distant–close and hot–cold he or she needs to be in relation to the patient in order to scaffold successfully the patient's ability to tolerate notions of trust and emotional intimacy. Patients not only contact or amplify memories of past abuses but may, in response to disappointments or the prospect of termination of CAT, enact negative procedures or enter negative self-states. The recognition of these negative states allows therapists to offer responses aiding their mitigation and assimilation. Suggesting or probing for memories of abuse is not part of CAT practice; if such memories are accessed, it is important to grant the patient the right to control the pace of disclosure or to attentively listen and witness. In general, patients go as far or as deep as they feel it is safe to go, and procedural change is often achieved without exploration of all that has been forgotten or repressed. But CAT therapists may find themselves on a knife's edge, poised between being experienced as intrusive on the one hand and indifferent on the other—a dilemma that is best shared with the patient. CAT therapists need to take every opportunity to suggest links with the higher-level, more general understandings of the patient's difficulties encapsulated in the SDR.

## The CAT Competency Model

CAT therapists need occupy a straddling position, with one foot in the therapeutic relationship connecting relationally with the patient and the other foot out of the therapy in an observing position, able to reflect in action on theory, potential ruptures, and enactments in the therapeutic relationship, and on their historical origins. In terms of the revision stage of CAT, some specific interventions may be of value; any technique aimed at procedural revision and integration may be employed, provided its relevance to the overall aim is clear; therefore, the change methods of CAT are catholic, client-centered, and always developed within the patient's ZPD (Kellett, 2012). Thus, for example, behavioral interventions to revise identified procedures, role playing to explore RRPs, and the use of drawing or writing as alternative expressions and sources of self-expression may all be helpful. The overall aim, however, remains the achievement of continuing awareness across states. Linked with this, the internalization of the therapeutic relationship as a model of a different reciprocal role patterns is crucial. Ultimately, the detailed "techniques" employed in CAT enable therapists to maintain a respectful human relationship with disturbed and disturbing patients.

Termination of CAT with deprived and damaged patients is always difficult; the use of predetermined time limits and reference to termination from the beginning does not make it simple/easy, but it does tend to prevent regressive dependency. Termination is especially difficult when the patient with PD has the fantasy of "perfect care" that has not been recognized and mapped. Patients with patients can never be given enough to compensate for their early abuse, pain, and hurts, but an intense and relational time-limited therapy can offer a powerful transformatory experience and manageable disappointment at the end, from which real change and more realistic hopes can stem. CAT at least aims to be a stable stepping-stone for the patient into the next phase of his or her life. For this to happen, the patient needs to take away from CAT an accurate and balanced memory that neither denies disappointment nor devalues what was achieved. The common return of symptoms during later sessions should be expected and calmly contained by the CAT therapist, with links made to the SDR, with earlier losses being kept in mind.

CAT is not a manualized therapy, but an "ideal model" of CAT work has been defined and empirically developed via the development of the Competence in CAT measure (CCAT; Bennett & Parry, 2004). CAT offers what has been recently called a "humanised skilled psychotherapy" (Tyrer, 2013); therefore, the competencies range from humanistic to technical. The CCAT was designed for use with whole-session audio recordings and has been found to be a useful supervision/training tool (Kellett & Bennett, 2016). The 10 domains of CAT competency are (1) phase-specific therapeutic tasks; (2) theory–practice links; (3) CAT-specific tools and techniques; (4) establishing and maintaining boundaries; (5) maintaining common factors and basic supportive good practice; (6) respect, collaboration, and mutuality; (7) naming and assimilation of warded-off problematic states and emotions; (8) making timely and appropriate links and hypotheses between therapy and the patient's past and other relationships, facilitating awareness of procedures in operation; (9) identifying and managing threats to the therapeutic alliance via identifying and managing in-session reciprocal role enactments; and (10) the therapist's awareness and management of his or her own reactions and emotions. The

CCAT has acceptable levels of interrater reliability and high internal consistency, and CCAT scores are significantly associated with quality of therapeutic alliance (Bennett & Parry, 2004). In relation to CCAT item 9 (identifying and managing threats to the therapeutic alliance), a rich vein of CAT research (using qualitative task analysis) refers to the ability of CAT therapists to engage in successful rupture repair sequences with patients (Bennett et al., 2006; Daly et al., 2010). The eight stages of CAT-informed rupture repair work are (1) acknowledgment of the rupture, (2) exploration (3) linking, (4) negotiation, (5) consensus, (6) further exploration, (7) new ways of relating, and (8) closure. In clinical practice, therapists often cycle between stages.

## Review of the CAT PD Outcome Evidence

### Overview

CAT has been slow to accumulate a satisfactory broad and disorder-specific evidence base, yet the quality of extant CAT outcome evidence is generally high (Calvert & Kellett, 2014). In part, this can be attributed to the fact that training and supervision in the model was initially championed over development of the evidence base (Ryle, Kellett, Hepple, & Calvert, 2014). It is also a consequence of the fact that internally valid outcome research such as randomized controlled trials (RCTs) have increasingly demanded adherence to treatment manuals. Therapeutic clinical input is not a standard factor analogous to medication and personality diagnosis, even using standardized procedures, and it bears an uncertain relation to the processes which therapy aims to influence. CAT involves the establishment of a unique relationship with each patient and the use of this by the therapist to apply theoretical understandings with the aim of supporting change rather than the delivery of "manualized, standardized and homogenized" input. Indeed, the evidence of "therapist effects" in RCTs and routine clinical practice (systematic variation in outcomes achieved by therapists) illustrates that therapy is not an interpersonally neutral and/or blandly technical endeavor (Castonguay & Hill, 2012).

It is generally agreed that psychotherapies for patients with the diagnosis of PD should be based on evidence that they are clinically effective (Higgitt & Fonagy, 2002), in order to improve both service design and commissioning, and to offer the patient a real choice.

Establishing a credible evidence base for any psychotherapy for PD is a complex endeavor, requiring critical evaluation and assimilation of typically diverse sources of outcome information (Barkham, Stiles, Lambert, & Mellor-Clark, 2010). There is a dilemma and tension between *effectiveness* studies completed in routine clinical practice with patients with PD and *efficacy* studies defining the outcomes derived from PD research trials (Donnenberg, Lyons, & Howard, 1999; Roth & Fonagy, 2005; Weston, Novotny, & Thompson-Brenner, 2004). Practice-based evidence (PBE) of effectiveness studies completed in routine clinical practice with patients with PD usefully contextualizes and benchmarks the results of trials of evidence-based practice (EBP; Bower & Gilbody, 2010; Gilbody & Whitty, 2002). The two methodological schools actually complement each other: PBE suffers from typically low internal validity (e.g., lack of randomization procedures and of checks regarding treatment integrity), while EBP approaches suffer from typically low external validity (e.g., excluding patients with comorbidity, which is the norm and not the exception in services). Considering the relative strengths and weaknesses of EBP and PBE for PD treatment facilitates the development of a robust and relevant PD modality specific evidence-base (Barkham & Mellor-Clark, 2003).

Calvert & Kellett's (2014) systematic review of the CAT pan-disorder evidence base noted that outcome studies (1) typically are of high quality (52%); (2) tend to be completed in complex populations (44%), with low dropout rates across studies; and (3) tend to be part of the PBE methodological tradition. Specific to the realm of PD, Mulder and Chanen (2013) noted that CAT particularly offers a valuable treatment option due to the following factors: (1) the practical nature of the CAT approach; (2) its short duration in comparison the other psychotherapies for PD; (3) the ease of obtaining training and supervision, due to the popularity of CAT with psychotherapists in clinical services; (4) the specified treatment duration having low cost implications; (5) evidence of efficacy from EBP style studies; (6) the explicitly relational approach; and finally (7) positive patient preference. When the outcomes of CAT EBP and PBE studies have been quantified across diagnoses, this has demonstrated a large effect size of 0.83 (Ryle et al., 2014), indicating that CAT is an effective intervention. It is worth noting that the evidence base for CAT with PD almost entirely consists of evaluations of individual treatment. The use and evaluations of CAT delivered in groups of patients with PD need attention. Calvert, Kellett, and Hagan (2015) benchmarked group CAT for survivors of child sexual abuse against other therapies and found that CAT produced a similar effect size and had a low dropout rate.

Our aim in this section has been to review the evidence for CAT in terms of treating PD by capturing the PBE and EBP evidence for each PD diagnosis. Table 27.1 details the CAT for PD evidence base by DSM-5 (APA, 2013) PD cluster and also in terms of whether the study used a PBE methodology in routine clinical practice or an EBP trial design. Within the CAT PBE style outcome methodologies, there is a hierarchy evident within the evaluations, from qualitative case studies to large group studies. Because the Clarke, Thomas, and James (2013) RCT of CAT was for PD regardless of cluster, this has been labeled as a Clusters A, B, and C EBP study. The studies are discussed in chronological order, and the main results and conclusions are presented.

### Cluster A: Paranoid Personality Disorder

Kellett and Hardy (2014) examined the effectiveness of CAT for a patient diagnosed with paranoid PD (PPD) and depression in a PBE-style study. The outcome methodology was a mixed methods single-case experimental design (SCED). The patient provided daily ratings of the presence and intensity of six target PPD variables throughout a time series of baseline (42 days), CAT intervention (161 days), and four-session follow-up phases (140 days). Standardized outcome measures were administered at assessment, termination, and final (6-month) follow-up. Results noted a significant reduction in suspiciousness and anxiety, with all target PPD measures (barring anxiety) extinguished by approximately the midpoint of the active treatment phase. No paranoid relapse occurred during the follow-up phase. Clinically significant improvements were recorded in terms of depression, general psychiatric symptomatology, and personality structure. The patient was interviewed about the change process to isolate the potential factors that had created change, and progress was attributed to CAT rather than to extraneous factors.

### Cluster B: BPD

In the first article to detail CAT with a patient with BPD, a PBE-style qualitative case description, Ryle and Beard (1993) suggested that CAT was effective for BPD, as it improved the patient's interpersonal functioning and reduced global distress and dissociation. Clinical improvements were also maintained at follow-up. In a PBE-style study promising outcomes at fol-

**TABLE 27.1. Summary of the CAT PD Evidence Base**

| | EBP methodology | PBE methodology |
|---|---|---|
| Cluster A | | |
| Paranoid personality disorder | | Kellett & Hardy (2013) |
| Cluster B | | |
| Borderline personality disorder | Chanen et al. (2008, 2009) | Ryle & Beard (1993); Duignan & Mitzman (1994); Ryle & Golynkina (2000); Wildgoose et al. (2001); Mace et al. (2006); Dasoukis et al. (2008); Livanos et al. (2008); Kellett et al. (2013) |
| Histrionic personality disorder | | Kellett (2007) |
| Cluster C | | |
| Obsessive–compulsive personality disorder | | Kosti et al. (2008) |
| Clusters A, B, and C | Clarke et al. (2013) | |

low-up for $N = 7$ patients (three with BPD and the remainder with a range of mainly PD issues) who had completed four one-to-one sessions leading to reformulation, then graduating into a 12-week group CAT, Duignan and Mitzman (1994) observed statistically significant change across a range of outcome measures between the start of the group phase and 1-month follow-up.

Further evidence for the effectiveness of CAT for BPD in routine practice was reported in Ryle and Golynkina's (2000) PBE study; $N = 27$ patients (69%) completed one-to-one CAT and contributed outcomes at 6-month follow-up. Significant pre- and posttreatment improvement was observed across all standardized measures over time. On completing CAT, 52% of patients were categorized as improved, 22% exhibited some level of change, and 26% were in stasis. Poorer outcome was associated with severity of BPD symptoms, unemployment, alcohol misuse, and self-injurious behavior. Approximately half the sample (52%) was deemed to require no further treatment. At 18-months post-CAT, there was evidence of continuing gains over time in patients with BPD.

Wildgoose, Clarke, and Waller (2001) evaluated the impact of CAT on dissociation, personality fragmentation, global distress, and interpersonal functioning in $N = 5$ patients with BPD, using a PBE-style methodology. At 9-month follow-up, $N = 4$ patients were classed as "recovered," while one had deteriorated. Mace, Beeken, and Embleton (2006) compared CAT and brief psychodynamic therapy (BPT) delivered by relatively inexperienced clinicians in a PBE-style methodology. Patients ($N = 17$) were allocated to treatment conditions following independent assessment and matched on various clinical factors. Findings suggest that both therapies produced improvements in mental health. The improvement rate was greater in BFT, but twice as many patients allocated to CAT were diagnosed with PD. Dasoukis and colleagues (2008) found that at 2-month follow-up from CAT, patients with BPD showed a statistically significant improvement across outcomes measures, and at 1-year follow-up, patients had maintained the achieved improvement. Livanos and colleagues (2008), in a study of $N = 57$ patients with BPD, demonstrated that at 2-month follow-up, the patients showed a statistically significant improvement on the Beck Depression Inventory, on an Anhedonia subscale score, as well as on the State–Trait Anxiety Inventory, compared to intake. Significantly fewer CAT patients were still anhedonic in comparison to pretherapy evaluation.

Chanen and colleagues (2008) conducted the first CAT study of PD in an RCT comparing CAT with manualized "good clinical care" (GCC) in adolescents with BPD attending a specialist early intervention service. Eighty-six adolescent patients were initially randomized, and 78 patients (CAT $N = 41$; GCC $N = 37$) provided follow-up outcomes. No significant differences were found between the trial arms in terms of psychopathology, parasuicidal behavior, and global functioning 2 years after completing interventions. There was some evidence, however, that adolescent patients treated with CAT improved more rapidly. No adverse effect were found for either treatment. Chanen and colleagues (2009) reanalyzed the data and compared findings in a quasi-experimental study design, comparing CAT and GCC in adolescents who received "historical treatment as usual" (H-TAU, $N = 32$). Participants completed measures on the level of borderline psychopathology, self-reported internalizing–externalizing difficulties, global functioning, frequency of self-harm behavior, and suicide attempts at baseline, and at 6-, 12-, and 24-month follow-up. Attempts were made to control for therapist effects by having the same therapists ($N = 3$) deliver CAT and GCC, and independent evaluations were made of treatment integrity. Results at final follow-up indicate that while all the interventions were successful in reducing BPD symptomatology, CAT produced the most marked improvement in externalizing difficulties and parasuicidal behavior.

Kellett, Bennett, Ryle, and Thake (2013) used a mixed method repeated measures PBE-type design to evaluate CAT with $N = 17$ adult patients with BPD. Four patients experienced clinically significant and reliable change, three patients experienced reliable improvement, and one patient reliably deteriorated. Analyzing outcomes at the group level showed statistically significant reductions in risk, dissociation, and psychological distress, with psychological improvements occurring early in treatment (i.e., the reformulation phase of CAT). Treatment integrity assessed using the CCAT (Bennett & Parry, 2004) indicated that 93% of sessions ($N = 70$) were competently delivered in routine practice. Furthermore, patients qualitatively attributed various personal changes to CAT rather than to other spurious positive life events.

Clarke and colleagues (2013) conducted an RCT comparing the efficacy of CAT for patients with a broader range of PDs ($N = 38$) with TAU ($N = 40$). All patients enrolled in the RCT had received at least one previous episode of therapy and were randomized according to whether they met diagnostic criteria for each PD cluster (A = 0, B = 18, C = 28, and mixed = 55). CAT treatment integrity was assessed and found to be sufficient. On completing CAT, 33% (9/27) of the patients no longer met diagnostic criteria for any PD, while all TAU patients (100%, 33/33) continued to meet criteria for at least one PD. Reliable change scores in the CAT patients noted that 42% (15/35) had either improved or recovered.

### Cluster B: Histrionic Personality Disorder

Kellett (2007) used a PBE-style SCED methodology with a patient diagnosed with histrionic PD (HPD) to evaluate the effectiveness of the CAT delivered. Psychometric measures were completed at assessment, end of treatment, and 6-month follow-up. Target variables constructed in line with DSM-IV diagnostic criteria for HPD were rated on a daily basis in a time series spanning baseline (21 days), CAT treatment (182 days) and follow-up (154 days) phases. Significant change in histrionic symptom intensity recorded over time demonstrated that CAT had a significant improvement on all target variables compared to baseline phase scores. Results indicated a more than 40% reduction in the majority of histrionic target variables during the treatment phase. Identity formation progression was maintained over the follow-up phase, although significant deterioration was observed in the patients' focus on physical appearance at the point of termination. Clinically significant improvements were recorded in terms of depression, general psychiatric symptomatology, and personality structure.

### Cluster C: Obsessive–Compulsive Personality Disorder

Kosti and colleagues (2008) showed that of $N = 64$ patients with obsessive–compulsive PD (OCPD) starting CAT, $N = 45$ patients completed therapy and attended the follow-up. Patients with OCPD receiving CAT showed a statistically significant improvement on Beck Depression Inventory total score, on the score of the Anhedonia subscale, as well as on the State and Trait scores of the State–Trait Anxiety Inventory, compared to the intake. Also, significantly fewer patients were still anhedonic in comparison to pretherapy evaluation.

### Discussion of the CAT-PD Evidence Base

CAT was conceptualized as a researchable therapy, relevant to any public sector delivery context (Ryle, 1995), and has increasingly been taken-up internationally in terms clinical practice and associated training and supervision (Margison, 2000; Ryle et al., 2014). This review of the PD evidence reported findings from two EBP RCTs, one quasi-experimental study, and 11 PBE-style studies of CAT conducted in routine clinical practice. Evidence is slowly accumulating for the promising utility of CAT in "hard to engage and treat" populations, with CAT being cited in the National Institute for Health and Clinical Evidence (NICE; 2009) guidelines for BPD.

### Future CAT PD Research

Developing a robust and relevant evidence base for any therapy requires integration of the findings from both EBP- and PBE-based studies (Barkham & Mellor-Clark, 2003). Further and coordinated evaluations of CAT treatment of PD are indicated to ensure continued commissioning, and the results from the trials also suggest that large-scale service evaluations of the effectiveness of CAT with BPD are the next indicated step. Future pragmatic treatment trials offer a methodology in keeping with the original research and service development aspirations of CAT. In randomized studies, comparing CAT against "active controls" (e.g., other modalities) will always be preferable to passive controls (e.g., wait-list controls). The further spread of EBP- and PBE-style studies are required across the PD diagnostic range, as most of the CAT evidence thus far is focal to treatment of BPD. Outcomes studies are sorely needed to evaluate outcomes for the CAT treatment of avoidant and dependent PD. CAT generates low treatment dropout rates across disorders; the reason for this needs to be identified (Calvert & Kellett, 2014). There is also a need to describe and isolate the mechanisms of change in CAT for PD. Some research suggests that the CAT-specific reformulation tools are associated with sudden gains in PD (Kellett & Hardy, 2014; Kellett, Simmonds-Buckley, & Totterdell,

2016). Building the evidence base for CAT with patients with PD requires further exploration of the impact of CAT-specific tools on outcomes. Eventually, deconstruction trials of the active ingredients may be possible in CAT for PD and there is a need to explore mediators and moderators of CAT outcome across the PD diagnoses. Certainly, all CAT PD outcome studies require truly long-term follow-up of patients to assess the durability of change.

## The Wider Organizational Role of CAT in the Management of PD

Only a small minority of patients with PD actually receive psychotherapy, but most spend some time in contact with psychiatric, forensic, or social agencies. In the absence of clear, shared understandings, staff members are all too easily drawn into unhelpful or actively collusive relationships with patients with PD. The theoretical model on which CAT is based emphasizes the permeability of the individual self and the crucial influence of the social and personal context provided. The collaborative ethos can be extended beyond individual therapy to other settings, and the jointly fashioned tools, notably diagrams, are accessible to staff members and patients as a basis for the maintenance of a humane, respectful working relationship. In a comprehensive service, CAT provides the opportunity for economical and effective interventions for less severe cases and may contribute to longer-term management involving day hospital, therapeutic community, and other inpatient care. By its provision of adequately detailed understandings of each individual patient, CAT reformulation can ensure that specific therapeutic inputs (e.g., behavioral programs or art therapy) are offered in ways supportive of the overall objective of aiding integration.

Although it was developed in the context of individual psychotherapy, CAT is being increasingly applied in other treatment modes and settings (Calvert & Kellett, 2014), particularly concerning the development and evaluation of contextual and team-based formulation (Carradice, 2013) as a means of helping organizational systems become more helpful and useful to the patient who is unsuitable for one-to-one or group psychotherapy. A five-session CAT consultancy model has been developed as a method of working collaboratively with mental health teams and patients to develop SDRs that map patients' current difficulties, procedures, and responses by the team. This therefore informs care planning for patients and shared understanding of the push and pull of dynamics between patients and teams. Dunn and Parry (1997) first reported the use of CAT reformulation as a basis for case management in a small inpatient unit for severely disturbed patients with BPD. Kerr (1999) described the use of CAT understandings in the management of a patient with BPD and introduced the notion of contextual reformulation to demonstrate parallels between the patient's procedures, problems within the staff group, and difficulties between the unit and other agencies. More recently, Kellett, Wilbram, Davies, and Hardy (2014) completed an RCT of the CAT team consultancy model. $N = 20$ patients in an Assertive Outreach Team were randomly allocated to either CAT consultancy or TAU. Three sessions of diagrammatic reformulation with care coordinators produced SDRs that were subsequently introduced to group supervision, in which the team discussed potential unhelpful enactments and a plan for team- and client-based exits based on the SDR. Although outcomes for patients were matched in each arm, the organizational outcomes evidenced a significantly improved team climate and more effective clinical and working practices in the team. Further dissemination and evaluation of the CAT consultancy model (as it is the main way the model has been adapted) is clearly indicated.

## Summary: The Distinguishing Features of CAT for PD

Although it shares features with other approaches, CAT has developed a distinct theory and specific methods (Ryle & Kerr, 2002). In regard to theory, the emphasis on the formation and maintenance of personality functioning through the understandings and activities shared with others offers a revision of object relations theories, with an emphasis on actual experience and socially derived meanings, as opposed to fantasy. This underlies the central importance accorded to the provision of a noncollusive therapy relationship. The MSSM describes the structural features of PD, which are derived from trauma-induced structural dissociation. The effect of treatment is understood to be due to the influence of the therapeutic relationship and to the creation within it of clear written and diagrammatic descriptions that represent, in Vygotskian terms, jointly elaborated interpsychological tools that, in due course, are internalized. The explicit framework provided by reformulation provides a safety within which an active and intense therapeutic relationship can be maintained, even by relatively inexperienced trainee therapists under close supervision. The time-limited basis of CAT is cost-effective and provides enough therapy for less severely disturbed patients. The contextual and team-based reformulation of individual patients can provide a basis for management in longer-term treatments and for coordinated care planning in institutional settings and community teams. Finally, CAT is starting to accumulate an expanding and convincing evidence base, but more research concerning the MSSM and large and controlled studies of PD outcome is required.

## Further Reading

The description offered in this chapter is, of necessity, brief. A full account of the CAT method applied to treating BPD and a discussion of its relation to other approaches is found in Ryle (1997) and case histories are provided there and in Ryle and Beard (1993), Dunn (1994) and Ryle and Kerr (2002). The model continues to be developed and new publications, applications to new patient groups, and new research are reported on the website of the Association or Cognitive Analytic Therapy (ACAT; www.acat.me.uk).

## REFERENCES

American Psychiatric Association. (2013). *Diagnostic and statistical manual of mental disorders* (5th ed.). Arlington, VA: Author.

Barkham, M., & Mellor-Clark, J. (2003). Bridging evidence-based practice and practice-based evidence: Developing a rigorous and relevant knowledge for the psychological therapies. *Clinical Psychology and Psychotherapy, 10,* 319–327.

Barkham, M., Stiles, W. B., Lambert, M. J., & Mellor-Clark, J. (2010). Building a rigorous and relevant knowledge base for psychological therapies. In M. Barkham, G. E. Hardy, & J. Mellor-Clare (Eds.), *Developing and delivering practice-based evidence.* Chichester, UK: Wiley.

Bennett, D., & Parry, G. (1998). The accuracy of reformulation in cognitive analytic therapy: A validation study. *Psychotherapy Research, 8,* 84–103.

Bennett, D., & Parry, G. (2004). A measure of psychotherapeutic competence derived from cognitive analytic therapy. *Psychotherapy Research, 14,* 176–192.

Bennett, D., Parry, G., & Ryle, A. (2006). Resolving threats to the therapeutic alliance in cognitive analytic therapy of borderline personality disorder: A task analysis. *Psychology and Psychotherapy: Theory, Research and Practice, 79,* 395–418.

Berrios, R., Kellett, S., Fiorani, C., & Poggioli, M. (2016). Assessment of identity disturbance: Factor structure and validation of the Personality Structure Questionnaire (PSQ) in an Italian sample. *Psychological Assessment, 28,* 27–35.

Bower, P., & Gilbody, S. (2010). The current view of evidence and evidence-based practice. In M. Barkham, G. E. Hardy, & J. Mellor-Clark (Eds.), *Developing and delivering practice-based evidence.* Chichester, UK: Wiley.

Boyes, M., Giordano, R., & Pool, M. (1997). Internalisation of social discourse: A Vygotskian account of the development of young children's theories of mind. In B. D. Cox & C. Lightfoot (Eds.), *Sociogenic perspectives on internalization.* Mahwah, NJ: Erlbaum.

Burkitt, I. (1995). *Social selves: Theories of the social formation of personality.* London: SAGE.

Calvert, R., & Kellett, S. (2014). Cognitive analytic therapy: A review of the outcome evidence base for treatment. *Psychology and Psychotherapy: Theory, Research and Practice, 87,* 253–277.

Calvert, R., Kellett, S., & Hagan, T. (2015). Group cognitive analytic therapy for female survivors of childhood sexual abuse. *British Journal of Clinical Psychology, 54,* 391–413.

Carradice, A. (2013). Five-session CAT consultancy: Using CAT to guide care planning with people diagnosed with personality disorder within community mental health teams. *Clinical Psychology and Psychotherapy, 20,* 359–367.

Castonguay, L. G., & Hill, C. H. (2012). *Transformation in psychotherapy: Corrective experiences across cognitive behavioral, humanistic, and psychodynamic approaches.* Washington, DC: American Psychiatric Association.

Chanen, A. M., Jackson, H. J., McCutcheon, L. K., Jovev, M., Dudgeon, P., Yuen, H. P., et al. (2008). Early intervention for adolescents with borderline personality disorder using cognitive analytic therapy: Randomised controlled trial. *British Journal of Psychiatry, 193,* 477–484.

Chanen, A. M., Jackson, H. J., McCutcheon, L. K., Jovev, M., Dudgeon, P., Yuen, H. P., et al. (2009). Early intervention for adolescents with borderline personality disorder: Quasi-experimental comparison with treatment as usual. *Australian and New Zealand Journal of Psychiatry, 43,* 397–408.

Clarke, S., Thomas, P., & James, K. (2013). Cognitive analytic therapy for personality disorder: Randomised controlled trial. *British Journal of Psychiatry, 202,* 129–134.

Daly, A.-M., Llewellyn, S., & McDougall, E. (2010). Rupture resolution in the cognitive analytic therapy for adolescents with borderline personality disorder. *Psychology and Psychotherapy: Theory, Research and Practice, 83,* 273–288.

Dasoukis, J., Garyfallos, G., Bozikas, V., Katsigiannopoulos, K., Voikli, M., Pandoularis, J., et al. (2008). Evaluation of cognitive-analytic therapy (CAT) outcome in patients with borderline personality disorder. *Annals of General Psychiatry, 7*(Suppl. 1), S108.

Delgado, S. V., Strawn, J. R., & Pedapati, E. V. (2014). *Contemporary psychodynamic psychotherapy for children and adolescents: Integrating intersubjectivity and neuroscience.* New York: Springer.

Donald, M. (1991). *Origins of the modern mind.* Cambridge, MA: Harvard University Press.

Donnenberg, G. R., Lyons, J. S., & Howard, K. I. (1999). Clinical trials versus mental health services research: Contributions and connections. *Journal of Clinical Psychology, 55,* 1135–1146.

Duignan, I., & Mitzman, S. (1994). Measuring individual change in patients receiving time-limited cognitive analytic group therapy. *International Journal of Short-Term Psychotherapy, 9,* 151–160.

Dunn, M. (1994). Variations in cognitive analytic therapy technique in the treatment of a severely disturbed patient. *International Journal of Short-Term Psychotherapy, 9,* 119–133.

Dunn, M., & Parry, G. (1997). A formulated case plan approach to caring for people with borderline personality disorder in a community mental health service setting. *Clinical Psychology Forum, 104,* 19–22.

Evans, M., Kellett, S., Heywood, S., Hall, J., & Majid, S. (2017). Cognitive analytic therapy for bipolar disorder: A pilot randomized controlled trial. *Clinical Psychology and Psychotherapy, 24*(1), 22–35.

Fairbairn, W. R. D. (1952). *Psychoanalytic studies of the personality.* London: Routledge & Kegan Paul.

Fonagy, P., & Target, M. (1997). Attachment and reflective function: Their role in self-organisation. *Development and Psychopathology, 9,* 679–700.

Gilbody, S., & Whitty, P. (2002). Improving the delivery and organisation of mental health services: Beyond the conventional randomised controlled trial. *British Journal of Psychiatry, 180,* 13–18.

Golynkina, K., & Ryle, A. (1999). The identification and characteristics of the partially dissociated states of patients with borderline personality disorder. *British Journal of Medical Psychology, 72,* 429–445.

Higgitt, A., & Fonagy, P. (2002). Clinical effectiveness. *British Journal of Psychiatry, 18,* 170–174.

Kellett, S. (2005). The treatment of dissociative identity disorder with cognitive analytic therapy: Experimental evidence of sudden gains. *Journal of Trauma and Dissociation, 6,* 55–81.

Kellett, S. (2007). A time series evaluation of the treatment of histrionic personality disorder with cognitive analytic therapy. *Psychology and Psychotherapy: Theory, Research and Practice, 80,* 389–405.

Kellett, S. (2012). Cognitive analytic therapy. In C. Feltham & I. Horton (Eds.), *The SAGE handbook of counselling and psychotherapy* (3rd ed.). London: SAGE.

Kellett, S. (2016). *Goodbye letter writing—worksheet for clients.* Sheffield, UK: University of Sheffield.

Kellett, S., & Bennett, D. (2016). Competency assessment during cognitive analytic supervision. In D. Pickvance (Ed.), *Cognitive analytic supervision: A relational approach* (pp. 144–162). London: SAGE.

Kellett, S., Bennett, D., Ryle, A., & Thake, A. (2013). Cognitive analytic therapy for borderline personality disorder: Therapist competence and therapeutic effectiveness in routine practice. *Clinical Psychology and Psychotherapy, 20,* 216–225.

Kellett, S., & Hardy, G. (2014). The treatment of paranoid personality disorder with cognitive analytic therapy: A mixed methods single case experimental design. *Clinical Psychology and Psychotherapy, 21,* 452–464.

Kellett, S., Simmonds-Buckley, M., & Totterdell, P. (2016). Testing the effectiveness of cognitive analytic therapy for hypersexuality disorder: An intensive time series evaluation. *Journal of Martial and Sexual Therapy, 6,* 1–16.

Kellett, S., Wilbram, M., Davis, C., & Hardy, G. (2014). Team consultancy using cognitive analytic therapy: A controlled study in assertive outreach. *Journal of Psychiatric and Mental Health Nursing, 21,* 687–697.

Kerr, I. B. (1999). Cognitive analytic therapy for borderline personality disorder in the context of a community mental health team: Individual and organisational psychodynamic implications. *British Journal of Psychotherapy, 15,* 425–438.

Kerr, I. B. (2001). Brief cognitive analytic therapy for post-acute manic psychosis on a psychiatric intensive care unit. *Clinical Psychology and Psychotherapy, 8,* 117–129.

Kerr, I. B., Finlayson-Short, L., McCutcheon, L. K., Beard, H., & Chanen, A. M. (2015). The "self" and borderline personality disorder: Conceptual and clinical consideration. *Psychopathology, 48,* 339–348.

Kosti, F., Adamopoulou, A., Bozikas, V., Katsigiannopoulos, K., Protogerou, C., Voikli, M., et al. (2008). The efficacy of cognitive-analytic therapy (CAT) on anhedonia in patients with obsessive–compulsive personality disorder. *Annals of General Psychiatry, 7*(Suppl. 1), S278.

Leighton, T. (1997). Borderline personality and substance abuse problems. In A. Ryle (Ed.), *Cognitive analytic therapy and borderline personality disorder: The model and the method.* Chichester, UK: Wiley.

Leiman, M. (1992). The concept of sign in the work of Vygotsky, Winnicott and Bakhtin: Further integration of object relations theory and activity theory. *British Journal of Medical Psychology, 65,* 209–221.

Leiman, M. (1994). The development of cognitive analytic therapy. *International Journal of Short-Term Psychotherapy, 9,* 67–82.

Leiman, M. (1995). Early development. In A. Ryle (Ed.), *Cognitive analytic therapy: Developments in theory and practice.* Chichester, UK: Wiley.

Leiman, M. (1997). Procedures as dialogic sequences: A revised version of the fundamental concept in cognitive analytic therapy. *British Journal of Medical Psychology, 70,* 193–207.

Leiman, M. (2000). Ogden's matrix of transference and the concept of sign. *British Journal of Medical Psychology, 73,* 385–400.

Livanos, A., Adamopoulou, A., Katsigiannopoulos, K., Bozikas, V., Voikli, M., Pandoularis, J., et al. (2008). Anhedonia in patients with borderline personality disorder: The efficacy of cognitive-analytic therapy (CAT). *Annals of General Psychiatry, 7*(Suppl. 1), S155.

Luborsky, L., & Crits-Christoph, P. (1990). *Understanding transference: The CCRT method.* New York: Basic Books.

Mace, C., Beeken, S., & Embleton, J. (2006). Beginning therapy: Clinical outcomes in brief treatments by psychiatric trainees. *Psychiatric Bulletin, 30,* 7–10.

Margison, F. (2000). Cognitive analytic therapy: A case study in treatment development. *British Journal of Medical Psychology, 73,* 145–149.

Marriott, M., & Kellett, S. (2009). Evaluating a cognitive analytic therapy service: Practice-based outcomes and comparisons with person-centred and cognitive-behavioural therapies. *Psychology and Psychotherapy: Theory, Research and Practice, 82,* 57–72.

Mead, G. H. (1972). *Mind, self, and society from the standpoint of a social behaviorist* (Edited and with an introduction by Charles W. Morris). Chicago: University of Chicago Press. (Original work published 1934)

Moran, P., Jenkins, R., Tylee, A., Blizard, R., & Mann, A. (2000). The prevalence of personality disorder among UK primary care attenders. *Acta Psychiatrica Scandanavia, 102,* 52–57.

Mulder, A., & Chanen, A. M. (2013). Effectiveness of cognitive analytic therapy for personality disorders. *British Journal of Psychiatry, 202,* 89–90.

National Institute for Health and Clinical Excellence (NICE). (2009). *Borderline personality disorder: Recognition and management* (Clinical Guideline 78). London: Author.

Ogden, T. H. (1983). The concept of internal object relations. *International Journal of Psychoanalysis, 64,* 227–241.

Oliviera, Z. M. R. (1997). The concept of role in the discussion of the internalization process. In B. D. Cox & C. Lightfoot (Eds.), *Sociogenic perspectives on internalization.* Mahwah, NJ: Erlbaum.

Pickvance, D. (Ed.). (2017). *Cognitive analytic supervision: A relational approach.* New York: Routledge.

Pollock, P. H., Broadbent, M., Clarke, S., Dorrian, A., & Ryle, A. (2001). The Personality Structure Questionnaire (PSQ): A measure of the multliple self-states model of identity confusion in cognitive analytic therapy. *Clinical Psychology and Psychotherapy, 8,* 59–72.

Pollock, P., Stowell-Smith, M., & Göpfert, M. (2006). *Cognitive analytic therapy for offenders: A new approach to forensic psychotherapy.* New York: Routledge.

Roth, A., & Fonagy, P. (2005). *What works for whom?: A critical review of psychotherapy research* (2nd ed.). New York: Guilford Press.

Ryle, A. (1975). *Frames and cages.* London: Sussex University Press.

Ryle, A. (1985). Cognitive theory, object relations and the self. *British Journal of Medical Psychology, 58,* 1–7.

Ryle, A. (1991). Object relations theory and activity theory: A proposed link by way if the procedural sequence model. *British Journal of Medical Psychology, 64,* 307–316.

Ryle, A. (1994). Projective identification: A particular form of reciprocal role procedure. *British Journal of Medical Psychology, 67,* 107–114.

Ryle, A. (1995). *Cognitive analytic therapy: Developments in theory and practice.* Chichester, UK: Wiley.

Ryle, A. (1997). *Cognitive analytic therapy and borderline personality disorder: The model and the method.* Chichester, UK: Wiley.

Ryle, A. (2007). Investigating the phenomenology of borderline personality disorder with the states description procedure: Clinical implications. *Clinical Psychology and Psychotherapy, 14,* 342–351.

Ryle, A., & Beard, H. (1993). The integrative effort of reformation: Cognitive analytic therapy with a patient with borderline personality disorder. *British Journal of Psychology, 66,* 249–258.

Ryle, A., & Golynkina, K. (2000). Effectiveness of time-limited cognitive analytic therapy of borderline personality disorder: Factors associated with outcome. *British Journal of Medical Psychology, 73,* 197–210.

Ryle, A., Kellett, S., Hepple, J., & Calvert, R. (2014). Cognitive analytic therapy at 30. *Advances in Psychiatric Treatment, 20,* 258–268.

Ryle, A., & Kerr, I. (2002). *Introducing cognitive analytic therapy: Principles and practice.* Chichester, UK: Wiley.

Sandler, J. (1976). Countertransference and role-responsiveness. *International Review of Psychoanalysis, 3,* 43–47.

Schacht, T. E., & Henry, W. P. (1994). Modelling recurrent relationship patterns with structural analysis of social behavior: The SASB-CMP. *Psychotherapy Research, 4,* 208–221.

Stern, D. N. (1985). *The interpersonal world of the infant.* New York: Basic Books.

Stiles, W., Barkham, M., Mellor-Clark, J., & Connell, J. (2008). Effectivesss of cognitive-behavioural, person-centered, and psychodynamic therapies in UK primary care routine practice: Replication with a larger sample. *Psychological Medicine, 36,* 677–688.

Strange, R., & Kellett, S. (2016). *Understanding and describing your past—worksheet for clients.* Sheffield, UK: University of Sheffield.

Treasure, J., Todd, G., Brolly, M., Tiller, J., Nehmed, A., & Denman, F. (1995). A pilot study of randomised trial of cognitive analytical therapy vs educational behavioral therapy for adult anorexia nervosa. *Behaviour Research and Therapy, 33,* 363–367.

Trevarthen, C., & Aitken, K. J. (2001). Infant intersubjectivity: Research, theory and clinical applications. *Journal of Child Psychology and Psychiatry, 42,* 3–48.

Tyrer, P. (2013). Psychotherapy made perfect. *British Journal of Psychiatry, 202,* 162.

Vygotsky, L. S. (1978). *Mind in society: The development of higher psychological processes.* Cambridge, MA: Harvard University Press.

Weston, D., Novotny, C., & Thompson-Brenner, H. (2004). The empirical status of empirically supported therapies: Assumptions, methods, and findings. *Psychological Bulletin, 130,* 631–663.

Wildgoose, A., Clarke, S., & Waller, G. (2001). Treating personality fragmentation and dissociation in borderline personality disorder: A pilot study of the impact of cognitive analytic therapy. *British Journal of Medical Psychology, 74,* 47–55.

# CHAPTER 28

# Cognitive-Behavioral Therapy

Kate M. Davidson

Cognitive-behavioral therapies (CBT) have the largest evidence base of all psychological therapies, having been subjected to systematic and rigorous assessment of its effectiveness in treating a wide array of mental and physical disorders (see The Matrix, 2015). Regardless of the type of disorder CBT is used to treat, the basic structure, characteristics, style of therapy, and theoretical assumptions are the same. The structure of therapy, such as agenda setting and experiments or assignments to test out a client's predictions of what might happen in real life, an open and collaborative client–therapist relationship, the sharing of the cognitive formulation, and assessment and interpretation of thoughts and beliefs, are all highly typical of CBT as applied across disorders.

CBT has evolved over time to meet increasing demand for psychological therapy and the needs of those with more complex disorders. This chapter describes the biopsychosocial model that underpins the cognitive therapies for personality disorders (PDs); explores the cognitive model of PD and the importance of dysfunctional schemas formed in early childhood; discusses differences in content and structure between the cognitive psychological therapies, especially between CBT for PD (CBTpd; Davidson, 2000, 2008) and schema-focused therapy (SFT; Young, Klosko, & Weishaar, 2003) to highlight critical change mechanisms; and reviews supporting evidence for CBTpd.

CBTpd was first described by Beck, Freeman, and Associates in 1990 and subsequently revised (Beck, Freeman, & Davis, 2004) to accommodate further therapeutic developments. Other notable developments that have shaped the field were Young's development of SFT (Young et al., 2003) and Davidson's (2000, 2008) development of CBTpd especially for antisocial and borderline PDs (Davidson, 2000, 2008). Young and colleagues (2003) introduced concepts such as early maladaptive schemas and schema modes and domains to provide a more elaborate theoretical framework to understand the problems encountered in treating PD. Although SFT departs from the cognitive therapy model in major ways that I discuss later, nonetheless, the main cognitive and behavioral strategies used in SFT are solidly grounded within CBT. CBTpd is more closely related to the Beckian framework; hence, it differs from SFT in terms of the model, the therapeutic relationship, structure, and content. Beck and Freeman's original 1990 book did not operationalize or specify therapy sufficiently for evaluation in randomized controlled trials (RCTs). Through single-case studies in which patients acted as their own controls (Davidson & Tyrer, 1996), CBT was refined and specified to make it possible to train therapists to delivery therapy in a consistent manner that became known thereafter as CBTpd. This therapy was then assessed in terms of efficacy in two RCTs for borderline PD

(BPD; Davidson, Norrie, et al., 2006; Davidson, Tyrer, et al., 2006) and antisocial PD (ASPD; Davidson et al., 2009).

## Theoretical Assumptions

How PDs arise is a matter of much academic and clinical interest. If we could understand how PD develops, we might be able to influence the course of its development. To date, multiple causes are implicated in the development of PD, and we have no single model that can integrate all the available evidence. Many factors are thought to contribute to the development of PD: genetics and temperament, neurobiological dysfunctions of emotional regulation and stress, childhood maltreatment and abuse, and attachment system problems. All of these factors have reinforced the idea that the development of emotional, cognitive, and behavioral patterns, what we call personality, is due to an interaction of nature and nurture. It is important to note that whatever factors give rise to PD, treatment outcome is much better than was originally thought. Although around half of people given a diagnosis of BPD improve sufficiently that they do not meet criteria for the disorder a decade or less after their first diagnosis, life events can worsen symptoms again, and comorbid problems are common (Zanarini, Frankenburg, Reich, & Fitzmaurice, 2012).

### Interaction of Environment and Biology

Cognitive therapies adopt a biopsychosocial model that assumes personality develops though an interaction of between genetic predispositions and environmental factors (Beck et al., 2004; Davidson, 2008; Kellogg & Young, 2006). Differences between individuals arise in part from unique, inherited biological predispositions (temperament) that influence how a child interacts with their early environment. Temperamental processes determine the infant's orientation toward the physical and social world in terms of positive affect, approach versus avoidance, anger and frustration, fearfulness, effortful control, and possibly affiliativeness (Rothbart, Adahi, & Evans, 2000). From the outset, the child's temperamental disposition interacts with the caregiver's ability to meet his or her needs, such as the caregiver's ability to soothe and stimulate him or her. This dynamic, two-way interaction varies depending on how each individual responds. The same caregiver may react differently to a baby who is alert and irritable compared to one that is less reactive and placid, and different babies may react differently to the same caregiver. As a result, differences in temperament lead to differences in experiences, particularly emotional experiences. As the child develops, multiple influences, of which temperament is only one factor, affect his or her ability to adapt to and cope with the environment, especially with other people. Even a temperamentally confident child may be overwhelmed by aversive experiences. Temperament may influence, but is not necessarily the dominant influence, on eventual adaptation.

Bowlby (1969) suggested that attachment relationships with the primary caregiver typically form at a very early stage, and the types of attachment formed play a significant role in determining relationship patterns in adulthood. A long-standing attachment relationship characterized by neglect, hostility, rejection, or threat leads to the development of the negative interpersonal schemas associated with PDs, including core beliefs resulting from unconditional, rigid, and pervasive schemas about self and others, such as "I am bad" and "Others will reject me." The operation of these schemas or beliefs leads to unstable and turbulent relationships in adulthood.

### Formation of Negative Core Beliefs

Beckian CBTpd emphasizes the role of assumptions or beliefs (Beck et al., 1990, 2004) and uses the term "schema" to refer to stable knowledge structures representing individuals' knowledge about themselves and their world that is highly idiosyncratic and personalized. Schemas are activated by events that resemble the original event that led to the formation of the schema. Thus, vulnerability to affective disturbance is due to the activation of negative schemas. For example, distress over the breakup of a relationship occurs because the event activates a schema concerned with interpersonal loss that leads to a negative affective response. This schema may then lead to the activation of related schemas concerned with themes of worthlessness and inadequacy. This diathesis–stress cognitive model is supported by both priming and longitudinal studies showing that depressive schemas become active under stressful conditions (Scher, Ingram, & Segal, 2005). In PD, negative schemas tend be activated on a more continuous basis because the individuals concerned become stressed in a wider number of situations, particularly interpersonal interactions, leading to frequent emotional states of hyperarousal or hypervigilance. This pattern of activation of schemas is therefore in contrast to that found in a symptomatic disorders, such as depression. In PD, schemas are hypervalent: They are the usual way of processing information that leads to more stable, inflexible, and rigid ways of thinking. This may account for the maintenance of the cognitive and emotional difficulties found in PD. The persistent activation of schemas leads to problems because the rigidity leads to a lack of adaptation to changes in the individual's environment.

Cognitive therapies also place importance on behavior. PD involves overdeveloped patterns of behavior that may lead to the underdevelopment of more adaptive patterns. For example, dependent PD (DPD) usually involves high levels of help-seeking behavior at the expense of patterns demonstrating independence and self-sufficiency. Beck and colleagues also suggest that certain key assumptions are associated with specific types of PDs, and that these assumptions serve to differentiate disorders. For example, in DPD, a dominant belief is "I need other people—specifically a strong person—in order to survive" and in ASPD a dominant belief might be "I need to look out for myself" or "I need to be the aggressor or I will be the victim" (Beck et al., 2004, p. 39).

The CBTpd model is similarly multifaceted in order accommodate the developmental impact of ongoing changes in biology, physiology, cognition, behavior, and social and emotion development (Davidson, 2008). However, the model emphasizes that development occurs in a family and social system embedded in a wider cultural context and gives prominence to the cognitive, emotional, and behavioral factors that are central to the child's development and shape adult self-identity, the perception of relationships and others, and coping responses (Davidson, 2008, p. 28). This model has implications for the practice of CBTpd because it requires a detailed, individualized narrative case formulation.

SFT (Young et al., 2003) differs from both Beckian cognitive therapy and CBTpd in two important respects: the emphasis placed on the role of early maladaptive schemas in the development of PDs and the concept of schema modes. "Early maladaptive schemas" are self-defeating emotional and cognitive patterns characterized by broad themes that comprise memories, emotions, cognitions, and bodily sensations regarding oneself and one's relationships to others. These schemas are formed by adverse childhood experiences and continue to be elaborated throughout an individual's lifetime. They are activated by similar experiences to those in childhood. Kellogg and Young (2006) note that this aspect highlights the psychodynamic aspect of Young's theory, particularly object relations and attachment theory (Ainsworth & Bowlby, 1991; Greenberg & Mitchell, 1983).

Early maladaptive schemas fall into five broad "domains": disconnection and rejection, impaired autonomy, impaired limits, other-directedness, and overvigilance and inhibition (Young et al., 2003). SFT also assumes that individuals with PD typically operate in schema modes that comprise a set of schemas that lead to pervasive patterns of thinking, emotions, and behavior. There are four broad modes of functioning: child mode, dysfunctional coping mode, dysfunctional parent mode, and last, healthy adult mode. Therapy seeks to strengthen the healthy adult mode to counteract maladaptive ways of functioning. The relative balance of child, parent, or coping modes differs across the different disorders.

Schema modes are also linked to dissociation: A dysfunctional schema mode is cut off to some degree from other modes. In the healthy adult mode, there is usually more integration of modes but in BPD, there may a shift between different aspects of self, with one aspect being split off from others. Figure 28.1 shows the

| Schema mode | Specific linked modes |
|---|---|
| Child | Vulnerable child<br>Angry child<br>Impulsive, undisciplined child<br>Happy child |
| Dysfunctional coping | Compliant surrenderer<br>Detached protector<br>Overcompensator |
| Dysfunctional parent | Punitive parent<br>Demanding parent |

**FIGURE 28.1.** Young's dysfunctional schema modes. From Young, Klosko, and Weishaar (2003). Adapted with permission from The Guilford Press

## Core Beliefs

CBTpd differs from Beck's model and SFT in that it does not assume that PDs are differentiated by a specific set of schemas or beliefs and it does not adopt the concept of schema mode. However, the concept of schema is used to account for the core unconditional beliefs about self and others. Beck (1967) introduced the concept of schema to CBT to describe cognitive structures that guide attention, code, and evaluate personal experience. Padesky (1994), like Beck, postulated that schemas (core beliefs) play a central role in the maintenance of chronic problems, and that the core beliefs associated with PD are expressed in unconditional terms. For example, "I am bad," a core belief commonly associated with BPD (Davidson, Norrie, et al., 2006) is used in an absolute or categorical way and often without awareness. This contrasts with conditional beliefs such as "If I do not do well at everything, I am a failure," typically found in disorders such as depression, and usually accessible through the stream of consciousness. We also found that other beliefs are strongly endorsed by those with BPD: In a group of 106 men and women, relatively high scores on the dimensions of mistrust and abuse, fears of abandonment, and social isolation were found on the Young Schema Questionnaire (Young, 1990), and lower scores on the entitlement dimension were found (Davidson, Norrie, et al., 2006).

CBTpd also makes greater use of individualized formulations of the client's core beliefs about self and others and associated behavioral strategies. The core beliefs, identified in an individual's life narrative, which is explored at the beginning of therapy, reflect deep schema structures rather than automatic thoughts that occur as a stream of thoughts in response to everyday situations. All cognitive theories agree that childhood traumatic experiences and problematic relationships make a major contribution to PDs by promoting the development of core beliefs about self and others that are attempts at avoiding, compensating for, or coping with these negative experiences and events. Thus, typical core beliefs associated with concerns of patients with BPD are about mistrust, failure, and emotional deprivation, and being undesirable or bad, or exploited. These beliefs lead to dysfunctional behavioral strategies to compensate for, avoid, or cope with them. CBTpd differs from other cognitive therapies by not prescribing the content or theme of a specific belief or set of beliefs that an individual may have developed. Rather, an individualized or "bespoke" formulation of problems is constructed through exploration of each patient's developmental experiences. However, CBTpd recognizes that specific types of PD are highly likely to share beliefs that have similar themes. For example, clients with BPD usually hold core beliefs that they are unlovable, defective, or inferior, and that others are threatening, uncaring, unpredictable, or abusive.

## Principal Intervention Strategies and Methods of CBTpd

CBTpd assumes that besides competency in CBT for other disorders, therapists treating personality disorder also need knowledge about the disorder and its general clinical management (see University College London [UCL], 2015). As noted, CBTpd involves a detailed assessment of PD and any coexisting condition, and working with the client to construct a narrative case formulation. Subsequently, emphasis is placed on engaging the client, and when appropriate significant others, and on helping the client to modify core beliefs, emotions, and unhelpful behavioral patterns.

### Phases of Therapy

Therapy is assumed to process through a series of stages: engagement, development of new cognitions and behaviors, and consolidation.

### Engagement

Client engagement is initially achieved through careful assessment of problems from a developmental perspective and the development of a written narrative formulation that is shared and agreed upon with the client. This stage typically takes about five sessions, but it can take longer with clients who are highly distressed or unfamiliar with therapy. Developing a coherent narrative formulation with individuals with antisocial behavior may take up to 10 sessions, since these clients tend to be wary of the process and anxious about disclosure, so that it takes time to build their trust. They also often have more difficulty than patients with BPD in describing childhood experiences.

The first phase aims to develop a narrative formulation that incorporates an agreed-upon understanding of the client's problems, core beliefs, and overdeveloped behaviors identified through a detailed developmental history. The formulation includes an explanation of why these beliefs developed and how they have affected the client's life, and forms the foundation for therapy. The formulation is written in a narrative style using everyday language. This helps to ensure that the therapist conveys an empathic understanding of the client's experience and difficulties, and that the therapist and client agree on what has led to the difficulties. The narrative formulation seeks to give a client a deeper psychological understanding of his or her past and current experience, including an explanation of why he or she developed the beliefs and problems to help him or her recognize how he or she is negatively influenced by the past. It also helps the therapy to proceed more smoothly and avoid "firefighting" because any future crisis can be readily understood within the context of the formulation. See Figure 28.2 for an extract of a CBTpd narrative formulation.

### Development of New Cognitions and Behaviors

The second stage of therapy focuses on working with the client to develop new ways of thinking about him- or herself and behaviors that strengthen these new ways of thinking. This stage typically lasts for several months and is the main focus of therapeutic change. In RCTs, we have found that significant and substantial change in thinking and behavior can be achieved in between 6 and 12 months (Davidson, Tyrer, et al., 2006; Davidson et al., 2009) even when there is a comorbid drug or alcohol problems in addition to the PD. The aim of this phase is to weaken core dysfunctional beliefs and develop more adaptive ways of thinking about self and other people. Associated with this change is practicing the new behaviors that have been historically underdeveloped and reducing the frequency and impact of overdeveloped behavioral strategies that are unhelpful. In-session (often cognitive- and emotion-focused) work is followed by related assignments to promote and practice change in behavior outside of therapy, and particularly behaviors that focus on improving relationships.

---

To Sarah:

We have now met on five occasions to talk in some depth about your past and your current problems. I think we have begun to have a better understanding of you, what led to you taking a serious overdose, and how you have been trying to cope in the past few years in difficult circumstances.

What we know about your early life:

From what you have described, your father had an alcohol problem that affected his mental health. He was "stormy" in temperament and seemed very inconsistent about whether he found you to be a "good or bad" girl. Regular contact with your father made you feel very low and hopeless. He was taciturn, blamed you for being a burden, and said it was your fault that he and your mother did not get on well. At other times, he seemed to take an interest in you, but only for so long. You say you did not know what to do to get his love and attention. Not seeing him for a while has allowed you to get some emotional distance from your relationship, but it has also been hard on you. You are aware that you may not have been to blame for what led to your parents' problems. You have had little to do with him since you were 20. You do not regret this, but you wish that you were able to have a full discussion with him about your relationship. He is still drinking heavily as far as you know.

Your mother was a quiet, shy woman who lacked confidence. She seemed to be very anxious when you were growing up, and you think she may have been taking prescribed medication for her "nerves." The atmosphere at home was often tense. You think this was due not only to your father's drinking but also because your mother was sometimes afraid of your father when he had been drinking. You think he may have been violent toward her. You found it hard to know what would please your mother and tried hard to please and make her life better, but you were never really able to do this. You think she may have loved you, but you were never really certain of this. You did worry that you were the reason for your parents' unhappiness. You began to worry that you were bad. Occasionally you tried to get your parents' attention by becoming very distressed, shouting at them, and crying, but this backfired and you were usually punished by your father for being attention seeking. You used to hide away in your bedroom and listen to your

*(continued)*

**FIGURE 28.2.** Extract from a CBTpd narrative formulation.

radio, hoping that you would not hear your parents argue or see your mother upset. She seemed to be preoccupied a lot of the time and rather distant from you. You became increasingly introverted, shying away from adults and from school friends. You say that you were afraid that other people would find out how "bad" you were. What is really very sad is that this shying away strengthened your view of yourself as being inadequate and bad. You began physically hurting yourself at the age of 12 to stop feeling the emotional pain you felt. You were all alone, and there really was nobody you thought you could speak to about how you felt.

It is clear that you have several very negative beliefs about yourself—that you are "no good," "a bad person" whom "nobody could ever love." We now understand that these beliefs developed from how you were treated as a child. It seems both your mother and father had mental health problems, and your father was dependent on alcohol. These problems were serious but not your responsibility. They seem to have led to your parents being unable to give you the nurturing and support that you needed as a child. Your father was largely emotionally absent from your life, even when you were a small child. He may even have been having problems with your mother before you were born. You wanted him to have a greater role in your childhood, and it is sad he did not, or could not, do this.

We also understand that your self-harming comes from a way of trying to cope with the emotional pain you suffered as a child and still feel to this day. Also, you have developed a pattern of relating to people that links to your belief that you are bad and unlikely to be loved. You seem to be reluctant to get involved with people unless you are sure they will like you. You often set tests of loyalty for people that show you some friendship. Unfortunately, this often backfires, and you get very upset if someone gets angry with you or, even worse in your view, does not call you back or contact you to see if you are OK. It reminds you of your mother's indifference. This is very upsetting for you and makes you feel very alone in the world. It is these beliefs and patterns of behavior that we will focus on in therapy. Together we will try to see if there is another way of thinking about yourself and of changing the way you relate to others (and yourself) that will make your life more worth living. You have already made some important

*(continued)*

**FIGURE 28.2.** *(continued)*

steps toward this by making links between the past and present. This understanding will be the platform from which we work together. The way we think about ourselves and other people is usually developed from what happens in our childhoods. When these are unhappy childhoods, the beliefs can take on a disproportionate weight. In your case, there was nobody to give you a more balanced sense of yourself as a child. We will talk more about this in the coming weeks.

Please let me know if you agree with what is in this note. It is my attempt at summarizing the understanding that we have reached in our sessions so far. You may wish to add to it or take things out. We can make changes to this at any time. . . .

**FIGURE 28.2.** *(continued)*

## Consolidation

The final phase of therapy, which usually lasts three to five sessions, is used to review progress, with the aim of consolidating and generalizing learning through homework assignments. At the end of therapy, the therapist summarizes progress in terms of new coping skills and new ways of thinking about self and others in the form of a letter given to the client. This process also includes a discussion and planning about how the client can continue to progress and strengthen his or her new ways of thinking and behavior when therapy ends. This final stage of therapy also deals with any difficulties the patient may have with endings due to the activation of earlier experiences of abandonment or rejection.

Some typical interventions in CBTpd are described. These reflect the collaborative style of CBTpd, as well as some of the cognitive and behavioral change strategies used in therapy to improve the client's quality of life and relationships.

### Helping Clients Regulate Their Emotions

In therapy we need to be able to help clients with PD understand and gain mastery of their emotions. This does not involve suppressing, ignoring, or avoiding emotions or the reasons why people are upset. Everyone needs to be able to express emotions appropriately and use effective strategies to cope better with personal problems and distressing situations. Emotions expressed in a dysregulated manner also occur in therapy sessions. The therapist and client can struggle to keep a therapy session on track if this happens, and it can interfere with progress in therapy.

As stated earlier, in CBTpd, a narrative formulation is developed to help clients understand their emotional distress, identify the emotions expressed, and describe underlying issues, some of which may be long-standing, with origins in childhood. Once the emotions are identified, the client is helped to manage his or her emotions in an appropriate and controllable way so that he or she can communicate effectively with others. Friends and family may feel overwhelmed and deskilled by emotional outbursts. As a result, they are often unable to help the client and may actually avoid him or her or become insensitive to the outbursts and close down communication in an attempt to cope. Unfortunately, this can make the client even more emotionally distressed and, being unable to obtain the help he or she craves, the client may respond by acting out. This leads others to react by seeking even greater physical and emotional distance from the client, creating a vicious cycle.

A therapist can help a client cope with high levels of emotional dysregulation in sessions in several ways. Taking on an opposite emotional stance can help calm the client. By behaving in an outwardly calm and controlled manner, keeping his or her voice low and speech slow, the therapist helps the client reach a more optimal level of emotional expression. Note that a CBTpd therapist would not use a cognitive strategy in the first instance in this situation. The therapist responds to the client's emotional distress with the behavioral expression of an opposite emotion. This is because the client is unlikely to be able to think more clearly at times of high emotionality. Levels of arousal are too high to think more rationally at these times. Once the client is calmer, giving some gentle feedback about what has happened is helpful, discussing how the client managed to gain more control of his or her emotions and recover a sense of perspective once he or she was calmer.

Sometimes those with PD avoid emotions and distressing topics, and appear to be rather underaroused or cut off from emotional reactions that would be appropriate to express. This may be an attempt to avoid experiencing distress, and clients may act in odd ways, jump from topic to topic, or appear sad while outwardly stating that they are relatively OK and coping. If this type of avoidance of emotions arises in therapy, the therapist should try to work on what issue might be bothering the client rather than focus on avoidance of emotions per se. In other words, we use a more cognitive strategy. The therapist may make a judgment about whether to gently point out that the client seems sad, even though the client may say that he or she is not, or the client may appear jumpy or unable to stick to a topic, but the therapist is not sure why the client feels like this or is behaving like this. The therapist can then move the session forward without belaboring the point that the client may be using avoidance. The therapist should remember to return to the issue at a later stage in therapy or even within the same session.

Often acknowledging emotional avoidance leads to discussion of what is upsetting the client. The therapist has gained an understanding of the main issues that distress the client through the formulation and may have an informed guess about what this might be. The therapist can ask about core beliefs that may be present at the time that may be related to what is being talked about or referred to in the session. The therapist may suggest which core belief of the client has been activated by a situation on the basis of information from the formulation and ask whether this is what has happened. This is an exploratory stance, assessing the situation and what it means for the client in terms of his or her core beliefs and emotional reaction to events. The client may also be reporting something that has occurred in the weeks between therapy sessions that has upset him or her. For example, the client may have been in contact with a member of his or her family and inadvertently reminded of abusive events that took place in the past. The client may feel ashamed about having been abused in childhood, believing that he or she was at fault for the abuse that took place. He or she may believe "I am bad" and "I am tainted by the past." The client has developed a behavioral strategy of avoidance to cope with these beliefs and associated feelings. This behavioral strategy is also operational in the therapy session, in which the client may wish to avoid discussing these beliefs due to feeing ashamed in front of the therapist.

### Working to Build More Adaptive Beliefs

One of the main tasks of cognitive therapy for other disorders is eliciting and modifying automatic thoughts. In depression, for example, clients are asked to pay attention to the stream of negative thoughts elicited by situations, mental images, or memories that result in, or arise from, dysphoric mood states. Negative automatic thoughts in depression center on the "negative cognitive triad," and the content of these thoughts is about the self, the world and the future. In CBTpd, the main cognitive task is identifying key core beliefs and modifying these, so that they become more adaptive, less rigid, and less absolute. Dysfunctional core beliefs in PD are manifestations of stable, underlying unconscious cognitive structures. In PDs, dysfunctional schemas are thought to have arisen in childhood and are assumed to be hypervalent in that they are likely to inhibit or dominate more functional adaptive schemas and beliefs. They are activated in a wide variety of situations, resulting in a consistent bias in the interpretation and meaning of events. These dysfunctional core beliefs concern central concepts about the self and other people. As such, they have a major impact on clients' interpersonal behavior in relationships. For example, the client who holds a belief that he or she is not loveable is unlikely to want to get close to others, and likely to expect rejection from others.

Changing core beliefs requires collection of information from the client's past experience and current life that can be evaluated in the light of a modified belief or an alternative, more adaptive, less rigid belief. The therapist's task is to lead an examination of the adaptiveness of the old core belief in the client's current life and through a collaborative process; to develop a new, more adaptive belief; or to modify a preexisting one. Then, through Socratic questioning, data that were previously ignored, negated, or distorted can be judged by the client for degree of fit with the new modified belief. This may be illustrated by Susan, who held a rigid and absolute belief that she was a "bad" and "useless" person. Her mother had left when Susan was 3 years old, and because her father, an offshore oil worker, had not been able to care for her, Susan had been emotionally neglected. She spent most of her childhood living with an aunt who was indifferent to her emotional needs, although Susan was looked after reasonably well in terms of her physical needs. She was intellectually above average but was not encouraged to work at school, and Susan fell behind her peers in terms of scholastic achievements and in sports. She made few friends, fearing that they would also show no interest, like her aunt and father. In therapy, it became evident that there was evidence that could have contradicted the view that Susan was useless and bad. For example, it was evident that one or two teachers had shown an interest in her and encouraged her to believe she could succeed. Susan's belief that she was useless had dominated her thinking, and she had not believed they were sincere in their alternative view of her. She believed that they felt sorry for her and were being "nice." The therapist examined this view more thoroughly, and it appeared that Susan had done well at school, at least in the classes of these "nice" teachers. Susan decided the teachers were doing their job well and not just being "nice" or feeling sorry for her, and that they were justified in telling her she was doing well on these occasions. The therapist and Susan documented this alternative view in a "test" of the validity of Susa's core belief across her lifetime so far. In the section they created on her school life, they documented that some teachers believed Susan was able and bright. More evidence across other periods of her life become evident as therapy progressed that helped modify and develop a new, more adaptive view of self—that she was "good enough" and at least "as good as anyone else." These included the experience of having passed her driving test, being picked for a team at work to do special duties, being good at art at school, and having her drawing be picked for a school Christmas card. Through therapy, Susan understood that she had ignored or rejected contrary evidence that could have supported a more adaptive view of herself. She also understood this was because her emotional needs had not been met as a child, and that this was not her fault. She had not been supported emotionally and encouraged to do well as a child. Her more adaptive view of herself helped her recognize some of her strengths and to capitalize on these to her benefit.

### Changing Overdeveloped Dysfunctional Behavioral Patterns

Individuals with PDs develop self-defeating behavioral patterns that are overdeveloped, to the detriment of other more adaptive patterns (Beck et al., 1990). Overdeveloped patterns of behavious represent attempts to cope and adapt to persistent dysfunctional early experiences. These schema-driven behavioral patterns may have been adaptive in a child's early environment, but as the child developed and entered into other relationships and explored different environments, they became self-defeating and dysfunctional, and needed to be changed. In order to achieve this, therapy has to focus explicitly on identifying and modifying behavioral strategies that are maladaptive and self-defeating. As a result, therapists need to be skilled at using behavioral change strategies, in addition to cognitive change strategies. New, more adaptive beliefs are unlikely to be maintained unless the client has also learned to change his or her behavioral strategies. By using an experimental model of treatment, the client gets the opportunity to learn and attempt new ways of behaving, to evaluate the impact of new behaviors, and to use the observable data to help in the modification of core beliefs. The main vehicle of change in therapy is the reworking of dysfunctional core beliefs and behavioral patterns (for further details, see Davidson, 2008).

## Similarities and Differences among the Cognitive Therapies

CBTpd is grounded in general cognitive therapy, especially Beck and colleagues' (1990) original extension of this treatment to personality disorder. However, in the subsequent revision of their approach, Beck and colleagues' (2004) position seemed to have moved closer to Young's SFT in terms of both conceptual assumptions about structure of PD and duration of treatment. Although they acknowledge that CBT can be carried out in approximately 1 year, they suggest that longer term change requires that client and therapist form an intensive corrective attachment relationship and that therapy be carried out once or twice weekly for up to 3 years. This proposal is consistent with the time frame used in the comparative study of SFT and transference-focused therapy by Giesen-Bloo and colleagues (2006). Consequently, this comparison of the cognitive therapies is largely confined to SFT and CBTpd. Figure 28.3 describes the main similarities and differences between SFT and CBTpd.

## Style and Structure

Some aspects of the style of therapy are similar in CBTpd and SFT. In both, therapists are active rather than passive, and both educate clients about their problems and how therapy can be helpful. The therapist takes an empirical approach with clients. Therapists help clients to assess and test out how realistic their core beliefs or schemas are, and how adaptive they are in clients' adult lives. In both therapies, clients are encouraged to make changes to their beliefs and behaviors to optimize their ability to adapt to their circumstances and live more fulfilling lives. Practical help is also provided in solving everyday problems that impede progress. Another shared aspect of CBTpd and SFT is that clients are encouraged to practice new ways of behaving to test out whether such changes are adaptive. Both also encourage generalization of new learning to everyday situations and discussion of these experiences in session.

CBTpd and SFT both conceptualize treatment as typically falling into three distinct phases. In both, the first phase involves constructing a shared formulation and gaining an understanding and commitment to treatment. Both also place emphasis on feelings and building empathy. The other phases involve changing thinking, emotional responses, and behavior, and an ending phase.

Despite these similarities, CBTpd and SFT also differ in style and structure. CBTpd retains the traditional cognitive therapy emphasis of setting an agenda at the beginning of each session and structuring therapy, whereas in SFT, sessions are less structured and a formal agenda is not necessarily set. These differences may reflect the shorter duration of CBTpd—1 year as opposed to several years.

## The Therapeutic Relationship

A major difference between CBTpd and SFT is in the way the therapeutic relationship is used as a vehicle for change. SFT emphasizes "limited reparenting" as a major way to effect change. Limited reparenting seeks to meet emotional needs that were not met in childhood and correct early maladaptive and toxic experiences. Young and colleagues (2003) place importance on the therapist meeting these needs now, so that the individual can become an emotionally healthier adult. However, they caution that it is *limited* reparenting. For example, in SFT, the therapist may give the client his or her home phone number to use in a crisis and may use self-disclosure in sessions as a way of meeting the client's emotional needs. In addition,

|  | SFT | CBTpd |
|---|---|---|
| Main influence | Beck, Freeman, & Associates (1990); Young et al. (2003) | Beck, Freeman, & Associates (1990); Davidson (2000); Padesky (1994) |
| Theoretical influences | Gestalt; emotion-focused therapies; object relations and psychodynamic approaches | CBT developmental psychology |
| Length of therapy | 3 years (circa 300 sessions) | 1 year (30 sessions) |
| Main change techniques | 1. Limited reparenting<br>2. Cognitive restructuring and education<br>3. Behavioral<br>4. Experiential imagery/dialogue work (Kellogg & Young, 2006) | 1. Shared narrative formulation<br>2. Cognitive<br>3. Behavioral |
| Mode and structure of therapy | Individual one-to-one sessions; less structure, no agenda; three phases:<br>1. Bonding and emotional regulation<br>2. Schema mode change<br>3. Development of autonomy | Individual one-to-one sessions; structured; three phases:<br>1. Initial formulation<br>2. Strengthen new ways of thinking of self and others and strengthen underdeveloped behaviors<br>3. Consolidation of beliefs and behaviors and ending |
| Cognitive level | Schema modes; especially early maladaptive schemas prescribed by theory | Core beliefs and assumptions about self and others determined through narrative "bespoke" formulation |
| Initial phase | 6 to 12 sessions | 5 to 10 sessions |
| Goal of initial sessions | Education about treatment; assessment of schemas | Education about treatment; developmental history taking to establish a written, agreed-upon narrative formulation |
| Therapeutic alliance | Collaborative; reparenting relationship; intensive relationship aimed at developing new secure attachment to correct for childhood experience (Beck et al., 2004, p. 201). | Collaborative; therapist warm, empathic, open, honest; recognition of and adherence to boundaries. |
| Goal of therapy | Meet the client's emotional needs that were not met in childhood | Develop new, more adaptive beliefs about self and others, and associated adaptive behaviors (underdeveloped beliefs) |
| Other therapeutic input | Possible group therapy experience | Can involve significant others, mental health team |

**FIGURE 28.3.** Main characteristics of CBTpd.

therapists may phone the client regularly and give him or her transitional objects if there is a short break in therapy. The therapist behaves in a manner that creates an atmosphere in therapy that is safe and accepting for the client. Creating a safe situation to enable a client to be able to express his or her feelings and beliefs about him- or herself to work on their beliefs and problems is in itself not unique to SFT, but the reparenting techniques are unique. The therapist's relationship with the client is very different and goes much beyond the collaborative relationship seen in CBTpd.

CBTpd does not use the concept of reparenting. Moreover, this type of therapeutic relationship is considered undesirable. The therapist's role in CBTpd is to work alongside the client and establish a collaborative relationship based on trust and openness, and not to take on a parental type of role. The therapist is active and interested in the client and his or her experiences. Questions about therapy and progress are answered in an open and straightforward manner. A CBTpd therapist does not assume to have the answers to a client's problems. Rather he or she encourages client to make their own judgments by demonstrating an air of curiosity and a stance toward problems that is not "all knowing."

Nevertheless, it is crucial that the CBTpd therapist be compassionate and sensitive to the client's emotional needs, but this is balanced by the therapist both encouraging the client's ability to change and being active in problem solving. Therapists are aware that clients with PD problems are likely to be exquisitely sensitive to signs of rejection or inauthenticity or lack of genuineness due to the problems the clients experienced in childhood. Therapists need to be clear with their clients that they may not always fully understand their subjective experiences, but they are trying to do so. Rather than potentially foster dependency on the therapist through reparenting, the therapist tries to increase the client's sense of self-efficacy and positive coping skills.

## Treatment Methods

There are interesting similarities and differences between CBTpd and SFT in treatment strategies and methods. Similarities reflect their common origins in cognitive therapy, their similar conceptions of the developmental origins of maladaptive beliefs and behavioral patterns, and similar understandings of the rigidity of these cognitions and behaviors that tend to be treated as if they were unalterable truths. Both therapies challenge this view but in slightly different ways. The agreed narrative formulation in CBTpd helps clients understand why they developed their core beliefs. This is an idiosyncratic individualized formulation is client specific, and it helps clients understand that these beliefs arose from childhood experiences, usually with caregivers, and that these beliefs may have made sense of these often highly dysfunctional and toxic experiences. In CBTpd, the usefulness and unhelpfulness of holding maladaptive core beliefs is examined, with particular attention to how these core beliefs operate in the present day, so that a fuller understanding can be reached about how they prevent the client from leading a better quality of life. Although SFT does this, the style in which this is done is different in both therapies. CBTpd may be thought of as being more collaborative in style and less prescriptive. The core beliefs may have been understandable in childhood, but in adulthood these beliefs may hinder the client's ability to be successful in work or relationships.

The client may have formed rules for living that are not only unsuitable to current circumstances but also when questioned about the rules, the client may not even value them. For example, one client believed that her mother's neglectful behavior and negative attitude toward her meant that she was "not worthy of love or affection" and was "defective" in some unspecified way that she could do little about correcting. While in therapy, she met a man she liked, who wanted to develop the relationship romantically, but she ended the relationship at that point because she was afraid he would find her unattractive and not worthy of love. She thought he would also find out that she was "bad and unable to have a relationship." She was very unhappy about ending the relationship but was too afraid to let it develop. When her fears were examined more fully, she said she wanted to share her life with someone even if having children would be too much responsibility for her, particularly given her awareness that her own mother had been unable to meet her needs. She would have liked to be able to discuss this with the man she liked, but she predicted that he would reject her if she did not want children for this reason. She came to value her opinion that she did not want children. She even thought that it would be worth the risk of being honest about this should she have another relationship.

A major distinction between CBTpd and both SFT and Beckian cognitive therapy is the emphasis the latter place on identifying and working with schema modes, especially with regard to what Young and colleagues (2003) call "doing battle" with the client's schemas. In this aspect, SFT seems to be more confrontational that CBTpd. Although CBTpd recognizes the need to restructure the schemas assumed to characterize each schema mode, the concept of mode is not considered necessary, and the therapeutic process is not considered one in which the therapist goes into battle with the core beliefs. CBTpd does not do "battle" with schemas. Instead, the core beliefs and accompanying dysfunctional behavioral patterns are established through the initial assessment phase and written into the agreed narrative formation. The client's core beliefs may be understandable given his or her early developmental experiences, particularly with caregivers who could not meet his or her emotional needs. These same core beliefs about self and others are no longer adaptive and prevent the person from optimal, healthy functioning in the here and now. So unlike SFT, CBTpd identifies and works with the core beliefs from the client's narrative. These core beliefs do not arise because a person has a PD; rather, the CBTpd model suggests that the beliefs arise because of the interaction between that individual and how he or she experienced the early environment. The beliefs become "core," that is, central to identity, due to the degree to which there is a fit between the beliefs and client's emotional reaction and behavior in relation to his or her childhood circumstances. CBTpd aims to help the client develop a better understanding of why he or she has developed these core beliefs about self and others, and the behavioral patterns that are a way of coping. If the formulation is not good enough in terms of explanatory power, then therapy is unlikely to proceed or succeed. The formulation should be both validating for the client and useful for spelling out what might need to change if the client is to live a more adaptive and positive life.

Both CBTpd and SFT make extensive use of standard cognitive techniques to help the client understand and overcome early maladaptive core beliefs, by helping the client recognize that these beliefs are inaccurate and require reassessment to see whether they fit with and are useful in the adult world inhabited by the client.

However, despite this emphasis on cognitive methods, SFT differs from CBTpd in using a wider range of techniques, some of which do not come from the CBT tradition. Besides the cognitive restructuring used by all cognitive therapies and the limited reparenting discussed previously, SFT also makes extensive use of experiential techniques drawn from Gestalt therapy and emotion–focused therapy. Clients are encouraged in the assessment phase and in the change phase of SFT to utilize imagery that reflects the early maladaptive schemas. Gestalt techniques, such as the two-chair technique, are used encourage and coach the client to overcome the maladaptive schema and answer back with more positive, healthier adaptive beliefs. Young and colleagues (2003) believe that this use of imagery work helps the client to move to an emotional rather than just an "intellectual" understanding of his or her schemas. CBTpd does not use these techniques, and instead uses cognitive and behavioral, here-and-now methods of change. CBTpd does challenge the client's view of past relationships, but it does so through memories of the past and how these memories fit with the core beliefs. CBTpd recognizes that past and current experiences and memories may be biased by the dominance of the core beliefs and associated schematic memory structures. CBTpd uses data logs, collects and summarizes new information, and revisits past memories, using careful questioning and discussion. Clients gain an understanding of how they have biased their view of self and others to fit with their core beliefs, and how this may have been unhelpful. New ways of thinking about self are strengthened through behavioral experiments in the real world. Sometimes clients find that even small changes in their behavior can bring about powerful new ways of thinking about self, others, and, of course, relationships.

## Summary of Evidence

This section deals only with the evidence supporting CBTpd (see Ryle & Kellett, Chapter 27, this volume, for studies of SFT). Most studies have evaluated the treatment of Cluster B PDs, most notably BPD (see Table 28.1). However, one trial that included patients with avoidant PD (Emmelkamp et al., 2006) found that patients who received CBT had a better outcome than those in a wait-list control, whereas the brief dynamic therapy group did no better than the wait-list control group.

### Borderline PD

Davison and colleagues (Davidson, Norrie, et al., 2006; Davidson, Tyrer, et al., 2006) investigated the comparative effects of CBTpd and treatment as usual (TAU) in an RCT trial involving 106 people with BPD attending community-based clinics in three centers across the U.K. National Health Service—in the BOSCOT trial, TAU varied between sites and individuals but was consistent with routine treatment in the U.K. National Health Service at the time. At 1-year posttherapy, CBTpd was superior to TAU in terms of a reduction in suicidal acts, anxiety, positive symptom distress, and dysfunctional beliefs. Mean total costs per patient in

TABLE 28.1. Outcome of CBTpd

| Personality diagnosis | No. of patients | Treatment comparison | Reference |
|---|---|---|---|
| Borderline | 86 | SFT-CBT vs. transferernce-focused therapy | Giesen-Bloo et al. (2006) |
| Borderline | 106 | CBTpd + TAU vs. TAU | Davidson, Norrie, et al. (2006); Davidson, Tyrer, et al. (2006) |
| Borderline | 65 | CBTpd vs. Rogerian supportive therapy | Cottraux et al. (2009) |
| Antisocial | 54 | CBTpd vs. TAU | Davidson et al. (2009) |
| Avoidant | 62 | CBT vs. brief dynamic therapy vs. WL control | Emmelkamp et al. (2006) |

Note. TAU, treatment as usual; WL, wait list.

the (CBTpd) group were also around one-third lower than for patients receiving TAU (Palmer et al., 2006). In a 6-year outcome study involving 82% of the original patients, over half the patients meeting criteria for BPD at entry into the study no longer did so, and the gains of CBTpd over TAU in reducing suicidal behavior were maintained. However, quality of life and affective disturbance remained poor in both groups. Length of hospitalization and cost of services were around two-thirds lower in the CBTpd group than in the TAU group.

Norrie, Davidson, Tata, and Gumley (2013) evaluated whether the amount of therapy and therapist competence had an impact on our primary outcome and the number of suicidal acts, using instrumental variables via regression modeling. These analyses suggested a relationship between the quantity and quality of therapy and suicidal behavior. The intention-to-treat estimate of approximately one suicidal act averted over 2 years approximately doubles when the patient was treated by more competent therapists and received over 15 therapy sessions. These findings underscore the importance of examining the effect of therapist competence and amount of therapy that may be required to improve adverse outcomes. Therapists competent in CBTpd were able to achieve changes clients' suicidal behavior in 20 or fewer sessions over 1 year, and this effect remained throughout the 2-year period.

A further study compared CBT with Rogerian supportive therapy (Cottraux et al., 2009). Both treatments took place over 1 year, and patients were followed up for a further year. The therapist established a collaborative relationship with the patient, and therapy was highly structured with the use of agendas and a focus on a specific theme. The therapy had elements of not only SFT and CBTpd but also some differences in that the main techniques were reformulation, reframing, reinforcing the patient's positive thoughts, and asking for feedback on the negative aspects of the therapy. The therapists analyzed the relationship between environmental cues, emotion, cognition, and dysfunctional behaviors, and gave patients a graphic representation of this to aid understanding. The patients were also helped to cope with and accept their emotions, and if posttraumatic stress disorder was present, then imaginal exposure techniques were used. Therapists confronted patients with their dysfunctional self-schemas via mental images or role playing rather similar to SFT, though reparenting techniques were not used. Cognitive therapy retained the patients in therapy for a longer time but no significant between-group differences were found in those who completed therapy. There was some evidence that those who received cognitive therapy showed an earlier positive effect.

## Antisocial PD

Davidson and colleagues (2009) carried out an exploratory randomized trial of CBT for men with ASPD living in the community to see whether it was possible to manage and retain people in treatment and whether the intervention was associated with health improvements and reductions in aggression. The trial took place in two U.K. cities: Glasgow and London. Fifty-two men with a diagnosis of ASPD with reported acts of aggression in the 6 months prior to the study were randomized to either TAU plus

CBT or TAU alone. We did not exclude ASPD participants who were abusing alcohol or drugs, which is likely to be common in this group. Of the men allocated to the treatment arm that received CBTpd, half were allocated to 6 months of CBTpd and the other half to 12 months. To determine the optimal components of therapy and the effect of the number of sessions on outcome, participants randomized to CBT received either 15 sessions of CBT over 6 months or 30 sessions of CBT over 12 months, each session lasting up to 1 hour. Everyone was followed up for 12 months. Change over 12 months of follow-up was assessed regarding acts of aggression, alcohol misuse, mental state, beliefs, and social functioning. The follow-up rate was 79%. At 1 year, both groups reported a decrease in acts of verbal or physical aggression. There were trends in the data in favor of CBT: a reduction in problematic drinking, improvements in social functioning, and more positive beliefs about others.

## Conclusion

The theoretical underpinnings of cognitive therapies and their structure, content, and style are adaptable enough to be suitable for the treatment of a wide variety of PDs. Cognitive therapies have been developed and have been the subject of rigorous assessment of efficacy in BPD and to a lesser degree in avoidant PD and ASPD. It would appear that cognitive therapies are helpful. This fits with the broader picture of psychological therapies for PDs, which all appear to be helpful at improving some problems associated with this group of disorders, with no single treatment being more effective than another. However, Young and colleagues' (2003) SFT is a very different form of cognitive therapy. The emphasis on limited reparenting, the use of Gestalt techniques, and the use of more psychodynamic concepts places this therapy along a path toward more psychodynamic approaches than those with their roots in cognitive and behavioral therapy. It is also a much lengthier and more intensive therapy than the other cognitive therapies, and for some people seeking help and for those providing services, this may be a disadvantage. When the effectiveness of shorter and more intensive psychological therapies is compared in terms of reducing two serious health outcomes—suicidal behavior and depression—no real differences between therapies are found (Davidson & Tran, 2013). It would seem appropriate, therefore, that therapists should deliver the least intensive interventions that provide these significant health gains.

## REFERENCES

Ainsworth, M., & Bowlby, J. (1991). An ethological approach to personality development. *American Psychologist, 46,* 333–341.

Beck, A. T. (1967). *Depression: Clinical, experimental, and theoretical aspects.* New York: Harper & Row.

Beck, A. T., Freeman, A., & Associates. (1990). *Cognitive therapy of personality disorders.* New York: Guilford Press.

Beck, A. T., Freeman, A., & Davis, D. D. (2004). *Cognitive therapy of personality disorders* (2nd ed.). New York: Guilford Press.

Bowlby, J. (1969). *Attachment and loss: Attachment.* New York: Basic Books.

Cottraux, J., Note, I. D., Boutitie, F., Milliery, M., Genouihlac, V., Nan Yao, S., et al. (2009). Cognitive therapy versus Rogerian supportive therapy in borderline personality disorder: Two year follow-up of a controlled pilot study. *Psychotherapy and Psychosomatics, 78,* 307–316.

Davidson, K. M. (2000). *Cognitive therapy for personality disorders: A guide for clinicians.* London: Arnold (Hodder).

Davidson, K. M. (2008). *Cognitive therapy for personality disorders: A guide for clinicians* (2nd ed.). Hove, UK: Routledge.

Davidson, K. M., Norrie, J., Tyrer, P., Gumley, A., Tata, P., Murray, H., et al. (2006). The effectiveness of cognitive behaviortherapy for borderline personality disorder: Results from the BOSCOT trial. *Journal of Personality Disorders, 20*(5), 450–465.

Davidson, K. M., & Tran, C. F. (2013) Impact of treatment intensity on suicidal behavior and depression in borderline personality disorder: A critical review. *Journal of Personality Disorders, 27,* 113–130.

Davidson, K. M., & Tyrer, P. (1996). Cognitive therapy for antisocial and borderline personality disorders: Single case series. *British Journal of Clinical Psychology, 35,* 413–429.

Davidson, K. M., Tyrer, P., Gumley, A., Tata, P., Norrie, J., Palmer, S., et al. (2006). Rationale, description, and sample characteristics of a randomised controlled trial of cognitive therapy for borderline personality disorder: The BOSCOT study. *Journal of Personality Disorders, 20*(5), 431–449.

Davidson, K. M., Tyrer, P., Tata, P., Cooke, D., Gumley, A., Ford, I., et al. (2009). Cognitive behavior therapy for violent men with antisocial personality disorder in the community: An exploratory randomised controlled trial. *Psychological Medicine, 39,* 569–578.

Emmelkamp, P. M. G., Benner, A., Kuipers, A., Feiertag, G. A., Koster, H. C., & van Apeldoorn, F. J. (2006). Comparison of brief dynamic and cognitive behavioral therapies in avoidant personality disorder. *British Journal of Psychiatry, 189,* 60–64.

Giesen-Bloo, J., Van Dyck, R., Spinhoven, P., Van Tilburg, W., Dirksen, C., & Van Asselt, T. (2006). Outpatient psychotherapy for borderline personality disorders: Randomised controlled trial of SFT vs transference-focused psychotherapy. *Archives of General Psychiatry, 63,* 649–658.

Greenberg, J. R., & Mitchell, S. A. (1983). *Object relations in psychoanalytic theory.* Cambridge, MA: Harvard University Press.

Kellogg, S., & Young, J. E. (2006). Schema therapy for borderline personality disorder. *Journal of Clinical Psychology, 62,* 445–458.

Norrie, J., Davidson, K. M., Tata, P., & Gumley, A. (2013). Influence of therapist competence and quantity of CBT on suicidal behavior and inpatient hospitalisation in a randomised controlled trial in borderline personality disorder: Further analyses of treatment effects in the BOSCOT study. *Psychology and Psychotherapy: Theory, Research and Practice, 86,* 280–293.

Padesky, C. A. (1994). Schema change processes in cognitive therapy. *Clinical Psychology and Psychotherapy, 1,* 267–278.

Palmer, S., Davidson, K. M., Tyrer, P., Gumley, A., Tata, P., Norrie, J., et al. (2006). The cost-effectiveness of cognitive behavior therapy for borderline personality disorder: Results from the BOSCOT trial. *Journal of Personality Disorders, 20*(5), 466–481.

Rothbart, M. K., Adahi, S. A., & Evans, D. E. (2000). Temperament and personality: Origins and outcomes. *Journal of Personality and Social Psychology, 78*(1), 122–135.

Scher, C. D., Ingram, R. E., & Segal, Z. V. (2005). Cognitive reactivity and vulnerability: Empirical evaluation of construct activation and cognitive diatheses in unipolar depression. *Clinical Psychology Review, 25,* 487–510.

The Matrix. (2015). Retrieved from *www.nes.scot.nhs.uk/education-and-training/by-discipline/psychology/the-matrix-(2015)-a-guide-to-delivering-evidence-based-psychological-therapies-in-scotland.aspx*.

University College London. (2015). Competency maps. Retrieved from *www.ucl.ac.uk/clinical-psychology/competency-maps/pd-map.html*.

Young, J. E. (1990). *Cognitive therapy for personality disorders: A schema-focused approach.* Sarasota, FL: Professional Resource Exchange.

Young, J., Klosko, J. S., & Weishaar, M. E. (2003). *Schema therapy: A practitioner's guide.* New York: Guilford Press.

Zanarini, M. C., Frankenburg, F. R., Reich, D. B., & Fitzmaurice, G. (2012). Attainment and stability of sustained symptomatic remission and recovery among patients with borderline personality disorder and Axis II comparison subjects: A 16-year prospective follow-up study. *American Journal of Psychiatry, 169,* 476–483.

# CHAPTER 29

# Dialectical Behavior Therapy

Clive J. Robins, Noga Zerubavel, André M. Ivanoff,
and Marsha M. Linehan

Dialectical behavior therapy (DBT) is a unique integration of behavior therapy, the principles and practice of Zen, and an overarching dialectical philosophy that guides the treatment. The treatment, developed by Marsha Linehan (1993a), evolved from many years of work with chronically suicidal women and has been well established as an empirically supported treatment for borderline personality disorder (BPD). DBT was developed to address the skills deficits of individuals with BPD, as well as the issues that lead therapists frequently to get stuck, go down blind alleys, and, in some cases, contribute to serious, even fatal, deterioration in the patient's well-being.

DBT is rooted firmly in the principles and practices of behavior therapy, including a strong emphasis on ongoing data collection during treatment, clearly defined target behaviors, a collaborative therapist–patient relationship, and the use of standard cognitive and behavioral treatment strategies. However, a distinctive characteristic of DBT is the emphasis on dialectics. The fundamental dialectic in DBT is the need for both acceptance and change. The therapist needs to fully accept the patient as he or she is and at the same time persistently push for and help the patient to change. The therapist also tries to develop and strengthen an attitude of acceptance toward reality on the part of the patient, as well as the motivation and ability to change what can be changed.

The fundamental treatment dialectic of acceptance and change is expressed through the two core sets of therapist strategies, validation and problem solving. DBT also involves a dialectic of communication style between a reciprocal, warm interpersonal style and a more irreverent style, and a dialectic in case management between consultation to the patient to help manage his or her environment on the one hand and direct environmental intervention by the therapist on the other. For patients with BPD, there are almost always serious skills deficits in emotion regulation, distress tolerance, and interpersonal domains. To facilitate both skills building and a focus on personal crises and skills application, separate skills training groups free up the individual therapist to help patients manage crises, reinforce the use of skills, and deal with motivational issues that interfere with using the skills they have.

## Scope and Focus: Domains of Psychopathology

DBT addresses problems associated with pervasive emotion dysregulation. Linehan conceptualized BPD criteria "either as a direct consequence of emotion dysregulation or as responses that function to modulate the aversive emotional states" (Linehan, Bohus, & Lynch, 2007, p. 584; see also Linehan, 1993a). Although originally developed for treatment of BPD, DBT may also be applied to many other disorders that are associated with difficulties in emotion regulation, including binge eating, bulimia, comorbid substance use, treatment-resistant depression, bipolar disorder, and attention-deficit/hyperactivity disorder (ADHD). We summarize the research findings later in this chapter.

## Treatment Stages and Targets

DBT consists of five stages: pretreatment and four active treatment stages: control, order, synthesis, and transcendence. Treatment goals are hierarchical within stages and determine the treatment agenda within and across sessions; each session agenda is based on the patient's behavior since the last session. It is the therapist's responsibility to remain mindful of treatment goals and to ensure that patient treatment activities are directed toward creating a life worth living.

### Pretreatment

The objectives of this stage are to orient patients to the philosophy and structure of treatment, and for therapist and patient to reach agreement on the goals of treatment. These goals are clearly prescribed: If patients are currently engaging in suicidal or other self-harming behaviors, they must agree that reducing or eliminating such behavior is the first priority. Patients must also agree not to kill themselves while they are in DBT. Although the coexistence of suicidal behaviors and desire to live is dialectically understood within DBT, treatment cannot progress beyond this target until it is under control. Obtaining explicit patient agreement is necessary prior to full participation in treatment; with patients who express reluctance to commit to DBT goals, ongoing pretreatment focuses on commitment-enhancing strategies. Becoming committed may entail numerous steps. DBT utilizes various strategies, including evaluating the pros and cons of commitment to DBT treatment, playing the devil's advocate, using "foot in the door" and "door in the face" techniques, and highlighting prior commitments and connecting them to current agreements. Therapists use basic principles of shaping (i.e., building on small steps toward larger commitments) and strong use of encouragement and reinforcement as commitment-enhancing strategies.

### Stage 1: From Behavioral Dyscontrol to Stability and Behavioral Control

For patients who enter treatment with severe behavioral dyscontrol, such as self-harm or substance abuse, DBT focuses initially on movement toward behavioral control. Suicide attempts, self-harming, and other life-threatening behaviors (e.g., harm to others) are primary targets addressed by increasing basic capacities (e.g., emotion regulation, self-control, connection to therapy) necessary to function in treatment. Goals include attaining a reasonable (immediate) life expectancy, control of behavior, stability, and tending to relationships with those who give help. The primary targets of Stage 1 are (1) decreasing behaviors involving self-harm, suicide, or violence toward others; (2) decreasing therapy-interfering behaviors; (3) decreasing serious quality-of-life-interfering behaviors; and (4) increasing skills needed to make life changes. We describe these skills in more detail later. During Stage 1 of standard DBT, treatment occurs in several modes: individual therapy, group skills training, telephone consultation, and team meetings, each of which is briefly discussed below.

### Individual Therapy

Weekly diary cards are used to collect ongoing information about target problems. Targets listed on the diary card are individually tailored but generally include suicidal behavior, ideation, and urges; self-harm; prescription, over-the-counter, and illicit drug use; binge eating; and general level of misery and other emotions. On the other side is a list of DBT skills for the patient to mark skills he or she has used. At the beginning of each individual session, the diary card is reviewed to identify priorities for that session's agenda. Patient self-monitoring via the diary card has a number of advantages over traditional memory-based narrative recall because it provides feedback and data; when completed daily, it may also increase the accuracy of reported events. Structurally, the diary card provides temporal detail about the relationship between maladaptive behaviors and emotional state.

All direct self-harm, suicide crisis behavior, intrusive or intense suicidal ideation, images or communications, and significant changes in ideation or urges to self-harm are addressed in individual therapy in the session that follows their occurrence. Self-harm, regardless of lethality or intent, is never ignored; these behaviors are good predictors of future lethal acts, may cause substantial harm, and, as primary DBT targets, must be brought under control before treatment can progress.

## Skills Training

DBT assumes that many problems experienced by patients who are chronically suicidal, self-harm, or engage in other behaviors characteristic of BPD result from a combination of motivational problems and behavioral skills deficits (i.e., lacking skills to regulate painful affect). For this reason, DBT emphasizes building skills to facilitate behavior change and acceptance. In DBT, four skills modules are taught sequentially in weekly skills training groups: mindfulness, interpersonal effectiveness, emotion regulation, and distress tolerance. Mindfulness skills are considered core skills; thus, this module is repeated, taking two sessions, between each of the other modules. The interpersonal effectiveness and distress tolerance modules take approximately 6 weeks each to complete, and the emotion regulation module, which is expanded significantly in the new edition of the skills manual (Linehan, 2014), now takes about 8 weeks. These skills are described in detail in the skills training manual (Linehan, 1993b, 2014). Groups use didactic instructions, modeled examples, coached rehearsal of new skills, feedback, and homework assignments.

Working in tandem, simultaneous group and individual components of treatment create dedicated time to learn much-needed skills and a separate context for coached individual application. This allows individual therapy to focus on priority target behaviors, as well as other crisis issues that patients with BPD frequently bring to session, without the pressure also to teach skill fundamentals. Group skills training has several advantages over individual skills training: Members practice together and learn from each other; skills practice is coached by an expert skills trainer; group membership often decreases real isolation and increases a patient's sense of feeling understood. Socially phobic patients or those who must begin skills training in individual sessions are moved to group skills training as soon as possible.

## Telephone Consultation

Between-session contact serves three functions in DBT: (1) to provide skills coaching *in vivo* to promote skills generalization, (2) to promote crisis intervention in a contingent manner, and (3) to provide an opportunity to resolve misunderstandings and conflicts that arise during therapy sessions, instead of waiting until the next session to deal with the emotions. Patients are oriented early in therapy to call their individual therapist for these reasons; inability to do so is viewed as therapy-interfering behavior and becomes a target. If patients are reluctant to call, planned calls are prescribed.

Consistent with viewing the therapist as coach for adaptive behavior, this contact must occur prior to any direct self-harm. If the patient has already engaged in such behavior, the therapist does not provide nonscheduled contact to the patient for 24 hours, limiting whatever contact may occur to management of safety. This provides reinforcement for adaptive coping and realistic consequences after the fact (i.e., "What help can I give you after you've already hurt yourself?") for maladaptive behavior.

## Consultation Team

DBT is best viewed as a treatment system in which the therapist applies DBT to patients while the consultation team simultaneously applies DBT to the therapist. Supervision and consultation are critical for therapists treating emotionally distressed, demanding, and often difficult patients. Clinicians experienced in treatment of BPD typically report that progress is often difficult and outcomes are relatively modest. In addition, some patients with BPD engage in behaviors that generate extreme stress in clinicians. Without ongoing supervision or consultation, clinicians working with this patient population can become extreme in their positions, blame the patient and themselves, and become less open to feedback from others about the conduct of their treatment. Accordingly, DBT requires that all therapists doing any part of this treatment must be part of a consultation team. Consultation to the therapist has several purposes, most importantly to ensure that the clinician remains in the therapeutic relationship and remains effective in that relationship. Validation of the therapist's reactions, feelings, and experiences in working with this extremely difficult population is combined with problem solving. The team also functions to improve treatment fidelity; therapist behavior that deviates from the model (e.g., defensiveness) is explicitly noted and corrective actions are suggested (Koerner, 2011).

### Stage 2: From Quiet Desperation to Nontraumatic Emotional Experiencing

Stage 1 may be thought of as guiding the patient from a state of loud desperation to a state of quiet desperation, and Stage 2 may be viewed as alleviating the patient's unremitting emotional desperation (Linehan, 1999). Stage 2 DBT addresses posttraumatic stress syndrome and may include remembering, exposure treatment, and accepting prior traumatic or emotionally important events. Individuals with BPD and comorbid posttraumatic stress disorder (PTSD) who complete 1 year of DBT have significantly poorer outcomes of intentional self-injury and BPD symptoms during 1 year of DBT (Barnicot & Priebe, 2013); thus, it is important to treat the PTSD in order for individuals to benefit fully from treatment. Once patients have the emotion regulation and distress tolerance skills needed to process emotionally scarring experiences, recent research shows that they may benefit from moving into PTSD treatment that overlaps with Stage 1 skills acquisition (Harned, Korslund, & Linehan, 2014). Stage 2 may therefore occur earlier in treatment than was originally anticipated. Harned and colleagues (2014) suggest that patient preparedness is indicated once serious maladaptive behaviors (i.e., suicide attempts, self-harm) have not occurred for 2 months, even in the face of relevant stressors. When the patient is prepared for such work, posttraumatic responses are targeted using a DBT prolonged exposure (DBT-PE) protocol (Harned et al., 2014). Although patients might enter Stage 2 with some suicidal ideation, entry into Stage 2 means they no longer engage in direct self-harm, buying guns for suicide, hoarding pills, or making other concrete plans for suicide.

### Stage 3: From Problems in Living to Ordinary Happiness and Unhappiness

Stage 3 treatment focuses on moving problems in living to the level of "ordinary" happiness and unhappiness, thereby attaining a higher quality of life. Targets include self-respect and achievement of personal goals. Patients cultivate an ongoing sense of connection to self, others, and life, synthesizing prior learning into mastery, self-efficacy, and a sense of personal values.

### Stage 4: From Incompleteness to Freedom and Capacity for Joy

Stage 4, a later addition (Linehan, 1999), addresses any lingering sense of incompleteness that continues after resolution of problems in living. Stage 4 goals include developing capacity for sustained joy and freedom from psychological imperatives by integrating past, present, and future; self and others; and accepting reality.

## Diagnosis, Assessment, and Formulation

Evaluation of whether an individual meets criteria for BPD is best accomplished by means of a structured diagnostic interview. However, simply establishing a diagnosis is of limited utility for DBT, and possibly for any psychotherapy. More important is to know the specific patterns of behavior that create difficulty for this particular individual, and what his or her maintaining variables are. Assessment in DBT therefore emphasizes day-to-day monitoring of target behaviors through the diary card and in-depth behavioral analysis of target behaviors. We have found that completion of diary cards is essential assessment throughout treatment, and the therapist is advised to continue having the patient complete them even when he or she has shown improvement and may not have had any suicidal, substance-abusing, or other high-priority target behaviors in some time. Without lying explicitly, patients with BPD frequently fail to mention the occurrence of such behaviors if they are not specifically asked about and/or monitored. Another helpful function is that diary cards enable the therapist to learn as much as possible about the patient's social context, including bringing in family members and significant others, for collateral information and to better understand these relationships. Many of the patient's problem behaviors occur within an interpersonal context, and the therapeutic relationship often provides an opportunity to identify subtle aspects of interpersonal problems; thus, the state of the therapeutic relationship, including the therapist's own contribution to it, is in need of ongoing assessment for clinically relevant information.

Case formulation is conducted through understanding the biosocial theory as it applies to the particular patient, delineating the problem behaviors within the hierarchical system, and identifying aspects of patient and therapist behavior that need to be addressed in order for treatment to be successful (see also Koerner, 2011; Linehan, 1993a).

## Theoretical Foundation of DBT

Two theoretical frameworks provide the foundation for DBT: (1) a biosocial theory of BPD, which helps the therapist to understand the patient's behaviors, and to know both how the patient needs to change and what he or she needs to learn; and (2) the core treatment principles, drawn from behavior therapy, Zen, and dialectical philosophy, which inform the therapist how to help bring about those changes. DBT includes assumptions that reflect the balance between acceptance (e.g., "Patients are doing the best they can," "Patients want to improve," and "Patients cannot fail in DBT") and change (e.g., "Patients may not have caused all of their own problems, but they have to solve them anyway" and "Patients need to do better, try harder, and be more motivated to change").

### Theory of Disorder: A Biosocial Theory of BPD

Biosocial theory proposes that BPD results from a series of transactions over time between a personal factor (i.e., emotion dysregulation) and an environmental factor (i.e., the invalidating environment). A patient who displays extreme emotional reactions may often receive invalidation of his or her experiences and behavior from others who have difficulty understanding his or her degree of intensity. The experience of being persistently invalidated, in turn, tends to increase emotional dysregulation and decrease learning of emotion regulation skills.

Difficulties in emotion regulation may occur because of a combination of two factors: an inherent emotional vulnerability and difficulty in modulating emotions. Emotional vulnerability may, in part, be biologically determined as temperament. The emotionally vulnerable person has low thresholds, rapid emotional reactions, and high-level reactions. High levels of emotion, in turn, lead to dysregulated cognitive processing, as they do for everyone. Unfortunately, most patients with BPD spend much of their time in a state of high arousal and are therefore frequently cognitively dysregulated. Emotional vulnerability also entails a slow return to baseline levels, which contributes to a high sensitivity to the next emotional stimulus. Difficulty modulating emotions is also a challenge for the patient with BPD. Basic research has found several tasks to be important for emotion modulation, including the abilities to reorient attention, inhibit mood-dependent action, change physiological arousal, experience emotions without escalating or blunting them, and to organize behavior in the service of non-mood-dependent goals. These all are skilled behaviors that, to a large degree, may be learned; for whatever reason, most patients with BPD have not learned them; therefore, an important aspect of treatment is teaching these skills.

An invalidating environment—one in which private experiences (i.e., emotions, thoughts) and overt behaviors are responded to as if they are invalid responses to events—also contributes to emotion dysregulation. Responses may be invalidated through punishment, rejection, and being ignored or overlooked, and they may be attributed to personal, undesirable characteristics. Furthermore, although emotional communication may be disregarded or punished, intense escalation may result in attention, meeting of demands, and other types of reinforcement. Finally, an invalidating environment may oversimplify the ease of achieving goals and problem solving. Possible consequences of pervasive invalidation include difficulties in accurately labeling emotions, regulating emotions, and trusting one's own experiences as valid. By oversimplifying problem solving, an invalidating environment does not teach problem solving, graduated goals, or distress tolerance; instead, one learns perfectionistic standards and self-punishment as a strategy to try to change one's behavior. Finally, reinforcement of only escalated emotional displays teaches the individual to oscillate between emotional inhibition and extreme emotional behavior.

### Fundamental Theoretical Constructs: Core Treatment Principles

DBT draws most of its treatment principles from three areas of knowledge: behavior therapy, Zen, and dialectical philosophy.

## Behavior Therapy

Principles of behavior therapy are primarily principles of learning. DBT assumes that many maladaptive behaviors, both overt and private (thoughts, feelings) are learned and therefore can be replaced by new learning. Three primary ways through which individuals learn are (1) "modeling," which involves learning through observation of others; (2) "operant conditioning," which refers to learning an association between a behavior and its consequences; and (3) "respondent conditioning," which involves a learned association between two stimuli. All three processes are central to understanding and changing maladaptive behavior. When consequences follow a behavior and result in a subsequent increase or decrease in that behavior, these are the operant (instrumental) conditioning processes of reinforcement and punishment, respectively. Extinction occurs when previously reinforced behavior is no longer reinforced and the behavior decreases. These principles are widely known and frequently employed systematically by parents, teachers, and others, but often they are not considered by therapists in relation to patient behaviors and therapist–patient interactions. Therapists need to avoid unwittingly reinforcing a maladaptive behavior by, for example, providing greater attention to patients when they engage in the behavior than when they do not. When more adaptive behavior is being learned, therapists must avoid punishing or failing to reinforce fledgling efforts because the behavior still falls short of the mark; instead, DBT therapists are constantly looking for opportunities to use shaping deliberately and contingently to provide interpersonal and other positive consequences to the patient's skillful behavior. In respondent (classical) conditioning, two stimuli become associated, so that a natural response to one becomes a learned response to the other (e.g., after being raped in a dark alley, being near a dark alley may provoke a full-force fear response). Positive but maladaptive associations may also be learned in this way, such as an association between the sight or touch of a knife used previously in self-harming and experiencing emotional relief.

## Zen

The introduction of principles from Zen practice into DBT came about largely because of the strong need for patients to develop an attitude of greater acceptance toward a reality that is often painful. Other spiritual traditions also provide valuable teachings on issues related to acceptance, but Zen particularly has developed methods for this. In DBT, the most essential Zen principles and practices include the importance of being mindful of the current moment, seeing reality without delusion, accepting reality without judgment, letting go of attachments that cause suffering, and finding the middle way. Zen is also characterized by the humanistic assumption that all individuals have an inherent capacity for enlightenment and intuitive truth, referred to in DBT as "wise mind."

## Dialectics

"Dialectics" refers to a process of synthesis of opposing elements, ideas, or events (i.e., thesis and antithesis). Individuals with BPD often exhibit extreme polarized beliefs and actions. DBT therapists model dialectical strategies and directly teach more balanced, synthesized, and dialectical patterns of thinking and behavior. A dialectical worldview permeates DBT treatment. In dialectical philosophy, reality is viewed as being whole and interrelated and at the same time as bipolar and oppositional, as in the opposing forces of subatomic particles. Reality is in continuous change, as its components transact with one another. This worldview is consistent with the transactional, systemic nature of the biosocial theory, and with the patient and therapist being in a dialectical relationship, transacting in ways that will inevitably lead to changes in both. Dialectics are also used to balance treatment strategies that are heavily change-oriented with others that are heavily acceptance-oriented. Balancing treatment does not mean watering down strong oppositions; rather, it frequently means firmly embracing both. Dialectical balance in treatment involves rapid movement from one type of strategy to another, a quality of movement, speed, and flow that is developed in the therapist through his or her own mindfulness practice. Finally, dialectical philosophy informs the treatment goals and skills taught in DBT, including the change-oriented goals of improving emotion regulation and interpersonal effectiveness and the more acceptance-oriented goals of learning mindfulness and the ability to tolerate distress. Patients need to learn to accept as much as they need to learn to change. Learning to accept is, of course, a change in itself.

## DBT Strategies

In DBT, change and acceptance strategies are woven together, integrated throughout the treatment, always in an effort to achieve a dialectical balance. A therapist doing DBT therefore strives to balance the use of acceptance and change strategies. Dialectical strategies are the overarching set of strategies that use the conflict of polarity to achieve synthesis. In core strategies, the key dialectic is between validation (acceptance) and problem solving (change).

### Dialectical Strategies

The most fundamental dialectical strategy is *balancing* all the other treatment strategies, as the needs of patient and situation constantly shift. Another is *entering the paradox,* where, much as in a Zen koan, the therapist simply highlights the constant paradoxes of life without attempting to explain them, modeling and teaching "both this and that" rather than "this or that." Another dialectical strategy is the use of *metaphor*. When collaboration has broken down, when the patient is feeling hopeless, or in many other situations, teaching, persuading, and making a point through metaphor often can be far more powerful than direct or literal communication. Patients with BPD seem to respond particularly well to metaphor, and a helpful metaphor may be revisited over the course of treatment. In *dialectical assessment,* the therapist continuously seeks to understand the patient in a situational context, regularly asking, "What is being left out?" Other dialectical strategies include *wise mind, extending, devil's advocate, making lemonade out of lemons,* and *allowing natural change* (see Linehan, 1993a).

### Core Strategies: Validation

Given both the important role invalidation plays in the biosocial theory underlying DBT and the frequency of self-invalidating behavior on the part of patients with BPD, it is natural that validation is one of the primary strategies employed by DBT therapists. For most people, before having someone help solve a problem, there is a need to feel that the other person understands the problem and acknowledges one's responses to it. This need may be particularly strong in persons diagnosed with BPD. Thus, validation from the therapist serves an important function in facilitating problem solving. Research shows that individuals who receive validating responses during stressor tasks experience significantly lower levels of negative affect, heart rate, and skin conductance over time in comparison to others who receive invalidating responses (Shenk & Fruzzetti, 2011). Thus, validation may be used to decrease emotional arousal on affective and physiological levels. Validation may also function to strengthen patterns of self-validation and combat self-invalidation, as well as to strengthen the therapeutic relationship or reinforce clinical progress. By "validation," we refer to communicating to the patient that his or her responses do make sense in the current context.

### Core Strategies: Problem Solving

In DBT, problem-solving strategies are the primary strategies for changing target behaviors and include procedures such as skills training, contingency management, observing limits, cognitive modification, and exposure. The elements of problem solving are divided here into a series of steps, though, in actual practice, these steps are usually interwoven rather than followed in linear fashion. First, the problem behavior must be fully understood. Such understanding involves *chain analysis* (described below). As a number of instances of a particular behavior are analyzed, therapist and patient together arrive at some insights about what factors maintain the behavior. This leads naturally to generating and evaluating various possible solutions in a *solution analysis.* Simply arriving at what would seem to be a helpful solution is not enough, however; it is also essential that the patient actively work toward the solution. This may require the therapist to employ didactic strategies or psychoeducation (about biological bases of depression, sleep, etc.). The patient needs to be clearly oriented to his or her role and expected behaviors not only in the treatment as a whole but also with regard to particular solutions generated for specific target behaviors. Finally, it is important to elicit an explicit verbal commitment from the patient to engage in the specific behaviors suggested by the solution analysis. Although such an explicit commitment does not guarantee that the behavior will occur, it does enhance the probability.

## Behavioral Chain Analysis

A key characteristic of behavior therapy that differentiates it from most other approaches is the use of behavioral analysis. The goal of behavioral analysis is to understand the factors that lead to or maintain the problem behavior. Rather than focusing on broad personality constructs or developmental antecedents, the focus is on first defining and describing the target behavior in an explicit and detailed manner, then attempting to understand the behavior in its current context by means of a chain analysis. Behavioral "chain" analysis identifies the problem, the internal (cognitive, affective, sensory) and external (social, contextual, physical environment) events preceding and causing the problem (antecedents and precipitants), and the consequences of engaging in the target behavior. DBT therapists inquire about consequences of problem behaviors, including affective consequences for the patient, interpersonal responses of others, and resulting environmental changes, as this may identify possible reinforcing factors and provide the therapist with opportunities to highlight negative consequences. In conducting a chain analysis, the object is to delineate as many links as possible. The more links in the chain, the more places there are that something different could occur in the future.

## Solution Analysis

Once the chain is clarified, the task becomes "solution analysis," identifying potential resources for solving the problem. Solution analyses include some combination of four sets of behavior therapy procedures: (1) skills training to address skills deficits that interfere with more adaptive responses; (2) contingency management strategies to address reinforcement that may support problematic behavior, or punishment that impedes skillful behavior; (3) cognitive modification procedures to address beliefs, attitudes, and assumptions that interfere with skillful behavior; and (4) exposure-based strategies to allow reduction in strong emotional responses that interfere with adaptive problem-solving attempts. An effective chain analysis need to be thorough, but the therapist needs to leave ample time in the session for conducting the solution analysis, he or she and must obtain a commitment from the patient to use these solutions as alternatives to the problem behavior if an urge or impulse arises in the future (Rizvi & Ritschel, 2014).

## Skills-Training Procedures

These procedures can teach new skills and also facilitate use of learned but unused skills. Acquired skills need to be strengthened and generalized across situations. The individual therapist and skills trainers may help the patient acquire skills by direct instruction, modeling (e.g., thinking out loud in front of the patient), self-disclosing his or her own use of skilled behaviors, and particularly through role-play and behavior rehearsal. Fledgling skills then need to be strengthened by further in-session behavior rehearsals and imaginal practice, as well as *in vivo* practice. The therapist needs to promptly reinforce any small movements toward more skilled behavior on the patient's part, even when this means reinforcing still unskilled behavior (i.e., shaping). Skills are also strengthened by direct feedback and coaching from the therapist, conveyed in a nonjudgmental manner focused on performance without inferred motives. Patients with BPD are particularly sensitive to critical feedback, yet such feedback often needs to be given, so it is best to surround it with positive feedback. Skills generalization is enhanced by *in vivo* behavior rehearsal assignments for homework, between-session telephone consultation, and procedures such as recording the therapy session for later review. Changing the environment so that it reinforces skilled behavior may also be necessary, for example, by having the patient make public commitments, or the therapist meeting with the patient and the patient's spouse or family.

## Contingency Management Procedures

The therapist tries to arrange for target-relevant adaptive behaviors to be reinforced, and for target-relevant maladaptive behaviors to be extinguished through lack of reinforcement or, if that does not work, through punishment. The primary reinforcer used by the DBT therapist is his or her behavior in relationship to the patient. The therapist observes and consciously directs, in a contingent manner, warmth versus coolness, closeness versus distance, approval versus disapproval, presence and availability versus unavailability, and other dimensions of his or her behavior in the relationship. For the therapeutic relationship to be used contingently, it must be highly valued by the patient. The DBT therapist works hard to establish a strong therapeutic relationship, developing an attachment between therapist and patient that is mutual and genuine, in order to be able to leverage the therapeutic relationship. Therapists also attend to contingencies in the patient's environment. Suggesting to the patient that maladaptive behavior may be maintained by reinforcement can be experienced as invalidating (e.g., "Are you saying that I injure myself in order to get support?"). It is helpful to discuss with the patient how reinforcement works regardless of intent or awareness, and that even unintended consequences still influence behavior.

As reinforcement and punishment are defined by their effects on behavior, they need to be determined for each particular patient. Although praise is a reinforcer for most people, some patients find praise aversive (e.g., they feel embarrassed, fear raised expectations). For most patients, therapist behaviors that are reinforcing include expression of approval, interest, concern and care, liking or admiring the patient, reassurance regarding the dependability of the relationship, direct validation, being responsive to patient requests, and increasing attention from, or contact with, the therapist. Therapists need to take care that they do not engage in reinforcing behaviors immediately following a patient's maladaptive behavior, even if it may be their natural urge to do so, or that they inadvertently make the behavior more apt to occur.

Punishment is used with great care in DBT because it can lead to strong emotional reactions that interfere with learning, strengthen a self-invalidating style, and fail to teach specific adaptive behavior. Nonetheless, it is sometimes necessary or helpful, usually when high-priority behavior is still occurring and is reinforced primarily by consequences that are not under the therapist's control, so that extinction cannot be used. Examples are the affect regulation that frequently accompanies self-harm and inpatient psychiatric admissions that may reinforce such behavior for some patients. The most common punishers in DBT are the therapist's disapproval, confrontation, or a reduction in therapist availability. With emotionally sensitive individuals, disapproval needs to be mild in order to be most effective. Care must be taken to punish specific behaviors rather than the person. Other punishment procedures used in DBT include overcorrection (doing the reverse behavior or undoing the effects of the behavior and going beyond that); taking a "vacation from therapy," in which access to the DBT individual therapist is made contingent on some commitment or change in behavior; and, as a last resort, termination from therapy.

### Observing Limits Procedures

Contingency management procedures are applied in DBT not only to behaviors that interfere with the patient's life but also to those interfering with the therapist's life. A patient's distressed call at midnight for skills coaching to resist urges to self-harm may be acceptable to the therapist, but probably not if it occurs numerous times each week. Rather than feeling guilty for attending to one's own needs rather than just the patient's, the DBT therapist must observe his or her own limits to prevent the otherwise likely burnout and dropout from treatment. The parameters of limits are not defined by DBT, but they are distinct to this therapist, with this patient, at this time, in this situation. Because there are no rules on which to fall back, therapists need to be self-aware, receptive to feedback from consultation team, and assertive with patients. Limits are often unknown until they are closely approached or crossed. Common areas for therapists to observe and to set limits with patients are frequency or utility of telephone calls, suicidal behavior, aggressive behavior, and patient's disengagement in treatment. We have found that when one's own limits are clearly delineated and described as something about oneself rather than patient pathology or what is best for the patient, and the behaviors that cross these limits are clearly specified in a nonjudgmental way, many battles over how the patient "should" behave can be resolved or avoided.

### Cognitive Modification Procedures

In DBT, thoughts, beliefs, assumptions, and expectations are seen as a category of behaviors that influence, and are reciprocally influenced by, transactions with emotional processes, overt behavior, and environmental factors. Standard cognitive therapy procedures are used in DBT; however, in DBT they are paired with an emphasis on first validating the wisdom in the patient's cognitions. The therapist stays alert for distortions of cognitive content and style. "Content" refers to negative automatic thoughts and maladaptive beliefs, attitudes, or schemas, such as viewing oneself as worthless, defective, unlovable, and vulnerable, and/or others as excessively admired, despised, or feared. Problems of cognitive style include dichotomous thinking and maladaptive allocation of attention (i.e., ruminating, dissociating). The therapist tries to help patients to change these problems by (1) teaching self-observation through mindfulness practice and written assignments; (2) identifying maladaptive cognitions and pointing to nondialectical thinking; (3) generating alternative, more adaptive cognitive content and style in session and for homework assignments; and (4) developing guidelines for when patients should trust rather than suspect their own interpretations, as self-validation is often also a goal.

DBT recognizes a special case of cognitive modification, *contingency clarification procedures*. It is extremely important that the patient understand the contingencies that currently operate in his or her life, including in the therapeutic relationship, and see how they influence his or her behaviors. Consistent use of contingencies and clear communication are the best response to patient difficulty learning or following rules.

### Exposure Procedures

One of the greatest successes of behavior therapy has been the treatment of many anxiety disorders. The core of these treatments involves repeated exposure to anxiety-provoking stimuli or situations, while ensuring that the normal escape or avoidance response does not occur. When these emotions are problematic in themselves, leading to maladaptive avoidance behavior, inhibiting the use of skills, or are associated with PTSD symptoms, exposure procedures may be useful. Central steps of exposure are to (1) orient the patient, often using a story or metaphor that illustrates the process; (2) provide nonreinforced exposure (i.e., exposure that does not meet with an outcome that could reinforce the emotional response); (3) block action and expressive tendencies associated with the problem emotion, especially behavioral or cognitive avoidance; and (4) enhance the patient's control over exposure as much as possible, such as by graduating intensity, as it is easier to tolerate aversive events when one experiences oneself as having some control.

Most of the change strategies used in DBT (and some of the acceptance strategies) may be viewed as involving emotional exposure. Exposure is extended in DBT to emotions other than anxiety, including guilt, shame, and anger. This exposure occurs when scrutinizing the patient's behavior and experience in a behavioral analysis; in skills training, such as practicing behaviors in interpersonal situations that generate discomfort; in contingency strategies, by exposure to therapist disapproval or approval that may set off feelings of shame or fear, anger, or pride; and in mindfulness practice, where the object may be to observe, in a nonjudgmental manner, the ebb and flow of one's thoughts or feelings. A thorough understanding of the importance of exposure for changes in emotional behavior helps therapists to take advantage of the innumerable opportunities that present themselves during all aspects of therapy sessions to work directly on patient's emotional reactions.

### Stylistic Strategies: Reciprocal and Irreverent Communication

Reciprocal communication is the modal stylistic strategy in DBT, used to convey acceptance and validation and to reduce the inherent patient–therapist power differential. Characterized by interest, genuineness, warm engagement, and responsiveness, it requires the therapist to take the patient's agenda and wishes seriously, and to respond directly to the content of the communications rather than interpreting or suggesting that either the content or the intent of the patient's communication is invalid. As an example, to the patient who states, "Today I really, really wish I were dead," one might reply, "I'm sorry to hear that; you must feel pretty awful" rather than "Let's get back to how you're going to talk with your family tonight." Therapists are encouraged to use self-involving self-disclosures such as pointing out the effects of the patient's behavior on the therapist in a nonjudgmental manner (e.g., "When you stare out the window instead of looking at me, it makes me think you don't want to work on these problems, and I feel like I'm working alone"), and letting patients know where they stand (e.g., "I'm concerned that we're not getting much done here today"). Personal self-disclosures are used to validate and model coping and normative responses.

"Irreverent communication," the dialectical alternative to reciprocal communication, involves a direct, confrontational, matter-of-fact, or "off-the-wall" style. Used to move the patient from a rigid stance to one that admits uncertainty and therefore promotes the potential for change, irreverent communication may be beneficial when therapist and patient are stuck or at an impasse. In addition to introducing an offbeat or potentially humorous moment, it may also occur when the therapist pays closer attention to indirect rather than direct communications. For example, to the patient who says, "I am going to kill myself!" the therapist might irreverently respond, "But I thought you agreed not to drop out of therapy!" Importantly, care is taken in observing effects of irreverent communication to avoid misuse, alienation, or invalidation. Whereas reciprocal communication is expected in most therapy approaches, irreverence is not included in most psychotherapy training, nor is it part of all therapists' natural communication styles. However, our experience has been that it is possible to learn irreverence by paying close attention to peers who are naturally irreverent, culling their behavior for responses that might fit or be tailored to fit, and practicing such responses in personal life and consultation group until they become genuine.

## Case Management Strategies

Case management strategies in DBT are important for enhancing skills generalization. More broadly defined than the traditional notion of case management, these strategies include consultation to the patient, environmental intervention, and consultation to the therapist.

### Consultation to the Patient

Therapists consult with patients about how to manage their social or professional networks, rather than consult with the network about how to manage patients. This skills-building focus fosters belief in patients' ability to learn more effective ways of intervening in their own environments. Consultation to the patient strategies begin by orienting the patient and the patient's social network to the approach, advising and coaching the patient about how to manage other professionals and other members of their interpersonal networks. Other professionals are given general information about DBT treatment but are not told how to treat the patient, and they are given details of treatment information only with the patient present. Therapists perform tasks for patients only when patients truly lack the skill and cannot learn it quickly enough to prevent an immediate adverse outcome.

### Environmental Intervention

Environmental intervention strategies include providing information to others independent of the patient, patient advocacy, and entering the patient's environment to provide assistance. Direct environmental intervention by the therapist is approved only under conditions in which the short-term gain is worth the long-term loss in learning. Examples of conditions requiring direct intervention are (1) when the patient is unable to act on his or her own and the outcome is very important (e.g., the suicidal patient who cannot tell his family he needs them to stay with him); (2) when the environment is intransigent and high in power (e.g., an application for social services that will automatically be denied without professional involvement); (3) when a patient's life risk or substantial risk to others is probable (e.g., high suicidality or risk of child abuse); (4) when direct intervention is the humane thing to do and will cause no harm and does not substitute passive for active problem solving (e.g., meeting with patients outside ordinary settings in a crisis); (5) when the patient is a minor (Linehan, 1993a).

### Consultation to the Therapist

Consultation to the therapist in the consultation team, the final component of DBT case management, has been previously described. Its purpose is to enhance the therapist's capabilities and motivation to stay within the treatment frame.

## The Therapeutic Relationship in DBT

We have touched on therapeutic relationship issues throughout this chapter. In this section, we highlight some of the contexts in which the therapeutic relationship is most evident or receives particular emphasis in DBT. One function of DBT theory is to help therapists understand and deal with effects of common BPD behaviors by influencing therapists' attitudes. For example, the biosocial theory concept of the invalidating environment leads naturally to the emphasis on validation strategies in the treatment. Similarly, the overarching position of dialectics leads the therapist to pay attention to dialectics, balance, and rapid movement back and forth on the teeter-totter on which the therapist sits with the patient.

Problematic interactions in the therapeutic relationship are directly targeted for change in DBT. These include a variety of therapy-interfering behaviors of both therapist and patient, which are a priority second only to life-threatening and self-harm behaviors. The secondary targets of DBT (e.g., self-invalidation, emotion dysregulation) frequently show up in session in response to patient–therapist interactions. These interactions are observed, analyzed collaboratively, and modified when possible.

Each mode of treatment has its own set of parameters for the therapeutic relationship. Relatively unique to DBT is the use of planned telephone or other consultation availability between sessions, which tends to generate a different type of therapeutic relationship than is prescribed in some treatments. DBT also emphasizes another therapeutic relationship, the one between the therapist and consultation team, which provides the support and guidance that is so helpful in work with this population.

Every treatment strategy suggests some form of therapeutic relationship, but we highlight several here. These include therapist as detective conducting behavioral analyses, therapist as model, therapist as teacher, therapist as reinforcer/punisher, and therapist as exposure stimulus, such as when the patient is exposed to threatening topics that he or she usually avoids. At the level of stylistic strategies, the therapist quite deliberately varies his or her interpersonal style. Reciprocal and irreverent styles are poles influencing the therapist's behavior and impacting the therapeutic relationship.

The dialectical strategy of *allowing natural change* to occur is different from emphasizing the need for structure and consistency in the treatment of patients with BPD. At the level of core validation strategies, a good therapeutic relationship is seen in DBT as having healing qualities of its own for many patients, although it is usually not sufficient for the goal of a life well worth living. The emphasis on validation itself, and particularly the use of cheerleading strategies, also sets DBT apart from some approaches.

DBT benefits from particular therapist characteristics. It requires the ability to behave and relate in various, often highly contrasting ways. The primary dimension on which DBT therapists strive to maintain dialectical balance is the dialectic of acceptance and change. An excessive orientation toward either is therapy-interfering behavior, yet strength in both may require development by the therapist, with the help of the team. Other variants of this acceptance–change dialectic are nurturing and taking care of the patient on the one hand and a benevolent demandingness of the patient on the other, and a compassionate flexibility regarding treatment parameters on the one hand and a nonmoving centeredness about treatment principles on the other.

## Summary of Empirical Evidence

DBT is generally considered the frontline treatment for BPD, and the American Psychological Association's website for empirically supported treatments (American Psychological Association, 2014) describes a strong research foundation for DBT. DBT was developed for treatment of chronically suicidal women with BPD, but it has now been shown to be effective in improving the lives of not only this population but also others (Neacsiu & Linehan, 2014). Although other studies are available, the research summarized here includes only randomized controlled trials (RCTs).

Many studies have demonstrated the efficacy of standard DBT with individuals meeting criteria for BPD. In comparison to treatment as usual (Koons et al., 2001; Linehan, Armstrong, Suarez, Allmon, & Heard, 1991; van den Bosch, Verheul, Schippers, & van den Brink, 2002), patient-centered therapy (Turner, 2000), and community treatment by nonbehavioral experts (Linehan et al., 2006), DBT has demonstrated reductions in suicidal behavior, hospitalizations, and other emotion regulation targets such as anger outbursts. On the other hand, some studies have not shown this extent of support with treatment of BPD in comparison to other treatments; in two RCTs, DBT reduced symptoms but without a significant difference from the effect of active treatment comparison groups (transference-focused therapy and supportive therapy: Clarkin, Levy, Lenzenweger, & Kernberg, 2007; general psychiatric management: McMain et al., 2009).

Studies have also shown the effectiveness of DBT with other clinical populations. Research supports the efficacy of standard DBT for patients with BPD and comorbid drug dependence

(Linehan et al., 1999, 2002; van den Bosch et al., 2002), for adults with binge-eating disorder (Safer, Robinson, & Jo, 2010), adults with Cluster B PD (Feigenbaum et al., 2011), suicidal college students (Pistorello, Fruzzetti, MacLane, Gallop, & Iverson, 2012), and adolescents with bipolar disorder (Goldstein et al., 2014). DBT has also been adapted for use in inpatient settings for BPD (Bohus et al., 2004) and for PTSD (Bohus et al., 2013).

In addition, some RCTs have examined adaptations of DBT skills training without individual therapy. These studies and have demonstrated efficacy for individuals with BPD (Soler et al., 2009), transdiagnostic emotion regulation (Neacsiu, Eberle, Kramer, Wiesmann, & Linehan, 2014), college students with ADHD (Fleming, McMahon, Moran, Peterson, & Dreessen, 2014) and Swedish adults with ADHD (Hirvikoski et al., 2011), bulimia (Safer, Telch, & Agras, 2001) and binge-eating disorder (Hill, Craighead, & Safer, 2011), treatment-resistant depression (Harley, Sprich, Safren, Jacobo, & Fava, 2008), and depressed older adults (Lynch, Morse, Mendelson, & Robins, 2003).

## REFERENCES

American Psychological Association. (2014). Society for Clinical Psychology (Division 12) webpage on research-supported psychological treatments. Retrieved from www.psychologicaltreatments.org.

Barnicot, K., & Priebe, S. (2013). Post-traumatic stress disorder and the outcome of dialectical behaviour therapy for borderline personality disorder. *Personality and Mental Health, 7,* 181–190.

Bohus, M., Dyer, A. S., Priebe, K., Krüger, A., Kleindienst, N., Schmahl, C., et al. (2013). Dialectical behaviour therapy for post-traumatic stress disorder after childhood sexual abuse in patients with and without borderline personality disorder: A randomised controlled trial. *Psychotherapy and Psychosomatics, 82,* 221–233.

Bohus, M., Haaf, B., Simms, T., Limberger, M. F., Schmahl, C., Unckel, C., et al. (2004). Effectiveness of inpatient dialectical behavioral therapy for borderline personality disorder: A controlled trial. *Behaviour Research and Therapy, 42,* 487–499.

Clarkin, J. F., Levy, K. N., Lenzenweger, M. F., & Kernberg, O. F. (2007). Evaluating three treatments for borderline personality disorder: A multiwave study. *American Journal of Psychiatry, 164,* 922–928.

Feigenbaum, J. D., Fonagy, P., Pilling, S., Jones, A., Wildgoose, A., & Bebbington, P. E. (2011). A real-world study of the effectiveness of DBT in the UK National Health Service. *British Journal of Clinical Psychology, 51,* 121–141.

Fleming, A. P., McMahon, R. J., Moran, L. R., Peterson, A. P., & Dreessen, A. (2015). Pilot randomized controlled trial of dialectical behavior therapy group skills training for ADHD among college students. *Journal of Attention Disorders, 19*(3), 260–271.

Goldstein, T. R., Fersch-Podrat, R. K., Rivera, M., Axelson, D. A., Merranko, J., Yu, H., et al. (2014). Dialectical behavior therapy (DBT) for adolescents with bipolar disorder: Results from a pilot randomized trial. *Journal of Child and Adolescent Psychopharmacology, 24,* 1–10.

Harley, R., Sprich, S., Safren, S., Jacobo, M., & Fava, M. (2008). Adaptation of dialectical behavior therapy skills training group for treatment-resistant depression. *Journal of Nervous and Mental Disease, 196,* 136–143.

Harned, M. S., Korslund, K. E., & Linehan, M. M. (2014). A pilot randomized controlled trial of dialectical behavior therapy with and without the dialectical behavior therapy prolonged exposure protocol for suicidal and self-injuring women with borderline personality disorder and PTSD. *Behaviour Research and Therapy, 55,* 7–17.

Hill, D. M., Craighead, L. W., & Safer, D. L. (2011). Appetite-focused dialectical behavior therapy for the treatment of binge eating with purging: A preliminary trial. *International Journal of Eating Disorders, 44,* 249–261.

Hirvikoski, T., Waaler, E., Alfredsson, J., Pihlgren, C., Holmström, A., Johnson, A., et al. (2011). Reduced ADHD symptoms in adults with ADHD after structured skills training group: Results from a randomized controlled trial. *Behaviour Research and Therapy, 49,* 175–185.

Koerner, K. (2011). *Doing dialectical behavior therapy: A practical guide.* New York: Guilford Press.

Koons, C. R., Robins, C. J., Tweed, J. L., Lynch, T. R., Gonzalez, A. M., Morse, J. Q., et al. (2001). Efficacy of dialectical behavior therapy in women veterans with borderline personality disorder. *Behavior Therapy, 32,* 371–390.

Linehan, M. M. (1993a). *Cognitive-behavioral treatment of borderline personality disorder.* New York: Guilford Press.

Linehan, M. M. (1993b). *Skills training manual for treating borderline personality disorder.* New York: Guilford Press.

Linehan, M. M. (1999). Development, evaluation, and dissemination of effective psychosocial treatments: Levels of disorder, stages of care, and stages of treatment research. In M. D. Glantz & C. R. Hartel (Eds.), *Drug abuse: Origins and interventions* (pp. 367–394). Washington, DC: American Psychological Association.

Linehan, M. M. (2014). *Skills training manual for treating borderline personality disorder* (2nd ed.). New York: Guilford Press.

Linehan, M. M., Armstrong, H. E., Suarez, A., Allmon, D., & Heard, H. L. (1991). Cognitive-behavioral treatment of chronically parasuicidal borderline patients. *Archives of General Psychiatry, 48,* 1060–1064.

Linehan, M. M., Bohus, M., & Lynch, T. R. (2007). Dialectical behavior therapy for pervasive emotion dysregulation: Theoretical and practical underpinnings. In J. J. Gross (Ed.), *Handbook of emotion regulation* (pp. 581–605). New York: Guilford Press.

Linehan, M. M., Comtois, K. A., Murray, A. M., Brown, M. Z., Gallop, R. J., Heard, H. L., et al. (2006). Two-year randomized controlled trial and follow-up of dialectical behavior therapy vs. therapy by experts for suicidal behaviors and borderline personality disorder. *Archives of General Psychiatry, 63,* 757–766.

Linehan, M. M., Dimeff, L. A., Reynolds, S. K., Comtois, K., Shaw-Welch, S., Heagerty, P., et al. (2002). Dialectical behavior therapy versus comprehensive validation plus 12-step for the treatment of opioid dependent women meeting criteria for borderline personality disorder. *Drug and Alcohol Dependence, 67,* 13–26.

Linehan, M. M., Schmidt, H., Dimeff, L. A., Craft, J. C., Kanter, J., & Comtois, K. A. (1999). Dialectical behavior therapy for patients with borderline personality disorder and drug dependence. *American Journal on Addictions, 8,* 279–292.

Lynch, T. R., Morse, J. Q., Mendelson, T., & Robins, C. J. (2003). Dialectical behavior therapy for depressed older adults: A randomized pilot study. *American Journal of Geriatric Psychiatry, 11,* 33–45.

McMain, S. F., Links, P. S., Gnam, W. H., Guimond, T., Cardish, R. J., Korman, L., et al. (2009). A randomized clinical trial of dialectical behavior therapy versus general psychiatric management for borderline personality disorder. *American Journal of Psychiatry, 166,* 1365–1374.

Neacsiu, A. D., Eberle, J., Kramer, R., Wiesmann, T., & Linehan, M. M. (2014). Dialectical behavior therapy skills for transdiagnostic emotion dysregulation: A pilot randomized controlled trial. *Behaviour Research and Therapy, 59,* 40–51.

Neacsiu, A. D., & Linehan, M. M. (2014). Borderline personality disorder. In D. H. Barlow (Ed.), *Clinical handbook of psychological disorders: A step-by-step treatment manual* (5th ed., pp. 394–461). New York: Guilford Press.

Pistorello, J., Fruzzetti, A. E., MacLane, C., Gallop, R., & Iverson, K. M. (2012). Dialectical behavior therapy (DBT) applied to college students: A randomized clinical trial. *Journal of Consulting and Clinical Psychology, 80,* 982–994.

Rizvi, S. L., & Ritschel, L. A. (2014). Mastering the art of chain analysis in dialectical behavior therapy. *Cognitive and Behavioral Practice, 21,* 335–349.

Safer, D., Robinson, A., & Jo, B. (2010). Outcome from a randomized controlled trial of group therapy for binge eating disorder: Comparing dialectical behavior therapy adapted for binge eating to an active comparison group therapy. *Behavior Therapy, 41,* 106–120.

Safer, D. L., Telch, C. F., & Agras, W. S. (2001). Dialectical behavior therapy for bulimia nervosa. *American Journal of Psychiatry, 158,* 632–634.

Shenk, C. E., & Fruzzetti, A. E. (2011). The impact of validating and invalidating responses on emotional reactivity. *Journal of Social and Clinical Psychology, 30,* 163–183.

Soler, J., Pascual, J. C., Tiana, T., Cebrià, A., Barrachina, J., Campins, M. J., et al. (2009). Dialectical behaviour therapy skills training compared to standard group therapy in borderline personality disorder: A 3-month randomised controlled clinical trial. *Behaviour Research and Therapy, 47,* 353–358.

Turner, R. M. (2000). Naturalistic evaluation of dialectical behavior therapy-oriented treatment for borderline personality disorder. *Cognitive and Behavioral Practice, 7,* 413–419.

van den Bosch, L., Verheul, R., Schippers, G. M., & van den Brink, W. (2002). Dialectical behavior therapy of borderline patients with and without substance use problems: Implementation and long-term effects. *Addictive Behaviors, 2,* 911–923.

# CHAPTER 30

# Mentalization-Based Treatment

Anthony W. Bateman, Peter Fonagy, and Chloe Campbell

## Origins of Mentalization-Based Treatment

Mentalization-based treatment (MBT) was originally developed in the 1990s for the treatment of patients with borderline personality disorder (BPD) in a partial hospital setting. More recently MBT has developed into an increasingly comprehensive approach to the understanding and treatment of personality disorders (PDs) in a range of clinical contexts. However, in this chapter, we focus on the use of MBT for its original purpose, the treatment of BPD.

Mentalizing is the capacity to understand ourselves and others in terms of intentional mental states. It includes an awareness of mental states in oneself or in other people, particularly when it comes to explaining behavior. That mental states influence behavior is beyond question. Beliefs, wishes, feelings, and thoughts, whether inside or outside our awareness, always determine what we do. Mentalizing involves a spectrum of capacities: Critically, this includes the ability to see one's *own* behavior as coherently organized by mental states, and to differentiate oneself psychologically from others. These capacities often tend to be conspicuously absent in individuals with a PD, particularly at moments of interpersonal stress.

The mentalization model was first outlined in the context of a large empirical study in which security of infant attachment with parents proved to be strongly predicted by the parents' security of attachment during pregnancy, but even more by parents' capacity to understand their own childhood relationships with their own parents in terms of states of mind (Fonagy, Steele, Steele, Moran, & Higgitt, 1991). This study paved the way for a systematic program of research demonstrating that the capacity to mentalize, which emerges in the context of early attachment relationships, is a key determinant of self-organization and affect regulation.

This early academic work on the theory of mentalizing coincided with the emergence of mentalizing as a developmental and clinical concept. The book *Affect Regulation, Mentalization, and the Development of the Self* (Fonagy, Gergely, Jurist, & Target, 2002) summarized the relationship between attachment and mentalizing, suggesting that the role of mentalizing—its acquisition and obstruction—should be understood as a central element of child social development. A link between abnormal development of social cognition during childhood and adult psychopathology was postulated as being mediated through mentalizing. Two further books (Bateman & Fonagy, 2004, 2006) established mentalizing as a core psychological process worthy of consideration when treating major psychiatric disorders and MBT as a psychotherapeutic orientation somewhere between psychodynamic and cognitive therapy. Recent work has expanded the clinical applications of mentalizing techniques, which are now being used for the treatment of posttraumatic stress disorder (Allen, 2001; Bleiberg & Markowitz, 2005); drug addiction (Bateman & Fonagy, 2009); eating disorders (Skårderud, 2007); emerging PD in adolescence (Bleiberg, 2001), particularly in those that self-harm (Rossouw & Fonagy, 2012); and with families in crisis (all this work is summarized in *Handbook of Mentalizing in Mental Health Practice*; Bateman & Fonagy, 2012). On a theoretical level, recent work on mentalizing has developed into a broad, multilevel understanding of development and psychopathology, integrating findings from clinical and developmental psychology with the biological processes involved in BPD (Fonagy & Luyten, 2016; Fonagy, Luyten, & Allison, 2015).

### Scope and Focus: General or Disorder-Specific Domains of Psychopathology

Our account of mentalizing and psychopathology focuses strongly on the development of the systems for social processes, which we consider to drive many higher-order social-cognitive functions underpinning interpersonal interaction, particularly in an attachment context. Four of these functions are of primary importance in understanding not only BPD but also many other severe PDs:

1. Affect representation and related affect regulation.
2. Attentional control, which also has strong links to the regulation of affect.
3. The dual arousal involved in maintaining an appropriate balance between mental function undertaken by the anterior and posterior portions of the brain.
4. Mentalization, a system for interpersonal understanding that is particularly relevant within the attachment system.

Because these capacities emerge in the context of the primary caregiving relationships experienced by the child, in addition to the child's constitutional vulnerabilities, they are affected by the quality of the child's social context, most notably, the attachment relationship. The developmental achievement of these capacities is particularly vulnerable to extremes of environmental deficiency, such as severe neglect, psychological or physical abuse, and maltreatment resulting in less child-initiated dyadic play (Valentino, Cicchetti, Toth, & Rogosch, 2011), empathy (Klimes-Dougan & Kistner, 1990), poor affect regulation (Kim & Cicchetti, 2010) and the struggle to understand emotional expressions (Shenk, Putnam, & Noll, 2013). Several PDs can be conceptualized as representing different types of failures in the mind's capacity to represent its own activities and contents, but here we focus on the model's theoretical and clinical application to BPD, where evidence is perhaps strongest (see Paris, Chapter 23, this volume, for a comprehensive review).

MBT, then, is almost unique as an integrative approach, in that it has a theoretical frame of reference that includes a developmental model, a theory of psychopathology, and a hypothesis about the mechanism of therapeutic change. We attempt briefly to explain these aspects of MBT in this chapter, particularly, our recent thinking on the structure of psychopathology and the process of therapeutic change, as well as an overview of treatment, from diagnosis and assessment to intervention strategies and methods.

### Overview of the Treatment Model

MBT is carefully structured, organized around the development of an attachment relationship with the patient, and offers a careful focus on the patient's internal mental processes, primarily of affect, as they are experienced moment by moment; it emphasizes the therapeutic relationship following principles of marking and contingency of affect states, with the active repair of ruptures in the relationship between patient and clinician (Bateman & Fonagy, 2006, 2009). The emphasis is on identifying the context in which serious breaks in mentalizing occur both in the personal life of the patient and in the sessions themselves, with the aim of restoring mentalizing and eventually enabling the patient to maintain mentalizing when, previously, it would have been lost. Core to this process is exploring mentalizing problems within the context of the individual attachment experiences that are activated within the patient–clinician relationship.

Importantly, the treatment is delivered according to a carefully constructed protocol that informs the clinician about how to manage common clinical situations following a number of basic principles and procedures, including the development of the following:

1. Collaborative process
2. Formulation of patient relational and mentalizing problems (evidenced through exploration of challenging behaviors) early in treatment, and a focus on those in each session.
3. General process
   a. Identification of nonmentalizing processes
   b. Monitoring of the state of affective arousal
   c. Identification of mentalizing polarities (see Morgan & Zimmerman, Chapter 10, this volume, for more details on the mentalizing polarities: automatic vs. controlled; self vs. others; external vs. internal; cognitive vs. affective).
4. Therapist stance
   a. "Not-knowing" stance of curiosity, authentic interest, responsiveness to internal states of mind
   b. Interventions consistent with the patient's mentalizing capacity
   c. Focus on maintaining clinician mentalizing
   d. Open-minded clinician
5. Trajectory of sessions: interventions are structured from empathic validation to exploration, clarification, and challenge through affect identification and affect focus, to mentalizing the relationship itself
6. A focus on contingency and marking of interventions
7. Explicit identification of clinician feelings related to the patient's mental processing

Treatment was originally organized around a partial hospital or weekly group plus individual therapy, but over the past few years, clinicians have offered less intensive treatment with either only group or only individual MBT. There is no clinical empirical basis in terms of outcomes for this reduction in format; the National Institute for Health and Clinical Excellence (NICE; 2009) Guidance for BPD in the United Kingdom concluded that there was indicative evidence that treatments combining two methods of delivery were superior to those offering treatment in a single modality. A pilot study of phased treatment is currently under way. Group plus individual MBT is offered for 6 months, followed by monthly individual sessions for a further 18 months.

## Diagnosis, Assessment, and Formulation

In the initial phase of MBT, the diagnosis of PD is discussed with the patient; a crisis plan is made, focusing on what the patient can do for him- or herself to reduce risk behavior; and a formulation of the patient's problems is discussed and agreed upon. Providing the diagnosis is an important process (Bateman & Fonagy, 2006). In doing so, the clinician emphasizes his or her own thinking about the key problem areas for the patient and how they coalesce, indicating a diagnosis of PD. Of significance is the requirement to present this in terms of the patient's history and current state, with the aim of stimulating the patient's reflection on his or her own state. The clinician is positive about outcomes, stating the evidence of gradual improvement over time and how treatment can bring forward these natural gains. This leads naturally toward a formulation that covers salient aspects of history, details of major current symptoms, behaviors, and social problems (housing, child protection, probation, court appearances), agreement on a hierarchy of these problem areas, features of attachment patterns and relationship problems, and the identification of significant processes leading to nonmentalization, along with the dominant modes of nonmentalization. This is done through the detailed exploration of events in which mentalizing has been lost (e.g., acts of self-harm, suicide attempts, or violence). Once this is complete, the clinician summarizes the material in a single-page document and discusses it with the patient, who develops it further. The aim is to collaboratively create a platform of understanding on which the treatment can be based. Over the course of treatment, the formulation is revisited by both patient and clinician, and modified as new evidence becomes apparent.

## Theoretical Foundations

### Theory of Disorder

The mentalizing approach aims to provide a comprehensive theoretical account of the phenomenology and origins of BPD from a developmental psychopathology perspective, leading to a more informed treatment approach (for more on the theory of mentalizing, see Fonagy & Luyten, Chapter 7, this volume). This fits with increasing interest over recent years in the developmental the origins of BPD (Arens et al., 2013; Bornovalova, Hicks, Iacono, & McGue, 2013; Chanen & McCutcheon, 2013; Stepp, Olino, Klein, Seeley, & Lewinsohn, 2013). The approach is strongly rooted within contemporary attachment theory. There are at least two strands of research supporting the link between BPD and attachment. The first strand has provided direct evidence for such a link by showing that BPD is associated with increased levels of insecure attachment styles, using both interview-based assessment of attachment such as the Adult Attachment Interview (AAI) and self-report measures. The second strand relates to attachment trauma (Allen, 2013). These views are congruent with general biopsychosocial models of BPD (Oldham, 2009), which assume that adverse childhood experiences and genetic factors interact to create a unique combination of biological factors (neurobiological structures and dysfunctions) and psychosocial factors (personality traits, personality functioning) that underpin BPD pathology.

According to attachment theory, the development of the self occurs in the affect regulatory context of early relationships, which requires consistent contingent and marked mother–infant interaction. To achieve normal self-experience, the infant requires its emotional signals to be accurately or contingently mirrored by an attachment figure (Gergely & Watson, 1996). In mirroring the infant, the caregiver must achieve more than mere contingency (in time, space, and emotional tone). The mirroring must be "marked" (e.g., exaggerated), in other words, slightly distorted, if the infant is to understand the caregiver's display as part of his or her emotional experience rather than an expression of the caregiver's experience. Not surprisingly, then, disorganization of the attachment system results in disorganization of self-structure. This underscores the need for treatment to be well structured and well coordinated if it is not to become iatrogenic.

In drawing up a mentalization developmental model of BPD in relation to childhood adversity, we suggest that two processes unfold, which have a cumulative effect.

1. We assume that the development of mentalization depends on the social co-construction of internal states between child and parents. Following from this, we hypothesize that early neglect and an early emotional environment incompatible with the normal acquisition of understanding oneself and others creates vulnerability for BPD.
2. We further hypothesize that subsequent brutality in an attachment context can disrupt mentalization as part of an adaptive adjustment to adversity when a child—whose early experiences of neglect have left him or her less resilient to deal with trauma—is in a state of helplessness in relation to those individuals (Fonagy, Steele, Steele, Higgitt, & Target, 1994; Stein, Fonagy, Ferguson, & Wisman, 2000).

In summary, we propose (Fonagy & Luyten, 2009) that early emotional neglect in particular, rather than physical or sexual abuse as such, predisposes an individual to developing BPD by limiting his or her opportunity to acquire mentalization and leaving the capacity to mentalize vulnerable to disruption under the influence of later stress.

## Fundamental Theoretical Constructs

### Disruptions in Mentalizing

Several factors can disrupt the normal acquisition and later deployment of mentalizing. Most important among these is psychological trauma early or late in childhood. Extensive evidence suggests that childhood attachment trauma undermines the capacity to think about mental states in giving narrative accounts of one's past attachment relationships and even in trying to identify the mental states associated with specific facial expressions. This may be due to (1) the defensive inhibition of the capacity to think about others' thoughts and feelings in the face of the experience of genuine malevolent intent of others and the overwhelming vulnerability of the child; (2) excessive early stress, which distorts the functioning of arousal mechanisms, causing the inhibition of orbitofrontal cortical activity (mentalizing) at far lower levels of risk than would be normally the case; (3) any trauma that arouses the attachment system (seeking for protection) and attachment trauma may do so chronically. In seeking proximity to the traumatizing attachment figure as a consequence of trauma, the child may naturally be further traumatized. The prolonged activation of the attachment system may be an additional problem because the arousal of attachment may have specific inhibitory consequences for mentalization, in addition to that which might be expected as a consequence of increased emotional arousal.

## Epistemic Trust and Epistemic Rigidity

Through the down-regulation of affect triggered by proximity seeking in the distressed infant, attachment not only establishes a lasting bond between child and caregiver, but it also opens a channel for information to be used for knowledge transfer between generations. This is well demonstrated in studies of cognitive styles associated with patterns of attachment in adulthood. Adult attachment insecurity is associated with a greater likelihood of cognitive closure, a lower tolerance for ambiguity, and a more pronounced tendency for dogmatic thinking (Mikulincer, 1997). Insecure individuals, who fear the loss of their attachment figures, also anxiously hold on to their initial constructions. Kruglanski (1989; Kruglanski & Webster, 1996; Pierro & Kruglanski, 2008) proposed the concept of "epistemic freezing," characterized by a tendency to defend existing knowledge structures even when they are incorrect or misleading (see also Fiske & Taylor, 1991).

Developmental adversity, and particularly attachment trauma (Allen, 2012, 2013), may trigger a profound destruction of trust. There may be other reasons, but once epistemic trust has been lost, its absence creates an apparent "rigidity," which is perceived by the communicator, who expects the recipient to modify his or her behavior on the basis of the information received and apparently understood; yet in the absence of trust, the capacity for change is absent. The information given by the communicator is not used to update the recipient's understanding. In terms of the theory of natural pedagogy (Csibra & Gergely, 2009), the person has a (temporarily) reduced capacity to learn from "teachers." From a therapist's standpoint, they have become "hard to reach" and potentially interpersonally inaccessible. Viewed another way, PDs in general may be seen as disorders of communication: Chronic epistemic vigilance limits the capacity to internalize available knowledge as something that is "safe" to use to organize behavior.

## The p Factor in Psychopathology

A striking challenge for attachment researchers is that little evidence has indicated a relationship between different attachment styles and particular forms of psychopathology. This lack of specificity may relate to compelling evidence presented by Caspi and colleagues (2013), suggesting that there is, in fact, a general psychopathology factor (p factor) in the structure of psychiatric disorders. In their longitudinal study based in Dunedin, New Zealand, Caspi and colleagues examined the structure of psychopathology from adolescence to midlife, examining dimensionality, persistence, co-occurrence, and sequential comorbidity. They found that psychiatric disorders were more convincingly explained by a hierarchical model that assumed disturbance to occur at a syndromal (e.g., mood disorder), spectral (e.g., internalizing), and overarching general psychopathology level. This last, the p factor score emerges when disorders are studied longitudinally, and it is associated with increased severity and chronicity. The p factor concept convincingly explains why discovering isolated causes, consequences, or biomarkers and specific, tailored treatments for psychiatric disorders has proved relatively elusive for the field.

The p factor is a statistical construct. The question that follows from this initial conceptualization is: What is it actually measuring? We have speculated (Fonagy et al., 2015) that the p factor may be an indication of a state of engagement with environmental influences, perhaps primarily genetically determined (Belsky, 2012), but conditioned by social experiences of maltreatment (Belsky et al., 2012): It culminates in a sense of general openness to environmental influence, potentially measured as epistemic trust. An individual with a high p factor score is one in a state of epistemic hypervigilance and chronic epistemic mistrust. A depressed patient with a low p factor may be relatively easy to reach in terms of treatment because he or she is open to social learning in the form of therapeutic intervention, whereas a depressed patient with a high p factor—suffering from high levels of comorbidity, longer-term difficulties, and greater impairment—will also demonstrate treatment resistance because of high levels of epistemic mistrust, or outright epistemic freezing. We consider it likely that such patients require more long-term therapy that enriches mentalization and is abundant in ostensive cues that will serve to stimulate epistemic trust and openness.

## Principles of Change

Mentalization in therapy is a generic way of establishing "epistemic trust" (trust in the authenticity and personal relevance of interpersonally transmitted information; Wilson & Sperber, 2012) between the patient and the therapist in a way that helps the patient to relinquish the rigidity that characterizes individuals with enduring personality pathology. The relearning of flexibility allows the patient to go on to learn, socially, from new experiences and achieve change in his or her understanding of social relationships and his or her own behavior and actions. The very experience of having our subjectivity understood—of being mentalized—is a necessary trigger for us to be able to receive and learn from the social knowledge that has the potential to change our perception of ourselves and our social world.

Feeling understood in therapy restores trust in learning from social experience (epistemic trust), but at the same time it also serves to regenerate a capacity for social understanding (mentalizing). Improved social understanding alongside increased epistemic trust makes life outside therapy a setting in which new information about oneself and about the world can be acquired and internalized. Ultimately, it may be that therapeutic change is not due to new skills or new insights gained in the consulting room, but rather to the capacity of the therapeutic relationship to create a potential for learning about oneself and others in the world outside of therapy.

In proposing that epistemic mistrust might constitute the p factor that underlies psychopathology, we also consider that the relearning of epistemic trust may be at the heart of effective therapeutic interventions. As discussed by Clark and colleagues (Chapter 20, this volume), we propose that there are three staged processes at work in the achievement of therapeutic change in the treatment of BPD: (1) the teaching and learning of content; (2) the reemergence of robust mentalizing; and (3) the reemergence of social learning beyond therapy. Mentalization is our route to garnering knowledge relevant to us and being able to use it across contexts, independent of the learning experience. Put simply, *the experience of feeling thought about in therapy makes us feel safe enough to think more accurately about ourselves in relation to our world and how other people think of us, opening the way to learning something new about that world and how we operate in it.*

## Principal Intervention Strategies and Method

### Engagement to Model

MBT begins with a 10–12 session introductory group (Karterud & Bateman, 2011) for 10 patients that combines psychoeducation with an experiential group process. Each session focuses on a specific topic, such as what mentalizing is, threats to mentalizing, PD, emotions, how to manage emotions, attachment that includes mapping of personal attachment relationships, and problems likely to be encountered in treatment. In each session, the patients undertake a series of structured exercises. Following completion of the group, patients are offered an individual session to review the work prior to being offered MBT organized around individual and group therapy on a weekly basis.

### Empathy and Support

Use of empathic statements is a way to deepen the rapport between patient and clinician and a powerful way to maintain mentalization by reducing arousal in the interpersonal interaction. Our clinical approach to empathy as a psychotherapeutic intervention follows from our understanding of the neurobiology of mentalizing and the developmental process of contingency (Watson, 1981). The therapeutic relationship is intrinsically an emotionally invested relationship in which the representation of the other person's mental state is closely linked to the representation of the self. This does not mean that the thoughts and feelings of self and other are identical; rather, they are highly contingent on each other. When two minds are experienced as having overlapping thoughts and feelings, and influencing each other, empathy is taking place. When two minds are experienced as having exactly the same thoughts and feelings (e.g., if both are in panic), self and other are assumed to merge. This is not empathy and, in the context of the therapeutic relationship, it is likely to be experienced as intrusive, arousing, and destabilizing of mentalization processes.

An empathic intervention in MBT is a clinical translation of the process of marking, in the context of contingent responsiveness. It has the hallmark of the other person's mind being the focus, and he or she experiences the interaction as such; the clinician demonstrates that he or she is in the mental shoes of the patient and able to understand the patient's feelings and emotions without being taken over by them. This is important because if the clinician experiences too high a level of personal distress linked to the emotions of the patient, he or she is likely to become partially self-oriented and therefore lack the ability to communicate full attention to the other's experience. Overall the person empathized with experiences compassion, understanding, care, and tenderness from the other person; there is a feeling of not being alone. It is a uniquely human experience, and it is more than sympathy. Sympathy is an expression of concern for the other through expression of comprehension of the other's plight or emotional state. The MBT clinician shows sympathy but is mostly concerned with empathic validation of the patient's experience.

From the point of view of developing a treatment strategy in a session starting with a focus on empathy, the clinician needs to come to a conclusion about the overall shape of the current relationship from the perspective of the patient. Broadly there are two possibilities:

1. A current relationship in which the patient conceives of the clinician as having a mental state highly contingent on that of the self—this is an empathic and validating relationship.
2. An interaction whose relationship representations suggest little contingency between the thoughts and feelings of the patient and the clinician—this is an unempathic and invalidating relationship.

If the first possibility is uppermost in a session, the clinician is in a position to develop a shared platform for exploring problems. If the second possibility is apparent, the clinician must actively work to establish an empathic and validating position before he or she can do anything else.

## Components of Empathy

In MBT, we ask the clinician to consider two components of empathy. The first identification with the feelings of the patient. The clinician recognizes the feeling, manages it in him- or herself, and is not taken over by it. In other words, he or she momentarily becomes sad, for example, but his or her mental process is not substantially affected by the feeling. For an empathic intervention to be effective in strengthening the therapeutic alliance, the patient needs to experience the clinician as recognizing the patient's emotional state, yet not be disturbed by it. Demonstrating this identification to the patient in a manner that shows the clinician has grasped the form and strength of the feeling, so that the patient "feels felt" is the difficult part. To do this, MBT requires the clinician to engage in a process that is described as "being ordinary" (Allen, Fonagy, & Bateman, 2008). If in doubt, the clinician should say to the patient what he or she would say to a good friend who was telling the same story while sitting in a café and he or she wanted to transmit a sense that he or she was "getting" the friend's emotional state (the café is important here because there is a social constraint, to some degree, on what one may say and how one may behave in that context!). The clinician has to mirror the friend's outrage, say, at her boyfriend's betrayal, without being equally disabled by the outrage. Yet the clinician's response cannot be wooden; to be so demonstrates a lack of the common humanity required to be supportive and empathic. Initially, a normalizing and validating response expressed with some feeling will suffice—"Anyone would feel like that under these circumstances. What on earth is he up to?"

The second part of empathy that the MBT clinician considers is that if the patient feels like this, what are the consequences of that feeling to the patient? So, for example, if the clinician is asking the patient to name a feeling he or she cannot name, this has an effect on the patient. Therefore, to be empathic, it is necessary to identify shame, for example, or annoyance, *and* how this leaves the patient feeling inadequate, which in turn has the effect of making the patient feel inferior to the clinician. Or, if a patient describes events that suggest to her that her boyfriend does not love her, this leaves her struggling with the *effect* of her *affect*; that is, she is an unlovable person.

For example, a patient, age 10 years, had wanted to see her older brother when he was hospitalized. She was not allowed to do so by the nurses and her parents because her brother was too ill. She protested strongly but with no effect. She did not see him for 2 months. When he returned home, he looked different because he had lost a considerable amount of weight, lost his hair, and was taking medication. She was upset that she had not been able to visit him and protested to her parents. They were unsympathetic. When describing all this during a session, she was upset and a little bitter. Having identified this, the clinician identified the effect that it had on her:

CLINICIAN: It is awful being a child in those situations [noting the affect], at the mercy of other people and so helpless and powerless [attempting to identify the effect that the affect and context had on her].

PATIENT: I never wanted people to have control over me ever again. I felt that they did not understand.

CLINICIAN: They probably didn't or at least they had no idea how powerless they were making you.

In this brief vignette, the clinician is identifying the effect that the upset had on her, which in this case was crucial for treatment. The patient was a person who insisted on autonomy from others but did so by making sure that she had no needs to be met by others. In MBT, therefore, the clinician identifies the emotional state of the patient and recognizes the effect it has—the *affect* and *effect*. This takes the empathic interaction beyond the simple identification of the feeling.

### Exploration and Clarification

As soon as the clinician senses that he or she and the patient have a shared affective platform through the empathic process, exploration and elaboration takes place, with the clarification of mental states. In addition, the clinician brings in some of his or her own thoughts about it. Clarification requires a reconstruction of events, but with an emphasis on the changing mental states, a tracing of process over time, and a recognition that decisions may in the end be capricious yet of value even if they turn out to be a mistake.

### Challenge

MBT recommends judiciously challenging the patient. This is a very important intervention when used sparingly. There are a number of indicators for challenge. First, it is considered specifically when a patient is interminably in nonmentalizing mode. This may be particularly the case if the patient is in prolonged pretend mode. Second, less direct attempts to rekindle mentalizing must have been ineffective. Third, the clinician believes that he or she is being excluded from the process—the "other" has no place in the mind of the patient. And fourth, the patient is in danger of believing his or her own narrative without question or reflection.

Challenge as an intervention in MBT has certain defining characteristics. It is nearly always outside the normal therapy dialogue, so it comes from "left field." It is a surprise to the patient and out of line with the current dialogue. The aim is for the patient to be suddenly derailed in his or her nonmentalizing process. If the intervention is successful, the clinician initiates a "stop-and-stand" moment to prevent the patient from continuing in the same mode.

For example, a female patient was engaged in a diatribe about the prison service and its ill-treatment of prisoners. She was highly aroused; she was shouting, ranting, and "reliving" her anger and rage in telling the story. Any interruption by the clinician resulted in a dismissive comment. At one point, the clinician looked out the window, wondering how to intervene and thinking that a challenge was necessary. As he looked out the window, the patient said, "Don't look out the window, you listen to me." So the clinician retorted that he could look and listen all at the same time, stating that he could multitask. Before the patient could respond, he said, "Do you know why I can multitask? It is because I am a man." At this point, the patient stopped, not knowing whether to laugh or to react contemptuously. So the clinician said that as a man, he could only multitask for a short time, so he exhorted her to rest for a moment so that they could both collect their thoughts.

This was a challenge; it was unexpected, it stopped the ranting, and the clinician was able to say that he was exhausted by all her talk and emotion, and that he thought it was better to sit back for a few minutes and rewind the session to start reflecting on what had happened that had led her to be sent to prison.

Once a stop-and-stand challenge is effective in halting nonmentalizing, it is important to rewind to the point at which either the patient or the clinician was mentalizing. Challenge is a very effective intervention when a patient is stuck in nonmentalizing mode.

## Identification of Affect and Affect Focus

Once the clinician and patient are able to maintain a mentalizing interaction, MBT suggests an increasing focus on affect and the interpersonal process characterized by the attachment strategies activated through the patient–therapist interaction. This has the effect of increasing emotional intensity and, if mentalizing is maintained under these conditions, the MBT clinician can move to mentalizing the relationship.

The purpose of focusing on affect in the interpersonal domain is to re-create the core sensitivity of people with BPD in the session itself. People with BPD are highly sensitive to interpersonal process; arousal in the interpersonal domain triggers much of the emotional dysregulation that in turn disrupts mental processing further. So MBT for BPD focuses on this area of sensitivity to generate more robust mentalizing around interpersonal processing. To do so, MBT starts by trying to identify an affect focus.

The affect focus is not simply labeling feelings, even though the *identification and labelling of feelings,* placing them in context, and understanding their disruptive influence and how they may lead to self-harm and other disruptive behaviors are all central to MBT. It is more a way of increasing the affective experience within the interpersonal relationship in the session. The affect focus is the clinical exemplification of moving the patient around one of the dimensions of mentalizing; it is an intervention designed to make explicit what is currently implicit within the patient–therapist relationship. It requires the clinician to recognize that both he or she and the patient are making unquestioned, jointly held, unspoken assumptions. So the clinician names the shared experience not as something that is arising solely from the patient but as a process that is shared between them without being characterized fully or explicitly.

For example, a patient was obviously anxious in a session, and he would manage his arousal by looking away from the clinician and turning his body sideways, falling silent, then saying, "Yeah, yeah, I don't know." Implicit in this interactive process was that, as the clinician asked questions, the patient's avoidant attachment strategies were activated along with increasing anxiety. As the clinician "probed," the patient "hid." The clinician was aware that the patient could become emotionally dysregulated to the extent of having to leave the session, so the clinician was wary of probing: Would another question generate too much arousal, leading to iatrogenic dysregulation? For his part, the patient wanted to be left alone but had become aware that he avoided intimate interactions with others. His significant relational problem in the formulation was isolation and loneliness.

At this point, MBT suggests that the clinician identify the shared dilemma related to the avoidant attachment strategies by making the anxiety implicit with the interaction more explicit. In this example, the clinician said, "We are both uncertain at the moment, I think. I am concerned that if I probe more, it will make things worse for you, yet this is an area of the problem that we have to explore more. It looks to me like you are kind of saying don't go further as well because it might not be safe to continue. But then I worry that I am leaving you alone and isolated. Where are you in this?"

The patient said that he was preoccupied with whether the clinician was going to stop asking him things or not. He didn't know whether he wanted him to do or not.

Having made this shared dilemma explicit, the clinician develops the mentalizing process around this affectively charged interpersonal area. To some extent, this is a rehearsal *in vivo* of an affectively salient interpersonal interaction that may derail the patient in their close relationships. Accurate identification of the current affectively salient focus allows the clinician to segue to mentalizing the relationship without clumsily disrupting the interpersonal process.

## The Treatment Relationship

The treatment relationship is a focus for MBT at a number of levels. The constant attention to collaboration, the development of an alliance through agreed-upon goals and shared focus, the empathic position of requiring the clinician to see things from the patient's perspective, and the focus on shared affective processes are all relational. Finally, we are often asked by both psychoanalytic and nonpsychoanalytic colleagues whether MBT recommends using the transference (Gabbard, 2006). Our standard reply is, "It all depends on what you mean by that phrase." If what is meant is a focus on the clinician–patient relationship in the hope that discussion concerning this relationship will contribute to the patient's well-being, the answer is a most emphatic "yes." If by transference one means the linking of the current pattern of behavior in the treatment setting to patterns of relationships in childhood and current relationships outside the therapeutic setting, then the answer is an almost equally emphatic "no." While we might well point to similarities between patterns of relationships in the therapy and in childhood or currently outside of the therapy, the aim of this is not to provide the patient with an explanation (insight) that he or she might be able to use to control his or her behavior pattern, but far more simply, it is just one other puzzling phenomenon that requires thought and contemplation, part of our general inquisitive stance aimed to facilitate the recovery of mentalization.

Thus, when we talk about "mentalizing the transference," this is a shorthand term for encouraging patients to think about the relationship they are in at the current moment. One of us (A. W. B.) prefers to name this level of intervention "mentalizing the relationship," primarily because it reminds the clinician to focus on the relational aspect of the interaction in the moment and not worry about causality and insight. The aim of mentalizing the relationship/transference is to create an alternative perspective by focusing the patient's attention on another mind, the mind of the clinician, and to assist the patient in the task of contrasting his or her own perception of him- or herself how he or she is perceived by another, by the clinician, or indeed by members of a therapeutic group.

### Mentalizing the Counterrelationship

MBT is explicit about managing and working with components of mentalizing the counterrelationship, or the countertransference. Working with the counterrelationship is part of the clinical translation of the self and other dimensions of mentalizing. Technically, the use of the counterrelationship in MBT borrows heavily from the work of Racker (1957, 1968).

Mentalizing the counterrelationship, by definition, links to the self-awareness of the clinician and often relies on the affective components of mentalizing. Some clinicians tend to default to a state of self-reference, whereby they consider most of what they experience in therapy as being relevant to the patient. This default mode needs to be resisted, and we clinicians need to be mindful of the fact that our mental states might unduly color our understanding of our patients' mental states, and that we tend to equate them without adequate foundation. Clinicians have to "quarantine" their feelings. How we "quarantine" informs the MBT technical approach to "countertransference," defined as those experiences, both affective and cognitive, that the clinician has in sessions, and that might further develop an understanding of mental processes. Feelings in the clinician are not considered initially as a result of projective processes, and the clinician must identify experiences clearly as his or her own; that is, they are "marked," and interventions using the countertransference are stated as the clinician's experience. They are "self" in contrast to "other."

The simplest way to release countertransference experience from quarantine without equating the clinician's feeling with that of the patient is to state "I" at the beginning of an intervention. Intriguingly, this seems to be difficult for clinicians, who understandably worry about violating therapeutic boundaries. Yet MBT does not suggest that clinicians start expressing their personal problems or start talking about any feeling that they might have in a session, whether relevant to the process or not. Rather, we maintain that the clinician's current experience of the process of therapy with the patient is to be shared openly to ensure that the complexity of the interactional process may be considered. Patients need to be aware that their mental processes have an effect on others' mental states, and that these, in turn, will influence the direction of the interaction.

### The Process of Treatment

MBT not only has an overall structure to the treatment program, described in detail elsewhere (Bateman & Fonagy, 2006), but it also identifies a trajectory for each session. In each session there is a recommended stepwise move from a supportive position toward a more relational subjective experiential process. MBT requires the clinician, as a general principle, to start from an *empathic and supportive* position before moving toward a more relational focus. So, the patient comes into the session and starts telling a story. MBT clinicians seek to demonstrate an empathic understanding of the story. In that sense, they use *empathic validation* as the starting point. Clinicians first need to find out the subjective truth of the patient's experience and to demonstrate that they have understood it from the patient's perspective. Only then can they "sit alongside the patient," so that they both start looking at their story and subjective experience from a shared vantage point.

In addition, the clinician manages process within the session by pacing the flow of the session. Technically, the clinician stops, explores, and rewinds the mentalizing process in the session itself, or stops, explores, and rewinds the content of the narrative by asking for more detail. If the patient's mentalizing is lost, the clinician stops and rewinds the session to a point at which mentalizing was apparent. From here, both patient and clinician "micro-slice the process" forward. The purpose of this strategy is to reinstate mentalizing when it has been lost or to promote its continuation in the furtherance of the overall goal of therapy, which is, to re-reiterate, to encourage the formation of a robust and flexible mentalizing capacity that is not prone to sudden collapse in the face of emotional stress. As a session moves forward, it is sometimes necessary either to pause to consider and explore the moment or to move it back to retrace the process or reexamine the content.

## Summary of Evidence

Different randomized control trials (RCTs) have tested the effectiveness of the MBT approach for patients with BPD. In an RCT of MBT for BPD in a partial hospital setting (Bateman & Fonagy, 1999, 2001), significant and enduring changes in mood states and interpersonal functioning were associated with an 18-month program. Outcome measures included frequency of suicide attempts and acts of self-harm; number and duration of inpatient admissions; service utilization; and self-report measures of depression, anxiety, general symptom distress, interpersonal function, and social adjustment. The benefits, relative to treatment as usual (TAU), were large, with a number needed to treat of around two, and were observed to increase during the follow-up period of 18 months. Analysis of participants' health care use suggested that day hospital treatment for BPD was no more expensive than general psychiatric care and showed considerable cost savings after treatment (Bateman & Fonagy, 2003). A follow-up study of patients with BPD 5 years after all treatment was completed and 8 years after initial entry into treatment compared patients treated with MBT and those receiving TAU. Those receiving MBT remained better over time than the TAU group. Superior levels of improvement were shown on levels of suicidality (23% in the MBT group vs. 74% in TAU group), diagnostic status (13 vs. 87%), service use (2 years vs. 3.5 years), and other measurements, such as use of medication, global function, and vocational status (Bateman & Fonagy, 2008).

Two well-controlled single-blind trials of outpatient MBT have been conducted with adults with BPD (Bateman & Fonagy, 2009) and adolescents presenting to clinical services with self-harm, the vast majority of whom met BPD criteria (Rossouw & Fonagy, 2012). In both trials, MBT was found to be superior to TAU in reducing self-harm, including suicidality, and depression. Importantly, in the Bateman and Fonagy (2009) trial, the control group received a manualized, highly efficacious treatment, and structured clinical management, but MBT was superior, particularly in the long run. Furthermore, improvements generated by MBT for adolescents (MBT-A) appear to have been mediated by improved levels of mentalization, reduced attachment avoidance, and assuagement in emergent BPD features: Groups in the MBT-A group showed a recovery rate of 44% compared to 17% in the TAU group (Rossouw & Fonagy, 2012).

Three more recent studies provide further support for MBT in patients with BPD. An RCT from Denmark investigated the efficacy of MBT versus a less intensive, manualized supportive group therapy, both delivered in combination with psychoeducation and medication, in patients diagnosed with BPD (Jørgensen et al., 2013). Patients were randomly allocated to MBT ($n = 58$) or the specialist combined treatment ($n = 27$). Both the combined MBT treatment and the less intensive supportive therapy brought about significant improvements on a range of psychological and interpersonal measures (e.g., general functioning, depression, and social functioning), as well as the number of diagnostic criteria met for BPD; effect sizes were large ($d = 0.5–2.1$). The combined MBT therapy was superior to the less intensive supportive group therapy only on therapist-rated Global Assessment of Functioning. No follow-up or cost-effectiveness data are available from this study. Furthermore, the same therapists conducted both treatments (there was therefore a high risk for spillover effects between the two treatments), and incomplete data were a significant limitation. In a further study from Denmark (Petersen et al., 2010), a cohort of patients treated with partial hospitalization followed by MBT group therapy showed significant improvements after 2 years on a range of measures, including Global Assessment of Functioning, hospitalizations, and vocational status, with further improvement at 2-year follow-up.

A naturalistic study by Bales and colleagues (2012) in The Netherlands investigated the effectiveness of an 18-month, manualized program of MBT in 45 patients diagnosed with severe BPD. There was a high prevalence of comorbidity of Axis I and Axis II disorders. Results showed significant positive change in symptom distress, social and interpersonal functioning, and personality pathology and functioning; effect sizes were moderate to large ($d = 0.7$–$1.7$). Also, these authors showed that care consumption (additional treatments and psychiatric inpatient admissions) decreased significantly during and after treatment. The lack of a control group in this study limits the ability to draw conclusions about the efficacy of the MBT intervention. A multisite randomized trial by the same group comparing intensive outpatient and partial hospitalization-based MBT for patients with BPD is currently under way.

In a naturalistic trial, Laurenssen and colleagues (2013) studied the feasibility and effectiveness of inpatient MBT-A for borderline symptoms in 11 female adolescents ages 14–18 years. Results showed significant decreases in symptoms, and improvements in personality functioning and quality of life 12 months after the start of treatment, with effect sizes between $d = 0.58$ and $1.46$, indicating medium to large effects. Furthermore, 91% of the adolescents showed reliable change on the Brief Symptom Inventory, and 18% moved to the functional range on this measure.

In conclusion, MBT offers an evidence-based framework for understanding the phenomenology of patients with BPD, and perhaps other PDs, along with a clinical intervention strategy based on that understanding. In so doing, the approach provides a clear therapeutic focus, enabling the clinician to monitor the therapeutic process in terms of (impending) mentalizing impairment and level of epistemic mistrust in the context of activation of the attachment system. Future work needs to refine this formulation and how it translates into more effective treatment methods.

# REFERENCES

Allen, J. G. (2001). *Traumatic relationships and serious mental disorders.* Chichester, UK: Wiley.

Allen, J. G. (2012). *Restoring mentalizing in attachment relationships: Treating trauma with plain old therapy.* Washington, DC: American Psychiatric Press.

Allen, J. G. (2013). *Mentalizing in the development and treatment of attachment trauma.* London: Karnac Books.

Allen, J. G., Fonagy, P., & Bateman, A. W. (2008). *Mentalizing in clinical practice.* Washington, DC: American Psychiatric Publishing.

Arens, E. A., Stopsack, M., Spitzer, C., Appel, K., Dudeck, M., Volzke, H., et al. (2013). Borderline personality disorder in four different age groups: A cross-sectional study of community residents in Germany. *Journal of Personality Disorders, 27,* 196–207.

Bales, D., Van Beek, N., Smits, M., Willemsen, S., Busschbach, J. J., Verheul, R., et al. (2012). Treatment outcome of 18-month, day hospital mentalization-based treatment (MBT) in patients with severe borderline personality disorder in The Netherlands. *Journal of Personality Disorders, 26,* 568–582.

Bateman, A., & Fonagy, P. (1999). Effectiveness of partial hospitalization in the treatment of borderline personality disorder: A randomized controlled trial. *American Journal of Psychiatry, 156,* 1563–1569.

Bateman, A., & Fonagy, P. (2001). Treatment of borderline personality disorder with psychoanalytically oriented partial hospitalization: An 18-month follow-up. *American Journal of Psychiatry, 158,* 36–42.

Bateman, A., & Fonagy, P. (2003). Health service utilization costs for borderline personality disorder patients treated with psychoanalytically oriented partial hospitalization versus general psychiatric care. *American Journal of Psychiatry, 160,* 169–171.

Bateman, A., & Fonagy, P. (2004). *Psychotherapy for borderline personality disorder: Mentalization-based treatment,* Oxford, UK: Oxford University Press.

Bateman, A. W., & Fonagy, P. (2006). *Mentalization based treatment for borderline personality disorder: A practical guide.* Oxford, UK: Oxford University Press.

Bateman, A., & Fonagy, P. (2008). 8-year follow-up of patients treated for borderline personality disorder: Mentalization-based treatment versus treatment as usual. *American Journal of Psychiatry, 165,* 631–638.

Bateman, A., & Fonagy, P. (2009). Randomized controlled trial of outpatient mentalization-based treatment versus structured clinical management for borderline personality disorder. *American Journal of Psychiatry, 166,* 1355–1364.

Bateman, A. W., & Fonagy, P. (Eds.). (2012). *Handbook of mentalizing in mental health practice.* Washington, DC: American Psychiatric Publishing.

Belsky, D. W., Caspi, A., Arsenault, L., Bleidorn, W.,

Fonagy, P., Goodman, M., et al. (2012). Etiological features of borderline personality related characteristics in a birth cohort of 12-year-old children. *Development and Psychopathology, 24,* 251–265.

Belsky, J. (2012). The development of human reproductive strategies: Progress and prospects. *Current Directions in Psychological Science, 21,* 310–316.

Bleiberg, E. (2001). *Treating personality disorders in children and adolescents: A relational approach.* New York: Guilford Press.

Bleiberg, K. L., & Markowitz, J. C. (2005). A pilot study of interpersonal psychotherapy for posttraumatic stress disorder. *American Journal of Psychiatry, 162,* 181–183.

Bornovalova, M. A., Hicks, B. M., Iacono, W. G., & McGue, M. (2013). Longitudinal twin study of borderline personality disorder traits and substance use in adolescence: Developmental change, reciprocal effects, and genetic and environmental influences. *Personality Disorders, 4,* 23–32.

Caspi, A., Houts, R. M., Belsky, D. W., Goldman-Mellor, S. J., Harrington, H., Israel, S., et al. (2013). The p factor: One general psychopathology factor in the structure of psychiatric disorders? *Clinical Psychological Science, 2,* 119–137.

Chanen, A. M., & McCutcheon, L. (2013). Prevention and early intervention for borderline personality disorder: Current status and recent evidence. *British Journal of Psychiatry Supplement, 54,* S24–S29.

Csibra, G., & Gergely, G. (2009). Natural pedagogy. *Trends in Cognitive Sciences, 13,* 148–153.

Fiske, S. T., & Taylor, S. E. (1991). *Social cognition.* New York: McGraw-Hill.

Fonagy, P., Gergely, G., Jurist, E., & Target, M. (2002). *Affect regulation, mentalization, and the development of the self.* New York: Other Press.

Fonagy, P., & Luyten, P. (2009). A developmental, mentalization-based approach to the understanding and treatment of borderline personality disorder. *Development and Psychopathology, 21,* 1355–1381.

Fonagy, P., & Luyten, P. (2016). A multilevel perspective on the development of borderline personality disorder. In D. Cicchetti (Ed.), *Development and psychopathology* (Vol. 3, 3rd ed., pp. 726–792). New York: Wiley.

Fonagy, P., Luyten, P., & Allison, E. (2015). Epistemic petrifaction and the restoration of epistemic trust: A new conceptualization of borderline personality disorder and its psychosocial treatment. *Journal of Personality Disorders, 29*(5), 575–609.

Fonagy, P., Steele, M., Steele, H., Higgitt, A., & Target, M. (1994). The Emanuel Miller Memorial Lecture 1992: The theory and practice of resilience. *Journal of Child Psychology and Psychiatry, 35,* 231–257.

Fonagy, P., Steele, M., Steele, H., Moran, G. S., & Higgitt, A. C. 1991. The capacity for understanding mental states: The reflective self in parent and child and its significance for security of attachment. *Infant Mental Health Journal, 12,* 201–218.

Gabbard, G. (2006). When is transference work useful in dynamic psychotherapy. *American Journal of Psychiatry, 163,* 1667–1669.

Gergely, G., & Watson, J. (1996). The social biofeedback model of parental affect-mirroring. *International Journal of Psycho-Analysis, 77,* 1181–1212.

Jørgensen, C. R., Freund, C., Boye, R., Jordet, H., Andersen, D., & Kjolbye, M. (2013). Outcome of mentalization-based and supportive psychotherapy in patients with borderline personality disorder: A randomized trial. *Acta Psychiatrica Scandinavica, 127,* 305–317.

Karterud, S., & Bateman, A. (2011). *Manual for mentaliseringsbasert psykoedukativ gruppeterapi (MBT-I).* Oslo, Norway: Gyldendal.

Kim, J., & Cicchetti, D. (2010). Longitudinal pathways linking child maltreatment, emotion regulation, peer relations, and psychopathology. *Journal of Child Psychology and Psychiatry, 51,* 706–716.

Klimes-Dougan, B., & Kistner, J. (1990). Physically abused preschoolers' responses to peers' distress. *Developmental Psychology, 25,* 516–524.

Kruglanski, A. W. (1989). *Lay epistemics and human knowledge: Cognitive and motivational bases.* New York: Plenum Press.

Kruglanski, A. W., & Webster, D. M. (1996). Motivated closing of the mind: "Seizing" and "freezing." *Psychological Review, 103,* 263–283.

Laurenssen, E. M., Feenstra, D. J., Busschbach, J. J., Hutsebaut, J., Bales, D. L., Luyten, P., et al. (2014). Feasibility of mentalization-based treatment for adolescents with borderline symptoms: A pilot study. *Psychotherapy, 51*(1), 159–166.

Mikulincer, M. (1997). Adult attachment style and information processing: Individual differences in curiosity and cognitive closure. *Journal of Personality and Social Psychology, 72,* 1217–1230.

National Institute for Health and Clinical Excellence. (2009). *Borderline personality disorder: Treatment and management* (Clinical Guideline 78). London: Author.

Oldham, J. M. (2009). Borderline personality disorder comes of age. *American Journal of Psychiatry, 166,* 509–511.

Petersen, B., Toft, J., Christensen, N., Foldager, L., Munk-Jørgensen, P., Windfeld, M., et al. (2010). A 2-year follow-up of mentalization-oriented group therapy following day hospital treatment for patients with personality disorders. *Personality and Mental Health, 4,* 293–301.

Pierro, A., & Kruglanski, A. W. (2008). "Seizing and freezing" on a significant-person schema: Need for closure and the transference effect in social judgment. *Personality and Social Psychology Bulletin, 34,* 1492–1503.

Racker, H. (1957). The meanings and uses of countertransference. *Psychoanalytic Quarterly, 26,* 303–357.

Racker, H. (1968). *Transference and countertransference.* London: Hogarth Press.

Rossouw, T. I., & Fonagy, P. (2012). Mentalization-based treatment for self-harm in adolescents: A randomized controlled trial. *Journal of the American Academy of Child and Adolescent Psychiatry, 51,* 1304–1313.

Shenk, C. E., Putnam, F. W., & Noll, J. G. (2013). Predicting the accuracy of facial affect recognition: The interaction of child maltreatment and intellectual functioning. *Journal of Experimental Child Psychology, 114,* 229–242.

Skårderud, F. (2007). Eating one's words: Part III. Mentalisation-based psychotherapy for anorexia nervosa—an outline for a treatment and training manual. *European Eating Disorders Review, 15,* 323–339.

Stein, H., Fonagy, P., Ferguson, K. S., & Wisman, M. (2000). Lives through time: An ideographic approach to the study of resilience. *Bulletin of the Menninger Clinic, 64,* 281–305.

Stepp, S. D., Olino, T. M., Klein, D. N., Seeley, J. R., & Lewinsohn, P. M. (2013). Unique influences of adolescent antecedents on adult borderline personality disorder features. *Personality Disorders, 4,* 223–229.

Valentino, K., Cicchetti, D., Toth, S. L., & Rogosch, F. A. (2011). Mother–child play and maltreatment: A longitudinal analysis of emerging social behavior from infancy to toddlerhood. *Developmental Psychology, 47,* 1280–1294.

Watson, J. S. (1981). Contingency experience in behavioral development. In K. Immelman, G. W. Barlow, L. Petriinovitch, & M. Main (Eds.), *Behavioral development: The Bielefeld Interdisciplinary Project.* Cambridge, UK: Cambridge University Press.

Wilson, D. B., & Sperber, D. (2012). *Meaning and relevance.* Cambridge, UK: Cambridge University Press.

# CHAPTER 31

# Schema Therapy

David P. Bernstein and Maartje Clercx

Schema therapy (also known as schema-focused therapy), an integrative form of psychotherapy that combines cognitive, behavioral, psychodynamic object relations, and experiential approaches (Rafaeli, Bernstein, & Young, 2011; Young, Klosko, & Weishaar, 2003), was developed as a treatment for (PDs) and other chronic forms of psychopathology, such as chronic depression and anxiety disorders. The focus of schema therapy is on modifying early, persistent, self-defeating patterns of thinking and feeling ("early maladaptive schemas"), maladaptive coping responses, and transient, maladaptive emotional states ("schema modes"). It is a moderate- to long-term form of psychotherapy that strives to produce genuine personality change, reducing the harmful consequences of PDs (e.g., suicidal and parasuicidal behavior and aggression directed toward others), and improving quality of life and feelings of subjective well-being (Young, 1990).

While schema therapy uses a variety of techniques to achieve these changes, a central emphasis is on the therapy relationship, in which the therapist attempts to provide for some of the unmet, early emotional/developmental needs of the patient (e.g., attachment, autonomy, boundaries) within appropriate limits, an approach known as "limited reparenting" (Rafaeli et al., 2011; Young et al., 2003). It is this quality of the therapy relationship, in which the therapist takes the role of "good enough parent" to the patient, that most distinguishes schema therapy from other therapies for PDs (e.g., Bateman & Fonagy, 2006; Linehan, 1993). While other therapies also emphasize the therapist's empathy and validation of the patient, in schema therapy, the therapist continually asks him- or herself, "What does this patient need at this moment: Safety, acceptance, autonomy, freedom to express himself, permission to be playful and spontaneous, limits and boundaries?" This persistent focus on the patient's emotional and developmental needs—along with the early maladaptive schemas that develop when these needs are insufficiently met in childhood; the emotional states (schema modes) that arise when schemas are triggered; and the integrative nature of the therapy itself—give schema therapy its distinctive character.

Considerable evidence supports the effectiveness and cost-effectiveness of schema therapy for the treatment of borderline personality disorder (BPD), when delivered via individual therapy (Giesen-Bloo et al., 2006; Van Asselt et al., 2008) and group therapy (Farrell, Shaw, & Webber, 2009) formats. In addition, more recent studies provide support for the effectiveness of schema therapy for patients with Cluster C PDs (Bamelis, Evers, Spinhoven, & Arntz, 2014), and preliminary support for forensic patients with Cluster B PDs (Bernstein et al., 2012) and patients with chronic depression (Renner et al., 2013).

In this chapter, we review the schema therapy conceptual model, along with treatment strategies and interventions, and the evidence base supporting its use for PDs and other treatment-resistant conditions.

## Conceptual Model

### Origins

Young developed schema therapy based on his experiences collaborating on Beck's (1979) early clinical trials of cognitive-behavioral therapy (CBT) for depression. Young (1990) observed that many of 20–30% of patients in these studies who responded poorly to CBT appeared to have PDs. For many patients with PDs, standard cognitive approaches such as correcting distorted cognitions (e.g., "all-or-nothing thinking") may feel irrelevant because their fundamental problems lie in the areas of self/identity disturbance, insecure attachment patterns, and past traumatic experiences (Young, 1994). Moreover, because of their mistrust and other relational difficulties, they find it difficult to engage in the kind of collaborative working relationship ("collaborative empiricism") on which cognitive therapy is predicated. Finally, many patients with PD exhibit emotional difficulties such as affective lability or avoidance of/detachment from emotions (Young, 1990), which are not addressed by standard cognitive techniques. Schema therapy was developed to overcome these difficulties. In comparison to standard CBT, it places greater emphasis on the therapy relationship to provide a "corrective emotional experience" in patients whose early attachments were often deficient. Schema therapy also incorporates experiential techniques to evoke and reprocess emotions, in addition to using standard cognitive techniques, and emphasizes the past origins of maladaptive behavior, especially traumatic experiences such as childhood abuse, neglect, and abandonment, in addition to focusing on present problems.

While the original schema therapy model focused on changing early maladaptive schemas and maladaptive coping responses (Young, 1990; see below), more recent developments focus on schema modes, extreme and fluctuating emotional states that are seen in severe PDs, such as BPD, narcissistic PD (NPD), and antisocial PD (ASPD) (Rafaeli et al., 2011). In schema mode work, the therapist tracks the fluctuations in the patient's modes and adjusts his or her interventions accordingly. All clinical trials supporting the effectiveness of schema therapy (Bamelis et al., 2014; Bernstein et al., 2012; Giesen-Bloo et al., 2006; Nadort et al., 2009; Renner et al., 2013; Van Asselt et al., 2008) have used this schema mode approach, leading to its widespread adoption among schema therapists in contemporary clinical practice.

### Scope and Focus

Schema therapy can be used with any PD or other chronic, treatment-resistant mood or anxiety disorder. However, rather than being a "one-size-fits-all" approach, it is a flexible system that may be individualized to each patient. In the initial phase of therapy, the therapist creates an individualized case conceptualization, using schemas and coping responses (or schema modes for severe PDs) as explanatory concepts that link the patient's developmental history to his or her past and current problems. The therapist then tailors interventions according to this model.

### Overview of the Treatment Model

In patients with less severe or less complex PDs, schema therapy typically lasts for 1–2 years, with therapy delivered on a once per week basis, and sometimes with decreasing frequency in the second year. In patients with more severe PDs, such as those with BPD, NPD, or ASPD, treatment is more intense, usually delivered twice a week, and it can last up to 3 years or longer (Young et al., 2003). This greater intensity is considered necessary to repair disturbed attachment patterns in these patients, in whom childhood trauma such as abuse, neglect, and abandonment prevented the development of secure bonds with caregivers (Bender, Farber, & Geller, 2001). Clinical trials support the notion that more intensive therapy is needed for these patients. While twice-per-week schema therapy, delivered for 3 years, was needed to promote recovery in outpatients with BPD (Giesen-Bloo et al., 2006; Nadort et al., 2009), a frequency of once a week for 40 sessions plus six optional booster sessions was sufficient for a less impaired group of patients with mostly Cluster C PDs (Bamelis et al., 2014). Farrell and colleagues (2009) found that a combination of individual and group schema therapy produced more rapid effects in patients with BPD, with large treatment gains observed in just 18 months. However, these findings should be considered tentative until a replication study, currently in progress (Dickhaut & Arntz, 2014), is completed.

Schema therapy consists of two phases: an assessment phase and case conceptualization phase, which usually last between six and 10 sessions, and a schema change phase (Young, 1990). In the first phase, the therapist uses multiple assessment methods to evaluate the patient's schemas and coping responses (or "schema modes"), linking them to their origins and current problems. This phase culminates in a case conceptualization that guides therapy and may be adapted over the course of therapy. In the schema change phase, the therapist targets the schemas and coping responses (or modes) in question, with the goal of bringing lasting relief from symptoms and other problems and improving well-being and quality of life. The therapist uses several therapeutic techniques to accomplish these changes. First, cognitive techniques are used to modify the distorted cognitions associated with schemas. Experiential techniques are used to modify the affective component of schemas. Behavioral techniques are implemented to change maladaptive behaviors. Finally there is the therapy relationship itself, in which the therapist provides limited reparenting, confronts the patient empathically about his or her self-destructive patterns ("empathic confrontation"), and sets limits, when necessary, on his or her destructive behavior (Rafaeli et al., 2011).

## Diagnosis, Assessment, and Formulation

### Assessment Process

In the initial phase of schema therapy, the therapist engages the patient in a collaborative process to assess schemas, maladaptive coping responses, and schema modes, and links to their developmental origins and current problems. This process culminates in a case conceptualization, which the therapist shares with the patient. Sometimes, the therapist presents the case conceptualization in simplified form, or decides to present it at a later time, when the patient's cognitive limitations (e.g., lower intelligence) or psychopathology (e.g., extreme mistrust) make this necessary. The case conceptualization serves as a "road map" for treatment, enabling the therapist to identify central unmet emotional and developmental needs, select and prioritize treatment targets, and plan interventions for early, middle, and late phases of therapy (Rafaeli et al., 2011; Young, 1990).

Multiple assessment methods are used to arrive at a case formulation. First, a life history interview is conducted to inquire about adverse life experiences in childhood and adolescence and other risk or protective factors (e.g., the child's innate temperament, a healthy attachment to a nonabusive parent). The patient then completes self-report questionnaires to assess schema therapy constructs, including early maladaptive schemas (e.g., Young Schema Questionnaire; Young & Brown, 1994), the origins of schemas (e.g., Young Parenting Inventory; Young, 1999), maladaptive coping responses (e.g., Rijkeboer, Lobbestael, Arntz, & Van Genderen, 2010), and schema modes (e.g., Schema Mode Inventory; Young et al., 2007). Imagery sessions are then conducted, in which patients are asked to close their eyes and recall a distressing experience with one of their parents. Because imagery is a powerful way of evoking emotions (Holmes & Mathews, 2005, 2010), it is particularly helpful for investigating early maladaptive schemas when patients lack insight or minimize or deny their presence on self-report questionnaires. Finally, the therapy sessions are an opportunity to observe situations that trigger the patient's early maladaptive schemas, his or her characteristic manner of coping with schema activation, and the resulting emotional states (schema modes) that occur during interaction with the therapist. When patients are hospitalized, additional sources of information are usually available, such as the patient's chart and observations of interactions on the ward. Combining information from multiple sources creates a full picture of the patient's problems and how they developed according to the schema therapy model.

### Psychoeducation

The assessment process is facilitated by the therapist teaching the patient the schema therapy "language" at the beginning of the therapy. In the original schema therapy approach, this language was that of early maladaptive schemas and maladaptive coping responses (Young, 1990). In the schema mode approach, it is the language of schema modes (Rafaeli et al., 2011). By explaining these concepts, the therapist makes the patient an active participant in the assessment process. Therapist and patient are able to explore the patient's history and problems together with a common vocabulary and set of ideas as a reference point. Sometimes, the therapist assigns self-help books (e.g., *Reinventing Your Life*; Young, Klosko, & Weishaar, 1993) that explain these concepts in accessible terms.

Simply going through this process of assessment and psychoeducation often brings patients relief, since they have a framework for understanding their difficulties for the first time.

## Theoretical Foundations
### Theory of Disorder
*Developmental Framework*

Schema therapy subscribes to a biopsychosocial theory of psychopathology that assumes that multiple risk and protective factors contribute to the child's development: innate temperament and biological predispositions; attachments to caregivers; family dynamics; adverse life experiences (e.g., child abuse, neglect, and abandonment); social interactions with peers; and opportunities and challenges at school and in other performance domains. Schema therapy does not propose a comprehensive theory of development. However, consistent with a developmental cascade model, risk and protective factors, and the interplay between them, are conceived as having "downstream" effects that facilitate or impede the child's ability to get his or her emotional needs met in adaptive ways. To the extent that these basic needs are met, the child develops in healthy directions. When these needs are significantly unfulfilled or frustrated, repetitive themes or patterns emerge in the form of early maladaptive schemas, which shape development in maladaptive ways. The central position of emotional needs in this theoretical account distinguishes schema therapy from other forms of therapy. While other therapies also highlight the importance of attachment relationships (Allen, 2012; Bateman & Fonagy, 2006) or the interplay between the child's biological temperament and adverse family environments (Linehan, 1993), schema therapy is unique in positing that emotional needs are the central driver of development.

*Emotional Needs*

According to the schema therapy model, five basic emotional needs are central to development (Young, 1990):

1. Attachment needs, including the need for safety, nurturance, attention, and validation
2. Autonomy needs, including the need for autonomy, independence, and identity
3. The need for the expression and validation of emotions
4. The need for spontaneity and play
5. The need for boundaries and limits

These basic needs are linked directly to the development of early maladaptive schemas, which are grouped into domains depending on the emotional needs to which they relate.

For example, five early maladaptive schemas may develop in response to unfulfilled or frustrated attachment needs: the abandonment/instability, mistrust/abuse, emotional deprivation, defectiveness/shame, and social isolation schemas. These schemas are classified together in the disconnection/rejection domain, which refers to the schemas that arise when attachment needs go unmet. The specific schemas that arise within this domain depend on the kinds of attachment failures that the child experienced. For example, the abandonment/instability schema is the expectation that one will inevitably be abandoned, especially in close relationships. This schema develops out of extreme or repeated experiences of loss, abandonment, or instability. It is most pronounced when children have experienced traumatic losses and dislocations, such as lack of stable caregivers due to mental illness or addiction; being repeatedly moved from one residential care facility, foster home, or relative to another, and so forth. In this way, early maladaptive schemas are mental representations that develop from real experiences in which basic emotional needs—in this case, the need for secure attachments—went unmet.

### Fundamental Theoretical Constructs
*Early Maladaptive Schemas*

"Early maladaptive schemas" are defined as repetitive themes or patterns that arise from a combination of adverse childhood experiences and a child's innate temperament, are elaborated over the course of a lifetime, and are self-defeating to a significant degree. Schema therapy describes 18 early maladaptive schemas (see Table 31.1), which are grouped into five larger schema domains:

1. Disconnection/rejection
2. Impaired autonomy and performance
3. Impaired limits
4. Other-directedness
5. Overvigilance/inhibition

**TABLE 31.1. Schema Domains and Early Maladaptive Schemas**

Disconnection and rejection

| | | |
|---|---|---|
| 1 | Abandonment/Instability | This schema involves the feeling that abandonment is inevitable. |
| 2 | Mistrust/Abuse | People with this schema expect that others will always lie to you; manipulate or take advantage of you; cheat, abuse, humiliate, or otherwise hurt you. |
| 3 | Emotional Deprivation | The schema is concentrated on the feeling that others will never be able to meet your core needs of emotional nurturance, protection and/or empathy. |
| 4 | Defectiveness/Shame | Within this schema, you have the feeling that you are inferior, bad, defective, or invalid in important aspects. |
| 5 | Social Isolation/Alienation | This schema involves feeling different, alienated, or like an outsider toward or around others. |

Impaired autonomy and performance

| | | |
|---|---|---|
| 6 | Dependence/Incompetence | The core characteristic of this schema is the feeling that you are incapable of handling everyday responsibilities without relying on the help of others. |
| 7 | Vulnerability to Harm or Illness | This schema involves having a large and unrealistic fear that harm, danger, or catastrophe is imminent and unavoidable. |
| 8 | Enmeshment/Undeveloped Self | In this schema the patient is excessively emotionally involved or so close to others that individuality or normal social development is lacking or absent. |
| 9 | Failure | The core feature of this schema is a feeling that you are a failure or will be a failure, and/or fundamentally inadequate in important areas of achievement. |

Impaired limits

| | | |
|---|---|---|
| 10 | Entitlement/Grandiosity | This schema involves feeling superior, entitled, and special, and/or that normal rules of social reciprocity do not apply to you. |
| 11 | Insufficient Self-Control/Self-Discipline | People with this schema experience severe difficulty or refuse to exercise self-control and lack frustration tolerance when trying to achieve goals. |

Other-directedness

| | | |
|---|---|---|
| 12 | Subjugation | This schema's core feature is relinquishing control to others in order to avoid anger, retaliation, or abandonment, or because you perceive (imaginary) you are being coerced. |
| 13 | Self-Sacrifice | This schema involves always trying to (voluntarily) fulfill other's needs at the expense of meeting your own needs. |
| 14 | Approval-Seeking/Recognition-Seeking | In this schema, the major focus is on gaining attention, approval, or recognition from others. |

Overvigilance and inhibition

| | | |
|---|---|---|
| 15 | Negativity/Pessimism | In this schema, the person is overly focused on life's negative aspects (e.g., death, loss, pain), while minimizing, overlooking, or ignoring positive aspects. |
| 16 | Emotional Inhibition | This schema involves excessively inhibiting your spontaneous actions, feelings, or communications. |
| 17 | Unrelenting Standards/Hyper criticalness | The core characteristic of this schema is the feeling that you must constantly strive to meet very high, internalized standards of behavior and performance. |
| 18 | Punitiveness | The schema mainly involves the feeling that you need harsh punishment for making mistakes. |

*Note.* From Keulen-de Vos, Bernstein, and Arntz (2014). Copyright 2014 by Wiley. Adapted by permission from Wiley.

Schemas were originally identified from clinical experience with psychotherapy patients and subsequently refined and confirmed in several factor analytic studies using versions of the Young Schema Questionnaire (Rijkeboer & Van den Bergh, 2006; Schmidt, Joiner, Young, & Telch, 1995; Welburn, Coristine, Dagg, Pontefract, & Jordan, 2002).

Early maladaptive schemas have several features. They consist of cognitions, affects, memories, and bodily sensations. They are triggered by specific situations and, when triggered, produce strong emotions, such as fear, sadness, anger, shame, or guilt. They filter information about the self, other people, and the world, and therefore lead to cognitive biases that result in the selective processing of information (Rafaeli et al., 2011). This can lead to the misinterpretation of situations in ways that are consistent with and therefore reinforce one's schemas. For example, an abandonment/instability schema may lead to the misinterpretation of ambiguous situations (e.g., a therapist is 5 minutes late in arriving for the patient's appointment) in ways that are consistent with the schema (e.g., "Now even my therapist isn't there for me when I need him!"). Early maladaptive schemas operate unconsciously, in the sense that most of mental processing is outside of the person's awareness. As a result, people are not usually aware that they have schemas or of the distortions they cause. Schemas developed early in life, in particular, act as "ground-truths," or deeply held convictions about the person himself (e.g., "I'm a loser"—defectiveness/shame schema), other people (e.g., "Other people will always hurt you"—mistrust/abuse schema), and the world (e.g., "Dangerous things can happen at any moment"—vulnerability to harm or illness schema). However, most patients can readily become aware of their schemas, a first step toward changing them.

The schema therapy model assumes that early maladaptive schemas are dimensional constructs that do not have one-to-one correspondences with different DSM-5 personality disorders (Jovev & Jackson, 2004). This assumption contrasts with Beck's model, which posits that each PD is characterized by a distinct and unique set of core beliefs (Beck, 1979).

## Maladaptive Coping Styles and Responses

When early maladaptive schemas are triggered, they produce strong emotions, accompanied by attempts at coping with this schematic activation. Three broad styles of maladaptive coping are recognized: schema surrender, schema avoidance, and schema overcompensation (Young, 1990). "Schema surrender" refers to (unconsciously) giving in to one's schemas. This usually means acquiescing to one's schemas in a dependent, passive, or submissive way. For example, surrendering to an abandonment schema might be evident when someone chooses a romantic partner who is rejecting or ambivalent. By (unconsciously) choosing a partner who triggers the abandonment schema, the patient leaves him- or herself in a helpless, dependent position, with a sense of loss and despair. "Schema avoidance" refers to avoiding people or situations that trigger one's schemas. For example, an individual may cope with an abandonment schema by avoiding romantic relationships altogether. Finally, "schema overcompensation" refers to doing the opposite of the schema. In practice, this often means taking the one-up position or turning the tables on the other person. For example, one may cope with an abandonment schema by rejecting or denigrating one's partner.

For each broad coping style, there are many specific types of maladaptive coping responses. For example, schema avoidance may be achieved by avoiding people or situations; by avoiding *thinking about* upsetting topics; or by using drugs, alcohol, or other compulsive behavior to block out feelings. Many people use more than one maladaptive coping style, though most have a predominant style, and these styles can shift over time or across situations. Not surprisingly, while coping styles are understandable attempts to protect one from the painful emotions associated with schemas, they usually end up perpetuating the schemas rather than resolving them in healthy ways.

## Schema Modes

Schema modes are the most recent development in the schema therapy conceptual model (Rafaeli et al., 2011). Early maladaptive schemas are trait-like entities, which means they are enduring features of the personality, developing in childhood and becoming elaborated over the lifespan. In contrast, schema modes are more state-like emotional entities, involving moment-to-moment fluctuations. Because patients with severe PDs often switch between extreme emotional states, it was necessary to develop a method, namely, schema mode work, to enable therapists to monitor these fluctuations and adjust their interventions accordingly. Schema mode work is typically used for patients with more severe PDs, such as BPD, NPD, or ASPD, or more generally, whenever the patient's schema modes would otherwise interfere with the therapy and impede progress (Rafaeli et al., 2011; see "Principal Intervention Strategies and Methods, and Process of Treatment").

Schema modes are the active state of early maladaptive schemas (Rafaeli et al., 2011). The combination of the schema, its associated cognitions and emotions, and coping responses constitute the schema mode. For example, imagine that someone with a strong abandonment schema is left by his or her partner or spouse. If the patient responds to these painful feelings in a helpless, passive, defeated way (surrendering coping response), the result is an Abandoned Child mode. In this emotional state, the patient feels *as if* he or she is an abandoned child. This is reflected in certain cognitions ("No one will ever stay with me"), emotions (loss, despair, and longing), and surrendering coping responses (e.g., spending hours or even days in bed crying, letting oneself be completely overwhelmed by the painful feelings). In contrast, a different coping response to the same abandonment schema could result in a different schema mode. For example, avoidant coping that involves blocking out feelings could lead to a state of emotional numbness referred to as Detached Protector mode. In this state, the person feels nothing. The patient is detached and emotionless. Thus, it is the combination of cognitions, emotions, and coping responses that determine the mode. A complete list of schema modes is presented in Table 31.2.

The schema mode approach was developed to treat patients with severe PDs who often switch between different emotional states (Lobbestael, Arntz, & Sieswerda, 2005; Young et al., 2003). For example, a patient with BPD may switch rapidly in a single session between states in which he or she is overwhelmed by painful feelings of abandonment (Abandoned Child mode), anger or rage (Angry Child mode), and extreme emotional detachment, which can even be of dissociative proportions (Detached Protector mode). When the patient is in one of these modes, it determines his or her thinking, feeling, and behavior to the exclusion of the other modes. Thus, a patient who is in the Detached Protector mode is not in touch with the painful feelings that he or she might have been experiencing just a few minutes earlier. In this way, the mode dominates his or her thinking, feeling, and behavior at that moment. The reason for the dissociation between modes is that people with severe PDs have poorly integrated personalities (Young et al., 2003). Most people have the capacity to reflect on and modulate their emotional responses. By contrast, people with BPD seem to lack this ability, especially when they are schematically triggered. In schema mode terms, they lack a strong Healthy Adult mode that can integrate their various emotional states, keeping them from going to extremes.

## Schema Mode Models

Young (1990) proposed that different PDs are characterized by different combinations of schema modes, a notion that has been confirmed by empirical research (Arntz, Klokman, & Sieswerda, 2005; Bamelis, Renner, Heidkamp, & Arntz, 2011; Lobbestael, Van Vreeswijk, & Arntz, 2008). The schema mode models for different PDs are often represented in the form of diagrams. For example, BPD is characterized by five main modes: Abandoned Child, Angry and Impulsive Child, Detached Protector, and Punitive Parent (Arntz et al., 2005). Most of the dynamics of these patients can be understood in terms of switches between emotional states: the intense feelings of abandonment that are triggered by real or perceived losses (Abandoned Child mode); relentless self-criticism (Punitive Parent mode); emotional numbness, an attempt to block out painful feelings, which in the extreme can take on a dissociative quality (Detached Protector mode); outbursts of anger or rage (Angry Child mode); and impulsive, self-destructive behavior (Impulsive Child mode). Note that suicidal and parasuicidal behavior can occur in different states: as a form of self-punishment when patients are overwhelmed with feelings of loss and self-loathing (Punitive Parent and Abandoned Child modes); a response to, or as an attempt to induce, emotional numbness (Detached Protector mode); or as a form of self-destructive angry and impulsive behavior (Angry and Impulsive Child modes). Thus, the function of the suicidal behavior depends on which mode the person is in at the time that it occurs.

## TABLE 31.2. Schema Modes

| | |
|---|---|
| Child modes | Involve feeling, thinking, and acting in a "child-like" manner |
| 1. Abused, Abandoned, or Humiliated Child (Vulnerable Child mode types) | When in this mode, one feels vulnerable and overwhelmed with feelings of anxiety, depression, shame, grief, or other painful feelings. |
| 2. Angry Child | People in this mode may throw a child-like temper tantrum. They are feeling and expressing anger excessively in response to real or perceived frustration, abandonment, hurt, or humiliation. |
| 3. Enraged Child | This mode is similar to the Angry Child mode; however, the patient loses control over anger and aggression and takes this feelings out on objects or humans. Patients often report being in a dissociative state ("Everything went black"). |
| 4. Impulsive Child | This mode involves trying to get one's needs met by acting impulsively. The person may be rebellious toward internalized parental modes or maltreatment. |
| 5. Undisciplined Child | People in this mode are unable tolerate limits of discipline or the resulting frustration. The person may act spoiled, want something right then and there, and not want to do anything he or she dislikes. |
| 6. Lonely Child | The feelings that dominate this mode are loneliness and emptiness. This mode is dominated by the feeling that no one can understand, soothe, or comfort, or make real contact with the person. |
| Avoidant and surrender coping modes | Involve attempts to protect the self from pain through maladaptive forms of coping |
| 7. Detached Protector | This mode involves detachment from emotions, feelings, and thoughts to shield oneself from pain. The person might be unaware, appear emotionally distant, and avoid getting close to others. The person might be, or claim to be, "feeling nothing." |
| 8. Detached Self-Soother/Self-Stimulator | In this mode, the person's objective is to distance or shield him- or herself from painful feelings, and he or she tries to reach this goal by engaging in repetitive, compulsive, addictive, or self-stimulating behaviors. The person is looking to calm or sooth him- or herself or to induce pleasurable or exciting sensations. |
| 9. Compliant Surrenderer | In this mode, people readily fulfill real or perceived needs, demands, or expectations of others. This might be because the other is perceived as more powerful than the self, to avoid pain or rejection, or as an attempt to get one's own needs met. |
| 10. Angry Protector | This mode involves keeping others, who are perceived as threatening or dangerous, at a distance by using a "wall of anger." Other than the Angry Child mode, the anger is quite controlled and serves a goal of "protecting" the self from others. |
| Maladaptive parent modes | Involve internalized dysfunctional parent "voices" |
| 11. Punitive, Critical Parent | This mode is very critical toward the self, criticizing and making the person feeling shame or guilt. Basically, it functions as an internalized critical or punishing parent. |
| 12. Demanding Parent | Like the Punitive Parent, this mode also involves an internalized parental voice. In the Demanding Parent mode, the person sets impossibly high standards and demands, keeps pushing him- or herself to do and achieve more, and is never satisfied with the self. |

*(continued)*

**TABLE 31.2.** *(continued)*

| | |
|---|---|
| Overcompensatory coping modes | Involve extreme attempts to compensate for feelings of shame, loneliness, or vulnerability |
| 13. Self-Aggrandizer mode | People in the Self-Aggrandizer mode are less concerned with the feelings of real contact with others than with keeping up appearances. A person in this mode feels more important, special, powerful, or overall superior compared to others. He or she exhibits self-aggrandizing behavior, categorizing the world in "top dog and bottom dog" fashion. |
| 14. Bully and Attack mode | A person in the Bully and Attack mode uses coercion, aggression, or threats to get what he or she wants. This might include dominant behaviors, feeling sadistic pleasure, or retaliation. |
| 15. Conning and Manipulative mode | People in this mode lie, manipulate, or con others to achieve specific goals, such as escaping punishment or victimizing others. |
| 16. Predator mode | This mode involves utilizing cold, ruthless, and calculating behaviors to eliminate real or perceived threat, obstacles, or enemies. |
| 17. Obsessive–Compulsive Overcontroller mode | The Obsessive–Compulsive mode, also called the Perfectionistic Overcontroller mode, involves ruminating, exercising extreme control and order, repetition, or rituals to divert attention from, or to protect oneself from real or perceived threat. |
| 18. Paranoid Overcontroller mode | The Paranoid Overcontroller tries to protect the self from real or perceived threat, and involves ruminating, exercising extreme control and order, repetition, or rituals. The Suspicious type is concerned with locating or uncovering hidden, real, or perceived threat. |

*Note.* From Keulen-de Vos, Bernstein, and Arntz (2014). Copyright 2014 by Wiley. Adapted by permission from Wiley.

### *Principles of Change*

Several change processes appear to be responsible for the effectiveness of schema therapy. First, the therapy relationship itself is considered the most important mechanism of change (Young, 1990). The therapist strives to form a genuine emotional bond with the patient, which is an essential goal, since many patients with PDs have histories of disturbed attachments. The therapist's limited reparenting counteracts early maladaptive schemas by providing for some of the patient's unmet emotional needs in an attachment relationship. Over time, these "corrective emotional experiences" with the therapist generalize, allowing the patient to develop more secure bonds with other people (Rafaeli et al., 2011).

Cognitive and experiential techniques enable the patient to reprocess the cognitive and affective components of early maladaptive schemas (Rafaeli et al., 2011). Cognitive techniques, such as cognitive restructuring and behavioral experiments, correct the cognitive distortions characteristic of early maladaptive schemas, allowing the patient to achieve perspective on his or her schemas. The patient is now able to recognize when his or her schemas are triggered and that his or her perceptions of situations are not realistic. For example, just because a patient's abandonment schema is triggered, this does not mean that the patient will actually be abandoned. Psychoeducation, such as teaching the patient about his or her early maladaptive schemas or schema modes, also increases insight into problems. Nevertheless, for most patients with PDs, changing the cognitive components of early maladaptive schemas is not sufficient. Although the patient understands intellectually that he or she has schemas, they can still cause painful emotions. For this reason, schema therapy uses experiential techniques such as imagery rescripting and chair work to reprocess the emotions associated with early maladaptive schemas (Rafaeli et al., 2011). For example, imagery techniques, which ask the person to close his or her eyes and allow images of specific situations to come to mind, have been shown to be more emotionally evocative than simply talking about the same situations (Holmes, & Mathews, 2005, 2010). Experiential techniques release painful emotions and facilitate the reprocessing of early maladaptive schemas because schema change is more likely to occur when cognitions are "hot" (i.e., emotionally triggered) than when they are "cold." These cognitive and experiential techniques lay the groundwork for behavioral change by modifying early maladaptive schemas before behavioral interventions are implemented.

## Principal Intervention Strategies and Methods, and Process of Treatment

### Treatment Relationship

In limited reparenting, the therapist provides for the patients' unfulfilled emotional needs within appropriate boundaries (Young et al., 2003). If patients missed out on warmth, attention, or validation, for example, the therapist attempts to provide it in genuine and appropriate ways. The therapist strives to be a real person with patients, showing care and compassion, and letting patients know that he or she is "there for them" when needed. At the same time, the therapist adjusts his or her style depending on the needs of the patient. For example, if a patient grew up in an emotionally distant family, the therapist seeks ways to provide warmth and attention. This may include, for example, encouraging the patient to share his or her enthusiasms (e.g., a love of film, sports, or animals), giving the therapist an opportunity to show genuine interest and pleasure in learning about an important aspect of the patient's life. The therapist also seeks opportunities to share him- or herself with the patient. The therapist has permeable boundaries, allowing the patient to experience him or her as he or she truly is, rather than keeping the patient at a distance that precludes genuine emotional contact. However, the therapist always stays within the professional role. For example, the clinician does not become a friend or confidant or engage in other dual relationships, nor does he or she self-disclose inappropriate information. On the other hand, in schema therapy, the therapist has the flexibility to share emotional reactions or anecdotes from his or her own life; offer guidance; and reach out to the patient in times of need, for example, by offering phone or e-mail contact between sessions. This persistent focus on the patient's emotional needs is the therapist's most powerful antidote for early maladaptive schemas that grew out of unfulfilled needs. Over time, as the patient experiences the partial fulfillment of these needs in the therapy relationship, he or she becomes more able to recognize them and get them met in his or her life outside of therapy. In effect, the patient learns to be a good-enough parent to him- or herself.

The therapy relationship is also the principal vehicle for confronting the patient about self-destructive patterns. In "empathic confrontation," the therapist confronts the patient in a compassionate way, showing understanding for the reasons that these patterns exist, while also pointing out their disadvantages (Young et al., 2003). Because these patterns are entrenched and occur automatically, without the patient's awareness, they need to be brought to the patient's attention persistently. When the patient pursues self-destructive relationships, undermines him- or herself by engaging in self-defeating behaviors, or behaves in ways that are destructive to others, the therapist points this out, making reference to the schemas and coping responses (or schema modes) that are responsible. When these patterns occur in the therapy sessions, empathic confrontation can be even more effective because the therapist can observe and confront them in the "here and now" of the therapy relationship. For example, when a patient arrives late for a session after having revealed something that caused feelings of shame in the previous session, the therapist confronts the early maladaptive schemas (e.g., defectiveness/shame) and avoidant coping behavior that may account for it. By using these concepts to understand the patient's behavior, the therapist is able to confront the patient in an objective, nonjudgmental way. The therapist strives for a balance between limited reparenting and empathic confrontation, providing for the patient's emotional needs and confronting the self-defeating patterns that stand in the way of their fulfillment (Young et al, 2003).

When patients engage in behaviors that violate the rights of the therapist (e.g., behaving in sexually inappropriate or demeaning ways); pose a danger to the therapist, the patient, or other people; or threaten to undermine therapy (e.g., missing sessions repeatedly without good reason), the therapist sets limits. In schema therapy, limit setting is done in a clear, firm, but personal way, for example, by disclosing the effects of the patient's behavior on the therapist (e.g., "The way you are speaking to me leaves me feeling uncomfortable"), and making reference to the needs and rights of the therapist and patient (e.g., "You and I both have the right to be and should be treated respectfully here"). If the patient has difficulty sticking to the limits, the therapist explains the consequences that he or she will impose, choosing consequences that are fitting and proportional to the behavior in question (e.g., "If you can't stop speaking to me in a disrespectful way, I'll need to stop the session").

### Cognitive, Behavioral, and Experiential Techniques

With patients with less severe symptoms, therapy unfolds in a relatively straightforward way. After the assessment phase, the therapist begins the process of changing schemas and coping responses (or modes; Young et al., 2003). Usually, cognitive techniques are introduced first, which help patients achieve some intellectual distance from their schemas. The therapist might use thought records, for example, to help patients recognize the early maladaptive schemas that get triggered in different situations, and challenge them with evidence. On the basis of these exercises, the therapist might create flash cards that patients can use to remind themselves of healthy, alternative cognitions in situations in which early maladaptive schemas are triggered.

The therapist then uses experiential techniques, such as imagery rescripting and role-playing exercises, to reprocess schemas at an emotional level. Imagery rescripting is used to explore the origins of schemas and modify them by asking the patient to close his or her eyes and call to mind an image of a recent, upsetting situation, essentially trying to reexperience it in a vivid way, in order to feel the emotions that were triggered. The therapist then asks the patient to let go of that image and let a new image come to mind. This image needs to be of a childhood situation that felt the same as the one that occurred in the present. Usually, this childhood situation involves the same early maladaptive schema that was triggered by the present situation, making the origins of the patient's reactions clear. The therapist then explores the past situation with the patient, focusing on the emotional needs that were frustrated or unmet. For example, the patient might describe a situation in which he or she was left alone for too long without parental attention, care, or supervision, leading to schemas such as emotional deprivation or abandonment. The therapist then asks the patient's permission to "enter" the image, providing some of what the child needed, for example, connection and safety. Imagery rescripting releases strong emotions and gives the patient the experience, in imagination, of having his or her core needs met. Patients often report feeling calmer after these exercises and being less susceptible to becoming triggered in comparable situations in the present.

Finally, behavioral techniques are used to disrupt self-destructive patterns. Role-playing exercises may be used during the sessions to let the patient practice healthier, alternative behaviors. Behavioral exercises may also be assigned to allow the patient to practice newly learned skills outside of the sessions. For example, for a patient who always feels like an outsider (Social Isolation schema), the therapist might create a behavioral hierarchy, having the patient gradually expose him- or herself to situations in which he or she can make contact with other people. Behavioral change is usually achieved more readily if the patient's schemas have already begun to change through cognitive and experiential techniques.

### Schema Mode Work

Schema mode work was developed for more severely disturbed patients who shift rapidly between emotional states or remain "stuck" in a state, unable to modulate their emotional responses (Rafaeli et al., 2011), which can block therapeutic progress. For example, a highly emotionally detached patient (Detached Protector mode) may spend session after session talking in a bland, superficial, or hyperrational way, avoiding feelings and personal issues. In schema mode work, the therapist tracks the patient's changing emotional states, altering interventions according to the mode that is currently active. Different states call for different kinds of interventions. For example, empathic confrontation is used with a patient in a highly detached state to make him or her aware that he or she is blocking out feelings. The therapist refers to the patient's modes as "sides of you" and invites the patient to create personalized labels for his or her different modes (e.g., "the wall" for the Detached Protector mode), making it easier to communicate about them (Rafaeli et al., 2011).

The goal of the therapist's mode interventions is to help the patient to change from emotional states that block out feelings to ones in which emotional pain is experienced directly (e.g., Vulnerable Child mode, Lonely Child mode) and is possible to reflect on these different states in a balanced and objective way (Healthy Adult mode). As the patient's modes are explored, the therapist invites the patient to understand their origins and function and highlights their advantages and disadvantages. Each mode is validated by noting its adaptive purpose, which usually involves protecting the patient from emotional pain. At the same time, the costs or disadvantages of the mode of functioning are emphasized in terms of the way they prevent the patient from satisfying his or her emotional needs. Various methods are used to explore and change the mode: for example, cognitive techniques, in which the therapist diagrams the patient's modes on a whiteboard and explains their development and functions; and experiential techniques, such as role playing and imagery rescripting, in which the patient experiences the modes emotionally, getting in touch with the modes that involve feelings of vulnerability, such as sadness, fear, and shame. It is these vulnerable sides of the patient that the therapist is trying to reach, so that the patient can reprocess the adverse childhood experiences that gave rise to them. When the patient is in a vulnerable state, the therapist is able to provide for some of the emotional needs the patient missed growing up (e.g., warmth, acknowledgment, and attention in a patient who experienced emotional deprivation). In this way, patients begin to modify and integrate the different schema modes, achieving greater balance and flexibility in their emotional states, and engaging in healthier forms of coping, so that they can get their emotional needs met in more adaptive ways (Young et al., 2003).

### Working with (Self-)Destructive Behaviors

Unlike some therapies, in which patients must make a contract to refrain from certain behaviors (e.g., refrain from making suicide attempts or calling the therapist outside of sessions), schema therapy makes no such preconditions that would lead to the exclusion of many patients with severe symptom levels. Instead, the therapist offers additional support where needed (e.g., letting the patient contact him or her between sessions) and fosters a therapeutic bond that helps the patient to bring destructive behavior under control. Using schema mode work, the therapist helps the patient conceptualize maladaptive behavior in terms of the schema modes that are triggered in different situations, leading to ineffective and self-defeating forms of coping (Young et al., 2003). For example, the therapist might help the patient to recognize and reduce the severity of his or her self-critical side (Punitive Parent mode), which, when triggered, leads to feelings of shame (Vulnerable Child mode) and escape into alcohol use (Detached Self-Soother mode). In this way, the therapist promotes the patient's healthy capacity to reflect on problems and adopt more adaptive coping behaviors (Healthy Adult mode). The therapist, when necessary, also sets limits on (self-)destructive behaviors. For example, the therapist might send the patient home if he or she comes to a session while under the influence of drugs or alcohol.

## Summary of Evidence

### Schema Therapy Conceptual Model

The schema therapy conceptual model is a heuristic one, having been developed from clinical experience to guide treatment (Young, 1990). However, there is increasing empirical support for the major tenets of the underlying model, including the concepts of early maladaptive schemas, maladaptive coping responses, and modes. Factor analytic studies support the idea that the early maladaptive schemas proposed by Young and colleagues (2007) represent distinct but intercorrelated factors. Schemas are associated with attachment difficulties and traumatic childhood experiences and show meaningful relationships to psychopathology (Bamelis et al., 2011; Jovev & Jackson, 2004) and mediating treatment response—changes in schemas account for treatment outcomes. However, the theory that schemas are grouped into schema domains based on specific needs has received less support (Hoffart et al., 2005; Jovev & Jackson, 2004).

In a recent test of the conceptual model, structural equation modeling was used to test the hypothesis that schema modes represent interactions between early maladaptive schemas and maladaptive coping responses. A large sample of patients and nonpatients completed questionnaires for early maladaptive schemas, maladaptive coping responses, and modes. Specific hypotheses were confirmed for all of the schema modes that were tested, showing that different coping styles (e.g., surrender, avoidance, and overcompensation) in combination with different schemas predicted different modes. This study provides a critical test linking the original model of early maladaptive schemas and coping responses to the more recent schema mode model (Rijkeboer et al., 2017).

Recent studies also have supported other central postulates about schema modes, such as the hypothesis that schema modes are evoked by environmental stimuli. In one study, patients with BPD or ASPD were shown a film fragment depicting childhood abuse and changes were assessed in their implicit cognitions, physiological responses, and self-reported schema modes (Lobbestael & Arntz, 2010). Consistent with predictions, patients with BPD and ASPD showed more self-abuse implicit associations following the film stimulus compared to other patients and healthy controls. However, only patients with BPD reported more explicit schema modes (i.e., Abused Child and Abandoned Child modes) and showed heightened physiological responses. In contrast, the patients with ASPD appeared to suppress their physiological responses and did not report more schema modes. These findings suggest that patients with BPD and ASPD cope with their abuse-related cognitions in different ways, resulting in different schema modes (Lobbestael & Arntz, 2010).

Other studies have tested the proposition that different PDs are characterized by different combinations of schema modes (i.e., schema mode models). For example, in one study, several hundred patients with PDs—avoidant (AVPD), dependent (DPD), obsessive–compulsive (OCPD), narcissistic (NPD), histrionic (HPD), or paranoid (PPD)—completed a questionnaire assessing schema modes (Lobbestael et al., 2008). The hypothesized combinations of modes were confirmed for each of the PDs. Other studies have confirmed that patients with BPD exhibit the four main schema modes hypothesized by Young and colleagues: Abused and Abandoned Child, Angry and Impulsive Child, Detached Protector, and Punitive Parent (Lobbestael et al., 2005). Other modes, such as Bully and Attack, also characterized patients with BPD. However, the evidence regarding the modes hypothesized for ASPD is mixed. One study found that patients with ASPD reported high scores on only the Angry Child and Healthy Adult modes, indicating a possible response bias (Lobbestael, Arntz, Löbbes, & Cima, 2009), whereas another found that patients with ASPD reported modes characterized by anger, impulsivity, and overcompensation (Lobbestael & Arntz, 2012).

Researchers have also investigated the relationship between schema modes and maladaptive behavior. For example, the relationship among schema modes, crimes, and aggressive incidents was investigated in hospitalized forensic patients with ASPD, BPD, NPD, or PPD. Schema modes were retrospectively assessed from descriptions of crimes in patients' files. As hypothesized, the events leading up to crimes were characterized by triggers involving vulnerable emotions such as sadness, fear, and shame (Vulnerable Child mode), as well as anger and impulsivity (Angry Child and Impulsive Child modes), and attempts to soothe emotions with substances (Detached Self-Soother mode). However, during the crimes themselves, patients' emotional states were characterized by increased anger and impulsivity, along with overcompensating modes involving aggression (Bully, Attack, and Predator modes). Moreover, these retrospectively assessed modes were significantly associated with different facets of psychopathy on the Psychopathy Checklist—Revised (PCL; Hare, 1991) and predicted future incidents of physical and verbal aggression in the forensic institution (Keulen-de Vos, Bernstein, & Arntz, 2014). These findings support the idea that an escalating sequence of schema modes plays an important role in criminal and aggressive behavior.

### Clinical Trials of Schema Therapy

#### Borderline Personality Disorder

The efficacy of schema therapy in treating BPD has been demonstrated in open trials, randomized clinical trials, and implementation studies. In an initial randomized clinical trial, 84 outpatients with BPD were given therapy twice per week for 3 years—either schema therapy or transference-focused therapy, a psychodynamic treatment—at four clinical centers in The Netherlands. Schema therapy retained a higher proportion of patients for the full duration of treatment (72 vs. 50%) and produced significantly larger reductions in self-harm behaviors and improvements in the personality features of the disorder (e.g., identity disturbance, unstable relationships, abandonment fears) and quality of life. These gains were maintained at 1-year follow-up, with 50% of the patients in the schema therapy condition judged to be recovered from their BPD symptoms and 70% showing clinically significant improvement (Giesen-Bloo et al., 2006). A cost-effectiveness study showed that schema therapy led to net cost savings in terms of days of hospitalization and other medical care and days of unemployment, relative to transference-focused psychotherapy (Van Asselt et al., 2008). In a subsequent implementation study without a control condition, the effectiveness of schema therapy with outpatients with BPD at 12 clinical centers was found to be comparable to that of the original study. Interestingly, Nadort and colleagues (2009) found that patients who were randomized to receive telephone contact with the therapist between sessions did not differ in treatment outcomes from those who did not.

In a study of group therapy for outpatients with BPD in the United States, schema therapy was found to be more effective than treatment as usual, with very large effect sizes after only one and a half years of treatment. Farrell and colleagues (2009) speculated that the delivery of schema therapy in a group format accounts for these strong effects. An international, multicenter randomized clinical trial is now in progress to determine whether these effects of group schema therapy can be replicated.

Recent meta-analyses suggest that schema therapy and mentalization-based therapy have the largest effect sizes for reducing BPD symptoms (Bateman, & Fonagy, 2008). However, clinical trials are needed comparing schema therapy to other major treatment alternatives for BPD (e.g., mentalization-based therapy, dialectical behavior therapy) to compare their effects directly.

### Other PDs

The effectiveness of schema therapy has recently been demonstrated in a multicenter randomized clinical trial of 323 outpatients with AVPD, DPD, OCPD, HPD, NPD, or PPD. Patients were offered 40 sessions plus six booster sessions of once-weekly schema therapy, client-centered therapy, or treatment as usual over a period of 2 years. At 1-year follow-up, schema therapy was found to be significantly more effective than either client-centered therapy or treatment as usual. Because most of the patients in the study had diagnoses of AVPD, DPD, or OCPD, the findings are most conservatively generalized to these mostly internalizing patients (Bamelis et al., 2014).

A structured, cognitive-behavioral form of group schema therapy has also produced significant improvements in symptoms in two open trials with patients with mixed PDs. However, randomized clinical trials of this form of group schema therapy have not yet been reported.

### Forensic Patients

Schema therapy is currently being tested in 103 forensic patients with ASPD, BPD, NPD, or PPD at seven forensic psychiatric hospitals ("TBS clinics") in The Netherlands. Nearly all of the patients are violent offenders with high levels of recidivism risk at the beginning of the study. An unusual feature of this study is that about 50% of the patients have high levels of psychopathy, which many experts consider to be an untreatable condition. The patients were randomly assigned to receive either 3 years of schema therapy or treatment as usual, which at each of these centers is typically a form of CBT. The patients were assessed repeatedly on multiple outcome variables, including recidivism risk, incidents during hospitalization, resocialization (i.e., permission to gradually reenter the community), PD symptoms, early maladaptive schemas, and schema modes. A 3-year posttreatment follow-up study is planned to assess actual recidivism.

Preliminary findings in the first 30 patients to complete the study show that schema therapy is outperforming treatment as usual in terms of retaining more patients in therapy, lowering recidivism risk more rapidly, and speeding patients' progress through the resocialization phase of treatment (Bernstein et al., 2012). Although these findings were not statistically significant in this small, preliminary sample, they have been maintained in reanalyses of the data with larger numbers of patients.

A 7-year case study of the first psychopathic patient to be treated with schema therapy, the patient showed significant reductions in recidivism risk and psychopathic symptoms and improvements in early maladaptive schemas and coping skills. At 3-year posttreatment follow-up, he had not recidivated, was continuously employed, and was living with his wife and their child (Chakhssi, Kersten, De Ruiter, & Bernstein, 2014).

### Summary

Taken together, these findings support the effectiveness of schema therapy for a range of

PDs, including BPD and PDs characterized by both internalizing (e.g., AVPD, DPD, OCPD, eating disorders, mood disorders) and externalizing (e.g., forensic patients with PDs) forms of psychopathology. Schema therapy appears to be particularly effective at retaining patients in treatment, a finding across all studies that is probably attributable to its use of limited reparenting to foster an attachment relationship. It has shown the ability to ameliorate the core personality features of PDs and to reduce the risk of maladaptive behaviors, such as self- and other-directed aggression. There is also evidence that it improves quality of life and is cost-effective, making up for the cost of delivering it by reducing the costs associated with the consequences of PDs. Although most of this evidence is from studies of patients with BPD, the studies of other PDs in general mental health and forensic populations are also quite promising, particularly in light of the limited treatment options for these patients. While further research on schema therapy is needed to replicate and extend these findings, the existing evidence already supports its use with a range of patients with PDs.

**REFERENCES**

Allen, J. G. (2012). *Restoring mentalizing in attachment relationships: Treating trauma with plain old therapy.* Washington, DC: American Psychiatric Publishing.

Arntz, A., Klokman, J., & Sieswerda, S. (2005). An empirical test of the schema mode model of borderline personality disorder. *Journal of Behavior Therapy and Experimental Psychiatry, 36,* 226–239.

Bamelis, L., Evers, S., Spinhoven, P., & Arntz, A. (2014). Results of a multicenter randomized controlled trial of the clinical effectiveness of schema therapy for personality disorders. *American Journal of Psychiatry, 171,* 305–322.

Bamelis, L. L., Renner, F., Heidkamp, D., & Arntz, A. (2011). Extended schema mode conceptualizations for specific personality disorders: An empirical study. *Journal of Personality Disorders, 25*(1), 41–58.

Bateman, A., & Fonagy, P. (2006). *Mentalization-based treatment for borderline personality disorder: A practical guide.* New York: Oxford University Press.

Bateman, A., & Fonagy, P. (2008). 8-year follow-up of patients treated for borderline personality disorder: Mentalization-based treatment versus treatment as usual. *American Journal of Psychiatry, 165,* 631–638.

Beck, A. T. (1979). *Cognitive therapy and the emotional disorders.* New York: International Universities Press.

Bender, D. S., Farber, B. A., & Geller, J. D. (2001). Cluster B personality traits and attachment. *Journal of the American Academy of Psychoanalysis, 29*(4), 551–563.

Bernstein, D. P., Nijman, H., Karos, K., Keulen-de Vos, M. E., de Vogel, V., & Lucker, T. (2012). Treatment of personality disordered offenders in The Netherlands: Initial findings of a multicenter randomized clinical trial on the effectiveness of schema therapy. *International Journal of Forensic Mental Health, 11,* 312–324.

Chakhssi, F., Kersten, G., De Ruiter, C., & Bernstein, D. P. (2014). Treating the untreatable: A single case study of a psychopathic patient treated with schema therapy. *Psychotherapy, 51*(3), 447–461.

Dickhaut, V., & Arntz, A. (2014). Combined group and individual schema therapy for borderline personality disorder: A pilot study. *Journal of Behavior Therapy and Experimental Psychiatry, 45*(2), 242–251.

Farrell, J., Shaw, I., & Webber, M. (2009). A schema-focused approach to group psychotherapy for outpatients with borderline personality disorder: A randomized controlled trial. *Journal of Behavior Therapy and Experimental Psychiatry, 40,* 317–328.

Giesen-Bloo, J., Van Dyck, R., Spinhoven, P., Van Tilburg, W., Dirksen, C., Van Asselt, T., et al. (2006). Outpatient psychotherapy for borderline personality disorder: Randomized trial of schema-focused therapy vs transference-focused psychotherapy. *Archives of General Psychiatry, 63,* 649–658.

Hare, R. D. (1991). *The Hare Psychopathy Checklist—Revised.* Toronto, ON, Canada: Multi-Health Systems.

Hoffart, A., Sexton, H., Hedley, H. M., Wang, C. E., Holthe, H., Haugum, J. A., et al. (2005). The structure of maladaptive schemas: A confirmatory factor analysis and a psychometric evaluation of factor-derived scales. *Cognitive Therapy and Research, 29*(6), 627–644.

Holmes, E. A., & Mathews, A. (2005). Mental imagery and emotion: A special relationship? *Emotion, 5*(4), 489–497.

Holmes, E. A., & Mathews, A. (2010). Mental imagery in emotion and emotional disorders. *Clinical Psychology Review, 30,* 349–362.

Jovev, M., & Jackson, H. J. (2004). Early maladaptive schemas in personality disordered individuals. *Journal of Personality Disorders, 18*(5), 467–478.

Keulen-de Vos, M. E., Bernstein, D. P., & Arntz, A. (2014). Schema therapy for offenders with aggressive personality disorders. In R. C. Tafrate & D. Mitchell (Eds.), *Forensic CBT: A practioner's guide* (pp. 66–83). Chichester, UK: Wiley-Blackwell.

Linehan, M. M. (1993). *Cognitive-behavioral treatment of borderline personality disorder.* New York: Guilford Press.

Lobbestael, J., & Arntz, A. (2010). Emotional, cognitive and physiological correlates of abuse-related stress in borderline and antisocial personality disorder. *Behaviour Research and Therapy, 48,* 116–124.

Lobbestael, J., & Arntz, A. (2012). The state dependency of cognitive schemas in antisocial patients. *Psychiatry Research, 198,* 452–456.

Lobbestael, J., Arntz, A., Löbbes, A., & Cima, M. (2009). A comparative study of patients and therapists' reports of schema modes. *Journal of Behavior Therapy and Experimental Psychiatry, 40*(4), 571–579.

Lobbestael, J., Arntz, A., & Sieswerda, S. (2005). Schema modes and childhood abuse in borderline and antisocial personality disorders. *Journal of Behavior Therapy and Experimental Psychiatry, 36,* 240–253.

Lobbestael, J., Van Vreeswijk, M. F., & Arntz, A. (2008). An empirical test of schema mode conceptualizations in personality disorders. *Behaviour Research and Therapy, 46,* 854–860.

Nadort, M., Arntz, A., Smit, J., Giesen-Bloo, J., Eikelenboom, M., et al. (2009). Implementation of outpatient schema therapy for borderline personality disorder with versus without crisis support by the therapist outside office hours: A randomized trial. *Behaviour Research and Therapy, 47,* 961–973.

Rafaeli, E., Bernstein, D. P., & Young, J. (2011). *Schema therapy: Distinctive features.* New York: Routledge.

Renner, F., van Goor, M., Huibers, M., Arntz, A., Butz, B., & Bernstein, D. P. (2013). Short-term group schema cognitive-behavioral therapy for young adults with personality disorders and personality disorder features: Associations with changes in symptomatic distress, schemas, schema modes and coping styles. *Behaviour Research and Therapy, 51,* 587–492.

Rijkeboer, M. M., Lobbestael, J., Arntz, A., & Van Genderen, H. (2010). *The Schema Coping Inventory.* Utrecht, The Netherlands: Universiteit Utrecht.

Rijkeboer, M. M., Lobbestael, J., Huisman-van Dijk, H. M., Koops, T., Zarbock, G., & Schonebaum, F. (2017). Coping styles mediate the relationship between schemas and schema modes. Manuscript in preparation.

Rijkeboer, M. M., & van den Bergh, H. (2006). Multiple group confirmatory factor analysis of the Young Schema-Questionnaire in a Dutch clinical versus non-clinical population. *Cognitive Therapy and Research, 30*(3), 263–278.

Schmidt, N. B., Joiner, T. E., Young, J. E., & Telch, M. E. (1995). The Schema Questionnaire: Investigation of psychometric properties and the hierarchical structure of a measure of maladaptive schemas. *Cognitive Therapy and Research, 19*(3), 295–321.

Van Asselt, A., Dirksen, C., Arntz, A., Giesen-Bloo, J., van Dyck, R., Spinoven, P., et al. (2008). Out-patient psychotherapy for borderline personality disorder: Cost-effectiveness of schema-focused therapy v. transference-focused psychotherapy. *British Journal of Psychiatry, 192,* 450–457.

Welburn, K., Coristine, M., Dagg, P., Pontefract, A., & Jordan, S. (2002). The Schema Questionnaire—Short Form: Factor analysis and relationship between schemas and symptoms. *Cognitive Therapy and Research, 26*(4), 519–530.

Young, J. E. (1990). *Cognitive therapy for personality disorders: A schema-focused approach.* Sarasota, FL: Professional Resource Exchange.

Young, J. E. (1999). *Young Parenting Inventory (YPI).* New York: Cognitive Therapy Centre.

Young, J. E., Arntz, A., Atkinson, T., Lobbestael, J., Weishaar, M. E., van Vreeswijk, M. F., et al. (2007). *The Schema Mode Inventory.* New York: Schema Therapy Institute. Available at *www.schematherapy.com/id49.htm.*

Young, J. E., & Brown, G. (1994). Young Schema Questionnaire. In J. E. Young (Ed.), *Cognitive therapy for personality disorders: A schema-focused approach* (2nd ed.). Sarasota, FL: Professional Resource Press.

Young, J. E., Klosko, J., & Weishaar, M. (1993). *Reinventing your life.* New York: Dutton Books.

Young, J. E., Klosko, J., & Weishaar, M. (2003). *Schema therapy: A practitioner's guide.* New York: Guilford Press.

# CHAPTER 32

# Transference-Focused Psychotherapy

John F. Clarkin, Nicole Cain, Mark F. Lenzenweger,
and Kenneth N. Levy

Transference-focused psychotherapy (TFP) is a theory driven, manualized, empirically supported treatment for patients with the categorical diagnosis of borderline personality disorder (BPD) and for the broader group of patients with borderline personality organization. Since many treatments are effective with patients with BPD, it is generally accepted that there are important common elements across these treatments and psychotherapeutic treatments in general (Laska, Gurman, & Wampold, 2013). In this chapter, we emphasize those aspects of TFP that go beyond the common therapeutic elements.

## Origins, Scope, and Focus

Object relations theory, deriving from Kleinian, as well as American object relations influences (Jacobson, 1964; Kernberg, 1984; Klein, 1957; Mahler, 1971), posits that the basic human drives and biological systems are always experienced in relation to a specific other, an object. TFP, a treatment approach based on object relations theory for patients with personality disorder (PD) was first manualized in 1999 (Clarkin, Yeomans, & Kernberg, 1999), and with further clinical and research experience we have expanded and refined the treatment (Clarkin, Yeomans, & Kernberg, 2006), and recently explicated the application of principles of treatment with multiple case examples (Yeomans, Clarkin, & Kernberg, 2015).

A major focus in the development of TFP has been on treatment of patients with severe PDs, especially BPD, as described by DSM-III (American Psychiatric Association [APA], 1980) and its successors. However, given the dysfunctions that cut across the PD categories and the resulting rampant comorbidity among these disorders, we have also focused on the aspects of treatment that are relevant across the less severe PDs (Caligor, Kernberg, & Clarkin, 2007). In fact, we have focused equally on the specific categories of PD as defined in DSM-5 (APA, 2013), and are concerned about the severity of key dimensions related to personality pathology that lead to levels of personality organization (neurotic and high- and low-level borderline organization).

## Overview of the TFP Treatment Model

Clinicians across treatment orientations as diverse as cognitive (Pretzer & Beck, 2004), metacognitive (Dimaggio, Semerari, Carcione, Procacci, & Nicolo, 2006), interpersonal (Benjamin, 2003; Cain & Pincus, 2016), attachment (Bateman & Fonagy, 2006; Levy, 2005; Meyer & Pilkonis, 2005), and object relations perspectives (Clarkin, Levy, Lenzenweger, & Kernberg, 2007) emphasize patients' representations of self and others as central to guiding interpersonal behavior. The conceptualizations of mental representations of self and others are variously referred to as cognitive–affective units, schemas, interpersonal copies, internal working models, and internalized object relations dyads, and in process terms such as reflective functioning. These self–other representations constantly appear either explicitly or by implication in therapy exchanges in which patients describe their relationship patterns with others to the therapist, and in patients' descriptions of their feelings and thoughts about the therapist.

In contrast to the general agreement about the centrality of mental representations of self–other and related interpersonal behavior, the manner in which psychotherapeutic treatment addresses these mental cognitive–affective units varies in important ways. Dialectical behavior therapy (DBT; Linehan, 1993) uses a predominantly instructional and cognitive approach to patient skills development. The mentalization-based treatment (MBT; Bateman & Fonagy, 2006) approach emphasizes the need to temper patient affect in therapy sessions. In contrast, the TFP model provides a treatment frame that allows the emergence of affect-driven perceptions of self and others (including the therapist). This model acknowledges the necessity of affect arousal in the sessions to provide a safe opportunity to modify extreme cognitions and related affects in the "hot" and immediate experience of others. This approach is consistent with current understanding of primitive affects and their contribution to numerous forms of psychopathology. As stated by Panksepp and Biven (2012, p. 445) emotion-focused therapeutic approaches are more effective than cognitive-behavioral approaches in promoting more lasting change: "The intense re-experiencing of emotional episodes opens up new treatment possibilities because it provides therapists an emotional 'closeness,' especially within a secure therapeutic alliance, that is optimal for therapeutic change." Key features of the contemporary object relations treatment model, known as TFP, include initial contract setting, a focus on disturbed interpersonal behaviors, both in the patient's current life and in relationship to the therapist, and the use of the process of interpretation (Caligor, Diamond, Yeomans, & Kernberg, 2009).

## Diagnosis, Assessment, and Formulation

The diagnosis of PD, both in general and in terms of specific categories, has undergone an evolution since DSM-III (APA, 1980). PDs in DSM-III were described using criteria that were a mixture of attitudes, emotions, and behaviors, with the clear intent of staying close to phenomenology in order to increase reliability of assessment. This phenomenological approach, admittedly very thin on theory, resulted in the often-noted problems and difficulties of transition from DSM-III to DSM-IV. The problems and shortcomings of the polythetic approach to the diagnosis of supposedly 10 distinct PD categories are largely captured in the excessive heterogeneity within a single specific PD among patients in one diagnostic category (see Lenzenweger, Clarkin, Yeomans, Kernberg, & Levy, 2008) and high levels of "comorbidity" (perhaps best described as co-occurrence or co-variation) across the PD.

In the progression from DSM-IV to DSM-5, there has been a perceptible shift in emphasis from categories of PD to dimensions of dysfunction. The movement behind the generation of DSM-5 was informed by focus on the biological underpinnings of psychiatric disorders suggestive of dysfunction at various levels of severity that span the diagnostic categories (Hyman, 2011). In order to capture domains of dysfunction, the architects of DSM-5 Section III introduced dimensional ratings of self- and other functioning and dimensional trait assessment.

We have long taken the dimensional approach to the specification of the primary domains of dysfunction in PD psychopathology. Our approach to the assessment and diagnosis of PD is consistent with but divergent somewhat from the approach taken by DSM-5 Section III. Based on the structural organizational approach to personality pathology advanced by Kernberg (1984), we have articulated a nosology of personality pathology with a related method of clinical assessment. Object relations theory combines a dimension of severity of pathology with a categorical or prototypical classification of three levels of personality organization (Clarkin et al., 2006; Kernberg & Caligor, 2005) (see Figure 32.1 and Table 32.1). This approach has the advantage of utilizing both the severity of personality pathology (by assessing the dimensions of identity, quality of object relations, defensive operations, social reality testing, aggression, and moral values), and categories of personal-

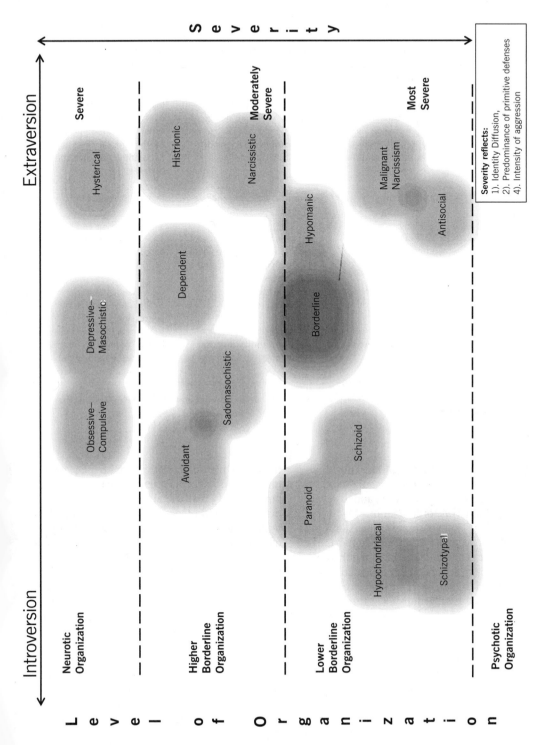

**FIGURE 32.1.** Structural organization of PD psychopathology. From Yeomans, Clarkin, and Kernberg (2015). Copyright © 2015 American Psychiatric Association. Reprinted by permission.

**TABLE 32.1. Dimensions and Categories of Personality Pathology**

| | High-level (neurotic) personality organization | Borderline personality organization | Low-level borderline personality organization |
|---|---|---|---|
| Identity | Investment in productive work or studies; coherent sense of self and others | Variable investment in work; superficial, vague, conflicted sense of self and others | Shifting, variable sense of self; poor sense of others; inability to invest |
| Quality of object relations | Friendships with depth of involvement; capacity for combining romance and sexuality; relationships that are reciprocal and enduring | Friendships are conflicted, at times superficial; intimacy limited by conflicts; views relationships in terms of need fulfillment | Friendships superficial, conflicted, chaotic; superficial attempts at intimacy or lacking; inability to combine romance and sexuality |
| Level of defenses | Advanced defenses | Primitive defenses such as splitting | Primitive defenses |
| Social reality testing | Relative accuracy in perceptions of self and others; accurate mentalization | Variable and at times inaccurate perceptions of self and others; lack of insight in how others see oneself | Variable and inaccurate perception of self and others |
| Aggression | Modulated and integrated anger | Verbal aggression | Verbal and potential physical aggression |
| Moral values | Integrated moral code; moral behavior | Some variability in moral behavior | Defective moral code to amoral; possibility of behavior against the law |

From Yeomans, Clarkin, and Kernberg (2015). Copyright © 2015 American Psychiatric Association. Reprinted with permission. All rights reserved.

ity organization going from high-level personality organization (i.e., neurotic organization), to middle or borderline organization, and to severe or low-level borderline organization.

This typology that combines dimensions and categories has received empirical support. We (Lenzenweger et al., 2008) utilized the theoretical model with an advanced latent structure statistical method known as "finite mixture modeling" to identify subgroups of patients with BPD. Three identified subgroups were characterized by different combinations of paranoid and suspicious orientation to others, aggressive attitudes and behavior, and antisocial behaviors and traits. These results have since been replicated (Hallquist & Pilkonis, 2012; Yun, Stern, Lenzenweger, & Tiersky, 2013), which suggests that the subtypes may be important to guide further efforts to understand underlying endophenotypes and genotypes.

The severity of the personality disorganization is as important as categorical diagnosis to treatment planning. Patients with PDs with a mild (neurotic) level of severity have a complex but generally realistic and accurate representation of self and others that enables them, albeit with some conflicts, to relate realistically to others and moderate their affect in interpersonal relations (see Table 32.1). In contrast, patients at a borderline level of PD severity have a biased internal representation of self and others, which leaves them with difficulties accurately perceiving the intentions of others, and confusion in goal-oriented self-direction. Patients with severe PD at low-level borderline organization not only have "identity diffusion," that is, polarized and distorted perceptions of self and others, but this is also combined with a more aggressive disposition, and minimal internal moral coherence. Treatment planning depends on the severity level of major domains of personality functioning in conjunction with the particular categorical level of personality organization.

## Clinical Assessment

The structural interview (Kernberg, 1984) is a clinical interview that combines a standard psychiatric assessment with an assessment of current personality functioning in order to arrive at a structural diagnosis. The structural interview begins with an exploration of the patient's symptoms and motivation for treatment. In listening to the patient's response to these opening questions, the interviewer develops an impression of the patient's mental state, extent and severity of symptoms, and an indication of the patient's attitude and motivation for treatment. In the assessment of patients with borderline organization, careful evaluation of suicidal and other self-destructive behaviors, eating disorders, substance abuse, and the nature and extent of depression are complicated and have direct implications for treatment selection. The interviewer then shifts the focus to the patient's representations of self, others, and relationship patterns with others. This process is informative in the evaluation of the presence or absence of identity consolidation or identity diffusion. Throughout the interview, the clinician is interested not only in the content of the patient's answers (e.g., patient is depressed, describes self as without intimate relations) but, most importantly, also in the form of the answers and any difficulties in responding that the patient demonstrates. The structural interview does not follow a totally predetermined order. Although the beginning and end are clear, the ways in which the interview develops and the diagnostic elements that become evident are less rigidly established, but depend on what emerges in the patient's self-presentation, and the diagnostician's response to this presentation.

## Semistructured Interview

To assist clinicians in utilizing this interview and ensure reliability for research purposes, the structural interview has been transformed into a semistructured interview, the Structured Interview of Personality Organization (STIPO; Horz, Clarkin, Stern, & Caligor, 2012; Stern et al., 2010), which consists of standardized questions and follow-up probes. As described by object relations theory, six domains of functioning are covered in the STIPO: identity (capacity to invest in work and recreation, sense of self, sense of others), quality of object relations (interpersonal relations, intimate relations and sexuality, internal working models of relationships), primitive defenses, coping and rigidity, aggression (self-directed and other-directed), and moral values.

The clinical usefulness of the STIPO can be compared to that provided by more conventional semistructured interviews of personality pathology such as the Structured Clinical Interview for DSM-IV Axis II (SCID-II), which is an almost literal review of the criteria for each PD that enables one to make a reliable DSM diagnosis (or diagnoses). In contrast, the STIPO provides dimensional ratings of six domains of personality functioning, with an indication of how these areas of functioning are reflected in the individuals' current life circumstances. Scores on these six domains provide a profile of the patient's functioning, with areas of adequate to inadequate functioning. The resulting profile can help the interviewer assess the closeness of the patient to prototypical descriptions of patients at a neurotic, high-, or low-level borderline organization.

## Theoretical Foundations

### Theory of the Disorder

There is growing consensus that the essential features of PD involve difficulties with self-identity and interpersonal dysfunction (Bender & Skodol, 2007; Gunderson & Lyons-Ruth, 2008; Horowitz, 2004; Livesley, 2001; Pincus, 2005). While a rather recent addition to the field via DSM-5 (Section III), this view has long been espoused in object relations theory (Kernberg, 1984). Several aspects of object relations theory contribute to its clinical usefulness. The theory addresses both the internal mental representations of self and other, and the related symptoms and observable behaviors. The theory provides a description of both normal and dysfunctional levels of personality organization. The relative strength and weaknesses across the domains of functioning contribute to tailoring intervention to the individual patient.

A major focus of object relations theory is real-time functioning, especially as the individual interacts with others. This focus on real-time functioning is consistent with advances in social-neurocognitive science (Clarkin & De Panfilis, 2013), and contributes to the understanding of the interpersonal dynamics between patient and therapist in the treatment situation.

Central to the object relations view of personality pathology is the interaction between observable behavior and internal mental structures representing self and others.

## Fundamental Theoretical Constructs

"Personality" is the integration of behavior patterns with their roots in temperament, cognitive capacities, character, and internalized value systems (Kernberg & Caligor, 2005). "Psychological structure" refers to a stable and enduring pattern of mental functions that organize the individual's behavior, perceptions, and subjective experience. "Internalized object relations" are the building blocks of psychological structures, and serve as the organizers of motivation and behavior. Internalized object relations dyads comprise a *representation of the self and a representation of other, linked by an affect* that provides focus and motivation. The internal representations of "self" and the "object" in the dyad are neither assumed to be totally accurate representations of the entirety of the self or the other nor are they totally accurate representations of actual interactions in the past. Rather, they are representations of self and other as they were experienced at specific, affectively charged moments in the past and processed by internal forces such as primary affects, defenses, and fantasies. Individuals with borderline personality organization are minimally aware of contradictory aspects of these representations, especially when they guide their behavior in peak moments of affective arousal.

The individual with a functional and satisfying personality organization operates with an integrated and coherent conception of self and significant others. With normal personality organization, the individual functions with a sense of continuity over time with self-esteem, a capacity to derive pleasure from relationships with others, and from commitments to work. There is a capacity to experience a range of complex and well-modulated affects without the loss of impulse control. A coherent and integrated sense of self contributes to the realization of one's capacities, desires, and long-range goals. Likewise, a coherent and integrated conception of others contributes to relations with others involving a realistic evaluation of others, empathy, and social tact. The healthy individual can "mentalize," that is, understand self and others in terms of intentions, motivations, and emotions. In addition to the ability to mentalize in general, the healthy individual can mentalize under peak affective states, and place momentary affect stimulation and related stimuli into a larger context that helps him or her maintain affect regulation and behavioral control in the moment. The combination of an integrated sense of self and of others contributes to mature interdependence with others, a capacity to make emotional commitments to others, while simultaneously maintaining self-coherence and autonomy.

In contrast, patients with PDs of varying degrees of severity manifest a combination of observable behaviors that are interpersonally disruptive, with internal symbolic representations of self and others that are dominated by extreme conceptions of self and others (i.e., sharp division of good and bad evaluations with extremes of affect; Lenzenweger, McClough, Clarkin, & Kernberg, 2012). The level of personality organization as it relates to the severity of PDs—from normal to neurotic to borderline to psychotic—is largely dependent on the degree of integration of the sense of self and others.

Object relations theory posits, as do the models maintained by many others (Fonagy, 1998; Gunderson & Lyons-Ruth, 2008; Paris, 2005; Zanarini & Frankenburg, 2007), that the combination and interaction of early social influences and genetic vulnerability are important etiological factors in BPD. The destructive effects of early sexual abuse occur in the history of some patients with BPD. However, the additional factors of caregiver neglect, indifference, and empathic failures have profound deleterious effects (Cicchetti, Beeghly, Carlson, & Toth, 1990; Westen, 1993). Children reared in these disturbed environments form insecure attachments with their primary caregivers that interfere with the development of capacities for effortful control and self-regulation. The internalization of conceptions of self and other are compromised by intense negative affect and defensive operations that distort the information system in an attempt to avoid pain and preserve islands of positive affect.

The link between early harsh treatment and later BPD has been confirmed by prospective studies (Carlson, Egeland, & Sroufe, 2009; Crawford, Cohen, Chen, Anglin, & Ehrensaft, 2009). Early maltreatment, maternal hostility, attachment disorganization, and family stress are predictive of social-cognitive difficulties at age 12, including disturbed repesentations of self. These disturbances in early adolescent self-representation were in turn linked to borderline symptoms at age 28. The study of 11,000 pairs of twins followed from birth to age 12 provides a prospective study of the diathesis–stress model of BPD (Belsky et al., 2012). The combination of genetic vulnerability, captured by family history of psychiatric illness, and the experience of early maltreatment was highly predictive of adult BPD status.

## Principles of Change

Prior to addressing the central question of therapeutic intervention and the possibility of change, one must consider the areas of stability in personality functioning, and the forces that contribute to this stability. It is commonly assumed that there is continuity between personality functioning and personality dysfunction. Although early evidence for this view was derived solely from correlational relationships between psychometric measures of normal personality and PD, today we have more integrated theories that posit underlying continuities between the domains of personality and PD using a neurobehavioral framework rooted in neurobiology (Depue & Lenzenweger, 2005; Lenzenweger & Depue, 2016). From this point of view, an empirically supported theory of personality functioning is a necessary foundation for progressing to a comprehensive understanding of personality dysfunction.

There are also other approaches to linking personality to PD (see Lenzenweger & Clarkin, 2005). One approach that we have found useful in considering linkages between normal personality and PD is the cognitive–affective processing model (CAP) of Mischel and Shoda (2008), an integrative model of personality functioning with empirical support. The model has been articulated in an effort to understand both the consistency of personality and the creativity of the individual in the specific situation. Central to this process model are distinct cognitive–affective units that capture an individual's encoding and construal of situations, beliefs about the world, affective tendencies, goals and values, and self-regulatory competencies. These cognitive–affective units are seen as existing in a structured network that mediates between the environmental situation and the individual's behavioral response. This theoretical model is able to capture intraindividual, interindividual, and group differences in personality, making it a compelling model for personality dysfunction.

There are some striking similarities between the CAPS model that grew out of the academic study of personality and personality functioning, and the object relations model that has emanated from the clinical evaluation and treatment of patients with difficulties in personality functioning. Most relevant to the present discussion of treatment of PDs is the central hypothesis of both theories that the mental representations of self and others are central to understanding behavioral consistency within a particular person–environment interaction.

In view of the crucial effects of disturbances in representations of self and other, with related negative effects in patients with borderline personality organization, the focus of TFP is on the systematic examination and eventual change in the self–other representations that the patient brings to the relationship with the therapist and is reflected in his or her current relationships. The goal of TFP is achievement of patient integration, that is, to arrive at representations of self and others that are balanced in the salience of positive and negative cognitions, accompanied by modulated rather than extreme affects, and balanced in terms of cooperative interpersonal behavior with others. This internal state of identity consolidation promotes emotion regulation and contributes to a cooperative, positive relationship with others.

## Principal Intervention Strategies and Methods

Kernberg (2016) has described four intervention strategies that are common to all psychodynamic treatments as interpretation, transference analysis, therapist stance of technical neutrality, and countertransference analysis. TFP is the application of these basic interventions modified specifically for patients with borderline personality organization. The goal of TFP is achieved by therapeutic interventions that are conceptualized as strategies, techniques, and tactics (see Table 32.2). *Strategies* are the overall approaches defining the sequential steps in the process of interpreting object relations that are activated in the transference. They describe the overall intentions of treatment and are best observed over the entire session or blocks of successive sessions. The *techniques* are the interventions used in the moment-to-moment interactions in the session. Finally, the *tactics* of TFP are the maneuvers that the therapist uses to lay the groundwork for using the process of interpretation.

**TABLE 32.2. Strategies, Tactics, and Techniques of TFP**

Strategies

- Defining the dominant object relations
- Observing and interpreting role reversals
- Observing and interpreting linkages between object relations dyads that defend against each other.
- Working through patient's capacity to experience a relationship differently in the transference and in current significant relationships

Tactics

- Negotiating the treatment contract
- Maintaining the frame of the treatment
- Choosing and pursuing priority themes to address in the material the patient is presenting
- Maintaining balance between expanding incompatible views of reality between patient and therapist, and establishing common elements of shared reality
- Regulating the intensity of affective involvement

Techniques

- Interpretive process
- Transference analysis
- Maintenance of technical neutrality
- Use of countertransference

---

Treatment begins with the negotiation of a verbal contract that enables the patient and therapist to create a consistent setting in which the relationships with others and their internal representations can be examined for their lack of reflection, polarized and affect laden extremes, and gaps in understanding. The focus of discussion and change is on the present, the current relationship with the therapist, and the here-and-now condition of the patient's daily life.

*Interpretation* is a major technique imbedded in the overall structure of the treatment. The stereotyped, oversimplified version of insight in a dynamic treatment is that the therapist interprets the patient's behavior, and the patient responds with sudden, astonished understanding and subsequent change in behavior. Nothing could be further from reality, as we describe later. Interpretation is a process carried out over time, titrated to the rise and fall of the patient's affective state, with the goal of expanding the patient's ability to put momentary perceptions of self and others in intense affective states into the larger context of the relationship pattern.

The patient's self and object representations are integrated through a process in which these representations are identified and labeled by the therapist, and traced as they contribute to the patient's experience of interpersonal relationships. When the patient has begun to recognize characteristic patterns of relating, and contradictory self and object images begin to reemerge in the relationship with the therapist, the therapist explores the patient's active effort to keep them separated and disruptive in interpersonal behavior.

## Treatment Relationship

TFP begins with several treatment contracting sessions in which the therapist describes the responsibilities of both therapist and patient if treatment is to be successful. Patient responsibilities include coming to scheduled sessions on time and talking as freely as possible about what is on the patients' mind. Therapist responsibilities include listening intently to the patient, and making comments when appropriate to assist the patient's understanding of self and others. In view of the fact that many patients with BPD are not involved in meaningful work, we have now included in the contracting process negotiation with the patient to obtain some form of work, even if it is voluntary work, to structure his or her day and potentially add to self-definition. In addition to these general aspects of contracting, there are specific ones based on the individual patient's clinical state and history of treatment. These especially involve potential suicidal acts and ways prior treatments have been aborted.

Once the treatment contract has been negotiated and accepted by both parties, the basic stance of a TFP therapist is therapeutic neutrality, that is, to maintain a position that does not join with the forces involved in the patients' internal conflicts. Rather, the TFP therapist fosters the patient's observation and understanding of his or her own conflicts, and allies with the patient's observing self. The careful encouragement by the therapist of the patient's capacity to articulate, observe, and reflect on his or her own conflicts is a major goal of treatment aimed at decreasing reflex action and increasing reflective self-observation.

Technical neutrality is often misunderstood as directing the therapist to be passive and maintain an uncaring, noncommittal attitude toward the patient. On the contrary, the TFP therapist conveys an interest and curiosity in understanding the patient's experience, and an expectation that the patient can change in ways that lead to a more productive and satisfying life. The therapist supports the healthy, self-observing part of the patient. One of the major benefits of treatment is an increase in the patient's ability to observe and reflect on his or her own feelings, thoughts, and behaviors.

The therapist's ability to diagnose, clarify, and interpret the dominant active transference paradigm at each point in the treatment is dependent on maintaining the position as a neutral observer. Since the dissociated affect-laden internal world of patients with BPD is complicated by extreme perceptions and affects, technical neutrality implies an equidistance between self and object representations in mutual conflict. The therapist takes a stance equidistant between mutually split off, all good and all bad, object relations dyads. It is these representations and dyads that become integrated in treatment.

## Process of Treatment

The process of treatment can be seen from the perspective of the progression of treatment interventions, and, in parallel fashion, from the perspective of the sequence of change in patients' behavior both in the sessions and in their everyday life. Of course, these two aspects of the process of the treatment are interactive and depend on each other.

### Process of TFP

The patient comes to treatment with not only a history of disturbed interpersonal relations but also a characteristic information-processing bias that will likely be demonstrated in the relationship with the therapist. TFP structures treatment in order to provide a safe setting in which these biases can be manifested, described in words, explored, understood, and eventually modified. The contracting process is crucial in creating this safe therapeutic space. The contract implies the possibility of a cooperative, productive relationship between two individuals, one who needs help and another who is willing to help. It is possible and very likely, however, that given the information-processing biases the patient brings to a new relationship, disagreement and conflict will arise.

It is the process of interpretation within the structure of the treatment frame that most defines TFP. There are four discernable levels of intervention in the interpretive process (Caligor et al., 2009), even though these are abstract representations of a complex process that is somewhat different with each patient. The first phase is defining the dominant object relations, that is, the implicit perceptions that the patient has of him- or herself in relationship to others, including the therapist. This dominant object relationship often takes the form of victim in the hands of a persecutor. The therapist brings attention to vagueness, omissions, and contradictions in the patient's depiction of self and others in conflict, and this can lead to further affective reactions on the part of the patient. Specific attitudes of the patient toward the therapist emerge, and it is the task of the therapist to put these confused reactions into words. This is done without calling into question the patient's experience. Done well, the statement of the dominant object relationship of patient to therapist helps contain the affect, and the patient feels understood.

The next phase in the interpretive process is observing and identifying role reversals of the object relations dyads exhibited by the patient. If, for example, the patient's perception of victim in the hands of a victimizer later shifts, so that the patient angrily attacks the therapist, the therapist becomes the victim of the verbal attack at the hands of the patient. It is the therapist's role, while maintaining therapeutic neutrality, to point out these instances and help the patient reflect on their meaning. Often, the patient is very aware of feeling like the victim in the hands of others but is not consciously aware of victimizing the other. By pointing out the role reversal, the therapist is introducing a new and different perspective on the patient's experience, inviting the patient to go beyond the immediate, concrete experience, to form cognitive connections between dimensions of experience that have been dissociated. This is a first step in suggesting to the patient that there is a representation of a relationship in his or her mind. This second phase enables the patient to appreciate that his or her transference experience is internal and symbolic, an invitation to the patient to observe the way his or her mind works and how it influences behavior.

In the third phase of interpretation, the connection between two contradictory object relations (typically, idealized and persecutory experiences of self and other) has been defensively dissociated. The therapist invites the patient to observe and reflect on the polarized and contradictory aspects of the experience. In the fourth phase, the therapist provides hypotheses about the meaning of the patient's transference experience.

## Process of Patient Change

There are discernable stages in the TFP treatment of BPD. Following assessment of both diagnostic criteria and level of personality organization, treatment contracting sets the stage for the early treatment phase in which threats to premature dropout, serious and potentially lethal behaviors, and patient criticism of the therapy and the therapist are common. Reduction in out-of-session self-destructive behavior is necessary for the major efforts to shift to understanding the intense underlying conflicted self–other representations that become salient in the therapeutic relationship.

The TFP therapist monitors both the process of the relationship between patient and therapist, and the patient's current ongoing adjustment to the environment. There may be disparities between the two, such as when the sessions are calm and filled with trivial material, and at the same time the patient is engaging in self-destructive behaviors (e.g., fights with supervisor at work, endangering employment) in daily life. A sign of progress in TFP is when the daily life is operating effectively, and the patient's dysfunctional representations of self and other are manifested in a conflicted relationship with the therapist, where they can be actively examined.

The usual progression of change that we have observed clinically is reduction of problem behaviors, followed by the patients' growing recognition of aggressive affects that can be "owned" rather than projected onto others. Gradually, there is a further modification in the representations of self and others, especially as manifested in the transference in the therapeutic relationship, and growing productive involvement in work and relationships in patients' daily lives. The capacity for intimate relationships is often the last domain to develop.

Treatment outcomes are not simple success or failure; rather, they involve a number of domains of functioning, with the possibility of successful change in one domain, with minimal change in another. We have stressed the interaction of observable behavior, organization, and functioning of the mental life of the patient, and underlying neurobiological processing. Given this complexity, change can occur in behavior, with or without change in the underlying organization of identity and moral values. TFP assumes the ambitious goal of not only bringing about symptomatic improvement but also increasing efficiency and satisfaction in work and profession, to help patients develop mature love relations in which eroticism and tenderness are integrated, and to enjoy a rich social life with friendship and social support.

## Summary of Evidence

We have taken a stepwise approach (Kazdin, 2004) to the empirical development of TFP. Development of a treatment manual was based on principles of intervention used by senior clinicians treating patients with BPD. Our approach from the beginning was that a manual that specified exactly the same detailed interventions for all patients would not be practical given the individuality of patients with BPD. Rather, we combined treatment principles with clinical vignettes illustrating the application of the principles across diverse therapeutic situations.

Evaluation of TFP began with an examination of the feasibility of delivering the treatment over 1-year duration and the ability of the treatment to reduce borderline symptomatology (Clarkin et al., 2001). Most subjects ($N = 17$; mean age 32.7 years) had more than one Axis I symptom disorder, and comorbid narcissistic and paranoid PDs were common. The 1-year dropout rate was low (19.1%), there were no suicides, and none of the treatment completers deteriorated or were adversely affected by the treatment. Compared to the year prior to treatment, study patients had significantly fewer psychiatric hospitalizations, fewer days of inpatient hospitalization, and a reduction in the number of suicide attempts.

## Randomized Controlled Trials

Based on these encouraging results we conducted a randomized controlled trial (RCT) that had elements of both efficacy and effectiveness studies. TFP was compared to DBT and a dynamically oriented supportive treatment (Clarkin et al., 2007). Like an efficacy study, patients were randomly assigned to treatments delivered by therapists trained in the respective treatments, with blind raters and reliably measured outcome variables. However, similar to effectiveness studies, patients with BPD with a range of severity were treated by community therapists in their own offices, and medication was prescribed by a study psychiatrist without standardized type or amount.

In view of the diversity of the patients with BPD and the different emphases of the three treatments, six domains of dysfunction were measured for change, with suicidality, aggression, and impulsivity as primary outcome domains, and anxiety, depression, and social functioning as secondary outcome domains. Individual growth curve analysis (Lenzenweger, Johnson, & Willett, 2004) was used to investigate change in the dimensions of symptoms and functioning over time. All three treatments showed significant change across multiple domains after 1 year of treatment, but some differences emerged among treatments. Both TFP and DBT were associated with improvement in suicidality. Only TFP was significantly associated with improvement in Barratt Factor 2 impulsivity, irritability, and verbal and direct assault. TFP had a broader scope of change: Significant change occurred in 10 of 12 variables across the six domains, in contrast to five of 12 variables for DBT, and six of 12 variables for supportive treatment.

In addition to symptom change, we hypothesized that TFP, with its therapeutic focus on perceptions of self and other, would result in changes in attachment organization and reflective functioning (RF; Levy et al., 2006). Patients receiving TFP improved significantly in narrative coherence on the Adult Attachment Interview (AAI), unlike those receiving other treatments. We also examined the influence of the three treatments on RF, the capacity to understand the behavior of oneself and others in terms of intentional mental states such as thoughts, feelings, and beliefs. As predicted, RF increased significantly in patients receiving TFT, whereas no change occurred with the other treatments.

The next step was to evaluate the effectiveness of TFP in a different cultural setting. Doering and colleagues (2010) conducted a two-site (Munich, Germany, and Vienna, Austria) RCT with efficacy and effectiveness components. Female patients with BPD ($N = 104$) were randomized to 1 year of either TFP or treatment by community therapists experienced in the treatment of BPD. The TFP psychotherapy group was significantly superior with regard to the number of DSM-IV BPD criteria at the end of treatment, with improvement in psychosocial functioning, reduction in suicide attempts, and number and duration of inpatient treatments during the 1-year treatment and number of premature dropouts (67.3 vs. 38.5%). In addition, patients in TFP showed superior improvement over the comparison group in personality organization and functioning.

### Empirically Derived Trajectories of Change

Using a subsample of the patients in the original RCT (Clarkin et al., 2007), we examined the domains of function as they changed across a treatment duration of 1 year (Lenzenweger, Clarkin, Levy, Yeomans, & Kernberg, 2012). Rather than focusing on endpoint/follow-up outcomes that do not capture the dynamic process of change, we examined baseline psychological predictors as they related to rates of change (i.e., change in variables measured multiple times on each patient during the course of 1 year of treatment) across domains of functioning. Selection of potential *predictors* of change was based on a neurobehavioral model (Depue & Lenzenweger, 2005), and an object relations model (Kernberg & Caligor, 2005) of severe personality pathology.

A principal component analysis (PCA) on the rate of change for 11 different dimensional measures of domains of change yielded three factors of change: aggressive dyscontrol, psychosocial adjustment (global functioning and social adjustment), and conflict tolerance (anxiety/depression and impulsivity). These results indicate that different areas of functioning and symptomatology change at different rates, and certain sets of variables change at the same rate (i.e., as a domain).

We examined the relations between baseline characteristics (predictors) and scores for each of the three domains of change. Lower pretreatment levels of negative affect and aggression were associated with more rapid clinical improvement in the domain of aggressive dyscontrol. Higher pretreatment identity diffusion was associated with more rapid clinical improvement in the global functioning domain. Lower initial levels of social potency were associated with more rapid improvement in anxiety/depression and impulsivity.

### Neurocognitive Functioning as a Measure of Change

Psychotherapy research will advance as the mechanisms of change become the target of intervention at both the psychological level

(Kazdin, 2007) and at the level of neural functioning (Insel & Gogtay, 2014). The hypothesized mechanism of change for BPD in TFP is increased affect regulation achieved through mentalization, that is, the ability of the patient to put momentary affect arousal, especially in social interactions, into a more benign and broader context (Levy et al., 2006). We hypothesized that as the patient experiences dominant object relations infused with negative and intense affect in the TFP sessions, the gradual analysis of the perception of self and others would modify the extreme cognitive–affective perceptions. These changes would be consistent with enhanced modification of responses in the amygdala by the prefrontal cortex.

In our preliminary neuroimaging study of TFP,[1] we used an emotional linguistic go/no-go task to investigate the processing of negative stimuli by female patients with BPD prior to and after a 1-year treatment episode with TFP. The aim of the study was to identify links between the phenomenology and neurocognitive/neurobiological domains underpinning BPD pathology before and after 1 year of TFP. Patients ($N = 10$) met the DSM criteria for BPD and, in addition, had an indication of affective dysregulation as manifested by high negative affect, low positive affect, and low constraint on the Multidimensional Personality Questionnaire (MPQ). Measures of psychological functioning at multiple points during the 1 year of treatment were combined with assessment of neurocognitive functioning pre- and posttreatment.

In terms of psychological functioning, the patients exhibited significant change over the course of 1 year of TFP, including reductions in affective lability, interpersonal sensitivity, and paranoia. They reported less intrusive and vindictive interpersonal problems and displayed overall higher levels of interpersonal warmth toward others. Importantly, at the end of 1 year of treatment, all patients in the study were employed, with significant changes in work functioning.

In a comparison of pretreatment and posttreatment functional magnetic resonance imaging (fMRI) scans, patients with BPD manifested a relative increase in activation in cognitive control regions (right anterior dorsal anterior cingulate cortex [ACC], dorsolateral prefrontal cortex [DLPFC], and frontopolar cortex [FPC]). Relative activation decreases were found in left ventrolateral PFC and hypocampus. These results demonstrated activation increases in emotion and cognitive control areas and relative decreases in areas associated with emotional reactivity and semantic-based memory retrieval. TFP may, in fact, mediate clinical symptom improvement in part by improving cognitive emotional control via increased engagement of dorsal ACC, posterior medial orbitofrontal cortex (OFC), FPC, and DLPFC activity. The effects of TFP may be mediated by top-down frontal control over limbic emotional reactivity and semantic memory processing systems. These results are consistent with those of other investigators (Goodman et al., 2014; Schnell & Herpertz, 2007) who have demonstrated the impact of DBT treatment programs for patients with BPD on neural functioning, consistent with an increase in emotion regulation.

## Conclusion

The PD field is in the interesting situation of having treatments informed by different theories of personality disordered functioning, all of which show significant improvement for patients' symptoms, but with no significant differences in outcome between them (Levy, Ellison, & Khalsa, 2012), and little effect on patients' functional level in work and intimate relations (see McMain, Guimond, Streiner, Cardish, & Links, 2012). In this context, Bateman (2012) has called for an increasingly coherent theory of PD that can be translated into an understanding of mechanisms of change that, in turn, could inform a precise treatment program. Future research may explicate which patients with specific domains of dysfunction would optimally respond to one of the available treatments. In addition, this matching of optimal treatment to specific patient may depend on research isolating the mechanisms of change in the various treatments across specific domains of functioning that involve the integration of neurocognitive functioning, internal subjective states of mind, and observable behavior. In the meantime, we suggest that TFP is a developed methodology for utilizing the patient–therapist

---

[1] The imaging and treatment of patients in TFP was done at Weill Cornell Medical College, New York City, Principal Investigator (P.I.) John Clarkin. The processing of the imaging data was done by David Silbersweig and his neuroimaging laboratory at Brigham and Women's/Faulkner Hospitals, Boston.

relationship in the exploration and change of patients' mental representations of self and other as they guide interpersonal behavior. Experience gained from the TFP methodology can be used in a total treatment approach or be integrated with other approaches in the treatment of patients with BPD (Clarkin, Yeomans, De Panfilis, & Levy, 2016).

## REFERENCES

American Psychiatric Association. (1980). *Diagnostic and statistical manual of mental disorders* (3rd ed.). Washington, DC: Author.

American Psychiatric Association. (2013). *Diagnostic and statistical manual of mental disorders* (5th ed.). Arlington, VA: Author.

Bateman, A. (2012). Treating borderline personality disorder in clinical practice. *American Journal of Psychiatry, 169,* 560–563.

Bateman, A., & Fonagy, P. (2006). *Mentalization-based treatment for borderline personality disorder.* Oxford, UK: Oxford University Press.

Belsky, D. W., Caspi, A., Aarseneault, L., Bleidorn. W, Fonagy, P., Goodman, M., et al. (2012). Etiological features of borderline personality related characteristics in a birth cohort of 12-year-old children. *Development and Psychopathology, 24,* 251–265.

Bender, D. S., & Skodol, A. E. (2007). Borderline personality as self-other representational disturbance. *Journal of Personality Disorders, 21,* 500–517.

Benjamin, L. S. (2003). *Interpersonal reconstructive therapy: An integrative personality-based treatment for complex cases.* New York: Guilford Press.

Cain, N. M., & Pincus, A. L. (2016). Treating maladaptive interpersonal signatures. In W. J. Livesley, G. S., Dimaggio, & J. F. Clarkin (Eds.), *Integrated treatment of personality disorder: A modular approach* (pp. 305–324). New York: Guilford Press.

Caligor, E., Diamond, D., Yeomans, F. E., & Kernberg, O. F. (2009). The interpretive process in the psychoanalytic psychotherapy of borderline personality disorder. *Journal of the American Psychoanalytic Association, 57,* 271–301.

Caligor, E., Kernberg, O. F., & Clarkin, J. F. (2007). *Handbook of dynamic psychotherapy for higher level personality pathology.* Washington, DC: American Psychiatric Publishing.

Carlson, E. A., Egeland, B., & Sroufe, L. A. (2009). A prospective investigation of the development of borderline personality symptoms. *Development and Psychopathology, 21*(4), 1311–1334.

Cicchetti, D., Beeghly, M., Carlson, V., & Toth, S. (1990). The emergence of the self in atypical populations. In D. Cicchetti & M. Beeghly (Eds.), *The self in transition: Infancy to childhood* (pp. 309–344). Chicago: University of Chicago Press.

Clarkin, J. F., & De Panfilis, C. (2013). Developing conceptualization of borderline personality disorder. *Journal of Nervous and Mental Disease, 201,* 88–93.

Clarkin, J. F., Foelsch, P. A., Levy, K. N., Hull, J. W., Delaney, J. C., & Kernberg, O. F. (2001). The development of a psychodynamic treatment for patients with borderline personality disorder: A preliminary study of behavioral change. *Journal of Personality Disorders, 15,* 487–495.

Clarkin, J. F., Levy, K. N., Lenzenweger, M. F., & Kernberg, O. F. (2007). Evaluating three treatments for borderline personality disorder: A multiwave study. *American Journal of Psychiatry, 164,* 922–928.

Clarkin, J. F., Yeomans, F., De Panfilis, C., & Levy, K. N. (2016). Strategies for constructing an adaptive self-system. In W. J. Livesley, G. Dimaggio, & J. F. Clarkin (Eds.), *Integrated treatment for personality disorders: A modular approach* (pp. 397–418). New York: Guilford Press.

Clarkin, J. F., Yeomans, F. E., & Kernberg, O. F. (1999). *Psychotherapy for borderline personality.* New York: Wiley.

Clarkin, J. F., Yeomans, F. E., & Kernberg, O. F. (2006). *Psychotherapy for borderline disorder: Focusing on object relations.* Washington, DC: American Psychiatric Publishing.

Crawford, T. N., Cohen, P. R., Chen, H., Anglin, D. M., & Ehrensaft, M. (2009). Early maternal separation and the trajectory of borderline personality disorder symptoms. *Development and Psychopathology, 21*(3), 1013–1030.

Depue, R. A., & Lenzenweger, M. F. (2005). A neurobehavioral model of personality disturbance. In M. F. Lenzenweger & J. F. Clarkin (Eds.), *Major theories of personality disorder* (2nd ed., pp. 391–453). New York: Guilford Press.

Dimaggio, G., Semerari, A., Carcione, A., Procacci, M., & Nicolo, G. (2006). Toward a model of self psychology underlying personality disorders: Narratives, metacognition, interpersonal cycles and decision-making processes. *Journal of Personality Disorders, 20,* 597–617.

Doering, S., Horz, S., Rentrop, M., Fischer-Kern, M., Schuster, P., Benecke, C., et al. (2010). Transference-focused psychotherapy v. treatment by community psychotherapists for borderline personality disorder: Randomized controlled trial. *British Journal of Psychiatry, 196,* 389–395.

Fonagy, P. (1998). Moments of change in psychoanalytic theory: Discussion of a new theory of psychic change. *Infant Mental Health Journal, 19*(3), 346–353.

Goodman, M., Carpenter, D., Tang, C., Goldstein, K., Avedon, J., Fernandez, N., et al. (2014). Dialectical behavior therapy alters emotion regulation and amygdala activity in patients with borderline personality disorder. *Journal of Psychiatric Research, 57,* 108–116.

Gunderson, J. G., & Lyons-Ruth, K. (2008). BPD's interpersonal hypersensitivity phenotype. *Journal of Personality Disorders, 22,* 22–41.

Hallquist, M. N., & Pilkonis, P. A. (2012). Refining the phenotype of borderline personality disorder: Diagnostic criteria and beyond. *Journal of Personality Disorders, 3,* 228–246.

Horowitz, L. M. (2004). *Interpersonal foundations of psychopathology.* Washington, DC: American Psychological Association.

Horz, S., Clarkin, J. F., Stern, B. L., & Caligor, E. (2012). The Structured Interview of Personality Organization (STIPO): An instrument to assess severity and change of personality pathology. In R. A. Levy, J. S. Ablon, & H. Kachele (Eds.), *Psychodynamic psychotherapy research: Evidence-based practice and practice-based evidence* (pp. 571–592). New York: Springer.

Hyman, S. E. (2011). Diagnosis of mental disorders in light of modern genetics. In D. Regier, W. Narrow, E. Kuhl, & D. Kupfer (Eds.), *The conceptual evolution of DSM-5* (pp. 3–18). Washington, DC: American Psychiatric Publishing.

Insel, T. R., & Gogtay, N. (2014). National Institute of Mental Health clinical trials: New opportunities, new expectations. *JAMA Psychiatry, 71,* 745–746.

Jacobson, E. (1964). *The self and the object world.* New York: International Universities Press.

Kazdin, A. E. (2004). Psychotherapy for children and adolescents. In M. J. Lambert (Ed.), *Bergin and Garfield's handbook of psychotherapy and behavior change* (5th ed., pp. 543–589). New York: Wiley.

Kazdin, A. E. (2007). Mediators and mechanisms of change in psychotherapy research. *Annual Review of Clinical Psychology, 3,* 1–27.

Kernberg, O. F. (1984). *Severe personality disorders: Psychotherapeutic strategies.* New Haven, CT: Yale University Press.

Kernberg, O. F. (2016). The basic components of psychoanalytic technique and derived psychoanalytic psychotherapies. *World Psychiatry, 15*(3), 287–288.

Kernberg, O. F., & Caligor, E. (2005). A psychoanalytic theory of personality disorders. In M. Lenzenweger & J. F. Clarkin (Eds.), *Major theories of personality disorder* (2nd ed., pp. 114–156). New York: Guilford Press.

Klein, M. (1957). *Envy and gratitude, a study of unconscious sources.* New York: Basic Books.

Laska, K. M., Gurman, A. S., & Wampold, B. E. (2014). Expanding the lens of evidence-based practice in psychotherapy: A common factors perspective. *Psychotherapy, 51*(4), 467–481.

Lenzenweger, M. F., & Clarkin, J. F. (Eds.). (2005). *Major theories of personality disorder* (2nd ed.). New York: Guilford Press.

Lenzenweger, M. F., Clarkin, J. F., Levy, K. N., Yeomans, F. E., & Kernberg, O. F. (2012). Predicting domains and rates of change in borderline personality disorder. *Personality Disorders: Theory, Research, and Treatment, 3,* 185–195.

Lenzenweger, M. F., Clarkin, J. F., Yeomans, F. E., Kernberg, O. F., & Levy, K. N. (2008). Refining the borderline personality disorder phenotype through finite mixture modeling: Implications for classification. *Journal of Personality Disorders, 22,* 313–331.

Lenzenweger, M. F., & Depue, R. A. (2016). Toward a developmental psychopathology of personality disturbance: A neurobehavioral dimensional model incorporating genetic, environmental, and epigenetic factors. In D. Cicchetti (Ed.), *Developmental psychopathology* (Vol. 3, pp. 1079–1110). New York: Wiley.

Lenzenweger, M. F., Johnson, M. D., & Willett, J. B. (2004). Individual growth curve analysis illuminates stability and change in personality disorder features: The longitudinal study of personality disorders. *Archives of General Psychiatry, 61,* 1015–1024.

Lenzenweger, M. F., McClough, J. F., Clarkin, J. F., & Kernberg, O. F. (2012). Exploring the interface of neurobehaviorally linked personality dimensions and personality organization in borderline personality disorder: The Multidimensional Personality Questionnaire and Inventory of Personality Organization. *Journal of Personality Disorders, 26,* 902–918.

Levy, K. N. (2005). The implications of attachment theory and research for understanding borderline personality disorder. *Development and Psychopathology, 17,* 959–986.

Levy, K. N., Ellison, W. D., & Khalsa, S. (2012, September). *Psychotherapy for borderline personality disorder: A multi-level menta-analysis and meta-regression.* Presented at the annual meeting of the European Society for the Study of Personality Disorders, Amsterdam, The Netherlands.

Levy, K. N., Meehan, K., Kelly, K., Reynoso, J., Weber, M., Clarkin, J. F., et al. (2006). Change in attachment patterns and reflective function in a randomized control trial of transference-focused psychotherapy for borderline personality disorder. *Journal of Consulting and Clinical Psychology, 74,* 1027–1040.

Linehan, M. M. (1993). *Cognitive-behavioral treatment of borderline personality disorder.* New York: Guilford Press.

Livesley, W. J. (2001). Conceptual and taxonomic issues. In W. J. Livesley (Ed.), *Handbook of personality disorders: Theory, research, and treatment* (pp. 3–38). New York: Guilford Press.

Mahler, M. (1971). A study of the separation–individuation process and its possible application to borderline phenomena in the psychoanalytic situation. *Psychoanalytic Study of the Child, 26,* 403–424.

McMain, S. F., Guimond, T., Streiner, D., Cardish, R. J., & Links, P. S. (2012). Dialectical behavior therapy compared with general psychiatric management for borderline personality disorder: Clinical outcomes and functioning over a 2-year follow-up. *American Journal of Psychiatry, 169,* 650–661.

Meyer, B., & Pilkonis, P. A. (2005). An attachment model of personality disorders. In M. F. Lenzenweger & J. F. Clarkin (Eds.), *Major theories of personality disorder* (2nd ed., pp. 231–281). New York: Guilford Press.

Mischel, W., & Shoda, Y. (2008). Toward a unified

theory of personality: Integrating dispositions and processing dynamics within the cognitive-affective processing system. In O. P. John, R. W. Robins, & L. A. Pervin (Eds.), *Handbook of personality: Theory and research* (3rd ed., pp. 208–241). New York: Guilford Press.

Panksepp, J., & Biven, L. (2012). *The archaeology of mind: Neuroevolutionary origins of human emotions.* New York: Norton.

Paris, J. (2005). Recent advances in the treatment of borderline personality disorder. *Canadian Journal of Psychiatry, 50*(8), 435–441.

Pincus, A. L. (2005). A contemporary integrative interpersonal theory of personality disorders. In M. F. Lenzenweger & J. F. Clarkin (Eds.), *Major theories of personality disorder* (2nd ed., pp. 282–331). New York: Guilford Press.

Pretzer, J. L., & Beck, A. T. (2005). A cognitive theory of personality disorders. In M. F. Lenzenweger & J. F. Clarkin (Eds.), *Major theories of personality disorder* (2nd ed., pp. 43–113). New York: Guilford Press.

Schnell, K., & Herpertz, S. C. (2007). Effects of dialectic-behavioral-therapy on the neural correlates of affective hyperarousal in borderline personality disorder. *Journal of Psychiatric Research, 41,* 837–847.

Stern, B. L., Caligor, E., Clarkin, J., Critchfield, C., Horz, S., Maccornack, V., et al. (2010). Structured Interview of Personality Organization (STIPO): Preliminary psychometrics in a clinical sample. *Journal of Personality Assessment, 92,* 35–44.

Westen, D. (1993). The impact of sexual abuse on self-structure. In *Rochester Symposium on Developmental Psychopathology: Disorders and dysfunctions of the self* (Vol. 5, pp. 223–250). Rochester, NY: University of Rochester Press.

Yeomans, F., Clarkin, J. F., & Kernberg, O. F. (2015). *Transference-focused psychotherapy for borderline personality disorder: A clinician's guide.* Washington, DC: American Psychiatric Publishing.

Yun, R. J., Stern, B. L., Lenzenweger, M. F., & Tiersky, L. A. (2013). Refining personality disorders subtypes and classification using finite mixture modeling. *Journal of Personality Disorders, 4,* 121–128.

Zanarini, M. C., & Frankenburg, F. R. (2007). The essential nature of borderline psychopathology. *Journal of Personality Disorders, 21,* 518–535.

# CHAPTER 33

# Systems Training for Emotional Predictability and Problem Solving

Nancee Blum, Donald W. Black, and Don St. John

Systems Training for Emotional Predictability and Problem Solving (STEPPS) is a manualized, cognitive-behavioral, skills-based group treatment program developed for adult outpatient clients with borderline personality disorder (BPD). The 20-week program combines psychoeducation and skills training with a systems component that is unique to STEPPS and provides members of the client's system, including family members, friends, and key professionals, with an understanding of the STEPPS approach and a common language to communicate clearly about BPD and the skills needed to manage symptoms.

Data show that STEPPS is effective and superior to treatment as usual in reducing symptoms (Black et al., 2008; Blum et al., 2008; Blum, Bartels, St. John, & Pfohl, 2002; Boccalon et al., 2012; Bos, van Wel, Appelo, & Verbraak, 2010; Freije et al., 2002; Harvey et al., 2010; van Wel et al., 2009). Surveys of patients and therapists showed high levels of acceptance (Blum, Pfohl, St. John, Monahan, & Black, 2002; Freije, Dietz, & Appelo, 2002). The manual has been adapted for the United Kingdom (Blum, Bartels, St. John, & Pfohl, 2009) and The Netherlands (van Wel et al., 2006). German, Dutch, and Italian translations are available, and a Spanish translation is in progress. STEPPS has been adapted for adolescents (Blum, Bartels, St. John, Pfohl, & Sussex NHS Foundation Trust, 2014). STEPPS has been implemented successfully in multiple settings, including residential treatment facilities, day treatment programs, and forensic settings (prisons and community corrections). The program is designated as an evidence-based treatment by the U.S. Substance Abuse and Mental Health Services Administration and listed on the National Registry for Evidence-Based Programs and Practices (www.nrepp.samhsa.gov).

The program was started in 1995 to meet the needs of ambulatory patients with BPD. Few programs were available, and traditional modes of therapy did not reduce deliberate self-harm, acting-out behaviors, or hospitalization rates. At that time, dialectical behavior therapy (DBT) was the only empirically supported treatment model available (Linehan, Armstrong, Suarez, Allmon, & Heard, 1991; Linehan, Heard, & Armstrong, 1993; Linehan, Tupek, Heard, & Armstrong, 1994), but its implementation was difficult in our setting and other outlying clinics: The 1-year treatment with weekly individual and group sessions was not feasible in rural states, where many patients live far away from mental health clinics and attendance is particularly difficult in winter months. We believed that a shorter and less labor-intensive program would be more appropriate. Since STEPPS was developed, other manualized treatments have become available, such as transference-focused therapy (Yeomans, Clarkin, & Kernberg, 2002) and mentalization-based therapy (Bateman & Fonagy, 1999, 2001, 2008), but we thought that they would also be difficult to implement in our setting.

After reviewing existing models, we chose to modify a program originally developed by Bartels and Crotty (1992). The theoretical orientation, systems approach, and actual content developed by Bartels and Crotty is fully incorporated into and expanded in the STEPPS manual. Although the psychoeducational approach suited our training and interests, we concluded that the length of the program and the manual required modification. Its *systems* approach was appealing: This involved teaching emotion regulation and behavioral skills to the patient and those in his or her system (i.e., persons with whom the patient regularly interacts and shares information about BPD). Members of the system are referred to as the "reinforcement team" and include family members, friends, and key professional care providers.

The program was lengthened from 12 weeks to 20 (22 weeks, if an optional screening session and a lesson specific to holiday stress are included), and specific client agendas were developed, including an increased use of algorithmic worksheets for specific situations clients might encounter. Detailed weekly lesson guidelines were also developed for group facilitators. The program has two phases—the basic 20-week skills group referred to as STEPPS (one 2-hour group meeting per week) and a twice-monthly advanced program called STAIRWAYS, which we describe later. STEPPS employs general psychotherapy principles and techniques, so it is readily used by therapists from varying educational and professional backgrounds, requiring little additional training. The program is intended to improve the effectiveness of the patient's ongoing treatment, which typically includes individual psychotherapy, pharmacotherapy, and case management. Patients are not required to drop their current therapist and adopt a specifically trained STEPPS therapist. We believe this is especially difficult for patients who have difficulty developing trust, and who experience feelings of abandonment (Gunderson, 1996) when asked to cut ties with existing supports.

## Theoretical Foundations

STEPPS builds on principles of cognitive-behavioral therapy (CBT) known to be effective in patients with BPD, including identifying and challenging distorted thoughts and specific behavioral change, combined with elements of schema-focused therapy (Beck, Freeman, & Davis, 2004; Young, 1994; Young, Klosko, & Weishaar, 2003). The systems approach was integrated to include the patient's social and professional support system, and to train both the patient and those in his or her system to respond more consistently and effectively using the STEPPS "language." The systems approach derives from family systems theory, which assumes that changing a system involves the whole family because family members tend to act in ways that maintain the status quo, even when it is dysfunctional. Minuchin (1974) developed structural family therapy to deal with dysfunctional family structures through education, behavioral techniques, and other directive approaches. STEPPS incorporates a workbook, materials to be shared with others in the support system, pocket-size skills cards, and other materials that are learning tools for both the client and his or her support system.

STEPPS assumes that the core deficit in BPD is the inability to regulate and manage emotional intensity. As a result, patients are frequently overwhelmed by intense emotional upheavals that drive them to seek relief through self-harm, impulsive and reckless behaviors, or substance misuse. The childhood history of individuals with BPD frequently includes inconsistent emotional support or even abuse by primary caregivers. This often leads therapists to focus treatment on identifying someone to "blame" for the disorder, an approach we believe is unproductive. Individuals with BPD do not consciously choose to have this disorder and, with rare exceptions, parents and other important caregivers do not consciously choose to create an abusive, inconsistent, and unsupportive childhood environment (Blum, Bartels, et al., 2002; Blum, Bartels, St. John, & Pfohl, 2012).

Providing education about BPD allows reinforcement team members to strengthen and support patients' newly learned skills and manage the tendency of persons with BPD to use "splitting" (i.e., externalizing their internal conflict by drawing others around them into taking sides against each other). Splitting, like other behaviors associated with BPD, is viewed not as an intentional act of aggression but as a learned or automatic response to the emotional intensity.

When patients enter treatment, they often view the term "borderline personality disorder" as pejorative and resist the diagnosis, while readily acknowledging its symptoms—more than one patient has asked, "What border am I on?" Bartels and Crotty (1992) suggested the term "emotional intensity disorder" (EID). Where the term "disorder" carries cultural stigma, EID has been translated to *emotional intensity difficulties*. EID may be easier for patients to accept, and it provides a more accurate description of their experiences. BPD and EID are used interchangeably throughout the manual. Regardless of terminology, there are advantages to reframing the client's understanding of BPD as a clinical disorder. Attention is diverted from a diagnostic term (BPD) that clients cannot change to a focus on learning skills to decrease the level of emotional intensity that produces problematic thoughts and behaviors that they can change. We encourage patients to see themselves as driven by BPD/EID to seek relief from painful emotions through desperate behaviors reinforced by negative and distorted thinking, both of which they can learn to change and master. One patient wrote in response to learning about her diagnosis, "I no longer think of BPD as a crippling diagnosis. Rather, I get to see the world from a greater perspective of joy, a deeper sadness of pain, a stronger emotion of anger, and a deeper sense of compassion. . . . Despite my many emotions about this illness, I now see life as an adventure to be lived rather than just survived."

## Systems Approach

The person entering therapy is often enmeshed in a system of unhealthy relationships that reinforce and support dysfunctional behavior even when friends and significant others are well intentioned. For example, the person experiencing a cognitive distortion that others dislike him or her may become irritated and behave in ways that turn the distortion into reality. This new reality serves to reinforce the cognitive distortions and maladaptive behavior that result.

Beginning with the first session, patients identify and use the previously described "reinforcement team," whose members agree to assist the patient in learning new skills. Patients are encouraged to enlist nonprofessionals, as well as professional care providers. The systems perspective emphasizes patients' responsibility for responding to their system more effectively and helps them to develop more realistic expectations of their support system. This also reduces the tendency to focus on seeking support from one individual (e.g., their individual therapist), who runs the risk of being alternately overidealized and devalued. For clients receiving individual therapy, we ask the therapist to support the program by reviewing the workbook materials provided to the client each week.

Patients are expected to become STEPPS experts and to teach their reinforcement team how to respond appropriately to them and their needs. They are encouraged to share what they learn in group and share appropriate handouts. Patients receive "Reinforcement Team" cards with specific instructions for team members about how to respond when contacted by the patient. The cards help to establish more consistent interactions between the patient and his or her support system by providing a common language. A 2-hour evening meeting is held for reinforcement team members, usually between Weeks 4 and 8 to help them to understand BPD, the format of STEPPS, and the language used to understand patient problems. Group members also attend this meeting to avoid the concern that the session is for reinforcement team members to "vent" frustrations and complaints about them. Reinforcement team members are instructed that their role is to reinforce and support the use of the skills taught in STEPPS. This empowers reinforcement team members to make more consistent and neutral responses, and to avoid the temptation to solve problems for, or provide therapy to, the patient. The central message is that the primary goal is on the *process* of reminding clients to use their STEPPS skills to reduce emotional intensity rather than on trying to respond to clients' perceptions of the event or situation that created the emotional intensity, which are usually distorted by their level of emotional reactivity. Reinforcement team members are instructed in how to use the cards that list the skills taught in STEPPS and specific questions to ask when contacted by the participant (e.g., "Where are you on the emotional intensity continuum?"; "Have you used your notebook?"; "What skill can you use in this situation?"; "How will you use it?"). Hearing the same consistent response from all members of the reinforcement team often decreases patients' emotional intensity. The ability to give a consistent and emotionally neutral response to patients may also decrease the emotional intensity of family members and others, who are often called on repeatedly to respond to the patient's perceived crises.

## Components of the STEPPS Program

STEPPS has three main components: (1) awareness of illness, (2) emotion management skills training, and (3) behavior management skills training. The number of lessons and a brief description of the content of each component are described below.

### Awareness of Illness Component

This component (Weeks 1 and 2) addresses misconceptions about the BPD label and increases awareness of the thought patterns, feelings, and behaviors that define the disorder (i.e., identifying these as symptoms of BPD/EID). Patients have often received numerous diagnoses in the past and are often confused about the term BPD. Patients frequently express relief that what they experience actually "has a name—BPD," and this diagnostic term applies to a group of patients similar to themselves; before they came into the room, they often believed they were the only ones. Through psychoeducation, patients learn that thoughts and behaviors can be changed, and feelings can be tolerated and managed. Patients often believe that they are fatally flawed, for which they may alternately blame themselves or others, and that they deserve to suffer. The ability to consider BPD to be treatable and that they can learn specific skills to help manage its consequences is an important precursor to change. If patients are firmly convinced that their lives will improve only if others change, or that they cannot learn the skills to manage the symptoms of their disorder (even in the absence of intellectual limitations), they may not be ready for STEPPS.

Patients are given a handout with the DSM-5 criteria for BPD and encouraged to provide examples of their own behavior that illustrate these criteria ("owning" the disorder). The second lesson introduces the idea of cognitive or thought filters, which is easier for patients to understand than the usual term of "schemas" (Young, 1999). Patients identify their dominant cognitive filters by completing a shortened version of Young's Schema Questionnaire, and learn that these long-held and long-practiced thought patterns about themselves, the world, and others have led to negative and distorted thoughts, feelings, and behaviors. STEPPS focuses on helping patients to identify their thought patterns and on learning skills to challenge the negative, unhelpful filters, and replace them with more positive and helpful thought patterns.

### Emotion Management Skills Training

This component teaches five basic skills (distancing, communicating, challenging, distracting, and managing problems) that help the person with BPD manage both the cognitive and emotional symptoms of the disorder. These skills help participants to predict the pattern of an emotional episode, anticipate stressful situations that may lead to increased emotional intensity with impulsive and/or self-destructive behaviors, and assist them in developing confidence in their ability to manage the illness. These five emotion management skills form the basic vocabulary for responding to the emotional intensity episodes, which we describe briefly.

*Distancing* (Week 3) involves noticing and acknowledging the increasing emotional intensity and describing its components (feelings, thoughts, and behaviors), then "taking a step back." This can be done with a physical action (e.g., moving to a different room) or a mental action (e.g., choosing to focus on a calming image or object, using deep breathing). In the session on distancing, a specific activity involves making a collage from pleasant images that clients cut from magazines and that can be carried in their STEPPS binder or folder, or put up on the wall where it is easily accessible. Beginning with Lesson 3, each session begins with a relaxation exercise, such as progressive muscle relaxation, visualization, and a variety of focusing activities, each starting with mindfulness breathing (a list of suggested relaxation exercises is included in the guidelines for the group leaders).

*Communicating* (Weeks 4 and 5) is described as "putting words on" the emotions that are experienced and also expanding participants' vocabularies. Clients often have a limited vocabulary, such as *sad, mad, glad*. One of the worksheets in this lesson asks the client to describe a list of emotions in a variety of ways, such as using a different word, a color, a sound, a physical sensation, an experience, and/or an action urge. The group setting is very helpful in stimulating responses for individuals who might have difficulty responding without helpful ideas from others in the group. The emotional intensity continuum (EIC) is introduced as part of this skill and is described as part of the group format of STEPPS.

*Challenging* (Weeks 6, 7, 8) teaches the STEPPS participant to recognize distorted and negative thoughts, and through the worksheets and homework assignments, to replace them with more rational and neutral or positive ones that are less likely to generate emotional intensity. As this skill develops, clients move away from their typical "all-or-nothing" perception of other people and situations.

*Distracting* (Weeks 9 and 10) gives individuals the opportunity to create a list of distracting activities to use during times of emotional intensity to allow time to pass until that intensity decreases. They work on prioritizing the list, and the five easiest or most accessible activities are written on a small card that they can carry (i.e., making the skills "portable"). Clients often have the expectation that someone outside of them (e.g., their therapist) will "rescue" them or direct them in how to respond to a situation. The ultimate goal of STEPPS is for persons with BPD/EID to recognize increasing emotional intensity and use their skills to manage the intensity on their own (or with only an occasional reminder from a member of their reinforcement team).

*Managing Problems* (Weeks 11 and 12) allows the client to state more clearly the problem and desired solution. This skill requires practice in generating alternative responses and evaluating the potential consequences of each response, narrowing the possible responses, and choosing to implement the best one. An event/ episode management worksheet guides clients through the process of identifying the advantages and disadvantages of a given response, resources that might be needed, and obstacles that might prevent the implementation of that response. They receive management worksheets to use through the remainder of the lessons.

### Behavior Management Skills Training

This component focuses on learning and relearning patterns of managing functional areas (e.g., eating, sleeping), and on keeping these areas under control during emotionally intense episodes. These eight behavioral skills (goal setting, eating, sleeping, exercise, leisure, physical health, abuse avoidance, and interpersonal relationships) are described briefly below. With BPD, disruptive interplay often occurs between emotionally intense episodes and the individual's social environment, which becomes increasingly nonempathic and unresponsive, leading many of these behavioral areas to break down. There is often a vicious cycle in which the functional behaviors deteriorate during times of emotional intensity, which leads to even greater emotional reactivity that further impacts the functional areas. For example, an emotional intensity episode may disrupt the patient's sleep pattern which in turn leads to greater inability to manage emotional intensity, which further disrupts sleep, and so forth. The patient completes a behavior questionnaire to assess and rank the severity of his or her problems in the previously mentioned areas.

*Introduction to Behavior Management* (Week 13) begins with a 40-item questionnaire that covers problematic lifestyle behaviors (eating, sleeping, exercise, etc.). This allows patients to see and rank specific areas of difficulty. Each patient chooses a specific problematic behavior (not necessarily the one that ranked highest in difficulty) and applies the goal-setting paradigm taught in Week 14.

*Goal Setting* (Week 14) teaches a systematic approach to identifying a main goal (chosen from the problem area identified in Week 13), listing specific subgoals, action steps, needed resources and possible obstacles, and progress monitoring forms. The patient works on this behavior and progress is monitored during the remaining weeks. The purpose of this lesson is to teach the *process* of setting a goal, which can then be applied to a variety of behavioral areas.

*Eating and Sleeping* (Week 15) presents information about healthy and unhealthy eating behaviors, helps patients identify on the emotional intensity continuum the level(s) at which eating difficulties occur, and asks patients to complete a food diary for the week. Information about healthy sleep behaviors and a sleep monitoring form are included in this lesson.

*Exercise, Leisure, and Physical Health Behaviors* (Week 16) identifies the primary benefits of various kinds of exercise (e.g., aerobic, strength, endurance), expanding the patient's repertoire of leisure activities and physical health behaviors (e.g., relationship with health care providers, adherence to recommendations, examining expectations about medication).

*Abuse Avoidance* (Week 17) applies skills to harmful behaviors (e.g., self-harm, self-destructive acts), using worksheets to clarify the pattern of thoughts, feelings, and behaviors, as well as how to ask for help. Information about relapse prevention is included in this lesson.

*Relationship Behaviors* (Weeks 18 and 19) provides practice in using STEPPS skills to increase interpersonal effectiveness and understanding appropriate relationship boundaries.

*Wrapping Up* (Week 20) celebrates the completion of STEPPS, and includes comparing the results of their current filter (schema) questionnaire to the one completed in Week 2, and evaluation of group content, format, and experience.

Several of the emotion management skills take more than one session to complete. In the behavior management section, some skills are combined into one session (e.g., eating and sleeping) to allow the program to be completed in 20 weekly sessions. In some settings, the length and frequency of the individual sessions are adjusted to the intellectual and/or functional level of group participants or the facility's schedule (e.g., residential treatment, forensic settings). For example, in a residential facility, it may be desirable to have two 1-hour sessions per week, and offer an optional weekly session for those who need help completing their homework. We are aware of a residential facility that offers a full year for those with lower intellectual functioning to complete the program. The program content is not changed, but each lesson may be broken into shorter segments. For those who have difficulty reading, a staff member or another resident can help the individual between sessions. This also allows facility staff members to become more familiar with STEPPS and how to reinforce what the resident is learning.

## Format of STEPPS

The suggested format in outpatient settings is a weekly, 2-hour classroom experience with two therapists and six to 10 patients. Patients receive a binder for their materials that they are asked to bring to each session. They are encouraged to share both the binder and the lesson materials with others in their system. The binders are considered resources to turn to in difficult times. STEPPS sessions have the feeling and look of a seminar or class, with clients at a table facing a board. Lesson concepts are facilitated by poetry, song recordings, art activities, and relaxation exercises. Suggested auxiliary materials and resources are listed in the facilitator guidelines for each lesson. Patients are encouraged to bring in materials, poems, or artwork they have created to reinforce the themes of the particular lesson.

## Structure of Sessions

Patients begin each session by completing the 15-item Borderline Evaluation of Severity over Time (BEST) scale to rate the intensity of their thoughts, feelings, and behaviors over the past week. This self-report instrument was developed for the STEPPS program to rate DSM-IV symptoms specific to BPD (Blum, Pfohl, et al., 2002; Pfohl, Blum, McCormick, St. John, & Black, 2009). The first draft of the BEST listed DSM-IV symptoms and asked patients to rate the amount of difficulty each had caused in the previous week (difficulty was rated on a scale from 1 to 5, with 1 being *little or no difficulty* and 5 being *extreme difficulty*). However, simply assigning a number to a criterion does not allow patients to separate thoughts and feelings from actual behaviors (e.g., patients may think about self-harming but not actually perform a self-harming act). Consequently, the final version of the BEST has three sections: (1) thoughts and feelings, (2) negative behaviors (e.g., substance abuse, self-harming behaviors, not attending therapy appointments), and (3) positive behaviors (e.g., keeping therapy appointments, choosing a positive behavior). By graphing BEST scores weekly, patients observe how symptom severity varies over time. They are also able to observe how the decreased frequency and intensity of emotional episodes relates to the increased use of the emotion management and behavior management skills. BEST scores also allow patients to monitor fluctuations in suicidal feelings and self-abuse urges, and behaviors, emotional intensity, and negative behaviors (e.g., substance abuse, abnormal eating behavior). It also allows them to monitor positive behaviors such as choosing a positive activity, keeping therapy appointments, and so forth, and how these are related to emotionality. After completing the BEST, a brief relaxation exercise follows. A variety of techniques are used so clients can find the ones that work best for them.

During the first few weeks, BEST scores are usually erratic but they start to fall after about 6 weeks. By the end of the 20 weeks, scores typically decrease significantly and fall within a much tighter range. In the first session, group leaders explain this to patients and "normalize" this as reflecting the erratic nature of BPD. This idea is further reinforced when patients read an essay contributed by a former STEPPS attendee, who describes her experience with the program and provides encouragement to those who are starting STEPPS.

Beginning with Week 4, the EIC scale is introduced and patients are asked to complete it daily by rating their emotional intensity on a scale from 1 to 5 (1—*feeling calm and relaxed*, 5—*feeling out of control*). They are also asked to summarize the percent of time spent at each level during the week. The scale allows patients to track changes over time and achieve a more balanced view of themselves—many are surprised by how much time that they are not at level 5. The EIC is also used to identify thoughts, feelings, maladaptive cognitive filters (schemas), physical sensations, action urges, and behaviors associated with each level of intensity.

By using the EIC consistently, patients become more adept at predicting the course of an emotional episode and anticipating situations that lead to destructive responses. The original EIC worksheet used weather symbols as metaphors represent their level of distress (1—sun shining, 2—partly cloudy, 3—cloud with rain, 4—dark cloud with thunder and lightning, 5—tornado). As STEPPS was disseminated to different geographic areas, we learned the tornado was not a universal metaphor. A volcano was suggested by another group. One STEPPS participant observed that she "had no more control over the weather than over her emotional intensity," and suggested pots on a stove (1—no heat under the pot, 2—some heat, 3—water starting to boil, 4—boiling harder, 5—boiling over). This has been adopted for subsequent groups, although all three designs are included in the manual. Finally, a skills monitoring card asks patients to indicate which skills they used in the previous week. The homework assignment is reviewed and the remainder of the session is devoted to the material for the current lesson.

Patients respond well to this structured approach. On one occasion when a group leader was delayed unexpectedly for 20 minutes, she arrived to discover the group had appointed one member to act as leader and the group was well into reviewing the EIC for each participant. We now invite a volunteer to review the EICs after the program has been running for four or five weeks. Patients often request to lead this portion of the group the following week. At other times, patients volunteer to lead the relaxation exercise. This helps patients acquire a greater feeling of competency about using the program themselves, helping others in the group, and disseminating information about the skills to reinforcement team members. It avoids the common perception that the professional group leader "has all the answers."

During a session, patients may try to reframe their emotional experience as the result of a personal or interpersonal problem. Although there are opportunities to respond to and share experiences relevant to the skills being taught, the structure of the STEPPS model does not allow the group to spend long periods of time focusing on a given group member who is experiencing a crisis. One effect of this is modeling how to acknowledge problems and offer support, yet impose reasonable limits on the scope of the interaction. Group facilitators are trained to reframe problems in the context of the disorder and its filters. Patients are reminded to "focus on the disorder, not the content."

One of our patients, a 19-year-old woman, reported the benefits she had gained from STEPPS: "STEPPS has made so many positive changes in my life. For the first time, I'm starting to figure out who I am. The biggest thing is that I am not angry all the time. I'm learning to deal with the big things in life and let the little trivial things slide, instead of everything making me angry. I'm learning to live all over again with a new set of rules for myself. Sometimes it's hard, but the new rules make my life a hell of a lot easier." She also stated that prior to STEPPS, she did not know there were "trivial things."

## Selection of Participants

### Referral

Some patients learn about STEPPS from previous participants and request the program, but we recommend a professional referral, which can serve as a screening tool. Although patients need not meet full criteria for BPD to enter a group, Van Wel and colleagues (2006) reported that persons with borderline traits who do not meet full criteria were more likely to drop out. Once 20–30 potential participants have been identified, they are invited to attend the next group to learn more about the program. By screening in a group context, facilitators may be able to more accurately assess the patient's ability to participate appropriately and share time with others in a group setting. In our experience, one-fourth to one-third of potential participants respond to the invitation, and one or two of them will not attend. Patients are asked to drop out with the option of joining a later group if they miss three consecutive sessions for reasons other than illness or bad weather.

### Selection and Assessment

It is preferable for clinicians to screen potential participants using a formal assessment. We also encourage clinicians to review information from referral sources. The STEPPS manual includes an optional Introductory/Intake Session that may be offered to prospective participants. Some settings require mandatory attendance at this session before a patient is admitted to a group. This allows a group member to experience a typical session (including a homework assignment, which must be completed and brought to the first lesson of the regular group) to see whether he or she is still interested in the full program. Another important aspect of assessment is an evaluation of the patient's ability to share time with others and to limit discussion of his or her own problems to the elements that serve the goals of STEPPS. The person's capacity for these attributes may often be gauged by his or her ability to allow the facilitator to direct discussion during the introductory screening. Those who cannot either focus on issues introduced by the facilitator or accept redirection may not be appropriate.

### Typical Group Composition

After the initial introductory session, approximately 12–14 prospective members are invited and typically eight to 12 of them actually join the group. It is common for one to three patients to drop out of the group, usually in the first 3 weeks. Some may ask to rejoin a future group when they feel more prepared to stay the course. Often each group includes one or two person who have attended a prior STEPPS group; some patients who have completed a group want to attend a new group to further consolidate their skills. This is useful to newcomers because it demonstrates hope and provides early leadership to the group.

### Exclusion

Individuals who are extremely narcissistic may not be suitable. Members must have some capacity to appreciate that others have problems and view them as equally serious or disturbing even though he or she may see those problems as different than or less challenging than his or her own. A key requirement is the ability to accept that another person's perception may differ from his or her own but nevertheless have validity. Ongoing substance misuse is counterproductive, and patients are asked to seek appropriate substance use disorder treatment either before attending STEPPS or concurrently. Similarly, those with severe eating disorder behaviors should be in an appropriate treatment program. Patients are instructed to inform those providers of their participation in STEPPS and are encouraged to share their materials. Furthermore, individuals who respond to conflict with physical threats or intimidation are not suitable because they are potential threats to the integrity of a group. This might be observed in patients with marked antisocial traits. That said, many STEPPS participants with mild antisocial traits have benefited from the program and did not disrupt the group process (Blum, St. John, et al., 2008).

An aggressive man may be threatening to women in the group. Some settings have separate groups for men and women. In a mixed-gender group, having at least two men increases the chance they will have sufficient common experiences to provide support for one another and reduce the perception that a single man represents the opinions and feelings of all men. Members are cautiously encouraged to use one another as reinforcement team members between sessions, once they feel safe in the group. They are encouraged to use the suggested responses on the skills card they give to their reinforcement team members.

### Group Facilitators

We recommend two group facilitators, both for practical reasons (if one facilitator is away, the group does not have to be canceled) and to reduce the tendency of persons with BPD to alternately overidealize and devalue individuals.

Group leaders should have graduate-level training in the social sciences and psychotherapy experience that includes cognitive-behavioral techniques. Facilitators are generally trained during a 2-day onsite workshop, with a provision for further Web-based (e.g., Skype) consultation or supervision, if desired. Further information about training may be obtained from one of the authors (N. B.). It is helpful (but not essential) to have a man and a woman as group leaders because this allows them to model relationship behaviors between genders. A male co-facilitator may also provide a healthy male role model and support male participants, who are usually in the minority. To maintain clear professional boundaries during sessions, facilitators do not sit at the table with participants; one is typically standing at the board and the other may be sitting to the side. In early sessions, facilitators are active and directive (e.g., handing out materials, writing patients' responses to the homework assignment on the whiteboard, or responding to patients' comments or questions by referring those issues to the others in the group for input). The level of facilitator activity decreases over time as patients gradually assume leadership by writing on the board and leading reviews of the EIC.

The primary tasks of facilitators are to maintain a psychoeducational format, adhere to facilitator guidelines, avoid involvement in individual issues and past traumas (i.e., avoid doing individual psychotherapy in a group setting), maintain focus on skills acquisition rather than content, encourage group cohesiveness, and facilitate participants' change of perspective from victims of BPD/EID to experts on managing their BPD symptoms. It is important that all members are treated similarly. Consequently, we suggest that facilitators avoid seeing group members individually unless there is a preexisting therapeutic relationship. In this case, patients are reminded (as part of the overall group guidelines reviewed in the first session) that issues discussed in individual therapy will not be discussed in the group sessions, unless the patient refers to an issue in the context of applying a STEPPS skill.

Facilitators should also avoid focusing on one patient's problems without generalizing them to the group and asking the group for assistance. The group should be involved in helping the patient use the skills being taught to avoid the therapist becoming "the expert" who is expected to resolve all issues. Facilitators must curb their tendency to respond to the expressed problems (i.e., content) and focus on the symptoms of BPD that drive the client's emotional responses.

Crises are common in patients with BPD and may easily derail the group process if not attended to appropriately. Crises are acknowledged and then managed by focusing attention on using skills (e.g., use of a crisis as an example of using the skill being taught in that session). Patients are referred to their individual therapist for long-standing personal issues. Individuals in imminent danger of self-harm or who are suicidal are removed from the group and referred to a professional reinforcement team member or emergency personnel. The referral is made quickly to avoid disrupting the group and the perception of special treatment. Otherwise, self-harm thoughts or behaviors are treated as unhelpful behaviors to be addressed using the skills being taught. A group facilitator observed, "I now look at patients with BPD differently and interact in a different way. I feel more competent to help them when they are in a crisis. My main response now is to listen, talk with them about how intense their feelings are, and ask what skills they can (and will) use to decrease the intensity."

Near the end of the group, usually at about Week 17, patients may express anxiety about the program ending and losing the weekly support of peers and leaders. Group leaders work to minimize the impact of these concerns by encouraging patients to continue using their reinforcement team. From the beginning, patients are encouraged to view STEPPS as a time-limited program to use their existing support system more effectively rather than viewing the program as a replacement for that system.

Patients receive information about options after STEPPS, which may include continuing with their current treatment (e.g., individual psychotherapy, pharmacotherapy, and case management), repeating STEPPS, or joining STAIRWAYS (described below). During STEPPS, some patients may resist homework assignments but eventually realize the benefits of practicing the skills (through homework or encouragement from other group members) when noticing improvement in other patients motivates them to engage in STEPPS with greater participation. Those who continue to have difficulty understanding or applying the skills may be encouraged (by the group leaders or another professional care provider) to repeat

STEPPS. This is reframed as "going through at a higher level" to avoid the perception of failing the group. Some patients ask to repeat a STEPPS group months to years later, to improve or refresh their skills.

## STAIRWAYS

STAIRWAYS is a 1-year follow-up group that meets twice a month. It consists of stand-alone modules to develop additional skills: **S**etting goals, **T**rying new things (goals like furthering education, employment), **A**nger management, **I**mpulsivity control, **R**elationship management (emphasis on conflict management), **W**riting a script (preparing for future stressors), **A**ssertiveness training, **Y**our choices (making healthy choices), and **S**taying on track (maintaining recovery and relapse prevention). STAIRWAYS follows a format similar to that of STEPPS. Participants continue to use previously learned skills to facilitate learning and applying new ones.

Once a STEPPS group begins, no additional patients are admitted because each skill builds on the previously learned ones. In STAIRWAYS, each module (some modules take two or three sessions) is discrete; clients who complete STEPPS and join STAIRWAYS receive an introductory packet of materials, then join at the beginning of any new module and stay in the program until they complete all the modules. In some settings, patients may attend repeated cycles of STAIRWAYS as an "aftercare" program or request to repeat sessions dealing with a particular skill when it is being offered. Each clinic or agency establishes its own policies in regard to repeating either STEPPS or STAIRWAYS.

## Case Vignette

"Cathy," a divorced woman in her late mid-40s, was referred after expressing suicidality during evaluation in another department. This was her first hospitalization at our hospital, although she had a long history of psychiatric treatment and more than 25 hospitalizations, beginning in her late teens. She had numerous past diagnoses, including attention-deficit/hyperactivity disorder (ADHD), bipolar disorder (sometimes Type I, other times Type II), alcohol dependence and abuse, and pathological gambling. Despite multiple examples of behavior patterns that met more than the required number of criteria for BPD, treatment records and her self-report did not mention BPD except for a notation of "borderline traits" from a recent hospitalization. Cathy estimated that she had spent 3–4 months per year in the hospital for the last 20 years.

She believed that frequent moves and changing schools during childhood fueled feelings of abandonment that were a recurrent theme in her adult life. She dated the onset of her problems to age 7 or 8, when she developed problems with anger control, such as putting her foot through a wall and picking on other children. She was disruptive in the classroom, could not sit still, and had learning problems. At age 10, she was seen by a psychologist who diagnosed ADHD, although her mother disputed the diagnosis, explaining that, at home, Cathy could read an entire book and put challenging picture puzzles together. Cathy's physician prescribed methylphenidate, and Cathy thought that this was the origin of her belief that solutions to her problems would come from external sources, including medication and health professionals.

She made the first of her estimated 25+ suicide attempts at age 10 by overdosing on the methylphenidate. Many of her attempts were described as gestures, but there were at least 6 serious attempts, one of which resulted in numerous fractures that led to chronic pain and difficulty walking. She began drinking alcohol at age 12, and continued using alcohol into her 20s, when she was jailed for public intoxication. Subsequently, she joined Alcoholics Anonymous (AA) and had been abstinent for more than 25 years. Gambling problems led to illegal behaviors including embezzlement, writing bad checks, and stealing money. She described relationships as stormy and unstable, initially viewing the person as flawless, and just as quickly becoming disillusioned. She often ended relationships because she believed the other person was preparing to leave her.

Cathy had a very limited response to a variety of medications. Antidepressants improved energy but also increased the risk of acting on suicidal thoughts. Mood stabilizers seemed to temper hypomanic episodes but not her daily mood swings.

Cathy showed many features of BPD, including sensitivity to abandonment, stormy relationships, impulsivity, suicidal gestures, affective instability, and anger dyscontrol. She also had symptoms suggesting additional diagnoses of major depression, bipolar disorder Type II, intermittent explosive disorder, alcohol dependence, pathological gambling, ADHD, and antisocial personality disorder, although BPD was considered the primary diagnosis.

Following discharge from the inpatient unit, Cathy was initially referred for individual therapy in the outpatient clinic and subsequently enrolled in STEPPS. The initial focus of individual therapy educated Cathy about BPD because this was the first time she had heard of the diagnosis. Her response was "This is the first diagnosis that really seems to fit." Her STEPPS-based therapy focused on accepting the reality of her symptoms and learning specific emotion management and behavior skills for dealing with them. This allowed a cognitive shift that took her beyond the futility of trying to assign blame to herself, others, or past events.

Cathy was seen for individual therapy every 2 weeks to reinforce what she was learning in STEPPS and help her to apply these skills in daily life. She used the EIC on a daily basis to monitor symptom severity and increase awareness of thoughts, feelings, cognitive filters, urges, and behaviors related to each level of severity. This allowed her to apply skills more effectively, leading to a decrease in time spent at Levels 4 and 5, at which destructive behaviors were most likely to occur.

Cathy worked on anger control and impulsivity by using *distancing* to notice the increase in emotional intensity and then "stepping back" by talking to a reinforcement team member, going to another room, or taking a drive. She became more adept at *communicating* her feelings and thoughts accurately, then used *challenging* to replace her distorted thoughts with more rational ones. She had several *distracting* activities (baking, needlework, and drawing) to decrease her emotional intensity. This allowed her to define the problem, identify the desired solution, consider a range of alternative responses, and evaluate the likely consequences of each response (*managing problems* skill).

She credited the *eating behavior skills* for helping her stop binge-eating episodes. Cathy attended weekly AA meetings and a gambling treatment group in her local community. She considered the group facilitator a member of her reinforcement team and stated, "I brought her my materials and taught her because she was unfamiliar with the program." Cathy was in a 2-year relationship with a man she described as a reinforcement team member "to a certain extent"; she was able to accept that his limited ability was due to his own health problems.

Cathy periodically discontinued her medications, sometimes due to financial problems, but at other times because of anger toward her physician or other professionals. One of her behavioral goals was to be more adherent to her medication regimen; she did this by making a chart to give herself a "gold star" sticker each day that she took her medications. She then took her charts to the individual therapy sessions and shared them with the STEPPS group members, who gave her positive feedback and also encouraged another group member with a similar goal. The *physical health skills* section helped her achieve a more realistic view of what her health care providers and medications could do. She observed, "My medications are like my crutches. They help, but they are not the fix-it answer." She achieved better control of her diabetes, and improved her relationships with health care providers.

Following STEPPS, Cathy completed STAIRWAYS. Individual sessions decreased to once a month or less, but she would e-mail periodically between appointments to "check in" and share some of her new activities (e.g., teaching a Sunday school class). She continued to attend AA meetings but stopped attending the gambling support group: Her gambling behaviors were limited to buying one lottery ticket per week for the past several years.

Cathy's hospitalizations decreased from 3–4 months a year to a total of 21 days in the 5 years after starting STEPPS. She saw an individual therapist once a month or less in her local community after STAIRWAYS. When the therapist moved, Cathy said, "I will miss her, but I know she is not abandoning me and I am not devastated." She has not been hospitalized for 16 years. She continues periodically to experience suicidal thoughts but states, "Now I know that is my disorder talking and not how I really feel or want to react."

Cathy has not been in regular treatment or taken psychotropic medications for 12 years. Two or three times per year, she e-mails to let us know how she is doing. She occasionally has symptoms of major depression and hypomania but feels she can manage these episodes with her emotion management and behavior skills. Cathy's mother told us that "Cathy is a totally different person since STEPPS. She is now responsible and accountable, and she is no longer impulsive."

## Summary of Evidence

The results of both uncontrolled and controlled studies consistently show that STEPPS leads to overall improvement, with specific improvement in many BPD symptom domains. A retrospective study of 52 patients (Blum, Pfohl, et al., 2002) showed significant improvement in BPD symptoms as measured by the BEST (Pfohl et al., 2009) and (Blum et al 2002) a significant decrease in depressive symptoms and negative affect. Similar results were obtained in a prospective study of women offenders (Black et al., 2008), and a larger study of 77 men and women (Black, Blum, & Allen, 2013). Additionally, in the latter study, offenders participating in STEPPS had fewer disciplinary infractions and suicidal behaviors.

In an early study from Holland, Freije and colleagues (2002) reported on 85 patients enrolled in STEPPS groups. Significant improvement was seen in ratings of anxiety, depression, and interpersonal sensitivity, and in BPD symptoms assessed using a Dutch version of the BEST. Both this study and that of Blum, Pfohl, and colleagues (2002) showed that patients and therapists were enthusiastic about the program and reported high levels of acceptance. A more recent study from the United Kingdom (Harvey, Black, & Blum, 2010) reported similar findings.

Randomized controlled trials of STEPPS and treatment as usual have been conducted in the United States and Holland. The Dutch study (van Wel et al., 2009) of 83 participants showed that those assigned to STEPPS experienced a greater reduction in BPD symptoms and greater improvement in mood. The U.S. study based on 124 participants (Blum et al., 2008), showed a similar reduction in BPD symptoms, improved mood, and fewer emergency department visits in participants assigned to STEPPS. Both studies concluded that STEPPS leads to broad-based improvements in the affective, cognitive, impulsive, and disturbed relationship domains, and that it also has a robust antidepressant effect. In the U.S. study, a 1-year follow-up showed no deterioration in these areas, and improvements were maintained.

## Conclusions

In most practice settings, STEPPS is utilized as one component of the overall outpatient treatment program that includes individual therapy, medication management as appropriate, and other individual or group treatment programs where indicated (e.g., substance abuse treatment, vocational rehabilitation).

This training approach has been adapted successfully for a variety of treatment settings, (e.g., inpatient units, residential facilities, substance abuse treatment, and correctional settings, including prisons and community corrections; Black et al., 2008, 2013; Black & Blum, 2011). On inpatient units, where the typical length of stay is a few days, the awareness of illness component may be used to assess the client's suitability for the full STEPPS program and to prepare the client to enter such a program. Boccalon and colleagues (2012, 2014) described its implementation on an Italian inpatient unit. Colleagues in the United Kingdom have adapted STEPPS for older adolescents (Blum et al., 2014; Harvey, Blum, Black, Burgess, & Henley-Cragg, 2014). The program length has been shortened to 18 weeks and includes a teaching component for parents and caregivers, who attend a separate weekly group at the same time as the adolescents. The program may be suitable for younger adolescents in some settings, and may be helpful in school settings in the future. A shorter, 13-week program consisting of three modules has been developed for use in the primary care settings (Blum et al., 2016).

In summary, STEPPS is a manual-based, short-term group therapy for the treatment of BPD. STEPPS combines cognitive-behavioral techniques and a systems component. The program was developed to augment, though not interrupt, a patient's current treatment regimen. STEPPS is relatively easy to learn and use, and it has been well accepted in a variety of settings.

## REFERENCES

Bartels, N., & Crotty, T. (1992). *A systems approach to treatment: The borderline personality disorder skill training manual.* Winfield, IL: EID Treatment Systems.

Bateman, A., & Fonagy, P. (1999). Effectiveness of partial hospitalization in the treatment of borderline personality disorder: A randomized controlled trial. *American Journal of Psychiatry, 15,* 1563–1569.

Bateman, A., & Fonagy, P. (2001). Treatment of borderline personality disorder with psychoanalytically oriented partial hospitalization: An 18-month follow-up. *American Journal of Psychiatry, 158,* 36–42.

Bateman, A., & Fonagy, P. (2008). Eight-year follow-up of clients treated for borderline personality disorder: Mentalization-based treatment versus treatment as usual. *American Journal of Psychiatry, 165,* 631–638.

Beck, A. T., Freeman, A., & Davis, D. D. (2004). *Cognitive therapy of personality disorders* (2nd ed.). New York: Guilford Press.

Black, D. W., & Blum, N. (2011, December). Taking STEPPS to address borderline personality disorder. *Corrections Today.*

Black, D. W., Blum, N., & Allen, J. (2013). STEPPS treatment in borderline offenders. *Journal of Nervous and Mental Diseases, 201,* 1–6.

Black, D. W., Blum, N., Eichinger, L., McCormick, B., Allen, J., & Sieleni, B. (2008). STEPPS: Systems Training for Emotional Predictability and Problem Solving in women offenders with borderline personality disorder in prison—a pilot study. *CNS Spectrums, 13,* 881–886.

Blum, N. S., Bartels, N. E., St. John, D., & Pfohl, B. (2002). *Systems Training for Emotional Predictability and Problem Solving Group Treatment Program for Borderline Personality Disorder.* Coralville, IA: Level One Publishing (Blums Books). Available at www.steppsforbpd.com.

Blum, N. S., Bartels, N. E., St. John, D., & Pfohl, B. (2009). *Systems Training for Emotional Predictability and Problem Solving (STEPPS UK): Group treatment program for borderline personality disorder.* Iowa City, IA: Level One Publishing (Blums Books). Available at www.steppsforbpd.com.

Blum, N. S., Bartels, N. E., St. John, D., & Pfohl, B. (2012). *Systems Training for Emotional Predictability and Problem Solving (Second Edition): Group treatment program for borderline personality disorder.* Iowa City, IA: Level One Publishing (Blums Books). Available at www.steppsforbpd.com.

Blum, N. S., Bartels, N. E., St. John, D., & Pfohl, B., with Harvey, R., & Sussex NHS Foundation Trust. (2016). *Systems Training for Emotional Predictability and Problem Solving (STEPPS EI): Group Treatment Programme for Managing Emotional Intensity Difficulties—Early Intervention.* Iowa City, IA: Level One Publishing (Blums Books). Available at www.steppsforbpd.com.

Blum, N. S., Bartels, N. E., St. John, D., & Pfohl, B., with Sussex NHS Foundation Trust. (2014). *Managing Emotional Intensity, A STEPPS Resource for Younger People (STEPPS YP).* Iowa City: Level One Publishing (Blums Books). Available at www.steppsforbpd.com.

Blum, N., Pfohl, B., St. John, D., Monahan, P., & Black, D. W. (2002). STEPPS: A cognitive-behavioral systems-based group treatment for outpatient clients with borderline personality disorder—a preliminary report. *Comprehensive Psychiatry, 43,* 301–310.

Blum, N., St. John, D., Pfohl, B., Stuart, S., McCormick, B., Allen, J., et al. (2008). Systems Training for Emotional Predictability and Problem Solving (STEPPS) for outpatient clients with borderline personality disorder: A randomized controlled trial and 1-year follow-up. *American Journal of Psychiatry, 165,* 468–478.

Boccalon, S., Alesiana, R., Giarolli, L., Franchini, L., Colombo, C., Blum, N., et al. (2012). Systems Training for Emotional Predictability and Problem Solving (STEPPS): Theoretical model, clinical application, and preliminary efficacy data in a sample of inpatients with personality disorders in comorbidity with mood disorders. *Journal of Psychopathology, 18,* 335–343.

Boccalon, S., Alesiana, R., Giarolli, L., Franchini, L., Colombo, C., Blum, N., et al. (2014). Systems Training for Emotional Predictability and Problem Solving (STEPPS): Program efficacy and personality features as predictors of drop-out—an Italian study. *Comprehensive Psychiatry, 55*(4), 920–927.

Bos, E. H., van Wel, B., Appelo, M. T., & Verbraak, M. J. P. M. (2010). A randomized controlled trial of a Dutch version of Systems Training for Emotional Predictability and Problem Solving for borderline personality disorder. *Journal of Nervous and Mental Disease, 198,* 299–304.

Freije, H., Dietz, B., & Appelo, M. (2002). Behandeling van de borderline persoonlijkheidsstoornis met de Vers: de Vaardigheidstraining emotionele regulatiestoornis [Treatment of the borderline personality disorder with VERS: The Skill Training emotional regulation disorder]. *Directive Therapies, 4,* 367–378.

Gunderson, J. (1996). The borderline client's intolerance of aloneness: Insecure attachments, and therapist availability. *American Journal of Psychiatry, 153,* 752–758.

Harvey, R., Black, D. W., & Blum, N. (2010). Systems Training for Emotional Predictability and Problem Solving (STEPPS) in the United Kingdom: A preliminary report. *Journal of Contemporary Psychotherapy, 40,* 225–232.

Harvey, R., Blum, N., Black, D. W., Burgess, J., & Henley-Cragg, P. (2014). Systems Training for Emotional Predictability and Problem Solving (STEPPS). In C. Sharp & J. Tackett (Eds.), *Handbook of borderline personality in children and adolescents* (pp. 415–429). New York: Springer.

Linehan, M. M., Armstrong, A. G., Suarez, A., Allmon, D., & Heard, H. L. (1991). Cognitive-behavioral treatment of chronically parasuicidal borderline clients. *Archives of General Psychiatry, 48,* 1060–1064.

Linehan, M. M., Heard, H. L., & Armstrong, H. E. (1993). Naturalistic follow-up of a behavioral treatment of chronically parasuicidal borderline clients. *Archives of General Psychiatry, 50,* 1971–1974.

Linehan, M. M., Tupek, D. A., Heard, H. L., & Armstrong, H. E. (1994). Interpersonal outcome of cognitive-behavioral treatment for chronically suicidal borderline clients. *American Journal of Psychiatry, 151,* 1771–1776.

Minuchin, S. (1974). *Families and family therapy.* Cambridge, MA: Harvard University Press.

Pfohl, B., Blum, N., McCormick, B., St. John, D., &

Black, D. W. (2009). Reliability and validity of the Borderline Evaluation of Severity Over Time: A new scale to measure severity and change in borderline personality disorder. *Journal of Personality Disorders, 23,* 281–293.

Van Wel, B., Bos, E. H., Appelo, M. T., Berendsen, E. M., Willgeroth, F. C., & Verbraak, M. J. P. M. (2009). De effectiviteit van de vaardigheidstraining Emotieregulatiestoornis (VERS) in de behandeling van de Borderlinepersoonlijkheidsstoornis: een gerandomiseerd onderzoek [The efficacy of the Systems Training for Emotional Predictability and Problem Solving (STEPPS) in the treatment of borderline personality disorder: A randomized controlled trial]. *Tijdschrift voor Psychiatrie, 51,* 291–301.

Van Wel, B., Kockmann, I., Blum, N., Pfohl, B., Heesterman, W., & Black, D. W. (2006). STEPPS group treatment for borderline personality disorder in The Netherlands. *Annals of Clinical Psychiatry, 18*(1), 63–67.

Yeomans, F. E., Clarkin, J. F., & Kernberg, O. F. (2002). *A primer for transference focused psychotherapy for the borderline patient.* Northvale, NJ: Jason Aronson.

Young, J. E. (1999). *Cognitive therapy for personality disorders: A schema-focused approach* (rev. ed.). Sarasota, FL: Professional Resource Press.

Young, J. E., Klosko, J., & Weishaar, M. E. (2003). *Schema therapy: A practitioner's guide.* New York: Guilford Press.

# CHAPTER 34

# Psychoeducation for Patients with Borderline Personality Disorder

Maria Elena Ridolfi and John G. Gunderson

In contrast with past practices, professionals are now more aware that patients have strengths and resources, need to be considered active participants in treatment, and may play an important role in enhancing change. As a result of these changes, it has become increasingly standard practice to share information with psychiatric patients and their families about the nature of their psychiatric disorders, and psychoeducational programs are now considered an important part of treatment. They have emerged as an effective, evidence-based, cost-effective type of intervention that has proved to be successful in treating many disorders, such as schizophrenia, bipolar disorder, major depression, eating disorders, and obsessive–compulsive disorder (Colom & Vieta, 2006; Dowrick et al., 2000; McFarlane, Dixon, Lukens, & Lucksted, 2003; Miklowitz, George, Richards, Simoneau, & Suddath, 2003; Peterson, Mitchell, Crow, Crosby, & Wonderlich, 2009; Tynes, Salins, Skiba, & Winstead, 1992). We present in this chapter an overview of the development and rationale for psychoeducation in general, and highlights the components and models of psychoeducational programs for borderline personality disorder (BPD).

## What Is Psychoeducation?

Psychoeducation provides information about various facets of a disorder, including symptoms, course, etiology, outcome, and prognosis, based on the premise that the more knowledgeable clients and their families are, the better the outcome for persons with the disorder and the less the burden on family members. The rationale for psychoeducation includes (1) patients' right to know about their disorder, (2) the need to increase awareness of BPD, (3) the need to reduce mystification and stigma, (4) its value in enlisting patients' intellectual strengths and curiosity in the service of recovery, (5) increasing active participation in treatment planning, and (6) establishing realistic hopes for change (see Ruiz-Sancho, Smith, & Gunderson, 2001).

Although previously clinical care seldom incorporated psychoeducation, social changes have resulted in a shift from the traditional hierarchical doctor–patient relationship to a more collaborative model in which patients and families are considered partners in the treatment (Solomon & Draine, 1995). Also, changes in the mental health system, starting with the deinstitutionalization movement in the 1960s, have resulted in a shift away from hospital-based treatment toward community-based treatment, which has made patients more responsible for their own care and increased the burden on families. With these changes, the nature of psychoeducation has broadened to embrace wider goals and includes learning skills and problem-solving techniques, and using guidelines for recovery and relapse prevention.

The term "psychoeducation" in its current form was introduced by Anderson, Hogarty, and Reiss in 1980 in the context of schizophrenia. Psychoeducation techniques borrow from several types of clinical practice, including cognitive-behavioral strategies, stress and coping models, social support models, and narrative approaches (Anderson et al., 1980; McFarlane et al., 2003). The demonstration of the value of interventions developed for Axis I disorders targeting either the patient or the family, supported by multiple randomized controlled trials (Colom et al., 2003, 2009; Dowrick et al., 2000; Miklowitz et al., 2003; Peterson et al., 2009; Rea et al., 2003; Rocco, Ciano, & Balestrieri, 2001), inspired the development of similar interventions for personality disorders (PDs). These developments were also encouraged by changing perspectives on the treatment of BPD. Since the 1970s, paralleling the larger shifts in psychiatry, changes in health care services and in the diagnostic construct itself have led to multimodal treatments resting heavily on the medical model of BPD as an illness.

Although psychoeducation is widely used with other mental disorders and was first proposed for use in treating BPD in the 1990s (Benjamin, 1993; Brightman 1992), our impression is that it is still not widely practiced or even seen as desirable. Also, in contrast to other disorders, the role of psychoeducation in managing BPD has received little research attention. To date, only one study has evaluated the efficacy of a solely psychoeducational approach (Zanarini & Frankenburg, 2008). Nevertheless, as with other disorders, the use of psychoeducation for patients with BPD has typically resulted in an upgrade in the quality of service delivery. It requires that the professionals become familiar with up-to-date information about BPD and its treatments and to have the facility for explaining it respectfully to patients and families. Furthermore, the process exposes the professional directly to a wide spectrum of questions and concerns about a complex and vexing disorder, rendering him or her unable to remain in the one-step-removed stance often assumed in psychotherapeutic care.

Psychoeducation, unlike psychotherapy or pharmacotherapies, can be delivered by individuals with no professional training or by individuals in recovery in either individual or group formats. Some programs have been developed specifically for patients, others are for family members, and still others are for both. Group interventions have multiple advantages: They are cost-effective; help social learning; allow role playing to learn and review skills; facilitate network building and social support; and by using peer feedback, they help to recognize specific patterns and normalize some experiences. The downside is that they are not easy to establish and sustain outside of busy clinical settings.

## Goals and Contents of Psychoeducation

Psychoeducation has many possible goals, although not all programs include them all.

1. To provide education about the disorder. Offering information about the disorder helps the patient to better understand certain interpersonal and behavioral patterns and helps to establish realistic expectations about course and treatment. It also respects the patient's right to know.
2. To strengthen the likelihood of complying with treatment.
3. To provide ongoing support. Psychoeducation may in fact reduce a patient's sense of isolation, providing the feeling of sharing similar difficulties and problems.

For several reasons, some clinicians continue to be reluctant to disclose the BPD diagnosis and discuss it with patients and family members. While trying to protect the patient and family from the consequences of the diagnosis, they are in fact colluding with the long-standing, highly stigmatizing, and ill-informed attitudes regarding the term. Missing the opportunity to openly and accurately educate, these clinicians keep the disorder in the shadows. The ongoing stigma stems from several causes. Rather than understanding that BPD has been validated as a diagnosis with both biological and environmental origins, and with characteristic features, the myth is perpetuated that it is not really an objective diagnosis with a biological basis. Also, clinicians do not always appreciate that longitudinal studies provide a more hopeful prognosis than previously realized, that the myth of a "life sentence" of doom and death is currently unaddressed. Rather than bringing outcomes research to light, showing clearly that there are several effective evidence-based therapies for BPD, the myth that "nothing works" is continued. It is true that pejorative terms such as "manipulative," "attention-seeking," "hateful," "self-centered," "needy," and "abusive" are associated with the diagnosis among the ill-informed, but to shy away from openly naming, and accurately educating people about BPD allows those damaging myths to go unaddressed. Psychoeducation is not possible without the disclosure of the diagnosis. Most patients and families are actually relieved and reassured to know that they what they have been struggling with is a medical condition, that they are not alone with the disorder and a body of knowledge is available about the disorder and its treatment.

In the following sections we discuss psychoeducational contents that clinicians can deliver to patients and families (based on Gunderson & Links, 2014; see Table 34.1). When delivering information, it is important to remember that many patients and families often have been blamed—or felt blamed—for the disorder, and are therefore very sensitive. Information should be delivered in a validating, sensitive, empathic, and nontechnical way that not only is clearly understandable and reliable but also eases the sense of guilt and conveys sense of hope.

## Diagnosis

For most patients and families, the diagnosis of BPD can represent relief and hope: relief from finally understanding what is wrong and that there are other people struggling with the same problems, and hope because now there may be a path out. Also, especially for patients who have gone already through several misdiagnoses and failed treatments, knowing that they have found a new diagnosis with hope for recovery can be reassuring and motivating. Others, however, may be distressed by knowing about the diagnosis if they think it means they are untreatable or distrustful. This occurs when the diagnosis has already been associated with "surplus-stigma" (i.e., that a person with BPD is violent or untreatable; Hoffman, Fruzzetti, & Bateau, 2007). For them, a more "biologically based" Axis I diagnosis would appear less threatening. Other patients, who have been previously mis- or underdiagnosed, might not want to hear about the BPD diagnosis because it challenges what had been diagnosed by cherished prior treaters. For them and for their families, the new diagnosis means that they have expended too much effort in the wrong direction.

Diagnosis may be disclosed by following the fifth edition of the *Diagnostic and Statistical Manual of Mental Health Disorders* (DSM-5; American Psychiatric Association [APA], 2013). Inviting both patients and families to discuss the presence or absence of different features of BPD is helpful because it involves the patient in making the diagnosis rather than having it assigned (Gunderson & Links, 2014). Another way to disclose the diagnosis involves the developmental perspective of the disorder as follows:

"Individuals suffering from BPD are born with a genetic predisposition to be very sensitive to signs of rejection and to be very emo-

**TABLE 34.1. Basic Themes for Psychoeducation**

*Borderline personality disorder (BPD) is significantly heritable* (~55%). This means that families need to customize their caregiving to accommodate the handicaps due to the borderline family member's genetic disposition.

*BPD is very sensitive to environmental stress,* especially interpersonal stressors (anger, rejection) or the lack of structure (inconsistent, unpredictable, ambiguous)—this means that patients get relief from structured and supportive environments. Neurobiological correlates involve elevated cortisol and opioids deficits.

*The brains of people with BPD have hyperreactive amygdala* (easily excited) *and underactive prefrontal cortex* (less cognitive/thinking inhibitions). Almost all effective therapies enhance prefrontal cortical activity, imposing thinking to evaluate perceptions and to control behaviors and feelings.

*Most patients with BPD have symptom remission* (about 50% by 2 years, 85% by 10 years) and once remitted, only 15% relapse. However, their symptom improvement is associated with only modest improvement in social adaptation (i.e., only about one-third achieve stable marriages or full-time employment by 10 years).

*There are multiple forms of empirically validated treatment for BPD.* All decrease self-harm, anger, depression, and use of hospitals, emergency departments, and medications. These treatments usually require 1–3 hours/week for a year or more by therapists with extensive training and ongoing supervision.

*The vast majority of patients with BPD improve without receiving these therapies.* Good Psychiatric Management (GPM) is usually sufficient. Treatment with intensive BPD-specific therapies should be sought for patients who do not respond.

*Note.* From Gunderson and Links (2014). Copyright © 2014 American Psychiatric Association. Reprinted by permission.

tional. This disposition negatively affects the parenting they receive and their perception of that parenting. They typically have grown up feeling that their parents did not give them the attention they needed or that they were untrustworthy or abusive. As adolescents or young adults they can make efforts to find somebody who can repair or make up for the childhood care they missed. When they think they have found it, they engage in emotionally intense, exclusive relationships, placing unrealistic expectations on the other person. People around them are expected to fill the void and provide what is painfully missed. While initially satisfying for both the individual with BPD and the other person, who at this stage is often idealized, these relationships are hard to maintain, stormy, and painful, often leading to frustration and rejection, or to real separation. When individuals with BPD feel rejected they frequently take any efforts, including clinging too long to harmful relationships or threatening to harm oneself, to avoid abandonment. When separation occurs they can react with anger or think that they deserve to be mistreated. The other person is no longer the rescuer but becomes the villain. Expressions of anger are often followed by secondary negative emotions such as shame or anger itself, and contribute to perceiving oneself as bad or even evil. Self-destructive behaviors can often occur within this context with the function to punish oneself for being "bad," to punish the other, and to relieve overwhelming emotions. Their extreme emotional pain, the tendency to blame others, and the self-destructive behaviors can evoke compassion, guilt, and protective attitudes in people around them. These reactions reinforce the borderline individual's unrealistic perception of mistreatment and the unrealistic expectations of being emotionally compensated for what he or she missed as a child. Impulsivity can also occur when individuals with BPD experience perceived or real separations. Behaviors such as substance or alcohol abuse, binge eating, and unprotected sex can temporarily relieve intense affects such as dysphoria, anxiety, or anger."

Regardless of the type of psychoeducational content, it is important to convey the message to both patients and families that, unfortunately, BPD is a condition that is frequently misunderstood and stigmatized: The pain and handicaps of individuals with BPD are often difficult to "read" from the outside. Their moodiness and failures in school or work are easily seen only as self-indulgent or manipulative. Hence, patients and families need to clarify that these are symptoms of a mental illness.

### Etiology

Information about etiology is often useful in constructively challenging parent blaming, which is still far too common, and helps to reduce the guilt and defensiveness that many parents feels about having a child with BPD. Thus, psychoeducation about etiology needs to convey the informative and destigmatizing message that BPD, like most psychiatric disorders, is associated with both a genetic disposition and adverse environmental factors, and that no single factor accounts for the disorder. Instead, in most cases, the disorder is due to a complex interplay between underlying vulnerability and environment. It is usually reassuring to both parents and patients to learn that there are genetic factors that make the person more vulnerable and sensitive to environmental stressors, and that there are biological underpinnings to the disorder. The downside is that this information might lead to the wrong assumption that something biological cannot be changed. Thus, it is helpful to explain that research indicates that the disorder can be treated successfully, and that psychotherapy can decrease amygdala hyperactivity—part of the disturbed neural circuitry underlying emotional dysregulation in BPD (Goodman et al., 2014).

When educating caregivers about environmental etiological factors, it is important to navigate the discussion carefully, so that they are informed but do not feel blamed. For example, when describing the meaning of "invalidating environment," it is important to emphasize that many, probably most, instances of invalidation result not from any malignant process but simply from mismatches between parental style and child temperament, or deficits in parenting skills or information. The professional can emphasize the fact that everyone is invalidated in life, and that we all often feel as if our environments do not confirm or corroborate our subjective experiences. It is likely that the parents of someone with BPD were invalidated significantly in their own lives and have been invalidated by their family member with BPD. These are typically transactional and transgenerational processes.

Still, while being sensitive to the possible damaging misinterpretations of what is meant by "invalidating environment," it is also important to provide our state-of-the-art understanding that, for an emotionally vulnerable individual, invalidation of a pervasive nature can contribute to problems in learning to regulate emotions.

Caregivers should understand that they may have played a significant, albeit unintentional, role in the development of the disorder: They did not intentionally choose to create an invalidating environment. Finally, they should be encouraged to actively participate in treatment for many reasons, including the opportunity to acknowledge their own role in the disorder and to contribute to recovery by making changes.

"Research has not yet discovered exactly how a person develops BPD, but genetic and environmental factors are both involved. Like in other major psychiatric disorders, BPD has a significant level of heritability (meaning inborn factors) (~55%). What is believed to be inherited it is not the disorder itself, but rather a genetic predisposition, 'temperament,' that makes it possible for a child to develop the disorder later on in life. Three predisposing temperaments, called phenotypes, are believed to be involved in the development of BPD: Affective (Emotional) Instability, Impulsivity, and Interpersonal Hypersensitivity. Neuroimaging studies show that people with BPD seem to have impairment in the area of the brain that regulates emotions. Also hormones, such as oxytocin and cortisol, seem to play a potential role in causing the disorder. Biological factors are not enough for the development of the disorder. Often patients report that their parents were neglectful, hostile, threatening, or even evil. While some patients with BPD clearly have traumatic childhood experiences (neglecting or abusive family), in many cases there is not a frankly traumatic environment, and siblings and even twins often report a more positive perception about caregiving. Moreover, BPD can develop without traumatic experiences, and traumatic experiences do not always lead them to develop BPD. The disorder seems often associated to a 'mismatched' interaction (e.g., a temperamentally emotional child might need an extraordinary calm and containing environment, which is hard to provide constantly). In conclusion, the exact causes of the disorder still need to be identified. What is clear is that neither patients with BPD nor their parents are responsible for the disorder."

## Course

When we deliver psychoeducation about the course, it is important to remember that patients and families may previously have been exposed to misleading information, often stemming from myths about the disorder (e.g., "BPD is a chronic illness"). They need to receive the more optimistic, albeit cautious, message that BPD is now considered to have a good prognosis that can also improve without treatment or the long-term treatments specifically designed for the disorder. It is also useful to inform them about the fact that longitudinal studies show more positive results than previously believed (Gunderson et al., 2011; Zanarini, Frankenburg, Reich, & Fitzmaurice, 2012). About 20% of individuals with BPD remit by 1 year, 50% by 2 years, and 85% by 10 years, and once remitted, only about 15% relapse (Gunderson et al., 2011). This message conveys hope, but it is also important to acknowledge that improved social functioning occurs far less frequently than symptomatic remission. Symptoms such as dysphoric feelings and self-harming behavior can respond more rapidly to treatment than do distrust and lack of vocational skills. Most individuals with BPD still have significantly diminished functioning, in school, work, and relationships after 10 years. Clearly, evidence-based therapies for BPD need to focus more on rehabilitation strategies and social learning, and to help patients to attain and maintain work roles. Patients and their families need to understand that staying in effective treatments will improve the likelihood and rate of recovery. Such treatments might contribute not only to decreased symptoms but also to improved quality of life.

## Treatment

Despite research documenting the efficacy of a variety of treatments for BPD, many patients and their families remain uninformed about therapy and its effectiveness. To counter these misunderstandings, therapists should always begin psychoeducation by communicating that recovery is possible (see Table 34.1) and that this can be expedited by the patient participation in assuming control over feelings and behaviors.

It is also helpful to provide information on the range of therapies available and how effective treatments often include multiple modalities, including family interventions, and that having a knowledgeable and trained primary clinician is the cornerstone of treatment.

*Psychotherapy*

The therapist should provide information about the different forms of evidence-based therapies (EBTs) and how patients often differ in their responses to these treatments. It is also useful to make participants aware of the fact that most therapies have important features in common, and that all decrease self-harm, hospitalizations, and access to emergency departments (Bateman & Fonagy, 1999, 2009; Clarkin, Levy, Lenzenweger, & Kernberg, 2007; Linehan, Armstrong, Suarez, Allmon, & Heard, 1991; Linehan, Heard, & Armstrong, 1993). It is even more useful for patients and their family members to know that one of the specialized therapies is not always needed and that often effective generalist models are available and can be provided by nonspecialists (Gunderson, 2016). More specific, intensive, and structured interventions should be reserved for patients who do not improve. Another important message is that recovery is not only related to the effectiveness of treatment but also to life events and environmental changes. Patients and families should be encouraged, regardless of the type of therapy, to seek clinicians who are nonjudgmental toward them, who like to work with them, and who have had experience in doing this work.

*Medications*

A key issue to address when discussing medications is the unrealistic expectations that some patients and family members place on pharmacotherapy. This is especially true when previous treatments have encouraged this hope or when they want to consider BPD a "brain disease" that should be treated only with medications. This can be addressed by providing a careful and realistic message about the limited effects of pharmacotherapy. Patients and family members should be informed that no medications have been officially approved for treatment of this disorder, although some may be useful in reducing symptoms such as depression, irritability, and impulsivity. However, they should be considered as playing an adjunctive role in treatment. They also need to be considered in the overall treatment of coexisting conditions, such as bipolar disorder or major depressive disorder. Patients and family members should also be informed about the dangers of polypharmacy, which is associated with an increased risk for multiple side effects (Zanarini et al., 2012).

When delivering psychoeducation about medications, it is important to get patient to collaborate in the process by actively discussing targets selected for treatment and explaining in detail the outcomes that may reasonably be expected, so that they do not have unreasonable expectations and become actively involved in monitoring the efficacy and side effects. This requires that patients be well-informed consumers. Some sources of information about medications are included in Appendix 34.1.

*Hospitalization*

The treatment history of many patients with BPD includes a repetitive and often unproductive cycle of repeated hospitalizations and emergency department visits. Psychoeducation may be useful in helping to break this cycle by providing information about the benefits and the downside of hospital admissions. The constructive use of hospitalization includes the chance for a brief period of stabilization and respite; conducting a thorough assessment of current dysfunction, including high-risk behavior; and the opportunity to work with the patient to develop or to readjust the outpatient plan. The downside of hospitalization includes the possibility that it will increase the individual's stigmatization in society; the tendency to reinforce escalated crisis behaviors in the long run by providing hospitalization in the short run; the removal of the patients from the contexts in which treatment needs to take hold; and the possibility that any learning in the hospital may not generalize to the outpatient setting. Furthermore, the patient who is exposed to frequent or lengthy hospitalizations may undergo institutionalization and even learn new problematic behaviors from other patients. Psychoeducation should convey the message that hospitalizations should usually be of short duration, should be restricted to severe crises management and sometimes medication major changes, and that they sometimes reflect problems in the outpatient care that need to be addressed.

## An Illustrative Program

Our current program delivers the kinds of information described using a closed group format of six weekly sessions, each lasting 90 minutes. The first hour of each session involves the presentation of didactic material based on a specific topic, with time for questions. The rest of the time is devoted to feedback and mutual support. We encourage socializing and lighter topics at the start and close of each meeting to keep the group pretty informal.

Groups include five to eight participants to ensure sufficient time to address individual concerns. We find that having more members makes it difficult to allow adequate attention for everyone, and less than five members diminishes the diversity of feedback. Groups are usually homogeneous relative to age in order to facilitate identification and sharing. A leader and a co-leader (both professionals) conduct the group. A peer facilitator, who has moved further in the journey of recovery, meets participants during the first session to share his or her experience and to give hope and support. Patients sit in circle facing a board, and they are provided didactic material to read at home. They are encouraged to share their lesson materials with family members, friends, and significant others. Family psychoeducation groups are also available for family members seeking more information and support.

The topics covered include (1) diagnosis (Sessions 1 and 2), (2) etiology; (3) course; and (4) treatment (Sessions 5 and 6). When delivering information, we use validation strategies and nontechnical terminology. Many clients report having had disappointing encounters with previous mental health providers: (1) receiving minimal information about the disorder; (2) being offered little hope for recovery, and (3) feeling blamed or criticized for their presenting problem behaviors. Thus, the main challenge is to replace misconceptions about BPD and sense of guilt with awareness, knowledge, and hope. At the end of the group, patients usually report that the program gave them a feeling of empowerment, clarity, and hope.

## Peer Psychoeducation

Peer-led psychoeducation has been found to be a useful and effective way to deliver the information patients need (Davidson, Chinman, Kloos, & Tebes, 1999; Mead & MacNeil, 2006). Service users who deliver such sessions often feel empowered in their own recovery journey and the increased sense of self-agency that they feel gets communicated to patients who are often reassured and motivated by hearing from others who have been in their position and recovered. The process reduces feelings of isolation and stigmatization. Research also shows that the process leads to improvements in community integration and social functioning (Forchuk, Martin, Chan, & Jensen, 2005; Lawn, Smith, & Hunter, 2008; Nelson, Ochocka, Janzen, & Trainor, 2006).

Two types of peer-led psychoeducation are currently available for BPD: (1) peer-led groups and (2) Web-based psychoeducational groups.

### Peer-Led Groups

Peer-led groups are conducted by a facilitator who is either well along the treatment pathway or has completed treatment. The value of these groups is that the facilitator can supplement information about the disorder and treatment with information about their own experiences in overcoming the challenges the disorder presents. Although such groups are commonly used in treating many mental disorders, they are often less available for people with BPD, especially in the United States, although such groups are available in Europe and Australasia. This may be because the interpersonal and emotion regulation difficulties associated with the disorder make it difficult to achieve and maintain the stability needed for an ongoing self-help group to function. Some patients may also avoid peer support groups as a way of "avoiding" acceptance of the diagnoses and because of concern about the stigma associated with the diagnosis. To date, the only peer support groups for BPD are the ones offered within Meetup, an online social network that facilitates offline group meetings, unified by a common interest, around the world (*www.meetup.com*). Another option is peer-led groups for individuals with psychiatric disorders offered by the National Alliance on Mental Illness (NAMI), whose peer-led groups include people with BPD but are not specifically designed for them. These groups are recovery-focused educational programs that incorporate educational presentations and discussion (*www.namiorg/peertopeer.com*).

## Web-Based Psychoeducational Groups

These days the Internet can be an excellent resource for peer psychoeducation, and plenty of online options are available for people with BPD. Some online groups are run by individuals in recovery, and other are designed for family members as well. Such groups can be the best way for some individuals with BPD to acquire information and support, either because they are unable to attend the in-person meetings, or because overwhelming emotional responses to the in-person context interfere with taking advantage of that context. There is also the problem that online messages are easily misinterpreted (Parks & Floyd, 1996). Misinformation may also be a problem. While some websites are helpful and reliable, others provide incorrect information, stigmatizing messages, and bad advice, possibly leading to a worsening of the disorder. Two reliable websites are BPDWORLD (*www.bpdworld.org*) and DBT Self Help (*www.dbtselfhelp.com*). BPDWORLD provides jargon-free educational material about the disorder along with online support. DBT Self Help, funded by a person in recovery, is structured around some dialectical behavior therapy (DBT) skills, with the goal of reinforcing the skills learned in the past and promoting acquisition and generalization of new ones. Another useful online psychoeducational option is the one represented by a series of clinician-led webinars offered by Mc Lean Hospital in Belmont, Massachusetts. These interactive webinars provide individuals and family members with an array of information specific to the disorder (*www.mcleanhospital.org/clinical-services/patient-and-family-resources?tab=borderline-personality-disorder-patient-and-family-education-initiative*).

Psychoeducational programs can be delivered in a manner that is more or less structured. The more structured versions are more classroom-like, following a formal curriculum, and may include practice assignments. Less structured curriculum versions may be delivered as an open forum that is intended to be supportive and flexible, revolving around the needs and interests of group members. Regardless of the way the program is structured, common elements usually include education about the disorder and the nature of treatment approaches, transmission of hope by offering the optimistic findings in studies on treatment and the longitudinal outcomes, advice and suggestions for coping with problematic aspects of the disorder, and sharing of resources that may prove useful to individuals and families in their pursuit of recovery.

## Conclusions

In contrast to those with other mental health disorders, patients with BPD and their families all too often are given neither the diagnosis nor are they provided with up-to date information, despite the considerable body of knowledge about the disorder and encouraging information about its treatment. It is important that clinicians become familiar with the latest information concerning BPD and convey this information in a respectful and destigmatizing way to patients and their families. By doing so, mental health professionals can both strengthen the likelihood of patients' compliance with treatment and be held accountable for high standards of service. Furthermore, although many EBTs for BPD include psychoeducational components, providing information about the disorder can be a useful and cost-effective approach whether or not patients receive BPD-specific treatments.

## APPENDIX 34.1. Psychoeducational Resources: Printed Materials, Websites, Videos, and Apps

### Printed Materials

**Publications authored by nonprofessionals: autobiographies, treatment histories, and self-help tools**

*Eclipses: Behind the Borderline Personality Disorder,* by M. F. Thornton (Monte Sano Publishing, 1997).—Written by a person recovering from BPD, this book offers an easy-to-read and informative account of the disorder and treatment with DBT in an inpatient setting.

*A Bright Red Scream: Self-Mutilation and the Language of Pain,* by M. Strong (Penguin Books, 1998).—A groundbreaking, comprehensive, and essential resource for people who self-harm.

*Surviving a Borderline Parent,* by K. Roth and F. B. Friedman (New Harbinger, 2003).—Step-by-step guidelines to understand and overcome the effects of being raised by a borderline parent.

*Get Me Out of Here—My Recovery from Borderline Personality Disorder* by R. Reiland (Hazelden, 2004).—Written by a person in recovery, this engaging memoir conveys a hopeful message to those suffering from BPD and their loved ones.

*The Buddha and the Borderline,* by K. VanGelder (New Harbinger, 2010).—A compelling memoir about both living with BPD and the process of recovery through DBT, Buddhism, and adventures in online dating.

*Remnants of a Life on Paper: A Mother and Daughter's Struggle with Borderline Personality Disorder,* by B. Tusiani, L. Tusiani, and P. Tusiani-Eng (Baroque Press, 2013).—An inspirational story of a woman suffering from BPD and her courageous family members.

**Publications authored by professionals: Didactic material and self-help tools**

*Stop Walking on Eggshells: Coping When Someone You Care about Has Borderline Personality Disorder,* by P. T. Mason and R. Krager (New Harbinger, 1998).—A compassionate, skill building guidance to help anyone in a relationship with someone suffering from BPD.

*Lost in the Mirror: An Inside Look at Borderline Personality Disorder,* R. Moskovitz (Taylor, 2001).—A valuable and compassionate resource for anyone seeking to understand the disorder.

*Borderline Personality Disorder Demystified: An Essential Guide for Understanding and Living with BPD,* by R. O. Friedel (Marlowe & Company, 2004).—A useful, wise, and compassionate guide for everyone seeking to understand BPD and learn about treatment.

*Understanding and Treating Borderline Personality Disorder: A Guide for Professionals and Families,* by J. G. Gunderson and P. D. Hoffman (American Psychiatric Publishing, 2005).—An informative and readable overview of current knowledge about BPD, written by experts, family members, and patients.

*Sometimes I Act Crazy: Living with Borderline Personality Disorder,* by J. J. Kreisman and H. Straus (Wiley, 2006).—A readable and practical guide offering different techniques to people affected by BPD and to those who love them.

*The Dialectical Behaviour Therapy Skills Workbook: Practical DBT Exercises for Learning Mindfulness, Interpersonal Effectiveness, Emotion Regulation and Distress Tolerance,* by M. McKay, J. C. Wood, and J. Brantley (New Harbinger, 2007).—A step-by-step, practical guide to better manage emotions through learning basic and more advanced DBT skills. Useful to support those who are in treatment and as a self-help manual.

*Overcoming Borderline Personality Disorder: A Family Guide for Healing and Change,* by V. Porr (Oxford University Press, 2010).—A readable and evidence-based guide for families to better understand and help those suffering from BPD.

*A BPD Brief,* by J. G. Gunderson (*www.borderlinepersonalitydisorder*).—A concise, informative summary of the diagnosis, origins, course, and treatment of BPD.

**Websites**

National Educational Alliance for Borderline Personality Disorder (NEA-BPD) (*www.borderlinepersonalitydisorder.com*).—This very well-organized, frequently updated, and exhaustive website is a comprehensive resource providing consumers, family members, and professionals with a full array of up-to-date information on BPD, including research on the disorder, along with links to videos of recent talks and workshops by leading experts in the field.

Treatment and Research Advancements Association for Personality Disorder (TARA APD) (*www.tara4bpd.org*).—Their website provides very useful, comprehensive information for consumers and family members about the disorder, including up-to-date research. It also includes a nationwide referral list for clinicians and treatment programs offering empirically validated treatments.

National Alliance on Mental Illness (NAMI) (*www.nami.org*).—This website provides information about BPD and includes a link to research articles on BPD. Suggestions on how to help relatives or friends who have BPD are also listed.

BPD Central (*www.bpdcentral.com*).—Geared primarily toward families, this website provides information and educational materials on BPD, as well as access to online support groups for family members.

BPDWORLD (*www.bpdworld.org*). This website provides jargon-free educational material about the disorder, along with online support.

DBT Self Help (*www.selfhelp.com*). Funded by a person in recovery in 2001, when very little information on DBT was available on the Web. It is structured around some DBT skills.

National Institute of Mental Health (NIMH) (*www.nimh.nih.gov/health/publications/borderline-*

*personality-disorder*).—This website presents a descriptive, educational overview of BPD, and tips on how to help a family member or friend diagnosed with the disorder. It also provides a link to learn about results of studies.

## Videos

Inspiring and vivid first-person accounts are videos featuring Amanda R. Wang (*www.youtube.com/user/rethinkbpd*).

*If Only We Had Known* is a five-video series—Understanding BPD, Causes of BPD, Diagnosing BPD, Treating BPD, and Coping with BPD—that provide useful and reliable educational materials to help individuals, families, and loved ones who live with borderline personality disorder (*www.bpdvideo.com*). Using the personal stories of families and insights from leading experts in the field, the disorder is explained in ways that are easy to understand.

## Apps

*DBT Diary Card:* Available on iTunes, this app was designed and created by a intensively trained psychologist in DBT.
*DBT Self Help:* Available on Androids.

Both are self-help tools structured around DBT skills.

## REFERENCES

American Psychiatric Association. (2013). *Diagnostic and statistical manual of mental disorders* (5th ed.). Arlington, VA: Author.

Anderson, C. M., Hogarty, G. E., & Reiss, D. J. (1980). Family treatment of adult schizophrenic patients: A psycho-educational approach. *Schizophrenia Bulletin, 6,* 490–505.

Bateman, A., & Fonagy, P. (1999). The effectiveness of partial hospitalization in the treatment of BPD: A randomized controlled trial. *American Journal of Psychiatry, 156,* 1563–1569.

Bateman, A., & Fonagy, P. (2009). Randomized controlled trial of outpatient mentalization-based treatment versus structured clinical management for borderline personality disorder. *American Journal of Psychiatry, 166,* 1355–1364.

Benjamin, L. S. (1993). *Interpersonal diagnosis and treatment of personality disorders,* New York: Guilford Press.

Brightman, B. K. (1992). Peer support and education in the comprehensive care of patients with borderline personality disorder. *Psychiatric Hospital, 23,* 55–59.

Clarkin, J. F., Levy, K. N., Lenzenweger, M. F., & Kernberg, O. F., et al (2007). Evaluating three treatments for borderline personality disorder: A multiwave study. *American Journal of Psychiatry, 164,* 922–928.

Colom, F., & Vieta, E. (2006). *Psychoeducation manual for bipolar disorder.* Cambridge, UK: Cambridge University Press.

Colom, F., Vieta, E., Martinez-Aran, A., Reinares, M., Goikolea, J. M., Benabarre, A., et al. (2003). A randomized trial on the efficacy of group psychoeducation in the prophylaxis of recurrences in bipolar patients whose disease is in remission. *Archives of General Psychiatry, 60,* 402–407.

Colom, F., Vieta, E., Sánchez-Moreno, J., Palomino-Otiniano, R., Reinares, M., Goikolea, J. M., et al. (2009). Group psychoeducation for stabilized bipolar disorders: 5-year outcome of a randomized clinical trial. *British Journal of Psychiatry, 194,* 260–265.

Davidson, L., Chinman, M., Kloos, B., & Tebes, J. K. (1999). Peer support among individuals with severe mental illness: A review of the evidence. *Clinical Psychology: Science and Practice, 6*(2), 165–187.

Dowrick, C., Dunn, G., Ayuso-Mateos, J. L., Dalgard, O. S., Page, H., Lehtinen, V., et al. (2000). Problem solving treatment and group psychoeducation for depression: Multicenter randomized controlled trial. *British Medical Journal, 321,* 1450.

Forchuk, C., Martin, M., Chan, Y., & Jensen, E. (2005). Therapeutic relationships: From psychiatric hospital to community. *Journal of Psychiatric and Mental Health Nursing, 12,* 556–564.

Goodman, M., Carpenter, D., Tang, C. I., Goldstein, K. E., Avedon, J., Fernandez, N., et al. (2014). Dialectical behavior therapy alters emotion regulation and amygdala activity in patients with borderline personality disorder. *Journal of Psychiatry Research, 57,* 108–116.

Gunderson, J. G. (2016). The emergence of a generalist model for treating borderline personality disorder patients. *American Journal of Psychiatry, 173*(5), 452–458.

Gunderson, J. G., & Links, P. (2014). *Handbook of good psychiatric management for borderline personality disorder.* Washington, DC: American Psychiatric Publishing.

Gunderson, J. G., Stout, R. L., McGlashan, T. H., Shea, M. T., Morey, L. C., Grilo, C. M., et al. (2011). Ten year course of borderline personality disorder: Psychopathology and function from the Collaborative Longitudinal Personality Disorders Study. *Archives of General Psychiatry, 68*(8), 827–837.

Hoffman, P. D., Fruzzetti, A. E., & Bateau, E. (2007). Understanding and engaging families: An education, skills and support program for relatives impacted by borderline personality disorder. *Journal of Mental Health, 16,* 69–82.

Lawn, S., Smith, A., & Hunter, K. (2008). Mental health peer support for hospital avoidance and early discharge: An Australian example of consumer driven and operated service. *Journal of Mental Health, 17*(5), 498–508.

Linehan, M. M., Armstrong, H. E., Suarez, A., Allmon, D., & Heard, H. L. (1991). Cognitive-behavioral treatment of chronically parasuicidal borderline patients. *Archives of General Psychiatry, 48*(12), 1060–1064.

Linehan, M. M., Heard, H. L., & Armstrong, H. E. (1993). Naturalistic follow-up of a behavioral treatment for chronically parasuicidal borderline patients. *Archives of General Psychiatry, 50*(12), 971–974.

McFarlane, W. R., Dixon, L., Lukens, E., & Lucksted, A. (2003). Family psychoeducation and schizophrenia: A review of the literature. *Journal Marital Family Therapy, 29,* 223–245.

Mead, S., & MacNeil, C. (2006). Peer support: What makes it unique? *International Journal of Psychosocial Rehabilitation, 10,* 29–33.

Miklowitz, D. J., George, E. L., Richards, J. A., Simoneau, T. L., & Suddath, R. L. (2003). A randomized study of family-focused psychoeducation and pharmacotherapy in the out-patient management of bipolar disorder. *Archives of General Psychiatry, 60,* 904–912.

Nelson, G., Ochocka, J., Janzen, R., & Trainor, J. (2006). A longitudinal study of mental health consumer/survivor initiatives: Part 1—literature review and overview of the study. *Journal of Community Psychology, 34*(3), 247–260.

Parks, M. R., & Floyd, K. (1996). Making friends in cyberspace. *Journal of Communication, 46,* 80–89.

Peterson, C. B., Mitchell, J. E., Crow, S. J., Crosby, R. D., & Wonderlich, S. A. (2009). The efficacy of self-help group treatment and therapist-led group treatment for binge eating disorder. *American Journal of Psychiatry, 166,* 1347–1354.

Rea, M. M., Tompson, M. C., Miklowitz, D. J., Goldstein, M. J., Hwang, S., & Mintz, J. (2003). Family-focused treatment versus individual treatment for bipolar disorder: Results of a randomized clinical trial. *Journal of Consulting and Clinical Psychology, 71,* 482–492.

Rocco, P. L., Ciano, R. P., & Balestrieri, M. (2001). Psychoeducation in the prevention of eating disorders: An experimental approach in adolescent schoolgirls. *British Journal of Medical Psychology, 74*(Pt. 3), 351–358.

Ruiz-Sancho, A., Smith, G., & Gunderson, J. G. (2001). Psychoeducational approaches. In W. J. Livesley (Ed.), *Handbook of personality disorders: Theory, research, and treatment* (pp. 460–474). New York: Guilford Press.

Solomon, P., & Draine, J. (1995). Subjective burden among family members of mentally ill adults: Relation to stress, coping, and adaptation. *American Journal of Orthopsychiatry, 65,* 419–427.

Tynes, L. L., Salins, C., Skiba, W., & Winstead, D. K. (1992). A psychoeducational and support group for obsessive–compulsive disorder patients and their significant others. *Comprehensive Psychiatry, 33,* 197–220.

Zanarini, M. C., & Frankenburg, F. R. (2008). A preliminary, randomized trial of psychoeducation for women with borderline personality disorder. *Journal of Personality Disorders, 22*(3), 284–290.

Zanarini, M. C., Frankenburg, F. R., Reich, D. B., & Fitzmaurice, G. (2012). Attainment and stability of sustained symptomatic remission and recovery among patients with borderline personality disorder and Axis II comparison subjects: A 16-year prospective follow-up study. *American Journal of Psychiatry, 169,* 476–483.

# CHAPTER 35

# Pharmacotherapy

Paul Markovitz

The field of pharmacotherapy of personality disorders (PDs) has grown tremendously since my review in the previous edition of the *Handbook* more than 15 years ago. The field has grown sufficiently that I review only double-blind, placebo-controlled trials in this chapter. The skepticism that pharmacological treatment of PD faced when the first edition was published has been replaced by greater acceptance. Converging lines of evidence from neuroimaging and biological studies unequivocally show structural and neurotransmitter anomalies in individuals with PDs, and further research suggests these physical abnormalities benefit from pharmacological interventions. As with any other medical illness—diabetes, cancer, heart failure, stroke—the treating clinician can improve the quality of an individual's life through the judicious use of medications. Unlike the aforementioned diseases, which are very well studied, pharmacological treatment of PD remains in its relative infancy, and paradigms for treatment are symptom based and rarely biologically based. The chapter focuses on the pharmacological treatment of borderline personality disorder (BPD) because no controlled trials are available on other PDs.

In this chapter I review and contextualize findings from controlled trials published since 2004, noting throughout the difference between statistically significant and clinically meaningful improvement. Throughout this review, I discuss the meaning of measured outcomes placed in context of treatment. Certain pharmacological modalities are better than others, and I make every attempt to describe these clearly to the clinician. The chapter summarizes evidence from controlled trials for the efficacy of major classes of treatment agents, including anticonvulsants, atypical antipsychotics, omega-3 fatty acids, and antidepressants. Next, I present considerations in interpreting results from meta-analyses. The chapter concludes with a discussion on treatment considerations.

## Anticonvulsants

I defer from calling these agents mood stabilizers, since they can be depressogenic for many (Gardner & Cowdry, 1986) and are more effective against irritability and anger than depression or impulsivity. Carbamazepine and valproate were reviewed in earlier work (Markovitz, 2001, 2004), and a new trial by Hollander, Swann, Coccaro, Jiang and Smith (2005) is added for completeness. Newer open-label trials of oxarbazepine (Bellino, Paradiso, & Bogetto, 2005) and lamotrigine (Preston, Marchant, Remherr, Strong, & Hedges, 2005; Weinstein & Jamison, 2007), appear in an Addendum at the end of the References. A trial of clonidine is also included (Philipsen et al., 2004), as it is more in line with an anticonvulsant in efficacy than its own subgroup.

### Lamotrigine

Tritt and colleagues (2005) conducted an 8-week, double-blind, placebo-controlled trial of lamotrigine in 27 female patients with BPD (18 lamotrigine and 9 placebo). The State–Trait Anger Expression Inventory (STAXI; Spielberger, Jacobs, Russell, & Crane, 1983) was the primary outcome measure. Lamotrigine proved superior to placebo in leading to reductions in State-Anger (transient anger intensity), Trait-Anger (frequency of angry feelings), Anger-Out (overt expression of aggression) and increased Anger-Control (constraint of overt anger expression). The medication was well tolerated, with only minor side effects, and patient retention was good. Only one patient in the active treatment group and two in the placebo group discontinued the trial before study completion. More recently, Reich, Zanarini, and Bieri (2009) conducted a 12-week double-blind, placebo-controlled trial of lamotrigine in 28 patients (15 lamotrigine and 13 placebo) with BPD. Doses were flexible and ranged from 25 to 275 mg/day, with a mean dose of 106.7 mg. Patients were also allowed to utilize one antidepressant during the study. Only 60% of the patients taking lamotrigine completed all 12 weeks of the trial. Three lamotrigine-treated patients developed a rash that necessitated study withdrawal. The data showed significant decreases in affective lability and impulsivity. Lamotrigine is an affective stabilizer, and performed effectively for the majority of the participants. Side effects were, however, problematic, as there was a potential Stevens–Johnson syndrome, which is a known side effect of lamotrigine. Considering the morbidity of BPD as a diagnosis, the risk–benefit ratio of lamotrigine use seems worthwhile in the group with reasonable monitoring and patient education.

Overall, findings suggest that lamotrigine is effective in reducing anger and aggression in patients with BPD. Both trials targeted a subset of patients with BPD showing difficulties with controlling anger, and lamotrigine was effective in accomplishing this.

## Topiramate

Topiramate is the most studied anticonvulsant in the treatment of BPD (Loew et al., 2006; Nickel et al., 2004, 2005). The trials evaluated outcomes for males and females separately, and examined aggression using the German version of the STAXI (Spielberger et al., 1983). Nickel and colleagues (2004) reported an 8-week trial that included a sample of 19 women taking topiramate titrated to 250 mg/day and 10 women in a matched placebo group. The topiramate group had a significant decrease in aggression, as measured by all scales on the STAXI except the Anger-In scale. Side effects were minimal, with weight loss being the most common. A study with an all-male sample compared patients on topiramate ($n = 22$) and a placebo group ($n = 20$), and found the same results as those found in women treated with topiramate described in Nickel and colleagues, in that all scores on the STAXI were significantly decreased except Anger-In. Topiramate was well tolerated, with weight loss being the primary side effect as in the earlier study. Both studies are interesting because they targeted a specific symptom of BPD that often proves to be one of the most difficult to treat. It also suggests the idea of targeting specific symptoms in BPD for treatment with specific drugs. This fits nicely with a medical model of the disease: Just as we treat cardiac disease with drugs tailored to fit specific symptoms (e.g., beta-blockers for arrhythmias, statins for high cholesterol, and calcium channel blockers for vasospasm following bypass surgery), treating specific symptoms in BPD with specific drugs appears to be an appropriate strategy. Both female and male participants were followed longitudinally over a period of 18 months after the trial was complete, and topiramate continued to provide ongoing benefit in the form of symptom reduction (Loew & Nickel, 2008; Nickel & Loew, 2008).

Loew and colleagues (2006) extended the work described earlier by investigating outcomes as assessed by the Symptom Checklist 90—Revised (SCL-90-R; Derogatis, 1994), the SF-36 Health Survey (Bullinger & Kirchberger, 1998), and the Inventory of Interpersonal Problems (IIP; Horowitz, Rosenbery, Baer, Ureno, & Villasenor, 1988) in 28 women with BPD taking a daily dose of 200 mg of topiramate and 28 women in a placebo group. All of the SCL-90-R subscale scores significantly improved except those measuring Obsessive–Compulsive, Depression, Paranoid Ideation, and Psychoticism subscales. The SF-36 scores showed significant improvement in all health-related quality-of-life subscales. The IIP showed significant diminution in scores on the Overly Autocratic, Socially Avoiding, Overly Quarrelsome, and Overly Expressive subscales. Conversely, scales measuring Overly Cold, Overly Submissive, Overly Exploitable, and Overly Nurturant features did not change. Significant differences emerged with respect to reported weight loss, with an average of 5.7 kg in the topiramate group and 1.4 kg in the placebo group. Significant improvement was reported for several BPD symptoms, with few side effects reported.

In summary, evidence from randomized trials suggest that anticonvulsants are an effective intervention for anger and aggression symptoms in patients with BPD. These symptoms are frequently difficult to treat, and all anticonvulsants show evidence of high levels of efficacy. Significant decreases in the Somatization subscale reported in Loew and colleagues (2006) also point to efficacy in an area affecting a large number of patients with BPD (Markovitz & Wagner, 1996). This is consistent with topiramate being approved for the purpose of treating migraines. In addition, antiepileptic drugs show efficacy in reducing symptoms of fibromyalgia, headaches, and migraines. I discuss the use of these agents in the comprehensive treatment of BPD in a later section.

## Atypical Antipsychotics

The preponderance of BPD treatment trials over the past decade has focused on the efficacy of atypical antipsychotics, due in part to the longstanding belief that BPD is in the neurochemical spectrum of bipolar disorder (Akiskal, 1981). Thus, agents known to improve symptoms of bipolar disorder should also be expected to work well in treating similar behaviors in the context of borderline pathology. Early open-label and placebo-controlled trials that were discussed in earlier reviews (Markovitz, 2001, 2004) are listed in the Addendum at the end of the References, as are newer open-label trials (e.g., Adityanjee et al., 2008). These articles are referenced for completeness and to provide context for the double-blind trials that followed. First, as a rule, the open-label trials reported markedly greater levels of efficacy than those reported in the double-blind, placebo-controlled trials. Second, and probably the main reason for the exponential growth of research, is the drive by the pharmaceutical industry to find a market for their drugs. The targeting of BPD was logical based on its breadth in the population, controlled data with older typical antipsychotics suggesting efficacy, and lack of any approved pharmacological treatment for BPD. Capturing this market would have been an economic windfall for any company that could do so. Unfortunately, the data from the double-blind, placebo-controlled trials are disappointing and do not argue convincingly for the use of these drugs or approval by the U.S. Food and Drug Administration (FDA) as first-line agents for the treatment of BPD.

Based on the initial positive reports in a handful of open-label trials and a few small double-blind trials, investigators moved forward on placebo-controlled trials of atypical antipsychotics. At the time this chapter was published in the first edition of this handbook, the sum total of all patients prescribed atypical antipsychotics for BPD reported in the literature was well under 100 (Markovitz, 2001). This number has now grown to almost 2,000. While the 20-fold increase in data is encouraging, it is still a very small sample for a disorder that affects many millions of people in the United States alone (Grant et al., 2008) and predicts the persistence of depressive disorders (Skodol et al., 2011). The number of double-blind trials using atypical antipsychotics to treat BPD is large enough that only these trials are reviewed here. Earlier open trials not previously reviewed are included for completeness in the Addendum. These include olanzapine (Hallmayer, 2003), quetiapine (Vileneuve & Lemelin, 2005), and risperidone (Friedel et al., 2008).

### *Aripiprazole*

Nickel and colleagues (2006) enrolled 52 patients (43 women and 9 men) in a 1:1 ratio in a double-blind, placebo-controlled trial comparing 15 mg aripiprazole to placebo over 8 weeks. A total of five participants met exclusion criteria, yielding a total sample size of 52, with 26 participants assigned to each of the aripiprazole and placebo groups. The results showed statistically significant decreases in scores on the Hamilton Depression Rating Scale (HAM-D; Hamilton, 1960), Hamilton Anxiety Rating Scale (HAM-A; Hamilton, 1959), SCL-90-R (Derogatis, 1994), and the STAXI (Spielberger et al., 1983). Individuals in the placebo group reported negligible levels of symptom change over the trial period. Self-injurious behavior decreased from seven of 26 observed participant cases to two of 26 observed at the end of the trial in the aripiprazole group. In contrast, there were five of 26 observations of self-injury reported at baseline and seven of 26 reported at the end of the study in the placebo group. Regarding attrition, five individuals withdrew, but it was unclear in which group(s) this occurred. Likewise, medication side effects were not reported, and no information is available as to whether this led to study dropouts. One interesting feature the authors note is that aripiprazole was not associated with any change on the SCL-90-R Somatization scale. The use of antidepressants and anticonvulsant agents tends to predict significant decreases on this scale. Finally, while decreases in self-injury were statistically significant, there were still clinically elevated scores on all other indices of psychopathology. At the end of the trial, the mean score on the HAM-D was $13.9 \pm 2.8$, the mean score on the HAM-A was $16.3 \pm 3.5$, and the STAXI scales remained elevated. The decreases in clinical syndrome scores are encouraging but suggest a minimal effect of the medication. It would have been more informative to see a quintile analysis of responders, as the data suggest that the top 25% of such participants likely had most of the gains. Analysis of this group could shed light on features predictive of response to atypical antipsychotics generally and aripiprazole in particular. Based on where and how this medication seems to work in individuals with BPD, it is probably best utilized as an augmentation modality for another primary agent.

## Olanzapine

The majority of the published controlled trials with atypical antipsychotics reports findings from the use of olanzapine. In all, 910 patients were studied in the five trials reviewed below. The first double-blind, placebo-controlled trial was reported by Bogenschutz and Nurnberg (2004). The 40 patients enrolled in the trial were randomized equally to either olanzapine or placebo. Only 23 participants completed the entire trial (10 in the olanzapine group and 13 in the placebo condition). Olanzapine dosage was 6.9 mg at study end versus a pseudodose of 10.2 mg for placebo. A Clinical Global Impression (CGI) score, comprising all nine criteria for BPD rated from 1 to 7, was the primary measure of efficacy (Clinical Global Impression Scale for BPD [CGI-BPD]; Perez et al., 2007). The olanzapine group showed a statistically significant decrease in CGI-BPD score of about 14 points versus 7 points in the placebo group. None of the nine individual items defining BPD had a significant mean-level reduction, with the exception of Inappropriate Anger. Weight gain was significantly higher in the olanzapine group, causing two patients to drop out of the trial, and two others discontinued due to sedation (20% of sample). All patients were included in the data analysis, with the last observation carried forward if they completed 2 weeks or more of the trial. This may have biased the outcome in a more positive manner. Regarding secondary outcome measures, the SCL-90-R showed no significant differences between the two groups. In addition, the HAM-A and HAM-D were not significantly different between the two groups at study end.

Although olanzapine was associated with significant improvement in some symptoms according to clinician report, patients' reports differed. The authors suggest that olanzapine may be an agent best used for short-term pharmacotherapy, as they noticed a decline in efficacy from 8 weeks (peak efficacy) to 12 weeks. Based on the average weight gain of 8 pounds, high dropout rate, and no patient-perceived difference versus placebo, as assessed by the SCL-90-R, the authors suggest that their positive findings needed to be interpreted with caution, and larger trials are needed to duplicate and extend their findings. Their astute observation of efficacy peaking at 8 weeks and declining thereafter was insightful in light of the studies that followed.

The pharmacological rationale underlying the Bogenschutz and Nurnberg (2004) trial was duplicated in two industry-sponsored multinational trials that were markedly larger than any BPD trials conducted to date. The first was a flexible-dose trial in a sample of 314 patients (Schulz et al., 2008) taking olanzapine ($n = 155$) or in a placebo group ($n = 159$) for 12 weeks, with a 1:1 ratio of assignment to either condition. Olanzapine dose ranged from 2.5 to 20 mg/day, and averaged 7.09 mg/day. Primary outcomes were measured by the Zanarini Rating Scale for Borderline Personality Disorder (ZAN-BPD; Zanarini, Vujanovic, et al., 2003), and secondary measures included the SCL-90-R (Derogatis, 1994), the Global Assessment of Functioning (GAF; American Psychiatric Association [APA], 2000), the Sheehan Disability Scale (SDS; Sheehan, Harnett-Sheehan, & Raj, 1996), the Overt Aggression Scale—Modified (OAS-M; Coccaro, Harvey, Kupsaw-Lawrence, Herbert, & Bernstein, 1991), and the Montgomery–Asberg Depression Rating Scale (MADRS; Montgomery & Asberg, 1979). There were no statistical differences in any outcome measures between the olanzapine and placebo-treated groups. Somnolence, sedation, increased appetite, and weight gain were significantly higher in the group taking olanzapine. The dropout rate was 48.4% in the olanzapine group and 38.4%

in the placebo group. The study was impressive in its size but failed to show any advantage for olanzapine over placebo on any measure.

Zanarini and colleagues (2011) reported a second trial, a fixed-dose, 12-week study comparing the efficacy of olanzapine versus placebo, and the results were similar to the Schulz and colleagues (2008) trial. This study involved 451 patients receiving olanzapine at 2.5 mg/day ($n = 150$, low-dose group), olanzapine 5–10 mg/day ($n = 148$, moderate-dose group) or placebo ($n = 153$). The primary outcome was measured by the ZAN-BPD (Zanarini, Vujanovic, et al., 2003) and secondary outcomes were assessed by the MADRS (Montgomery & Asberg, 1979), the OAS-M (Coccaro et al., 1991), the GAF (APA, 2000), the SCL-90-R (Derogatis, 1994), and the SDS (Sheehan et al., 1996). There were no significant differences on ZAN-BPD scores between the low-dose olanzapine group and placebo at the 12-week study endpoint. Participants in the moderate-dose olanzapine group showed a significantly greater decrease in ZAN-BPD scores from baseline to trial end compared to the placebo group, but the effect size was modest. Similar to the Bogenschutz and Nurnberg (2004) study, the highest level of change in the high-dose group was seen at study midpoint (Week 6), with a less robust response versus placebo thereafter. Individual items of the SDS, OAS-M, and the SCL-90-R total score also showed statistical improvement versus placebo at the end of the trial. There were no significant differences in scores between groups on the MADRS or GAF. Weight gain and somnolence were significantly higher in both low- and moderate-dose olanzapine groups. The authors refer to the response to 5–10 mg olanzapine dose as "clinically modest" and note that the risk of side effects, particularly weight gain, needs to be balanced against response.

Both of the described studies are impressive in clinical design and magnitude but report modest results. The data from both trials provide evidence of efficacy for some individuals with BPD treated with olanzapine. A reanalysis of the data looking at quintile response would be enlightening and might provide a better picture of the responsive group. This would aid in selecting which patients with BPD to treat with olanzapine and possibly other atypical antipsychotics. There is little question that some patients with BPD benefit from olanzapine, but it is not clear from the studies available how many and how to identify individuals who may derive benefit from this medication in clinical practice.

Ultimately, clinicians want to know which patient characteristics predict a higher likelihood of response to a particular medication class. The two trials just described failed to show any clinically meaningful benefit of olanzapine over placebo; moreover, a significant number of side effects were reported in the olanzapine groups. In summary, should a clinician choose an atypical antipsychotic to aid in the treatment of BPD, the evidence suggests that olanzapine is one of the least favored agents because of the side effect profile.

Zanarini, Frankenburg, and Parachini (2004) conducted an 8-week, industry-sponsored, randomized trial of fluoxetine ($n = 14$) versus olanzapine ($n = 16$) versus fluoxetine plus olanzapine ($n = 15$) in female patients with BPD who were free of major depression at entry into the trial. Ratings consisted of the OAS-M, MADRS, GAF, and Hollingshead Two Factor Index of Social Position (Hollingshead, 1965). There were no patient self-rating scales included to assess user satisfaction. All three groups showed a substantial decrease in scores on the OAS-M and MADRS. The olanzapine and fluoxetine combination product resulted in larger improvements and was superior to fluoxetine statistically. The dose of fluoxetine was $15.0 + 6.5$ in the fluoxetine-alone group (maximum dose of 30 mg), and this may have been part of the reason for underwhelming results with fluoxetine, as it was a lower dose than that shown to be associated with a response in patients with BPD in prior trials (see Markovitz, 2001, for a review). Olanzapine dosage varied between 2.5 and 7.5 mg/day ($3.2 \pm 1.5$). Attrition was low, with over 90% of patients completing the 8-week trial. Reported weight gain was statistically higher in the olanzapine group. As with the Schulz and colleagues (2008) and the Zanarini and colleagues (2011) trials, results indicated that olanzapine led to significant symptom reduction for some patients, but it is not clear from the information reported which presenting symptoms predict response. It is also clear from the effect sizes in all these trials that symptom improvement was modest for the all treatment cohorts. Finally, with respect to the Zanarini and colleagues (2004) study, without a placebo control group, it is difficult to clearly evaluate overall efficacy of any of the three treatment groups.

The final randomized trial of interest in relation to olanzapine is a 12-week study reported by Soler and colleagues (2005). This trial consisted of 60 patients, with 30 participants each assigned to receive dialectical behavior therapy

(DBT) plus olanzapine or placebo. The majority of individuals were taking benzodiazepines, antidepressants, or mood stabilizers at baseline. The olanzapine group received dosages between 5 and 20 mg/day, averaging 8.83 mg/day. This group showed a greater decrease in depressive symptoms, anxiety symptoms, and impulsivity/aggressive symptoms compared to placebo. There was also a trend toward significant decreases in self-injury and suicide attempts. The reported level of weight gain by the end of the study was significantly higher in the olanzapine group, averaging about 6 pounds compared to less than a pound in the placebo group. The results are the first to evaluate the efficacy of olanzapine plus psychotherapy, and the results are encouraging. The olanzapine plus DBT group improved more over the 3-month trial than the placebo plus DBT group, pointing to the same synergism seen in therapy plus medication trials in major depression. Another possibility is that olanzapine augmented the antidepressant therapy received by 80% ($n = 24$) of the olanzapine group. Antidepressant augmentation with atypical antipsychotics is well documented, including the use of olanzapine (Marangell, Johnson, Kertz, Zboyan, & Martinez, 2002; Shelton et al., 2001). The findings were encouraging, as this study the first attempt to evaluate in BPD what has been evaluated in depression, namely, combining pharmacotherapy and psychotherapy. Because of the prevalence of BPD, more trials like this are needed. Since there are few dosing guidelines established in the field of BPD pharmacotherapy, trials such as these are even more difficult, in part due to the uncertainty regarding appropriateness of the dose and class of pharmacotherapy provided.

The evidence from all the previously summarized trials suggests that olanzapine is beneficial for some patients with BPD. In every trial, olanzapine outperformed placebo in associations with symptom reduction, although not all outcome indices reached significant levels of reduction. This speaks to the heterogeneity of BPD and suggests that a proportion of patients with borderline pathology (well less than a majority) have a form of the disorder that may benefit from treatment with atypical antipsychotics. It is imperative to evaluate the characteristics of responders in predicting significant treatment gains with olanzapine. Based on low responsivity versus placebo, loss of efficacy with time, and significant side effects, olanzapine is probably not a particularly good medication to use in BPD longitudinally.

## Ziprasidone

Pascual and colleagues (2008) conducted a double-blind, placebo-controlled trial of ziprasidone in which the CGI-BPD was the primary measure. Secondary outcomes were assessed by the HAM-D, HAM-A, Brief Psychiatric Rating Scale (BPRS), SCL-90-R, Barratt Impulsiveness Scale (Barratt, 1995), and the Buss–Durkee Inventory (Buss & Durkee, 1957). Patients were randomized to either receive ziprasidone ($n = 30$) with a dose range of 40–200 mg/day (84.1 mg/day ± 54.8 was average dose) or placebo ($n = 30$). Seventeen patients (57%) left the ziprasidone group prior to study completion at 12 weeks, and 14 individuals (47%) dropped out of the placebo condition. Treatment responses to ziprasidone and placebo were clinically identical. The authors discuss reasons behind the null findings; however, the reported data are similar to those seen in all the other controlled trials focusing on atypical antipsychotics. There is either a small subgroup of patients with BPD who respond to atypical antipsychotics or the drugs are simply not effective when studied versus placebo.

In terms of other atypical antipsychotic medications, risperidone, clozapine, quetiapine, paliperidone, and asenapine have had no double-blind, placebo-controlled trials or new trials reported since the last comprehensive review (Markovitz, 2004). Overall, the entire group of atypical antipsychotic medications is probably best avoided as a first-line agent in treating BPD, as evidence of efficacy is relatively modest. As previously noted, a distinction may be made between statistical and clinically meaningful significance. The vast majority of patients with BPD I have treated are smart enough to know whether a medication is helping them or not. If they do not believe it is, they stop it. That is what is seen in the above trials; even in short-term use of the atypical antipsychotics, compliance is low, and patient-perceived improvement (e.g., as measured by the SCL-90-R) is lacking. This unequivocally leads to noncompliance. Compounding the problem with these agents are the side effects, which outweigh the small gains. There is likely a place for these agents, but to augment other pharmacological interventions that unequivocally show a more robust response and better side effects profile.

Looking at all the recent controlled trials, the impressive investigation of atypical antipsychotics as a primary treatment in BPD appears to be planned by pharmaceutical company marketing rather than actual results.

## Omega-3 Fatty Acids

The use of omega-3 fatty acids to decrease aggression was first studied by Hamazaki and colleagues in 1996. This study examined the effects of docosahexaenoic acid (DHA) on healthy university students over a 3-month period. Half the group started taking DHA and half started on placebo at the end of summer vacation. During the time students were administered DHA, they were evaluated at the end of a rigorous school semester through the use of a picture test showing scenes that should cause frustration. The students taking DHA had statistically less "extraggression," defined as frustration leading to enhanced readiness to be aggressive toward external trigger factors. The data from this study helped lead to the addition of DHA and/or ethyl-eicosapentaenoic acid (EPA) for treatment of patients with bipolar disorder (Stoll et al., 1999) or recurrent major depression (Nemets, Stahl, & Belmaker, 2002) as augmenting agents. In both cases there was benefit from the omega-3 fatty acids.

Use of these agents in patients with BPD was first undertaken by Zanarini and Frankenburg (2003) and used as monotherapy in 20 women receiving 1 g of EPA daily, and 10 women receiving placebo. There were no side effects of note associated with EPA use, and there was statistical improvement between the placebo and active treatment groups, as measured by the OAS-M and MADRS scores, the only two measures used in the trial. The reported magnitude of change was moderate, but the side effects to the medication were benign; hence, it could easily be argued that it makes sense to utilize EPA in all patients with BPD as either a monotherapy or an augmenting agent.

In another study, Hallahan, Hibbeln, Davis, and Garland (2007) screened and followed 49 patients presenting to the accident and emergency department with self-harm, 35 of whom had a diagnosis of BPD (71%). The authors completed ratings on the Beck Depression Inventory (BDI; Beck, Ward, Mendelson, Mock, & Erbaugh, 1961), HAM-D, OAS-M for Suicidality and Aggression, Immediate and Delayed Memory Tasks (IMT/DMT; Dougherty, Marsh, & Mathias, 2002) for Impulsivity, and the Perceived Stress Scale (PSS; Cohen, Kamarch, & Mermelstein, 1983) and a measure of daily stresses over the 12-week trial (Daily Hassles and Uplifts Scale [DHUS]; Kanner, Coyne, Schaefer, & Lazarus, 1981). Patients ($n = 22$) received DHA (0.9 g/day) and EPA (1.2 g/day) or placebo ($n = 27$). At the onset of the trial, 26 patients (53%) were on antidepressants, and this increased to 33 individuals (67%) by the end of the trial. BDI, HAM-D, PSS, and DHUS scores all improved significantly over the course of the trial. Indices measured by the OAS-M and IMT/DMT did not show improvement. The authors noted that improvements were seen entirely in the affective spectrum, and that the Zanarini and Frankenburg (2003) study found improvement in aggression. Reasons for this discrepancy are not clear, but both studies did demonstrate benefit for patients with BPD who took omega-3 fatty acids to reduce depressive symptoms.

More recently, Bellino, Bozzatello, Rocca, and Bogetto (2014) conducted an extremely interesting study involving 43 patients treated with valproate, then randomized them in a 12-week, double-blind, placebo-controlled trial to receive either placebo or EPA (1.2 g/day) and DHA (0.8 g/day). The group receiving the essential fatty acids showed greater reductions in self-injury, impulsivity, and anger outbursts on the Borderline Personality Disorder Severity Index (BPDSI) total score compared to the placebo group, and side effects were minimal in both conditions. The authors noted that treatment with omega-3 fatty acids is an easy and beneficial addition to therapy with the anticonvulsant valproate, and was utilized in their treatment setting. They could not, however, explain why they saw no decrease in depression in this trial in contrast to the prior two trials. The take-away message from all the trials summarized earlier is that EFA helped reduce symptoms. In a study with a small sample size, positive changes are noteworthy. Just as one would not expect similar studies to show identical changes in the HAM-D, CGI, or SCL-90-R, one would, however, expect at least evidence of a trend toward change in the predicted direction. This is exactly what Bellino and colleagues reported, corroborating the benefit of EFA in the treatment of BPD.

In summary, findings suggest the use of EFA is consistently associated with treatment gains.

Financial cost and side effects are minimal, and they are an easy addition to treatment. Many patients would rather take a dietary supplement than a medication, and for those patients who are unwilling to take a medication, this is a suitable alternative.

## Antidepressants

There are no published trials of antidepressants used to treat BPD since our last review 12 years ago. Open trials of interest included duloxetine (Bellino, Paradiso, Bozzatello, & Bogetto, 2010) and transdermal selegiline (Markovitz, 2012). My colleagues and I recently completed a 12-week, double-blind, placebo-controlled trial of transdermal selegiline in BPD and some of the data are presented here.

Selegiline is a monoamine oxidase inhibitor, and these agents are known to be effective treatment for BPD (Cowdry & Gardner, 1988; Klein, 1968). We felt that transdermal delivery had advantages over the oral medications previously studied, since the transdermal selegiline largely bypasses the gastric system, necessitating a need for lower doses of medication, and less inhibition of the gastric and hepatic monoamine oxidase systems. This in turn markedly reduces the risks of tyramine interactions as a side effect. We anecdotally found little to no weight gain in our open-label trial (Markovitz, 2012), and wanted to examine whether this feature also emerged in our double-blind trial. This in turn would improve compliance longitudinally in the group. Dosing is simple, since the starting dosage is the same as the ending dosage. Last, we wanted to see the efficacy of the selegiline in a random collection of individuals with BPD, and we went out of our way to recruit patients receiving treatment in mental health centers compared to our earlier trials examining individuals with active but lesser forms of BPD, gleaned from our private practice. The individuals had a Diagnostic Interview for Borderline Personality—Revised (Zanarini, Gunderson, Frankenburg, & Chauncey, 1989) scale score of $9.2 \pm 1.2$ for the group as a whole.

Since the overlap of BPD and bipolar disorder is so prevalent, we only enrolled patients who satisfied criteria for both diagnoses based on lifetime ratings of the Structured Clinical Interview for DSM-IV Axis I and II Disorders (SCID-I and SCID-II). Most industry-sponsored trials for bipolar disorder claim to exclude patients with BPD, but no structured interview is administered to measure BPD and see whether it is present. It would be similar to excluding abnormal thyroid results without measuring a thyroid level. My suspicion is that the trials would likely never fill if the structured interviews for BPD were done. It is not an either–or scenario, but what to do if both are present. Because the two disorders are so closely aligned diagnostically, I felt it would be reasonable to see how both responded simultaneously to the same treatment. The literature notes poor response to antidepressants in patients with bipolar disorder, but studies have suggested the monoamine oxidase inhibitors (MAOIs) are effective in this group.

Thirty evaluable patients were enrolled and randomized in a 2:1 ratio to receive 12 mg transdermal selegiline daily or placebo. Patients needed to complete at least 6 weeks of treatment to be part of the data analysis, and early terminators were replaced in the trial. There were four dropouts on placebo and two on selegiline, for a total of 36 patients enrolled. The primary outcome measure was the Hopkins Symptoms Checklist 90—Revised. The HAM-D, SDS, CGI Clinician, and CGI Patient were all measured at each visit.

The data were analyzed using a quadrille analysis. The top one-third of the patients in the trial had a decrease in their SCL-90-R scores of $135.1 \pm 65.7$ points versus the entire placebo group reduction of $28.9 \pm 46.8$ points. The $p$ value for the differences in mean response $t$-test with unequal variances was 0.0047 (see Table 35.1). Similar results were seen with the HAM-D as a secondary measure. The active medication group had a $13.1 \pm 7.8$ point reduction in their score and the placebo group $4.7 \pm 2.4$. The $p$ value for the differences in mean response $t$-test with unequal variances was 0.029. Similar results were seen on all of the other scales utilized.

These results showed transdermal selegiline to be very effective for the top one-third of the group. This confirmed the results seen in prior studies in BPD or BPD-like illnesses. The structured clinical intakes for Axis I and Axis II disorders mirrored the results seen in our fluoxetine trials with multiple Axis I and Axis II diagnoses. Like our venlafaxine trial, Axis III morbidity for migraines, headaches, irritable bowel syndrome, restless leg syndrome, fibromyalgia, premenstrual syndrome, and neurodermatitis were high, with over 90% of pa-

**TABLE 35.1. Hopkins Symptoms Checklist Scores for Placebo versus Active Medication**

Two-sample $t$-test with unequal variances

| Group | Obs | Mean | Std. Err. | Std. Dev. | [95% Conf. Interval] | |
|---|---|---|---|---|---|---|
| 0 | 7 | −28.85714 | 24.85714 | 65.76582 | −89.68038 | 31.96609 |
| 1 | 8 | −135.123 | 16.54479 | 46.79572 | −174.2472 | −96.0028 |
| combined | 15 | −85.53333 | 19.93319 | 77.20091 | −128.2858 | −42.78089 |
| diff | | 106.2679 | 29.8598 | | 40.31723 | 172.2185 |

| diff = mean (0) − mean (1) | | $t = 3.5589$ |
|---|---|---|
| Ho: diff = 0 | Satterthwaite's degrees of freedom = 10.6947 | |
| Ha: diff < 0 | Ha: diff = 0 | Ha: diff > 0 |
| Pr $(T < t)$ = .9977 | Pr $(|T|) > |t|)$ = .0047 | Pr $(T > t)$ = .0023 |

*Note.* The test compares placebo (Group 0) to active (Group 1) patients by looking at the score change between the second visit and the last visit in the data for the top one-third of responders to active drug only. The patients receiving the active drug did respond more than patients receiving placebo (an improvement of 135.1 points vs. 28.9 points for the placebo patients). The $p$-value highlighted below for the differences in mean response $t$-test for samples with unequal variances was .0047.

tients having one or more of these diagnoses. The symptoms resolved in the vast majority of responders.

No placebo-controlled trials of other antidepressants have been conducted in the past decade. This underscores the situation faced in BPD research: The field is largely driven by pharmaceutical industry funding, as can be seen by scanning the funding disclosure information in the vast majority of the aforementioned trials. The market for antidepressants is already well defined. In addition, since many of the branded agents have generic counterparts, it makes little sense for any of the pharmaceutical companies to fund trials in BPD, since there will be little return on investment no matter how well the trial is conducted. The use of antidepressants in BPD requires further investigation to demonstrate their appropriateness in clinical use. As almost two-thirds of patients with recurrent major depression have comorbid BPD (Skodol et al., 2011) on face value it would seem these agents are effective in depressed patients with BPD. Data for dosing with selective serotonin reuptake inhibitors (SSRIs), serotonin–norepinephrine reuptake inhibitors (SNRIs), and MAOIs in BPD are inadequate.

Concomitantly, in many of the aforementioned trials, patients were utilizing antidepressants along with the particular agent under study. This suggests that researchers appreciate that some benefit is derived from these agents. Earlier data supports this, but newer trials are lacking in number, which in turn artificially skews data analysis done on treatment modalities (see below).

## Meta-Analysis

Meta-analyses of randomized controlled trials are important for clinicians in making sense of the current literature. These important contributions present an intriguing perspective on what studies the industry has chosen to fund. As an example, every olanzapine trial described earlier was funded by the drug's manufacturer. There is nothing inherently wrong with this, and it is encouraging that the pharmaceutical industry is willing to investigate pharmacotherapy of BPD. However, the sheer number of patients enrolled in these trials tends to produce findings that often, due to the increased power to detect even small effects, are disproportionate to findings from smaller pharmacotherapy trials reported for other classes of medication. It is essential for clinicians to know what the data show in the literature, and it is also important to know what is missing from the literature and, ultimately, the meta-analysis. For example, both large olanzapine trials reported null findings (Schulz et al., 2008; Zanarini et al., 2011). Likewise, side effects are not included as part of the meta-analyses, so weight gain and lethargy do not show up as part of the data consideration.

For these reasons inadequately or understudied medications will not accumulate the evidence base required to be considered effective treatment interventions. Antidepressants are poorly studied in the treatment of BPD, for example, and require further study to prove or disprove their efficacy. Based on the biochemistry of BPD, earlier trials, and the ongoing use of antidepressants in many of the above trials (Hallahan et al., 2007; Soler et al., 2005; Tritt et al., 2005), clinicians believe they are effective, but inadequate data exist to quantify the effect of antidepressants.

## Discussion

BPD is a syndrome, like diabetes or hypertension, that includes multiple behavioral problems subsumed under the same diagnosis. Different features associated with BPD respond in varying ways to medications administered. For example, some of the studies reviewed in this chapter suggest that anger control issues may be better addressed with antiepileptic drugs but, again, this may not be the case for some individuals. Depression, likewise, may initially be treated with antidepressants, but these may be inferior to anticonvulsants or antipsychotics. There simply are not enough data from which to draw definitive conclusions. Thus, despite the various meta-analyses reported in the literature, there is no way to determine the most effective treatment for individual patients. The available trials provide guideposts, but they are far from definitive. Clearly, not all the patients respond to the particular agent under investigation in any trial. It is my view that if a particular type of agent fails to elicit a positive response, it makes sense to change the class of medication, just as one would if treating an infection with penicillin, or major depression with an SSRI. Ultimately, this involves treating the brain like an organ that has logical behaviors flowing from the disease process. For example, if the patient has mood swings, brief psychotic episodes, depression, headaches, migraines, and fibromyalgia, it is more appropriate to use a medication that conceptually addresses all of these symptoms and their common neurochemical underpinning.

This concept, "parsimony of diagnosis," is a more logical way to treat any illness. The idea is that individuals have one disease process with many symptoms. Thus, an antidepressant that addresses serotonergic deficits, or an anticonvulsant that addresses these symptoms, makes the most sense in the aforementioned case. Neuroleptics potentially address some of the symptoms—brief psychotic episodes and depression—but not the others. In the case of BPD, treating the illness in each patient as a single neurochemical malady makes the most sense. This is not to say every patient will improve completely on a single medication, but like a cardiac patient or asthmatic patient, a single medication should be the cornerstone of treatment and provide most of the benefit one is hoping to achieve. Since there are different biological types of BPD, the cornerstone of treatment will differ in many of the patients. Additional medications may be added for fine-tuning in the same way sleep medications, modafinil, or low-dose antipsychotics are added to antidepressants to augment the positive effects of the primary agent.

All of the pharmacotherapy trials of BPD, positive or negative, have helped to define productive treatments. When I initially reviewed the literature 15 years ago, the paucity of well-controlled trials was tacitly accepted in the field. Now, well-controlled trials are *de rigeur* in the field. Open-label trials provide data to move forward with controlled trials, or at least allow clinicians to utilize agents in their patients when better defined treatments have failed to provide effective relief. Nevertheless, a tremendous amount remains to be done. Most of the trials are small, and even fewer investigate dose–response measures. The olanzapine trials did everything one could ask for in a trial. Unfortunately, they did not show enough efficacies to argue for chronic use in BPD. Topiramate treatment showed a marked response, but the dosing tended to lie in the lower range, and makes one wonder whether higher dosages would result in higher efficacy in some cases. These are not criticisms of the articles but simply a critique of where we must go in the field. Larger trials with variable doses, as in the olanzapine trial, are needed. Since so many patients with recurrent depression have BPD (Skodol et al., 2011), and these patients are excluded from routine depression trials, we do not know how to dose antidepressants to treat them. As an example, the fluoxetine antidepressant trials in BPD used 40 mg/day as the maximum dose (Salzman et al., 1995; Simpson et al., 2004). Would 60 or 80 mg have worked better? In our unpublished double-blind trial using fluoxetine, all patients were given 80 mg, and the response was much more robust (Markovitz, 2001). Trials defining dosages of medication that are maximally beneficial and safe need to be done.

While minimal space has been dedicated in this chapter to discussion of noncontrolled trials, all contributions to the field, including noncontrolled trials, are important and listed in the appropriate addendum. The evidence reviewed from the controlled trials show statistically meaningful change in certain patients with BPD. Most individuals, however, have a far from complete response. Some patients do not respond at all to the better studied medications. From articles I have written and reviewed, most of the total drug effect seen is by the top 25% of responders. The open trials provide direction as to where we should go to treat our patients who do not respond to better studied pharmacotherapy, and indicate how we can augment partial responders, and where the research should be directed in the future. If topiramate, for example, reduces the expression of hostility but fails to lessen depressive symptoms, which other agent(s) are likely to be effective? The open trials provide clinicians alternatives to the medications already used, and suggest possible ways of combining pharmacotherapies to best treat patients. There are no approved treatments of BPD, and the best interventions are based on treating known neurochemical anomalies in the CNS. Most studies point to a serotonergic anomaly in BPD or in symptom clusters occurring together and commonly in BPD (Markovitz, 2001). I feel that effective treatment should be addressed with this in mind. I respect the information gleaned by the meta-analyses but also recognize that the results are dependent on the data being analyzed. Pharmaceutical companies are providing the majority of financing for trials in BPD, not governmental agencies. Because the former are profit oriented, they tend to conduct trials of products still under patent. Furthermore, there is no reason to conduct comparative trials with alternative products to show superiority or even equivalency of their products. Since no approved treatment for BPD exists, any positive signal elicited in a clinical trial can be claimed as a sign of efficacy. The two large olanzapine trials (Schulz et al., 2008; Zanarini et al., 2011), while well designed, are examples of this. In other contexts, these randomized controlled trials (RCTs) would be considered failures or negative trials. Yet the positive findings available are data that can be used in a meta-analysis to justify efficacy of atypical antipsychotics, when, in real life, they offer little benefit and abundant side effects. The very magnitude of the industry-funded study slants the results of meta-analyses to proffer a more favorable position for these agents than merited. On a personal level, after my associates and I published our venlafaxine open-label data, the manufacturer informed us that our proposed double-blind, placebo-controlled trial had been rejected because of risk. Our research group assumed that this meant the risk of very ill patients with BPD harming themselves or committing suicide. We rewrote the protocol with safeguards, and resubmitted it, only to find out that the risk was not to patients as we were initially informed but to the possibility of the study not having as robust findings as those in our open-label trial. Since the open-label trial was already published and defined a new treatment modality (SNRI) for BPD, the company saw no reason to invest in a trial that might not work or even if it did, simply corroborate the original data. There were no plans to move forward on a new drug indication and FDA approval, so the financial risk was not worthwhile. Thus, what we have found to be the most efficacious starting modality in BPD (SNRI therapy), has no chance of ever being funded. The net result is that the literature will consist of newer agents under patent that have some level of efficacy, but are overrepresented in data analyses. Hopefully, newer National Institute of Mental Health programs under way for BPD will address the gap existing in the literature.

## Treatment

A thorough review of the current literature revealed that no unified pharmacotherapy treatment paradigm for BPD can be identified. While the APA Guidelines (2001) include treatment modalities, the already dated guidelines are based on information that has become available over the past 14 years. The treatments offered to patients must minimize short- and long-term side effects. When I reviewed the double-blind or open trials for this chapter, it was easy to see that dropout rates are fairly high, averaging at least 25–35%. Medications are obviously not effective if they are not taken, and minimizing side effects to which the patient is exposed enhances the chances of compliance and beneficial outcomes. The model is based on the neurochemistry of BPD, and treats BPD as behavioral sequelae flowing from aberrant central nervous system (CNS) wiring and/or neurochemistry (Brambilla et al., 2004) arising from the underlying disease (Figure 35.1).

Treating the brain as an organ is the premise behind our paradigm. Our center has been treating BPD almost exclusively for the past 20 years, and ordering the following treatment has been found to be effective. The majority of patients respond favorably to SNRI medication. These medications have higher efficacy in depression than SSRIs, less sexual dysfunction, less weight gain, and less asthenia. This side effect profile improves compliance over the long-term, which is essential to adequate pharmacotherapy. The correct dose is probably found over a range, but we titrate up every 5 days until carbohydrate craving resolves when present. We have treated many thousands of patients over the past decade with BPD, and over 90% of them have carbohydrate craving. Carbohydrate consumption causes an insulin surge, which in turn causes all the neutral amino acids except tryptophan to be preferably taken up by muscles. Tryptophan is the precursor of serotonin, and when more serotonin is needed in the brain, tryptophan is taken up by the neutral amino acid uptake system. Carbohydrate craving enriches the uptake for tryptophan over the other neutral amino acids by increasing the relative amount of tryptophan versus the other neutral amino acids. This is why one sees carbohydrate craving in many types of BPD, depression, most eating disorders, and fibromyalgia. Elimination of this symptom is a good clinical marker for adequacy of effect/dose of medication in the brain. Underdosing the SNRI may still result in a measureable decrease in BPD symptoms, but the individual frequently notes ongoing carbohydrate craving. This is analogous to giving a type 1 diabetic a too low dose of long-acting insulin every day. Ketones will be eliminated, but patients will continue to drink copious amounts of liquids in an attempt to eliminate excess glucose from the bloodstream. They are using two medications, insulin and water, in the body's attempt to get to homeostasis. The same thing happens in BPD. Inadequacy of SNRI dose results in the patient continuing to eat carbohydrates to compensate for inadequate serotonin levels in the brain, or whatever the serotonin serves as a proxy for in the brain. Venlafaxine extended release at 450 mg/day, duloxetine at 120 mg/day, and desmethyl-venlafaxine at 300–400 mg/day have proven highly effective in this

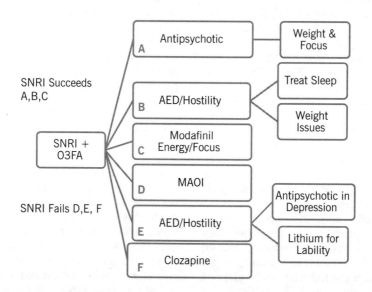

**FIGURE 35.1.** Treatment schemas for pharmacotherapy in BPD. The paradigm assumes all patients will be started on a serotonin–noradrenaline reuptake inhibitor (SNRI) and omega-3 fatty acid (O3FA). If treatment is effective, augmentation for further effect can be done with an antipsychotic (A) for augmentation to address depression, an antiepileptic drug (AED) (B) if anger or hostility remains, or modafinil (C) if energy and/or concentration are issues. If SNRI treatment fails, options for therapy include monoamine oxidase inhibitors (MAOIs) (D) to address depression, somatization, anxiety, and lability; AEDs (E) for aggression and rage; or clozapine (F) for lability and aggression.

group. If simple serotonin reuptake inhibition were the modality through which these agents were working, the dosages are excessive. Lower dosages, however, almost never work in BPD. We routinely start an essential fatty acid (EFA) with the SNRI, and this seems to improve outcome without increasing side effects.

The SNRI medications routinely take 3–5 days to begin working once an effective level has been reached. The carbohydrate craving goes away almost immediately when this level is achieved. Somatic complaints tend to diminish rapidly after this and usually resolve in 2 weeks or so. Mood lability is largely gone by 4 weeks. Depression seems to diminish between Weeks 4 and 5 and anxiety between Weeks 6 and 8. Sleep is the last component to improve, and this takes about 12 weeks. Poor sleep is treated aggressively with standard sleeping agents. Partial efficacy of SNRI medications is addressed (see Figure 35.1) with either low-dose antipsychotics (A) for depression or antiepileptic drugs for hostility and aggression (B). Concentration and energy issues are common in the group, and these are addressed with modafinil (C) whenever possible because of lack of habituation and abuse potential. Nausea, if it occurs at the initiation of medication, can be treated by dissolving 30 mg of mirtazapine in water, and taking 15–30 ml of the solution at night to blockade 5-HT$_3$ receptors for 3–5 days.

Not all patients respond to SNRI medications. If one looks at the CNS as an electrical circuit, there are different places the wire may be broken, resulting in BPD. Inadequate levels of neurotransmitters may be addressed by SNRI, but they may also be too low for SNRI to work. MAOIs (D in Figure 35.1), particularly transdermal selegiline, have proven highly effective in this group at 12 mg/day. Dietary restrictions are essentially nil with this medication, and weight gain is very low. To further illustrate, an individual would be required to eat almost a kilogram of blue cheese at a single sitting to have even a 10-mm increase in blood pressure. This makes long-term compliance easier. The MAOI medications tend to be highly energizing as a group, and are very effective for somatization, anxiety, and lability. Just as in depression, the same problems exist in patients with BPD and substance abuse, particularly stimulants, and the MAOI medications are best avoided in this group. The major issue with the MAOI is a very slow onset of action. These drugs routinely take 4–8 weeks to achieve some level of efficacy, and many patients are too acutely ill to wait this long. This is particularly true for hospitalized patients. On the positive side, MAOIs seem to have the highest and broadest level of efficacy, and a database to support efficacy in BPD (Cowdry & Gardner, 1988; Klein, 1967, 1968; Soloff et al., 1993).

If SNRI and MAOI medications fail, antiepileptic agents (E in Figure 35.1) are the next best choice. These agents have benefits but also are limited in their ability to address depression and anxiety. They can be augmented with either antipsychotics or lithium to enhance efficacy. Unfortunately, the antiepileptics can be depressogenic and in our cohort are less well tolerated than antidepressants. Furthermore, adding atypical antipsychotics and/or lithium decreases compliance even further.

Finally, clozapine is occasionally used for BPD (F in Figure 35.1). The lethargy and weight gain seen with the medication are highly problematic, but clozapine unequivocally can benefit a small cohort of patients with BPD. This medication is almost always the last one utilized because of the side effects, cost, and issues with weekly blood monitoring.

When all is said and done, it is unlikely that many patients with BPD will respond fully to any single agent discussed in this chapter. First, if the illness is structural in nature, and data suggest that it is, it borders on impossible to change strong neurological connections in the brain. Even worse, if connections are missing or have died, even less can be done (Bramilla et al., 2004). Second, most systemic illnesses are not fully alleviated or addressed by a single medication. It is illogical to think a brain disease such as BPD will be any different. Finally, there is a learned component of the illness, just as there is muscle atrophy with a casted arm resulting from a broken bone. It would be foolhardy to think that the addition of a medication could allay this learned component, and that is where therapy fits into the schemas once the underlying illness is treated.

The pharmacological treatment data are encouraging, but a great deal remains to be done. Although no specific treatment for BPD addresses the needs of this group, data regarding anticonvulsants are probably the strongest and show diminishing lability and anger, but even here there is only a 25% improvement. Neuroleptics have shown limited efficacy in controlled trials, and would now appear to be a dead end as the primary agent for long-term treatment. The initially promising data of antidepressants in open and small controlled trials have not been further investigated or extended in larger clinical trials, albeit they are frequently utilized with other agents or as a primary modality. They address the neurochemistry of the disease better than any other medication group. Dietary EFA supplements have improved outcomes but leave many symptoms of BPD unaddressed. Yet perspective clearly shows there is progress in the field.

Predicting the future is difficult, and it is not an easy task to know where the field is headed. When I began my residency in the mid-1980s, obsessive–compulsive disorder and social anxiety were considered PDs, and not biological illnesses. As neurochemical findings and pharmacological treatments arose for these two anxiety disorders, they transitioned from what were then Axis II disorders to Axis I disorders. It is likely that BPD will make the same transition over the next decade, and like the aforementioned anxiety disorders, successful treatments will be the cornerstones of making this happen. Based on patients coming to our center and responding very favorably to treatment, most were diagnosed as having some type of bipolar disorder, and informed antidepressants were contraindicated. The use of the appropriate antidepressant agents markedly reduced their illness burden. It is my hope that future trials will be conducted using adequate doses of antidepressant medications to treat patients with bipolar/borderline symptoms and evaluate what works best.

## ACKNOWLEDGMENTS

It is not often that one gets a chance to thank people who have impacted one's view and education, and chapters like this afford one of these opportunities. First, I want to thank Mark Woyshville, MD, for helping me understand the idea of parsimony of diagnosis. I recall the conversation from 30 years ago as if it were yesterday. It made treatment of my patients easier and more effective, and explained the comorbidity seen in most psychiatric diseases. I also thank Susan Wagner, MA, for introducing me to cognitive-behavioral therapy 30 years ago and how it helps patients with BPD. My heartfelt thanks to John Livesley, MD, PhD, for allowing me to write this chapter. After being outside of academia for so long, I appreciate the faith he showed. Finally, my appreciation and never-ending love to my wife Ginger for everlasting support and encouragement in my work in this field. Having someone support your endeavors, especially during the hard times, makes everything easier as you move toward your goal.

## REFERENCES

Adityanjee, A., Romine, A., Brown, E., Thuras, P., Lee, S., & Schulz, S. C. (2008). Quetiapine in patients with borderline personality disorder: An open-label trial. *Annals of Clinical Psychiatry, 20,* 219–226.

Akiskal, H. S. (1981). Subaffective disorders: Dysthymic, cyclothymic, and bipolar II disorders in the "borderline" realm. *Psychiatric Clinics of North America, 4,* 25–46.

American Psychiatric Association. (2000). Global assessment of functioning (GAF) scale. In *Diagnostic and statistical manual of mental disorders* (4th ed., text rev., pp. 32–34). Washington, DC: Author.

American Psychiatric Association. (2001). Practice guidelines for treatment of borderline personality disorder. *American Journal of Psychiatry, 158*(Suppl.), 10.

Barratt, E. S. (1995) Impulsiveness and aggression. In J. Monahan & H. J. Steadman (Eds.), *Violence and mental disorder: Development of risk assessment* (pp. 61–79). Chicago: University of Chicago Press.

Beck, A. T., Ward, C. H., Mendelson, M., Mock, J., & Erbaugh, J. (1961). An inventory for measuring depression. *Archives of General Psychiatry, 4,* 561–571.

Bellino, S., Bozzatello, P., Rocca, G., & Bogetto, F. (2014). Efficacy of omega-3 fatty acids in the treatment of borderline personality disorder: A study of the association with valproic acid. *Journal of Psychopharmacology, 28*(2), 125–132.

Bogenschutz, M. P., & Nurnberg, H. G. (2004). Olanzapine versus placebo in the treatment of borderline personality disorder. *Journal of Clinical Psychiatry, 65,* 104–109.

Brambilla, P., Soloff, P. H., Sala, M., Nicoletti, M. A., Keshavan, M. S., & Soares, J. C. (2004). Anatomical MRI study of borderline personality disorder patients. *Psychiatry Research, 131,* 125–133.

Bullinger, M., & Kirchberger, I. (1998). *SF-36 Health Survey (Fragebogen zum Gesundheitszustand) (SF-36).* Goettingen, Germany: Hogrefe.

Buss, A. H., & Durkee, A. (1957). An inventory for assessing different kinds of hostility. *Journal of Consulting Psychology, 21,* 343–349.

Coccaro, E. F., Harvey, P. D., Kupsaw-Lawrence, E., Herbert, J. L., & Bernstein D. P. (1991). Development of neuropharmacologically based behavioral assessments of impulsive aggressive behavior. *Journal of Neuropsychiatry and Clinical Neuroscience, 3*(Suppl.), 44–51.

Cohen, S., Kamarch, T., & Mermelstein, R. (1983). A global measure of perceived stress. *Journal of Health and Social Behavior, 24,* 385–396.

Cowdry, R. W., & Gardner, D. L. (1988). Pharmacotherapy of borderline personality disorder: Alprazolam, carbamazepine, trifluoperazine, and tranylcypromine. *Archives of General Psychiatry, 45,* 111–119.

Derogatis, L. R. (1994). *Symptom Checklist-90-Revised (SCL-90-R).* New York: Pearson.

Dougherty, D. M., Marsh, D. M., & Mathias, C. W. (2002). Immediate and delayed memory tasks: A computerized behavioral measure of memory, attention, and impulsivity. *Behavioral Research Methods, Instruments and Computers, 34,* 391–398.

Gardner, D. L., & Cowdry, R. W. (1986). Development of melancholia during carbamazepine treatment in borderline personality disorder. *Journal of Clinical Psychopharmacology, 6,* 236–239.

Grant, B. F., Chou, S. P., Goldstein, R. B., Huang, B., Stinson, F. S., Saha, T. D., et al. (2008). Prevalence, correlates, disability, and comorbidity of DSM-IV borderline personality disorder: Results from the Wave 2 National Epidemiologic Survey on Alcohol and Related Conditions. *Journal of Clinical Psychiatry, 69,* 533–545.

Hallahan, B., Hibbeln, J. R., Davis, J. M., & Garland, M. R. (2007). Omega-3 fatty acid supplement in patients with recurrent self harm: Single-centre double-blind randomized controlled trial. *British Journal of Psychiatry, 190,* 118–122.

Hamazaki, T., Sawazaki, S., Itomura, M., Assoka, E., Nagao, Y., Nishimuro, N., et al. (1996). The effect of docosahexaenoic acid on aggression in young adults. *Journal of Clinical Investigation, 97,* 1129–1133.

Hamilton, M. (1959). The assessment of anxiety states by rating. *British Journal of Medical Psychology, 32,* 50–55.

Hamilton, M. (1960). A rating scale for depression. *Journal of Neurology, Neurosurgery, and Psychiatry, 23,* 56–62.

Hollander, E., Swann, A. C., Coccaro, E. F., Jiang, P., & Smith, T. B. (2005). Impact of trait impulsivity and state aggression on divalproex versus placebo response in borderline personality disorder. *American Journal of Psychiatry, 162,* 621–624.

Hollingshead, A. B. (1965). *Two factor index of social position.* New Haven, CT: Yale University Press.

Horowitz, L. M., Rosenbery, S. E., Baer, B. A., Ureno, G., & Villasenor, V. S. (1988). Inventory of interpersonal problems: Psychometric properties and clinical applications. *Journal of Consulting and Clinical Psychology, 56,* 885–892.

Kanner, A. D., Coyne, J. C., Schaefer, C., & Lazarus, R. S. (1981). Comparison of two modes of stress measurement: Daily hassles and uplifts versus major life events. *Journal of Behavioral Medicine, 4,* 1–39.

Klein, D. F. (1967). Importance of psychiatric diagnosis in prediction of clinical drug effects. *Archives of General Psychiatry, 16,* 118–126.

Klein, D. F. (1968). Psychiatric diagnosis and a typology of clinical drug effects. *Psychopharmacolgia, 13,* 359–386.

Loew, T. H., & Nickel, M. K. (2008). Topiramate treatment of women with borderline personality disorder: Part II. An open 18-month follow-up. *Journal of Clinical Psychoparmacology, 28,* 355–357.

Loew, T. H., Nickel, M. K., Muehlbacher, M., Kaplan, P., Nickel, C., Kettler, C., et al. (2006). Topiramate treatment for women with borderline personality disorder: A double-blind placebo-controlled study. *Journal of Clinical Psychopharmacology, 26,* 1–6.

Marangell, L. B., Johnson, C. R., Kertz, B., Zboyan, H. Z., & Martinez, J. M. (2002). Olanzapine in the treatment of apathy in previously depressed participants maintained with selective serotonin reuptake inhibitors: An open-label, flexible dose study. *Journal of Clinical Psychiatry, 63,* 391–395.

Markovitz, P. J. (2001). Pharmacotherapy. In W. J. Livesley (Ed.), *Handbook of personality disorders: Theory, research, and treatment* (pp. 475–493). New York: Guilford Press.

Markovitz, P. J. (2004). Recent trends in the pharmacotherapy of personality disorders. *Journal of Personality Disorders, 18,* 90–101.

Markovitz, P. J. (2012, October). *Transdermal selegiline in the treatment of borderline personality disorder (BPD): An open label trial in 58 patients treated for 3 years.* New York: Institute for Psychiatric Services.

Markovitz, P. J., & Wagner, S. (1996). Venlafazine in the treatment of borderline personality disorder. *Psychopharmacology Bulletin, 31,* 773–777.

Mongomery, S. A., & Asberg, M. (1979). A new depression scale designed to be sensitive to change. *British Journal of Psychiatry, 134,* 382–389.

Nemets, B., Stahl, Z., & Belmaker, R. H. (2002). Addition of omega-3 fatty acid to maintenance medication treatment for recurrent unipolar depressive disorder. *American Journal of Psychiatry, 159,* 477–479.

Nickel, M. K., & Loew, T. H. (2008). Treatment of aggression with topiramate in male borderline patients: Part II. 18 month follow-up. *European Psychiatry, 23,* 115–117.

Nickel, M. K., Muehlbacher, M., Nickel, C., Kettler, C., Gil, F. P., Bachler, E., et al. (2006). Aripiprazole in the treatment of patients with borderline personality disorder: A double-blind, placebo-controlled study. *American Journal of Psychiatry, 163,* 833–838.

Nickel, M. K., Nickel, C., Kaplan, P., Lahmann, C., Muhlbacher, M., Tritt, K., et al. (2005). Treatment of aggression with topiramate in male borderline patients: A double-blind, placebo-controlled study. *Biological Psychiatry, 57,* 495–499.

Nickel, M. K., Nickel, C., Mitterlehner, F. O., Tritt, K., Lahmann, C., Leiberich, P. K., et al. (2004). Topiramate treatment of aggression in female borderline personality disorder patients: A double-blind, placebo-controlled study. *Journal of Clinical Psychiatry, 65,* 1515–1519.

Pascual, J. C., Soler, J., Puigdemont, D., Perez-Egea, R., Tiana, T., Alvarez, E., et al. (2008). Ziprasidone in the treatment of borderline personality disorder: A double-blind, placebo-controlled, randomized study. *Journal of Clinical Psychiatry, 69,* 603–608.

Perez, V., Barrachina, J., Soler, J., Pascual, J. C., Campins, M. J., Puigdemont, D., et al. (2007). The Clinical Global Impression Scale for Borderline Personality Disorder patients (CGI-BPD): A scale sensible to detect changes. *Actas Españolas de Psiquiatría, 35,* 229–235.

Reich, D. B., Zanarini, M. C., & Bieri, K. A. (2009). A preliminary study of lamotrigine in the treatment of affective instability in borderline personality disorder. *International Clinical Psychopharmacology, 24,* 275–279.

Salzman, C., Wolfson, A. N., Schatzberg, A., Looper, J., Henke, R., Albanese, M., et al. (1995). Effect of fluoxetine on anger in symptomatic volunteers with borderline personality disorder. *Journal of Clinical Psychopharmacology, 15,* 23–29.

Schulz, S. C., Zanarini, M. C., Baterman, A., Bohus, M., Detke, H. C., Trzaskoma, Q., et al. (2008). Olanzapine for the treatment of borderline personality disorder: Variable dose 12-week randomized double-blind placebo-controlled study. *British Journal of Psychiatry, 193,* 485–492.

Sheehan, D. V., Harnett-Sheehan, K., & Raj, B. A. (1996). The measurement of disability. *International Clinical Psychopharmacology, 11*(Suppl. 3), 89–95.

Shelton, R. C., Tollefson, G. D., Tohen, M., Stahl, S., Gammon, K. S., Jacobs, T. G., et al. (2001). A novel augmentation strategy for treating resistant major depression. *American Journal of Psychiatry, 158,* 131–134.

Simpson, E. B., Yen, S., Costello, E., Rosen, K., Begin, A., Pistorello, J., et al. (2004). Combined dialectical behavior therapy and fluoxetine in the treatment of borderline personality disorder. *Journal of Clinical Psychiatry, 65,* 379–385.

Skodol, A. E., Grilo, C. M., Keyes, K. M., Geier, T., Grant, B. F., & Hassin, D. S. (2011). Relationship of personality disorders to the course of major depressive disorder in a nationally representative sample. *American Journal of Psychiatry, 168,* 257–264.

Soler, J., Pascual, J. C., Campins, J., Barrachina, J., Puigdemont, D., Alvarez, E., & Perez, V. (2005). Double-blind, placebo-controlled study of dialectical behavior therapy plus olanzapine for borderline personality disorder. *American Journal of Psychiatry, 162,* 1221–1224.

Soloff, P. H., Cornelius, J. R., George, A., Nathan, S., Perel, J. M., & Ulrich, R. F. (1993). Efficacy of phenelzine and haloperidol in borderline personality disorder. *Archives of General Psychiatry, 30,* 377–385.

Spielberger, C., Jacobs, G., Russell, S., & Crane, R. (1983). Assessment of anger: The State–Trait Anger Scale. In J. N. Bucher & C. S. Speilberger (Eds.), *Advanced personality assessment* (Vol. 3, pp. 89–131). Hillsdale, NJ: Erlbaum.

Stoll, A. L., Severus, W. E., Freeman, M. P., Rueter, S., Zbovan, H. A., Diamond, E., et al. (1999). Omega 3 fatty acids in bipolar disorder: A preliminary double-blind, placebo-controlled trial. *Archives of General Psychiatry, 56,* 407–412.

Tritt, K., Nickel, C., Lehmann, C., Leiberich, P. K., Rother, W. K., Loew, T. H., et al. (2005). Lamotrigine treatment of aggression in female borderline-patients: A double-blind, placebo-controlled study. *Journal of Psychopharmacology, 19,* 287–291.

Zanarini, M. C., & Frankenburg, F. R. (2003). Omega-3 fatty acid treatment of women with borderline personality disorder: A double-blind, placebo-controlled pilot study. *American Journal of Psychiatry, 160,* 167–169.

Zanarini, M. C., Frankenburg, F. R., & Parachini, E. A. (2004). A preliminary, randomized trial of fluoxetine, olanzapine, and the olanzapine–fluoxetine combination in women with borderline personality disorder. *Journal of Clinical Psychiatry, 65,* 903–907.

Zanarini, M. C., Gunderson, J. G., Frankenburg, F. R., & Chauncey, D. L. (1989). The Revised Diagnostic Interview for Borderlines: Discriminating BPD from other Axis II disorders. *Journal of Personality Disorders, 3*(1), 10–18.

Zanarini, M. C., Schulz, S. C., Detke, H. C., Tanaka, Y., Zhao, F., et al. (2011). A dose comparison of olanzapine for the treatment of borderline personality disorder: A 12-week randomize, double-blind, placebo-controlled study. *Journal of Clinical Psychiatry, 72,* 1353–1362.

Zanarini, M. C., Vujanovic, A. A., Parachini, E. A., Boulanger, A., Frankenburg, F. R., & Hennen, J. (2003). Zanarini Rating Scale for Borderline Personality Disorder (ZAN-BPD): A continuous measure of DSM-IV borderline psychopathology. *Journal of Personality Disorders, 17,* 233–242.

## ADDENDUM FOR ANTIDEPRESSANTS

### Duloxetine

Bellino, S., Paradiso, E., Bozzatello, P., & Bogetto, F. (2010). Efficacy and tolerability of duloxetine in the treatment of patients with borderline personality disorder: A pilot study. *Journal of Psychopharmacology, 24,* 333–339.

### Transdermal Selegiline

Markovitz, P. J. (2012, October). *Transdermal selegiline in the treatment of borderline personality disorder (BPD): An open label trial in 58 patients treated for 3 years.* New York: Institute for Psychiatric Services.

## ADDENDUM FOR ATYPICAL ANTIPSYCHOTICS

### Aripiprazole

Bellino, S., Paradiso, E., & Bogetto, F. (2008). Efficacy and tolerability of aripiprazole augmentation in sertraline-resistant patients with borderline personality disorder. *Psychiatry Research, 161,* 206–212.— Twenty-one patients started the trial, 16 completed it, and nine responded.

Mobascher, A., Mobascher, J., Schlemper, G., Winterer, G., & Malevani, J. (2006). Aripiprazole pharmacotherapy of borderline personality disorder: A series of three consecutive case reports. *Pharmacopsychiatry, 39,* 111–112.—Three patients started and two completed the trial.

Nickel, M. K. (2007). Aripiprazole treatment of patients with borderline personality disorder. *Journal of Clinical Psychiatry, 68,* 1815–1816.—Eighteen-month follow-up of 22 patients using aripiprazole.

## Asenapine

Martin-Blanco, A., Patrizi, B., Villatta, L., Gasol, X., Gasol, M., & Pascual, J. C. (2014). Asenapine in the treatment of borderline personality disorder: An atypical antipsychotic alternative. *International Clinical Psychopharmacology, 29*(2), 120–123.—Twelve patients entered the trial and nine completed the full 8 weeks.

## Clozapine

Benedetti, F., Sforzini, L., Columbo, C., & Smeraldi, E. (1998). Low-dose clozapine in acute and continuation treatment of severe borderline personality disorder. *Journal of Clinical Psychiatry, 59,* 103–107.—Twelve patients started and 12 completed the trial.

Chengappa, K. N. R., Ebeling, T., & Kang, J. S. (1999). Clozapine reduces severe self-mutilation and aggression in psychotic patients with BPD. *Journal of Clinical Psychiatry, 60,* 477–484.—Seven patient case reports.

Frankenburg, F. R., & Zanarini, M. C. (1993). Clozapine treatment of borderline personality patients: A preliminary study. *Comprehensive Psychiatry, 34,* 402–405.—Fifteen longitudinal patient case studies presented.

Swinton, M. (2001). Clozapine in severe borderline personality disorder. *Journal of Forensic Psychiatry, 12,* 580–591.—Case report of five patients.

## Olanzapine

Hallmayer, J. F. (2003). Olanzapine and women with borderline personality disorder. *Current Psychiatry Reports, 63,* 241–244.

Hough, D. W. (2001). Low-dose olanzapine for self-mutilation behavior in patients with borderline personality disorder. *Journal of Clinical Psychiatry, 62,* 296–297.—Two case reports.

Schulz, S. C., Camlin, K. L., Berry, S. A., & Jesberger, J. A. (1999). Olanzapine safety and efficacy inpatients with borderline personality disorder and comorbid dysthymia. *Biological Psychiatry, 46,* 1429–1435.—Eleven patients were evaluable.

Zanarini, M. C., & Frankenburg, F. R. (2001). Olanzapine treatment of female borderline personality disorder patients: A double-blind, placebo-controlled pilot study. *Journal of Clinical Psychiatry, 62,* 849–854.—Nineteen patients on olanzapine and nine patients on placebo at entry, and eight olanzapine-treated patients and one placebo-treated patient completed all 24 weeks of the study.

## Paliperidone

Bellino, S., Bozzatello, P., Rinaldi, C., & Bogetto, F. (2011). Paliperidone ER in the treatment of borderline personality disorder: A pilot study of efficacy and tolerability. *Depression Research and Treatment, 2011,* Article ID 680194.—Eighteen patients entered the trial and 14 completed the 12-week assessment.

## Quetiapine

Adityanjee, A., Romine, A., Brown, E., Thuras, P., Lee, S., & Schulz, S. C. (2008). Quetiapine in patients with borderline personality disorder: An open-label trial. *Annals of Clinical Psychiatry, 20,* 219–226.—16 patients entered and nine completed an 8-week trial.

Adityanjee, A., & Schulz, S. C. (2002). Clinical uses of quetiapine in disease states other than schizophrenia. *Journal of Clinical Psychiatry, 63*(Suppl. 13), 32–38.—Ten patients entered the trial and six completed it.

Bellino, S., Paradiso, E., & Bogetto, P. (2006). Efficacy and tolerability of quetiapine in the treatment of borderline personality disorder: A pilot study. *Journal of Clinical Psychiatry, 67,* 1042–1046.—Fourteen patients entered the trial and 11 completed it.

Hilger, E., Barnas, C., & Kasper, S. (2003). Quetiapine in the treatment of borderline personality disorder. *World Journal of Biological Psychiatry, 4,* 42–44.—Two patient case reports.

Perrella, C., Carrus, D., Costa, E., & Schifano, F. (2007). Quetiapine for the treatment of borderline personality disorder: An open-label study. *Progress in Neuropsychopharmacology and Biological Psychiatry, 31,* 158–163.—Twenty-nine patients started and 23 completed the trial.

Vanden Eynde, F., De Saedeleer, S., Naudis, K., Day, J., Vogels, C., van Heeringen, C., et al. (2009). Quetiapine treatment and improved cognitive functioning in borderline personality disorder. *Human Psychopharmacology, 24,* 646–649.—Forty-one patients started and 32 completed a 12-week trial.

Vanden Eynde, F., Senturk, V., Naudis, K., Vogels, C., Bermagie, K., Thas, O., et al. (2008). Efficacy of quetiapine for impulsivity and affective symptoms in borderline personality disorder. *Journal of Clinical Psychopharmacology, 28,* 147–155.—Forty-one patients started and 32 completed the trial.

Villeneuve, E., & Lemelin, S. (2005). Open-label study of atypical neuroleptic quetiapine for treatment of borderline personality disorder: Impulsivity as main target. *Journal of Clinical Psychiatry, 66,* 1298–1303.

### Risperidone

Friedel, R. O., Jackson, W. T., Huston, C. S., May, R. S., Kirby, N. L., & Stoves, A. (2008). Risperidone treatment of borderline personality disorder assessed by a borderline personality disorder-specific outcome measure: A pilot study. *Journal of Clinical Psychopharmacology, 28,* 345–347.

Khouzam, H. R., & Donnelly, N. J. (1997). Remission of self-mutilation in a patient with borderline personality during risperidone therapy. *Journal of Nervous and Mental Disease, 195,* 349.—One patient case report.

Rocca, P., Marchiaro, L., Cocuzza, E., & Bogetto, E. (2002). Treatment of borderline personality disorder with risperidone. *Journal of Clinical Psychiatry, 63,* 241–244.—Fifteen patients began and 13 completed the study.

Szigethy, E. M., & Schulz, S. C. (1997). Risperidone in co-morbid borderline personality disorder and dysthymia. *Journal of Clinical Psychopharmacology, 17,* 326–327.—One patient case report.

### Ziprasidone

Pascual, J. C., Madre, M., Soler, J., Barrachina, J., Campins, M. J., & Alvarez, E. (2006). Injectable atypical antipsychotics for agitation in borderline personality. *Pharmacopsychiatry, 39,* 117–118.—Twenty patient case reports; 12 patients began and nine completed a 2-week trial.

Pascual, J. C., Olier, S., Soler, J., Barrachina, J., Alvarez, E., & Perez, V. (2004). Ziprasidone in the acute treatment of borderline personalit disorder in psychiatric emergency services. *Journal of Clinical Psychiatry, 65,* 1281–1283.—Twelve patients began and nine completed a 2-week trial.

## ADDENDUM FOR ANTICONVULSANTS

### Lamotrigine

Preston, G. A., Marchant, B. K., Remherr, F. W., Strong, R. E., & Hedges, D. W. (2004). Borderline personality disorder in patients with bipolar disorder and response to lamotrigine. *Journal of Affective Disorders, 7,* 297–303.—Retrospective analysis of 35 patients with comorbid bipolar disorder.

Weinstein, W., & Jamison, K. L. (2007). Restrospective case review of lamotrigine use for affective instability of borderline personality disorder. *CNS Spectrums, 12,* 207–210.—Review of charts of 13 women with BPD openly treated.

### Oxcarbazepine

Bellino, S., Paradiso, E., & Bogetto, F. (2005). Oxcarbazepine in the treatment of borderline personality disorder: A pilot study. *Journal of Clinical Psychiatry, 66,* 1111–1115.—Seventeen patients entered and 13 completed a 12-week open-label trial.

### Valproate

Hollander, E., Swann, A. C., Coccaro, E. F., Jiang, P., & Smith, T. B. (2005). Impact of trait impulsivity and state aggression on divalproex versus placebo response in borderline personality disorder. *American Journal of Psychiatry, 162,* 621–624.

## ADDENDUM FOR OTHER MEDICATIONS

### Clonidine

Philipsen, A., Richter, H., Schmahl, C., Peters, J., Rusch, N., Bohus, M., et al. (2004). Clonidine in acute aversive inner tension and self-injurious behavior in female patients with borderline personality disorder. *Journal of Clinical Psychiatry, 65,* 1414–1419.

# CHAPTER 36

# A Treatment Framework for Violent Offenders with Psychopathic Traits

Stephen C. P. Wong

Psychopathy is characterized by a constellation of aberrant personality traits pertaining mainly to the affective and interpersonal domains that, taken together, are often described as a personality disorder (PD). Individuals who are psychopathic and violence prone are challenging to manage and treat. Despite significant advances in the assessment and treatment of PD, the assessment and prediction of recidivism, and offender rehabilitation,[1] there is, as yet, no generally acceptable treatment approach for such individuals.[2] An integration of these areas of research and practice may shed some light on how best to offer them effective treatment and services to reduce the risk of violence. This is the goal of this chapter.

## Assessment of Psychopathy

The point of departure of the current conception of psychopathy is Cleckley's (1976) description of the construct. The assessment of psychopathy is covered extensively elsewhere in this volume, so it is not repeated here. For my purposes in this chapter, I use the Psychopathy Checklist–Revised (PCL-R; Hare, 2003) as the operational definition of psychopathy.

## Overview of the Treatment Literature

The therapeutic nihilism about psychopathy is illustrated by Suedfeld and Landon (1978): A "review of the literature suggests that a chapter on effective treatment should be the shortest in any book concerned with psychopathy. In fact, it has been suggested that one sentence would suffice: No demonstrably effective treatment has been found" (p. 347). There is also a lack of well-designed studies on the topic. A narrative review found very few treatment evaluation studies that satisfy even minimal requirements for such studies (Wong, 2000). Others echoed with similar sentiments: "The treatment of psychopaths [is] . . . short on quality and long on lore" (Simourd & Hoge, 2000, p. 269). Although a meta-analysis of 42 studies found some evidence of successful intervention (Salekin, 2002), it was criticized on methodological grounds (Harris & Rice, 2006) because many studies did not include a control group and failed to include an objective measure of psychopathy. A systematic review also pointed to the poor state of the psychopathy treatment literature and highlights the absence of evidence

---

[1] "Offender rehabilitation" refers to services provided to offenders to reduce the risk of or actual reoffending. The services may vary from formal clinical interventions to offender case management processes, and so forth.

[2] "Offender" is a generic term that refers to those who have had contact with or are held by law in the criminal justice or forensic mental health systems.

suggesting psychopathy is untreatable (D'Silva, Duggan, & McCarthy, 2004). In essence, there are so few well designed studies that it is difficult to draw meaningful conclusions about what if any treatment is efficacious. In a more recent review, Salekin, Worley, and Grimes (2010) reported that some recent studies show positive treatment outcomes. This review also highlighted that no systematic evidence shows that treatment can make psychopaths worse or that they are untreatable, as previously suggested (see Harris, Rice, & Cormier, 1991). Nevertheless, there is no clear indication of what model or approach is likely to be useful in treating violence-prone psychopathic offenders.

Although psychopathy is a PD, many, if not all, individuals with the disorder come into contact with the forensic mental health or the criminal justice systems as a result of their criminality and violence rather than their PD. Their release from custody or involuntary detention is usually contingent on reducing their risk of violence and antisocial behaviors. As such, a major treatment goal is to reduce violence, which is the focus of this chapter. Here, "violence" is defined as behaviors that can or are expected to lead to significant physical or psychological harm to others (see Wong & Gordon, 2006, p. 288). Deliberate self-harm is excluded.

## Treatment of PD: Generic and Specific Factors

Systematic reviews of treatment efficacy demonstrate that treatments for PD are effective. Livesley (2003, 2007a, 2007b) concluded that most therapies have comparable efficacy (see also Introduction to Part VII), which suggests that effective therapies share some common or generic factors, such as establishing therapeutic alliance or positive engagement between therapists and clients (also see Beck, Freeman, & Davis, 2004; Livesley, Dimaggio, & Clarkin, 2015) that predicate change. Besides generic factors, most therapies also address the individual's specific concerns; for those with psychopathic and violence concerns, there is likely be a broad range of problems. A problem-based assessment can then match treatment with specific problem areas; this has been referred to as the "specific factors" in PD treatment (Livesley, 2007a, 2007b).

The generic–specific model of treatment is congruent with Palmer's (1996) distinction between nonprogrammatic and programmatic factors in offender rehabilitation. "Nonprogrammatic factors" are essentially generic factors, whereas "programmatic factors," including targeted interventions such as prosocial skills development and/or cognitive-behavioral skills training, correspond to specific factors. Other researchers have made similar suggestions (see Jesness, Allison, McCormick, Wedge, & Young, 1975, pp. 153–154, cited by Wong & Hare, 2005, p. 49). The generic–specific model for conceptualizing the treatment of PDs also converges with the risk–need–responsivity (RNR) framework widely used in offender rehabilitation (Andrews & Bonta, 1994–2010). McGuire (2008) concluded that the RNR framework is currently the best validated model, based on a review of 70 meta-analyses on offender rehabilitation. The relevance of the RNR principles to the treatment of PD in general and antisocial PD (ASPD) in particular was also alluded to by Andrews and Bonta (2010). The responsivity principle parallels general change mechanisms, and the risk and need factors share many similarities with specific interventions. Given the significant crossover between Livesley's generic–specific and Andrews and Bonta's RNR framework, it is possible to integrate the treatment of psychopathy, a PD, with recidivism reduction, a cornerstone in offender rehabilitation.

## Psychopathy, Violence, and Violence Reduction Treatment

Extensive evidence from prospective follow-up studies and meta-analyses show that psychopathic traits (higher scores on the PCL-R) are related to violence and antisocial behavior (Edens, Campbell, & Weir, 2007; Walters, 2003). Although the PCL-R total score predicts violence, results from a meta-analysis (Yang, Wong, & Coid, 2010) show that Factor 1 (F1) scores (Interpersonal/Affective) and Factor 2 (F2) scores (Impulsive/Antisocial) differ in predictive efficacy: Chronic antisocial and unstable behaviors captured by F2 significantly predicted violence recidivism (with an area under the curve [AUC] of about .65), whereas psychopathic personality traits, captured by F1 predicted violence at no better than chance (AUC of .56 ;95% confidence interval [CI] overlapping with .5). These results were replicated in a meta-analysis of sex offenders for sexual, violent, and general recidivism (Murrie, Boccaccini, Caperton, & Rufino, 2012) and in a non-Aboriginal and Aboriginal sample using violent, nonviolent, and general recidivism as outcomes (Olver, Neumann, Wong, & Hare, 2013). Meta-analyses also failed to show significant interactions between F1 and F2; that is, differences in magnitudes of one factor did not influence the magnitude of the other factor (Kennealy, Skeem, Walters, & Camp, 2010).

The evidence suggests that when treating violent psychopathic offenders, it is important to decompose the disorder into its components, and that violence reduction treatment should be primarily directed at behavioral characteristics (F2), since focusing on moderating F1 features is unlikely to be effective in reducing violence as F1 features are not associated with violence. However, this does not mean that the Interpersonal/Affective features can be ignored because F1 traits are closely linked to treatment interfering and noncompliant behavior and poor treatment outcome, including treatment dropout. Psychopathic offenders assessed using the PCL-R were resistant and unmotivated toward treatment, showed little treatment improvement, and had high dropout rates (Ogloff, Wong, & Greenwood, 1990). Higher PCL-R scores were associated with poorer outcome in a sample of offenders with PD, treated in a highly secure forensic mental health setting (Hughes, Hogue, Hollin, & Champion, 1997) and with higher treatment attrition, noncompliance with drug tests, and inconsistent program attendance in a sample of female substance abusers. Other studies examining treatment response as a function of F1 and F2 scores found that F1 traits are strongly associated with treatment-interfering behaviors in male offenders convicted of violent and sexual offences and were participating in a therapeutic community-based treatment program (Hobson, Shine, & Roberts, 2000). In another study, F1 (particularly the affective facet) together with being unmarried uniquely predicted program attrition (Olver & Wong, 2011). In summary, treatment directed at changing the F1 core psychopathic personality traits is unlikely to result in the reduction of violence, whereas treatment directed at changing chronic antisocial and poorly regulated behaviors (F2) may bring about reductions in violence. That said, it is also essential to manage F1-related treatment-interfering behaviors to maintain program integrity.

The literature on whether F1 and F2 are changeable on their own or with treatment is limited. Harpur and Hare (1989) showed that the magnitude of F2 decreased with age (F2 scores went from 13 to 4, a reduction of 67%, from late adolescence to about age 60 years) which is similar to the well-known age–crime curve (see Blonigen, 2010), while F1 remained at similar levels across the same age range. This means that psychopathy as measured by the PCL-R total score will appear to decrease with age due to a decrease in F2 rather than F1 features. Given its strong links with recidivism, F2 can be conceptualized as a proxy for an extended pattern of antisocial behavior. The offender rehabilitation literature has shown that treatments such as skills-based and cognitive-behavioral methods can reduce reoffending and antisocial behaviors. In the next section I describe a model for violence reduction in the treatment of individuals with psychopathic traits.

## A Model for Violence Reduction Treatment of Individuals with Psychopathic Traits

The treatment of violence proneness in individuals with psychopathic traits can be conceptualized within a two-component model based on the PCL-R two factor conceptualization of psychopathy. The model is consistent with the generic–specific framework in the treatment of PD and the RNR principles in offender rehabilitation (also see Wong, Gordon, & Gu, 2007; Wong, Gordon, Gu, Lewis, & Olver, 2012). Within this model, the objective of treatment is to reduce the risk of violence and antisocial behaviors rather than to effect changes in the core psychopathic personality features.

The interpersonal component (IC) of the two-component model addresses PCL-R F1 interpersonal and affective features. The treatment implications of the IC emphasize the importance of engaging and motivating the individual, establishing therapeutic alliance, managing and containing treatment-interfering behaviors, and maintaining professional boundaries such that the treatment program can be delivered as planned; that is, to maintain program integrity. The IC for treating psychopathy is analogous to the generic factor proposed for the treatment of PD in general (Livesley, 2007a, 2007b) and is closely aligned with the responsivity principle of the RNR model of offender rehabilitation (Andrews & Bonta, 1994–2010).

Component 2 of the model is the criminogenic component (CC), which addresses F2 behaviors of the PCL-R. The treatment implications of the CC are that effective treatment should be directed toward the individual's problem areas or criminogenic needs that are closely associated with violence and antisocial behaviors as assessed by the PCL-R. Addressing these problem areas should reduce the risk of future violence. The CC is analogous to the specific factor proposed by Livesley (2007a, 2007b) in the treatment of offenders with PD and with the risk and need principles of the RNR model for offender rehabilitation (Andrews & Bonta, 1994–2010).

The two-component model was developed by integrating three main bodies of literature: the assessment of psychopathy; the treatment of PD, especially for offenders with PD; and the rehabilitation of offenders to reduce reoffending—the so-called "what works" literature, together with appropriate program delivery and management strategies. Treatment of offenders, especially for those with histories of violence and psychopathic traits, often takes place in high security and complex custodial environments with myriad rules and regulations, and many disciplines working together to try to achieve goals that may not always be complementary to each other. Even with well-conceptualized treatment programs, the delivery of treatment can be very challenging in such complex environments and, if not well implemented, often can threaten the integrity of the program.

### Component 1: Interpersonal Component

The treatment implications of the IC are to engage offenders in a functional working relationship or alliance in order to motivate them to engage in treatment and to manage treatment-interfering behaviors. Each of these interrelated issues is discussed below.

*Motivating the Unmotivated*

"Psychopathy" is almost synonymous with "lack of motivation for change." Some would say there is no better example of an oxymoron than that of a treatment-motivated psychopath! Individuals with psychopathy are not *intrinsically* motivated to change, since, by definition, those who refuse to accept responsibility for their actions, see themselves as superior and lack empathy (essentially F1 traits), are unlikely to have an intrinsic need for change. There may be *extrinsic* reasons for wanting to change, such as an opportunity for release, reduce security, or other short-term benefits. These externally based or, in some cases, "talking the talk" motivations, which may appear to be disingenuous, shallow, or insincere, are quite frequently what one has to work with, at least at the beginning. As such, intrinsic motivation for change should not be stipulated as a prerequisite for entry into treatment (also see Livesley, 2007a, p. 219); otherwise, we can easily put psychopaths in a catch-22 situation: If they have no intrinsic motivation to change, they cannot be accepted for treatment, and, without treatment, they will likely not be intrinsically motivated. Being intrinsically or sincerely motivated for treatment is tantamount to expressing a willingness to collaborate and work with treatment providers to address entrenched personal problems and to form a functional interpersonal working relationship with the therapist to work on issues that may be deeply threatening or alien to the self. Psychopathic personality traits are the antithesis to such undertakings and, if a psychopath, in fact, is so motivated, he or she would have already made significant personality changes for the better. As such, taking psychopaths into treatment only when they are intrinsically motivated is tantamount to only offering treatment to those who have already improved and may not require an intensive regime of treatment. An IC treatment objective is to work with the individual to develop some intrinsic motivation to learn prosocial behavior starting with extrinsic motivation.

Motivational interviewing techniques (Miller & Rollnick, 2012) are often used to facilitate engagement in resistant and unmotivated clients by attending to four key principles: (1) expressing empathy, (2) developing discrepancies, (3) rolling with resistance, and (4) supporting self-efficacy. The approach is useful in working with psychopaths who appear to be unmotivated and resistant, who project blame, are argumentative, and constantly engage in one-upmanship. Expressing empathy may not come easily to some therapists because of the horrendous acts that some psychopaths have committed. However, maintaining professionalism may alleviate some personal reactions and help therapists maintain objectivity. Developing discrepancy by focusing on the difference between the way the person is as opposed to how he or she would like to be is often the key to opening the door ever so slightly for the person to recognize and want to change his or her self-defeating behaviors.

At best, motivation or getting the individual to buy-in, is achieved by building on small gains. Rolling with resistance and avoiding argumentation are particularly useful approaches with psychopathic individuals, who are highly adept in drawing the therapist into meaningless debates, thereby gaining control of the situation and sidestepping relevant issues. The goal for the therapist is to redirect away the many meaningless challenges and provocations while always keeping the treatment goal in mind. Although reinforcement contingencies are similar to therapies often used with nonpsychopathic individuals, managing the therapeutic interactions with psychopathic individuals can be quite different from their nonpsychopathic counterparts. Building an effective working alliance with psychopathic individuals often is more difficult than with individuals with other types of PDs, and a strong alliance is rarely attained. Resistance is best managed by taking a step back (rolling with resistance) and trying another approach, or simply planting the seed, with the intent of taking the approach up again later when the alliance is better developed. Within a more robust and trusting working alliance, a more direct approach can be tried. The therapist must be very goal oriented, find the path of least resistance to get to the goal, and avoid the many traps and distractions on the way (see Wong, 2016, for a more extensive discussion in this area).

### Building Working Alliances

The concept of working alliance can be decomposed into three domains: bond, task, and goal (see Bordin, 1979, 1994; Horvath & Greenberg, 1994). In treatment, therapist and client work collaboratively on shared treatment *tasks* (specific factors) to reach the agreed and shared *goals* (specific factors), sustained by positive affective regard or *bond* (generic factors) between them. The bond is often considered key in a good working alliance. However, psychopathic individuals with callous, unemotional traits have difficulty maintaining affective bonds. They also tend to generate strong countertransference reactions that further hinder alliance formation. For example, the tendency to use affective "words" in superficial ways, such as saying that they are "so sorry" without the affective "music" or showing genuine affect (see McCord & McCord, 1964) can reinforce perception of the individual's lack of sincerity and inability to engage, leading therapists and other staff members to conclude that further therapeutic work is unlikely to be helpful, which can then precipitate treatment failure. Olver and Wong (2011) reported that the affective facet of the PCL-R and marital status uniquely predicted treatment dropout in a sex offender program with a number of psychopathic offenders. Such therapeutic nihilism can readily become a self-fulfilling prophecy.

Therapists should not consider the difficulty that psychopathic individuals have in establishing a therapeutic bond as an indicator of treatment failure or noncompliance. It is still possible to work collaboratively and productively with these individuals in setting goals and working toward attaining them within a respectful, supportive, functional, and professional working alliance, even though a full therapeutic bond cannot be achieved. An individual with high PCL-R scores may not fully fit the callous–unemotional prototype often attributed to them. Though uncommon, it is mathematically possible to have a PCL-R total score of 32 (about the 91st percentile) with all eight F1 items being scored as *may be*. This suggests caution in only considering the PCL-R total score without reading both the total, F1, and F2 scores carefully before drawing inferences about an individual's psychopathic personality. Tasks and goals are discussed in detail in the section on criminogenic components (Component 2) as they pertain to problem areas linked to violence and antisocial behavior.

### Containing Treatment-Interfering Behavior and Maintaining Professional Boundaries

The maintenance of professional boundaries is a special challenge when working with forensic clients. Many offenders grew up in chaotic families and social environments, and experienced physical or sexual abuse that deprived them of appropriate role models to help them learn to set limits and to maintain and respect boundaries. Boundary problems are exacerbated by interpersonally exploitative traits such as lying, conning, manipulation, and narcissism, and by the failure to take responsibility for one's actions (Wong & Hare, 2005). These traits give rise to serious treatment-interfering behavior that tends to evoke strong negative reactions from staff members, leading to staff splitting, boundary violations, and even the demoralization of entire treatment teams, which compromises treatment integrity. If individuals with psychopathy are to be managed effectively, therapists need to prepare for, and learn to manage, their own internalized reactions such as feelings of despair, helplessness, or externalizing reactions (e.g., lashing out) or unprofessional liaisons. In essence, therapists need to be inoculated against such treatment-inferring behaviors. In addition, building and mending the alliance can occur if the therapist manages such reactions adequately. Some of the approaches presented below designed to promote a collaborative working relationship while minimizing the likelihood of boundary violation are abstracted from Bowers (2002), Doren (1987), and Wong and Hare (2005).

First, therapists need to maintain objectivity, a nonjudgmental approach, and avoid labeling or demonizing psychopathy. It often helps if psychopathic personality is viewed as a maladaptive variant of common personality traits (Widiger & Lynam, 1998) rather than a distinct entity unrelated to normal personality variation. It is also important to dispel the idea that psychopathy is untreatable or that treatment can make psychopaths worse. Although these ideas are not supported by the empirical literature, they are still common beliefs that can undermine therapist morale and foster negative reactions.

Second, to counteract the manipulative and staff-splitting maneuvering that often occurs when working with psychopathic individuals, it is advisable for staff members to work as a cohesive team rather than individually, to reduce staff vulnerability to such behavior. The use of small treatment teams of three or four members can lessen the occurrence of staff splitting. The team can also provide support and debriefing opportunities to staff members when working with psychopathic individuals. For those who have to work in solo practices, it is advisable to seek supervision and debriefing from a colleague on a regular basis.

Third, it is key to recognize and repair staff splitting proactively by being aware of deviations from the group's or one's own usual clinical practices and be willing to point them out within the team in a constructive and caring manner. Staff members may wish to form a buddy system (dyads or triads) for the purpose of monitoring one another's behaviors on boundary issues. Always maintain open lines of communication by sharing with one another and with the team information about one's perception of the psychopath's treatment plan and progress. Convincing a staff member to keep small secrets is a grooming tactic often used by psychopaths and may be the beginning of a slippery slope. The limits of confidentiality have to be clearly articulated and agreed to by all staff members and shared with the offender. Follow structured and clear treatment processes and objectives, and be mindful of deviation from usual practices. Treatment of psychopathy requires a structured and clearly articulated plan or pathway that should be followed by all staff members. Be wary of dramatic improvements.

### Component 2: Criminogenic Component

The criminogenic component entails identifying specific problems of the psychopathic individual that are closely associated with violence, then establishing the best way to treat them.

### Criminogenic Features

The criminogenic component is linked to PCL-R F2, which includes items such as a parasitic lifestyle and a lack of long-term goals, which are changeable, and early behavioral problems and juvenile delinquency, which are unchangeable. The F2, like the overall PCL-R, was not developed to guide violence reduction in treatment. To capture the underlying variance of this factor for treatment purposes, it is essential to identify dynamic risk that can be reduced through treatment and in turn lead to a reduction in violence and antisocial behavior (see Wong et al., 2007). It is preferable to use a risk assessment tool such as the Violence Risk Scale (VRS; Wong & Gordon, 1999–2003, 2006), which was developed as a dynamic risk assessment and treatment planning tool based on RNR principles. The VRS has six static and 20 dynamic risk predictors; can be used to identify risk of violence (Risk principle), treatment targets (Need principle), treatment readiness (Responsivity principle); and measures risk change, recognizing that risk is dynamic. Staff ratings of the dynamic predictors (0, 1, 2, 3) indicate the relative strength of association between the predictor (e.g., criminal attitude) and violence, with higher ratings indicating a stronger association with violence. Thus ratings of 2 or 3 are treatment targets. Examples of the dynamic predictors include antisocial attitudes and beliefs (e.g., loathing of law abiding behaviors, justification of antisocial behaviors), emotion dysregulation (e.g., excessive anger, irritability), violent lifestyle (e.g., gang affiliation), aggressive interpersonal interaction style, substance use, and so forth.

The individual's readiness for treatment of each treatment target is then assessed by staff members using a modified version of the stages of change model (Prochaska, DiClemente, & Norcross, 1992) to establish a pretreatment baseline measure (e.g., at the Contemplation stage). At the conclusion of treatment, the stage of change for each treatment target is reassessed. Risk reduction is indicated by progression through the stages of change (e.g., from Contemplation to Action) and translated into a quantitative reduction in violence risk. The pretreatment stage of change can be used to guide the selection of appropriate intervention strategies, matched to the level of treatment readiness, the posttreatment risk level and the stage of change can be used to guide posttreatment risk management (Wong & Gordon, 2004).

The dynamic items of the VRS correlate significantly with F2 ($r = .80$, $p < .001$), thus capturing a significant portion of F2 variance in predicting violent recidivism (AUC = .75; Wong & Gordon, 2006). As an illustration, at pretreatment, after undergoing assessment with the VRS, each program participant has an individualized set of dynamic risk factors specifying the thoughts, feelings, behaviors, living conditions, and so on, that may put him or her at risk for reoffending; they are his or her individualized treatment targets. Figure 36.1 is a profile of the VRS dynamic items, showing the percentages of individuals who identified each item as a treatment target in samples of general and psychopathic offenders. Although psychopathic offenders identified more risk factors as treatment targets than general offenders, the types of risk factors endorsed by the two groups were quite similar. There is also evidence suggesting that positive changes in VRS dynamic predictors in psychopathic offenders (mean PCL-R = 26), who had participated in violence reduction treatment, were linked to reduction in violent recidivism in the community (Lewis, Olver, & Wong, 2013; Olver, Lewis, & Wong, 2013). In summary, dynamic predictors assessed by the VRS can be used to identify treatment needs.

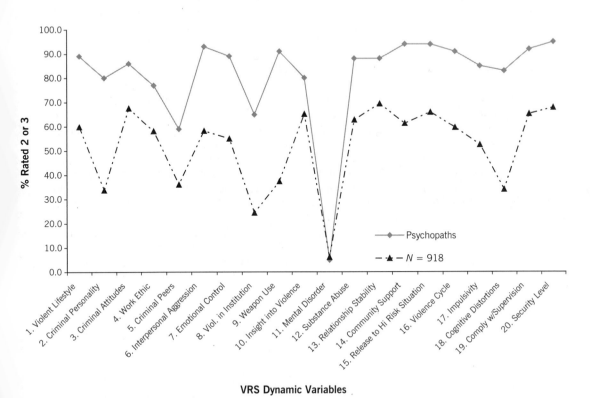

**FIGURE 36.1.** Dynamic risk profile assessed using the VRS. From Wong and Gordon (2006). Copyright © 2006 American Psychological Association. Adapted by permission.

Dynamic predictors are changeable and the reductions in risk assessed by the dynamic predictors at postreatment have been shown to link to a reduction in violence in the community after release from incarceration. I discuss these findings in more detail later.

Although dynamic risk assessment tools provide a systematic way to identify the treatment needs of offenders with psychopathic traits, a combination of dynamic risk assessment and clinical case formulation is the preferred approach. Some psychopathic individuals, especially the outliers among them, tend to have atypical treatment needs that even specialized risk assessment tools may not identify.

## Treatment Options

Having identified what to treat, the next step for the clinician is to identify the best treatment approach. Here, treatment is understood broadly to include either an organized set of interventions delivered by clinicians that are either empirically supported or rationally derived (e.g., the psychotherapies and pharmacotherapy) or structured, module-based programs such as general counseling, case work, education, and occupational training delivered by nonclinicians (e.g., prison or correctional officers) or a combination of both. Although there is some evidence that structured skill-based approaches are effective in reducing reoffending (Lipsey, 2009), specific studies of effectiveness of the various psychotherapies are limited. Whereas a variety of therapies have been evaluated in randomized controlled trials (RCTs), only one RCT study was conducted with a focus on antisocial personality disorder (see below) and none on psychopathy. Individual studies on treatment efficacy for psychopathy are largely confined to psychodynamic therapy, therapeutic community (TC) approaches and cognitive-behavioral and skills-based interventions (see Salekin, 2002; Salekin et al., 2010; Wong, 2000 for summary). Over the last six decades, treatment of psychopathy has shifted from most psychodynamic psychotherapies to TCs and CBTs and the gradual merging of the latter two (see Wong, Stockdale & Olver, in press).

## Psychodynamic Therapy

Gabbard (2004, p. 2) defined long-term psychodynamic psychotherapy as "a therapy that involves careful attention to the therapist–patient interaction, with thoughtfully timed interpretation of transference and resistance embedded in a sophisticated appreciation of the therapist's contribution to the two-person field." Although widely used in some settings, the efficacy of psychodynamic interventions for psychopathy has not been demonstrated, but this is due more to a lack of evidence than to evidence of lack of efficacy. Both a meta-analysis of 11 RCTs evaluating psychodynamic psychotherapy with patients with PDs (Leichsenring, 2010) and a Cochrane Systematic Review of psychological interventions for ASPD (Gibbon et al., 2010) noted the absence of RCTs on ASPD or psychopathic PD. The only evaluation of the efficacy of psychodynamic therapy with ASPD and co-occurring substance abuse did not use offending behaviors as outcomes (Woody, McLellan, Luborsky, & O'Brien, 1985). However, a meta-analysis of the effectiveness of psychodynamic psychotherapy and cognitive-behavioral therapy (CBT) for PDs generally reported similar efficacies for the two therapies (Leichsenring & Leibing, 2003).

The efficacy of psychodynamic therapy for treating violence associated with psychopathy should also be considered in the context of Stone's (2010) discussion of the factors that can compromise the treatment of PD with psychodynamic therapy. Stone listed 10 issues: (1) impaired reflective capacity or concreteness of thought; (2) ego fragility; (3) poor empathic capacity; (4) impulsivity, especially if aggravated by substance abuse; (5) arrogance, grandiosity, contemptuousness, entitlement, and exploitativeness; (6) lying, deceitfulness, callousness, conning behavior, and lack of remorse; (7) dismissive attachment style; (8) bitterness, indiscretion, shallowness, vindictiveness, sensation seeking; (9) controlling and taking pleasure in the suffering of others; and (10) marked rigidity of personality. Since most if not all these features characterize the psychopathic personality, Stone's analysis suggests that psychodynamic therapy for psychopathy is fraught with problems, although it should be noted that the problems Stone raises are equally applicable to other forms of psychotherapy. Even if psychodynamic therapies could successfully address F1 personality features, and personality features (not violence) are what such therapies are tailored to address, the outcome would not lower violent risk because F1 features are not linked to future violence.

## Cognitive and Cognitive Behavioral/Skills-Based Therapy

Cognitive therapists tend to adopt a more "pragmatic" approach to treating psychopathy and ASPD by focusing on improving moral and social behavior through enhancement of cognitive functioning, with a view toward essentially helping the client to progress from being self-serving and self-centered to taking into account others' feelings or perspectives. These improvements may lead to a reduction in institutional misconduct or repeated reinstitutionalization (Beck et al., 2004). Beck and colleagues (2004) stressed the importance of skills development in addressing deficits in perspective taking, impulse control, emotional regulation, frustration tolerance, communication and assertiveness, consequential thinking and, of course, cognitive restructuring. In the treatment of psychopathy, cognitive therapy, CBT, and skills-based approaches as well as more recent iterations of TCs (see Wong et al., in press) have many common attributes. As such, these treatment approaches are considered together.

An extensive literature, often referred to as the "what works" literature, based on meta-analyses and narrative reviews (Andrews et al., 1990; Gendreau, 1996; Gendreau & Ross, 1979; Lipsey, 2009; Lipsey & Wilson, 1998) shows consistent evidence of the efficacy of some treatments in reducing reoffending, criminality, and antisocial behaviors among offenders, including many with ASPD (50–80%; Fazel & Danesh, 2002; Hare, 2003) and psychopathy (4.5–15%; Hare, 2003). Especially important is McGuire's (2008) review of 70 meta-analyses of offender treatment outcome studies between 1985 and 2007, and additional studies with primary data concluding that "there is sufficient evidence currently available to substantiate the claim that personal violence can be reduced by psychosocial interventions " (p. 2577) and that "emotional self-management, interpersonal skills, social problem solving and allied training approaches show mainly positive effects with a reasonably high degree of reliability." (p. 2591). This conclusion is consistent with an earlier meta-analysis demonstrating that behaviorally oriented treatment focused on criminogenic needs and delivered to high-risk cases in well-structured programs reduced recidivism (Andrews al., 1990). An additional meta-analysis of 548 independent study samples, reported between 1958 and 2002, compared different types of counseling and skills-building approaches among juvenile offenders, not all of whom showed psychopathic traits (Lipsey, 2009). Although behavioral and cognitive-behavioral approaches had the largest absolute reduction in recidivism, the differences between different treatment approaches were not statistically significant. In addition, no significant differences were obtained between the different subtypes of intervention within different broad treatment philosophies such as counseling vs skill building vs multiple coordinated services such as case management. The lack of differences may be due, in part, to the lack of power (Lipsey, 2009).

Overall, the meta-analytic evidence favors using a cognitive-behavioral skill-based treatment approach to reduce the risk of recidivism among offender populations. Although the evidence suggests that no single treatment approach within the CBT skills-based framework is clearly superior, it does not imply that one should not use a rationally derived process to justify the inclusion or exclusion of aspects of treatment that are better suited to different offender need profiles or management requirements. In other words, besides attending to empirical evidence, it is also important to be sensitive to the needs of the individual and the treatment environment. One size just does not fit all.

The National Institute of Health and Clinical Excellence (NICE), a part of the National Health Service in the United Kingdom, publishes guidelines for the treatment of various health and mental health conditions. One of the guidelines is for the treatment of ASPD (2009) with associated references and comments on the treatment of psychopathy; the guidelines were derived from a review of the literature on treatment efficacy rather than on any particular theoretical approach. For those with ASPD and/or psychopathy and a history of offending behaviors, the guidelines recommend using cognitive-behavioral group-based approaches to reduce offending behaviors; no mention was made about the use of psychodynamic treatment approaches. The NICE guidelines are also similar to RNR principles in recommending that attention be given to clients' needs and responsivity. Finally, they recommend that pharmacological interventions should not be routinely used in treating ASPD or associated aggression, anger, and impulsivity.

Treatment methods also need to accommodate different types of violent behavior such as nonsexual, sexual, and domestic violence. Returning to the two-component framework of treatment discussed earlier, Component 1 strategies and methods are applicable to all types of violent behaviors. The differences among treatments lie in Component 2 methods. For example, with sexual violence, considerable attention needs to be given to assessing and treating sexual deviancy, in addition to treatment for general criminality and violence using appropriate dynamic risk tools to identify treatment targets. In all, for individuals with psychopathic traits, there is, as yet, no comprehensive violence reduction treatment approach with clear and replicable evidence of efficacy.

## Treatment Delivery

Besides actual treatment methods, treatment delivery and maintaining treatment integrity are also key considerations because treatment integrity can be readily compromised when treating psychopathy. Hence, attention needs to be given to the use and organization of multidisciplinary teams, the coordination of the delivery of different components of the treatment program, and management support for the program.

### The Multidisciplinary Team

Although a multidisciplinary team approach can enrich treatment by providing different professional perspectives and expertise, it needs to be implemented in a collaborative and focused manner. The team, despite its multidisciplinary nature, must share and support a clearly articulated and conceptualized treatment model in order for all disciplines to work together toward a common goal. Since the treatment of psychopathy is still controversial and a consensus treatment model acceptable to all disciplines is lacking, a multidisciplinary approach may result in a diversity of opinions about treatment methods and delivery; as Donald R. Gannon states, "When facts are few, experts are many." The worst case scenario occurs when different disciplines work in silos, with little communication or coordination among them, leading to the different interventions and components being delivered in a confusing and inconsistent manner. Poor communication within the team, open disagreements among team members, and turf wars among disciplines provide fertile ground for individuals with psychopathy to split and manipulate staff members. Such disagreement and dissention lead to demoralized, isolated staff members lacking in direction or with burnout, increasing the likelihood of boundary violations and disruption of treatment consistency and program integrity.

Such problems can be avoided by the adoption of explicitly defined set of common treatment strategies and goals acceptable to all disciplines and team members. This lays the foundation for consistent treatment delivery, which is then implemented by way of clearly defined individualized treatment plans for achieving set goals that are collaboratively formulated between offenders and treatment providers. All disciplines should participate in and commit to the above process. The level of staff communication and agreement, along with collaborative decision making, promotes integration within the treatment team and allows the entire team to speak with one voice—an "all roads should lead to Rome" sort of approach that makes splitting of the team more difficult. An example of an effective multidisciplinary approach is the philosophy of the multisystemic therapy (MST), a social-ecological and evidence-based intervention to reduce antisocial behaviors in high-risk youth that has been shown to be effective (Henggeler, Schoenwald, Borduin, Rowland, & Cunningham, 1998).

A challenge faced by multidisciplinary teams in forensic settings is to integrate and reconcile treatment and security requirements. Within prison or forensic mental health facilities, treatment needs to be delivered within a safe and secured environment. Understandably, security staff[3] do not have the same work objectives as treatment staff and, at times, they may work at odds with one another. Resolving conflicts between the security and the treatment requirements is always challenging because the two disciplines have different background, training, and work objectives. However, unless the two practices are well coordinated, offenders can be caught in the middle, which compromises treatment delivery and integrity.

---

[3] This role may be assumed by nursing staff in some forensic mental health facilities.

## Multi-Intervention Treatment

Most program participants are likely to have multiple criminogenic needs (see Figure 36.1) requiring interventions with multiple treatment targets. This raises the question of how best to arrange the delivery of such treatments to meet the multiple needs of the individual. In some programs, each need (e.g., substance use, antisocial attitudes, and maladaptive cognitions) has a designated intervention or module, and offenders are required to participate sequentially in a number of different treatment modules to address their different problem areas: a cafeteria type approach to treatment delivery. An alternative and oft used arrangement is for individuals to attend different types of established therapies (e.g., dialectical behavior therapy and schema therapy) or different therapy groups developed locally to address specific problems. Both approaches to program deliver can lead to disjointed and poorly coordinated treatment. The myriad interventions often are poorly integrated and confusing to participants because of the differences in problem conceptualization and therapy terminologies in particular when treatment teams and staff members have limited communication with one another. Offenders are sometimes required to re-do a certain module, such as a motivation and engagement module, or undergo an additional reassessment simply because that is the way that particular "therapy course" is set up with little or no regard to what was done prior. Such approaches also tend to encourage staff members to be competitive rather than collaborative leading to treatment being therapy-focused (e.g. therapy A vs B) or discipline-focused (e.g. psychology vs psychiatry) rather than program objective-focused: violence reduction. In such sliced-salami-like treatment approaches, in which the whole is often obscured by its parts, offenders may find it difficult to integrate the many sources of information and guidance offered to them. Sequencing of the interventions becomes unwieldy, unresponsive to the needs of the offender, and time consuming, thus increasing program cost. For example, if anger control is a pressing issue but the relevant module is scheduled for an inappropriate future date, such intervention cannot be provided to the offender as needed and in a timely manner.

Although an eclectic combination of different interventions may be needed to treat the diverse pathologies and criminogenic needs of offenders with psychopathic traits, the interventions should be delivered in an integrated and coordinated way. Such an eclectic approach does not "mean that multiple interventions can be delivered as separate and unrelated modules. A curriculum approach that assigns patients to an array of modules tailored to their individual problems is inappropriate because it offers little opportunity to . . . bring about the integration needed to address core self and interpersonal problems" (Livesley, 2007b, p. 33).

To bring about integration in a violence reduction program, the thread of violence reduction should run all the way through all programming for the offender. Program designers need to pause and consider how each therapy, module, and even daily activities contribute to the overall program objective of violence reduction so as to bring about a meaningful and rational integration of program activities within the local environment. There is no one-size-fit-all approach as much depends on resource availability and local conditions, but see Wong and Gordon (2006) and Wong, Gordon, and Gu (2007) for discussions on these issues.

## Management and Institutional Support

A treatment program for offenders is usually a part of a larger organization, and successful implementation requires support from its parent organization. Several researchers have identified a number of correlates of successful program implementation that Harris and Smith (1996) condensed into three key conditions for success (Ellickson & Petersilia, 1983; Petersilia, 1990; also see Wong & Hare, 2005, pp. 52–53). First, the closer the fit of the goals and objectives between a program and the parent organization, the better the chance of success. Second, commitment to the program at all levels of the system is necessary, from external stakeholder to senior governance to program manager to frontline staff. The program must also have a clear line of authority: There should be no ambiguity about who is in charge. Third, appropriate resources must be consistently made available to the program. Results of a number of meta-analytic studies support these views (Andrews et al., 1990; Lipsey, 2009; Lipsey & Cullen, 2007; Lipsey & Wilson, 1998). At times, a somewhat less efficacious but better implemented program outperformed a more efficacious but less well-implemented program. As Lipsey (2009, p. 145) put it after a review of the efficacy of different juvenile programs, "It does not take a magic bullet program to impact recidivism, only one that is well made and well-aimed."

Though program implementation is an important consideration, Andrews and colleagues (1990) have argued that effective programs needs to follow certain rules. The more the program adheres to RNR principles, the larger the effect size in relation to recidivism reduction. This relationship holds in programs that have high, medium, and low levels of integrity while programs with higher integrity have larger effect sizes than those with lower integrity (Andrews & Bonta, 2010).

A systematic assessment of the integrity of correctional rehabilitation programs can be carried out using the Correctional Program Assessment Inventory (CPAI; Gendreau & Andrews, 1994; Gendreau & Andrews, 2001; cited in Andrews & Bonta, 2010). This tool evaluates the adherence of correctional programs to eight domains indicative of program integrity: (1) organizational culture reflecting the agency's goals, ethical standards, outreach and self-evaluations; (2) program implementation/ maintenance; (3) management and staff characteristics; (4) offender risk and needs assessment practices; (5) program adherence to RNR characteristics; (6) staff interpersonal and relationship skills levels; (7) interagency communication; and (8) pre- and postprogram evaluation of outcomes.

A CPAI score can be used to assess the link between program integrity and reoffending. Lowenkamp (2004, cited by Andrews & Bonta, 2010) in a survey of community correctional facilities including both halfway houses and community correctional facilities, with a total of 13,221 offenders, found that the total CPAI score correlated positively with the effect sizes of recidivism ($r = .41$). Overall, the evidence suggests that maintaining program integrity is very important to ensure program efficacy.

### Evaluating Change

In custodial settings, offenders' problem behaviors often take on different appearances or even go totally underground because of close monitoring and punishment for misbehavior. Psychopathic offenders are no exception, and the literature is rife with examples of how individuals with psychopathy can con and manipulate their way through treatment. Progressing from "talking the talk to walking the walk" is a challenge for such offenders, and it is also challenging for staff to assess the validity of the walk. For example, a child molester who used the Internet to lure his victims may resort to viewing and masturbating to images of children in magazines, and the psychopath who swindled and defrauded others may turn into a jailhouse lawyer. The presence of these offense analogue behaviors (OABs) are indications that the underlying criminogenic behavior is unchanged, though no illegal act or harm has been perpetrated nor institutional rules broken. Treatment should target OABs that are proxies of the individual's criminal behavior, and meaningful changes that lead to risk reduction should be shown by the reduction of OABs and their replacement with prosocial, adaptive offense reduction behaviors (ORBs) (see Gordon & Wong, 2009, 2010). It is unusual for OABs to simply disappear without being replaced by something else, since OABs satisfy specific needs, although they can be suppressed temporarily due to situational demands. Hence, sustainable prosocial changes are unlikely unless dysfunctional OABs are replaced by consistent, generalizable prosocial adaptive ORBs. Staff members must be vigilant in observing the presence of both OABs and ORBs in assessing change and risk reduction. The suppression of OABs without establishing corresponding ORBs may account for the enigmatic observations that some psychopaths may be considered by staff members to be model inmates in custody, yet they go on to commit a serious offense upon release into the community.

Systematic assessment of treatment changes, for example, using the VRS, is based on assessing the decrease in OABs and the increase in ORBs. These changes have been shown in program outcome evaluations to be related to reduction in violence in the community after long-term follow-up, as discussed below.

### Treatment Outcome Evaluations

Recent studies with better research methodologies have examined the responses of psychopathic offenders to effective contemporary treatments. Olver and Wong (2009) used the VRS—Sexual Offender version (VRS-SO) to measure changes in risk in adult male sex offenders with psychopathy who received a cognitive-behavioral-based sex offender treatment program shown to be effective in reducing sexual and violent recidivism (Nicholaichuk,

Gordon, Gu, & Wong, 2000; Olver, Wong, & Nicholaichuk, 2009). Treatment led to a reduction in sexual and violent recidivism in the community in a 10-year follow-up after controlling for sexual offender risk, PCL-R scores, and length of follow-up. The findings were similar to those reported by Looman, Abracen, Serin, and Marquis (2005), suggesting that significant psychopathic traits did not prevent participants from benefiting from treatment.

In a separate study, high-risk violence-proned and psychopathic nonsexual offenders were treated in violence-reduction-focused cognitive-behavioral treatment based on the RNR model and followed up for about 4 years in the community (Lewis, Olver, & Wong, 2013; Olver, Lewis, & Wong, 2013). Reductions in risk, assessed with the VRS, were associated with reduction in violent recidivism. The objective of both studies was to determine whether risk changes for treated offenders are linked to recidivism change, and as such, no control group was used.

A comparison of a treatment and a matched control group was used to assess treatment effects on psychopathic offenders (PCL-R = 28; $n$ = 32 for both groups) with a case-matched control design (Wong, Gordon, Gu, Lewis, & Olver, 2012). Treatment was similar to that used in the Lewis and colleagues (2012) study. The two groups were matched for PCL-R total, F1 and F2 scores, length of follow-up, risk level, age, and past criminal histories. Trends were all in the predicted directions, but there was no significant difference between violent and nonviolent recidivism rates (probably due to power issues because of small sample sizes), but those in the treated group who reoffended received significantly shorter sentences (less than half the lengths), which suggests that they committed less serious offenses than their untreated counterparts. The results suggest that treatment reduces the seriousness of reoffending, thus supporting a harm reduction effect. Although more well-designed studies are needed, these results provide some evidence that treatment can reduce violence and aggression in psychopathic offenders.

## Conclusion

Although the literature on the outcome of treating psychopathy is limited, converging evidence suggest that psychopathy is not untreatable, and treatment can be effective in reducing reoffending risks. Such risk reduction is not contingent on modifying psychopathic personality traits. However, a viable and evidence-based model to guide treatment of psychopathy is still lacking, and this chapter attempts to address the gap. While it is too soon to conclude that psychopathic personality is as "treatable" as some other PDs, there is room for cautious therapeutic optimism. Therapeutic nihilism, which is so pervasive in this area of forensic work, is not justified.

## ACKNOWLEDGMENT

This chapter is a revised version of Wong (2016). Adapted with permission of The Guilford Press.

## REFERENCES

Andrews, D. A., & Bonta, J. (1994–2010). *The psychology of criminal conduct* (1st to 5th eds.). Cincinnati, OH: Anderson.

Andrews, D. A., Zinger, I., Hoge, R. D., Bonta, J., Gendreau, P., & Cullen, F. T. (1990). Does correctional treatment work?: A clinically relevant and psychologically informed meta-analysis. *Criminology, 28,* 369–404.

Beck, A. T., Freeman, A., & Davis, D. D. (2004). *Cognitive therapy of personality disorders* (2nd ed.). New York: Guilford Press.

Blonigen, D. (2010). Explaining the relationship between age and crime: Contributions from the developmental literature on personality. *Clinical Psychology Review, 30*(1), 89–100.

Bordin, E. S. (1979). The generalizability of the psychoanalytic concept of the working alliance. *Psychotherapy, Theory, Research, and Practice, 16,* 252–260.

Bordin, E. S. (1994). Theory and research on the therapeutic working alliance: New directions. In A. O. Horvath & L. S. Greenberg (Eds.), *The working alliance* (pp. 13–37). New York: Wiley.

Bowers, L. (2002). *Dangerous and severe personality disorder: Response and role of the psychiatric team*. London: Routledge.

Cleckley, H. (1976). *The mask of sanity* (5th ed.). St. Louis, MO: Mosby.

Daffern, M., Jones, L., & Shine, J. (Eds.). (2010). *Offence paralleling behaviour: An individualized approach to offender assessment and treatment*. Chichester, UK: Wiley.

Doren, D. M. (1987). *Understanding and treating the psychopath*. Toronto, ON, Canada: Wiley.

D'Silva, K., Duggan, C., & McCarthy, L. (2004). Does treatment really make psychopaths worse?: A review of the evidence. *Journal of Personality Disorders, 18,* 163–177.

Edens, J. F., Campbell, J. S., & Weir, J. M. (2007). Youth psychopathy and criminal recidivism: A meta-analysis of the psychopathy checklist measures. *Law and Human Behavior, 31*(1), 53–75.

Ellickson, P., & Petersilia, J. (1983). *Implementing new ideas in criminal justice*. Santa Monica, CA: RAND.

Fazel, S., & Danesh, J. (2002). Serious mental disorder in 23000 prisoners: A systematic review of 62 surveys. *Lancet, 359,* 545–550.

Gabbard, G. O. (2004). *Long-term psychodynamic psychotherapy: A basic text*. Washington, DC: American Psychiatric Publishing.

Gendreau, P. (1996). The principles of effective intervention with offenders. In A. Harland (Ed.), *Choosing correctional options that work* (pp. 117–130). Thousand Oaks, CA: Sage.

Gendreau, P., & Andrews, D. A. (1994). *The correctional program assessment inventory* (6th ed.). St. John, NB, Canada: St. John College, University of New Brunswick.

Gendreau, P., & Ross, R. R. (1979). Effective correctional treatment: Bibliotherapy for the cynics. *Crime and Delinquency, 25,* 463–489.

Gibbon, S., Duggan, C., Stoffers, J., Huband, N., Völlm, B. A., Ferriter, M., et al. (2010). Psychological interventions for antisocial personality disorder. *Cochrane Database Systematic Reviews, 6,* CD007668.

Gordon, A., & Wong, S. C. P. (2009). *OAB and ORB guide*. Unpublished manuscript. Saskatoon, Canada: Psynergy Consulting.

Gordon, A., & Wong, S. C. P. (2010). Offense analogue behaviours as indicator of criminogenic need and treatment progress in custodial settings. In M. Daffern, L. Jones, & J. Shine (Eds.), *Offence paralleling behaviour: An individualized approach to offender assessment and treatment* (pp. 171–184). Chichester, UK: Wiley-Blackwell.

Hare, R. D. (2003). *The Hare Psychopathy Checklist—Revised* (2nd ed.). Toronto, ON, Canada: Multi-Health Systems.

Harpur, T. J., & Hare, R. D. (1994). The assessment of psychopathy as a function of age. *Journal of Abnormal Psychology, 103,* 604–609.

Harris, G. T., & Rice, M. E. (2006). Treatment of psychopathy: A review of empirical findings. In C. J. Patrick (Ed.), *Handbook of psychopathy* (pp. 555–572). New York: Guilford Press.

Harris, G. T., Rice, M. E., & Cormier, C. A. (1991). Psychopathy and violent recidivism. *Law and Human Behavior, 15,* 625–637.

Harris, P., & Smith, S. (1996). Developing community corrections. In A. T. Harland (Ed.), *Choosing correctional options that work* (pp. 183–222). Thousand Oaks, CA: SAGE.

Henggeler, S. W., Schoenwald, S. K., Borduin, C. M., Rowland, M. D., & Cunningham, P. B. (1998). *Multisystemic treatment of antisocial behavior in children and adolescents*. New York: Guilford Press.

Hobson, J., Shine, J., & Roberts, R. (2000). How do psychopaths behave in a prison therapeutic community? *Psychology, Law, and Crime, 6,* 139–154.

Horvath, A. O., & Greenberg, L. S. (Eds.). (1994). *The working alliance*. New York: Wiley.

Hughes, G., Hogue, T., Hollin, C., & Champion, H. (1997). First-stage evaluation of a treatment programme for personality disordered offenders. *Journal of Forensic Psychiatry, 8*(3), 515–527.

Jesness, C., Allison, T., McCormick, P. M., Wedge, R. F., & Young, M. L. (1975). *Cooperative Behavior Demonstration Project: Final Report to the Office of Criminal Justice Planning*. Sacramento: California Youth Authority.

Kennealy, P., Skeem, J., Walters, G., & Camp, J. (2010). Do core interpersonal and affective traits of PCL-R psychopathy interact with antisocial behavior and disinhibition to predict violence? *Psychological Assessment, 22*(3), 569–580.

Leichsenring, F. (2010). Evidence for psychodynamic psychotherapy in personality disorders: A review. In J. F. Clarkin, P. Fonagy, & G. O. Gabbard (Eds.), *Psychodynamic psychotherapy for personality disorder: A clinical handbook* (pp. 421–437). Washington, DC: American Psychiatric Association.

Leichsenring, F., & Leibing, E. (2003). The effectiveness of psychodynamic psychotherapy and cognitive–behavioral therapy in personality disorder: A meta-analysis. *American Journal of Psychiatry, 160,* 1223–1232.

Lewis, K., Olver, M., & Wong, S. C. P. (2013). The Violence Risk Scale: Predictive validity and linking changes in risk with violent recidivism in a sample of high risk offenders with psychopathic traits. *Assessment, 20,* 150–164.

Lipsey, M. W. (2009). The primary factors that characterize effective interventions with juvenile offenders: A meta-analytic overview. *Victims and Offenders, 4,* 124–147.

Lipsey, M. W., & Cullen, F. T. (2007). The effectiveness of correctional rehabilitation: A review of systematic reviews. *Annual Review of Law and Social Science, 3,* 279–320.

Lipsey, M. W., & Wilson, D. B. (1998). Effective intervention for serious juvenile offenders: A synthesis of research. In R. Loeber & D. Farrington (Eds.), *Serious and violent juvenile offenders: Risk factors and successful interventions* (pp. 313–345). Thousand Oaks, CA: SAGE.

Livesley, W. J. (2003). *Practical management of personality disorder*. New York: Guilford Press.

Livesley, W. J. (2007a). Common elements of effective treatment. In B. van Luyn, S. Akhtar, & W. J. Livesley (Eds.), *Severe personality disorder* (pp. 211–239). New York: Cambridge University Press.

Livesley, W. J. (2007b). The relevance of an integrated approach to the treatment of personality disordered offenders. *Psychology, Crime and Law, 13*(1), 27–46.

Livesley, W. J., Dimaggio, G., & Clarkin, J. F. (Eds.).

(2015). *Integrated treatment for personality disorder: A modular approach.* New York: Guilford Press.

Looman, J., Abracen, J., Serin, R., & Marquis, P. (2005). Psychopathy, treatment change, and recidivism in high-risk, high-need sexual offenders. *Journal of Interpersonal Violence, 20,* 549–568.

McCord, W., & McCord, J. (1964). *The psychopath: An essay on the criminal mind.* Princeton, NJ: Van Nostrand.

McGuire, J. (2008). A review of effective interventions for reducing aggression and violence. *Philosophical Transactions of the Royal Society B: Biological Sciences, 363,* 2577–2597.

Miller, W. R., & Rollnick, S. (2012). *Motivational interviewing* (3rd ed.). New York: Guilford Press.

Murrie, D. C., Boccaccini, M. T., Caperton, J., & Rufino, K. (2012). Field validity of the Psychopathy Checklist—Revised in sex offender risk assessment. *Psychological Assessment, 24*(2), 524–529.

National Institute of Clinical Excellence. (2009). *Antisocial personality disorder: Treatment, management and prevention.* London: Author.

Nicholaichuk, T., Gordon, A., Gu, D., & Wong, S. (2000). Outcome of an institutional sexual offender treatment program: A comparison between treated and matched untreated offenders. *Sexual Abuse: Journal of Research and Treatment, 12*(2), 137–153.

Ogloff, R. P., Wong, S., & Greenwood, A. (1990). Treating criminal psychopaths in a therapeutic community program. *Behavioral Sciences and the Law, 8,* 181–190.

Olver, M. E., Lewis, K., & Wong, S. C. P. (2013). Risk reduction treatment of high-risk psychopathic offenders: The relationship of psychopathy and treatment change to violent recidivism. *Personality Disorders: Theory, Research, and Treatment, 4,* 160–167.

Olver, M. E., Neumann, C. S., Wong, S. C. P., & Hare, R. D. (2013). The structural and predictive properties of the Psychopathy Checklist—Revised in Canadian aboriginal and non-aboriginal offenders. *Psychological Assessment, 25,* 167–179.

Olver, M. E., & Wong, S. C. P. (2009). Therapeutic responses of psychopathic sexual offenders: Treatment attrition, therapeutic change, and long term recidivism. *Journal of Consulting and Clinical Psychology, 77,* 328–336.

Olver, M. E., & Wong, S. C. P. (2011). Predictors of sex offender treatment dropout: Psychopathy, sex offender risk, and responsivity implications. *Psychology, Crime and Law, 17*(5), 457–471.

Olver, M., Wong, S. C. P., & Nicholaichuk, T. P. (2009). Outcome evaluation of a high intensity inpatient sex offender treatment program. *Journal of Interpersonal Violence, 24*(3), 522–536.

Palmer, T. (1996). Programmatic and nonprogrammatic aspects of successful intervention. In A. T. Harland (Ed.), *Choosing correctional options that work* (pp. 131–182). Thousand Oaks, CA: SAGE.

Petersilia, J. (1990). Conditions that permit intensive supervision programs to survive. *Crime and Delinquency, 36,* 126–145.

Prochaska, J. O., DiClemente, C. C., & Norcross, J. C. (1992). In search of how people change: Applications to addictive behaviours. *American Psychologist, 47,* 1102–1114.

Salekin, R. (2002). Psychopathy and therapeutic pessimism: Clinical lore or clinical reality? *Clinical Psychology Review, 22,* 79–112.

Salekin, R., Worley, C., & Grimes, R. (2010). Treatment of psychopathy: A review and brief introduction to the mental model approach for psychopathy. *Behavioral Sciences and the Law, 28,* 235–266.

Simourd, D. J., & Hoge, R. D. (2000). Criminal psychopathy: A risk-and-need perspective. *Criminal Justice and Behavior, 27*(2), 256–272.

Stone, M. (2010). Treatability of personality disorder: Possibilities and limitations. In J. F. Clarkin, P. Fonagy, & G. O. Gabbard (Eds.), *Psychodynamic psychotherapy for personality disorders: A clinical handbook* (pp. 391–420). Washington, DC: American Psychiatric Association.

Suedfeld, P., & Landon, P. B. (1978). Approaches to treatment. In R. D. Hare & D. Schalling (Eds.), *Psychopathic behavior: Approaches to research* (pp. 347–376). Chichester, UK: Wiley.

Walters, G. D. (2003). Predicting institutional adjustment and recidivism with the Psychopathy Checklist factor scores: A meta-analysis. *Law and Human Behavior, 27,* 541–558.

Webster, C. K., Douglas, D. E., Eaves, D., & Hart, D. (1997). *HCR-20 assessing risk for violence: Version II.* Burnaby, BC, Canada: Mental Health, Law and Policy Institute, Simon Fraser University.

Widiger, T. A., & Lynam, D. R. (1998). Psychopathy and the five-factor model of personality. In T. Millon, E. Simonsen, M. Birket-Smith, & R. D. Davis (Eds.), *Psychopathy: Antisocial, criminal, and violent behaviors* (pp. 171–187). New York: Guilford Press.

Widiger, T. A., Simonsen, E., Sirovatka, A. J., & Regier, D. A. (2006). *Dimensional models of personality disorder.* Washington, DC: American Psychiatric Publishing.

Wong, S. (2000). Treatment of criminal psychopath. In S. Hodgins & R. Muller-Isberner (Eds.), *Violence, crime and mentally disordered offenders: Concepts and methods for effective treatment and prevention* (pp. 81–106). London: Wiley.

Wong, S. (2016). Treatment of violence-prone individuals with psychopathic personality traits. In W. J. Livesley, G. DiMaggio, & J. F. Clarkin (Eds.), *Integrated treatment for personality disorders* (pp. 345–376). New York: Guilford Press.

Wong, S., & Gordon, A. (1999–2003). *The Violence Risk Scale.* Unpublished manuscript, Department of Psychology, University of Saskatchewan, Saskatoon, Canada.

Wong, S. C. P., & Gordon, A. (2004). A Risk-Readiness

Model of post-treatment risk management. *Issues in Forensic Psychology, 5,* 152–163.

Wong, S., & Gordon, A. (2006). The validity and reliability of the Violence Risk Scale: A treatment friendly violence risk assessment scale. *Psychology, Public Policy and Law, 12*(3), 279–309.

Wong, S., Gordon, A., & Gu, D. (2007). The assessment and treatment of violence-prone forensic clients: An integrated approach. *British Journal of Psychiatry 190,* S66–S74.

Wong, S. C. P., Gordon, A., Gu, D., Lewis, K., & Olver, M. E. (2012). The effectiveness of violence reduction treatment for psychopathic offenders: Empirical evidence and a treatment model. *International Journal of Forensic Mental Health, 11,* 336–349.

Wong, S., & Hare, R. D. (2005). *Guidelines for a psychopathy treatment program.* Toronto, ON, Canada: Multihealth Systems.

Wong, S. C. P., Stockdale, K. C., & Olver, M. E. (in press). Violence reduction treatment of psychopathy. In P. Sturmey (Ed.), *The Wiley handbook of violence and aggression.* Hoboken, NJ: Wiley.

Woody, G. E., McLellan, A. T., Luborsky, L., & O'Brien, C. P. (1985). Sociopathy and psychotherapy outcome. *Archive of General Psychiatry, 42,* 1081–1086.

Yang, M., Wong, S. C. P., & Coid, J. (2010). The efficacy of violence prediction: A meta-analytic comparison of nine risk assessment instruments. *Psychological Bulletin, 136*(5), 740–767.

# CHAPTER 37

# Integrated Modular Treatment

W. John Livesley

In the equivalent chapter in the first edition of this handbook I noted that no single approach or theory has a monopoly on the treatment of personality disorder (PD), and that many treatment methods are effective in changing at least some components of the disorder. This led to the suggestion that "an integrated approach using a combination of interventions drawn from different approaches, and selected where possible on the basis of efficacy, may be the optimal treatment strategy" (Livesley, 2001, p. 570). Subsequent developments support this contention. As new therapies have become available and outcome studies have increased, it has become increasingly apparent that these therapies are effective but do differ in efficacy, making the case for transtheoretical and transdiagnostic treatment even stronger (Livesley, Dimaggio, & Clarkin, 2015).

The original chapter presented a conceptual framework for organizing integrated treatment and selecting interventions. In the intervening years, this framework has been elaborated, based on new empirical and conceptual developments. Unfortunately, it became necessary to give integrated treatment a name, since proponents of most therapies often claim that their approach is also integrated, even though it is based on a single therapeutic model. The term integrated modular treatment (IMT) was selected to capture the intent of developing an eclectic approach that could be applied flexibly to meet the diverse needs of individual patients. In giving integrated treatment a name, the intent was not to propose yet another therapy for PD that could be represented with a three-letter acronym but rather to propose a way to combine the effective ingredients of all current therapies.

IMT is proposed as an evidence-based, patient-focused, transtheoretical approach that uses an eclectic array of treatment principles and methods. This chapter outlines the basic structure of IMT, beginning with a brief overview of the approach, followed by a discussion of the rationale for integration based on the results of outcome studies and the limitations of current treatments. The general literature on psychotherapy integration is then examined to identify strategies found to be useful in integrating therapies. The rest of the chapter describes the different components of IMT, and shows how generic change mechanisms can be used to establish the basic structure of treatment, and how an eclectic array of interventions can be added to this structure and delivered in a coordinated and coherent way.

## Overview of IMT

Given the importance of basing therapy on an explicit conceptual structure noted by Critchfield and Benjamin (2006), IMT has a clearly defined structure consisting of two conceptual frameworks. The first specifies the nature of normal and disordered personality, the impairments that are treatment targets, and the origins and development of these impairments.

The framework is designed to organize clinical information so as to facilitate case formulation and treatment planning. A key part of this framework is the organization of impairments into four functional domains that become the targets for specific interventions: symptoms, problems with regulation and modulation of behavior and experience, interpersonal problems, and self/identify pathology. The second framework conceptualizes treatment in terms of (1) the interventions needed to treat these impairments and (2) the phases through which treatment progresses.

Interventions are organized into modules, each consisting of interrelated interventions designed to achieve a given outcome. Modules are divided into *general treatment modules* that are based on change mechanisms common to all effective therapies, and *specific treatment modules* consisting of interventions drawn from all therapies to treat a specific problem, such as difficulty self-regulating emotions or deliberate self-injury. The distinction between general and specific treatment modules is important. General modules form the basic structure of therapy and are used with all patients throughout treatment. They are designed to establish the within-therapy and within-patient conditions necessary for change by focusing on building a structured, consistent, and validating treatment process, a collaborative alliance, and enhancing patient motivation and self-reflection. Specific modules are added to this structure as needed to treat the problems of individual patients. Consequently, the specific modules used vary according to patient need and the issues that are the focus of treatment at a given moment. Specific modules are only used when the conditions established by the general modules are met, most notably, a satisfactory alliance and when the patient is motivated to change. If these conditions are not in place, general interventions are used to promote the alliance and build a commitment to change.

The treatment process is conceptualized as progressing through five phases: (1) safety, which is primarily concerned with ensuring the safety of the patient and others; (2) containment, which is concerned with the resolution of crises and the containment of symptomatic distress and behavioral dysregulation; (3) regulation and modulation, which primarily focuses on increasing the self-regulation of emotions and impulses; (4) exploration and change, which is largely concerned with restructuring maladaptive interpersonal schemas and interpersonal patterns; (5) integration and synthesis, which focuses primarily on helping patients to construct a more adaptive self-system and a more satisfying life. Each phase primarily addresses a specific domain of impairment using appropriate specific treatment modules. This structure organizes and coordinates the use of specific interventions. The safety and engagement phases deal with the symptom domain. The goals of these phases are to ensure safety, contain symptoms, promote greater stability, and engage the patient in therapy. With a reduction in crises and the achievement of greater stability, therapy progresses to the regulation and modulation phase, with a focus on improving self-management of emotions and impulses. The exploration and change phase primarily addresses the interpersonal domain, and the integration and synthesis phase focuses on the self domain.

## Rationale for Integrating Therapies

The Introduction to Part VII suggested that evidence indicated that therapies for PD do not differ substantially in efficacy, and they are not more effective than either good clinical care or supportive therapy provided strong grounds for integrating them. Currently there are no scientific reasons either to select one therapy over another or to use a specialized therapy rather than good care or supportive therapy. Nevertheless, many therapists continue to use their favorite method and more expensive specialized treatments even as first-line treatments. It might be argued that this does not matter because all therapies produce similar results. However, there are serious problems with this argument.

First, the specialized therapies are generally more expensive than either supportive therapy or good clinical care, a serious problem that limits treatment availability. Second, since all therapies are effective, all must include effective components. Thus, exclusive reliance on one therapy would lead to some effective interventions not being used simply because they are parts of different therapeutic models. Third, current therapies do not provide comprehensive treatment of all aspects of personality pathology because most are based on conceptual models that assume PD is primarily caused by a single specific impairment that then largely determines the focus and scope of therapy. Since most cases of PD show a wide range of impairments, exclusive use of a single therapy could well lead to some problems not being addressed because they are not considered core features of the disorder. Finally, current therapies have limited effectiveness: Even after successful treatment, many patients have substantial residual problems. Moreover, early dropout is relatively common, with roughly one-fourth of patients terminating therapy early, a figure that is substantially higher in some studies.

One obvious way to address these problems is to adopt an integrative and transtheoretical approach that uses all effective treatment methods regardless of the theoretical lineage. This may seem a challenging task because the conceptual models underlying current therapies often seem incompatible with each other. However, once the importance of integration is recognized, the task of selecting and combining effective interventions is not as difficult as it first appears—interventions taken from different therapies can be easily combined, provided that interventions are separated from their theoretical context (Livesley, 2012). Nevertheless, treatment cannot be based simply on an eclectic array of treatment methods; these interventions also need to be coordinated and sequenced. This is the issue addressed in this chapter, beginning with a consideration of how traditional routes to psychotherapy integration can help to integrate PD treatments.

## Routes to Psychotherapy Integration

The general psychotherapy literature describes three routes to integration: common factors, technical eclecticism, and theoretical integration (Norcross & Newman, 1992). The *common-factors approach,* which uses principles of change common to all therapies, is based on the well-established finding that different therapies are equally effective (Beutler, 1991; Luborsky, Singer, & Luborsky, 1975) and that common factors account for much of outcome change. Since treatments for personality disorder also do not differ in efficacy, the common-factors approach is an obvious starting point for integration. Common change mechanisms have a relationship and supportive component and a technical component that provides opportunities to learn and test new skills (Lambert, 1992; Lambert & Bergen, 1994). The emphasis on building the treatment relationship makes the general factors approach particularly relevant to treating PD because an impaired capacity for relationships is a central feature of the disorder (Livesley, 1998, 2003a, 2003b; Livesley, Schroeder, Jackson, & Jang, 1994), and most therapies emphasize the importance of managing the treatment relationship and using it as a vehicle for change.

*Technical eclecticism* involves selecting the best intervention or combination of interventions from diverse treatment models. Most experienced therapists show a form of technical eclecticism that Stricker (2010) calls "assimilative integration"—they use an eclectic set of interventions taken from various therapies, even though they primarily subscribe to a specific model. Besides being consistent with the practices of expert clinicians, technical eclecticism is also relevant to integrating PD therapies because most therapies incorporate effective interventions and a wide variety of methods are needed to cover all domains of personality pathology.

The *theoretical integration* pathway seeks to create a more effective model by integrating the underlying theories of therapeutic change of different therapies (Norcross & Newman, 1992; Stricker, 2010). Although theoretical integration is an ultimate goal, it is probably not a current option because of the inherent limitations of contemporary theories of PD and personality change. Current treatment models are not sufficiently well developed or comprehensive enough to form the basis for theoretical integration. There are, however, some opportunities for greater theoretical integration that are worth exploring, most notably, the concept of cognitive structure (Eells, 1997; Gold, 1996) because most therapies incorporate the notion that cognitive representations of the self and others are important components of personality (Holt, 1989) and a large component of treatment is concerned with restructuring cognitive structures that are variously referred to as object relationships, cognitive schemas (Beck, Davis, & Freeman, 2015), self- and object representations (Gold, 1996), and working models (Bowlby, 1980).

Currently, a combination of the common factors and technical eclecticism offers the most obvious starting point for integration. This suggests a two-component treatment model consisting of interventions that operationalize generic change mechanisms and more specific interventions selected from all effective therapies to provide comprehensive coverage of all components of PD (Livesley, 2003a, 2003b).

## Framework for Conceptualizing PD

Effective treatment requires an explicit conception of the disorder in order to organize the complex psychopathology of individual cases in the systematic way needed to construct a formulation, identify targets for change, and organize therapy. Without such a scheme, it is easy to overlook problems and to miss the nuances of important aspects of the patient's psychopathology. This conceptual framework also needs to incorporate an understanding of normal personality because this helps to clarify both the nature of personality pathology and the changes that treatment needs to bring about. The framework proposed has four components. First, PD is considered to have two main components: features common to all forms of disorder and features that delineate different disorders, such as borderline personality disorder (BPD) and antisocial personality disorder (ASPD) (Livesley, 1998, 2003a, 2003b). Second, personality is conceptualized as a loosely organized dynamic system. Third, the basic building blocks of personality are assumed to be cognitive–emotional–personality schemas that are used to encode and appraise events and initiate response sequences. These schemas are a primary focus of intervention for most therapies. The final component is a description of the etiology and development of PD. Although a detailed description of the conceptual model of PD is beyond the scope of this chapter, the main features are described briefly because this framework impacts all aspects of treatment, including targets for change and intervention strategies.

### *Two-Component Structure of PD*

Current nosological developments such as the fifth edition of the *Diagnostic and Statistical Manual of Mental Disorders* (DSM-5; American Psychiatric Association, 2013) and the proposed revisions to the *International Classification of Diseases* (ICD-11; Tyrer et al., 2011) distinguish between those features that are common to all forms of disorder and the specific features of different diagnoses. This distinction is clinically useful because the general features of PD have a substantial impact on treatment, and severity predicts outcome better than specific diagnoses (Crawford, Koldobsky, Mulder, & Tyrer, 2011). Clinical descriptions of the general features typically refer to difficulty in establishing a coherent self or identity and chronic interpersonal dysfunction (Livesley et al., 1994). This structure gives rise to a different way to approach treatment than that adopted by the specialized therapies. Rather than developing therapies for specific disorders such as BPD or ASPD, IMT emphasizes the importance of organizing therapy around methods needed to treat the pathology common to all disorders. This transdiagnostic approach allows for more economical treatment delivery, since the core component is used with all PDs. This strategy is also useful because core self and interpersonal pathology have a major impact on treatment by hindering alliance formation, creating boundary problems, impeding motivation, and causing difficulty setting and achieving long-term goals. Consequently, a critical therapeutic issue is to define the basic strategy for treating core pathology. This is where the common factors are helpful. An emphasis on a treatment relationship provides the support, empathy, and validation needed to manage core pathology, while also reducing the risk of activating unstable emotions and maladaptive behavior patterns in ways that impede treatment.

### *Personality System*

Personality is conceptualized as a complex system with multiple interacting components or subsystems. Four subsystems figure prominently in treatment: (1) the regulatory and modulatory system used to self-regulate emotions, impulses, and intentional action; (2) the trait system; (3) the interpersonal system, and (4) the self-system. Personality is assumed to develop around heritable traits that represent clinically important differences among individuals with PD. As traits develop, they influence the emergence of the self- and interpersonal systems. These systems are conceptualized as knowledge structures that organize information about the self and others into the schemas used to interpret and respond to events. Thus, the self is conceptualized as a body of knowledge composed of self-schemas that are progressively elaborated and enriched during development. At the same time, connections develop among these schemas to form a matrix. The connections established among self-schemas give rise to the subjective experience of personal unity that characterizes adaptive personality functioning (Livesley, 2003b; Toulmin, 1978). The more extensive and complex these connections are, the greater is the sense of integration and coherence (Horowitz, 1998).

As development proceeds, the integration of the self-system extends beyond connections among self-schemas with the construction of a global self-narrative. This is an important aspect of the self. The hallmark of an adaptive personality system is the establishment of a coherent sense of self and identity. Humans are storytelling, meaning-seeking, interpretive beings who seek to understand their experiences, emotions, moods, and personal qualities by constructing and reconstructing interpretative narratives (Stanghellini & Rosfort, 2013). Once formed, these narratives organize diverse experiences into an overarching understanding of our lives and the world we occupy that helps to integrate and regulate personality functioning. The interpersonal system similarly consists of schemas representing other people and the interpersonal world that are organized when needed into representations of others and our relationship with them.

The emergence of the self- and interpersonal systems depends on an array of basic cognitive processes for combining and integrating information, and on metacognitive processes used to understand the mental states of oneself and others (Dimaggio, Semerari, Carcione, Nicolò, & Procacci, 2007; Fonagy, Gergely, Jurist, & Target, 2002). The personality system also includes regulatory and modulatory mechanisms that control emotions and impulses, and coordinate action.

The idea of personality as a system is an important part of the conceptual framework of IMT for several reasons. First, it moves the conception of PD away from static representation based on a fixed set of criteria to a more dynamic and interactive model that forces us to think about personality as a whole and as a process rather than a list of criteria. Second, it helps to ensure that treatment is based on a comprehensive assessment that takes into account patients' assets as well as their liabilities, and that all aspects of personality pathology are addressed in therapy. Third, the idea of personality as a system draws attention to the organization and coherence of adaptive personality functioning and how this is disturbed in PD. At the highest level of description, PD is probably best characterized as disorganization and lack of coherence in the personality system. However, many current therapies neglect this overarching problem and focus on specific impairments such as emotional dysregulation, or specific problems with maladaptive schemas or dysfunctional modes of thought. These problems are important treatment targets, but they are not the whole story. Outcome and longitudinal studies clearly show that even with symptomatic improvement, the lives of many patients continue to be troubled and unsatisfying, and social adjustment often remains poor. To address these problems, we need to think about how to help patients to create a way of living that is satisfying and rewarding. To do this, we need to promote more integrated personality functioning and a more coherent self-structure.

Finally, the notion of personality as a system has practical utility in organizing treatment. It provides a scheme for organizing the different features of personality pathology into different domains of dysfunction that can then be used to identify specific interventions and subsequently to organize therapy. PD extends to all personality subsystems, giving rise to four major domains of functional impairment (Livesley, 2003b; Livesley & Clarkin, 2015b; see also Clarkin, Livesley, & Meehan, Chapter 21, this volume):

1. Symptoms such as distress, dysphoria, self-harm, dissociative behaviors, and quasi-psychotic symptoms.
2. Regulation and modulation problems involving difficulty self-regulating emotions, impulses, and intentional behavior. Impaired regulatory mechanisms may involve either undercontrol of emotions and impulses leading to the emotional lability associated with borderline and antisocial pathology or overcontrol leading to emotional constriction, as observed in patients with schizoid, avoidant and compulsive features.
3. Interpersonal problems involving maladaptive schemas, difficulty with intimacy and attachment, conflicted interpersonal patterns, and unstable relationships.
4. Self- or identity problems, involving a poorly developed self-system, maladaptive self-schemas, difficulty regulating self-esteem, a poorly integrated and unstable sense of self or identity, and failure to construct an adaptive and coherent self-narrative.

It will be noted that the trait system is not included as a separate domain. This is simply because dysfunctional traits are largely manifested through the other domains.

Decomposing global diagnoses into domains is useful in selecting specific interventions and establishing the sequence in which they will be used in therapy. Work on the stability of normal personality and clinical experience suggests that domains differ in stability and how they respond to therapy (Tickle, Heatherton, & Wittenberg, 2001). The symptom domain is the most responsive, and many symptoms fluctuate naturally over time. The regulatory and modulatory domain tends to be more stable but appears to respond well to most of the specialized therapies and often changes before other aspects of personality pathology. The interpersonal domain is somewhat more intractable, so that even after completing treatment, many patients have poor social adjustment. The self/identity domain seems the most resistant to change. Thus, domains may be organized into a sequence according to their stability and responsiveness to treatment: symptoms → regulation and modulation → interpersonal → self/identity. Since domains are also linked to specific treatment methods, this sequence may also be used to organize and coordinate the specific intervention modules. This allows therapy to be organized into phases in which the most changeable domains are addressed first because this increases the probability of progress early in therapy. This structure enables use of an eclectic array of interventions in an organized and coordinated way, as will be discussed in detail later.

### Cognitive Structure of Personality

Many of the theories underlying current therapies share the assumption that personality involves structures that are largely cognitive in nature. Although the terms used to refer to these cognitive structures vary substantially across theories, terms such as "schemas," "object relationships," "working models," and "mental representations" share the common assumption that cognitive structures are important building blocks of personality, and that treatment is largely a matter of changing these structures to make them more adaptive. The main difference in how the cognitive structures are conceptualized is whether they are considered to be purely cognitive in nature or whether they also have an emotional component. For example, traditional cognitive-behavioral therapy (CBT) assumes that they are purely cognitive, whereas object relationship theory assumes that they include an emotional component. The assumption underlying the integrated perspective being proposed is that these units are cognitive–emotional systems (Mischel & Shoda, 1995). They are referred to here as "personality schemas," since this term has a long tradition in psychology and cognitive science, and is defined as constellations of related ideas, expectations, memories, and emotions.

Within IMT, the personality schema is an important transtheoretical construct that links psychodynamic and cognitive approaches to PD. Schemas are assumed to form the basic structure of the trait, regulatory, interpersonal, and self-systems. It was noted earlier that the self may be viewed as a body of self-referential knowledge consisting of schemas that are used to construct different images of the self and a global self-narrative. PD typically involves a poorly developed self that consists of relatively few self-schemas that are poorly integrated, leading to a fragmented and unstable sense of self. Treatment largely involves promoting greater self-knowledge and enriching the repertoire of self-schemas and promoting their integration. Similarly, the interpersonal system schemas are used to construct representations of others. With PD, a limited array of interpersonal schemas are available, leading to relatively stereotyped and poorly integrated representations of others. As with self-pathology, treatment goals include greater differentiation and integration of the person's conceptions of others. Traits also have a substantial cognitive component. During development, traits are shaped by environmental events. This occurs through the elaboration of schemas that influence the way traits are activated and expressed. For example, a trait such as dependency involves an array of schemas that influences the individual's perception of his or her ability to cope in a given situation and the need for support from others. Gradually these schemas give rise to relatively fixed ways of appraising and responding to situations. Treatment of maladaptive traits largely involves restructuring the schema component.

Given the important role that schemas play in all aspects of personality functioning, considerable time is spent during therapy discussing the schemas associated with different personality subsystems and how schemas are shaped by developmental experiences. The central role of schemas means that a general treatment task is to help patients to recognize and restructure maladaptive schemas across the different domains of personality dysfunction and to understand how these schemas are linked to symptoms and recurrent problems.

## Etiology and Development

A coherent treatment model needs to incorporate an understanding of etiology and development because these influence how change is conceptualized and the selection of treatment methods. As documented in Part IV of this volume, PD arises from the interaction of multiple genetic and environmental influences, each having a relatively small effect, and develops along multiple pathways. These conclusions account for the enormous heterogeneity of PD and hence the need for a flexible approach that allows treatment to be tailored to the needs of individual patients as opposed to a fixed treatment protocol for use with all patients.

Evidence of the heritability of personality features also raises questions about the optimal way to manage maladaptive traits, the main source of individual differences in PD. It is not that heritable traits cannot be changed; rather, the repetitive interplay between genetic and environmental influences may constrain the extent to which traits can be changed with treatment. Although many therapies give the impression that all aspects of personality are amenable to change, this is probably not the case. For example, it seems unlikely that patients with high levels of traits such as anxiousness, emotional lability, or submissiveness will become calm and relaxed or highly assertive with treatment. However, it may be possible to modulate the way these traits are expressed and to help patients to accept their basic traits and use them more adaptively.

An understanding of the developmental consequences of psychosocial adversity also helps to identify intervention targets and shape treatment strategies. Adversity has widespread effects on both the structure and contents of personality. At a structural level, it leads to difficulty developing a coherent self, integrated representations of others, and well-defined interpersonal boundaries. Hence, it is important to include treatment methods that promote integration and self-development. At a content level, adversity leads to maladaptive schemas and modes of thought. Especially important for identifying treatment targets is the way adversity exerts a lasting effect on adjustment through the formation of maladaptive schemas that shape the person's understanding of self, others, and the world. Although a wide range of maladaptive schemas are associated with PD, particularly common are schemas associated with distrust, the unpredictability and unreliability of others and the world; lack of personality efficacy and agency, involving powerlessness, passivity, and vulnerability; and low self-esteem, inferiority, and incompetence. The prevalence of these schemas suggests that besides attempting to restructure them using specific interventions, is it also important to establish a treatment process that provides an ongoing corrective experience that challenges these beliefs. Thus, schemas related to distrust, unpredictability, invalidation, and powerlessness, and lack of agency and self-efficacy, point, respectively, to the importance of a treatment process that provides support, empathy, consistency, and validation, and builds motivation, competency, and mastery. This is an important point: In IMT, many aspects of personality pathology are addressed not only directly with appropriate interventions but also by providing a treatment process that provides ongoing experiences that counter these beliefs.

## General Treatment Modules

Since IMT proposes that treatment is organized around interventions that implement generic change mechanisms, a major task in developing integrated therapy is to translate these mechanisms into interventions tailored to the requirements of treating PD. In the previous edition of the *Handbook,* common change mechanisms were operationalized through four general strategies: building and maintaining a collaborative working relationship, maintaining a consistent therapeutic process, validation, and building and maintaining motivation to change. These strategies were subsequently elaborated to place greater emphasis on enhancing self-reflection and metacognitive functioning generally, processes that are common across all therapies (Livesley, 2011). The initial effort also did not place sufficient emphasis on the importance of a structured treatment process. Consequently, common mechanisms were subsequently parsed into six general treatment modules: structure, treatment relationship, consistency, validation, self-reflection, and motivation (Livesley, 2017; Livesley & Clarkin, 2015a). The first four modules (structure, relationship, consistency, and validation) establish the within-therapy conditions needed for change, whereas the remaining modules (self-reflection and motivation) establish the within-patient conditions for change.

## Module 1: Structure

All effective treatments are highly structured, with a clearly defined treatment model and therapeutic frame. The latter consists of the therapeutic stance and treatment contract, which together create the conditions for change by establishing the structure needed to ensure a consistent process. The "stance" refers the interpersonal behaviors, attitudes, responsibilities, and activities that determine how the therapist relates to the patient. This establishes therapeutic climate by shaping patient–therapist interaction and defining how the therapist approaches treatment. The evidence suggests that most appropriate stance for treating PD provides support, empathy, and validation so as to engage the patient in a collaborative treatment process (Livesley, 2003b).

As most therapies emphasize, the therapeutic contract is fundamental to a structured treatment process. Negotiation of the contract begins toward the end of assessment, with the therapist working collaboratively with the patient to establish treatment goals. Discussion of what the patient wants from treatment communicates the idea that treatment is a collaborative process for which the patient and therapist share responsibility. It also implies a goal-orientated approach, a characteristic of effective treatments. The rest of the contract consists of an explicit understanding of how treatment goals will be achieved and the role of both patient and therapist in the process. The contract also includes agreement on the practical arrangements for treatment—the frequency and duration of sessions and expectations about the length of treatment. The treatment contract orients the patient to treatment and helps to create the safe and consistent environment needed to contain emotional reactivity and build motivation.

## Module 2: Treatment Relationship

If there is an essential ingredient to successful treatment, it is the establishment and maintenance of a collaborative working relationship (Horvath & Greenberg, 1994). This provides support, builds motivation, and predicts outcome. With PD, considerable effort is usually needed to build a truly collaborative relationship and, in some ways, effective collaboration is more the result of effective treatment than a prerequisite for treatment.

Luborsky's (1984) explication of the principles of psychoanalytic psychotherapy offers therapists a useful practical model. Luborsky suggested that alliance has two components: (1) a perceptual–attitudinal component linked to therapist credibility, in which the patient sees the therapy and the therapist as helpful and him- or herself as accepting help; and (2) a relationship component, in which the patient sees therapist and patient working collaboratively for the patient's benefit. The maintenance of an effective alliance also requires that any breakdown in the relationship—what are often called "alliance ruptures"—are dealt with in a timely way. Thus, we can think of the relationship module as consisting of three components: (1) build credibility; (2) maintain collaboration; and (3) repair alliance ruptures. Each submodule is made up of relatively straightforward interventions that need to be delivered consistently throughout therapy.

To form a working relationship, patients need to believe that treatment can work, and that the therapist is helpful and competent. The first submodule, credibility, builds the alliance by (1) generating optimism and confidence about the value of treatment that is conveyed by a professional manner that indicates respect, understanding, and support; (2) educating patients about their problems and how therapy can be helpful; (3) communicating understanding and acceptance through reflective listening; (4) demonstrating support for the patient's treatment goals; (5) communicating realistic hope; (6) recognizing progress; and (7) acknowledging areas of competence.

Interventions forming the second submodule, building collaboration, (1) recognize the patient's use of skills and knowledge learned in therapy, which helps to build the patient–therapist bond; (2) build a connection with the patient through the use of language that recognizes the patient–therapist bond and collaboration (as Luborsky [1984] noted, the use of words such as "we" and "together" are simple ways to cement the relationship); (3) refer to shared experiences in therapy; and (4) emphasize how the patient and therapist are engaged in a collaborative search for understanding.

The third module is concerned with repairing ruptures to the alliance. The crucial role of the alliance in the change process requires that the alliance be monitored throughout treatment and that any deterioration be dealt with promptly. When monitoring the alliance, it should be noted that it is the patient's opinion about the alliance, not the therapist's, that predicts outcome. Any disruption in the therapeutic relationship should be dealt with in an empathic rather than a confrontational and interpretive manner. The strategy for dealing with ruptures to the alliance developed by Safran and colleagues (Safran, Crocker, McMain,& Murray, 1990; Safran, Muran, & Samstag, 1994), which emphasizes that alliance ruptures are opportunities to change dysfunctional interpersonal schemas, is particularly relevant to treating PD (see Tufekcioglu & Muran, 2015). Their approach to managing alliance ruptures requires the following steps:

*Step 1:* Notice "rupture markers"—changes in the relationship and rapport.
*Step 2:* Draw the patient's attention to the decreased rapport in an empathic and noncritical way.
*Step 3:* Explore the rupture and the maladaptive schemas involved.
*Step 4:* Validate the patient's description of his or her experience, an important step that requires therapists to be frank and nondefensive about their part in causing the rupture.
*Step 5:* If these steps are not effective, discuss how the patient is avoiding recognizing and exploring the rupture.

This sequence provides an opportunity to apply several change processes: By noticing and discussing the rupture, the therapist demonstrates empathy, models cooperation, teaches interpersonal problem-solving skills, and communicates the idea that interpersonal problems can be understood and resolved.

## Module 3: Consistency

Effective outcome depends on the therapist's ability to maintain a consistent treatment process (Critchfield & Benjamin, 2006), and patients who respond well to treatment often note that therapist consistency contributed to their improvement (Livesley, 2007). "Consistency" is defined simply as adherence to the frame of therapy, which is why it is important to have a clearly defined treatment model and to spend time establishing the treatment contract. The treatment model and contract provide a frame of reference that helps the therapist to identify deviations from the frame by either patient or therapist. Such violations are relatively common when treating PD and, like alliance ruptures, they are best dealt with promptly.

However, a consistent treatment process does not imply therapist inflexibility. Flexibility is often needed to manage the complexity of personality pathology effectively, especially when managing crises and when the patient feels stuck. Successful management of these situations may require changes to the treatment frame, such as additional appointments or telephone contact. What matters is that the frame not be changed lightly and then only after careful consideration of whether the change is necessary and what short- and long-term effects it is likely to have on the patient, the treatment relationship, coping capacity, and so on.

Challenges to consistency arise from multiple factors, such as unstable emotions, neediness, fearfulness, distrust, and fears of rejection. Patients also tend to test the therapist's ability and resolve to be consistent. Although this is not surprising given the dysfunctional relationships that many have experienced, it nevertheless means that an important therapeutic task is to set limits in a way that does not impair the supportive and empathic stance. Effective limit setting typically requires the therapist to act promptly when a violation occurs by drawing attention to the problem in a way that invites the patient to recognize what he or she is doing. A common problem is that therapists wait too long to address frame violations, then only address the problem when strong feelings are aroused in both parties. Such delays are often due to countertransference problems, such as fear of causing a further deterioration in the alliance, although effective limit setting usually strengthens the alliance, or difficulty believing that limit setting can actually help to contain aggressive and self-destructive behavior. The reasons for noncompliance are then explored while the therapist also explains the purpose of the limit. This process needs to be handled in a firm but supportive and validating way, without argument or debate (Livesley, 2017).

## Module 4: Validation

Validation is a key ingredient of the common factors approach and therapies ranging from self psychology (Kohut, 1971) to DBT (Linehan, 1993). "Validation" may be defined as recognition and affirmation of the patient's experiences: the nonjudgmental acknowledgment and acceptance of the authenticity of the patient's feelings and experience (Livesley, 2003b). Validation contributes to successful treatment by creating an empathic and supportive process that strengthens the alliance, while also countering self-invalidating ways of thinking that result from developmental adversity. Acceptance, and hence validation, are often conveyed more by an attentive and accepting attitude than by specific statements. Validation is closely linked to "empathy," which refers to the therapist's understanding of the mental state of the patient. Validation occurs when the therapist conveys this understanding to the patient in a way that indicates acceptance of his or her feelings.

The general purpose of validation is to help patients to understand their experiences and responses (Linehan, 1993; see Robins, Zerubavel, Ivanoff, & Linehan, Chapter 29, this volume). Linehan (1993) described three steps leading to validation: (1) listening and observing actively and attentively; (2) accurately reflecting back to the patient his or her feelings, thoughts, and behaviors; and (3) direct validation. The first two steps are part of most forms of therapy. Linehan considers the third step, direct validation, specific to dialectical behavior therapy (DBT). Here the therapist communicates to the patient that his or her responses make sense within the context in which they occur. Linehan recommends that therapists search for the adaptive and coping significance of behavior, then communicate this understanding to their patients. Such interventions are part of a more therapeutic general strategy involving a search for meaning that is especially important when treating PD because most patients find their lives and experiences inexplicable, which often causes further distress and self-derogation. Consequently, explanations that the patient's behavior is understandable in terms of his or her history or basic physiological and psychological mechanisms help to reduce self-blame and promote construction of more adaptive narratives about the patient's life and experiences. For example, patients who blame themselves for not coping better because they dissociate, or because their thinking becomes confused when stressed, can be offered information about the way intense anxiety affects performance.

The specific component of the search for meaning that Linehan (1993) emphasizes is *to help the patient recognize that problem behaviors may be adaptive*. That is, actions previously considered either inexplicable or to be manifestations of pathology may actually represent the only way to cope with the problem available to the patient, given his or her life experiences. While not all behavior is explicable in this way, this is a useful form of validation for behaviors that make adaptive sense. For example, patients who self-mutilate when faced with intolerable feelings find it helpful to recognize that such acts may have been the only way to terminate intolerable feelings that the patient had available at the time.

A useful form of validation is to recognize and support strengths and areas of competence, such as recognizing that a patient is able to attend sessions regularly despite a chaotic life style or manages to hold down a part-time job despite severe problems. This approach seems to be most effective if areas of successful coping are not examined in detail, but are instead recognized as achievements on which to build. It is also helpful to draw attention to personal qualities that are helpful or that the person can draw on in therapy. This is another way that the concept of personality system is useful—it draws attention to the more adaptive aspects of personality functioning. For example, a moderate level of compulsivity may make patients more conscientious about pursuing treatment. Although patients often dismiss such characteristics, a discussion of their strengths during or shortly after the contracting stage often contributes to engagement and helps to counter feelings of alienation and demoralization. Patients also often find it easier to talk about their problems when their assets are recognized. Nevertheless, acknowledging competence should be approached carefully: Patients can easily interpret such interventions as indications that the therapist is insensitive to their pain or minimizing their distress.

## Module 5: Self-Reflection

The general treatment strategies may involve not only interventions that enhance the alliance and the treatment process but also those that promote in patients the mental states needed for successful change, especially self-reflection and motivation. Most therapies encourage patients to develop a better understanding of how they think, feel, and act by helping them to become more aware of the links between their problem behaviors and the events that trigger them, and the thoughts, feelings, and resulting actions activated by these events (Critchfield & Benjamin, 2006). Therapy may be thought of as a process of collaborative description, with patient and therapist working to enhance the patient's self-knowledge and self-awareness by using open-ended questions, focusing on inner mental processes and states, decomposing global experiences into their components, and integrating self-knowledge by providing summary statements that draw together different experiences, thoughts, feelings, and actions, and by constructing narratives (Livesley, 2003b, 2017).

The extent and depth of self-knowledge depends on self-reflection: the capacity to think about and understand one's own thoughts and feelings including why one acts in a given way. An important feature of human cognition is that we are not only aware—but we are also aware of our awareness. Impaired self-reflection limits self-knowledge because many forms of self-understanding require the person to reflect on his or her mental processes. This ability also underlies self-regulation and contributes to integrated personality functioning. Also, higher-order regulatory structures such as the self are constructed in part by reflecting on and reorganizing experience. This is why self-reflection is a prerequisite for change—many changes come about because patients restructure the meaning attributed to life events and their impact.

Most patients are acutely aware of their inner experience, especially negative feelings, but have difficulty reflecting on this experience. This is most apparent in patients who have been traumatized. These patients often ruminate endlessly about their experiences. Although this can create the impression that they are engaged in therapeutic work, nothing changes because they simply reexperience their pain without reflecting on, and therefore processing, what happened.

The centrality of self-reflection to change is recognized by most treatments for PD, although a variety of terms are used to describe the same processes, such as the traditional concept of "psychological mindedness" and more recent elaborations of this construct, such as "mentalization" to refer to the capacity to understand the mental processes of self and others and to see behavior as linked to intentions (Bateman & Fonagy, 2004). It also relates to the concept of "meta-cognitive processes," which refers to the processes involving in "thinking about thinking." Here, self-reflection is used to encompass these ideas because it is readily understood and lacks the theoretical connotations of other terms.

Self-reflective thinking is promoted by a therapeutic style that piques patients' interest in the nature and reasons for their actions and stimulates curiosity about how their minds work. In the process, self-knowledge increases, and patients begin to view themselves more objectively. The process is encouraged by the therapist adopting a reflective questioning style that encourages patients to go beyond simply describing events, by drawing their attention to the reasons for their experiences and actions and encouraging them to think more deeply about the reasons behind their feelings and actions.

Self-reflection is limited by the cognitive rigidity that characterizes PD (see Fonagy & Luyten, Chapter 7, this volume). Patients tend to act in relatively fixed and stereotyped ways partly because these are well-established patterns and partly because they tend to see events in rigid ways and have difficulty recognizing that alternative interpretations of events are possible. Cognitive rigidity is reduced and self-reflection is enhanced by challenging these fixed ways of seeing and responding to events, and by encouraging patients to look at situations from different perspectives and to consider alternative ways of looking at what happened.

### Module 6: Motivation: Build and Maintain Motivation for Change

A second instrumental component of the general strategies is to build a commitment to change. Although patients need to be motivated to seek help and engage in therapeutic work, psychosocial adversity often causes intense passivity and pessimism about the prospects of change. Consequently, patients have difficulty motivating themselves to do the work needed to change. This requires therapists to become skilled in building motivation and to make extensive use of motivation-enhancing techniques and methods of interviewing (Miller & Rollnick, 2002; Rosengren, 2009).

When a commitment to change is lacking, little is gained from pressing on with specific interventions designed to bring about change because they are unlikely to be effective and the therapist's persistence will probably damage the alliance and increase emotional reactivity. Instead, it seems more effective to deal with therapeutic impasses in a supportive and flexible way that acknowledges how change is difficult (Linehan, Davison, Lynch, & Sanderson, 2006). When patients feel stuck, it seems best to recognize and thereby validate both how difficult it is to change and any fears the patient may have about the consequences of change. Little is achieved with more confrontational methods that directly challenge resistance to change.

Motivation is influenced by other generic interventions, especially the alliance, which should be reviewed whenever motivational problems arise. Motivation is also enhanced by a goal-focused approach that seeks to define and address patient concerns early in therapy. It is also useful to encourage patients to set modest goals at the outset of treatment because these are more likely to be attained, and nothing builds motivation better than success. For example, rather than setting the goal of stopping deliberate self-harm, the patient may be encouraged initially to try to postpone acting on the urge to self-injure for a short time and progressively increase this interval until the patient manages to abort some episodes. Any success in attaining such goals, such as resisting the urge to self-harm for, say, 10 minutes, is recognized and used to build motivation, strengthen the alliance, and promote self-efficacy. With these small steps, the goal is to help patients to "own" the change process and begin reinforcing themselves when their efforts are successful. Motivation is also enhanced by maintaining a focus on change, monitoring progress toward attaining goals, and reviewing progress regularly to remind patients about their goals and that therapy is about making changes.

Developments in motivational interviewing report that talking about change increases the likelihood of attempts to implement change (Miller & Rollnick, 2013; Rosengren, 2009). Patients should be encouraged talk about the changes they would like to make and about their hopes and goals. Any spontaneous talk about change or the need for change should be reinforced. The kind of talk that is particularly effective in increasing motivation is in reference to changing specific behaviors or problems. Patients often talk generally about the need to change because everything is wrong with their lives. This kind of talk is not as effective as talking about making specific changes. Hence, when patients make general comments about the need to change, they need to be encouraged to focus on specific changes, such as being more active, reducing self-harm, managing their anger better, and so on. It also helps if patients talk about making changes now rather than as something they need to do sometime in the future.

In everyday life, discontent is a powerful motivator of change (Baumeister, 1991, 1994). People only think about making changes when they are discontented with the way things are. Discontent is often aroused by relatively minor incidents that suddenly change how people see themselves and their situation. Occasionally, this occurs in therapy when patients suddenly realize that they need to change. Some years ago, a patient suddenly became enraged in a session, jumped up, swept everything off my desk, and rushed from the room. It happened so quickly that I did not have time to react. Later she told me that when she rushed out of the building, she suddenly realized what she had done. She stopped dead in her tracks and told herself that she had to stop behaving in this way because it was wrecking her life. In an instant, she decided she had to make some changes. She stopped abusing alcohol and street drugs and began to work more determinedly at making changes and controlling her moods.

Although such events are rare, discontent can be used to build motivation when a specific incident causes a patient to think more about what he or she is doing. Modest levels of discontent can be promoted by exploring the negative consequences of maladaptive behavior. This is especially effective if the discontent can be linked to the hope that therapy can help the patient to change. Discontent builds the initial intent to change, but it is hope of success that translates the intent into action. Hope is also promoted by reminding patients of other changes they have made and by helping them to recognize that other options are available.

### Specific Treatment Modules

The second component of IMT derived from technical eclecticism consists of interventions selected to treat specific problems and impairments. A comprehensive repertoire of interventions culled from all effective therapies is required to treat all aspects of personality pathology. The challenge of technical eclecticism is how to use an eclectic array of interventions with diverse theoretical origins in a coordinated way without therapy becoming disorganized and therapist and patient becoming confused by the use of multiple interventions. This is a significant risk because the wide-ranging psychopathology of PD usually leads to a patient raising multiple problems in most sessions. Since not all can be addressed at once, therapists need guidelines about the problems that should be given priority and how to sequence the use of specific intervention modules. Earlier, it was suggested that this problem can be managed in two ways: first, by decomposing global diagnoses such as BPD or ASPD into domains of functional impairment (symptoms, regulation and modulation impairments, interpersonal problems, and self/identify problems), then selecting the most appropriate interventions to treat each domain, a process that systematically links treatment goals and methods, and second, by dividing the overall process of therapy into phases, with each phase focusing primarily on a single domain so that domains are addressed sequentially.

## Domains of Impairment and Specific Intervention Modules

Ideally, interventions should be selected on the basis of efficacy. However, outcome studies have not progressed to identifying the most effective way to treat the different components of PD. Consequently, interventions are selected by extrapolating from the limited studies available and from a rational analysis of what interventions are likely to be most useful in treating a specific problem. Figures 37.1–37.4 illustrate some of the interventions derived from current therapies that therapists may wish to consider when treating the different domains of personality dysfunction when implementing integrated treatment.

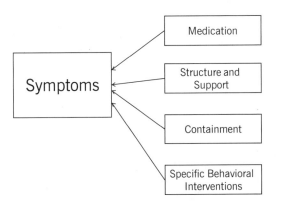

**FIGURE 37.1.** Symptom domain and intervention modules.

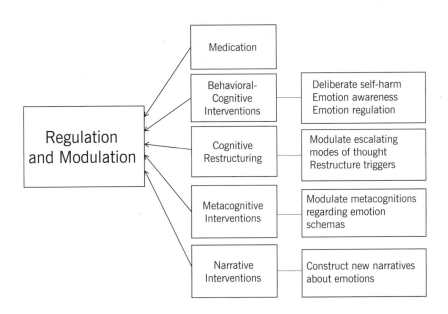

**FIGURE 37.2.** Regulation and modulation domain and intervention modules.

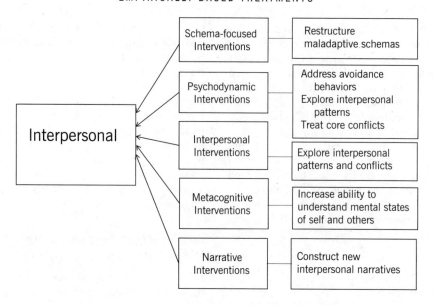

**FIGURE 37.3.** Interpersonal domain and intervention modules.

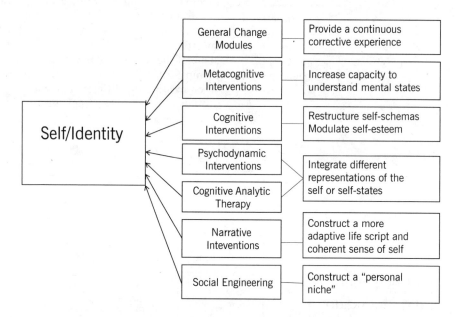

**FIGURE 37.4.** Self domain and intervention modules.

## Phases of Therapeutic Change

Since therapy for PD can be complex, the overall process is easier to understand if treatment is divided into phases. IMT conceptualizes therapy in terms of five phases:

1. Safety: Immediate interventions to ensure the safety of the patient and others when treatment begins in a crisis state.
2. Containment: Having ensured safety, the next phase is to contain behavioral reactivity and emotional distress.
3. Regulation and modulation: Once a measure of stability and containment is achieved, treatment gradually focuses more on building emotional control and decreasing self-harm and suicidality by improving self-regulation skills and strategies.
4. Exploration and change: With increased emotional control, therapeutic attention turns to exploring and changing the maladaptive cognitions and ways of thinking that underlie dysfunctional interpersonal patterns. This includes exploration and change of conflicted patterns of interpersonal relationships and the maladaptive traits contributing to these behaviors, and work on the interpersonal consequences of adversity and trauma.
5. Integration and synthesis: As treatment progresses, attention gradually shifts to helping the patient to develop a more integrated sense of self and identity, and a more satisfying and rewarding lifestyle.

Although general treatment strategies are used in each phase, specific interventions usually differ across phases. Consequently, the phases of change scheme offers a plan for using an eclectic combination of interventions, with a general progression from more structured to less structured methods.

### Phase 1: Safety

When treatment begins with the patient in a decompensated crisis state, the immediate goal is to ensure the safety of the patient and others. Following an appropriate assessment, safety is largely achieved by providing structure and support through outpatient treatment or crisis intervention service, or occasionally, through brief inpatient treatment. The treatment methods used during this phase are based largely on the general treatment modules and involve providing the support and structure the patient needs to resolve the crisis. Specific interventions are not normally used because the patient is usually too distressed to use anything more than simply supportive methods. The exception is the use of medication to manage symptoms and settle distress.

### Phase 2: Containment

With most cases, the safety phase quickly progresses to the containment phase, enabling the treatment goal to be extended to containing and settling emotional and behavioral instability, and helping the patient to regain behavioral control. The safety and containment phases are essentially different aspects of crisis management. At this point in treatment, the concern is to return the patient to the precrisis level of functioning as soon as possible, reduce the frequency of crises, minimize the escalation of psychopathology that is a common outcome of crisis management in some settings, and engage the patient in treatment.

The therapist continues to rely on general treatment methods that are largely delivered through containment interventions. Containment is based on the idea that in an acute emotional crisis, the patient's primary concern is to obtain relief from distress, and that relief comes from feeling a connection with someone who understands (Joseph, 1983; Links & Bergmans, 2015; Livesley, 2003b; Steiner, 1994). Having someone acknowledge how dreadful he or she feels is usually sufficient to provide the support needed to regain control. Thus, in crises, the therapist's task is to make a connection with the patient and acknowledge his or her distress by listening attentively and reflecting back an understanding of the patient's feelings and experiences. Containment interventions are most effective if they are short and focus on the emotional component of the patient's immediate concerns rather than on factual details of the events triggering the crisis. Besides providing understanding, it is also helpful to avoid interventions that hinder containment, such as lengthy attempts to clarify feelings, attempts to explain or interpret the reasons for the crisis, failure to acknowledge distress, and discussion of coping strategies. At these times, it is best to keep things simple and not to try to accomplish too much.

Since dysregulated emotions are destabilizing, emotional arousal needs to be managed and modulated. Containment interventions are useful throughout therapy. The first indications of the adverse effects of heightened arousal are difficulty thinking, losing track of what is being discussed, feeling confused, and difficulty concentrating. These behaviors should not be managed as if they are purely defensive actions or indications of resistance, but rather as indications that emotional arousal is overwhelming cognitive processes and hence as an indication of the need to discontinue current interventions and switch to containment interventions until emotional control is regained. This approach uses the treatment relationship to regulate emotional arousal until the patient has developed the capacity to self-regulate emotions.

### Phase 3: Regulation and Control

Increased behavioral and emotional stability are usually accompanied by an improved alliance and increased motivation that allow therapy to progress to the regulation and control phase by gradually incorporating interventions drawn from specific treatment modules to increase emotional regulation skills and reduce deliberate self-harming behavior and suicidality. The primary goal of this phase is to enhance emotion regulation—the ability to control the occurrence, intensity, experience, and expression of emotions (Gross & Thompson, 2007) by (1) increasing knowledge about emotions and emotional dysregulation; (2) increasing awareness of emotional experience; (3) teaching emotion regulating skills and strategies; and (4) increasing emotional processing capacity. Each goal is associated with a specific module and hence a specific set of submodules and interventions. The complexity of these goals lends itself well to a transtheoretical modular approach that uses interventions from various therapies including DBT, CBT, schema-focused therapy (SFT), acceptance-based therapies, and narrative therapies.

The impaired emotional control may involve either under- or overcontrol. Emotional dyscontrol is a central feature of patients with personality features that span the DSM diagnoses of BPD, ASPD, narcissistic PD, and dependent PD. Therefore, I discuss this in more detail than emotional overcontrol or constriction, which is more a feature of schizoid and obsessive–compulsive PDs. The extent to which both forms of emotional dysregulation pathology cuts across traditional clinical diagnoses illustrates the value of a mechanism-based, transdiagnostic approach.

### Emotional Dysregulation

Improvements in unstable and dysregulated expression of emotions requires enhancement of skills in monitoring, appraising, and modulating emotional responses (Nolen-Hoeksema, 2012). It also requires that patients be educated about the value of emotions and the diverse effects of emotional lability, and that they be helped to develop an enhanced capacity to process emotional experiences. This requires a wide range of interventions that may be organized into four modules: psychoeducation; awareness, self-regulation, and emotion processing.

PATIENT EDUCATION

This module provides information about the adaptive functions and origins of emotions, how intense emotions affect thought and action, and the role of emotions in normal personality functioning. This information is useful because patients tend to hold erroneous beliefs about their emotions. Because their emotions are so intense, many assume that feelings are harmful and are best supressed or avoided. These ideas can be countered with information on the adaptive functions of emotions and how emotions provide the information we need to understand and organize our experience of the world and our interactions with it. Emotional tolerance often increases with the realization that emotions provide information about what is frightening and should be avoided and what is pleasant or interesting and worth pursuing, and that without emotions, life would be bland and uninteresting. This can be linked to information about how emotions are necessary to communicate and interact effectively with others. It also helps to point out just how difficult it is to interact with people who do not show much emotion. Besides information about how emotions help us to adapt to our world, information is also needed about how intense, unstable emotions interfere with information processing by making it difficult to think clearly.

The psychoeducation module is not intended to be delivered all at once or through a designated number of sessions. It seems to work best if the information is imparted gradually as different aspects of the patient's emotional life come to the fore in treatment, so as to avoid overwhelming patients with too much information especially when they are still relatively unstable and vulnerable to information overload.

## AWARENESS

This module consists of interventions that increase the ability to identify feelings, track emotions, have a present-focused awareness of emotions, and tolerate and accept emotions.

*Identifying and Labeling Emotions.* Improved emotional regulation begins with the patient learning to recognize, identify, and label emotions. This is challenging because many patients experience a complex mixture of negative feelings but have difficulty disentangling the specific emotions involved. Also, many patients are intensely self-focused and are therefore acutely aware of their distress but have little awareness of the origins of their distress or how distress and anger can mask feelings of sadness, fearfulness, and shame. The therapeutic task is to unpack these emotional states by helping patients to recognize the specific emotions involved as the first step toward transforming an intense self-focus into greater self-awareness, and later into greater self-reflection on the causes and consequences of emotional experiences.

*Tracking Emotions and Emotional Responses.* While learning to identify emotions, patients can also learn to track the flow of their emotional responses by exploring the event–emotional response–consequences sequence used by cognitive therapy. Although patients often insist that nothing triggers their distress and that it usually occurs spontaneously, it is important that they identify triggers as the first step toward controlling emotional reactions. Since most emotional reactions are triggered by interpersonal events, such as a perceived rejection or humiliation, the process also begins to increase patients' understanding of the interpersonal factors linked to intense emotions.

Following identification of triggering events, emotional arousal is explored in terms of the thoughts, behaviors, and additional feelings activated by the initial reaction. Connection of triggering events, emotions, and the consequences of emotional arousal begins to make experiences more meaningful, while also integrating events and experiences that may have been considered unrelated. At the same time, patients are also helped to recognize how self-talk in the form of self-criticism, rumination, and catastrophizing escalates their distress. Finally, attention focuses on identifying the short-term and long-term consequences of emotional states. Although patients usually recognize the short-term consequences of responses to reduce distress, such as deliberate self-injury, they are less aware of the long-term effects of intense emotions on self-esteem and their lives and relationships.

*Developing Moment-by-Moment Awareness of Emotions.* The capacity for emotional self-regulation depends on the development of present-focused or moment-to-moment nonjudgmental awareness of emotions—the capacity to observe experiences objectively as they occur (Barlow et al, 2011; Kabat-Zinn, 2005a, 2005b). Patients with severe emotional dysregulation lack this ability. Instead, they tend to "fuse" with their experience (Hayes, Strosahl, & Wilson, 1999) so that the experience defines who they are at that moment as opposed to being a transient feeling state, and they have difficulty decentering from the experience and viewing it objectively.

Present-focused awareness is helpful because initial emotional responses to events are often useful (e.g., feeling fear in response to a threat), but subsequent reactions are often more judgmental and self-critical (Barlow et al., 2011). Hence, it is important to distinguish the initial emotion from the subsequent cascade of other emotions and reactions. Recognition of the usefulness of initial emotional responses helps to reinforce psychoeducation about the adaptive value of emotions and promotes tolerance and self-compassion. The task is to help patients to attend to these reactions and observe the flow of inner experience without evaluating it. Since judgmental and self-critical reactions to emotional responses are common in patients with PDs, it is often helpful to explore specific events that evoke strong emotions in order to promote a more detached way of observing what happened rather than simply reliving events.

Several therapies stress the value of mindfulness exercises in promoting present-focused awareness, and it may be useful to include these interventions at this point (Kabat-Zinn, (2005a, 2005b; Ottavi, Passarella, Pasinetti, Salvatore, & Dimaggio, 2015) to promote this ability and help control tendencies to ruminate over humiliations, rejections, wrongs, and embarrassments suffered at the hands of others. Although mindfulness is often taught as a separate exercise, it is readily incorporated into the treatment process. This is useful because the process of patient and therapist working collaboratively is often as helpful as the skills themselves, and any improvement in mindfulness skills may be used to build the alliance and promote self-efficacy.

*Promoting Emotion Acceptance and Tolerance.* The increased emotional awareness and nonjudgmental momentary focus on experience needed for emotion regulation require tolerance and acceptance of negative feelings without self-criticism. Acceptance and tolerance are important because emotional arousal is automatic and outside of our control. However, we can self-regulate the intensity and persistence of the emotions aroused, but it usually requires that we accept our emotions rather than trying to avoid or suppress them. We also need to tolerate distress long enough to implement self-regulation skills and strategies. Acceptance and tolerance are promoted by encouraging patients to examine and hold negative emotions as they occur in therapy. Although patients often seek to avoid such feelings and promptly suppress them when they arise, they often reveal their feelings fleetingly by changes in facial expression and other nonverbal responses that can be used to focus the patient's attention on these transient states.

Tolerance is also built by the patient modeling the therapist's empathic and nonjudgmental response to his or her emotions. At this point in therapy, it is often useful to incorporate some of the methods used in acceptance and commitment therapy to foster greater self-compassion, something that is often poorly developed in patients with emotion dysregulation, especially in the context of a history of abuse.

*Countering Emotional Avoidance.* Emotional dysregulation is usually linked to cognitive and behavioral strategies to suppress and avoid emotions. As with self-talk, patients are often unaware of these behaviors. The problem is managed initially by drawing the patient's attention to how he or she tends to avoid painful feelings. Some patients readily recognize that they act in this way but others are almost totally oblivious. Subsequently, attention is focused on helping patients to recognize how they avoid emotion first in therapy and later in everyday situations, by doing things such as rapidly changing a topic when emotions are triggered, using distracting behaviors, avoiding eye contact, refusing to talk about emotive topics, deliberately suppressing feelings, or refocusing attention to positive thoughts or events. It is also useful to incorporate a psychoeducational component by explaining the consequences of avoidance, especially how avoidance limits awareness and self-understanding, and prevents the person from learning how to manage feelings more effectively, and how suppressed and avoided feelings do not disappear but rather often emerge in an even stronger form.

SELF-REGULATION

A wide range of interventions is available for therapists to draw on to build emotion regulation skills because treatment development has largely focused on BPD. A few of the simpler and most readily applied methods are described for illustrative purposes.

*Self-Soothing and Distraction.* Skills acquisition is usually introduced early in treatment with relatively simple interventions such as self-soothing and distraction to reduce distress and subsequently is supplemented with more complex interventions that require more training. Self-soothing is probably the first self-regulating strategy children learn by internalizing the soothing actions of caregivers. The process seems to go awry in patients with emotional dysregulation, so that the capacity to self-soothe becomes impaired. Early in therapy, a similar process occurs when the therapist uses containment interventions to settle and soothe the patient's distress. Over time, this process is internalized to promote self-soothing skills. Distraction is also often introduced during crisis management to reduce distress and manage deliberate self-injury. To be effective, self-soothing and distraction need to be used in early stages of emotional arousal, before emotions escalate out of control, which is a further reason to focus on increasing emotional awareness. Since patients are often unable to recall what to do when distressed, it is useful to work with them to compile a list of suitable activities to which they can refer when they first notice something is amiss.

Therapists need to be clear about the purpose in using simple behavioral ways of manage distress. Besides providing some immediate relief, the intent is to demonstrate to the patient that feelings can be controlled in order to reduce the sense of pessimism that nothing can be done to change these feelings and begin to enhance feelings of self-efficacy.

*Grounding Techniques.* Another simple but effective way to manage intense, panic-like anxiety, especially when associated with dissociation, is to use grounding methods. Intense anxiety leads to an intense self-focus and loss of contact with surroundings that escalate panic and dissociation. Simple exercises that increase sensory input and decrease self-focus help to control these reactions. This is most easily achieved by sitting in a chair and concentrating on the sensations caused by placing one's feet firmly on the ground, feeling a solid object (e.g., the arms of the chair), and concentrating on objects in the environment. This increases sensory input and diverts attention from painful inner experience. With more intense dissociative reactions, it may necessary to increase sensory input using tasks such as balancing exercises that require greater concentration and hence reduce the focus on inner experience. The technique is also easy to teach to significant others who can then coach the patient in using the method when he or she begins to dissociate. This is useful because significant others often do not know what to do on these occasions, which adds to the panic and distress.

*Relaxation.* Relaxation training is especially useful in managing the anxious/fearful component of emotional dysregulation. Although a wide variety of methods are available, simple methods such as breath training involving slow abdominal breathing is often best because many patients lack the resources and motivation to use more complex methods. If initially introduced during a session when the patient is anxious and rapport is satisfactory, it nearly always has immediate benefits. This can then be used to encourage the patient to practice regularly between sessions. Since relaxation is easy to use in everyday situations, it can also be used to manage any emotional reaction such as fear, stress, assumed slights, anger, and jealousy.

*Attention Control.* The ability to shift attention from unpleasant thoughts and feelings rather than ruminating about them is an integral part of self-regulation that is usually impaired in those with dysregulated emotions as part of a general problem with executive functioning (Lenzenweger, Clarkin, Fertuck, & Kernberg, 2004). Attention control can be improved by using an extension of the relaxation exercise to teach patients to switch attention from painful thoughts and feelings to a more pleasant and relaxing image using an exercise based on systematic desensitization (Wolpe, 1958). In systematic desensitization, fear evoked by a specific stimulus is progressively decreased by presenting the stimulus at a low level of intensity while encouraging relaxation. A similar procedure is used to desensitize fear responses to traumatic stimuli and promote attention control.

First, the stimulus triggering distress and dissociation is identified, which may be a specific characteristic manifested by an abuser such as a facial feature or words the perpetrator used, situations that evoke traumatic memories, or the memories themselves. Next, the patient is asked to imagine a pleasant scene which is used to help the patient to relax. Once relaxation is achieved the patient is asked to think about the triggering stimulus. Emotional arousal is monitored and the patient is asked to divert attention back to the pleasant scene as soon as anxiety increases to ensure that he or she can be helped to relax successfully. This may only be a matter of seconds. The therapist then talks the patient through the relaxation exercise until relaxation is achieved. The process is then repeated several times. As the capacity to tolerate distress and shift attention increases, the time that the patient is asked to focus on the traumatic stimulus is gradually increased. With some patients, it is necessary to construct a hierarchy of stimuli or memories that evoke intense distress and dissociation and each is sensitized in turn because the main trigger generates overwhelming distress. Once the patient understands the process and is able to regulate distress, he or she can begin to practice between sessions. As with the grounding exercise, some patients also benefit from involving significant others. Intent is not just to desensitize traumatic stimuli but also to strengthen attention control and to demonstrate to the patient that painful thoughts and feelings can be managed.

*Treating Escalating Cognitions.* As noted earlier, distress is often exacerbated by self-talk ranging from constant self-criticism to thoughts about being unable to cope, and by intolerable feelings and chronic suicidal ideation that are usually so automatic that the patient is barely aware of them. Hence, change begins by increasing awareness of these thoughts and their effects. Subsequently, patients are encouraged to restructure these thoughts using standard cognitive therapy interventions. Although such interventions are not as effective in treating PDs as other disorders (Bernstein & Clercx, Chapter 31, this volume; Dimaggio, Popolo, Carcione, & Salvatore, 2015; Layden, Newman, Freeman, & Morse, 1993; Young, Klosko, & Weishaar, 2003), simple methods such as disputing dysfunctional thoughts and examining the evidence supporting a belief are often helpful.

EMOTION PROCESSING

Enhancement of emotional processing capacity is often neglected by therapies that focus heavily on building emotion regulation skills. Although such skills are important, it is also useful to enhance the capacity to reflect on emotions and their consequences, and to promote construction of higher-order meaning systems and narratives to provide an additional level of self-regulation. The concern is also to restore the informational value of emotions and to facilitate the integration of emotions with other personality processes. This work requires interventions drawn from several therapies besides the cognitive-behavioral methods that have dominated the therapeutic repertoire so far. The promotion of self-reflection now assumes even greater significance; hence, it is useful to incorporate methods used in MBT and metacognitive therapy at this point. It also becomes increasingly important to incorporate a narrative therapy component (Angus & McLeod, 2004) to help patients to construct the new scripts needed to understand the meaning and function of emotion in their mental lives.

*Promoting More Flexible Emotional Responses.* Emotional dysregulation tends to lead to emotions being expressed in a fixed and all-or-nothing manner due in part to the intensity of the feelings involved and in part to the tendency to react to emotional events in a rigid, stereotyped fashion. There is also a tendency to treat emotions as if they are enduring states rather than processes that fluctuate. Hence, it is helpful for patients to understand that *emotions are processes* that wax and wane, and that even painful feelings are transient. Seeing emotions in this way opens up the possibility of expressing emotions differently. This is enhanced by helping patient to become more *flexible in how they interpret emotional events*. Patients tend to assume that their interpretations of events are correct and the only possible way to understand the event (Dimaggio et al., 2015). Consequently, many patients are initially closed to the idea that events can be interpreted from different perspectives, and that other response options are possible. This is where mentalizing interventions are useful: Along with interventions that promote self-reflection, mentalizing interventions encourage patients to view things in different ways and to see events from other people's points of view. This in turn helps them to understand how emotions are intertwined with their interpersonal lives. This change of perspective makes it possible to recognize that emotions are evoked by not only external events but also internal processes such as interpersonal schemas. This recognition opens up the possibility of greater flexibility in interpreting and responding to events. Greater flexibility in emotional expression is also encouraged by promoting the idea that emotions are experiences, not actions, and that patients may experience but not necessarily express emotions, and even if expressed, this does not need to be in an all-or-nothing way.

*Increasing Emotional Range.* Intense dysregulated emotions are primarily confined to negative emotions such as anger, anxiety, distress, sadness, and shame, and rarely involve positive emotions such as happiness, joy, delight, and interest (Sadikaj, Russell, Moskovitz, & Paris, 2010; Stepp, Pilkonis, Yaggi, Morse, & Feske, 2009). When emotional lability decreases with treatment, there is often a sense of emotional emptiness or flatness because positive emotions rarely increase to fill the gap. This problem often prevents patients from making the most of the changes they have made. Negative emotions cause people to withdraw and live more constricted lives, and even when negative emotions decrease, this constricted way of living continues because the positive emotions people need in order to be more outgoing and engaged with the world do not automatically increase. Unfortunately, it is difficult to stimulate positive emotions. Instead, they seem to occur naturally with therapeutic improvement. The exception is the development of a sense of interest. As patients improve, they often begin to talk about things that interest them, often in response to incidental events. Thus, patients often recall things that have interested them in the past or comment about something they would like to do. When this happens in therapy, it is important to reflect and nurture the interest no matter how minor in order to promote reengagement with the world and as a step toward promoting positive emotions.

*Constructing More Adaptive Narratives.* Humans are meaning-seeking, interpretive beings who seek to understand their life experiences, mental states, and personal characteristics by constructing and reconstructing meaningful narratives (Ricoeur, 1981; Stanghellini & Rosfort, 2013). These narratives are important: They give meaning to people's lives by offering a broad perspective on events that promote integration and coherence and help to self-regulate action and emotion. During development, narratives are constructed about diverse aspects of life, including the nature and value of emotions, what triggers them, and one's ability to cope with them. If these beliefs or schemas are positive, they help to regulate emotions. When they are negative, they exacerbate distress, as illustrated by the negative self-talk that often accompanies intense distress. As the regulation and modulation phase of treatment begins to give way to the exploration and change phase, it is useful to spend some time helping patients to construct more adaptive narratives that incorporate the idea that emotions are useful sources of pleasure and satisfaction and allow them to see their emotions in the broader context of their lives and relationships. This happened with one patient, a student who, after being fearful of her anxiety for some time, suddenly realized that modest levels of anxiety helped her to work more effectively. The essential point is that a comprehensive approach to treating unstable emotions requires both the acquisition of appropriate skills and the construction of narratives capable of regulating emotions and integrating them with other personality processes.

## Emotional Constriction

The literature on treating constricted emotional expression is sparse compared with that on emotional dysregulation because little attention has been given to treating forms of PD associated with this pattern (e.g., schizoid and obsessive–compulsive PDs). It is also more difficult to treat: It is easier to teach emotional regulation and modulation than to promote emotional expression, something noted when discussing the challenges of encouraging positive emotions in emotionally dysregulated individuals. Emotional constriction varies in nature and intensity according to its associated traits. When associated with obsessive–compulsive tendencies, the picture is one of constraint: Emotions are suppressed and avoided to maintain orderliness and structure. The situation is different when emotional constriction is associated with socially avoidant features. In this case, emotions are not only contained and suppressed but also rarely experienced, and then only in muted form. It is as if the basic personality pattern is to avoid social contact, and since emotions facilitate and often initiate social interaction, they are not experienced, or if experienced, they are not expressed.

Less severe forms of emotional constriction involving suppression, avoidance, and overcontrol is often easier to treat using modified versions of the same modules used with emotional dysregulation. Patient education is important to counter beliefs about the harmful and disruptive effects of emotion and to increase awareness of the role of emotion in social interaction. Emotional awareness is increased by drawing attention to minor changes in expression and tone of voice in session and helping the patient to reflect on his or her thoughts at the time. Whereas, with emotional dysregulated individuals, the broad strategy in dealing with the scenarios discussed in therapy is to focus on details to help identify emotional triggers and the emotions aroused, the opposite strategy is used with emotional constriction by focusing more on general impressions and reactions than on detail because attention to detail and facts is a form of emotional avoidance.

With these patients, emotional constriction is part of a general need for control. As patients come to accept that control is useful only if they are able to control their control, and that it is not useful when their control controls them, the overall impact of their controlling strategies decreases, leading to the occurrence of transient emotional experiences in session. These events offer an opportunity to explore the feelings involved and associated thoughts, and to encourage the patient to "hold" the feelings as a way to build tolerance and acceptance. The goal is to promote the idea that emotions are useful and even enjoyable experiences that can occur without loss of control. Ultimately, this idea needs to become part of a new narrative that recognizes the benefits of emotions and incorporates the idea that emotions can be used and managed.

Emotional constriction as part of a more socially avoidant or schizoid pattern is more difficult to treat. In the more severe cases, in which the emotional constriction involves inhibited emotional expression and the almost total absence of feelings associated with avoidance of social interaction, therapeutic change is likely to be limited and it may be best to focus on helping the patient to accept his or her basic personality structure and to find a comfortable niche compatible with his or her personality. For example, one such patient, who was extremely emotionally inhibited and indeed expressed puzzlement about what emotions are, enjoyed gambling and was good at it because nothing distracted him. He found satisfying work as a dealer in a casino. Having a job boosted his self-esteem, and the work itself gave the impression that he was socializing even though he only interacted with clients. His lack of emotion was in fact useful because it allowed him to concentrate on the cards. With less severe cases, management is similar to that described for emotional constriction associated with more compulsive traits. The main difference is that even more attention is given to the therapeutic alliance. Trust is essential for the patient to begin experiencing even the most modest emotional arousal in therapy. However, inhibitedness and lack of emotional responsiveness make it difficult to build an effective treatment process (Dimaggio et al., 2012). This requires considerable therapist tolerance and patience. It also requires assiduous avoidance of actions that appear to be either pressuring or intrusive. Such patients are often highly sensitive to both, so that many of the things therapists do routinely are experienced as too pressuring or intrusive, or even invasive. Hence, social distance and closeness need to be managed carefully.

### Phase 4: Exploration and Change

As emotion regulation improves and the treatment focus gradually shifts to interpersonal problems, this shift is usually heralded by a change of focus from acquiring skills to enhancing emotion processing capacity, which inevitably involves greater attention to the interpersonal aspects of emotional arousal. An increasingly interpersonal focus leads to therapy becoming more complex and less structured in order to manage the greater complexity and diversity of interpersonal problems compared to problems involving emotion dysregulation. The scope of interventions, which progressively broadened during the regulation and control phase with the addition of mentalizing and narrative methods, now broadens further with the incorporation of interpersonal and psychodynamic methods needed to address the breadth and nuances of interpersonal pathology. These changes place additional demands on the therapist. Previously, it was possible to deal with relatively specific and readily apparent emotional impairments with well-defined interventions. The complexity and diversity of interpersonal problems makes therapy less predictable because the problems and issues raised vary considerably within and across sessions.

The goal of this phase is to explore and change the interpersonal pathology that underlies symptoms and problems and impedes adaptation. This requires restructuring maladaptive schemas, modifying repetitive maladaptive interpersonal patterns, and resolving conflicted relationships. However, with increased attention on interpersonal issues, the psychosocial adversity associated with these problems also becomes a major therapeutic issue. At this point in therapy, emotion regulation will have improved sufficiently for these issues to be addressed more systematically.

Although the interpersonal impairments associated with PD differ widely across patients, three broad constellations of features are clinically important: (1) the emotional dependency constellation seen in DSM-5 BPD and related PDs largely consists of insecure attachment, submissiveness–dependency, and interpersonal fearfulness; (2) the dissocial/psychopathic constellation involves callousness, hostility and aggression, impulsivity and recklessness, disregard for social norms, and a tendency toward grandiosity; and (3) the socially avoidant constellation consists of restricted emotional expression and social avoidance. It is beyond the scope of this chapter to discuss the treatment of each constellation. However, the management of these constellations uses four general strategies that are described briefly to illustrate the coordinated use of an eclectic set of interventions: (1) psychoeducation about schemas and interpersonal problems; (2) a general framework for restructuring maladaptive interpersonal schemas and associated behavior patterns; (3) the application of this approach to treating maladaptive patterns; and (4) the construction of more adaptive interpersonal narratives.

## Psychoeducation

Earlier discussion of the framework for conceptualizing PD that underpins IMT noted that an integrative feature of current therapies is the assumption that personality schemas are important building blocks of personality. Hence, as with other therapies, a large component of IMT involves restructuring schemas. Schemas were encountered earlier when discussing ways to increase emotional regulation when it was suggested that attention be given to changing schemas that escalate distress. However, schema restructuring only really comes to the fore during the exploration and change phase, when considerable time is devoted to changing maladaptive interpersonal and self-schemas. Hence, it is useful to provide patients with information about the nature of schemas and how they function. If this information was not already provided, then it should be discussed earlier in the current phase.

Patients need to understand that a "schema" is a set of beliefs, ideas, feelings, and memories linked by a common theme, and although people may not be aware of their schemas, schemas have a strong influence on their thoughts, feelings, and actions. They also need to understand that schemas are stable and self-perpetuating because people tend to notice things that are consistent with their beliefs and ignore things that are not, and they tend to act in ways that cause others respond in ways that confirm their beliefs. Thus, individuals who believe that people cannot be trusted react to interpersonal situations with caution and suspicion, causing others to be wary, which then confirms the initial belief that people are untrustworthy. Patients also need to understand how schemas are also perpetuated by avoiding actions and situations that may lead to experiences that are inconsistent with the schema. As a result, schema-based fears are rarely tested. This is common with individuals whose fear of social embarrassment causes them to avoid social interactions, so that they do not have the opportunity to learn that this rarely happens, and that if it does, it can be managed.

## General Approach to Treating Maladaptive Schemas and Behavior Patterns

Since this phase of treatment focuses on restructuring maladaptive schemas and behavior patterns, it is useful for therapists to have a general model for treating them. This is provided by modifying Prochaska and DiClemente's naturalistic description of the way addictive behaviors change (DiClemente, 1994; Prochaska, & DiClemente, 1983; Prochaska, DiClemente, & Norcross, 1992; Prochaska, Norcross, & DiClemente, 1994). They described a six-stage process: (1) *Precontemplation,* in which there is no clearly defined intention to change; (2) *Contemplation,* which emerges when the person becomes aware of a problem and begins to contemplate about dealing with it; (3) *Preparation,* which combines the decision to change with actual steps that lead to action; (4) *Action,* which involves serious efforts to change; (5) *Maintenance,* in which gains are consolidated; and (6) *Termination,* which occurs when change is well established, without fear of relapse. This model brings order to the change process because each stage involves a set of tasks that need to be accomplished before treatment can proceed to the next stage. For example, during the first stage of problem recognition, the patient's task is to describe and acknowledge problems and commit to change, whereas the therapist's task is to help the patient to feel sufficiently secure to recognize problems. This structure is useful when planning how to help patients change a maladaptive schema such as rejection sensitivity or a behavioral pattern such social avoidance. However, with PD, the model may be simplified to a four-stage process: problem recognition, exploration, acquisition of alternatives, and generalization and maintenance.

### STAGE 1: RECOGNITION AND COMMITMENT TO CHANGE

This stage involves identifying a problematic schema or pattern and affirming a commitment to change. This step is needed because patients are often unaware of their schemas and habitual patterns, and even when these features are recognized, patients do not always see the need to change them. Recognition involves first drawing the patient's attention to a particular problem such as rejection sensitivity, then encouraging the patient to identify the different ways the schema or behavior is expressed. This process combines the traditional emphasis of psychodynamic methods on recognizing broad patterns of relating to others with CBT's emphasis on behavioral analysis to identify specific actions and the factors that reinforce them. The recognition process usually leads naturally to establishing a commitment to change, although sometimes this may involve a lengthy discussion of the costs and benefits of continuing to act in this way as opposed to changing.

## STAGE 2: EXPLORATION

Schema or pattern exploration involves identifying the different ways it is expressed and how it influences experience and action. This process increases self-knowledge and patients begin to integrate diverse feelings, cognitions, and behaviors into a common theme that enables them to recognize patterns to their behavior and experiences that they may not have recognized. Thus, concerns about losing a parent, worrying intensely if one's spouse is a little late returning from work, worries about a romantic partner leaving, or an urgent need to be with a significant other when something goes wrong are all part of the attachment insecurity that links these experiences. This process also helps patients to recognize that many of their actions arise from inner beliefs and not from the actions of others. This is an important step in initiating change. As Critchfield and Benjamin (2006) noted, linking schemas to the symptoms and problems that caused the patient to seek treatment is a crucial part of the change process.

Exploration also promotes recognition of the links among different schemas. Schemas are organized into clusters, so that the arousal of one schema tends to arouse others in the same cluster. In order to change interpersonal behavior, patients need to be able to recognize and track the flow of schema arousal and the impact of schemas on emotions and actions, much as they learned to track emotional arousal. For example, an event that activates the schema that a romantic partner may leave may then activate the schema "he or she does not care about me," and hence the schema "he or she does not love me," and ultimately the higher-order schema "I am unlovable." Exploring schemas and patterns in this way inevitably leads to a discussion of their developmental origins. Although IMT assumes that change is primarily achieved by modifying maladaptive processes as they occur in the present rather than through insight into their developmental origins, many patients need to understand why these problems developed. This often is useful because it provides a perspective on problems that helps patients to make sense of their lives. Later we will see how this helps them to construct a more adaptive narrative. Finally, an important part of exploration is to help patients to understand the processes that help to maintain and reinforce maladaptive schemas and patterns.

## STAGE 3: SCHEMA AND PATTERN CHANGE

The process of restructuring schemas, modifying interpersonal patterns, generating alternative responses, and acquiring new behaviors often takes time because the understanding generated by exploration does not automatically lead to change. Hence, during this process, therapists need to monitor motivation closely and intervene promptly when motivation declines or frustration mounts. Therapists often need to be flexible in how they manage any difficulties the patient may have in implementing change (Critchfield & Benjamin, 2006).

Many of the interventions used during this phase are based on the various cognitive, behavioral, emotional, and interpersonal methods traditionally used by the cognitive therapies, supplemented by interpersonal and narrative interventions. Extensive use is also made of the treatment relationship as a vehicle for examining and changing maladaptive schemas in a way that is similar to psychodynamic therapy.

*Cognitive Strategies.* Although, as noted, the standard cognitive interventions that are the cornerstone of traditional CBT are generally considered to be less effective when treating PD compared to other disorders (Bernstein & Clercx, Chapter 31, this volume; Davidson, 2008; Layden et al., 1993; Rafaeli, Bernstein, & Young, 2011). Nevertheless, interventions such as disputing dysfunctional thoughts, examining the evidence supporting a belief, and promoting greater flexibility in schema usage are three simple techniques that patients find useful and readily adopt.

*Behavioral Strategies.* As with cognitive methods, behavioral interventions seem to work best if they are relatively simple, especially early in therapy. When schemas are maintained through behavioral avoidance, it is often helpful use gradual exposure to avoided situations to test the validity of fears and negative expectations. For example, avoidant individuals who avoid social interactions due to a fear of ridicule may be encouraged to talk to another person for a few moments in a no-risk situation and note how the other person responds. Over time, the range of situations may be extended and the duration of conversation increased. Or dependent–submissive individuals who feel the need to always agree to another person's suggestions or requests lest the person get angry can be encouraged to say "no" occasionally and note the effect this has on other people and feelings about the self. This requires patients to act against the schema-based rules, hence testing the validity of their assumptions. Other schemas are maintained by the patient acting in ways that elicit confirming responses from others. For example, fear of rejection often causes individuals to be cautious and hold back in relationships, which increases the probability of the other person acting in a rejecting way. In many instances, it is important to reduce anxiety about trying out new behaviors by rehearsing the behavior in therapy, by role playing or rehearsing in imagination, or by helping the patient find an appropriate way to say something.

*Interpersonal Strategies.* At this point in therapy, the therapeutic relationship provides a major vehicle for changing core schemas and maladaptive interpersonal patterns (Bernstein & Clercx, Chapter 31, this volume; Young et al., 2003). The general treatment modules of IMT incorporate this change mechanism by creating a collaborative, consistent, and validating treatment process that continuously challenges and restructures core schemas and ways of relating related to distrust, abandonment and rejection, neglect, defectiveness, cooperation/control, predictability, and reliability schemas, and by focusing on building motivation and competency, which help to modulate passivity, lack of self-efficacy, and powerlessness. In addition, core schemas and interpersonal patterns are invariably enacted in the context of the treatment relationship, where they can be explored and restructured. Although this work began in the earlier phases of treatment, it assumes a more consistent focus during this phase, and the work proceeds at greater depth because exploration of interpersonal problems leads to more frequent activation of core schemas in context of the treatment relationship.

*Emotional Strategies.* Although some forms of cognitive therapy seek to change schemas using emotional methods such as role playing and psychodrama, they are not used extensively in IMT because intense emotional arousal is potentially destabilizing, especially with severe forms of PD. If used at all, they are confined to later phases of treatment. Nevertheless, work on interpersonal problems inevitably evokes intense feelings that need to be addressed. Initially, the focus is on containing emotional intensity evoked by these schemas and memories of painful events. Later, as emotional control increases and resilience improves, a graduated approach is used, with the therapist managing the intensity of emotional arousal so that the patient is not overwhelmed. The goal is not to encourage intense cathartic reactions but rather to help the patient to assess and express painful feelings in tolerable doses to drain some of the intensity of emotions attached to core schemas while maintaining emotion regulation. Often all that this requires is a straightforward psychodynamic approach that focuses attention on the feelings associated with schema arousal and the memories evoked, and deals with any avoidant or defensive behavior evoked by painful memories.

## STAGE 4: CONSOLIDATION AND GENERALIZATION

The final stage in changing a specific schema or behavior pattern is to ensure that changes are consolidated and generalized to everyday situations. This requires persistent encouragement to apply what was learned in treatment to specific events in everyday life and a review of the experience. Successful implementation of change often requires changes in the patient's current situation when this threatens to impede progress. Also, patients are often reluctant to implement changes when these threaten to disrupt relationships with significant others. Therapists often need to be flexible in how they manage these situations. Sometimes, conjoint sessions with significant others are needed to help them to accommodate changes in the patient's behavior. On other occasions, patients need help in managing their social relationships more effectively, which may involve learning new skills or learning how to adjust their interactions with others. With other patients, it may be necessary to encourage more radical changes to the social environment when ongoing social relationships actually help to perpetuate problems.

### Treating Maladaptive Traits

Since many maladaptive schemas and behavior patterns are linked to maladaptive traits, change often requires some modification of these traits. However, traits are heritable entities that are relatively stable once formed due to the way they are constructed, and they are reinforced by the repetitive interplay of genetic and environmental influences. Since radical changes in basic traits are difficult to achieve, it may be more productive to help patients to modulate the way their basic traits are expressed by helping them to accept and tolerate their basic personality attributes in much the same way that they were helped to tolerate their emotions. This is a useful strategy with patients who are self-critical and blame themselves for having certain qualities. This often allows patients to reflect on their qualities and find more adaptive ways to express them.

Traits can be modified in terms of the frequency and intensity with which they are expressed. With many patients, the problem is not necessarily the traits themselves but rather their rigidity or the way they are expressed. An obvious example is compulsivity. Even relatively high levels of this trait can be adaptive in situations where attention to detail, conscientiousness, or orderliness is helpful. Problems only arise when compulsivity is expressed in a rigid and inflexible way. This strategy is most effective with emotional traits such as anxiousness and emotional lability, which can be regulated by teaching the patient appropriate skills, such as stress management. However, it can also be used with other traits by helping patients to change the way they perceive and interpret situations, so that fewer situations are considered relevant to the trait. Earlier, the value of helping patients to become more discriminating in how situations are interpreted was discussed, as a way to modulate schemas. This can also be used to modulate trait expression. For example, highly submissive, "people-pleasing" individuals can be helped to interpret some requests by others as unreasonable or inconvenient. They can also be taught assertiveness skills as a way to modulate these tendencies.

Patients may be helped to find more adaptive ways to express their basic dispositions. For example, some patients with DSM-5 BPD or ASPD are highly sensation-seeking individuals who use a variety of ways to meet their needs for stimulation, such as substance abuse, somewhat deviant lifestyles, or even precipitating crises in their relationships with significant others. However, more healthy individuals with the same need for stimulation may meet this need in more adaptive ways, such as an active lifestyle, constructive risk taking in the work situation, participation in stimulating sporting activities, and so on. Hence, those who express this trait in maladaptive ways may often be helped to shift to more adaptive ways to satisfy these needs.

### Constructing More Adaptive Interpersonal Narratives

As I discussed when considering emotion regulation, the higher-order meaning systems and narratives that people construct play an important part in regulating and integrating different aspects of personality functioning. The mental health field tends to neglect narrative, and most specialized therapies for PD make little mention of the topic, although narratives are an important part of normal personality study (McAdams, 1994; McAdams & Pals, 2006) and narrative methods in psychotherapy are gaining recognition (Angus & McLeod, 2004). Narratives make an important contribution to coherent personality functioning by providing an integrated perspective of past, present, and future. Narratives about interpersonal experiences also help to integrate these experiences and modulate their impact on current relationships. Hence, an important part of the later phases of therapy is the construction of more adaptive narratives, an issue that is considered later when discussing the construction of an adaptive self-narrative.

### Phase 5: Integration and Synthesis

The final phase of therapy focuses on the construction of a more integrated self-system. Systematic work on these issues probably occurs with relatively few patients, since most therapies terminate once emotion regulation improves and some initial work on interpersonal problems is completed. Nevertheless, this phase is important if patients are to be helped to live more satisfying lives because the evidence suggests that even after successful treatment, many patients still have serious problems with social adjustment. This phase of therapy differs from earlier phases: It is less concerned with analyzing and restructuring already existing behaviors and schemas and more concerned with synthesizing a new self-structure. This is achieved in three main ways: (1) integrating different self-representations; (2) constructing a more adaptive life script or narrative; and (3) creating a personal niche that permits a more satisfying way of living.

### Integrating Different Self-Representations

A common feature of PD is a fragmented and unstable self-structure. With PD, connections within the self-referential knowledge that forms the basis for an emerging self do not develop as they do in healthy individuals, leaving a set of disjointed self-representations. This is most clearly observed in BPD and related pathology. In the more severe forms, patients experience distinct self-states, each involving a specific cluster of thoughts, feelings, and interpersonal behavior. An important task for this phase of treatment is to integrate and reconcile these different self-states by exploring these states as they emerge in therapy and the therapeutic narrative, and helping patients to recognize their different self-states and identify both the factors that lead to a switch from one state to another and any factors that are common to these states.

### Promoting a Coherent Self-Narrative

At different points in therapy, patients are helped to construct new narratives about their experiences, emotions, and relationships. Now, the task is to combine these narratives into a more global self-narrative that is integrated with other aspects of personality functioning. This is not achieved in a structured or formal way; rather, it occurs in a more opportunistic manner as events occur inside and outside therapy that create an opportunity to draw things together in narrative form. Such opportunities are more readily recognized if the therapist keeps in mind the task of developing a new narrative and has a broad conception of the structure and function of effective narratives. Self-narratives organize experiences into a global account of a person's life that explains who the person is and how he or she came to be this way, by building connections among life experiences, personality features, and behavior, and showing how they are related across time (Livesley, 2017). The narrative adds to the sense of integration and personal unity that is an inherent feature of adaptive personality functioning. Effective self-narratives incorporate scripts that make knowledge about events and situations accessible the patient in managing the problems of everyday living. They also help to regulate emotions and behavior, and are essential to the establishment and attainment of long-term goals. Most self-narratives also include a vision for the future—a sense of the person the patient would like to be—that adds to the patient's sense of personal unity by extending the self into the future.

#### REMINISCING ABOUT THERAPY

During this phase of treatment, considerable time is spent reviewing therapy in order to consolidate changes to ensure that they are generalized to everyday life. Reminiscing about therapy deepens the therapeutic relationship and promotes the trust needed to develop a new self-view and way of living. Reminiscing also activates the storytelling mode that makes people more expansive and open to new ideas and alternative constructions. As events in therapy are reviewed, opportunities arise to connect events across time and highlight changes that contribute to a new sense of self. Throughout therapy, narratives were constructed about specific problems and impairments, a process that began with the case formulation, which represents the therapist's initial understanding of the patient's life and disorder. This understanding formed the first step toward constructing a new self-narrative. As treatment proceeded, new narratives were constructed to help patients understand their crises, emotional experiences, and interpersonal problems. As these narratives are recalled, they can be combined into a more coherent self-narrative that integrates the understanding gained in treatment into a global, autobiographical sense of self.

#### PROVIDING SUMMARIES

Narrative construction can sometimes be facilitated by the therapist offering summary statements that draw things together, offering a broad perspective on a set of problems or events. The idea is not to provide patients with a tailor-made sense of identity but rather to draw together material discussed in therapy in a way that offers them a different perspective that can trigger further exploration and discussion. Used judiciously, this intervention can be effective when patients are struggling or feel stuck. To be effective, the summary has to be presented as a stimulus for discussion and as something for patients to think about and change, so that it feels authentic.

#### ENCOURAGING ACTION THAT CONSOLIDATES SELF-DEVELOPMENT

The behavioral experiments used in CBT to test existing or alternative beliefs may also be used to foster self-development and narrative construction. For example, one patient who was working on the narrative of her future self—the kind of life she would like to have—encountered difficulty because she was convinced that she was too incompetent to realize her ambitions, especially as they related to her career. She held this belief despite making substantial changes, which included successfully completing higher-level education and being successful in a demanding job. She was particularly concerned about having to make presentations to her colleagues because she feared that they would think her incompetent. She eventually agreed to a behavioral experiment that involved making a brief presentation to a few immediate colleagues. After rehearsing the presentation several times, she felt comfortable enough to proceed. To her surprise, it went well. Besides using the success to begin restructuring the incompetency schema, she also used the event to begin constructing a new self-narrative that included her hopes for the future and the realization that she did not need to be so cautious and fearful in her dealings with work colleagues.

## INCORPORATING CHANGES INTO SELF-NARRATIVES

The previous example also illustrates the importance of ensuring that the changes made in therapy are actually incorporated into a new self-narrative. The patient in question had made extensive changes that transformed her from consistently being in a decompensated crisis state and unable to work to coping well with a demanding career. However, these changes had little impact on her core belief that she was incompetent and less capable that all her peers. Even with successes like the one described, it took considerable therapeutic effort to ensure that they were incorporated into her sense of self.

### Getting a Life, Constructing a Personal Niche

Patients with PD tend to live restricted lives that offer few opportunities for satisfaction and personal growth. Successful treatment involves helping them to "get a life" that is worth living. This requires not only changes in how patients act and think about themselves but also support in constructing an environment that supports their progress and provides sources of fulfillment and opportunities for self-expression. The idea of helping patients to construct a rewarding environment is neglected by many therapies because the environment is usually assumed to be something separate from the person. However, healthy individuals actively create a congenial personal niche (Willi, 1999) by selecting situations and individuals to create a social world that meets their needs, abilities, talents, and aspirations. Patients rarely manage to do this. Rather than constructing satisfying niches, they occupy worlds that maintain their problems and offer little by way of satisfaction. Rather than constructing niches that offer opportunities for self-expression, they continually struggle to mold themselves to the perceived expectations of others. However, niche construction is important: A long-term follow up of untreated patients found that those who did well had managed to establish a niche that provided security and a sense of identity (Paris, 2003).

Helping patients to create a personal niche begins with helping them to recognize the need to get a life—something that most intuitively understand—and that an alternative lifestyle is an option. It then requires the therapist to recognize opportunities that enable the patient to build a new life. Some of the more general things that therapists can also do to encourage niche construction are to promote activity, encourage the pursuit of interests, and encourage engagement with the community.

Activity is important for niche construction: The more active patients are, the greater their chances of encountering situations and activities that are interesting and rewarding. Early in therapy, activity is encouraged to introduce structure into everyday routines. Later, activity is encouraged to challenge maladaptive schemas and try out new ways of behaving. Inevitably, increased activity makes patients more engaged with their world, which creates opportunities for self-development. Therapists need to be alert to these opportunities and encourage patients to pursue them. Therapists should be especially alert to any expression of interest because this provides an inroad to new behaviors and the development of a new social life. It does not matter what the interest is, it is the pursuit of an interest that matters because it promotes positive feelings and increases activity, which creates further opportunities for niche development. For example, one patient in her mid-40s, who had made good progress in managing her emotions, noted spontaneously that she had always been interested in embroidery and quilting but had never had the opportunity. With the therapist's encouragement, she joined a neighborhood group. The group went for coffee after the meeting, so she rapidly built a small social circle. The group meet regularly in a community center, and the patient became interested in other community activities; her social circle increased further, so that she felt less isolated.

The example illustrates how a chance event—the casual mention of an interest—led to a chain of events that helped the patient to begin constructing a new niche.

Since the social life of most patients shrinks, an important aspect of recovery involves helping patients to rebuild social networks. Social networks are important because they create a sense of belonging and a connection to one's world that contributes to the sense of stability that is an important part of identity. It is interesting how often patients who are beginning to feel better comment about the need to be more involved in their community, and how many volunteer with agencies such as local foodbanks. These seem to be healthy developments that signify a more outward-looking attitude and the emergence of feelings of communion with the world.

## Concluding Comments

The intent behind this chapter is not to develop another form of therapy to be evaluated in a randomized controlled trial but rather to present a framework for conceptualizing and delivering integrated therapy that uses all effective treatment methods. At the same time, the framework is designed to be sufficiently flexible to accommodate new methods that have been shown to be effective. Hence, the intervention component of IMT may be expected to evolve as new evidence emerges. The specific treatment modules are likely to be the most variable component given growing recognition of the need for research on both the mechanisms of change and the interventions that are most effective in treating specific problems and impairments. The general treatment modules are likely to be modified more gradually as more effective ways are found to apply generic mechanisms to the treatment of PD.

## REFERENCES

American Psychiatric Association. (2013). *Diagnostic and statistical manual of mental disorders* (5th ed.). Arlington, VA: Author.

Angus, L., & McLeod, J. (2004). Toward an integrative framework for understanding the role of narrative in psychotherapy process. In L. E. Angus & J. McLeod (Eds.), *The handbook of narrative and psychotherapy: Practice, theory and research* (pp. 367–374). Thousand Oaks, CA: SAGE.

Barlow, D. H., Farchione, T. J., Fairholme, C. P., Ellard, K. K., Boieseau, C. L., Allan, L. B., et al. (2011). *Unified protocol for transdiagnostic treatment of emotional disorders.* Oxford, UK: Oxford University Press.

Bateman, A., & Fonagy, P. (2004). *Psychotherapy for borderline personality disorder: Mentalization-based treatment.* Oxford, UK: Oxford University Press.

Baumeister, R. F. (1991). *Meanings of life.* New York: Guilford Press.

Baumeister, R. F. (1994). The crystallization of discontent in the process of major life change. In T. F. Heatherton & J. L. Weinberger (Eds.), *Can personality change?* (pp. 281–297). Washington, DC: American Psychological Association.

Beck, A. T., Davis, D. D., & Freeman, A. (2015). *Cognitive therapy of personality disorders* (3rd ed.). New York: Guilford Press.

Beutler, L. E. (1991). Have all won and must all have prizes?: Revisiting Luborsky et al.'s verdict. *Journal of Consulting and Clinical Psychology, 59,* 226–232.

Bowlby, J. (1980). *Attachment and loss: Sadness and depression.* London: Hogarth Press.

Crawford, M. J., Koldobsky, N., Mulder, R., & Tyrer, P. (2011). Classifying personality disorder according to severity. *Journal of Personality Disorders, 25,* 321–330.

Critchfield, K. L., & Benjamin, L. S. (2006). Integration of therapeutic factors in treating personality disorders. In L. G. Castonguay & L. E. Beutler (Eds.), *Principles of therapeutic change that work* (pp. 253–271). New York: Oxford University Press.

Davidson, K. (2008). *Cognitive therapy for personality disorders* (2nd ed.). New York: Routledge.

DiClemente, C. C. (1994). If behaviours change, can personality be far behind? In T. F. Heatherton & J. L. Weinberger (Eds.), *Can personality change?* (pp. 175–198). Washington, DC: American Psychological Association.

Dimaggio, G., Popolo, R., Carcione, A., & Salvatore, G. (2015). Improving metacognition by accessing autobiographical memories. In W. J. Livesley, W. G. Dimaggio, & J. F. Clarkin (Eds.), *Integrated treatment for personality disorder: A modular approach* (pp. 173–193). New York: Guilford Press.

Dimaggio, G., Salvatore, G., Fiore, D., Carcione, A., Nicolò, G., & Semerari, A. (2012). General principles for treating the over-constricted personality disorder: Toward operationalizing technique. *Journal of Personality Disorders, 26,* 63–83.

Dimaggio, G., Semerari, A., Carcione, A., Nicolò, G., & Procacci, M. (2007). *Psychotherapy of personality disorders: Metacognition, states of mind, and interpersonal cycles.* London: Routledge.

Eells, T. D. (2010). History and current status of case formulation. In T. D. Eells (Ed.), *Handbook of psychotherapy case formulation* (2nd ed., pp. 3–32). New York: Guilford Press.

Fonagy, P., Gergely, G., Jurist, E. L., & Target, M.

(2002). *Affect regulation, mentalization, and the development of the self.* New York: Other Press.

Gold, J. R. (1996). *Key concepts in psychotherapy integration.* New York: Plenum Press.

Gross, J. J., & Thompson, R. A. (2007). Emotional regulation: Conceptual foundations. In J. J. Gross (Ed.), *Handbook of emotion regulation* (pp. 3–24). New York: Guilford Press.

Hayes, S. C., Strosahl, K. D., & Wilson, K. G. (1999). *Acceptance and commitment therapy: An experiential approach to behavioral change.* New York: Guilford Press.

Holt, R. R. (1989). *Freud reappraised: A fresh look at psychoanalytic theory.* New York: Guilford Press.

Horowitz, M. J. (1998). *Cognitive psychodynamics.* New York: Wiley.

Horvath, A. O., & Greenberg, L. S. (Eds.). (1994). *The working alliance.* New York: Wiley.

Joseph, B. (1983). On understanding and not understanding: Some technical issues. *International Journal of Psychoanalysis, 64,* 291–298.

Kabat-Zinn, J. (2005a). *Coming to our senses: Healing ourselves and the world through mindfulness.* New York: Hyperion.

Kabat-Zinn, J. (2005b). *Full catastrophe living: Using the wisdom of your body and mind to face stress, pain, and illness* (15th anniversary ed.). New York: Delta Trade Paperback/Bantam Dell.

Kohut, H. (1971). *The analysis of the self.* New York: International Universities Press.

Lambert, M. J. (1992). Psychotherapy outcome research: Implications for integrative and electical therapists. In J. C. Norcross & M. R. Goldfried (Eds.), *Handbook of psychotherapy integration* (pp. 94–129). New York: Basic Books.

Lambert, M. J., & Bergen, A. E. (1994). The effectiveness of psychotherapy. In A. E. Bergin & S. L. Garfield (Eds.), *Handbook of psychotherapy and behavior change* (4th ed., pp. 143–189). New York: Wiley.

Layden, M. A., Newman, C. F., Freeman, A., & Morse, S. B. (1993). *Cognitive therapy of borderline personality disorder.* Needham Heights, MA: Allyn & Bacon.

Lenzenweger, M. F., Clarkin, J. F., Fertuck, E. A., & Kernberg, O. F. (2004). Executive neurocognitive functioning and neurobehavioral systems indicators in borderline personality disorder: A preliminary study. *Journal of Personality Disorders, 18,* 421–438.

Linehan, M. M. (1993). *Cognitive-behavioral treatment of borderline personality disorder.* New York: Guilford Press.

Linehan, M. M., Davison, G. C., Lynch, T. R., & Sanderson, C. (2006). Techniques factors in treating personality disorders. In L. G. Castonguay & L. E. Beutler (Eds.), *Principles of therapeutic change that work* (pp. 239–252). New York: Oxford University Press.

Links, P. S., & Bergmans, Y. (2015). Managing suicidal and other crises. In W. J. Livesley, G. Dimaggio, & J. F. Clarkin (Eds.), *Integrated treatment for personality disorder: A modular approach* (pp. 197–210). New York: Guilford Press.

Livesley, W. J. (1998). Suggestions for a framework for an empirically based classification of personality disorder. *Canadian Journal of Psychiatry, 43*(2), 137–147.

Livesley, W. J. (2001). A framework for an integrated approach to treatment. In W. J. Livesley (Ed.), *Handbook of personality disorders: Theory, research, and treatment* (pp. 570–600). New York: Guilford Press.

Livesley, W. J. (2003a). Diagnostic dilemmas in the classification of personality disorder. In K. Phillips, M. First, & H. A. Pincus (Eds.), *Advancing DSM: Dilemmas in psychiatric diagnosis* (pp. 153–189). Arlington, VA: American Psychiatric Association Press.

Livesley, W. J. (2003b). *Practical management of personality disorder.* New York: Guilford Press.

Livesley, W. J. (2007). Integrated therapy for complex cases of personality disorder. *Journal of Clinical Psychology, 64,* 207–221.

Livesley, W. J. (2012). Moving beyond specialized therapies for borderline personality disorder: The importance of integrated domain-focused treatment. *Psychodynamic Psychiatry, 40*(1), 47–74.

Livesley, W. J. (2017). *Integrated modular treatment for borderline personality disorder.* Cambridge, UK: Cambridge University Press.

Livesley, W. J., & Clarkin, J. F. (2015a). Diagnosis and assessment. In W. J. Livesley, G. Dimaggio, & J. F. Clarkin (Eds.), *Integrated treatment for personality disorder: A modular approach* (pp. 51–79). New York: Guilford Press.

Livesley, W. J., & Clarkin, J. F. (2015b). A general framework for integrated modular treatment. In W. J. Livesley, G. Dimaggio, & J. F. Clarkin (Eds.), *Integrated treatment for personality disorder: A modular approach* (pp. 19–47). New York: Guilford Press.

Livesley, W. J., Dimaggio, G., & Clarkin, J. F. (2015). *Integrated treatment for personality disorder: A modular approach.* New York: Guilford Press.

Livesley, W. J., Schroeder, M. L., Jackson, D. N., & Jang, K. L. (1994). Categorical distinctions in the study of personality disorder: Implications for classification. *Journal of Abnormal Psychology, 103,* 6–17.

Luborsky, L. (1984). *Principles of psychoanalytic psychotherapy.* New York: Basic Books.

Luborsky, L. (1994). Therapeutic alliances as predictors of psychotherapy outcomes: Factors explaining the predictive success. In A. O. Horvath & L. S. Greenberg (Eds.), *The working alliance* (pp. 38–50). New York: Wiley.

Luborsky, L., Singer, B., & Luborsky, L. (1975). Comparative studies of psychotherapies. *Archives of General Psychiatry, 32,* 995–1008.

McAdams, D. P. (1994). Can personality change?: Levels of stability and growth in personality across the life span. In T. F. Heatherton & J. L. Weinberger

(Eds.), *Can personality change?* (pp. 299–313). Washington, DC: American Psychological Association Press.

McAdams, D. P., & Pals, J. L. (2006). A new Big Five: Fundamental principles for an integrative science of personality. *American Psychologist, 61,* 204–217.

Miller, W. R., & Rollnick, S. (2002). *Motivational interviewing: Preparing people for change* (2nd ed.). New York: Guilford Press.

Miller, W. R., & Rollnick, S. (2013). *Motivational interviewing: Helping people change* (3rd ed.). New York: Guilford Press.

Mischel, W., & Shoda, Y. (1995). A cognitive-affective system theory of personality: Reconceptualizing situations, dispositions, dynamics, and invariance in personality structure. *Psychological Review, 102,* 246–268.

Nolen-Hoeksema, S. (2012). Emotion regulation and psychopathology: The role of gender. *Annual Review of Clinical Psychology, 6,* 161–187.

Norcross, J. C., & Newman, J. C. (1992). Psychotherapy integration: Setting the context. In J. C. Norcross & M. R. Goldfried (Eds.), *Handbook of psychotherapy integration* (pp. 3–45). New York: Basic Books.

Ottavi, P., Passarella, T., Pasinetti, M., Salvatore, G., & Dimaggio, G. (2015). Adapting mindfulness for treating personality disorder. In W. J. Livesley, G. Dimaggio, & J. F. Clarkin (Eds.), *Integrated treatment for personality disorder: A modular approach* (pp. 282–302). New York: Guilford Press.

Paris, J. (2003). *Personality disorders over time.* Washington, DC: American Psychiatric Publishing.

Prochaska, J. O., & DiClemente, C. C. (1983). Stages and processes of self-change of smoking. *Journal of Consulting and Clinical Psychology, 51,* 390–395.

Prochaska, J. O., DiClemente, C. C., & Norcross, J. C. (1992). In search of how people change. *American Psychologist, 47,* 1102–1114.

Prochaska, J. O., Norcross, J. C., & DiClemente, C. C. (1994). *Changing for good: The revolutionary program that explains the six stages of change and teaches you how to free yourself from bad habits.* New York: Morrow.

Rafaeli, E., Bernstein, D. P., & Young, J. (2011). *Schema therapy: Distinctive features.* New York: Routledge.

Ricoeur, P. (1981). The narrative function. In P. Ricoeur (Ed.), *Hermeneutics and the human sciences* (J. B. Thompson, Ed., & Trans.) (pp. 165–181). Cambridge, UK: Cambridge University Press.

Rosengren, D. B. (2009). *Building motivational interviewing skills: A practitioner workbook.* New York: Guilford Press.

Sadikaj, G., Russell, J. J., Moskowitz, D. S., & Paris, J. (2010). Affect dysregulation in individuals with borderline personality disorder: Persistence and interpersonal triggers. *Journal of Personality Assessment, 92*(6), 490–500.

Safran, J. D., Crocker, P., McMain, S., & Murray, P. (1990). Therapeutic alliance rupture as a therapy event for empirical investigation. *Psychotherapy, 27,* 154–165.

Safran, J. D., Muran, J. C., & Samstag, L. N. (1994). Resolving therapeutic alliance ruptures: A task analytic investigation. In A. O. Horvath & L. S. Greenberg (Eds.), *The working alliance: Theory, research, and practice* (pp. 225–255). New York: Wiley.

Stanghellini, G., & Rosfort, R. (2013). *Emotions and personhood.* Oxford, UK: Oxford University Press.

Steiner, J. (1994). Patient-centered and analyst-centered interpretations: Some implications of containment and countertransference. *Psychoanalytic Quarterly, 14,* 406–422.

Stepp, S. D., Pilkonis, P. A., Yaggi, K. E., Morse, J. Q., & Feske, U. (2009). Interpersonal and emotional experiences of social interactions in borderline personality disorder *Journal of Nervous and Mental Disease, 197,* 484–491.

Stricker, G. (2010). A second look at psychotherapy integration. *Journal of Psychotherapy Integration, 20,* 397–405.

Tickle, J. J., Heatherton, T. F., & Wittenberg, L. G. (2001). Can personality change? In W. J. Livesley (Ed.), *Handbook of personality disorders: Theory, research, and treatment* (pp. 242–258). New York: Guilford Press.

Toulmin, S. (1978). Self-knowledge and knowledge of the "self." In T. Mischel (Ed.), *The self: Psychological and philosophical issues* (pp. 291–317). Oxford, UK: Oxford University Press.

Tufecioglu, S., & Muran, J. C. (2015). A relational approach to personality disorder and alliance rupture. In W. J. Livesley, G. Dimaggio, & J. F. Clarkin (Eds.), *Integrated treatment for personality disorder: A modular approach* (pp. 123–147). New York: Guilford Press.

Tyrer, P., Crawford, M., Mulder, R., Blashfield, R., Farnam, A., Fossati, A., et al. (2011). The rationale for the reclassification of personality disorder in the 11th revision of the *International Classification of Diseases* (ICD-11). *Journal of Personality and Mental Health, 5,* 246–259.

Willi, J. (1999). *Ecological psychotherapy.* Seattle, WA: Hogrefe & Huber.

Wolpe, J. (1958). *Psychotherapy by reciprocal inhibition.* Stanford, CA: Stanford University Press.

Young, J. E., Klosko, J. S., & Weishaar, M. E. (2003). *Schema therapy: A practitioner's guide.* New York: Guilford Press.

# Author Index

Aaronson, C. J., 126
Abbass, A., 466
Abbass, A. A., 134
Abbot, E. S., 48
Abbott, R. D., 222
Abi-Dargham, A., 258
Ablow, J. C., 311
Abracen, J., 641
Abraham, K., 7
Achenbach, T. M., 78, 159, 349, 353
Ackerman, R. A., 345, 347
Ackerman, S. J., 412
Adahi, S. A., 513
Adams, G. R., 115
Adityanjee, A., 613
Adler, J. M., 115, 130
Afifi, T. O., 129
Agam, G., 244
Aggen, S. H., 241, 429
Agosti, V., 463
Agras, W. S., 463, 539
Agrawal, H. R., 126
Ahn, H., 134
Ainsworth, M., 514
Aitken, K. J., 492
Ajchenbrenner, M., 127
Ajdacic-Gross, V., 129
Akhtar, S., 108, 113, 115, 116, 118
Akiskal, H., 420
Akiskal, H. S., 420, 613
Aksan, N., 330, 434
Albert, U., 461, 463
Aldea, M. A., 469
Alexander, J., 77
Alexander, M. S., 7, 192
Alexander, R., 18
Alimohamed, S., 378
Allen, J., 597
Allen, J. G., 126, 133, 542, 544, 545, 547, 558
Allen, J. J., 433

Allen, J. P., 319
Allen, J. S., 288
Allen, T. A., 233, 309, 316
Allik, J., 93
Allison, E., 133, 542
Allison, T., 630
Allmon, D., 483, 538, 586, 605
Allport, G. W., 37, 103, 374, 375
Alnaes, R., 461
Aluja, A., 77, 348
Alvares, G. A., 262
Amato, P. R., 302, 303
Amin, F., 258
Amirthavasagam, S., 246, 272
Anckarsater, H., 463
Anderluh, M., 470
Anderluh, M. B., 463
Andershed, H., 240, 327, 427, 428, 429, 448, 450, 452
Anderson, C. M., 600, 601
Anderson, J. L., 80, 81, 162, 353, 431
Anderson, S., 288
Andreasen, N. C., 11
Andrews, B. P., 427, 448
Andrews, D. A., 453, 454, 630, 631, 632, 637, 639, 640
Andrews, G., 242
Anglin, D. M., 576
Angus, L., 664, 670
Ansell, E., 459
Ansell, E. B., 211, 345, 373, 380, 461, 463, 467, 470, 471
Ansseau, M., 465
Antonowitz, D. H., 453, 454
Appelo, M., 586
Appelo, M. T., 586
Appels, C., 146, 291
Aragona, M., 4, 7
Arató, M., 256
Arens, E. A., 544
Aristotle, 271

Arkowitz-Westen, L., 368
Armbrust, M., 485
Armor, D. J., 468
Armstrong, A. G., 586
Armstrong, H. E., 483, 538, 586, 605
Arnau, R. C., 142
Arndt, S., 317
Arnett, J. J., 215
Arnett, P. A., 452
Arnott, B., 132
Arnsten, A. F. T., 259
Arntz, A., 101, 102, 104, 141, 142, 143, 144, 145, 146, 147, 148, 149, 150, 231, 291, 292, 294, 484, 555, 556, 557, 559, 561, 563, 567
Arsal, G., 427, 449, 450
Asberg, M., 252, 253, 256, 614, 615
Ashton, M. C., 40, 77, 80, 348, 349
Aspán, N., 286
Aston-Jones, G., 260
Atkinson, G., 348
Aubin, E., 110
Aucoin, K. J., 328
Auerbach, J. S., 130
Augustine, J. R., 272
Aycicegi, A., 94, 465
Aycicegi-Dinn, A., 148, 465
Ayearst, L., 80, 81, 353
Azzoni, A., 462

Baca-Garcia, E., 260
Bachelor, A., 387
Baer, B. A., 612
Baer, L., 467
Bagby, R. M., 57, 80, 81, 216, 346, 353, 437
Bagner, D. M., 324
Bahl, N., 286
Bailey, G. R., Jr., 466
Bailor-Jones, D. M., 19
Baird, A. A., 432
Baker, B. R., 260

# Author Index

Bakermans-Kranenburg, M. J., 143
Baldessarini, R. J., 261
Bales, D., 552
Balestrieri, M., 601
Baleydier, B., 95
Ball, S., 60
Ball, S. A., 142
Ballard, C. G., 261
Ballenger, J. C., 253
Balsis, S., 208, 210, 215, 231, 314, 467
Baltes, P., 199
Bamelis, L., 555, 556, 568
Bamelis, L. L., 561, 566
Bamelis, L. L. M., 143, 148, 484
Banducci, A. N., 158
Banerjee, G., 96
Banki, C. M., 256
Barbas, H., 273
Barber, J. P., 466, 470
Barch, D. M., 161
Barelds, D. P., 41
Bargh, J. A., 130
Bar-Haim, Y., 145
Barker, E. D., 330
Barkham, M., 343, 503, 506
Barlow, D. H., 661
Barnicot, K., 530
Barnow, S., 130, 146, 148
Baron, M., 175, 178, 180, 181, 182, 183, 184, 185
Barone, L., 126
Barratt, E. S., 616
Barrett, E., 338, 369, 374
Barry, C. T., 449
Bartak, A., 82, 483
Bartels, N., 587, 588
Bartels, N. E., 481, 586, 587
Bartko, J., 257
Bartolo, T., 331
Bartz, J., 263
Baruch, D. E., 128
Baskin-Sommers, A. R., 431, 432
Bastiaansen, L., 64, 216
Bateau, E., 602
Bateman, A., 110, 117, 123, 124, 125, 127, 133, 134, 380, 388, 422, 481, 483, 541, 542, 546, 547, 551, 555, 558, 568, 571, 572, 582, 587, 605, 655
Bateman, A. W., 123, 133, 223, 481, 541, 542, 543, 550
Bates, J. E., 132, 216, 316, 317
Batstra, L., 157
Battle, C. L., 464
Bauer, L. O., 434
Bauman, Z., 108
Baumeister, R. F., 103, 656
Bayles, K., 132
Bazanis, E., 284, 288, 289, 290
Beard, C., 149
Beard, H., 492, 504, 508
Beauchaine, T. P., 127, 420
Beauregard, M., 277, 278
Beblo, T., 276, 286, 287, 290
Bech, M., 294
Bechara, A., 288
Beck, A. T., 28, 51, 130, 142, 302, 377, 421, 466, 481, 482, 512, 513, 514, 515, 519, 520, 521, 556, 560, 571, 587, 617, 630, 637, 647
Beck, J. S., 466
Becker, C., 255, 256

Becker, D., 109
Becker, S. P., 325, 329
Beebe, B., 132
Beeghly, M., 128, 576
Beeken, S., 505
Beeney, J. E., 210
Beers, C., 48
Beevers, C. G., 148
Bègue, L., 255
Belin, D., 272
Bell, R., 255
Bellino, S., 617
Bellodi, L., 463
Belmaker, R. H., 244, 617
Belsky, D. W., 315, 317, 545, 577
Belsky, J., 132, 545
Bender, D. S., 58, 62, 64, 82, 126, 130, 350, 355, 465, 556, 575
Benecke, C., 114
Benish, S. G., 134
Benjamin, L. S., 28, 32, 204, 337-338, 339, 342, 343, 394, 395, 396, 397, 398, 399, 400, 401, 403, 405, 408, 409, 410, 411, 412, 413, 445, 484, 571, 601, 645, 653, 655, 668
Bennett, D., 490, 497, 500, 501, 502, 503, 505
Bennett, D. C., 325, 326, 328, 329, 497
Benning, S. D., 344, 428, 429, 430, 431, 433, 437, 446-447, 448, 449, 452
Benson, J., 262
Benson, K. T., 83
Berenbaum, H., 164
Berenson, K. R., 209
Berenz, E. C., 317
Berg, E. A., 286
Bergeman, C., 304
Bergen, A. E., 647
Bergeman, C., 304
Bergman, A., 117
Bergmans, Y., 659
Berk, M. S., 421
Berkson, J., 203
Berlin, H., 291
Berman, M. E., 255, 256
Berman, S., 465
Berman, S. L., 110
Bermudo-Soriano, C. R., 260
Bernat, E., 428, 429, 432
Bernat, E. M., 160, 428, 433, 447
Bernbach, E., 132
Bernstein, D., 143, 150
Bernstein, D. P., 60, 61, 73, 91, 143, 219, 221, 231, 357, 462, 482, 555, 556, 559, 563, 567, 568, 664, 668, 669
Bernstein, I. H., 209
Bernstein D. P., 614
Berridge, C. W., 259
Berrios, G. E., 5, 6, 89
Berrios, R., 492
Bertillon, J., 49
Bertilsson, L., 253, 256
Bertsch, K., 150, 263
Berzonsky, M. D., 115
Besser, A., 469
Betan, E., 116
Beurel, E., 262
Beutel, M. E., 277
Beutler, L. E., 367, 377, 378, 388, 484, 647
Bezirganian, S., 219

Bhui, K. S., 95
Bieling, P. J., 469
Bieri, K. A., 612
Birbaumer, N., 432, 433
Birgenheir, D. G., 143
Biven, L., 572
Bjork, J., 290
Bjork, J. M., 291
Black, D. W., 175, 179, 180, 181, 182, 183, 184, 185, 186, 192, 287, 481, 586, 591, 597
Blackburn, R., 452
Blagov, P. S., 329
Blagys, M. D., 412
Blair, J., 447
Blair, K., 447
Blair, K. S., 274
Blair, R. J., 328
Blair, R. J. R., 324, 325, 326, 328, 329, 431, 432, 434, 436
Blais, M. A., 412
Blake, C. A., 324
Blanchard, E. B., 175, 178, 181, 182, 183, 184, 185
Bland, R. C., 175, 182, 186, 190
Blankstein, K., 469
Blashfield, R. K., 8, 12, 13, 20, 48, 52, 53, 55, 59, 60, 63, 72, 156, 345
Blatt, S. J., 108, 117, 130, 131, 469
Blazer, D., 174
Bledowski, C., 273
Bleiberg, E., 542
Bleiberg, K. L., 542
Blennow, K., 257, 258
Blizard, R., 491
Block, J., 38, 338
Blonigen, D., 631
Blonigen, D. M., 344, 429, 433, 435, 437, 447, 448, 452
Bloo, J., 143
Bloom, C., 342
Blos, P., 117
Blud, L., 453
Bluhm, C., 109
Blum, N., 176, 179, 354, 481, 586, 591, 593, 594, 597
Blum, N. S., 481, 586, 587
Bo, S., 221
Boccaccini, M. T., 630
Boccalon, S., 586, 597
Bódi, N., 286
Bodin, S. D., 449
Bodlund, O., 461
Boergers, J., 469, 470
Bogenschutz, M. P., 614, 615
Bogetto, F., 461, 617
Bogg, T., 468
Boggs, C. D., 461
Bohleber, W., 108, 110
Bohman, M., 303
Bohus, M., 30, 158, 274, 527, 539
Bolton, D., 3, 4, 10, 11, 19
Bolton, R., 124
Bond, A. J., 255
Bond, M. H., 92
Bondi, C. M., 469
Bonelli, R. M., 273
Bongar, B., 378
Bonge, D. R., 412
Bonelli, R. M., 273
Bonta, J., 453, 630, 631, 632, 640
Boomsma, D. I., 239, 244

Booth, A., 302, 303
Booth-LaForce, C., 126
Bordin, E. S., 633
Borduin, C. M., 222, 638
Born, M. P., 80, 349
Bornovalova, M. A., 128, 315, 317, 544
Bornstein, R. F., 28, 30, 58, 59, 60, 61, 63, 66, 345, 369, 376
Borroni, S., 116
Bortolato, M., 255
Bortolitti, L., 4
Bos, E. H., 157, 586
Boschen, M. J., 60
Bouchard, T. J., Jr., 239, 242
Bouffard, L. A., 453
Bourne, H. R., 252
Bower, P., 503
Bowers, L., 634
Bowlby, J., 126, 330, 331, 400, 513, 514, 647
Bowler, J. L., 42
Bowler, M. C., 42
Bowles, D. P., 127
Boyd, J. H., 156, 157
Boyd, S., 53
Boyd, S. E., 341
Boyes, M., 492
Bozzatello, P., 617
Bradley, B., 129, 316
Bradley, B. P., 145, 292
Bradley, M. M., 432
Bradley, R., 59, 130
Brakoulias, V., 460
Brambilla, P., 274, 623
Brand, M., 289
Brandt, D., 199
Braun, C. M., 291
Breen, M., 59
Bremner, J. D., 274, 275
Brennan, J., 330, 331
Bretherton, I., 403
Brewer, M. B., 111, 117
Brightman, B. K., 601
Brill, H., 52
Brinded, P. M. J., 176
Brislin, S. J., 326, 332, 426, 431, 437, 445, 446
Britner, P. A., 132
Broadbent, K., 294
Broadbent, M., 492
Broks, P., 343
Bromberg, P. M., 113, 114
Brook, J. S., 107, 143, 219
Broome, M. R., 4
Brouwers, P., 284
Brown, E. C., 222
Brown, G., 557
Brown, G. K., 421
Brown, G. L., 253, 254, 257, 259
Brown, J. S., 464
Brown, L., 253, 254, 255, 257, 259
Brown, M. Z., 422
Browne, A., 304
Bruce, K. R., 470
Bruce, S., 253
Brunner, R., 231
Brunnlieb, C., 262
Bryk, A. S., 199
Bryson, S., 463
Buchanan, R. W., 286
Buchel, C., 272

Buchheim, A., 263, 276
Buckley, P. J., 376
Budge, S. L., 483
Budhani, S., 325
Bullinger, M., 612
Bunge, S. A., 277
Burgess, J., 597
Burgess, J. W., 284, 285
Burke, J. D., 219
Burkhardt, M., 285
Burkitt, I., 493
Burnam, M., 461
Burnett, L., 435
Burt, S. A., 332, 429
Burton, A., 148
Busch, A. J., 83
Bush, G., 273, 288
Bushnell, J. A., 176
Buss, A. H., 616
Busschbach, J. J., 221, 462
Busschbach, J. J. V., 352, 483
Bustamante, M. L., 290
Butcher, G., 465
Butti, G., 461
Byrd, A. L., 232

Cadoret, R. J., 317
Cahill, B. S., 342
Cahill, M. A., 453
Cain, N., 481, 571
Cain, N. M., 163, 345, 380, 461, 470, 571
Caldwell-Harris, C. L., 94, 148, 465
Caligor, E., 108, 110, 115, 130, 374, 379, 388, 571, 572, 575, 576, 579, 581
Callander, L., 469
Calliess, I. T., 91
Calvert, R., 490, 503, 504, 506, 507
Calvo, R., 464
Cameron, A. Y., 485
Camp, J., 450, 453, 631
Campbell, C., 481, 541
Campbell, J. S., 630
Campbell, L., 292
Campbell, W. K., 58, 60, 61, 147, 345
Camps, F. E., 252
Cannon, W., 271
Cantor-Graae, E., 95
Caperton, J., 630
Caplan, P. J., 54
Carcione, A., 110, 466, 571, 649, 664
Carcone, D., 284, 285, 286, 288
Cardish, R. J., 582
Cardon, L. R., 238, 241
Carey, G., 239
Carlson, E. A., 128, 318, 576
Carlson, E. N., 210, 345
Carlson, S. R., 429, 431, 433, 435
Carlson, V., 576
Carpenter, C., 284, 286
Carpenter, L. L., 129
Carr, A. C., 350
Carr, S. N., 142, 144
Carradice, A., 507
Carré, J. M., 264
Carson, D. S., 262
Carson, R., 403
Carter, C. S., 273
Carter, N., 463
Cartwright, N., 19
Carvalho, G. B., 271
Carver, C. S., 103, 374, 375

Casillas, A., 77, 342
Caspi, A., 159, 199, 217, 243, 244, 245, 302, 310, 311, 314, 316, 317, 318, 319, 358, 545
Cassidy, J., 302, 304, 397
Castonguay, L. G., 134, 378, 484, 503
Catalano, R. F., 222
Cath, D. C., 244
Cattell, R. B., 37, 39
Cauffman, E., 324, 328, 329
Cavedini, P., 463
Cecero, J. J., 142
Cecil, C. A., 327
Cellucci, T., 128, 144
Cervone, D., 374
Chakhssi, F., 143, 568
Chamberlain, S. R., 463
Champion, H., 631
Chan, F., 129, 330
Chan, Y., 606
Chanen, A., 231
Chanen, A. M., 6, 171, 206, 215, 216, 219, 220, 221, 222, 223, 231, 288, 423, 483, 492, 503, 504, 505, 544
Chang, L. Y., 305
Chapman, A., 128, 144
Chapman, A. L., 289, 465, 467
Chapman, G. L., 453
Chapman, J., 325
Chauncey, D., 73
Chauncey, D. L., 618
Chavez, J. X., 450
Chavira, D. A., 461
Cheavens, J. S., 467
Chelminski, I., 221, 342, 420, 461, 467
Chemerinski, E., 63
Chen, C., 93
Chen, H., 143, 219, 576
Chen, S. E., 420
Chen, S. W., 97
Chen, Y., 97
Chentsova-Dutton, Y. E., 159
Cheslow, D., 464
Chess, S., 434
Chin, E. D., 115, 130
Chinman, M., 606
Chipuer, H. M., 242
Chirkov, V., 96
Chittams, J., 466
Chmielewski, M., 75, 80, 81, 353
Cho, D. Y., 274
Choi-Kain, L. W., 127, 132, 260
Church, A. T., 41, 92
Churchill, W., 421
Ciano, R. P., 601
Cicchetti, D., 128, 192, 218, 223, 231, 301, 309, 310, 316, 542, 576
Cima, M., 143, 146, 147, 567
Cipriano-Essel, E., 401
Cjaza, C., 302
Claes, L., 471
Clancy, S. A., 293
Clare, A. W., 465
Claridge, G., 343
Clark, C. R., 260
Clark, D. B., 219
Clark, L. A., 10, 57, 59, 60, 61, 63, 65, 72, 75, 76, 77, 78, 80, 81, 82, 155, 156, 159, 160, 171, 188, 216, 220, 313, 314, 315, 337, 338, 341, 342, 343, 345, 346, 347, 352, 353, 354, 355, 356, 357, 358, 370, 373, 446, 459, 463, 469, 546

Clark, M. A., 469
Clark, M. S., 93
Clark Barrett, H., 127
Clarke, S., 483, 492, 504, 505, 506
Clarkin, J., 286
Clarkin, J. F., 3, 14, 16, 20, 21, 58, 63, 66, 74, 109, 114, 115, 116, 118, 130, 157, 198, 274, 338, 346, 367, 369, 372, 373, 376, 377, 378, 379, 381, 383, 386, 388, 481, 483, 538, 571, 572, 573, 575, 576, 577, 580, 581, 582, 583, 587, 605, 630, 645, 649, 652, 663
Cleare, A. J., 255
Cleckley, H., 5, 7, 63, 91, 324, 344, 426, 430, 431, 432, 445, 446, 447, 452, 629
Clercx, M., 482, 555, 664, 668, 669
Cloninger, C. R., 12, 72, 103, 243, 244, 251, 303, 348, 370, 373
Clum, G. A., 470
Coatsworth, J. D., 319
Coccaro, E., 259, 264
Coccaro, E. F., 231, 232, 245, 251, 253, 254, 255, 256, 257, 259, 261, 262, 264, 289, 611, 614, 615
Coffey, H. S., 32
Cohen, J., 176
Cohen, J. D., 260
Cohen, M. S., 192
Cohen, P., 107, 129, 143, 176, 199, 201, 202, 216, 218, 219, 221, 223, 231, 302, 315, 319
Cohen, P. R., 576
Cohen, R. P., 115
Cohen, S., 617
Coid, J., 90, 95, 175, 177, 180, 181, 182, 183, 184, 185, 186, 187, 188, 189, 190, 191, 422, 630
Coid, J. W., 462
Coifman, K. G., 209
Cole, P. M., 272
Coles, M. E., 463
Colledge, E., 328
Collier, D., 470
Collins, L. M., 199
Colom, F., 600, 601
Colwell, L. H., 450
Comai, S., 258, 261
Compton, W. M., III, 91
Comtois, K. A., 422
Conger, R. D., 209
Conners, C. K., 288, 290
Connolly, D. A., 293
Connolly Gibbons, M. B., 470
Conroy, D., 381
Conroy, D. E., 381
Constantine, D., 256, 275
Constantino, M. J., 399
Contopoulos-Ioannidis, D. G., 161
Conway, M. A., 293
Cooke, D. J., 91, 94, 344, 428, 448, 450
Cooley, W. W., 414
Coolidge, F. L., 315, 320, 342
Coon, H. M., 93
Cooper, J. A., 261
Cooper, L. D., 208, 467
Cooper, T. B., 254
Coplan, J. D., 260
Copp, O., 48
Corbitt, E. M., 55, 184
Corenthal, C., 192
Coric, V., 261

Coristine, M., 560
Cormier, C. A., 453, 630
Cornelius, J., 258
Cornelius, J. R., 219, 283
Cornell, A. H., 325
Correll, J., 147
Corriveau, K. H., 133
Corte, C., 113
Coryell, W., 179, 184, 187, 189, 190, 192, 461
Coryell, W. H., 73, 175, 179, 180, 181, 182, 183, 185, 186, 192
Cosmides, L., 17, 18
Costa, P., 91
Costa, P. T., 57, 162, 198, 240, 242, 244, 251, 311, 420, 468
Costa, P. T., Jr., 37, 40, 41, 61, 74, 75, 80, 160, 162, 313, 343, 346, 348, 369, 370
Cottaux, P., 485
Cotton, H. A., 48
Cottraux, J., 524
Coussons-Read, M., 264
Cowan, C. P., 311
Cowan, P. A., 311
Cowan, T., 469
Cowdry, M., 284
Cowdry, R. W., 256, 257, 261, 262, 283, 286, 611, 618, 623
Cox, B., 469
Cox, D., 450
Coyle, J. T., 261
Coyne, J. C., 617
Craig, J. M., 239
Craig, S. G., 233, 324, 331
Craighead, L. W., 539
Cramer, V., 90, 176, 422, 461, 462
Crandell, L. E., 128, 132
Crane, R., 611
Crawford, A., 469
Crawford, C. B., 241
Crawford, M., 91, 216, 221
Crawford, M. J., 14, 20, 65, 83, 220, 337, 369, 485, 648
Crawford, T. N., 107, 129, 175, 176, 180, 181, 182, 183, 184, 185, 186, 189, 193, 199, 218, 219, 302, 315, 319, 576
Crego, C., 47, 61, 62, 66, 346
Crick, N. R., 223, 231, 313, 314
Cristea, I. A., 483
Critchfield, K. L., 338, 339, 394, 397, 399, 412, 413, 484, 645, 653, 655, 668
Crits-Christoph, K., 466
Crits-Christoph, P., 497
Crocker, P., 653
Cromer, T. D., 387
Cronbach, L. J., 12
Cropley, V. L., 259
Crosby, R., 469
Crosby, R. D., 600
Cross, B., 330
Crotty, T., 587, 588
Croughan, J., 174, 175
Crow, S. J., 600
Crowe, S. F., 328
Crowell, S., 420
Crowell, S. E., 115, 127
Csernansky, J. G., 465
Csibra, G., 135, 545
Cuevas, L., 77
Cullen, F. T., 639
Cummings, J. L., 273

Cundiff, J. M., 115
Cunningham, P. B., 638
Curtin, J. J., 431, 432
Cushing, G., 400
Cuthbert, B. N., 155, 163, 275, 432
Cuzder, J., 284
Czaja, S. J., 129
Cziko, A. M., 247

Dadds, M. R., 324, 325, 326, 327, 330, 331, 332
Dagg, P., 560
Dahl, A., 55
Dalgleish, T., 294
Daly, A.-M., 490, 503
Daly, E., 337, 341
Daly, E. J., 347
Damasio, A., 271, 288
Damasio, H., 288
Dammann, G., 113, 114
Damsa, C., 95
Dandreaux, D. M., 325
Danesh, J., 637
Darby, D., 287
Darwin, C., 27, 36
Dasoukis, J., 504, 505
Daversa, M. T., 330
Davidson, K., 378, 481, 482, 484, 668
Davidson, K. M., 482, 484, 512, 513, 514, 515, 516, 520, 521, 523, 524, 525
Davidson, L., 606
Davidson, R. J., 272, 275
Davis, C., 507
Davis, D., 377
Davis, D. D., 28, 130, 302, 512, 587, 637, 647
Davis, G. C., 420
Davis, H., 290
Davis, J. M., 617
Davis, K. L., 104, 158, 251, 258, 259, 303, 420
Davis, R. D., 17, 25, 302, 337
Davis, W., 56
Davis, W. W., 55
Davison, G. C., 656
Dawkins, R., 14
Dawson, D. A., 175, 177
Dawson, M. E., 433
De Almeida, R. M. M., 257
De Boeck, P., 148
De Bold, J. F., 257
De Bolle, M., 218, 231, 314, 346
De Bonis, M., 148
De Clercq, B., 77, 216, 217, 218, 220, 231, 312, 313, 314, 319, 346, 349
de Decker, A., 294
De Dreu, C. K., 263
De Fruyt, F., 64, 77, 79, 80, 81, 216, 217, 218, 220, 231, 312, 313, 314, 349
De Fruyt, F. D., 346
de Jong, J., 257
de Jong, P. J., 147
de los Cobos, J. C. P., 256
de Moor, M., 244
De Panfilis, C., 575, 583
De Pauw, S. S. W., 311, 312
De Raad, B., 41
de Reus, R. J., 459, 461
de Reus, R. J. M., 342
De Roover, K., 41
de Rosnay, M., 127

De Ruiter, C., 568
de Vries, R. E., 80, 349
Deal, J. E., 317
Decety, J., 435
Decker, H. S., 53
Decuyper, M., 217, 220, 346
DeFife, J. A., 116, 318
DeFries, J. C., 238, 241
Delgado, S. V., 492
Delis, D. C., 286
DelVecchio, W. F., 74, 198, 199, 217, 218, 314, 358
Delville, Y., 262
Demetriou, C. A., 326
Dennett, D. C., 18
Denys, D. A., 463
Depue, R. A., 211, 251, 577, 581
Derefinko, K. J., 446
Derks, E. M., 239
Derksen, J. J., 264
Derogatis, L. R., 613, 614, 615
Derringer, J., 60, 76, 80, 162, 246, 350, 353, 373, 437
DeRubeis, R. J., 142
Descartes, R., 27
d'Espine, M., 49
DeStefano, J., 220
DeWolf, M. S., 132
Dexter, C., 128
DeYoung, C. G., 75, 310, 311, 312, 468
Di Pierro, R., 380
Diaconu, G., 462
Diamond, A., 110
Diamond, D., 572
Diamond, J., 464
Dickhaut, V., 556
Dickinson, A., 272
DiClemente, C. C., 410, 635, 667
Diedrich, A., 460
Diener, E., 242
Dietz, B., 586
Dietzel, R., 144
Digman, J. M., 311, 469
Dikman, Z. V., 433
DiLalla, D. L., 239
Dimaggio, G., 110, 369, 466, 571, 630, 645, 649, 661, 664, 666
Dinan, T. G., 465
Dindo, L., 431, 432, 433, 452
Dinn, W. M., 148, 285, 286, 287, 290, 291, 465
Distel, M. A., 422
Ditzen, B., 263
Diwadkar, V., 274, 277
Dixon, L., 600
Dodge, K. A., 222
Dodson, M. C., 332
Doering, S., 483, 581
Dolan, C. V., 239
Dolan-Sewell, R. T., 155, 158
Dolcos, F., 292
D'Olio, C., 464
Dombrovski, A. Y., 272
Domes, G., 145, 146, 148, 274, 293, 327
Donald, M., 492
Donaldson, D., 469
Donegan, N. H., 275
Donnellan, M. B., 347
Donnelly, J., 452
Donnenberg, G. R., 503
Donoghue, K., 329, 330

Dopp, A. R., 222
Doren, D. M., 634
Dorovini-Zis, K., 253
Dorrian, A., 492
Doss, A. J., 222
Dougherty, D., 290
Dougherty, D. D., 277
Dougherty, D. M., 291, 617
Dougherty, J. W. D., 25
Douglas, K. S., 449, 453
Downey, G., 209
Dowrick, C., 600, 601
Dowson, J. H., 192, 284, 288
Draguns, J. G., 20, 52
Draine, J., 600
Drake, R. E., 175, 178, 181, 183, 184, 185, 186, 188, 191
Dreessen, A., 539
Dreessen, L., 142, 144, 146, 149
Drevets, W. C., 272
Drieling, T., 470
Driessen, M., 274, 284, 286
Drislane, L. E., 427, 428, 430, 431, 433, 436, 438, 447, 449, 452
Dritschel, B., 148
Druecke, H. W., 284
Drye, R. C., 7
D'Silva, K., 630
Duggan, C., 630
Duignan, I., 504, 505
Duke, A. A., 255
Duman, R. S., 260
Dumenci, L., 353
Duncan, G. J., 204
Duncan, S., 449
Dunn, A. J., 259
Dunn, M., 507, 508
Dupré, J., 17, 19
Durbin, C. E., 358, 430
Durkee, A., 616
Durrant, C., 245
Durrett, C., 369
Durrett, C. A., 60, 173, 188, 251, 446
Dvorak-Bertsch, J. D., 431, 432, 433
Dyck, M., 148
Dye, D. A., 40
Dyer, A., 158
Dymond, R. F., 130

Eaton, N. R., 10, 315, 357, 370
Eaton, W. W., 176
Eaves, L. J., 239, 306
Eber, H. W., 37
Eberle, J., 539
Ebner-Priemer, U., 209, 210, 274
Ebner-Priemer, U. W., 274, 421
Ebstein, R. P., 262
Ebsworthy, G., 292
Eccleston, E. G., 252
Edelen, M. O., 467
Edell, W., 109
Edell, W. S., 114
Edens, J. F., 427, 450, 453, 630
Edmundson, M., 342, 346
Eelen, P., 294
Eells, T. D., 647
Egan, S. J., 469
Egeland, B., 128, 318, 576
Egner, T., 288
Ehlert, U., 470
Ehrensaft, M., 576

Ehrensaft, M. K., 129
Einstein, A., 28
Eisen, J., 468
Eisen, J. L., 459, 463
Eisenberg, N., 316, 317, 318
Eisenlohr-Moul, T., 255
Ekman, P., 275
Ekselius, L., 158, 461
Elklit, A., 294, 342
Ellickson, P., 639
Elliot, A. J., 374
Ellis, C. G., 55
Ellison, W. D., 582
Elmore, K., 110
Elzinga, B. M., 274
Embleton, J., 505
Emmelkamp, P. M., 459, 461
Emmelkamp, P. M. G., 342, 523, 524
Emmons, R. A., 345
Emond, C., 469
End, A., 432
Endicott, J., 52, 54, 175, 178
Endrass, T., 288
Enero, C., 466
Engel, S. G., 471
Enns, M., 469
Epstein, M., 449
Erbaugh, J., 617
Erbaugh, J. K., 51
Erickson, T. M., 470
Eriksen, B. A., 288
Eriksen, C. W., 288
Erikson, E., 103
Erikson, E. H., 108, 110, 116
Erikson, M., 453
Erlenmeyer-Kimling, L., 175, 179, 181
Erni, T., 109
Ersche, K. D., 246
Erzegovesi, S., 463
Esteller, À., 437, 449
Estes, W. K., 208
Etkin, A., 288
Eureligs-Bontekoe, E., 149
Evans, D. E., 311, 513
Evans, M., 490
Evans, R. W., 286
Everitt, B. J., 272
Evers, S., 555
Evers, S. M. A. A., 143, 484
Ewalt, J., 52
Ewles, C. D., 453
Exner, J. E., 283
Eynan, R., 64
Eysenck, H. J., 74, 78, 92, 348, 370, 373
Eysenck, M. W., 348, 370
Eysenck, S. B., 92
Eysenck, S. B. G., 74

Fabiano, E. A., 453
Fabrega, H., Jr., 88, 89, 92, 97
Fabrigar, L. R., 39
Fagiolini, A., 273
Fairbairn, W. R. D., 489
Falkenstrom, F., 135
Fan, J., 128, 276
Fang, C. M., 113
Fanning, J. R., 231, 232, 251, 255
Fanti, K. A., 326, 329
Faraone, S. V., 236, 237
Farber, B. A., 556
Farell, J. M., 325

Farmer, R. F., 343, 467
Farr, W., 49
Farrell, J., 555, 556, 568
Farrell, J. M., 483
Farrington, D., 450
Farrington, D. P., 462
Fava, G. A, 164
Fava, M., 539
Fawcett, J., 62
Fazekas, H., 328
Fazel, S., 637
Fearon, P., 126
Fearon, P. R. M., 132
Fedorov, C., 287, 291
Feeney, J., 116
Feenstra, D. J., 118, 221, 352
Fehr, E., 263, 435
Feigenbaum, J. D., 539
Feighner, J. P., 52
Feighner, J. P, 419
Feiler, A. R., 239
Feinberg, T. E., 131
Feinstein, A. R., 156
Feldman, R., 284
Feline, A., 148
Fenton, W., 284
Ferguson, C. J., 198, 217, 314
Ferguson, K. S., 127, 544
Ferguson, N., 15
Fergusson, D. M., 302, 304, 423
Fernyhough, C., 132
Ferrer, E., 209
Ferris, C. F., 254, 262
Fertuck, E. A., 274, 286, 663
Feske, U., 664
Few, L. R., 76, 79, 80, 83, 163, 351, 354, 355
Fiedler, E. R., 231, 342
Fiester, S. J., 54
Fineberg, N. A., 463, 465, 471
Finkelhor, D., 302, 304
Finlayson-Short, L., 492
Finn, J. A., 77, 80, 343
Fiorani, C., 492
Fiore, D., 466
First, M., 56, 175, 178, 394
First, M. B., 55, 57, 59, 63, 158, 164, 176, 342, 346, 354, 405, 409, 445
Fischbacher, U., 263, 435
Fish, E. W., 257, 259, 262
Fishbein, D. H., 254
Fishler, P. H., 350
Fiske, S. T., 545
Fitzmaurice, G., 207, 423, 513, 604
Fitzmaurice, G. M., 127, 421
Fitzpatrick, C. M., 427
Fitzpatrick, M., 220
Flanagan, E., 55, 59
Flanagan, E. H., 48
Flashman, L. A., 284
Fleiss, J. L., 52, 59, 397
Fleming, A. P., 539
Fletcher, P. C., 273
Flett, G. L., 469
Flint, J., 245
Flor, H., 433
Florentino, M. C., 470
Florsheim, P., 412
Floyd, K., 607
Flynn, C. A., 469
Foa, E. B., 463
Foelsch, P. A., 113, 115, 116

Foley, D. L., 231
Folstein, M. F., 157
Fonagy, P., 101, 102, 103, 110, 117, 123, 124, 125, 126, 127, 128, 129, 130, 131, 132, 133, 134, 222, 377, 380, 388, 422, 481, 483, 495, 503, 541, 542, 543, 544, 545, 547, 550, 551, 555, 558, 568, 571, 572, 576, 587, 605, 649, 655
Fontaine, N. M., 327
Forbush, K. T., 159
Forchuk, C., 606
Ford, J. D., 325
Forgan, G., 470
Forman, E. M., 421
Forman, J. B., 53
Forner, F., 461
Forrester, B., 378
Forsman, A., 257, 258
Forth, A. E., 427, 448, 449
Fossati, A., 109, 116, 126, 304
Foulds, G. A., 9
Fournier, J. C., 142
Fowles, D., 452
Fowles, D. C., 429, 431, 432, 433, 434, 444
Fox, N. A., 317
Fradley, E., 132
Fraley, R. C., 126, 198
Frances, A., 109, 156
Frances, A. J., 53, 54, 55, 56, 62, 65, 445
Francis, A. J., 142, 144
Frank, H., 304
Frank, J. B., 134
Frank, J. D., 134
Frankenburg, F., 73
Frankenburg, F. R., 199, 207, 343, 357, 421, 423, 513, 576, 601, 604, 615, 617, 618
Frankenhuis, W. E., 127
Frankle, W. G., 256
Franklin, M. E., 464
Franzen, N., 150
Fredrikson, M., 158
Freedman, M. B., 32
Freedman, R., 62
Freeman, A., 28, 130, 302, 377, 466, 481, 512, 521, 587, 637, 647, 664
Freeman, R., 463, 464
Freije, H., 586, 597
Freud, S., 198, 271, 467
Freyberger, H. J., 130
Frick, P., 436
Frick, P. J., 219, 324, 325, 326, 327, 328, 329, 331, 332, 427, 428, 429, 431, 433, 434, 435, 446, 448, 449
Friedel, R. O., 257
Friedman, H. S., 469
Friendship, C., 453, 454
Friesen, W. V., 275
Fruzzetti, A. E., 533, 539, 602
Fujita, F., 242
Fujita, M., 259
Funder, D. C., 198
Furmark, T., 94, 158
Furnham, A., 461

Gabbard, G., 549
Gabbard, G. O., 636
Gabriel, S., 255
Gabrieli, J. D., 277
Gabrielsen, G., 221
Gadamar, H.-G., 9
Gallagher, E. F., 469

Gallagher, N. G., 148, 465
Gallagher-Thompson, D., 378
Gallop, R., 539
Galton, F., 36
Gamer, M., 263
Gamez, W., 74, 163
Gannon, D. R., 638
Gao, Y., 129, 330
Garcia, L. F., 77
Garcia, O., 77
García-Herráiz, M. A., 260
Gardner, C. O., 459
Gardner, D., 284, 286
Gardner, D. L., 256, 261, 262, 611, 618, 623
Gardner, F., 333
Garfield, S. L., 410
Garland, M. R., 617
Garrett, C. J., 454
Garyfallos, G., 463
Gasperi, M., 430
Gatchel, R. J., 453
Gaudiano, B. A., 485
Gaughan, E. T., 77, 345, 349, 427
Gawronski, B., 146
Gay, M., 54
Geiger, T. C., 313
Gelernter, J., 245
Gelfand, D. M., 400
Geller, J. D., 556
Gendreau, P., 452, 637, 640
George, E. L., 600
George, K., 262
George, L., 174
Gergely, G., 126, 129, 131, 135, 541, 544, 545, 649
Gerra, G., 259
Gershon, S., 253
Ghaemi, S. N., 420
Ghera, M. M., 317
Gibbon, M., 175, 178, 342, 346, 354, 405, 445
Gibbon, S., 636
Giesen-Bloo, J., 143, 376, 481, 483, 520, 524, 555, 556, 567
Gilbert, F., 435
Gilbody, S., 503
Gill, A. D., 326
Gillanders, D. T., 481
Gillberg, C., 463
Gillberg, I. C., 463
Gilligan, C., 34
Gilmore, M., 109
Giordano, R., 492
Gizer, I. R., 436
Gjerde, L. C., 464
Glas, G., 109, 110
Glauser, D., 95
Gleason, M. E. J., 345
Gleaves, D. H., 468
Glick, B., 453
Glick, D. M., 277
Glover, N., 346
Glueck, E., 179
Glueck, J., 179
Gobbi, G., 258
Goddard, L., 148
Goggin, C., 452
Gogtay, N., 582
Gold, J., 284
Gold, J. M., 286

Gold, J. R., 647
Gold, L., 283
Goldberg, D., 159
Goldberg, L. R., 37, 39, 74, 343, 348
Goldberg, M. G., 318
Goldberg, T. E., 164
Golden, L. S., 453
Goldin, P. R., 277
Golding, I., 461
Goldman, B. N., 114
Goldsmith, H. H., 241
Goldstein, A. P., 453
Goldstein, M., 275
Goldstein, R. B., 179
Goldstein, T. R., 539
Goldweber, A., 324, 328
Golynkina, K., 497, 504, 505
Goodman, G. S., 128
Goodman, M., 272, 582, 603
Goodwin, F. K., 253, 254, 257, 420
Goodyer, I., 294
Göpfert, M., 495
Goradia, D., 274
Gordon, A., 447, 630, 631, 634, 635, 639, 640, 641
Gordon, H. L., 432
Gordon, H. M., 293
Gordon, O. M., 463
Gordon, R. S., Jr., 221
Gore, W. L., 60, 61, 63, 75, 76, 80, 346
Gorman, J. M., 260
Gosden, N. P., 221
Gosling, S. D., 198, 217
Gosling, S. M., 311, 315
Goth, K., 113, 115
Gotlib, I. H., 292
Gottesman, I. I., 160, 239, 472
Gould, T. D., 160, 472
Goyer, P. F., 253, 275
Graetz, B. W., 429
Granic, I., 470
Granstrom, F., 135
Grant, B. F., 90, 131, 157, 175, 177, 180, 181, 182, 183, 184, 185, 186, 187, 188, 189, 190, 191, 422, 461, 613
Grant, J. E., 460, 461, 462
Gratz, K. L., 128, 318
Gray, J. A., 21, 311
Gray, J. R., 310, 311
Gray, R. D., 230
Grazioplene, R. G., 75
Green, B. A., 142
Greenberg, B. D., 244
Greenberg, J. R., 514
Greenberg, L. S., 633, 652
Greenberg, R. P., 350
Greene, A. L., 461, 462
Greene, R. L., 239
Greenwald, A. G., 147
Greenwood, A., 631
Greer, P. J., 256, 275
Gremaud-Heitz, D., 108
Greve, K. W., 461
Grienenberger, J., 132
Grienenberger, J. F., 132
Griffiths, P. E., 230
Grilo, C., 109
Grilo, C. M., 73, 205, 206, 207, 221, 462, 463, 467, 468
Grimes, R., 630
Grimm, K. J., 208

Grinker, R. R., 7
Grob, G. N., 48, 49
Grosjean, B., 261
Gross, J. J., 271, 272, 277, 660
Gross, J. N., 434
Grosse Holtforth, M., 163
Gruen, R., 178
Gruenberg, A. M., 179
Gruenberg, E. M., 52
Gu, D., 447, 631, 639, 641
Guastella, A. J., 262
Guiducci, V., 126
Guimond, T., 582
Gulbinat, W., 49
Gumley, A., 524
Gunderson, J., 73, 126, 163, 223, 587
Gunderson, J. G., 55, 56, 58, 61, 62, 63, 66, 126, 127, 201, 202, 207, 209, 210, 218, 303, 318, 343, 357, 419, 420, 421, 422, 423, 461, 463, 468, 482, 575, 576, 600, 602, 604, 605, 618
Gupta, R. C., 261
Gupta, S., 262
Gurman, A. S., 571
Gurtman, M., 403
Gurvits, I. G., 264
Guttman, H., 288, 305, 306, 420
Guzder, J., 304, 305, 422
Guze, S. B., 12, 13, 14, 459
Gvirts, H. Z., 288, 290
Gyra, J., 466

Haaland, V. Ø., 288, 289
Habke, A. M., 469
Hagan, T., 504
Haggerty, R. J., 221
Haigler, E. D., 76
Hajcak, G., 160
Hakimi, S., 262
Hakkaart-van Roijen, L., 462
Hakstian, A. R., 428, 448
Hall, C. S., 345
Hall, J., 490
Hall, J. R., 160, 428, 430, 431, 433, 447
Hall, R. E., 95
Hallahan, B., 617, 620
Haller, J., 260
Hallion, L. S., 149
Hallmayer, J., 461
Hallquist, M. N., 58, 170, 197, 208, 210, 216, 574
Halmi, K. A., 469
Halperin, J. M., 255
Halverson, C. F., 317
Hamagami, F., 208
Hamby, S. L., 302
Hamer, D. H., 244, 245
Hamilton, M., 613
Hamilton, W. D., 132
Han, M. H., 274
Hansen, D. J., 302
Happé, F. G., 435
Harbeck, S., 485
Hardt, J., 302
Hardy, G., 504, 506, 507
Hare, R. D., 47, 56, 63, 324, 332, 344, 427, 428, 431, 432, 445, 446, 447, 448, 449, 450, 451, 453, 567, 629, 630, 631, 633, 634, 637, 639
Haring, M., 469
Hariri, A. R., 245, 264, 317

Harkness, A. R., 74, 77, 78, 80, 160, 162, 314, 343, 370
Harlan, E. T., 317, 434
Harley, R., 539
Harlow, H., 399, 403
Harned, M. S., 530
Harnett-Sheehan, K., 614
Harpur, T. J., 324, 427, 428, 448, 631
Harralson, T. L., 305
Harris, C. L., 465
Harris, G. T., 427, 453, 629, 630
Harris, P., 639
Harris, P. L., 127
Harrison, J., 337, 341
Hart, S., 450
Hart, S. D., 324, 427
Harter, S., 375
Hartkamp, N., 412
Hartwell, N., 470
Harvey, A. G., 292
Harvey, P. D., 614
Harvey, R., 586, 597
Hasin, D. S., 175, 177, 180, 182, 183, 184, 185, 186, 188, 189, 190, 191
Haslam, N., 357
Hathaway, S. R., 74
Hauger, R. L., 254
Hautzinger, M., 285
Hawes, D. J., 330, 331, 332
Hawkins, J. D., 222
Hawley, K. M., 222
Hayes, S. C., 661
Hayward, M., 188
Hazlett, E. A., 128, 274
Healey, B. J., 350
Heard, H. L., 483, 538, 586, 605
Heatherton, T. F., 650
Heaton, N., 400
Heaton, R. K., 286
Hecht, H., 470
Heck, A., 245
Heeringa, S. G., 177
Heidkamp, D., 143, 561
Heim, A. K., 113, 115
Heim, C., 263
Heinrichs, M., 263, 327, 435
Heldmann, M., 262
Helgeland, M. I., 219
Hellerstein, D. J., 463
Helzer, J. E., 58, 174, 175
Hempel, C. G., 13, 27, 33
Hemphill, J., 448
Hemphill, J. F., 453
Henderson, H. A., 317
Hendricks, C. M., 465
Hendrickse, J., 80, 349
Hendriks, T., 149
Hengartner, M. P., 129
Henggeler, S. W., 638
Henley-Cragg, P., 597
Hennen, J., 199, 207, 261, 357
Henriques, G. R., 421
Henry, W. P., 497
Henson, R. N., 273
Hentschel, A. G., 352, 355, 382
Hepple, J., 503
Herbert, J. L., 614
Herbst, J. H., 244
Herkov, M. J., 55, 59
Herman, J. L., 231, 305, 420
Hermann, C., 433

Hermans, D., 294
Herpertz, S., 284
Herpertz, S. C., 21, 146, 150, 263, 274, 275, 278, 582
Herr, N. R., 113
Hertler, S. C., 468
Herzhoff, K., 220, 231, 312
Heslegrave, R., 291
Hesselbrock, V. M., 434
Hettema, J. M., 242
Heun, R., 179, 180, 461
Hewitt, P. L., 469, 470
Hewlett, W. A., 465
Heywood, S., 490
Hiatt, K. D., 452
Hibbeln, J. R., 254, 617
Hickie, I. B., 262
Hickling, E. J., 178
Hickling, F. W., 90
Hicks, A., 53
Hicks, B. M., 161, 315, 325, 329, 344, 428, 429, 433, 434, 447, 448, 450, 451, 452, 544
Higgitt, A., 123, 126, 127, 503, 544
Higgitt, A. C., 132, 541
Hill, C. H., 503
Hill, D. M., 539
Hill, K. G., 222
Hilsenroth, M. J., 387, 412
Hipwell, A. E., 218, 219, 423
Hirschfeld, R. M., 56
Hirschfeld, R. M. A., 345
Hirvikoski, T., 539
Hobson, J., 631
Hobson, R. P., 128, 132
Hochhausen, N. M., 289
Hodgins, S., 291, 429
Hoekstra, H. A., 80
Hoermann, S., 274
Hoerst, M., 261
Hoertel, N., 190
Hoffart, A., 566
Hoffman, P. D., 602
Hofmann, S. G., 149
Hofmann, V., 132
Hofmans, J., 64, 216
Hofstadter, D. R., 290
Hogan, R., 39
Hogarty, G. E., 600
Hoge, R. D., 453, 629
Hoglend, P., 412
Hogue, T., 631
Holder, J., 127
Holker, L., 292
Holland, A. S., 126
Hollander, E., 260, 261, 611
Hollenstein, T., 470
Hollin, C., 631
Hollingshead, A. B., 615
Holmes, A., 245
Holmes, B. M., 126
Holmes, E. A., 557, 564
Holmes, S. E., 143
Holmqvist, R., 135
Holt, R. R., 647
Hood, J., 274
Hooley, J. M., 148, 208, 293
Hopwood, C. J., 60, 63, 82, 158, 163, 201, 206, 207, 211, 242, 347, 358, 369, 373, 374, 380, 388, 437
Hornblow, A. R., 176

Horowitz, L. M., 575, 612
Horowitz, M. J., 104, 649
Horowitz, M. J. E., 28
Horvath, A. O., 633, 652
Horz, S., 575
Hörz, S., 108, 116
Hoshino-Browne, E., 147
Hourtane, M., 148
Houston, R. J., 461
Howard, A., 330
Howard, K. I., 503
Hoyer, J., 116
Huang, Y., 58, 175, 177, 181, 182, 183, 185, 186, 187, 189, 190, 191, 216
Huckabee, H., 290
Hudson, J. I., 303
Hughes, G., 631
Hügli, C., 113
Huibregtse, B. M., 317
Hull, J. W., 109, 116
Hulsey, T. L., 305
Hummelen, B., 63, 467, 468, 471
Hunter. K., 606
Huprich, S. K., 58, 59, 63, 66, 350, 467
Hur, Y. M., 239
Hurlemann, R., 263
Hurt, S. W., 109, 114
Hutsebaut, J., 118, 221, 352
Hwu, H. G., 305
Hyare, H., 145
Hyde, A. L., 381
Hyde, L. W., 317, 318, 333
Hyler, S., 175, 180
Hyler, S. E., 73, 82, 346
Hyman, S. E., 11, 15, 47, 59, 64, 161, 572

Iacono, W. G., 159, 160, 161, 315, 429, 431, 433, 447, 448, 452, 544
Iannone, V. N., 286
Imel, Z. E., 134
Inbar, M., 149
Ingram, R. E., 514
Innis, R. B., 259
Insel, T., 155, 163, 437
Insel, T. R., 47, 59, 64, 65, 395, 582
Intoccia, V., 60, 345
Ioannidis, J. P. A., 26, 161
Irle, E., 274, 284, 285
Irwin, W., 275
Isabella, R. A., 132
Iscan, C., 73, 91, 357
Isoma, Z., 329
Israel, A. C., 156
Israel, S., 262
Ivanoff, A. M., 481, 527, 654
Ivanova, M. Y., 92, 353
Iverson, K. M., 539
Iwawaki, S., 92
Izzo, R. L., 454

Jablensky, A., 11, 12, 49, 164
Jackson, D., 77, 78
Jackson, D. N., 10, 12, 13, 91, 237, 239, 343, 348, 370, 385, 647
Jackson, H. J., 142, 220, 222, 560, 566
Jackson, P. L., 435
Jacob, G. A., 145, 274
Jacobo, M., 539
Jacobs, G., 611
Jacobs, K. L., 12, 13, 14, 72, 417
Jacobsen, B., 258

Jacobsen, T., 132
Jacobson, E., 116, 571
Jaffe, J. H., 254
Jahng, S., 177, 421
Jambrak, J., 331
Jamerson, J. E., 80
James, K., 483, 504
James, W., 101, 109, 198, 217, 271
Janca, A., 175, 180, 342
Jane, J. S., 342, 461
Jang, K., 305
Jang, K. L., 10, 18, 75, 161, 162, 216, 231, 235, 237, 239, 240, 251, 315, 338, 350, 352, 356, 370, 374, 385, 422, 647
Janzen, R., 606
Jardri, R., 161
Jaspers, K., 5, 6
Jenkins, R., 491
Jensen, E., 606
Jesness, C., 630
Jiang, P., 261, 611
Jilek-Aall, L., 96
Jo, B., 539
Johansson, P., 428, 452, 484
John, O. P., 35, 39, 80, 198, 217, 311, 315
John, S. L., 427
Johnson, A. M., 239
Johnson, C. R., 616
Johnson, F., 464
Johnson, J. G., 107, 129, 143, 199, 206, 211, 218, 219, 231, 302, 313, 315, 319
Johnson, M. D., 208, 357, 581
Johnson, T., 95, 369
Joiner, T. E., 428, 451, 560
Joiner, T. E., Jr., 464
Joireman, J., 347
Joksimovic, L., 470
Jones, A., 342
Jones, A. P., 435, 436
Jones, B., 148, 294
Jones, D. K., 375
Jonkman, S., 272
Joormann, J., 292
Jordan, C. H., 147
Jordan, S., 560
Jørgensen, C. R., 101, 103, 107, 108, 109, 110, 111, 113, 114, 115, 116, 118, 130, 294, 483, 484
Jose, A., 57
Joseph, B., 659
Joseph, S., 284
Joshua, S., 53
Jouriles, E. N., 332
Jovev, M., 142, 220, 221, 560, 566
Joyce, A. S., 368, 484
Joyce, P. R., 91, 176
Judd, P. H., 284, 285, 286, 287
Jung, E., 113
Jurist, E., 129, 541
Jurist, E. L., 649
Jutai, J. W., 432

Kabat-Zinn, J., 661
Kaess, M., 219, 231
Kagan, J., 199, 304
Kahn, R. E., 325, 326, 329
Kahneman, D., 15
Kaiser, D., 145
Kakuma, T., 116
Kalisch, R., 288
Kalpin, A., 466

Kalyvoka, A., 461
Kamarch, T., 617
Kamen, C., 345
Kamphuis, J. H., 64, 352, 382
Kanner, A. D., 617
Kaplan, E., 286
Kaplan, U., 96
Karkowski-Shuman, L., 242
Karno, M., 461
Karpiak, C. P., 338, 339, 394
Karpman, B., 325, 326, 446, 451
Karterud, S., 63, 467, 485, 546
Kasen, S., 129, 143, 199, 218, 219, 302, 315
Kashani, J., 143
Kass, F., 54
Kathmann, N., 288
Katsuragi, S., 245
Kaufman, E., 115
Kavoussi, R. J., 254, 255
Kazdin, A. E., 580, 582
Keefe, R. S., 283
Keeley, J. W., 48
Keller, F., 290
Keller, M., 56
Keller, M. B., 57
Kellert, S. H., 19
Kellett, S., 104, 481, 489, 490, 491, 492, 496, 500, 502, 503, 504, 505, 506, 507, 523
Kellman, D., 180
Kellman, H. D., 73
Kellogg, S., 513, 514, 521
Kelly, K., 132
Kelly, M. M., 129
Kelly, T. M., 275, 305
Kemmelmeier, M., 93
Kempf, L., 262
Kendall, J. P., 284
Kendall, P. C., 157
Kendell, R. E., 11, 47, 48, 49, 51, 52, 55
Kendler, K., 52, 59
Kendler, K. S., 4, 8, 10, 14, 18, 19, 25, 62, 63, 66, 78, 161, 164, 175, 179, 180, 181, 182, 183, 184, 185, 239, 240, 241, 242, 306, 429, 436, 459, 464
Kennealy, P., 631
Kennealy, P. J., 257, 428, 453
Kent, J. M., 260
Kenyon, A. R., 262
Kerber, K., 283
Kéri, S., 286
Kerig, P. K., 325, 326, 328, 329, 330, 332
Kern, M. L., 469
Kernberg, O., 481
Kernberg, O. F., 7, 56, 58, 62, 102, 108, 110, 111, 114, 115, 116, 117, 118, 130, 285, 286, 374, 375, 377, 378, 379, 382, 387, 388, 419, 483, 538, 571, 572, 573, 574, 575, 576, 577, 581, 587, 605, 663
Kernis, M. H., 114
Kerr, I., 495, 496, 501, 507, 508
Kerr, I. B., 492, 507
Kerr, M., 319, 427, 428, 450, 452
Kersten, G., 568
Kertz, B., 616
Kessler, R. C., 78, 90, 91, 156, 157, 174, 175, 176, 177, 182, 183, 205, 208, 422, 460
Kety, S. S., 258
Keulen-de Vos, M. E., 559, 563, 567
Keune, N., 149

Khalsa, S., 582
Kiehl, K. A., 427, 432
Kierkegaard, S., 109
Kiesler, D. J., 370, 373
Kim, J., 316, 542
Kim, J. J., 93
Kim, Y., 96, 343
Kimbrel, N. A., 304
Kim-Cohen, J., 218
Kimonis, E. R., 324, 325, 326, 328, 329, 330, 333, 449
Kimpara, S., 367, 388
Kindt, M., 149
Kinead, B., 264
King, R., 285, 286, 287, 290
King-Casas, B., 272
Kiraly, I., 135
Kirchberger, I., 612
Kirk, S. A., 72
Kirkpatrick, T., 286
Kirrane, R., 258
Kirrane, R. M., 259
Kirsch, P., 327
Kischka, U., 291
Kiser, L. J., 132
Kistner, J., 542
Kitayama, S., 88, 93
Kitzman, H., 222
Kjelsberg, E., 219
Klahr, A. M., 332
Klebe, K. J., 342
Klein, D. F., 623
Klein, D. N., 219, 358, 462, 544
Klein, M., 571
Klein, M. H., 342, 403, 405
Kleindienst, N., 158
Klerman, G. L., 4, 8, 11, 156, 468
Kliem, S., 485
Klimes-Dougan, B., 542
Klinger, T., 180, 461
Klokman, J., 143, 561
Klonsky, E., 210
Klonsky, E. D., 231, 345
Kloos, B., 606
Klosko, J., 555, 557, 587
Klosko, J. S., 114, 142, 377, 481, 512, 514, 664
Kluckhohn, C., 16, 17
Knaack, A., 330
Knafo, A., 262
Knobloch-Fedders, L. M., 400
Knutelska, M., 260
Ko, J. Y., 420
Koch, J., 5
Koch, J. L., 445
Koch, W., 256
Kochanska, G., 317, 328, 330, 434
Koelen, J. A., 350
Koenigsberg, H., 420, 421
Koenigsberg, H. W., 264, 273, 275, 276
Kohut, H., 7, 30, 102, 374, 654
Koldobsky, N., 14, 83, 337, 369, 485, 648
Kolisetty, A. P., 115, 130
Kongerslev, M., 221
Kongerslev, M. T., 221, 231
Koons, C. R., 483, 538
Koot, H. M., 220, 313, 314, 319
Köppen, D., 274
Korfine, L., 148, 173, 180, 208, 293

Korsgaard, C. M., 113
Korslund, K. E., 530
Kosfeld, M., 263, 435
Kosson, D. S., 427, 432, 449, 450, 451, 452
Kosterman, R., 222
Kosti, F., 504, 506
Kotov, R., 74, 159, 163
Koutoufa, I., 461
Kozak, M. J., 163
Kraemer, H. C., 463
Kraepelin, E., 5, 7, 420, 445
Kraft, M., 347
Krakauer, I., 466
Kramer, J. H., 286, 290
Kramer, M., 49, 52, 449
Kramer, M. D., 430, 433, 437, 449
Kramer, R., 539
Krämer, U., 262
Kramp, P., 221
Kranzler, H., 245
Krasnoperova, E., 292
Kraus, A., 276
Kraus, M. W., 247
Kremers, I., 294
Kremers, I. P., 148, 294
Kretschmer, E., 5, 7
Kringlen, E., 90, 176, 422, 461, 462
Kröger, C., 485
Kroger, J., 116
Kroll, J., 283
Krueger, R., 58, 83
Krueger, R. F., 10, 12, 13, 14, 58, 59, 60, 61, 62, 63, 65, 72, 75, 76, 77, 78, 80, 82, 104, 105, 155, 157, 158, 159, 160, 161, 162, 163, 178, 205, 208, 210, 215, 216, 231, 251, 313, 314, 315, 344, 350, 351, 353, 354, 357, 370, 373, 417, 428, 429, 430, 431, 433, 434, 435, 437, 444, 447, 449, 451, 452, 459
Kruglanski, A. W., 545
Krukowski, R. A., 353
Kruse, J., 134, 483
Kucharski, L. T., 449
Küchenhoff, J., 108
Kuhl, E. A., 57, 72, 162, 163
Kuhlman, D. M., 347
Kuhlman, M., 348
Kuhn, T. S., 3, 4, 26, 45
Kullgren, G., 461
Kunert, H. J., 284, 287, 289, 290, 295
Kunst, H., 116
Kuo, J., 274
Kuperminc, G. P., 469
Kupfer, D., 62
Kupfer, D. J., 57, 72, 162, 163, 273, 394
Kupsaw-Lawrence, E., 614
Kurcz, M., 256
Kushner, M. G., 460, 461
Kushner, S. C., 216, 217, 220, 313
Kushner, S. K., 220
Kutchins, H., 72
Kvist, K., 285
Kyrios, M., 466

Lab, S. P., 454
Ladouceur, C. D., 272, 273
Lahey, B. B., 159, 163, 219
Lam, J., 287
Lambert, M., 387
Lambert, M. J., 503, 647
Lambert, W., 305

Lampard, A. M., 135
Lampert, C., 464
Landenberger, N. A., 453, 454
Landgraf, R., 263
Landon, P. B., 629
Landrø, N. I., 288, 289
Lane, M., 205, 208
Lane, M. C., 90, 176, 422, 460
Lang, A. R., 433, 451
Lang, P. J., 275, 432
Lange, C., 274, 284
Lapierre, D., 291
Lapointe, L., 469
Laporte, L., 220, 288, 305, 306, 420, 423
Larson, C. L., 272, 432
Larson, D. G., 283
Larsson, H., 240, 327, 330, 436
Larstone, R., 352, 382
Larstone, R. M., 233, 324
Laruelle, M., 258, 260
Laska, K. M., 571
Lasko, N. B., 293
Laurenssen, E. M., 552
Laverdiere, O., 127
Lavy, E., 145
Lawn, S., 606
Lawrence, K. A., 288
Lawrence, T., 259
Layden, M. A., 664, 668
Lazare, A., 468
Lazarus, R. S., 617
Lazarus, S. A., 232
Le Strat, Y., 190
Leadbeater, B. J., 469
Leary, M. R., 101, 109
Leary, T., 32, 373, 399
LeBel, E. P., 146
Lee, C. K., 91
Lee, C. L., 94
Lee, K., 40, 77, 80, 348, 349
Lee, R., 254, 259, 261, 263, 264, 289
Lee, S., 145
Lee, S. H., 88, 94
Lee, T., 95
Lee, Z., 452
Legris, J., 287, 288, 289
Leibenluft, E., 215, 324
Leibing, E., 134, 483, 636
Leichsenring, F., 116, 134, 483, 636
Leighton, T., 499
Leiman, M., 491, 492, 499
Leising, D., 10, 369, 370, 388
Leistico, A. R., 429
Lejuez, C. W., 128, 158
Lelchook, A. M., 469
Lenane, M., 464
Lenane, M. C., 464
Lengua, L. J., 316, 317
Lenzenweger, M., 286
Lenzenweger, M. F., 3, 90, 116, 170, 173, 175, 176, 180, 181, 182, 183, 185, 186, 187, 188, 189, 190, 191, 193, 197, 198, 199, 205, 206, 208, 209, 210, 211, 216, 251, 274, 343, 357, 422, 460, 481, 483, 538, 571, 572, 574, 576, 577, 581, 605, 663
Leon, A. C., 470
Leonard, H. L., 464
Lerner, H., 283
Lerner, P., 283
Lesch, K. P., 245

Lesser, J. C., 255
Lester, D., 253
Leukefeld, C., 437
Leung, D. W., 289
Levander, S., 427, 450
Levant, R. F., 412
Levenik, K., 397
Levenson, M. R., 427, 429
Levin, J. D., 109
Levine, D., 274
Levine, M. D., 218
Levy, A. K., 318
Levy, D., 132
Levy, K. N., 114, 116, 126, 481, 483, 538, 571, 572, 581, 582, 583, 605
Leweke, F., 134
Lewinsohn, P. M., 219, 221, 462, 544
Lewis, G., 245
Lewis, K., 447, 631, 635, 641
Lewke, F., 483
Leyton, M., 256, 291
Lezak, M., 286
Lezak, M. D., 283
Lichtenstein, P., 240, 242, 327
Lichtermann, D., 179, 180, 461
Lida-Pulik, H., 148
Lidberg, L., 253, 254, 257, 259
Lieb, K., 30
Lieberman, J. A., 175, 179
Liebowitz, M. R., 463
Light, K. J., 461, 464
Light, R. H., 286
Li-Grining, C. P., 317
Lilenfeld, L. R., 464, 469
Lilienfeld, S. O., 74, 156, 157, 160, 343, 344, 427, 429, 433, 434, 446, 448, 449
Limosin, F., 190
Limson, R., 254, 256, 257
Lin, M. H., 434
Linares, D., 324
Linde, J. A., 220, 313
Lindner, R. M., 427, 445
Lindstrom, E., 461
Linehan, M., 274
Linehan, M. M., 28, 30, 114, 127, 278, 292, 303, 304, 305, 377, 378, 387, 388, 420, 421, 422, 481, 483, 527, 529, 530, 531, 533, 537, 538, 539, 555, 558, 572, 586, 605, 654, 656
Links, P., 422, 602
Links, P. S., 64, 287, 288, 291, 582, 659
Linnaeus, C., 27
Linnoila, M., 254, 257
Linnoila, V. M., 254
Linville, P. W., 42
Lipsey, M. W., 453, 454, 636, 637, 639
Lis, E., 305, 422
Little, G. L., 453
Liu, T., 264
Livanos, A., 504, 505
Livesley, W. J., 3, 10, 12, 13, 16, 18, 20, 21, 40, 57, 58, 59, 60, 61, 62, 63, 64, 66, 72, 75, 77, 78, 83, 91, 101, 102, 103, 114, 130, 161, 162, 216, 217, 237, 239, 240, 241, 251, 303, 305, 313, 337, 338, 343, 346, 348, 350, 352, 355, 356, 357, 367, 369, 370, 372, 374, 375, 377, 381, 382, 383, 385, 386, 388, 420, 422, 483, 484, 575, 630, 631, 632, 639, 645, 647, 648, 649, 651, 652, 653, 654, 655, 659, 671
Llewellyn, S., 490

Loas, G., 345
Löbbes, A., 567
Lobbestael, J., 101, 102, 104, 141, 143, 146, 147, 148, 231, 557, 561, 567
Lochman, J. E., 325
Lochner, C., 463
Lock, J., 463
Locke, J., 5
Locker, A., 132
Loeber, R., 219, 423
Loehr, A., 346
Loevinger, J., 12, 13, 72
Loew, T. H., 612, 613
Loft, H., 261
Logan, C., 452
Lohnes, P. R., 414
Lohr, N., 283
Lombardi, A. J., 470
Lombardi, D. N., 470
Loney, B. R., 328
Longino, H. E., 19
Looman, J., 641
Loos, W., 178
López, R., 431, 433, 437, 449
Lopez-Ibor, J. J., 256
Loranger, A., 90
Loranger, A. W., 53, 55, 90, 156, 173, 175, 176, 177, 179, 180, 199, 202, 205, 208, 342, 358, 422, 460
Lorenz, A. R., 289, 447, 452
Lösel, F., 454
Louden, J. E., 428, 452
Lowe, J. R., 377
Lowy, M., 253
Lowyck, B., 127, 377, 380
Lozovsky, D., 254
Luborsky, L., 484, 497, 636, 647, 652
Lucas, P. B., 256, 286
Lucey, J. V., 465
Lucksted, A., 600
Lucy, M., 431, 447
Lüdtke, O., 358
Ludwig, J., 204
Lukens, E., 600
Lumley, C., 469
Luscomb, R. L., 470
Luu, P., 273, 288
Luyckx, K., 108
Luyten, P., 101, 102, 103, 117, 123, 124, 125, 126, 127, 128, 130, 131, 133, 377, 380, 542, 544, 655
Lykken, D. T., 431, 432, 446, 452
Lynam, D. R., 60, 61, 63, 75, 77, 83, 163, 344, 346, 349, 427, 437, 446, 448, 449, 452, 468, 469, 634
Lynch, K. G., 305
Lynch, T. R., 289, 467, 527, 539, 656
Lyons, J. S., 503
Lyons, M., 175, 180
Lyons, M. J., 173, 179
Lyons-Ruth, K., 126, 575, 576
Lyons-Ruth, R., 420, 422
Lyoo, I. K., 274

MacCallum, R. C., 39
MacDonald, K., 92
Mace, C., 504, 505
Macfie, J., 231
Machleidt, W., 91
MacIntyre, J., 62
Mack, J. M., 325

Mackaronis, J. E., 412
MacKenzie, D. L., 453
MacKillop, J., 83, 163
MacKinnon, R. A., 54, 376
MacLane, C., 539
MacLeod, C., 149, 292
MacNeil, C., 606
Madeddu, F., 304, 380
Maffei, C., 116, 304
Magnus, K., 242
Magnuson, K. A., 204
Mahler, M., 117, 571
Maier, W., 175, 179, 180, 181, 182, 183, 184, 185, 186, 189, 190, 461
Main, M., 126, 127
Maina, G., 461
Maj, M., 157
Majid, S., 490
Major, L. F., 253
Malik, M. L., 378
Malinovsky-Rummell, R., 302
Malinow, K., 49
Malone, K. M., 275
Malone, S. M., 160, 433
Malouff, J. M., 74
Mancebo, M. C., 459, 463
Manetti, A., 190
Mangine, S., 55
Manhem, A., 257
Manly, J. T., 316
Mann, A., 491
Mann, J. J., 253, 259, 275
Mansfeld, E., 110
Mansour, K. M., 262
Marangell, L. B., 616
Marble, A., 412
Marci, C. D., 277
Marcia, J. E., 107, 108
Marcus, D. K., 427
Margison, F., 506
Marinangeli, M. G., 461
Marion, B. E., 449
Markon, K., 47
Markon, K. E., 58, 60, 61, 62, 65, 75, 76, 77, 80, 82, 157, 159, 160, 161, 162, 163, 205, 216, 251, 313, 350, 353, 373, 428, 437, 449, 452, 469
Markovitz, P., 482, 611
Markovitz, P. J., 611, 613, 615, 616, 618, 620, 621
Markowitz, J. C., 542
Marks, D. J., 255
Markus, H. R., 88, 93
Marquis, P., 641
Marriott, M., 490
Marsee, M. A., 324, 428, 433, 434, 435, 446
Marsh, A., 431, 432
Marsh, A. A., 432, 434
Marsh, D. M., 617
Marshall, P. J., 317
Martin, K., 465
Martin, M., 606
Martin, T. A., 37, 80
Martinez, J. M., 616
Marvin, R. S., 132
Marziali, E., 274
Marzialli, E., 114
Marzuk, P. M., 470
Maser, J., 73, 91, 357
Masley, S. A., 481
Maslin, C. A., 132

Maslow, A. H., 367
Mason, N. S., 255
Masten, A. S., 319
Masterson, J. F., 117
Mathe, A., 264
Matheny, A. P., 316
Mathews, A., 149, 292, 557, 564
Mathias, C. W., 461, 617
Mathiesen, B. B., 232, 283, 284, 285, 287, 288
Matthies, S., 289
Mattia, J. I., 157, 173
Mattis, S., 376
Matusiewicz, A. K., 158
Maudsley, H., 5
Maughan, B., 218, 301, 302, 330
Maurex, L., 288, 289, 294
Maxwell, J. C., 28
Maxwell, K., 347
May, J. V., 48
Maynard, R. E., 148
McAdams, D. P., 17, 110, 310, 317, 318, 319, 374, 670
McAleavey, A. A., 134
McArdle. J. J., 241
McBride, P. A., 253
McBurnett, K., 446
McCarthy, G., 292
McCarthy, K. S., 470
McCarthy, L., 630
McClearn, G. E., 238, 239, 242
McCloskey, M. S., 255, 259, 289
McClough, J., 376
McClough, J. F., 576
McClure, E. B., 215
McClure, M. M., 148
McCord, J., 427, 430, 445, 633
McCord, W., 427, 430, 445, 633
McCormick, B., 591
McCormick, C. M., 264
McCormick, P. M., 630
McCrae, R., 91
McCrae, R. R., 37, 39, 40, 41, 74, 75, 80, 92, 162, 198, 240, 242, 244, 311, 343, 346, 348, 369
McCrory, E. J., 327
McCutcheon, L., 220, 423, 544
McCutcheon, L. K., 219, 220, 221, 223, 492
McDavid, J. D., 199
McDermut, W., 341
McDonald, R., 332
McDougall, E., 490
McFarlane, W. R., 600, 601
McGee, B., 469
McGhee, D. E., 147
McGilloway, A., 95
McGlashan, T., 109, 209
McGlashan, T. H., 114, 157, 357, 423, 460, 462, 463
McGorry, P. D., 220
McGrother, C. W., 469
McGue, M., 159, 160, 161, 315, 429, 433, 544
McGuire, J., 630, 637
McGuire, M., 179
McHugh, P. R., 157
McKay, D., 148
McKinley, J. C., 74
McLaron, M. E., 429
McLellan, A. T., 636
McLeod, J., 664, 670

McMahon, R. J., 332, 539
McMain, S., 653
McMain, S. F., 287, 483, 485, 538, 582
McNally, R. J., 293, 304
McNaughton, N., 311
McNulty, J. L., 77, 78, 80, 162, 314, 343
McRae, K., 277
McWilliams, N., 28, 130
Mead, G. H., 491
Mead, S., 606
Meaney, M. J., 399
Measelle, J. R., 311
Medawar, P. B., 3
Mednick, S. A., 129, 330
Meehan, K. B., 16, 338, 367, 373, 649
Meehl, P. E., 9, 12, 26, 33, 158, 230
Meeren, M., 148, 294
Mehlum, L., 222
Meier, M. H., 317
Meins, E., 128, 130, 132
Meissner, S. J., 109
Mejia, V. Y., 433
Mellor-Clark, J., 503, 506
Mellsop, G., 53
Meltzer, C. C., 255, 256, 275
Meltzer, H. Y., 253
Mendelson, M., 51, 617
Mendelson, T., 539
Menninger, K., 48
Mensebach, C., 286, 293
Merckelbach, H., 294
Merikangas, K., 174, 193
Merikangas, K. R., 176, 394
Mermelstein, R., 617
Merson, S., 95
Mertens, I., 146, 291
Mervielde, I., 77, 216, 311, 312, 313, 349
Messier, C., 272
Messnick, S., 237
Mestel, R., 338, 339, 394, 402, 408, 409
Metzger, L. J., 293
Meyer, A., 48
Meyer, B., 127, 148, 571
Meyer, G. E., 148
Meyer, J. H., 255
Meyer-Lindenberg, A., 262, 327
Michel, M. K., 272
Michels, R., 376
Michie, C., 344, 428, 448, 450
Miczek, K. A., 257, 259, 262
Middeldorp, C. M., 244, 245, 246, 247
Midgley, N., 134
Miklowitz, D. J., 600, 601
Mikulincer, M., 130, 545
Miles, S. R., 48
Miller, D. J., 427
Miller, J. D., 58, 60, 61, 75, 77, 83, 163, 344, 345, 346, 349, 427, 437
Miller, K., 262, 367, 388
Miller, L. C., 375
Miller, P. R., 55, 59
Miller, S. R., 255
Miller, W. R., 632, 655, 656
Millon, T., 17, 25, 28, 34, 35, 39, 44, 48, 56, 74, 90, 302, 305, 337, 342, 374, 461, 467
Mills, J., 93
Mills, S., 262
Mills-Koonce, W. R., 132
Mineka, S., 148, 155, 157, 465
Minges, J., 179
Minuchin, S., 587

Minzenberg, M. J., 128, 276, 284
Mischel, W., 374, 380, 388, 577, 650
Mitchell, D., 447
Mitchell, D. G. V., 325, 328
Mitchell, J., 469
Mitchell, J. E., 600
Mitchell, S. A., 514
Mitropoulou, V., 258
Mitton, M. J. E., 287, 291
Mitzman, S., 504, 505
Mlačić, B., 41
Mock, J., 617
Mock, J. E., 51
Modell, A. H., 117
Modestin, J., 108, 109
Moeller, F., 290
Moeller, F. G., 254
Moeller, G., 291
Moffitt, T. E., 159, 222, 245, 324, 436
Mogg, K., 145, 292
Moltó, J., 431, 437, 449
Monahan, P., 586
Monarch, E. S., 284, 285, 287, 288
Mongomery, S. A., 614, 615
Monroe, S. M., 233, 303
Montanes, S., 431
Moon, H.-S., 93
Mooney, M. E., 460, 461
Moore, D. S., 327
Moore, T. M., 254, 256
Mor, N., 149
Moran, G. S., 132, 541
Moran, L. R., 539
Moran, P., 188, 219, 221, 491
Moretti, M. M., 233, 324, 331
Morey, L., 59, 72, 346, 459
Morey, L. C., 58, 64, 75, 82, 83, 84, 206, 207, 210, 216, 342, 350, 351, 352, 358, 380, 437, 461, 463, 468
Morf, C. C., 374
Morgan, A. B., 433, 434
Morgan, B., 264
Morgan, T. A., 75, 169, 173, 345, 543
Moritz, S., 146, 148
Morrell, W., 463
Morris, A. S., 329, 434
Morse, J. Q., 58, 208, 346, 466, 539, 664
Morse, S. B., 664
Moser, J. S., 430
Moskowitz, D., 421
Moskowitz, D. S., 209, 210, 368, 421, 664
Moss, E., 132
Moss, H. B., 254
Mrazek, P. J., 221
Muderrisoglu, S., 59
Mulder, A., 503
Mulder, R., 14, 83, 91, 223, 337, 369, 483, 485, 648
Mulder, R. T., 65, 88, 89, 91, 96, 216, 221, 373
Mullen, P. E., 302, 423
Müller, M., 129
Mullins-Sweatt, S., 61, 346, 427
Mullins-Sweatt, S. N., 38, 40, 55, 60, 61, 80
Munafo, M. R., 245
Muñoz, L. C., 328
Muñoz, R. A., 52
Munroe-Blum, H., 114
Münte, T. F., 262
Muran, J. C., 653
Murphy, D. L., 244

Murphy, G., 52
Murphy, J. M., 91
Murphy, S. E., 277, 278
Murray, H., 399
Murray, H. A., 16, 17, 283
Murray, J. B., 283
Murray, K. T., 317, 434
Murray, L., 328
Murray, P., 653
Murray-Close, D., 314
Murrie, D. C., 427, 630
Myers, E. M., 142
Myers, J., 78, 161
Myers, J. M., 242

Nadort, M., 556, 568
Nagy, G., 358
Nandi, D. N., 96
Nandi, P., 96
Nandi, S., 96
Napolitano, L., 148
Naragon-Gainey, K., 80
Narrow, W., 62
Narrow, W. E., 57, 72, 162
Nash, M. R., 305
Nater, U. M., 260
Nathan, P. J., 259
Naumann, L. P., 35, 311
Nduaguba, M., 180, 190, 193
Neacsiu, A. D., 113, 114, 538, 539
Neale, M. C., 78, 161, 238, 239, 241, 242
Nee, J., 53
Neeleman, J., 157
Neff, C., 173, 180
Neiderhiser, J. M., 242
Nelson, E. E., 215
Nelson, G., 606
Nelson, L. D., 160, 447
Nelson-Gray, R. O., 304
Nemeroff, C. B., 262, 264
Nemets, B., 617
Nesse, R. M., 19
Nesselroade, J., 199, 204
Nesselroade, J. R., 239
Nestadt, G., 157, 174, 175, 182, 183, 184, 185, 462
Nettles, M. E., 97
Neumann, C. S., 47, 344, 427, 428, 447, 448, 631
Neumann, I. D., 263
New, A. S., 128, 134, 245, 253, 254, 256, 272, 275, 276, 483
Newcorn, J. H., 255
Newman, C. F., 664
Newman, J. C., 647
Newman, J. P., 289, 428, 431, 432, 447, 450, 452
Newman, M. G., 470
Newman, S. C., 186
Newton, J., 469
Newton-Howes, G., 65, 216, 217, 218, 220, 221, 223
Ng, R. M., 466
Nicholaichuk, T., 640
Nicholaichuk, T. P., 641
Nichols, K. E., 317, 434
Nickel, M. K., 612, 613
Nicolo, G., 110, 466, 571
Nicolò, G., 649
Nieuwenhuis, S., 260
Ninan, T., 256

Nobs, M., 148, 294
Nolen-Hoeksema, S., 660
Noll, J. G., 542
Norcross, J. C., 134, 410, 635, 647, 667
Norcross, J. N., 378
Nordahl, H. M., 464
Nordin, C., 261
Norman, W. T., 37, 39
Norrie, J., 482, 484, 513, 515, 523, 524
Northoff, G., 18, 131
Norton, G. R., 469
Novotny, C., 503
Novotny, C. M., 157
Noyes, R., 158, 179
Ntzani, E. E., 161
Nunnally, J. C., 209
Nurnberg, H. G., 614, 615
Nutche, J., 274
Nuutila, A., 254

Oakley-Browne, M. A., 176
Ober, B. A., 286
Oberson, B., 109
O'Brien, B. S., 446
O'Brien, C. P., 636
Obsuth, I., 331
Ochoa, E., 59
Ochocka, J., 606
Ochsner, K. N., 272, 277
O'Connor, B. P., 75, 160, 216
O'Connor, R., 470
O'Connor, S., 434
Odbert, H. S., 37
Oesterle, S., 222
Ofrat, S., 72, 353
Ogden, T. H., 491
Ogle, C. M., 128
Ogloff, R. P., 631
Oh, K. J., 93
Oh, K. S., 88
Oiler, M. R., 337, 341
Okada, M., 342, 346
O'Keane, V., 254, 256, 465
Oldfield, V. B., 463
Oldham, J., 73, 180
Oldham, J. M., 58, 72, 73, 82, 83, 126, 157, 175, 179, 544
Olds, D. L., 222
O'Leary, K. M., 274, 283, 284, 285, 286, 287
Olino, T. M., 544
Oliver, B. R., 330
Olivier, B., 255
Oliviera, Z. M. R., 492
Olson, B. D., 317, 319
Olson, D. R., 80
Olson, L. A., 427, 444
Oltmanns, T. F., 115, 130, 148, 210, 215, 231, 314, 342, 345, 346, 461, 465
Olver, M., 635, 641
Olver, M. E., 447, 631, 633, 635, 636, 640, 641
Olvet, D. M., 160
Ono, Y., 244
Onyett, S., 95
Oorschot, M., 150
Oquendo, M. A., 259, 275
Ormel, J., 159, 163
Ormrod, R. K., 302
Orr, S., 262
Orr, S. P., 262

Oshri, A., 223
Ossorio, A. G., 32
Ost, L. G., 467
Ottavi, P., 661
Owen, A. M., 289, 290
Owen, M. T., 126
Owens, M. J., 264
Oyama, S., 230
Oyserman, D., 93, 94, 110, 111

Padesky, C. A., 515, 521
Pagan, J. L., 342
Pagano, M. E., 223, 463
Page, A. C., 346
Palm Reed, K., 485
Palmer, S., 524
Palmer, T., 630
Pals, J. L., 17, 310, 317, 318, 319, 374, 670
Panchanathan, K., 127
Panksepp, J., 18, 572
Panzak, G. L., 254
Papp, Z., 256
Parachini, E. A., 615
Paradise, A. W., 114
Pardini, D. A., 325, 330
Pare, C. M. B., 252
Parent, S., 132
Paris, J., 8, 58, 63, 66, 90, 91, 95, 96, 129,
    134, 170, 209, 210, 220, 232, 246, 251,
    254, 260, 284, 287, 288, 291, 301, 302,
    303, 304, 305, 306, 316, 357, 368, 419,
    420, 421, 422, 423, 542, 576, 664, 672
Park, J. H., 408
Park, R. J., 294
Parke, R. D., 198
Parker, G., 304, 338, 351, 369, 373
Parks, M. R., 607
Parry, G., 490, 497, 500, 502, 503, 505, 507
Partridge, T., 128
Pasalich, D., 331
Pasalich, D. S., 330, 332
Pascual, J. C., 95, 616
Pasinetti, M., 661
Passarella, T., 661
Pastor, M., 431
Patrick, C. J., 160, 161, 241, 257, 325, 326,
    332, 344, 426, 427, 428, 429, 430, 431,
    432, 433, 434, 435, 436, 437, 438, 444,
    445, 446, 447, 448, 449, 450, 451, 452
Patsiokas, A. T., 470
Patterson, C. M., 432
Paulhus, D. L., 92, 344, 427, 429, 448
Paus, T., 215
Pavlovic, Z., 258
Pavot, W., 242
Pearce, J. M. S., 4
Pearson, C. A., 468
Pearson, G., 325
Pearson, K., 36
Peat, J. K., 222
Pedapati, E. V., 492
Pedersen, G., 63, 467
Pedersen, N. L., 239, 242
Peeters, F., 294
Pepper, C. M., 143
Perez, M., 464
Perez, V., 614
Perez-Fuentes, G., 301
Perez-Rodriguez, M. M., 260
Perlin, J., 220
Perline, R., 253

Perry, J., 109
Perry, J. C., 199, 231, 305, 374
Pervin, L. A., 42
Peschardt, K. S., 325
Peters, J., 272
Peters, K. R., 146
Petersen, B., 552
Petersen, I. T., 316
Petersilia, J., 639
Peterson, A. P., 539
Peterson, C. B., 600, 601
Peterson, J. B., 75, 468
Petruzzi, C., 461
Petty, F., 261
Pfohl, B., 109, 175, 176, 179, 192, 193, 354,
    460, 462, 481, 586, 587, 591, 597
Philippot, P., 292
Philipsen, A., 289
Phillips, B. C., 42
Phillips, K., 62, 316
Phillips, K. A., 56, 420
Phillips, L., 51
Phillips, M. L., 272, 273
Phillips, T. R., 430, 433, 436, 449
Piacentini, J. C., 464
Piasecki, T. M., 159
Pick, O., 113
Pickett, K., 131
Pickles, A., 219
Pickvance, D., 501
Pierro, A., 545
Pilkonis, P., 58, 59, 60, 62, 63, 66
Pilkonis, P. A., 148, 199, 208, 210, 218, 343,
    346, 423, 469, 571, 574, 664
Pincus, A., 75
Pincus, A. L., 58, 60, 61, 62, 63, 66, 74,
    126, 163, 208, 211, 343, 345, 347, 373,
    374, 380, 381, 401, 469, 470, 571, 575
Pincus, H., 56
Pincus, H. A., 55, 57
Pinderhughes, E. E., 332
Pine, D. S., 215, 324, 325
Pine, F., 117
Pinel, P., 444
Pins, D., 161
Pinto, A., 459, 461, 462, 463, 465, 467,
    468, 469
Piper, W. E., 368, 484
Pistorello, J., 539
Pitman, R. K., 293
Pittenger, C. K., 261
Pleydell-Pearce, C. W., 293
Plomin, R., 126, 238, 239, 242, 243, 304,
    327, 330, 436
Plutchik, R., 114, 271
Poggioli, M., 492
Polaschek, D. L., 446
Polich, J., 160
Pollak, J. M., 461, 467
Pollock, B. G., 80, 81, 353
Pollock, P., 495, 497
Pollock, P. H., 492
Pollock, V. E., 305
Pontefract, A., 560
Pool, M., 492
Poole, J. H., 284
Popolo, R., 664
Popper, K. R., 45
Porges, S. W., 398
Porporino, F. J., 453
Porter, S., 325, 326, 330, 333

Portera, L., 470
Porteus, S. D., 290
Posner, M., 287
Posner, M. I., 273, 288, 311
Posternak, M. A., 157
Potegal, M., 262
Potenza, M. N., 471
Potter, J., 198, 217, 311, 315
Pouchet, A., 161
Poulton, R. G., 242
Powell, N., 325
Powers, A. D., 129
Poy, R., 431, 437, 449
Poythress, N. G., 427, 428, 449, 451, 452
Prado, C. E., 328
Prescott, C. A., 78, 161, 242, 459
Presly, A. J., 7
Presnall, J. R., 346
Preti, E., 380
Pretzer, J., 145, 146
Pretzer, J. L., 377, 571
Price, J. C., 255
Price, K., 252
Price, L. H., 129
Priebe, K., 158
Priebe, S., 530
Pritchard, J. C., 5, 445
Procacci, M., 110, 571, 649
Prochaska, J. O., 134, 410, 635, 667
Proietti, J. M., 343
Pryor, L. R., 345
Przybeck, T., 243
Przybeck, T. R., 243, 251, 370
Pull, C., 55
Putnam, F. W., 542
Putnam, K. M., 271, 272, 275

Qin, P., 131
Quas, J. A., 128
Queern, C., 286
Quilty, L. C., 80, 81, 216, 353, 437, 468
Quine, W. V. O., 33
Quinlan, D. M., 469
Quinsey, V. L., 427
Quinton, D., 219
Quirion, R., 59

Rabe-Hesketh, S., 463, 470
Rabung, S., 134
Racker, H., 550
Rader, T. J., 284
Radua, J., 272
Raes, F., 294
Rafaeli, E., 209, 555, 556, 557, 560, 561,
    563, 565, 668
Rahm, B., 273
Raine, A., 129, 219, 254, 330, 343, 433, 436
Raj, B. A., 614
Raja, M., 462
Ram, N., 208, 381
Ramel, W., 277
Ramesar, R., 247
Ramos-Fuentes, M. I., 260
Rapee, R. M., 93, 94
Rapoport, J. L., 464
Raskin, R. N., 345
Rasmussen, S. A., 459, 463
Rastam, M., 463
Ratcliff, K. S., 174, 175
Rauch, S. L., 277
Raudenbush, S. W., 199

Ray, J., 325
Rea, M. M., 601
Read, S. J., 375
Realo, A., 93
Reardon, K., 220
Rebar, A. L., 381
Reddington, A., 465
Reed, G. M., 220
Reeves, M., 142
Refseth, J. S., 134
Regier, D., 394
Regier, D. A., 57, 72, 162, 163, 174, 175, 178, 182, 183, 190, 305, 419, 450
Reich, D. B., 199, 207, 423, 513, 604, 612
Reich, J., 158, 175, 180, 181, 182, 183, 184, 185, 186, 189, 190, 191, 192, 193
Reich, W., 7
Reichborn-Kjennerud, T., 161, 315, 464
Reid, T., 294
Reider, R., 180
Reisch, T., 274
Reiss, D. J., 601
Reitan, R. M., 286
Remington, M., 192
Renneberg, B., 148, 288, 294
Renner, F., 143, 555, 556, 561
Rentrop, M., 291
Renwick, S. J. D., 452
Repetti, R. L., 126
Ressler, K. J., 129
Revelle, W., 148, 465
Reynolds, S., 155
Reynolds, S. K., 346
Reynolds, S. M., 60, 63, 160, 343
Rhee, S. H., 436
Rhines, H. M., 330
Rhodes, T., 324, 325
Rice, K. G., 469
Rice, M. E., 427, 453, 629, 630
Richards, J. A., 600
Ricoeur, P., 665
Riddell, A. D. B., 346
Ridolfi, M. E., 482, 600
Riemenschneider, A., 108
Rigozzi, C., 91
Rijkeboer, M. M., 557, 560, 567
Rijsdijk, F. V., 327
Rilling, J. K., 262
Rimmele, U., 470
Rinck, M., 147
Rind, B., 304
Riolo, S. A., 318
Risch, N., 245
Riso, L. P., 469
Ritschel, L. A., 534
Rizvi, S. L., 534
Ro, E., 77, 80, 81, 313, 352, 353, 354, 355, 356
Robbins, T. W., 272
Roberts, A., 90, 177, 422
Roberts, B. W., 74, 198, 199, 210, 217, 218, 302, 314, 315, 319, 358, 359, 468
Roberts, R., 631
Robertson, A., 253
Robertson, C. D., 304
Robinowitz, C., 62
Robins, C. J., 481, 527, 539, 654
Robins, E., 12, 13, 14, 52, 459
Robins, L., 7, 303
Robins, L. N., 56, 156, 174, 175, 305, 427, 445

Robins, R. W., 198, 199
Robinson, A., 539
Robinson, D., 453
Robinson, G. E., 247
Robinson, K. D., 453
Robinson, P., 133
Rocca, G., 617
Rocco, P. L., 601
Roche, M. J., 381
Rodgers, S., 129
Rodriguez, G., 324
Rodriguez, M. A., 113
Rodríguez-Santos, L., 260
Roffman, J. L., 277
Rogers, C. R., 130, 134
Rogers, J. H., 157
Rogers, R. D., 289
Rogosa, D., 199
Rogosch, F. A., 128, 223, 309, 316, 542
Rohde, P., 219, 462
Rohlfing, J. E., 470
Roisman, G. I., 126, 319
Rollnick, S., 632, 655, 656
Rolls, E., 291
Romanoski, A. J., 157, 174
Ronchi, P., 463
Ronningstam, E., 58, 60, 61, 63, 66
Ronningstam, E. F., 28
Rooke, S. E., 74
Roose, S. P., 278
Rorschach, H., 283
Rosell, D. R., 255
Rosenbery, S. E., 612
Rosenfield, D., 332
Rosengren, D. B., 655, 656
Rosenhan, D. L., 8, 52
Rosenthal, D., 258
Rosenthal, R., 203
Rosfort, R., 649, 665
Rosnick, L., 73, 180
Rosnow, R. L., 203
Ross, R. R., 453, 454, 637
Ross, S. R., 429
Rossi, A., 461
Rossi, G., 64, 216, 342
Rossier, J., 77, 91, 348
Rössler, W., 129
Rossouw, T. I., 222, 542, 551
Roth, A., 503
Rothbart, M. K., 216, 311, 316, 317, 434, 513
Rothschild, L., 342, 461
Rothweiler, J. R., 399
Rounsaville, B. J., 25, 57, 162
Rousseau, D., 132
Roussos, P., 63
Rowe, D. C., 304
Rowe, J. B., 273
Rowland, M. D., 638
Rubinstein, T. J., 431
Rubio, G., 291
Ruff, R., 284, 285, 286, 287
Ruff, R. M., 286
Rufino, K., 630
Ruge, J., 130
Ruggero, C., 82, 163
Ruggero, C. J., 420
Ruigrok, P., 244
Ruiz, M. A., 74
Ruiz-Sancho, A., 600
Rule, N., 220

Ruocco, A. C., 232, 246, 272, 274, 283, 284, 285, 286, 287, 288, 289, 290, 295
Rüsch, N., 261, 274
Ruscio, A. M., 149
Rush, B., 445
Rushton, J. P., 34
Russakoff, L.M., 175, 179
Russell, J., 288, 306, 420
Russell, J. J., 209, 210, 368, 664
Russell, S., 611
Russell-Archambault, J., 421
Rutherford, B. R., 278
Rutherford, E., 292
Rutter, M., 7, 218, 219, 301, 302, 303, 306, 374, 423
Ryan, R. M., 96
Ryder, A. G., 57
Ryle, A., 104, 114, 481, 489, 490, 491, 492, 495, 496, 497, 501, 503, 504, 505, 506, 507, 508, 523

Saavedra, A. S., 286
Sabbarton-Leary, N., 4
Sabol, S. Z., 244
Sachsse, U., 274, 284
Sadikaj, G., 209, 664
Sadler, L., 222
Safer, D., 539
Safer, D. L., 539
Safran, J. D., 653
Safren, S., 539
Sahakian, B., 463
Saintong, J., 132
Saiz-Ruiz, J., 256
Sakado, K., 470
Sala, M., 274
Salekin, R., 452, 629, 630, 636
Salekin, R. T., 330, 429, 431, 449, 453
Salet, S., 146
Salins, C., 600
Salkovskis, P. M., 463
Salmon, K., 326
Salmon, T. W., 48
Salvatore, G., 661, 664
Salzman, C., 620
Samaco-Zamora, M. C., 17, 25, 337
Samenow, S. E., 453
Sameroff, A. J., 218
Samstag, L. N., 653
Samuel, D. B., 60, 61, 73, 80, 82, 83, 163, 216, 313, 342, 346, 358, 468
Samuel, S., 108, 113, 115, 118
Samuels, J., 175, 176, 180, 181, 182, 183, 184, 185, 186, 189, 190, 191, 463, 464
Samuels, J. F., 157
Sanderson, C., 14, 346, 369, 388, 656
Sanderson, C. J., 74
Sandler, J., 496
Sanislow, C. A., 155, 208, 468
Sanislow, C. A., III, 469
Sansone, R. A., 465
Sartorius, N., 47, 49, 55, 175, 180, 342
Sass, H., 284
Sato, T., 91
Saucier, G., 41, 44
Saudino, K. J., 242, 315, 316
Saulsman, L. M., 346
Savitz, J., 247
Sawyer, A. M., 222
Sawyer, A. T., 149
Sawyer, M. G., 429

Sayer, A. G., 199
Saykin, A. J., 285
Saykin, A. S., 284
Scalia-Tomba, G. P., 253
Scarpa, A., 254
Schacht, T. E., 497
Schaefer, C., 617
Schaefer, E., 32, 399
Schaefer, E. S., 399
Schafer, R., 108
Schalling, D., 252
Scheier, M. F., 103, 374, 375
Schell, A. M., 433
Scher, C. D., 514
Schermerhorn, A. C., 316
Schilling, L., 150
Schinka, J. A., 74
Schippers, G. M., 538
Schlüter-Müller, S., 113
Schmahl, C., 30
Schmahl, C. G., 274, 275, 276
Schmeck, K., 113
Schmidinger, I., 263
Schmidt, F., 74, 163
Schmidt, N. B., 560
Schmitt, T. A., 59
Schmitt, W., 452
Schmitt, W. A., 452
Schmitz, N., 412
Schneider, K., 5, 6, 7
Schnell, K., 21, 278, 582
Schobre, P., 150
Schoenwald, S. K., 638
Schotte, C., 64, 216
Schotte, C. K., 463
Schouten, E., 142, 146
Schramm, A. T., 319
Schroeder, M. L., 10, 39, 91, 237, 240, 370, 647
Schuermann, B., 288, 289
Schulenberg, J. E., 218
Schulsinger, F., 258
Schulz, K. P, 255
Schulz, P. M., 258
Schulz, S. C., 257, 258, 614, 615, 619, 621
Schulze, L., 146, 274
Schumacher, J. A., 255
Schuppert, H. M., 222
Schuster, J. P., 190
Schutte, N. S., 74
Schutzbach, C., 95
Schwartz, J. L. K., 147
Schwartz, S. J., 108
Schwarz, J., 285
Scott, L. N., 126
Seeley, J. R., 219, 462, 544
Seeman, T. E., 126
Segal, D. L., 342
Segal, Z. V., 514
Segarra, P., 431, 437, 449
Sellbom, M., 430, 431 433, 436, 437, 447, 449, 465
Selten, J. P., 95
Seltzer, M. H., 466
Semerari, A., 110, 466, 571, 649
Seo, D., 257, 264
Serafini, G., 264
Seres, I., 286
Serin, R., 641
Sestoft, D., 221
Sexton, M. C., 305

Shafran, R., 469
Shahar, G., 469
Shalev, I., 262
Shallice, T., 290
Shamay-Tsoory, S. G., 263
Shapiro, D., 375, 465, 467
Shapiro, J. L., 337, 341
Sharma, L., 469
Sharma, P., 463
Sharp, C., 231, 319
Shaver, P. R., 130, 302, 304, 397
Shaw, D. M., 252
Shaw, D. S., 317
Shaw, I., 555
Shaw, I. A., 483
Shea, M., 205, 206, 207
Shea, M. T., 55, 56, 155, 358, 469
Shedler, J., 58, 59, 60, 61, 63, 66, 130
Sheehan, D. V., 614, 615
Sheehy, M., 54
Sheese, B. E., 311
Sheldon, A., 466
Sheldon, K. M., 374
Shelton, R. C., 616
Shenk, C. E., 533, 542
Sher, K. J., 177, 421
Sherry, S. B., 469
Shields, S. M., 77, 80, 343
Shine, J., 631
Shiner, R., 231
Shiner, R. L., 216, 217, 219, 223, 233, 309, 310, 311, 312, 313, 314, 315, 316, 317, 318, 319
Shmueli-Goetz, Y., 126
Shoda, Y., 374, 380, 388, 577, 650
Shrout, P. E., 58, 216
Sieberer, M., 91
Siegal, B. V., 258, 259
Siegrist, J., 470
Sieswerda, S., 143, 146, 148, 149, 291, 292, 561
Siever, J., 104
Siever, L., 126, 258
Siever, L. J., 63, 128, 158, 245, 246, 251, 252, 255, 258, 259, 263, 264, 272, 275, 276, 303, 420
Sigvardsson, S., 303
Silberschmidt, A. L., 314
Silbersweig, D., 274, 275, 276, 283, 582
Silbersweig, D. A., 277
Silk, K. R., 199, 207, 271, 272, 275, 283, 357
Silva, P. A., 159, 217
Silverman, J., 258
Silverman, M. H., 104, 105, 155
Simenson, J. T., 342
Simeon, D., 253, 254, 260, 263
Simmonds-Buckley, M., 506
Simms, E. E., 80
Simms, L. J., 10, 77, 80, 81, 220, 313, 342, 350, 357, 370
Simoneau, T. L., 600
Simons, A. D., 233, 303
Simonsen, E., 13, 47–48, 58, 61, 74, 77, 78, 83, 162, 221, 231, 232, 283, 284, 285, 288, 294, 342, 370, 417
Simourd, D. J., 629
Simpson, E. B., 620
Simpson, H. B., 461, 462, 463
Simpson, S. G., 481
Singer, B., 484, 647

Singer, J. D., 199
Singer, M. T., 283, 419, 421
Sisemore, T. B., 142
Sivakumaran, T., 463
Sjodin, A.-K., 258
Sjödin, I., 261
Sjöstrand, L., 256
Skårderud, F., 542
Skeem, J., 324, 328, 431, 631
Skeem, J. L., 329, 428, 446, 450, 452, 453
Skiba, W., 600
Skinner, H. A., 12, 13
Skodol, A., 58, 59, 60, 61, 62, 64, 65, 66, 175, 180, 219
Skodol, A. E., 53, 58, 59, 60, 61, 62, 63, 64, 72, 73, 76, 80, 82, 83, 84, 111, 124, 126, 130, 156, 162, 199, 216, 218, 219, 220, 223, 350, 351, 353, 373, 437, 459, 461, 471, 575, 613, 619, 620
Skodol, A. W., 319
Skowron, E. A., 401
Slade, A., 132
Slade, T., 159
Slaney, R. B., 469
Slaughter, J. R., 143
Slof-Op, M. C. T., 245
Slovic, P., 15
Slutske, W. S., 317
Smack, A., 220
Smith, A., 606
Smith, G., 110, 600
Smith, L., 260
Smith, L. E., 56
Smith, L. K., 469
Smith, P., 452
Smith, R. S., 302
Smith, S., 639
Smith, S. S., 450, 452
Smith, T. B., 261, 611
Smith, T. E., 350
Smith, T. L., 338, 339, 342, 394, 405
Sneed, J. R., 107, 319
Snyder, J., 470
Soderstrom, H., 257, 258
Soegaard, U., 285
Soeteman, D. I., 462, 483
Soler, J., 539, 615, 620, 623
Sollberger, D., 108, 109, 111, 116, 118
Soloff, P. H., 232, 255, 256, 258, 271, 274, 275, 277, 305, 369
Solomon, P., 600
Solomon, R. C., 271
Someah, K., 367, 388
Sookman, D., 209, 368, 421
Sorabji, R., 109
Sorbye, O., 412
Sorenson, S., 461
Soto, C. J., 35, 217, 311, 315
Sourander, A., 452
South, S. C., 10, 148, 315, 357, 370, 461, 465
Southwick, S. M., 260
Spain, S. E., 449
Specht, M. W., 128, 144
Spence, S. H., 94
Spencer, S. J., 147
Sperber, D., 132, 133, 546
Sperling, M. B., 350
Sperry, L., 466
Spielberger, C., 611, 612, 613
Spinelli, S., 399

Spinhoven, P., 143, 148, 149, 294, 484, 555
Spirito, A., 469
Spitzer, C., 130
Spitzer, R., 180
Spitzer, R. L., 52, 53, 54, 55, 56, 58, 59, 156, 175, 178, 405, 445
Sponheim, S. R., 314
Spoont, M. R., 254
Sprich, S., 539
Sprock, J., 284, 286, 287, 289
Srivastava, S., 80, 198, 217
Sroufe, L. A., 128, 310, 318, 576
St. John, D., 481, 586, 587, 591, 593
Stacey, R. S., 252
Stacks, A. M., 128
Staebler, K., 146
Stahl, Z., 617
Stanford, M. S., 461
Stanghellini, G., 649, 665
Stangl, D., 175, 179, 192
Stanley, B., 263, 264, 274
Stanley, J. H., 449
Stanley, M., 252, 253
Starcevic, V., 460
Starke, D., 470
Startup, M., 294
Stasik, S., 75, 80, 81, 353
Stattin, H., 319, 427, 450
Stauffer, O., 95
Steele, H., 126, 127, 132, 541, 544
Steele, M., 127, 132, 541, 544
Steiger, H., 470
Steil, R., 158
Stein, D. J., 19, 286, 287, 465
Stein, H., 127, 544
Stein, J. L., 262
Stein, K. F., 113
Steinberg, L., 215
Steiner, J., 659
Steinglass, J. E., 461
Stengel, E., 51, 52
Stennett, B., 60
Stepp, S. D., 58, 208, 218, 219, 232, 423, 544, 664
Stern, A., 419
Stern, B., 115, 379
Stern, B. L., 108, 574, 575
Stern, D. N., 110, 492
Stern, E., 277
Stevens, A., 285
Stevenson, H. W., 93
Stewart, J. W., 463
Stewart, S. E., 342
Stickle, T. R., 326
Stigler, S., 199
Stiglmayr, C., 288
Stiles, T. C., 403, 464, 466
Stiles, W. B., 110, 503
Stinson, F. S., 187
St.-Laurent, D., 132
Stockdale, K. C., 636
Stoffers, J., 420
Stoffers, J. M., 216
Stoll, A. L., 617
Stone, M., 7, 636
Stone, M. H., 423
Stoolmiller, M., 470
Stopa, L., 144
Storch, E. A., 462
Stouthamer-Loeber, M., 423
Stowell-Smith, M., 495

Strack, S., 343
Strahan, E. J., 39
Strange, R., 500
Strauss, J. L., 466
Strawn, J. R., 492
Streiner, D., 582
Strengl, D., 109
Stricker, G., 350, 647
Strickland, C. M., 431, 437, 447, 449
Strimpfel, J. M., 231
Stringer, D., 220, 313
Stringer, D. M., 313
Strober, M., 463, 464
Strosahl, K. D., 661
Strotmeyer, S. J., 275
Stuart, S., 461
Suarez, A., 483, 538, 586, 605
Suddath, R. L., 600
Suedfeld, P., 629
Sullivan, E. A., 450
Sullivan, G. M., 260
Sullivan, H. S., 399
Summerfield, D., 96
Susman, V. L., 175, 179
Sutandar-Pinnock, K., 469
Sutton, S. K., 452
Svaldi, J., 289
Svartberg, M., 403, 466
Svrakic, D., 243
Svrakic, D. M., 251, 370
Swann, A., 290
Swann, A. C., 261, 291, 611
Swanson, M. C., 186
Swartz, M., 174, 175, 183, 189, 191
Swedo, S. E., 464
Swiergiel, A. H., 259
Swirsky-Sacchetti, T., 284, 285, 286, 287
Swogger, M. T., 451, 452
Szasz, T. S., 52

Tackett, J. L., 6, 158, 159, 171, 210, 215, 216, 217, 219, 220, 221, 223, 231, 251, 312, 313, 314, 316, 318, 319, 349, 429
Takeichi, M., 91
Takemoto-Chock, N. K., 469
Tang, C. Y., 128, 276
Tang, Y., 311
Tangney, J. P., 101, 109
Tannock, R., 287
Target, M., 126, 127, 129, 130, 131, 495, 541, 544, 649
Tasca, G. A., 135
Tata, P., 292, 524
Tatar, J. R., 329
Tatsuoka, M. M., 37
Tau, M., 258
Taub, N. A., 469
Taylor, A. E., 178
Taylor, J., 142
Taylor, M. A., 481
Taylor, M. L., 469
Taylor, S. E., 126, 262, 263, 545
Tchanturia, K., 463, 470
Teasdale, J., 294
Tebartz van Elst, L., 274
Tebes, J. K., 606
Tekin, S., 273
Telch, C. F., 539
Telch, M. E., 560
Tellegen, A., 78, 80, 287, 319, 348
Tempelmann, C., 262

ten Haaf, J., 148
Tengström, A., 429
Tenney, N. H., 463
Terburg, D., 264
Teta, P., 347
Teti, D. M., 400
Teti, L. O., 272
Tewes, U., 285
Thái, S., 429
Thake, A., 505
Thatcher, D. L., 219
Thede, L. L., 315, 342
Theobald, E., 148, 294
Thimm, J. C., 144
Thomaes, K., 277
Thomas, A., 434
Thomas, G. V., 55
Thomas, K. M., 60, 63, 80, 81, 82, 129, 163, 353, 437
Thomas, P., 161, 483, 504
Thompson, A., 429
Thompson, K., 222, 223
Thompson, K. N., 6, 171, 215, 231
Thompson, L., 378
Thompson, M., 325
Thompson, R., 262
Thompson, R. A., 271, 272, 660
Thompson, R. R., 262
Thompson-Brenner, H., 157, 503
Thomsen, M. S., 232, 283, 284, 285, 286, 288
Thoren, P., 253
Thorndike, E. L., 203
Thornton, D., 453
Thornton, L. C., 325
Thorsteinsson, E. B., 74
Thurston, A., 429
Tickle, J. J., 650
Tielbeek, J. J., 436
Tiersky, L. A., 574
Tillfors, M., 158
Timmerman, M. E., 41
Tolfree, R. J., 150
Tomko, R. L., 177, 421
Tomlinson-Keasey, C., 198
Tondo, L., 261
Tooby, J., 17, 18
Toomey, J. A., 449
Toplak, M., 287, 288
Torgersen, S., 90, 175, 176, 180, 181, 182, 183, 184, 185, 186, 190, 191, 219, 241, 242, 422, 460, 461, 462, 464
Toth, S., 576
Toth, S. L., 128, 542
Totterdell, P., 506
Toulmin, S., 375, 649
Tracey, T. J., 470
Tracey, T. J. G., 470
Tracy, J., 256
Tragesser, S. L., 343
Trainor, J., 606
Tran, C. F., 525
Trapnell, P. D., 92
Träskman, L.; 253, 256
Traskman-Bendz, L., 252, 253
Trautwein, U., 358
Travers, C., 285, 286, 287, 290
Travers, R., 453
Travis, M. J., 273
Treasure, J., 463, 470, 499
Treeby, M. S., 328

Trestman, R. L., 258
Trevarthen, C., 492
Triandis, H. C., 88, 93, 94, 95
Tricou, B. J., 253
Triebwasser, J., 63, 272
Trikalinos, T. A., 161
Tritt, K., 611, 620
Troisi, A., 17
Tromofovitch, P., 304
Tromp, N. B., 220, 313, 314, 319
Trull, T., 343, 369
Trull, T. J., 57, 59, 60, 162, 173, 175, 177, 180, 181, 182, 183, 184, 185, 186, 187, 188, 189, 190, 191, 199, 209, 210, 251, 346, 421, 422, 437, 446
Trzesniewski, K. H., 198
Tsai, G. E., 261
Tschacher, W., 274
Tsuang, D. W., 236, 237
Tsuang, M. T., 236, 237
Tuck, J. R., 253
Tuckey, M., 132
Tufekcioglu, S., 653
Tull, M. T., 128, 318
Tupek, D. A., 586
Turecki, G., 462
Turkheimer, E., 9, 17, 210, 230, 231, 342, 345, 346, 461
Turkheimer, E. F., 210
Turnbull-Donovan, W., 469
Turner, H. A., 302
Turner, R. M., 538
Tversky, A., 15, 25
Tylee, A., 491
Tynes, L. L., 600
Tyrer, F., 469
Tyrer, P., 7, 14, 47, 48, 59, 65, 72, 77, 83, 90, 91, 95, 174, 177, 192, 216, 220, 221, 337, 343, 355, 369, 420, 422, 482, 502, 512, 513, 516, 523, 524, 648
Tyrer, P. J., 65
Tyrka, A. R., 129

Uher, R., 245
Ulbert, R., 412
Uliaszek, A. A., 288, 469
Ullrich, S., 90, 177, 422, 462
Unckel, C., 285
Unoka, Z., 286
Unterrainer, J. M., 290
Upmanyu, V. V., 470
Ureno, G., 612
Üstün, T. B., 177
Uzefovsky, F., 262

Vadi, M., 93
Vaidyanathan, U., 160, 325, 428, 431, 433, 447
Vaillant, G. E., 175, 178, 181, 183, 184, 185, 186, 188, 191, 374
Valentino, K., 542
Van Asselt, A., 555, 556, 568
van Asselt, A. D., 483
van Calker, D., 470
Van De Wiele, L., 77
van den Berg, J. F., 342
van den Bergh, H., 560
van den Bosch, L., 538, 539
van den Brink, W., 538
Van den Broeck, J., 162
van den Hout, M. A., 145, 149

van den Noortgate, W., 218, 231, 314
Van der Does, A., 294
Van der Does, A. J. W., 148, 294
van der Kolk, B. A., 231, 305
Van Der Merwe, L., 247
Van Dyck, R., 294
Van Essen, D. C., 161
Van Genderen, H., 557
Van Heeringen, C., 77
van Honk, J., 264
van IJzendoorn, M. H., 132, 143
van Kampen, D., 80, 348, 349
Van Leeuwen, K., 77, 216, 218, 231, 312, 313, 314, 349
Van Leeuwen, K. G., 311
Van Limbeek, J., 118
van Megen, H. J., 463
van Oorschot, R., 255
van Praag, H. M., 256
van Reekum, R., 286, 287, 291
Van Ryzin, M. J., 401
van Vreeswijk, M. F., 149, 561
van Wel, B., 586, 592, 597
van Wijk-Herbrink, M., 143
van Wijk-Herbrink, M. F., 143
Van Zalk, M., 319
Van Zalk, N., 319
Vanderbleek, E. N., 337, 341
Vandereycken, W., 471
Vanman, E. J., 433
Vaquero-Lorenzo, C., 260
Varga, S., 9
Varghese, F., 53
Vazire, S., 210, 345
Vaz-Leal, F. J., 260
Veen, G., 148
Venables, N., 431, 433
Venables, N. C., 428, 431, 433, 434, 436, 437, 438, 447, 451
Venables, P. H., 129, 330
Venta, A., 231, 319
Verbeke, L., 314
Verbraak, M. J. P. M., 586
Verheul, R., 10, 58, 60, 63, 64, 73, 82, 83, 115, 116, 118, 148, 221, 313, 352, 368, 374, 382, 462, 483, 538
Vermetten, E., 274
Vermote, R., 127, 377, 380
Vernon, P. A., 18, 162, 216, 231, 235, 237, 239, 240, 251, 385, 422
Verona, E., 428, 450
Vertommen, H., 471
Vertommen, S., 146, 291
Vezina, P., 261
Viding, E., 126, 219, 324, 327, 330, 435, 436
Viechtbauer, W., 74, 198, 217, 315, 358
Vieta, E., 600
Vignoles, V. L., 108
Villasenor, V. S., 612
Villemarette-Pittman, N. R., 461, 471
Vincent, G. M., 453
Vinogradov, S., 284, 465
Virgilio, J., 253
Virkkunen, M., 254, 257, 259, 262
Vitale, J., 450
Vitale, J. E., 452
Voderholzer, U., 460
Vollebergh, W. A. M., 159
von Ceumern-Lindenstjerna, I.-A., 293
von dem Knesebeck, O., 470
von Eye, A., 132

von Knorring, L., 461
Voss, W. D., 452
Vrshek-Schallhorn, S., 464
Vujanovic, A. A., 343, 614, 615
Vurro, N., 380
Vygotsky, L. S., 491, 492

Wachs, T. D., 316, 317
Wade, T. D., 469
Wager, T. D., 278
Wagner, A., 252
Wagner, D. V., 222
Wagner, S., 613
Wakefield, J. C., 338, 356, 374
Walcott, G., 90
Waldman, I., 219
Waldman, I. D., 156, 436
Walker, E. F., 128
Wall, P. M., 272
Wall, T. D., 431, 433, 437, 447
Waller, G., 505
Waller, N. G., 80
Waller, R., 324, 330, 333
Walsh, D., 175, 179
Walsh, K. W., 287
Walsh, Z., 452
Walter, M., 114
Walters, G., 631
Walters, G. D., 452, 453, 630
Walton, H. J., 7
Walton, J. C., 262
Walton, K. E., 74, 198, 217, 315, 358, 468
Wampold, B. E., 134, 571
Wang, K. T., 469
Wang, M., 315, 316
Wang, Z., 435
Ward, C. H., 51, 617
Warner, J. C., 60
Warner, L., 109
Warner, M. B., 218, 461, 468
Waterhouse, B. D., 259
Waters, A., 144
Waters, C. K., 19
Waters, F., 164
Watson, C., 57
Watson, D., 60, 65, 74, 75, 76, 78, 79, 80, 81, 155, 159, 160, 162, 163, 216, 251, 313, 350, 353, 354, 373, 437
Watson, D. B., 353
Watson, J., 544
Watson, J. S., 546
Watters, E., 96
Weaver, T., 220
Webber, M., 555
Webber, M. A., 483
Weber, C., 469
Weber, E. U., 461
Webster, D. M., 545
Wechsler, D., 283, 284, 285
Wedge, R. F., 630
Wedig, M., 421
Weertman, A., 142, 146, 147
Wegener, D. T., 39
Weinberg, I., 420
Weinberger, D. R., 164
Weinstein, L. N., 252
Weir, J. M., 630
Weisbrod, M., 148, 294
Weishaar, M., 555, 557
Weishaar, M. E., 114, 142, 377, 481, 512, 514, 587, 664

## Author Index

Weiss, D. J., 350
Weiss, L. G., 77
Weissman, M., 174, 193
Weissman, M. M., 174, 179, 394
Weisz, J. R., 222
Welburn, K., 560
Welch, S. S., 274
Wells, J. E., 175, 176, 182, 183, 190
Wender, P. H., 258
Wentz, E., 463
Werble, B., 7
Werner, E. E., 302
Wessel, I., 148, 294
Westen, D., 59, 108, 113, 115, 116, 130, 157, 283, 318, 368, 576
Westenberg, H. G., 463
Weston, C. G., 318
Weston, D., 503
Wetzel, R. D., 243
Wetzler, S., 57
Whalen, D. J., 218, 220
Wheatman, S. R., 114
Wheaton, M. G., 459
Whitaker, D. J., 114
Whitcomb, J. M., 342
White, C. N., 303, 420
White, R., 277
White, S. F., 324, 325, 428, 432, 433, 434, 435
Whitehead, C., 370
Whitehead, J. T., 454
Whiteside, S. P., 469
Whitfield, C., 247
Whitlock, F. A., 5
Whitty, P., 503
Widaman, K., 198
Widaman, K. F., 209
Widiger, T., 13
Widiger, T. A., 8, 10, 38, 40, 47, 48, 53, 54, 55, 56, 57, 58, 59, 60, 61, 62, 63, 64, 66, 73, 74, 75, 76, 77, 78, 80, 82, 83, 109, 157, 160, 162, 184, 216, 251, 313, 341, 342, 343, 346, 349, 368, 369, 370, 377, 417, 420, 427, 437, 446, 468, 634
Widom, C., 302
Widom, C. S., 129, 329
Widows, M. R., 344, 427, 429, 446, 448, 449
Wiesmann, T., 539
Wiggins, J., 75
Wiggins, J. S., 239, 370, 373, 399
Wilberg, T., 63, 467
Wilbram, M., 507
Wilcock, G. K., 261
Wilder, J., 203
Wildgoose, A., 504, 505
Wilkinson, R., 131
Wilkinson-Ryan, T., 108, 115
Willett, J. B., 199, 208, 210, 211, 357, 581

Willi, J., 672
Williams, G., 289
Williams, J. B., 156
Williams, J. B. W., 52, 53, 54, 55, 175, 178, 405, 445
Williams, J. M. G., 294
Williams, K., 222
Williams, K. M., 344
Williams, O. B., 378
Wilson, D., 132, 133
Wilson, D. B., 453, 454, 546, 637, 639
Wilson, E. O., 34
Wilson, K. G., 661
Wilson, P. T., 52, 56
Winfield, I., 174
Wingenfeld, K., 276
Wink, P., 347
Winstead, D. K., 600
Winston, A., 466
Winter, D., 292
Wirtz, P. H., 469, 470
Wisman, M., 127, 544
Witkiewitz, K., 332
Wittenberg, L. G., 650
Wolkowitz, O. M., 257
Wolpe, J., 663
Wonderlich, S., 469
Wonderlich, S. A., 600
Wong, S., 453, 629, 630, 631, 633, 634, 635, 636, 639, 641
Wong, S. C. P., 428, 447, 482, 629, 630, 631, 633, 635, 636, 637, 640, 641
Wood, D., 319, 358
Wood, P. K., 177, 421
Woods, K., 314
Woodward, N. D., 259
Woody, G. E., 636
Woolfenden, S. R., 222
Wootton, J. M., 446
Worley, C., 630
Wormworth, J. A., 39, 240
Wozniak, J., 261
Wright, A. G., 80, 81, 82, 373
Wright, A. G. C., 76, 78, 163, 170, 197, 208, 210, 211, 343, 350, 437
Wu, K. D., 77, 342
Wyche, M. C., 129
Wygant, D. B., 431, 447, 449

Yager, J., 62
Yaggi, K. E., 664
Yalch, M. M., 163
Yancey, J. R., 434, 438
Yang, J., 90
Yang, M., 90, 177, 422, 630
Yao, J. K., 254
Yates, W., 158, 180, 190, 193
Yeh, E. K., 305
Yen, S., 273

Yeomans, F., 118, 483, 571, 573, 583
Yeomans, F. E., 116, 377, 388, 481, 571, 572, 581, 587
Yeung, D. P. H., 252
Yik, M. S., 92
Yildirim, B. O., 264
Yochelson, S., 453
Yoder, C. Y., 284
Young, D., 221, 420
Young, J., 512, 514, 520, 521, 522, 523, 525, 555, 668
Young, J. C., 329
Young, J. E., 114, 142, 143, 144, 146, 377, 466, 481, 513, 514, 515, 521, 555, 556, 557, 558, 560, 561, 563, 564, 565, 566, 567, 587, 589, 664, 669
Young, L. J., 435
Young, M. L., 630
Young, S. E., 433, 451
Yovel, I., 148, 465
Yue, D. N., 292
Yun, R. J., 574

Zaboli, G., 289
Zachar, P., 12, 14, 19, 25
Zak, P. J., 263, 435
Zakzanis, K. K., 246, 272
Zanarini, M., 73, 343
Zanarini, M. C., 30, 127, 157, 199, 201, 202, 207, 209, 288, 292, 303, 304, 342, 357, 420, 421, 422, 423, 513, 576, 601, 604, 605, 612, 614, 615, 617, 618, 619, 621
Zanna, M. P., 147
Zboyan, H. Z., 616
Zeier, J. D., 431
Zeigler-Hill, V., 142
Zelkowitz, P., 284
Zerubavel, N., 481, 527, 654
Zetzsche, T., 274
Zheng, W., 91
Ziegenbein, M., 91
Ziegler, S., 433
Zigler, E., 51
Zilboorg, G., 48
Zimmerman, D. J., 260
Zimmerman, M., 53, 58, 59, 60, 62, 63, 66, 73, 109, 157, 169, 173, 174, 175, 176, 179, 180, 181, 182, 183, 184, 185, 186, 187, 189, 190, 192, 198, 208, 209, 341, 342, 354, 358, 420, 423, 461, 467, 543
Zimmerman, M. E., 221
Zimmermann, J., 10, 83, 351, 369, 370, 388
Zimowski, M., 199
Zink, C. F., 262
Zoccolillo, M., 219
Zonderman, A. B., 244
Zuckerman, M., 347, 348
Zuroff, D. C., 209, 368, 469
Zweig-Frank, H., 304, 305, 422, 423

# Subject Index

Note. *f* or *t* following a page number indicates a figure or a table.

Abandoned Child mode, 561, 562*t*. *See also* Schema mode
Abandonment, 370, 559*t*, 560
Abuse, 128–129, 144, 219, 559*t*. *See also* Childhood experiences
Acceptance, 527, 532–533, 586, 662
Acceptance and commitment therapy (ACT), 467
Activity, 672–673
Adaptation, 17–18, 127, 374–375
Addiction, 499, 667. *See also* Substance abuse
Addiction personality disorder, 50*t*
Adolescence.
   antisocial personality disorder and, 433
   assessment and, 449–450
   Big Five personality model and, 216–217
   borderline personality disorder and, 293
   callous–unemotional (CU) traits and, 324–325, 330
   development of identity and, 116
   developmental psychopathology model and, 233, 319–320
   diagnosis and, 220–221
   dialectical behavior therapy (DBT) and, 539
   dimensional approaches and, 313
   identity diffusion and, 113–114, 116
   mentalization-based treatment (MBT) and, 222, 551
   obsessive–compulsive personality disorder and, 463
   overview, 215, 220, 231
   personality impairment and, 318–319
   personality traits and, 310–314, 312*t*, 315
   precursor signs and symptoms, 218–220
   prevalence and, 221
   psychoeducation and, 603–604
   stability and change and, 217–218

Adult Attachment Interview (AAI), 126, 544, 581
Adulthood
   antisocial personality disorder and, 433
   Big Five personality model and, 216–217
   development of identity and, 116
   developmental psychopathology model and, 319–320
   dimensional approaches and, 313
   early intervention and, 221–222
   overview, 215
   perfectionism and, 469
   personality impairment and, 319
   personality traits and, 310–314, 312*t*, 314, 315
   prevalence and, 221
   stability and change and, 217–218
   *See also* Developmental factors
Affect
   diagnosis and, 30–31
   identification and focus of, 549
   mentalization and, 124, 125*f*. *See also* Mentalization
   numbing and, 326, 561
   regulation of, 576
   representation of, 542
   schema-focused therapy (SFT) and, 560
Affective instability (AI), 104–105, 246, 252, 417, 421, 422
Affiliation, 41, 370*t*, 371*t*, 435, 446
Age, 190, 193
Agency, 101, 109–110
Aggression
   antisocial personality disorder and, 429, 436, 451
   assessment and, 373, 379–380
   borderline personality disorder and, 275
   callous–unemotional (CU) traits and, 233, 324, 325–326, 332–333
   genetic factors and, 246

   historical overview of classification systems and, 50*t*
   neurotransmitter function and, 252, 253–254, 256, 257–258, 259–260, 261–262
   overview, 104–105, 417
   pharmacotherapy and, 611–612, 616, 617, 623
   psychopathy and, 428
   risk factors and, 219
   systems training for emotion predictability and problem solving (STEPPS) and, 593
   trait assessment and, 370
   transference-focused psychotherapy (TFP) and, 574*t*
Agreeableness
   cultural factors and, 91–92
   developmental factors and, 312, 312*t*
   developmental psychopathology model and, 319–320
   five-factor model (FFM) and, 39–40
   overview, 41–42, 74
   traits relevant to personality disorders, 315
   *See also* Five-factor model (FFM)
Alcohol Use Disorder and Associated Disabilities Interview Schedule—DSM-IV (AUDADIS-IV), 175*t*, 177
Alternative FFM measure (A-FFM), 348
Alternative Five, 77*t*
Alternative Model
   assessment and, 344, 350–354, 357, 359, 373
   guide to, 80–83, 81*t*
   obsessive–compulsive personality disorder and, 460
   overview, 26, 27, 40, 41–42
   theoretical orientations and, 31
   transference-focused psychotherapy (TFP) and, 572
   *See also Diagnostic and Statistical Manual of Mental Disorders* (DSM-5)

Altruistic behavior, 374–375
Anger
  antisocial personality disorder and, 434
  cognitive analytic therapy (CAT) and, 499
  interpersonal reconstructive therapy (IRT) and, 396
  neurotransmitter function and, 257
  pharmacotherapy and, 611–612, 617
  psychoeducation and, 603
  schemas and, 560, 561
Angry Child mode, 561, 562t. See also Schema mode
Angry Protector mode, 562t
Anhedonia, 59–60, 505
Anorexia nervosa, 463, 499. See also Eating disorders
Antagonism
  antisocial personality disorder and, 446
  developmental factors and, 313
  developmental psychopathology model and, 319–320
  dimensional approaches and, 77t
  factor hierarchy and, 78f
  overview, 417
Antagonism (ANT) versus agreeableness domain, 76
Anticonvulsants, 611–613, 628. See also Pharmacotherapy
Antidepressants, 618–620, 623, 624, 626. See also Pharmacotherapy; Selective serotonin reuptake inhibitor (SSRI)
Antiepileptics, 622f, 623. See also Pharmacotherapy
Antipsychotics, 623, 626–628. See also Atypical antipsychotics; Pharmacotherapy
Antisocial behaviors
  callous–unemotional (CU) traits and, 233, 325–326, 333
  cognitive-behavioral therapy for PDs (CBTpd) and, 515–516
  comorbidity and, 160
  cultural factors and, 90–91
  neurotransmitter function and, 252, 256–257, 259–260
  risk factors and, 219
  treatment and, 482
  See also Antisocial personality disorder (ASPD); Violence
Antisocial personality disorder (ASPD)
  assessment and, 368, 447–450, 448t
  borderline personality disorder and, 420
  callous–unemotional (CU) traits and, 233, 325
  childhood and adolescence and, 220, 305
  classification systems and, 47–48
  clinical correlates and, 186, 187, 189
  cognitive-behavioral therapy for PDs (CBTpd) and, 512, 513, 524–525, 524t
  comorbidity and, 159, 160, 163, 450–451
  course and outcomes and, 452–453
  cultural factors and, 90–91
  demographic correlates, 189–191
  developmental factors and, 215
  developmental psychopathology model and, 317
  diagnosis and, 368
  dimensional approaches and, 446–447

early conceptualizations of, 5
  early intervention and, 222
  emotion regulation and, 273
  epidemiology and, 173, 174, 176, 178, 193
  etiology and, 431–437
  future editions of classification systems and, 63–64
  genetic factors and, 240
  historical overview of, 50t, 51–52, 426–427, 444–445
  integrated approach and, 381
  interpersonal reconstructive therapy (IRT) and, 394–395
  interpretational bias and, 147
  neurotransmitter function and, 252, 254
  overview, 417, 426–429, 444, 445–446, 648
  parental psychopathology and, 303
  prevalence, 182, 183t, 184, 450
  risk factors and, 219
  schema-focused therapy (SFT) and, 556, 561, 567
  structural analysis of social behavior (SASB) model and, 405, 406t–407t, 409t
  subdimensions of, 429, 437–438
  subtypes of psychopathy and, 451–452
  treatment and, 453–454, 484, 630
  triarchic model, 429–431
  violence reduction treatment and, 636, 637–638
  in young people, 221
  See also Psychopathy
Antisocial Process Screening Device (APSD), 427, 428, 448t, 449
Antisocial psychopathic personality disorder, 50t
Antisocial reaction personality disorder, 50t
Anxiety
  antisocial personality disorder and, 452
  assessment and, 385
  callous–unemotional (CU) traits and, 325, 326
  comorbidity and, 160
  diagnostic classification and, 21
  factor hierarchy and, 79
  genetic factors and, 244
  interpersonal reconstructive therapy (IRT) and, 396
  mentalization and, 126
  neurotransmitter function and, 252, 257
  overview, 104–105, 371t, 417
  perfectionism and, 469
  personality impairment and, 319
  pharmacotherapy and, 616, 623
  structural analysis of social behavior (SASB) model and, 408–409, 409t
  trait assessment and, 370, 370t
  transference-focused psychotherapy (TFP) and, 581
  See also Anxiety disorders
Anxiety disorders
  antisocial personality disorder and, 450–451
  attentional bias and, 145
  borderline personality disorder and, 420
  comorbidity and, 159, 187
  neurotransmitter function and, 260
  obsessive–compulsive personality disorder and, 463
  parental psychopathology and, 303

risk factors and, 219
  schema-focused therapy (SFT) and, 556
  structural analysis of social behavior (SASB) model and, 408–409, 409t
  See also Anxiety
Approval needs, 370t, 372t, 559t
Arginine vasopressin (AVP), 262–263. See also Neurotransmitter systems
Arousal
  cognitive-behavioral therapy for PDs (CBTpd) and, 517–518
  comorbidity and, 163
  mentalization and, 125f, 126, 542, 544–545
  neurotransmitter function and, 259
Assertiveness, 446, 637
Assessment
  Alternative Model and, 350–354
  antisocial personality disorder and, 427, 447–450, 448t
  Big Five personality model and, 216
  borderline personality disorder and, 287–291
  characterizing personality dysfunction, 368–375, 370t, 371t–372t
  cognitive analytic therapy (CAT) and, 491–492, 492
  cognitive-behavioral therapy for PDs (CBTpd) and, 515
  cultural factors and, 97
  diagnostic classification and, 21, 22
  dialectical behavior therapy (DBT) and, 530–531
  dimensional approaches and, 77t
  DSM-5-III Trait Model and, 80–82, 81t
  emotion regulation and, 277
  epidemiology and, 191–192
  five-factor model (FFM) and, 74–76, 77t
  future research and, 354–359
  identity diffusion and, 115
  interpretational bias and, 146
  longitudinal studies and, 198, 202, 203, 204, 209–210
  mentalization and, 126, 543
  methods for, 375–387, 377t, 383t, 386t
  neuropsychological mechanisms and, 284–287, 295
  overview, 337–339, 341–344, 342t–343t, 359, 367, 388–389
  psychopathy and, 447–450, 448t, 629
  schema-focused therapy (SFT) and, 523, 557, 557–558
  systems training for emotion predictability and problem solving (STEPPS) and, 593
  transference-focused psychotherapy (TFP) and, 572–575, 573f, 574t
  treatment and, 387–388
  validity and, 11–14
  violence reduction treatment and, 634–636, 635f, 640
  See also Assessment measures; Diagnosis
Assessment measures
  Alternative Model and, 350–354
  cognitive analytic therapy (CAT) and, 491–492
  list of, 342t–343t
  new or revised instruments, 344–350
  overview, 341–344
  See also Assessment; individual measures

Assumptions, 141–142, 513–515, 514f
Attachment
  anxious attachment, 126
  attachment needs, 370t, 371t, 558
  attachment relationships, 124
  borderline personality disorder and, 422
  callous–unemotional (CU) traits and, 324–325, 330–331
  childhood adversity and, 127–129
  deactivating strategies, 126
  epistemic trust and, 132–133
  hyperactivating strategies, 126
  identity and, 112t
  interpersonal reconstructive therapy (IRT) and, 399, 410
  mentalization and, 103, 126–127, 132–133, 541–542, 544–545
  overview, 417
  schema-focused therapy (SFT) and, 558
  theoretical orientations and, 32
  transference-focused psychotherapy (TFP) and, 576–577, 581
Attachment figures
  interpersonal reconstructive therapy (IRT) and, 396–397, 398, 410
  mentalization and, 124, 132, 545
Attachment theory, 302–303, 514
Attachment-based perspectives, 229
Attention seeking, 59–60
Attentional bias, 145–146, 145f, 149, 292–293. See also Biases; Cognitive biases
Attentional Network Test (ANT), 287–288
Attentional processes
  antisocial personality disorder and, 434
  borderline personality disorder and, 287–288, 294–295
  integrated modular treatment and, 663
  mentalization-based treatment (MBT) and, 542
  neurobiological factors and, 272–273
  neurotransmitter function and, 259
  overview, 19, 141–142
Attention-deficit/hyperactivity disorder (ADHD), 159, 261, 528, 539
Atypical antipsychotics, 613–617, 626–628. See also Pharmacotherapy
Autobiographical memory, 145f, 293–294. See also Memory processes
Automatic mentalizing, 124, 125f. See also Mentalization
Automatic thoughts, 518–519
Autonomy, 32, 112t, 113, 558, 559t
Avoidance
  avoidant attachment, 370t
  avoidant modes, 562t
  cognitive-behavioral therapy for PDs (CBTpd) and, 518
  integrated modular treatment and, 662, 665, 666
  obsessive–compulsive personality disorder and, 460
  overview, 142–143
  trait assessment and, 370t
  See also Social avoidance
Avoidant personality disorder (AVPD)
  clinical correlates and, 186
  cognitive theories and, 142
  comorbidity and, 158
  cultural factors and, 90, 93–94

demographic correlates, 189–191
developmental factors and, 216
epidemiological studies, 178, 179
five-factor model (FFM) and, 76
genetic factors and, 240
historical overview of classification systems and, 52
interpersonal reconstructive therapy (IRT) and, 394–395, 409–410, 413
interpretational bias and, 146
memory bias and, 149
obsessive–compulsive personality disorder and, 463
overview, 34–35, 417
prevalence, 184, 185t
schema-focused therapy (SFT) and, 567, 568, 569
structural analysis of social behavior (SASB) model and, 409t
Awareness, 589, 661–662

Beck Depression Inventory (BDI), 505
Behavior
  antisocial personality disorder and, 433, 438
  behavioral control, 528
  callous–unemotional (CU) traits and, 324–325, 332
  cognitive-behavioral therapy for PDs (CBTpd) and, 516, 519–520
  confident-narcissistic personality and, 35t
  cultural factors and, 88, 89, 96
  development of new behaviors in CBTpd, 516
  identity and, 112t, 116
  immigration and modernization and, 95–96
  integrated modular treatment and, 654, 667–669, 671–673
  overview, 28–29
  risk factors and, 219
  schemas and, 561, 564
  violence reduction treatment and, 633–634, 640
  See also Antisocial behaviors; Conduct problems; Criminal behavior
Behavioral classification, 92
Behavioral diagnostic criteria, 30–31. See also Diagnostic classification
Behavioral genetics, 315–316, 435–436. See also Genetic factors
Behavioral inhibition, 311, 316–317
Behavioral interventions
  behavior modification approaches, 453, 516, 519–520, 668–669
  behavior skills training, 590–591
  behavioral experiments, 523, 563, 671–672
  chain analysis, 534
  integrated modular treatment and, 657f
  overview, 527, 531, 532
  schema-focused therapy (SFT) and, 557, 565
Behavioral responses, 259
Behavioral theory, 30
Belief-Desire Reasoning Task, 127–128
Beliefs, 79, 141–142, 142f, 150, 518–519. See also Core beliefs
Between-session contact, 529

Biases
  attentional bias and, 145–146, 145f, 149, 292–293
  borderline personality disorder and, 293–294
  cognitive biases and, 144–148, 145f, 560
  longitudinal studies and, 202–203
  memory bias, 148–149
  memory bias and, 293–294
  overview, 150
  schema-focused therapy (SFT) and, 560
Big Five personality model
  cultural factors and, 91–92
  developmental factors and, 216–217, 311–312, 312t, 313
  developmental psychopathology model and, 319–320
  lexical hypothesis and, 42–43
  overview, 26, 37–44, 93
  See also Five-factor model (FFM)
Binge-eating disorder (BED), 467, 528, 539. See also Eating disorders
Biological factors
  antisocial personality disorder and, 433
  callous–unemotional (CU) traits and, 326–327, 330–331
  case formulation and, 398–399
  childhood adversity associated with mental disorders and, 302
  cognitive analytic therapy (CAT) and, 492
  comorbidity and, 160–164
  developmental psychopathology model and, 319
  future directions in, 246–247
  interpersonal reconstructive therapy (IRT) and, 398–399, 410
  moral development and, 329
  obsessive–compulsive personality disorder and, 464
  overview, 17–18, 229, 232–233, 513
  personality traits and, 310
  trait assessment and, 370
  See also Neurobiological factors
Biophysical domain, 28–29, 35t, 44
Biopsychosocial models, 126, 558
Biosocial theory, 127, 243–244, 531, 532–533, 537–538
Bipolar affective disorder (BPAD), 247
Bipolar disorder
  borderline personality disorder and, 420
  cognitive analytic therapy (CAT) and, 491
  dialectical behavior therapy (DBT) and, 528, 539
  identity diffusion and, 113
  pharmacotherapy and, 617, 618–619
Bivariate models, 104–105, 155–156, 158–159, 158t
Boldness, 446–447, 451
Borderline Evaluation of Severity over Time (BEST) scale, 591–592
Borderline personality disorder (BPD)
  assessment and, 368, 379
  attentional bias and, 145
  childhood adversity associated with, 303–306
  clinical correlates and, 186, 187, 188
  clinical implications, 423

cognition and emotion interactions and, 292–294
cognitive analytic therapy (CAT) and, 491, 494–503, 495f, 498f, 504–506, 504t, 507
cognitive flexibility and, 286–287
cognitive theories and, 150, 151
cognitive-behavioral therapy for PDs (CBTpd) and, 512, 523–524, 524t, 525
comorbidity and, 157, 158, 163
coping styles and, 143
critique of the BPD construct, 419–421
cultural factors and, 90
demographic correlates, 189–191
developmental factors and, 215, 217
diagnosis and, 31, 368
dialectical behavior therapy (DBT) and, 527, 530, 531, 538–539
early conceptualizations of personality disorder and, 5
early intervention and, 222
emotion regulation and, 273, 274–276, 277, 278
epidemiological studies, 174
epidemiology and, 176, 178, 179, 422
etiology and, 230, 422–423
five-factor model (FFM) and, 75–76
genetic factors and, 240, 315–316
historical overview of, 50t, 52, 55, 419
identity and, 108–109, 114, 115–116
integrated approach and, 381
interpersonal reconstructive therapy (IRT) and, 394–395, 409–410
interpretational bias and, 146
longitudinal studies and, 210
measuring discrete cognitive abilities, 287–291
memory bias and, 148–149
mentalization and, 124–125, 125f, 126, 129, 131, 132, 134
mentalization-based treatment (MBT) and, 541, 542, 544, 546, 549, 551, 552
neuropsychological mechanisms and, 232, 274–276, 283–284, 284–287, 294–295
neurotransmitter function and, 252, 253, 254, 257, 260, 261–262, 263
obsessive–compulsive personality disorder and, 462, 463, 470
outcomes and course of, 423
overview, 28, 123, 417, 620, 648
pharmacotherapy and, 611–624, 619t, 622f
prevalence, 182, 183t
psychoeducation and, 600–609, 602t
risk factors and, 219
schema-focused therapy (SFT) and, 555, 556, 561, 567–568
stability and change and, 315
structural analysis of social behavior (SASB) model and, 405, 406t–407t, 409t
systems training for emotion predictability and problem solving (STEPPS) and, 586–587, 588, 589, 590, 592–595
theoretical orientations and, 30
transference-focused psychotherapy (TFP) and, 571, 574, 578, 580–581, 582–583
treatment and, 278, 482, 483–484
in young people, 231
Borderline personality features, 94–95, 102–103, 108–109, 114, 574t
Boundaries, 558, 633–634
Brief psychodynamic therapy (BPT), 505
Bulimia, 528, 539. See also Eating disorders
Bully and Attack mode, 563t
Buss-Durkee Hostility Inventory (BDHI), 254

C1AB chains, 398, 408, 409, 412
Callousness
 antisocial personality disorder and, 446, 451
 factor hierarchy and, 79
 interpersonal reconstructive therapy (IRT) and, 394–395
 overview, 76
 trait assessment and, 370t
 violence reduction treatment and, 636
 See also Callous–unemotional (CU) traits
Callous–unemotional (CU) traits
 antisocial personality disorder and, 433, 434, 435, 436, 437
 assessment and, 449–450
 attachment process and, 330–331
 clinical features, 325–326
 emotional processing and, 327–328
 environmental and genetic influences, 327
 etiology and, 326–327
 future directions and, 332–333
 moral development and, 328–329
 overview, 233, 324–325, 333
 parenting and, 330
 psychopathy and, 428
 trauma and, 329–330
 treatment and, 331–332
 See also Callousness
Cambridge Gambling Task, 289
Caregiving, 132–133, 325, 328, 330–331. See also Parenting
Case conceptualization, 163, 557
Case formulation
 assessment and, 367, 377–378
 dialectical behavior therapy (DBT) and, 530–531, 531
 integrated approach and, 381
 interpersonal reconstructive therapy (IRT) and, 395–399, 409–410, 413
 mentalization-based treatment (MBT) and, 543
 overview, 388
 reliability, specificity, and sensitivity of, 397–398
 schema-focused therapy (SFT) and, 557–558
 transference-focused psychotherapy (TFP) and, 572–575, 573f, 574t
Case management, 483–484, 537, 639–640
Categorical approaches to classification
 antisocial personality disorder and, 451–452
 assessment and, 357–359, 367, 389
diagnosis and assessment and, 368
future research and, 83–84
limitations of, 72–74
neurotransmitter function and, 264
See also Classification systems
Causal factors, 149, 230. See also Etiology
Chain analysis, 533, 534
Challenging the patient, 548, 590
Change
 comorbidity and, 162–164
 dialectical behavior therapy (DBT) and, 527, 532–533
 integrated modular treatment and, 646, 655–656, 658f, 659, 666–670, 672
 mentalization-based treatment (MBT) and, 546
 overview, 650
 principles of change, 546, 563–564, 577
 schema-focused therapy (SFT) and, 563–564
 transference-focused psychotherapy (TFP) and, 577, 580, 581
 violence reduction treatment and, 640
 See also Change in personality disorders
Change in personality disorders
 assessment and, 357–359
 cognitive analytic therapy (CAT) and, 494
 developmental psychopathology model and, 320
 longitudinal studies and, 205–208, 207f
 overview, 197, 208–211, 217–218
 traits relevant to personality disorders, 314–315, 316
 See also Change; Course of personality disorders
Child Psychopathy Scale (CPS), 427, 448t, 449
Childhood
 antisocial personality disorder and, 433, 434–435
 assessment and, 449–450
 Big Five personality model and, 216–217
 borderline personality disorder and, 291
 callous–unemotional (CU) traits and, 324–325, 326, 333
 development of identity and, 116–117
 developmental psychopathology model and, 233, 319–320
 diagnosis and, 220–221
 differentiating traits from other aspects of personality functioning, 318
 dimensional approaches and, 313
 obsessive–compulsive personality disorder and, 462
 overview, 215, 220, 231
 perfectionism and, 469
 personality and, 310–314, 312t, 318–319
 precursor signs and symptoms, 218–220
 prevalence and, 221
 psychoeducation and, 602–604
 stability and change and, 217–218
 traits relevant to personality disorders, 314, 315, 316–317
 See also Childhood experiences; Developmental factors

Childhood experiences
  associated with mental disorders, 301–303
  associated with personality disorders, 303–306
  callous–unemotional (CU) traits and, 325, 333
  cognitive-behavioral therapy for PDs (CBTpd) and, 518
  developmental psychopathology model and, 320
  gene–environment interactions and, 306
  mentalization and, 126, 127–129, 544–545
  overview, 232–233, 306
  personality impairment and, 319
  precursor signs and symptoms, 218–219
  psychoeducation and, 602–604
  schemas and, 144
  transference-focused psychotherapy (TFP) and, 576–577
  *See also* Childhood
Children in the Community Self-Report Scales (CIS-SR), 175*t*, 176–177
Children in the Community Study (CIC), 200–208, 200*t*, 218, 219, 221
Circumplex model, 29, 29*f*, 32–33, 36*f*
Classification systems
  comorbidity and, 162–164
  cultural factors and, 88, 89
  epidemiology and, 173–174
  epistemic choices for structuring, 26–29
  five-factor model (FFM) and, 38
  future directions and, 63–65, 83–84
  historical overview of, 48–63, 50*t*
  overview, 25–26, 47–48, 65–66
  transference-focused psychotherapy (TFP) and, 572
  *See also* Diagnosis; Diagnostic classification; Dimensional approaches to classification; *individual diagnostic manuals and their editions*
Clinical assessment. *See* Assessment
Clinical correlates, 186–189, 192–193
Clinical interviews
  measures for, 342*t*–343*t*
  overview, 376, 377*t*, 380, 389
  schema-focused therapy (SFT) and, 557
  stability and change and, 357–358
  structural interview, 378–380
  transference-focused psychotherapy (TFP) and, 574–575
  *See also* Assessment
Clinical utility of PD categories, 72, 73–74
Clinician factors
  assessment and, 375–376, 388–389
  integrated modular treatment and, 652–654
  interpersonal reconstructive therapy (IRT) and, 412
  mentalization-based treatment (MBT) and, 550–551
  schema-focused therapy (SFT) and, 564–565
  systems training for emotion predictability and problem solving (STEPPS) and, 593–594
  violence reduction treatment and, 633–634
  *See also* Therapist stance

Cluster A personality disorders, 219, 504, 504*t*. *See also individual personality disorders*
Cluster B personality disorders, 219, 252, 504–506, 504*t*, 555. *See also individual personality disorders*
Cluster C personality disorders, 219, 504*t*, 506, 555, 556. *See also individual personality disorders*
Cognitive analytic therapy (CAT)
  borderline personality disorder and, 494–503, 495*f*, 498*f*
  case example of, 496–497
  early intervention and, 222
  features of, 493–494
  integrated modular treatment and, 658*f*
  outcome evidence and, 503–507, 504*t*
  overview, 481–482, 483–484, 489–492, 507–508
  theoretical orientations and, 492–493
Cognitive biases, 144–148, 145*f*, 560. *See also* Biases
Cognitive functioning, 104–105, 283–284, 420, 422
Cognitive interventions
  assessment and, 377–378
  integrated modular treatment and, 657*f*, 658*f*, 668
  schema-focused therapy (SFT) and, 563–564, 565
Cognitive modification, 533, 535–536
Cognitive processes
  cognitive disorganization, 246
  cognitive distortion, 535–536, 563
  cognitive dysregulation, 370*t*, 371*t*, 385
  comorbidity and, 163
  development of new cognitions in CBTpd, 516
  diagnosis and, 30–31
  flexibility, 124–125, 286–287, 295
  integrated modular treatment and, 663–664
  interactions of with emotion, 292–294
  mentalization and, 124, 125*f*
  overview, 28–29, 149, 277
  schema-focused therapy (SFT) and, 560
  schemas and, 132, 650–651
  self and, 102–103
Cognitive psychology, 110–111
Cognitive restructuring, 466, 563, 637, 657*f*
Cognitive theory
  causal status and, 149
  clinical implications, 149–150
  cognitive biases and, 144–148, 145*f*
  overview, 30, 31–32, 44, 141–143, 142*f*, 150–151
Cognitive therapy
  assessment and, 377–378
  comparisons among the cognitive therapies and, 520, 521*f*
  medical model and, 19
  obsessive–compulsive personality disorder and, 466
  treatment methods, 522–523
  violence reduction treatment and, 637–638
Cognitive-affective processing (CAP) system, 388, 452, 577
Cognitive-behavioral therapy (CBT)
  antisocial personality disorder and, 453–454
  comparisons among the cognitive therapies and, 520, 521*f*

  emotion regulation and, 278
  integrated modular treatment and, 657*f*
  interpersonal reconstructive therapy (IRT) and, 410, 411*f*, 412
  intervention strategies and methods of, 515–520, 516*f*–517*f*
  obsessive–compulsive personality disorder and, 466
  overview, 143, 150, 512–513, 650
  research support for, 523–525, 524*t*
  schema-focused therapy (SFT) and, 556, 568
  systems training for emotion predictability and problem solving (STEPPS) and, 587
  theoretical orientations and, 513–515, 514*f*
  treatment methods, 522–523
  violence reduction treatment and, 636, 637–638
  *See also* Cognitive-behavioral therapy for PDs (CBTpd)
Cognitive-behavioral therapy for PDs (CBTpd)
  comparisons among the cognitive therapies and, 520, 521*f*
  overview, 481–482, 484, 512–513, 525
  research support for, 523–525, 524*t*
  theoretical orientations and, 513–515, 514*f*
  therapeutic relationship and, 520–522
  treatment methods, 522–523
  *See also* Cognitive-behavioral therapy (CBT)
Coherence, 112*t*, 116, 118, 131–132
Collaboration
  cognitive analytic therapy (CAT) and, 490–491
  cognitive-behavioral therapy for PDs (CBTpd) and, 521–522
  dialectical behavior therapy (DBT) and, 537
  integrated modular treatment and, 652–653, 654–655
  mentalization-based treatment (MBT) and, 543, 549–550
  violence reduction treatment and, 638, 639
Collaborative Longitudinal Study of Personality Disorders (CLPS)
  assessment and, 357–358
  emotion regulation and, 273
  historical overview of classification systems and, 59, 60
  methodological differences among studies, 201–208
  obsessive–compulsive personality disorder and, 461, 462–463, 468
  overview, 200*t*, 201, 210
Collectivism
  cultural factors and, 94–95, 97
  future directions and, 97–98
  identity and, 108
  individualism-collectivism cultural syndrome and, 93–94
  modernization and, 95
Commitments, 112*t*–113*t*, 667
Common factor approaches, 134, 647–648
Communication, 134–136, 536–537, 589–590, 637, 652
Communities that Care system, 222

Comorbidity
  antisocial personality disorder and, 450–451
  assessment and, 357
  biological factors and, 160–164
  borderline personality disorder and, 420
  change and, 162–164
  clinical correlates and, 186–189
  cognitive analytic therapy (CAT) and, 499–500
  diagnosis and assessment and, 339
  dialectical behavior therapy (DBT) and, 528, 538–539
  interpersonal reconstructive therapy (IRT) and, 409–410
  limitations of categorical approaches and, 72, 73
  mentalization-based treatment (MBT) and, 545
  neurotransmitter function and, 260
  obsessive–compulsive personality disorder and, 463
  overview, 156–160, 158t, 192–193
  risk factors and, 219
  structural analysis of social behavior (SASB) model and, 403, 408–409, 409t, 413
  See also Co-occurance of PD and other mental disorders
Comparative Psychotherapy Process Scale (CPPS), 412
Competence in CAT measure (CCAT), 502–503, 505–506
Complication/scar model, 158, 158t. See also Bivariate models
Composite International Diagnostic Interview (CIDI), 175t, 176
Compulsive personality disorder, 34–35, 50t
Compulsivity
  developmental factors and, 312t, 313–314, 319–320
  diagnostic classification and, 20–21
  dimensional approaches and, 77t
  overview, 417
  trait assessment and, 370t
  validity and, 13–14
Computerized Adaptive Test of Personality Disorder (CAT-PD), 350
Conduct disorder
  antisocial personality disorder and, 429, 436, 446
  comorbidity and, 159
  developmental factors and, 216
  parental psychopathology and, 303
  See also Conduct problems
Conduct problems
  antisocial personality disorder and, 433, 436
  callous–unemotional (CU) traits and, 326, 332–333
  overview, 371t
  trait assessment and, 370t
  See also Behavior; Conduct disorder
Confident-narcissistic personality, 35, 35t
Conners' Continuous Performance Test–II (CPT), 288, 290–291
Conscientiousness
  antisocial personality disorder and, 434–435
  cultural factors and, 91–92
  developmental factors and, 311–312, 312t, 316–317, 319–320
  obsessive–compulsive personality disorder and, 468–469
  overview, 41–42, 74, 371t, 417
  personality traits and, 315, 370t
  See also Five-factor model (FFM)
Consolidation, 379, 517, 669–670
Constraint, 311–312, 417, 469
Construct Repertory Test (CRT), 42–43
Consultation, 529–530, 537
Containment, 646, 657f, 659–660
Contempt towards others, 446, 636
Contextual influences, 316–317, 320
Contingency management, 533, 534–535, 546–547
Control, 470, 636, 660–666
Controlled mentalizing, 124, 125f. See also Mentalization
Co-occurance of PD and other mental disorders, 104–105. See also Comorbidity
Cooperativeness, 244, 374–375
Coping styles
  assessment and, 379–380
  callous–unemotional (CU) traits and, 325
  clinical implications, 150
  cognitive biases and, 145f
  cognitive-behavioral therapy for PDs (CBTpd) and, 518
  memory bias and, 149
  overview, 19, 142–143
  schema-focused therapy (SFT) and, 557, 560
CORDS label, 397, 398, 409–410, 413
Core beliefs, 141–142, 142f, 513–515, 514f, 518, 522–523. See also Beliefs
Core Conflict Relationship Theme (CCRT), 497
Cortisol functioning, 260, 262
Countertransference, 497, 550
Course of personality disorders
  antisocial personality disorder and, 452–453
  borderline personality disorder and, 423, 604
  developmental psychopathology model and, 320
  obsessive–compulsive personality disorder and, 462–463
  overview, 170–171, 208–211, 217–218, 223, 231
  psychoeducation and, 604
  See also Change in personality disorders; Longitudinal studies; Outcomes; Stability of personality disorders
Criminal behavior
  antisocial personality disorder and, 452–453
  neurotransmitter function and, 254, 259–260
  overview, 629
  treatment and, 629–641, 635f
  violence reduction treatment and, 631–632, 634–638, 635f
  See also Antisocial behaviors; Behavior; Violence
Cultural factors
  classification systems and, 89
  clinical considerations, 97
  DSM personality disorders across, 90–91
  five-factor model (FFM) and, 39–40
  future directions and, 97–98
  identity and, 107–108
  immigration and modernization and, 95–96
  individualism-collectivism cultural syndrome and, 93–94
  overview, 41, 88–89, 96–97
  personality and cultural interactions and, 94–95
Cyclothymic personality disorder, 50t, 52

Daily diary card. See Diary cards
Dangerous behavior, 324–325
Danish Adult Reading Test (DART), 285
Deceitfulness, 394–395, 429, 636
Decision making, 288–290, 294–295, 375–376
Deductive theory, 31–32
Defense mechanisms, 114, 379, 574t
Demographics correlates, 189–191, 192–193
Dependency, 13–14, 345, 373, 385, 559t, 650, 666
Dependent personality disorder (DPD)
  clinical correlates and, 186, 189
  cognitive-behavioral therapy for PDs (CBTpd) and, 514
  comorbidity and, 158
  demographic correlates, 189–191
  epidemiological studies, 178
  five-factor model (FFM) and, 76
  genetic factors and, 240
  historical overview of classification systems and, 50t, 52, 59–60, 61
  interpretational bias and, 146
  overview, 28, 417
  prevalence, 184, 185t
  schema-focused therapy (SFT) and, 567, 568, 569
  structural analysis of social behavior (SASB) model and, 409t
  theoretical orientations and, 30, 32–33
Depression
  antisocial personality disorder and, 450
  borderline personality disorder and, 420
  cognitive analytic therapy (CAT) and, 504
  cognitive-behavioral therapy for PDs (CBTpd) and, 515, 525
  comorbidity and, 157, 159
  cultural factors and, 94–95
  dialectical behavior therapy (DBT) and, 528, 539
  emotion regulation and, 277
  genetic factors and, 244
  interpersonal reconstructive therapy (IRT) and, 396
  memory bias and, 294
  negative thoughts and, 519
  neurotransmitter function and, 257, 260
  obsessive–compulsive personality disorder and, 461, 463
  perfectionism and, 469
  pharmacotherapy and, 256, 277–278, 616, 617, 618–619, 620, 623
  schema-focused therapy (SFT) and, 555, 556
  structural analysis of social behavior (SASB) model and, 408–409, 409t
  transference-focused psychotherapy (TFP) and, 581

Depressive personality disorder (DPD), 32–33, 56–57, 221
Detached Protector mode, 561, 562*t*. *See also* Schema mode
Detached Self-Soother/Self-Stimulator mode, 562*t*
Detachment, 76, 77*t*, 78*f*, 325, 373
Developmental factors
 antisocial personality disorder and, 432–435, 433
 borderline personality disorder and, 422–423
 callous–unemotional (CU) traits and, 332, 333
 childhood adversity and, 127–129, 301
 cognitive analytic therapy (CAT) and, 492–493
 cognitive theories and, 150
 early intervention and, 221–223
 identity and identity diffusion and, 107–108, 114, 116–117, 118*f*
 interpersonal reconstructive therapy (IRT) and, 398
 mentalization and, 124, 127–129, 133, 542, 545
 moral development and, 328–329
 overview, 17–18, 32, 215, 223, 229–233, 651
 personality and, 215–217, 310–314, 312*t*
 precursor signs and symptoms, 218–220
 prevalence and, 221
 risk factors and, 218–220
 schema-focused therapy (SFT) and, 558
 stability and change and, 217–218
 temperament and, 215–216
 traits relevant to personality disorders, 314–319
 *See also* Adolescence; Adulthood; Childhood; Personality development
Developmental psychopathology model
 overview, 232–233, 309–310, 319–320
 personality traits and, 310–314, 312*t*
 role of personality traits and, 317–319
 traits relevant to personality disorders, 314–319
Diagnosis
 antisocial personality disorder and, 445–446, 451–452
 approaches to, 367, 368–373, 370*t*, 371*t*–372*t*
 borderline personality disorder and, 419–422, 494–495
 case formulation and, 397
 cognitive analytic therapy (CAT) and, 491–492
 cognitive heuristics and, 15
 cultural factors and, 96, 97
 dialectical behavior therapy (DBT) and, 530–531
 DSM era and, 7–8
 early conceptualizations of personality disorder and, 6
 epidemiology and, 193
 essentialism and, 14–15
 future research and, 83–84
 genetic factors and, 235–236
 historical overview of classification systems and, 48–49
 immigration and, 95
 limitations of categorical approaches and, 72–74
 longitudinal studies and, 198
 measures for, 342*t*
 medical model and, 9–11
 mentalization-based treatment (MBT) and, 543
 neurotransmitter function and, 264
 outcomes and, 170–171
 overview, 22, 231, 337–339, 382
 psychiatric syndromes and, 155–156
 psychoeducation and, 601–603, 602*t*
 schema-focused therapy (SFT) and, 557–558
 structural analysis of social behavior (SASB) model and, 403, 405–408, 406*t*–407*t*
 transference-focused psychotherapy (TFP) and, 572–575, 573*f*, 574*t*
 validity and, 11–14
 in young people, 220–221
 *See also* Assessment; Classification systems; *individual personality disorders*
Diagnostic and Statistical Manual of Mental Disorders (DSM)
 antisocial personality disorder and, 445
 borderline personality disorder and, 419
 comorbidity and, 156–157, 162–164
 cultural factors and, 90–91, 96
 diagnostic classification and, 21
 early conceptualizations of personality disorder and, 6–7
 evolution of, 28
 five-factor model (FFM) and, 38
 medical model and, 9–11
 overview, 7–8, 25–26, 169–170, 171
 theoretical orientations and, 34–35
 validity and, 13–14
Diagnostic and Statistical Manual of Mental Disorders (DSM-I), 49, 50*t*, 51
Diagnostic and Statistical Manual of Mental Disorders (DSM-II), 50*t*, 51–52, 426
Diagnostic and Statistical Manual of Mental Disorders (DSM-III)
 antisocial personality disorder and, 426–427
 assessment and, 341
 borderline personality disorder and, 419
 childhood and adolescence and, 220
 comorbidity and, 156–157
 DSM era and, 7–8
 early conceptualizations of personality disorder and, 6–7
 epidemiology and, 173–174, 174, 175*t*, 176
 historical overview of classification systems and, 50*t*, 52–53, 56
 medical model and, 9–10
 obsessive–compulsive personality disorder and, 461
 overview, 4, 25–26
Diagnostic and Statistical Manual of Mental Disorders (DSM-III-R)
 antisocial personality disorder and, 427
 comorbidity and, 156–157
 DSM era and, 7–8
 epidemiology and, 173, 174, 175*t*, 176
 historical overview of classification systems and, 50*t*, 53–54, 56
 obsessive–compulsive personality disorder and, 460, 461
 theoretical orientations and, 31
Diagnostic and Statistical Manual of Mental Disorders (DSM-IV)
 antisocial personality disorder and, 427
 assessment and, 341
 borderline personality disorder and, 419
 cognitive theories and, 150–151
 comorbidity and, 156–157, 159
 DSM era and, 7–8
 epidemiology and, 173, 174, 175*t*, 176–177
 five-factor model (FFM) and, 38, 39–40, 75
 genetic factors and, 241–242
 historical overview of classification systems and, 50*t*, 55–57
 medical model and, 9–10
 obsessive–compulsive personality disorder and, 459–460, 461, 462–463, 467–468, 471
 structural analysis of social behavior (SASB) model and, 403
 theoretical orientations and, 30–31, 31, 32–33
 transference-focused psychotherapy (TFP) and, 572, 581
 validity and, 14
Diagnostic and Statistical Manual of Mental Disorders (DSM-IV-TR)
 comorbidity and, 156–157, 161
 DSM-5 and, 63–64
 future editions and, 64, 65
 historical overview of classification systems and, 50*t*, 57
 longitudinal studies and, 198
 obsessive–compulsive personality disorder and, 461
 theoretical orientations and, 31
Diagnostic and Statistical Manual of Mental Disorders (DSM-5)
 antisocial personality disorder and, 427, 429, 436, 437, 444, 445–447
 assessment and, 337–338, 341, 344, 389
 borderline personality disorder and, 419, 421, 494–495
 callous–unemotional (CU) traits and, 326
 childhood and adolescence and, 220
 cognitive heuristics and, 15
 cognitive theories and, 142, 150–151
 comorbidity and, 159, 162–164
 cultural factors and, 88–89
 developmental factors and, 312–313
 developmental psychopathology model and, 233, 309, 319, 320
 diagnosis and, 21, 221, 337–338
 differentiating traits from other aspects of personality functioning, 318
 DSM era and, 7–8
 early conceptualizations of personality disorder and, 6–7
 epidemiology and, 174, 177–178
 five-factor model (FFM) and, 38, 39–40, 76, 78–80, 78*f*, 80*t*
 future editions and, 63–64, 65
 genetic factors and, 246
 historical overview of classification systems and, 50*t*, 57–63
 identity and, 108–109

interpersonal reconstructive therapy
   (IRT) and, 394–395, 413
lexical hypothesis and, 42
longitudinal studies and, 198
medical model and, 10–11
mentalization and, 130
obsessive–compulsive personality
   disorder and, 459–460, 471
overview, 26, 47–48, 648
psychiatric syndromes and, 155
psychoeducation and, 602
psychopathology and, 101, 428
schema-focused therapy (SFT) and,
   560
systems training for emotion
   predictability and problem solving
   (STEPPS) and, 589
theoretical orientations and, 31, 32–33
transference-focused psychotherapy
   (TFP) and, 572
*See also* Alternative Model
Diagnostic classification
   comorbidity and, 162–164
   cultural factors and, 90–92
   DSM-5-III Trait Model and, 80–82, 81*t*
   epidemiology and, 173–174
   future research and, 83–84
   limitations of categorical approaches
      and, 72–74
   overview, 20–22, 65–66, 169–170
   theoretical orientations and, 30–31
   *See also* Classification systems;
      *individual diagnostic manuals and
      their editions*
Diagnostic Interview for Borderlines—
   Revised (DIB-R), 421
Diagnostic Interview Schedule (DIS),
   175*t*, 176
Dialectical behavior therapy (DBT)
   diagnosis, assessment, and formulation
      and, 377–378, 377*t*, 387–388,
      530–531
   domains of psychopathology and,
      527–528
   emotion regulation and, 278
   obsessive–compulsive personality
      disorder and, 467
   overview, 481–482, 483–484, 527
   research support for, 538–539
   strategies, 533–537
   systems training for emotion
      predictability and problem solving
      (STEPPS) and, 586
   theoretical foundation of, 531–533
   therapeutic relationship and, 537–538
   transference-focused psychotherapy
      (TFP) and, 572, 580–581
   treatment stages and targets, 528–530
Dialectical behavior therapy prolonged
   exposure (DBT-PE) protocol, 530.
   *See also* Dialectical behavior therapy
   (DBT)
Dialectics, 531, 532–533, 537–538
Dialogic sequence analysis (DSA), 499
Diary cards, 387–388, 528–529, 530–531
Diathesis–stress model, 232–233, 303, 306,
   513–514
Dichotomous thinking, 147–148
Differential diagnosis, 403, 405–408,
   406*t*–407*t*. *See also* Diagnosis
Differentiation, 375, 382, 384

Digit Symbol subtest, 284
Dimensional approaches to classification
   advantages to, 74
   antisocial personality disorder and,
      437–438, 446–447
   assessment and, 357–359, 369–373,
      370*t*, 371*t*–372*t*
   comorbidity and, 163
   cultural factors and, 91–92
   developmental factors and, 313, 320
   diagnosis and, 369–373, 370*t*, 371*t*–372*t*
   future research and, 83–84
   genetic factors and, 236–237, 236*f*, 237*f*
   limitations of categorical approaches
      and, 72–74
   neurotransmitter function and, 264
   overview, 43–44, 72
   transference-focused psychotherapy
      (TFP) and, 572
   *See also* Classification systems;
      Five-factor model (FFM); Trait-
      dimensional model
Dimensional Assessment of Personality
   Pathology (DAPP), 77*t*, 239–240,
   241
Dimensional Assessment of Personality
   Pathology—Basic Questionnaire
   (DAPP-BQ), 217, 370
Dimensional Personality Symptom Item
   Pool (DIPSI), 77*t*, 217, 349
Dimensional trait model, 60–61. *See also*
   Trait models
Disability, 356–357
Disagreeableness, 312, 312*t*, 313–314
Disconnection, 558, 559*t*
Disease model, 3–4, 26, 31
Disinhibition
   antisocial personality disorder and, 429,
      433–434, 434, 435, 446, 451
   assessment and, 373
   dimensional approaches and, 77*t*
   factor hierarchy and, 78*f*
   obsessive–compulsive personality
      disorder and, 471
Disinhibition (DIS) versus
   conscientiousness domain, 76
Dispositional dimensions, 437–438
Disruptive behavior disorder, 63–64, 219
Dissocial behavior
   diagnostic classification and, 20–21
   integrated modular treatment and, 666
   overview, 417
   trait assessment and, 370*t*
   validity and, 13–14
Dissociative symptoms
   childhood adversity and, 305
   cognitive analytic therapy (CAT) and,
      493–494, 497
   identity diffusion and, 114
   neurotransmitter function and, 260
   schema mode and, 561
Distraction, 590, 662–663
Distress, 126, 330
Dopamine system, 244, 257–259. *See also*
   Neurotransmitter systems
DSM-5 Clinicians' Personality Trait Rating
   Form (DSM-5 CPTRF), 354
DSM-5 Personality and Personality
   Disorders Work Group (PPDWG)
   comorbidity and, 162
   five-factor model (FFM) and, 76

future editions and, 63–64
historical overview of classification
   systems and, 58, 59–63
overview, 66
DSM-5 Section III Alternative Model for
   PD. *See* Alternative Model
DSM-5 Work Groups, 459
DSM-5-III Informant Personality Trait
   Rating Form (DSM-5 IPTRF), 354
DSM-5-III Trait Model, 78–79, 78*f*, 80–84,
   80*t*, 81*t*
Dyssocial reaction personality disorder,
   50*t*
Dysthymia, 56–57

Early experiences. *See* Childhood
   experiences
Early intervention, 221–223. *See also*
   Interventions
Early maladaptive schemas (EMSs),
   142–143, 144, 558–560, 559*t*
Eating disorders
   borderline personality disorder and,
      420
   cognitive analytic therapy (CAT) and,
      499
   dialectical behavior therapy (DBT) and,
      528, 539
   identity diffusion and, 113, 114
   obsessive–compulsive personality
      disorder and, 463, 467, 469
   perfectionism and, 469
   schema-focused therapy (SFT) and, 569
Eccentric perceptions, 79, 373
Ecological momentary assessment (EMA)
   strategies, 381, 421
Effortful control, 386*t*, 434, 576
Egocentrism, 370*t*, 371*t*
Ego-identity, 111, 113, 114, 115, 636. *See
   also* Identity
EIC scale, 592, 594
Elemental Psychopathy Assessment (EPA),
   427
Emotion regulation
   assessment and, 388
   cognitive-behavioral therapy for PDs
      (CBTpd) and, 517–518
   dialectical behavior therapy (DBT) and,
      532–533, 539
   personality impairment and, 318–319
   psychotherapy and pharmacotherapy
      and, 277–278
   skills training and, 222
Emotional abuse, 128–129. *See also*
   Childhood experiences
Emotional dysregulation
   borderline personality disorder and,
      420–421
   cognitive-behavioral therapy for PDs
      (CBTpd) and, 517–518
   diagnostic classification and, 20–21
   integrated modular treatment and,
      660–665
   overview, 417
   validity and, 13–14
Emotional intensity disorder (EID), 588,
   590
Emotional interventions, 669
Emotional processing, 232, 246, 271–272,
   327–328, 664–665
Emotional reactivity, 370*t*, 371*t*, 664–665

Emotional regulation
  cognitive processing in BPD and, 277
  dialectical behavior therapy (DBT) and, 527, 531
  dysregulation in patients with PD, 273
  in healthy subjects, 272–273
  integrated modular treatment and, 664–665
  neuroimaging studies in BPD and, 274–276
  neuropsychological mechanisms and, 274
  overview, 232, 271–272
  parental psychopathology, 303
  skills training and, 589–590, 591
  trait assessment and, 369–370, 370$t$
  violence reduction treatment and, 637
Emotional unstable personality disorder, 50$t$
Emotions
  dialectical behavior therapy (DBT) and, 530
  inhibition and, 559$t$
  instability and, 312$t$, 313
  integrated modular treatment and, 661–662
  intensity and, 370$t$, 371$t$
  interactions of with cognition, 292–294
  lability, 79, 370$t$, 385
  overview, 271–272
  schema-focused therapy (SFT) and, 560
Empathy
  antisocial personality disorder and, 435, 446
  callous–unemotional (CU) traits and, 327
  interpersonal reconstructive therapy (IRT) and, 395
  mentalization-based treatment (MBT) and, 546–548, 550–551
  overview, 371$t$
  schema-focused therapy (SFT) and, 564
  trait assessment and, 370$t$
  triarchic model and, 430
  validation and, 550–551
  violence reduction treatment and, 636
Empirically based treatments, 367, 481–485, 566–568, 602$t$
Engagement, 515–516, 545, 546
Entitlement, 373, 559$t$, 636
Environmental factors
  antisocial personality disorder and, 429, 435–437
  callous–unemotional (CU) traits and, 326–327
  childhood adversity and, 127, 301–303
  cultural factors and, 92, 94–95
  developmental psychopathology model and, 320
  dialectical behavior therapy (DBT) and, 531, 533
  genetic factors and, 237, 239, 306
  mentalization and, 127, 132, 545
  overview, 229, 513
  personality and, 242–243, 319
  psychoeducation and, 602–604, 602$t$
  risk factors and, 219
  traits relevant to personality disorders, 316
  twin studies and, 239
  violence reduction treatment and, 638
  *See also* Family factors

Epidemiologic Catchment Area Study (ECA), 90–91, 174, 176
Epidemiology
  assessment and, 191–192
  borderline personality disorder and, 422
  childhood adversity and, 306
  epidemiological studies, 174–180, 175$t$
  longitudinal studies and, 198
  obsessive–compulsive personality disorder and, 462
  overview, 169–171, 173–174, 192–193
  *See also* Prevalence
Epigenetics, 333. *See also* Genetic factors
Episodic memory, 285–286, 294–295. *See also* Memory processes
Epistemic choices, 26–29, 45
Epistemic distrust, 103–104
Epistemic hypervigilance, 130, 135, 136
Epistemic openness, 134
Epistemic rigidity, 545
Epistemic trust, 123, 130, 132–133, 135–136, 545
Epistemic vigilance, 130, 133
Equifinality, 233, 309
Error detection, 272–273
Error-related negativity (ERN), 160, 433
Etiology
  borderline personality disorder and, 422–423, 603–604
  callous–unemotional (CU) traits and, 326–327
  moral development and, 329
  obsessive–compulsive personality disorder and, 464–465
  overview, 229–233, 651
  psychoeducation and, 603–604
  *See also* Biological factors; Causal factors; Psychosocial factors
Evaluation bias, 145$f$, 147–148, 149
Event-related potentials (ERPs), 160, 433
Evidence-based approach to personality disorder, 417–418
Evidence-based practice (EBP), 503–507, 504$t$
Evidence-Based Practice in Psychology (EBPP), 412–413
Evidence-based psychotherapies
  borderline personality disorder and, 605
  cognitive-behavioral therapy for PDs (CBTpd) and, 523–525, 524$t$
  interpersonal reconstructive therapy (IRT) and, 412–413
  mentalization and, 134, 551–552
  overview, 482
  psychoeducation and, 605, 607
  systems training for emotion predictability and problem solving (STEPPS) and, 597
  transference-focused psychotherapy (TFP) and, 580–582
  *See also* Treatment; *individual treatment approaches*
Evolutionary factors
  cultural factors and, 92, 98
  diagnostic classification and, 21
  five-factor model (FFM) and, 39
  mentalization and, 131
  overview, 17–18, 27, 34–35, 44
Experiential techniques, 563–564, 565
Exploitativeness, 370$t$, 371$t$, 446, 636
Exploration, 548, 646, 659, 666–670

Explosive aesthenic personality disorder, 50$t$, 52
Exposure approaches, 277, 463, 530, 533, 536
External features of self, 124, 125$f$
Externalizing spectrum (ES) model, 451
Externalizing Spectrum Inventory (ESI), 430–431
Externalizing symptoms
  comorbidity and, 159, 187
  cultural factors and, 97
  factor hierarchy and, 78$f$
  obsessive–compulsive personality disorder and, 470
  schema-focused therapy (SFT) and, 569
Extraversion
  cultural factors and, 91–92
  developmental factors and, 311, 312$t$
  developmental psychopathology model and, 319–320
  future editions of classification systems and, 65
  overview, 41–42, 74
  transference-focused psychotherapy (TFP) and, 573$f$
  *See also* Five-factor model (FFM)
Eysenck Personality Questionnaire (EPQ), 74, 77$t$, 240

Factor analysis
  antisocial personality disorder and, 429
  assessment and, 373
  developmental factors and, 217
  five-factor model (FFM) and, 39
  lexical hypothesis and, 42
  overview, 36–37, 417
  schema-focused therapy (SFT) and, 566
Factor hierarchy, 78–79, 78$f$
Factor models, 35–44, 36$f$
Failure, 559$t$
Family factors
  borderline personality disorder and, 420
  childhood adversity associated with mental disorders and, 301–303
  dysfunctional families, 303–304
  epidemiological studies, 179–180
  genetic analyses, 237–243
  obsessive–compulsive personality disorder and, 464
  personality impairment and, 318–319
  risk factors and, 218–220
  traits relevant to personality disorders, 315–317
  *See also* Environmental factors; Genetic factors
Fast Track program, 222
Fear
  antisocial personality disorder and, 437
  fear-based disorders, 159
  mentalization and, 126
  neurotransmitter function and, 252
  schema-focused therapy (SFT) and, 560
  triarchic model and, 430
Fearlessness, 325, 327, 433, 434–435, 437
Fight–flight–freeze process, 142–143. *See also* Coping styles
Fight–flight–freeze system (FFFS), 311
Five Dimensional Personality Test (5DPT), 77$t$, 348
Five-factor model (FFM)
  classification systems and, 61–62, 65
  cultural factors and, 91–92

developmental factors and, 216–217, 311–312, 312t
developmental psychopathology model and, 233
obsessive–compulsive personality disorder and, 460, 468–469
overview, 37–44, 43–44, 74–76, 77t
trait assessment and, 370
traits described in DSM-5 and, 76, 78–80, 78f, 80t
*See also* Agreeableness; Big Five personality model; Conscientiousness; Extraversion; Neuroticism; Openness to Experience
Flexibility, 132, 494, 495f, 664
Forensic treatment settings, 499, 568, 569
Functional impairments, 21, 337, 373, 461–462
Functional magnetic resonance imaging (fMRI). *See* Neuroimaging technologies

Galton, Sir Francis, 36
Game of Dice Task, 289–290
Gamma-aminobutyric acid (GABA), 260–262. *See also* Neurotransmitter systems
Gender, 112t, 189–190, 193, 293, 315
Gene–environment interactions, 306. *See also* Environmental factors; Genetic factors
General Assessment of Personality Disorders (GAPD), 352
Generalization, 669–670
Generalized anxiety disorder (GAD), 159, 216, 463. *See also* Anxiety disorders
Genetic factors
 antisocial personality disorder and, 433, 435–437
 callous–unemotional (CU) traits and, 325, 327, 333
 developmental psychopathology model and, 315–316, 317, 320
 future directions in, 246–247
 gene–environment interactions and, 306
 genetic analyses, 237–243
 identifying putative genes, 243–246
 interpersonal reconstructive therapy (IRT) and, 399
 mentalization and, 126
 obsessive–compulsive personality disorder and, 464
 overview, 17–19, 161, 217, 229, 231, 235, 247
 phenotype, 235–237, 237f, 238f
 psychoeducation and, 603–604
 traits relevant to personality disorders, 315–316
 *See also* Family factors; Phenotypic features
Genomewide association (GWA) studies, 436
Gift of Love (GOL), 396–397, 398, 410, 412
Global Assessment of Functioning (GAF) score, 369, 551
Glutamate, 260–261. *See also* Neurotransmitter systems
Goals
 assessment and, 384
 dialectical behavior therapy (DBT) and, 530, 532–533

identity and, 108–109, 112t
integrated modular treatment and, 652, 656
personality impairment and, 318
systems training for emotion predictability and problem solving (STEPPS) and, 590
violence reduction treatment and, 633
Go/no-go task, 277, 290–291
Grandiosity, 59–60, 79, 559t, 636
Group treatments
 dialectical behavior therapy (DBT) and, 527, 529
 mentalization-based treatment (MBT) and, 552
 obsessive–compulsive personality disorder and, 466
 peer psychoeducation, 606–607
 psychoeducation and, 606
 schema-focused therapy (SFT) and, 555, 568
 systems training for emotion predictability and problem solving (STEPPS) and, 591–595
Growth hormone (GH), 259–260
Guilt, 467, 560

Hare Self-Report Psychopathy Scale (SRP-III), 427, 430–431
Harm avoidance, 243–244, 245
Helping Young People Early (HYPE) program, 222
Heterogeneity
 borderline personality disorder and, 419
 callous–unemotional (CU) traits and, 325, 332
 diagnosis and assessment and, 368
 limitations of categorical approaches and, 72, 73
 longitudinal studies and, 207–208, 207f
 mentalization and, 126
Hexaco Dark Triad, 40–41
Histrionic personality disorder (HPD)
 clinical correlates and, 186, 187, 188
 cognitive analytic therapy (CAT) and, 504t, 506
 demographic correlates, 189–191
 emotion regulation and, 273
 epidemiological studies, 176
 future editions of classification systems and, 63–64
 genetic factors and, 240
 historical overview of classification systems and, 50t, 59–60
 overview, 28
 prevalence, 182, 183–184, 183t
 schema-focused therapy (SFT) and, 567, 568
 structural analysis of social behavior (SASB) model and, 405, 406t–407t, 409t
 theoretical orientations and, 32–33
Honesty-Humility, Emotionality, Extraversion, Agreeableness, Conscientiousness, Openness (HEXACO), 26, 40–41, 42, 43–44, 77t, 349–350
Hospitalization, 605. *See also* Inpatient treatment
Hostile-dominance, 370t, 371t, 469
Hostility, 394–395, 623

Human Connectome Project, 161
Hybrid model, 64, 65, 163, 357, 373

Identification of feelings, 549, 661
Identity
 assessment and, 379, 386t
 clinical implications, 118–119
 definitions of, 110–113, 112t–113t
 development of, 116–117, 118f
 integrated approach and, 381, 658f
 layers of, 111
 mentalization and, 130, 131
 overview, 103, 107–109, 649
 personality impairment and, 318
 schema-focused therapy (SFT) and, 558
 the self and, 109–110
 transference-focused psychotherapy (TFP) and, 574t, 575
 *See also* Identity diffusion; Self; Self-concept
Identity diffusion
 assessment and, 379
 clinical implications, 118–119
 development of, 116–117, 118f
 inferred self and, 102–103
 mentalization and, 130
 overview, 108–109, 112t–113t, 113–116
 *See also* Identity
Imagery work, 523, 557, 563–564, 565
Immigration, 95–96, 97
Implicit Association Test (IAT), 147
Implicit processes, 146–147
Impulse control, 94–95, 386t. *See also* Impulsivity
Impulsive Child mode, 561, 562t. *See also* Schema mode
Impulsivity
 antisocial personality disorder and, 429, 433, 446, 452
 assessment and, 373
 borderline personality disorder and, 275, 420–422, 423
 callous–unemotional (CU) traits and, 325, 327
 genetic factors and, 246
 identity and, 113, 114
 interpersonal reconstructive therapy (IRT) and, 394–395
 mentalization and, 126
 neurotransmitter function and, 252, 253–254, 256–257, 261
 obsessive–compulsive personality disorder and, 469
 overview, 104–105, 371t
 pharmacotherapy and, 616, 617
 psychoeducation and, 603
 risk factors and, 219
 schema mode and, 561
 trait assessment and, 370t
 transference-focused psychotherapy (TFP) and, 581
 violence reduction treatment and, 636
Inadequate personality disorder, 50t, 52
Individual differences, 20, 42, 310–311
Individual therapy, 465, 507, 528–529
Individualism, 93–94, 93–95, 97–98
Individuation process, 117
Inductive approach, 27–28, 42–45
Inductive-lexical-factor-trait tradition, 36–37
Inferred self, 102–103

Informants in assessment, 191–192, 220–221, 353–354, 354. *See also* Assessment
Information processing, 141–142, 144–148, 145*f*, 246
Inhibition
  developmental psychopathology model and, 316–317
  neurotransmitter function and, 252
  obsessive–compulsive personality disorder and, 471
  overview, 104–105, 370*t*, 371*t*
  schema-focused therapy (SFT) and, 558, 559*t*
Inpatient treatment, 116, 499, 605. *See also* Treatment
Insecure attachment
  mentalization and, 127–128, 545
  overview, 371*t*, 417
  trait assessment and, 370*t*
  validity and, 13–14
  *See also* Attachment
Insight-oriented approach, 465–466
Integrated Family Intervention for Child Conduct Problems, 332
Integrated modular treatment
  assessment and, 377*t*
  containment phase, 646, 659
  exploration and change phase, 646, 659, 666–670
  integration and synthesis phase, 646, 659, 670–673
  overview, 645–648, 673
  regulation and modulation phase, 646, 659, 660–666
  safety phase, 646, 659
  treatment modules, 651–657, 657*f*, 658*f*
  *See also* Integrated treatment approach
Integrated treatment approach
  assessment and, 381–387, 383*t*, 386*t*
  interpersonal reconstructive therapy (IRT) and, 410–412, 411*f*
  mentalization-based treatment (MBT) and, 542
  overview, 16–17, 373–375, 483
  rationale for, 646–647
  routes to, 647–648
  *See also* Cognitive analytic therapy (CAT); Integrated modular treatment
Integration
  assessment and, 379, 383*t*, 384
  clinical definition of PD and, 375
  integrated modular treatment and, 646, 659, 670–673
  *See also* Integrated treatment approach
Intelligence
  assessment and, 283–284
  comorbidity and, 159
  developmental factors and, 312, 312*t*, 319–320
  overview, 41–42
  risk factors and, 219
Interdependence, 94–95
Intermittent explosive disorder (IED), 275
Internal features of self, 124, 125*f*
Internalizing symptoms
  cognitive analytic therapy (CAT) and, 494
  comorbidity and, 159
  factor hierarchy and, 78*f*

obsessive–compulsive personality disorder and, 470
schema-focused therapy (SFT) and, 569
Internalizing–externalizing model, 105, 159–160
International Affective Picture System (IAPS), 275, 276, 277
*International Classification of Diseases* (ICD), 96, 419
*International Classification of Diseases* (ICD-6), 49, 51
*International Classification of Diseases* (ICD-8), 51–52
*International Classification of Diseases* (ICD-9), 52–53
*International Classification of Diseases* (ICD-10), 47–48, 55–57, 220, 408, 421
*International Classification of Diseases* (ICD-11)
  assessment and, 355, 356
  early diagnosis and, 221
  epidemiology and, 174
  historical overview of classification systems and, 57–63
  overview, 47–48, 65, 648
  psychopathology and, 101
International Classification of Functioning, Disability, and Health (ICF), 356
International Personality Disorder Examination (IPDE), 90, 175*t*, 176, 180, 198
Internet-based treatment, 607
Interpersonal Dependency Inventory (IDI), 345
Interpersonal diagnostic criteria, 30–31. *See also* Diagnostic classification
Interpersonal factors
  adaptive impairment and, 374–375
  assessment and, 384–385, 386*t*
  borderline personality disorder and, 420–421
  callous–unemotional (CU) traits and, 324
  dialectical behavior therapy (DBT) and, 530–531
  emotion regulation and, 278
  expectations and, 132
  integrated approach and, 374, 381, 658*f*, 666, 672–673
  interpersonal circle and, 32–33, 43–44, 370
  intervention and, 669
  mentalization and, 126, 131–132
  obsessive–compulsive personality disorder and, 469
  overview, 28–29, 44, 107–108, 123, 648, 649
  problems with, 13–14, 338, 383*t*, 384–385
  sensitivity, 257
  violence reduction treatment and, 631
  *See also* Social factors
Interpersonal psychotherapy (IPT), 277, 278, 658*f*
Interpersonal reconstructive therapy (IRT)
  case formulation and, 395–399
  comorbidity and, 408–409, 409*t*
  diagnosis and assessment and, 339
  evidence-based practice and, 412–413
  natural biology in, 398–399

overview, 394–395, 413
structural analysis of social behavior (SASB) model and, 399–408, 400*f*, 402*f*, 404*f*, 406*t*–407*t*
treatment model, 409–412, 411*f*
Interpersonal theory, 30, 377*t*, 380–381
Interpretation
  cognitive biases and, 145*f*
  integrated modular treatment and, 664
  overview, 141–142
  personality impairment and, 318–319
  transference-focused psychotherapy (TFP) and, 578, 579
Interpretational bias, 145*f*, 146–147, 149
Interventions
  callous–unemotional (CU) traits and, 331–332
  cognitive-behavioral therapy for PDs (CBTpd) and, 515–520, 516*f*–517*f*
  cultural factors and, 97
  DBT strategies, 533–537
  diagnosis and, 220–221, 337
  early intervention and, 221–223
  integrated modular treatment and, 652–653, 656–657, 657*f*, 658*f*, 668–669
  mentalization-based treatment (MBT) and, 543, 546–549
  schema-focused therapy (SFT) and, 563–566
  transference-focused psychotherapy (TFP) and, 577–578, 578*t*
  violence reduction treatment and, 632–634
  *See also* Treatment; *individual treatment approaches*
Interviews, clinical. *See* Clinical interviews
Intimacy, 112*t*, 395, 460
Intrapsychic level, 35*t*
Introjections, 117, 401
Introversion, 312*t*, 313, 319–320, 417, 573*f*
Inventory of Callous and Unemotional Traits (ICU), 329, 448*t*, 449–450
Iowa Gambling Task (IGT), 288–289
Irreverent communication, 536–537
Irritability, 255, 429, 581

Labeling of feelings, 549, 661
Language processing, 284–285
Law of initial values, 203–204
Learning
  borderline personality disorder and, 295
  cognitive analytic therapy (CAT) and, 494, 501
  neurotransmitter function and, 260
  personality impairment and, 318–319
Leary circle, 32–33
Level of Personality Functioning Scale (LPFS), 82, 83, 351, 355, 430–431
Levenson Self-Report Psychopathy Scale (LSRP), 427
Lexical models, 36–37, 42–43, 44
Lifestyle habits, 590–591
Limits, 558, 559*t*
Linnaeus, Carl, 27
London Parent–Child Project, 127–128
Lonely Child mode, 562*t*
Longitudinal course of personality disorder. *See* Course of personality disorders

Longitudinal studies
  designing, 199
  methodological differences among studies, 201–208, 207t
  overview, 197–198, 209–210, 217
  overview of four major studies of PD, 199–201, 200t
  See also Course of personality disorders
Longitudinal Study of Personality Disorders (LSPD), 199–201, 200t, 201–208
Loss, feelings of, 561

Major depressive disorder (MDD), 157, 159, 277, 294. See also Depression
Maladaptive beliefs, 141–142, 142f, 560. See also Beliefs
Maladaptive coping styles, 560. See also Coping styles
Maltreatment
  associated with mental disorders, 301–303
  callous–unemotional (CU) traits and, 325, 331
  mentalization and, 128–129, 545
  risk factors and, 219
  schemas and, 144
  See also Childhood experiences
Manic-depression concept, 420
Manipulativeness, 79, 373, 394–395, 446
Marital status, 190–191, 193
Masochistic personality disorder, 35, 54
McLean Study of Adult Development (MSAD), 200t, 201, 201–208, 211
Meaning, sense of, 384, 649
Mean-level stability, 206–207, 315, 320. See also Stability of personality disorders
Meanness, 434, 435, 436, 446, 451. See also Callous–unemotional (CU) traits
Measure of Disordered Personality Functioning (MDPF), 351–352
Medical model
  alternative versions of, 16, 19–20
  cultural factors and, 89
  influence of, 14–15
  overview, 3–4, 8–11, 26
  theoretical orientations and, 31
  validity and, 11–14
  See also Disease model
Medications. See Pharmacotherapy
Memory processes
  borderline personality disorder and, 285–286, 293–294, 295
  cognitive biases and, 145f
  development of identity and, 117
  memory bias, 148–149, 293–294
  neurotransmitter function and, 259, 260
  overview, 19, 141–142
  schema-focused therapy (SFT) and, 560
Mental disorders, 301–303. See also individual disorders
Mental representations, 115, 271, 318–319, 572, 575
Mental states, 104, 133
Mentalization
  approach to personality disorders and, 124–127, 125f
  assessment and, 380, 386t
  attachment and, 103, 126–127
  childhood adversity and, 127–129

clinical implications, 133–136
cognitive theories and, 150
development of identity and, 117
disruptions in, 544–545
epistemic trust and, 132–133
integrated modular treatment and, 655, 665
overview, 104, 109–110, 123–124, 136
the self and, 129–132
transference-focused psychotherapy (TFP) and, 576
See also Mentalization-based treatment (MBT); Self-reflective thinking
Mentalization-based treatment for adolescents (MBT-A), 222, 551–552
Mentalization-based treatment (MBT)
  assessment and, 377t
  diagnosis, assessment, and formulation and, 543
  integrated modular treatment and, 664
  intervention strategies and methods of, 546–549
  overview, 133–134, 481–482, 483–484, 541–543
  process of, 550–551
  research support for, 551–552
  theoretical orientations and, 543–544
  therapeutic relationship and, 549–550
  transference-focused psychotherapy (TFP) and, 572
Metacognitive processes, 373, 657f, 658f
Metacognitive therapy, 466–467, 664
Millon Clinical Multiaxial Inventory (MCMI), 77t
Millon Inventory of Personality Styles (MIPS), 77t
Millon's model, 39, 43–44, 74
Mindfulness skills, 529, 536, 661–662, 664
Minnesota Multiphasic Personality Inventory (MMPI), 74, 239, 254
Mistrust, 373, 559t. See also Trust
Modulatory system, 648, 649, 657f, 659, 660–666
Molecular genetics, 436. See also Genetic factors
Monoamine oxidase inhibitors (MAOIs), 618, 619, 622f, 623. See also Antidepressants; Pharmacotherapy
Mood affective disorder (MAD), 259–260
Mood disorders
  antisocial personality disorder and, 450
  borderline personality disorder and, 420
  cognitive analytic therapy (CAT) and, 499
  comorbidity and, 187
  epidemiological studies, 179–180
  historical overview of classification systems and, 56–57
  obsessive–compulsive personality disorder and, 461–462
  schema-focused therapy (SFT) and, 556, 569
Mood Disorders Work Group, 56–57
Mood stabilizers. See Pharmacotherapy
Moral development, 328–329
Moral reconation therapy (MRT), 453
Moral values, 379–380, 574, 574t
Motivation, 632–633, 655–656
MRI studies. See Neuroimaging technologies

Multidimensional Personality Questionnaire (MPQ), 242–243, 287, 582
Multidisciplinary team, 638
Multifinality, 233, 309
Multiple self-states model (MSSM)
  case example of, 496–497
  cognitive analytic therapy (CAT) and, 495–496, 498f, 507–508
  research support for, 497
  screening and, 499
Multisource Assessment of Personality Pathology (MAPP), 345–346
Multisystemic therapy (MST), 638
Multivariate models, 105, 159–160, 247

Narcissism
  assessment and, 345, 347–348
  callous–unemotional (CU) traits and, 326
  coping styles and, 142
  inferred self and, 102–103
  overview, 372t
  psychopathy and, 428
  theoretical orientations and, 30
  trait assessment and, 370t
Narcissistic personality disorder (NPD)
  assessment and, 347–348
  demographic correlates, 189–191
  five-factor model (FFM) and, 75–76
  genetic factors and, 240
  historical overview of classification systems and, 52, 59–60, 61
  interpersonal reconstructive therapy (IRT) and, 394–395
  interpretational bias and, 147
  obsessive–compulsive personality disorder and, 463
  overview, 28, 35, 35t
  prevalence, 182–183, 183t
  schema-focused therapy (SFT) and, 556, 561, 567, 568
  structural analysis of social behavior (SASB) model and, 405, 406t–407t, 409t
  in young people, 221
Narcissistic Personality Inventory (NPI), 345
Narratives
  historical overview of classification systems and, 59
  integrated modular treatment and, 657f, 658f, 664, 665, 671
  narrative formation, 515–516, 516f–517f
  narrative psychology, 110
  overview, 18–19
  See also Self-narrative
National Comorbidity Survey (NCS), 156–157, 176
National Comorbidity Survey Replication (NCS-R)
  cultural factors and, 90
  epidemiological studies, 176
  gender and, 189
  longitudinal studies and, 205
  obsessive–compulsive personality disorder and, 460–461
  overview, 157
National Epidemiologic Survey on Alcohol and Related Conditions (NESARC), 177, 189, 460–461

Natural biology, 398–399, 410. *See also* Biological factors
Negative affectivity
  antisocial personality disorder and, 452
  developmental factors and, 313, 319–320
  dimensional approaches and, 77*t*
  factor hierarchy and, 78*f*
  mentalization and, 126
  overview, 417
Negative core beliefs, 513–515, 514*f*
Negative emotionality, 316–317, 446
Negativistic depressive personality disorder, 50*t*
Negativistic personality disorder, 33, 35
Negativity, 147–148, 559*t*
Neglect, 128–129, 219, 304. *See also* Childhood experiences
NEO Five-Factor Inventory (NEO-FFI), 162
NEO Personality Inventory (NEO PI, NEO PI-R, and NEO-PI-3)
  environmental factors and, 242
  five-factor model (FFM) and, 74, 75–76
  genetic factors and, 240, 245
  obsessive–compulsive personality disorder and, 468–469
  overview, 37, 346–347
Neo-Kraepelinian movement, 4, 8, 19, 156, 157
Neurobiological factors
  antisocial personality disorder and, 433, 433–434, 435, 438
  borderline personality disorder and, 420
  callous–unemotional (CU) traits and, 326
  emotion regulation and, 272–273, 274–276
  genetic factors and, 246
  interpersonal reconstructive therapy (IRT) and, 395
  mentalization-based treatment (MBT) and, 546
  obsessive–compulsive personality disorder and, 464–465, 469–470
  overview, 18–19, 229, 251–252
  pharmacotherapy and, 621–623, 622*f*
  psychoeducation and, 602*t*
  transference-focused psychotherapy (TFP) and, 581–582
  *See also* Biological factors; Neurotransmitter systems
Neurogenesis, 244. *See also* Genetic factors
Neuroimaging technologies
  comorbidity and, 161
  emotions and, 271, 274–276, 277
  genetic factors and, 246
  neurotransmitter function and, 252, 255–256, 264
  transference-focused psychotherapy (TFP) and, 582
Neuroleptics, 623–624. *See also* Pharmacotherapy
Neuropsychological mechanisms
  borderline personality disorder and, 232, 283–284, 287–295
  cognition and emotion interactions and, 292–294
  emotion regulation and, 274
  measuring discrete cognitive abilities and, 287–291

neuropsychological testing using conventional test batteries, 284–287
  obsessive–compulsive personality disorder and, 465
  overview, 18–19, 229, 283, 294–295
  psychoeducation and, 602*t*
  transference-focused psychotherapy (TFP) and, 581–582
Neurotic personality organization, 108–109
Neuroticism
  assessment and, 379
  cultural factors and, 91–92
  developmental factors and, 216, 311, 312*t*, 316–317, 319–320
  five-factor model (FFM) and, 41
  genetic factors and, 245
  obsessive–compulsive personality disorder and, 468–469
  overview, 74, 417
  traits relevant to personality disorders, 315
  transference-focused psychotherapy (TFP) and, 574*t*
  *See also* Five-factor model (FFM)
Neurotransmitter systems
  emotion regulation and, 277–278
  genetic factors and, 244
  overview, 229, 231–232, 251–252, 264
  *See also* Dopamine system; Gamma-aminobutyric acid (GABA); Glutamate; Neurobiological factors; Norepinephrine; Serotonin system
Niche expression, 672–673
NIMH Research Domain Criteria (RDoC). *See* Research Domain Criteria (RDoC)
Nonsuicidal self-injury (NSSI), 253. *See also* Self-harm
Norepinephrine, 244, 259–260. *See also* Neurotransmitter systems
Normal personality
  assessment and, 358–359
  emotion regulation and, 272–273
  integrated approach and, 374
  overview, 16–17
  personality impairment and, 319
  stability and change and, 217–218
  trait assessment and, 370
Norwegian Institute of Public Health Twin Panel, 240
"Not otherwise specified" (NOS) designation, 72, 73, 211
Novelty seeking, 243–244, 324–325, 327
Numbness, 326, 561
Nurse Family Partnership program, 222

Object relations, 132, 379, 574*t*, 578, 579–580
Object relations theory
  Alternative Model and, 350
  borderline personality disorder and, 30
  cognitive analytic therapy (CAT) and, 489
  cognitive-behavioral therapy for PDs (CBTpd) and, 514
  identity diffusion and, 114
  overview, 30
  transference-focused psychotherapy (TFP) and, 571, 572, 575, 576, 577
Observing limits, 533, 535

Obsessive–compulsive disorder (OCD)
  comorbidity and, 159, 160
  emotion regulation and, 277
  obsessive–compulsive personality disorder and, 461, 463
  pharmacotherapy and, 624
Obsessive–Compulsive Overcontroller mode, 563*t*
Obsessive–compulsive personality disorder (OCPD)
  clinical correlates and, 186, 187, 188
  cognitive analytic therapy (CAT) and, 504*t*, 506
  construct validity and, 467–468
  cultural factors and, 90, 94–95
  demographic correlates, 189–191
  epidemiological studies, 176
  etiology and, 464–465
  five-factor model (FFM) and, 76
  genetic factors and, 240
  historical overview of classification systems and, 50*t*
  interpersonal reconstructive therapy (IRT) and, 394–395, 409–410, 413
  interpretational bias and, 146, 147
  neurotransmitter function and, 253–254
  overview, 417, 459–463, 471–472
  prevalence, 184, 185, 185*t*
  schema-focused therapy (SFT) and, 567, 568, 569
  structural analysis of social behavior (SASB) model and, 409
  theoretical orientations and, 30
  traits linked to, 468–471
  treatment and, 465–467, 471–472
Occupation, 191, 193, 356
Older adults, 539. *See also* Adulthood
Omega-3 fatty acids, 617–618, 622*f*. *See also* Pharmacotherapy
Openness to Experience
  cultural factors and, 91–92
  developmental factors and, 312, 312*t*, 319–320
  dimensional approaches and, 77*t*
  five-factor model (FFM) and, 39–40
  overview, 41–42, 74
  *See also* Five-factor model (FFM)
Oppositional behavior, 370*t*, 372*t*
Oppositional defiant disorder (ODD), 159, 331–332
Orderliness, 41, 370*t*, 372*t*, 467, 468–469
Organic personality disorder (OPD), 285
Other-orientation, 34–35, 124, 125*f*, 558, 559*t*
Other-representations, 379, 388
Outcomes
  antisocial personality disorder and, 452–453
  borderline personality disorder and, 423
  cognitive analytic therapy (CAT) and, 503–507, 504*t*
  interpersonal reconstructive therapy (IRT) and, 413
  overview, 170–171, 649
  risk factors and, 218–219
  transference-focused psychotherapy (TFP) and, 580
  treatment and, 484–485
  violence reduction treatment and, 640–641
  *See also* Course of personality disorders

Overcompensation, 142–143, 563t
Overgeneralization, 147–148
Overvigilance, 558, 559t
Oxytocin (OXT), 262, 263, 327. *See also* Neurotransmitter systems

Paranoid Overcontroller mode, 563t
Paranoid personality disorder (PPD)
  clinical correlates and, 186, 188
  cognitive analytic therapy (CAT) and, 504, 504t
  coping styles and, 143
  demographic correlates, 189–191
  epidemiological studies, 178, 179
  future editions of classification systems and, 63–64
  genetic factors and, 240
  historical overview of classification systems and, 50t, 59–60
  obsessive–compulsive personality disorder and, 463
  prevalence, 180, 181t, 182
  schema-focused therapy (SFT) and, 567, 568
  structural analysis of social behavior (SASB) model and, 409t
  theoretical orientations and, 30, 32–33
Parasuicidality, 90. *See also* Suicidality
Parental Bonding Instrument (PBI), 304
Parental factors, 302, 303, 330. *See also* Family factors; Parenting
Parent–child relationships, 218, 330–331, 332, 435, 470
Parenting
  associated with personality disorders, 304
  callous–unemotional (CU) traits and, 325, 330–331, 333
  developmental psychopathology model and, 316–317
  moral development and, 328
  overview, 32
  personality impairment and, 318–319
  psychoeducation and, 602–604
Parenting interventions, 332. *See also* Interventions; Treatment
Passive-aggressive personality disorder (PAPD)
  clinical correlates and, 188
  demographic correlates, 190–191
  historical overview of classification systems and, 49, 50t
  interpersonal reconstructive therapy (IRT) and, 409–410
  neurotransmitter function and, 254
  prevalence, 184, 185t
  structural analysis of social behavior (SASB) model and, 409t
Pathological identity, 112t–113t. *See also* Identity
Pathological Narcissism Inventory (PNI), 347–348
Pathoplasty/exacerbation, 158, 158t. *See also* Bivariate models
Perceptions, 104–105, 376, 581
Perfectionism, 460, 469–470
Performance impairment, 558, 559t
Perinatal factors, 218–219
Personality
  cognitive structure of, 650–651
  course of personality disorders and, 210–211

cultural interactions and, 94–95
developmental factors and, 215, 215–217
developmental psychopathology model and, 233
diagnosis and assessment and, 338–339
differentiating traits from other aspects of personality functioning, 317–318
environmental factors and, 242–243
five-factor model (FFM) of, 37–44
individualism-collectivism cultural syndrome and, 93–94
mentalization and, 126, 131, 132
overview, 44–45, 648–650
theoretical orientations and, 33–34
Personality and Personality Disorders Work Group (PPDWG), 356
Personality Assessment Inventory, 380
Personality Assessment Schedule (PAS), 77t
Personality constructs and dispositions, 18–19
Personality development, 114, 492–493. *See also* Developmental factors
Personality Diagnostic Questionnaire (PDQ), 175t, 180, 192
Personality Diagnostic Questionnaire–4 (PDQ-4), 90
Personality Disorder Beliefs Questionnaire (PDBQ), 146
Personality Disorder Examination (PDE), 175t
Personality Disorders and Relational Disorders Work Group, 57
Personality disorders in general, 3–14, 15–20, 648–651. *See also individual disorders*
Personality functioning
  Alternative Model and, 350–352
  assessment and, 355, 378–381
  developmental factors and, 318–319
  historical overview of classification systems and, 50t, 58–59
  integrated approach to characterizing, 373–375
  overview, 26
  *See also* Personality traits
Personality Inventory for DSM-5 (PID-5), 76, 78–79, 78f, 162, 178, 353
Personality Inventory for DSM-IV (PID-IV), 90
Personality Psychopathology Five (PSY-5), 77t, 78, 79, 460
Personality Structure Questionnaire (PSQ), 491–492
Personality traits
  assessment and, 352–354, 355, 385–387, 386t
  in childhood, adolescence, and adulthood, 312t
  cultural factors and, 91–92
  developmental psychopathology model and, 310–314, 320
  historical overview of classification systems and, 50t
  integrated modular treatment and, 669–670
  role of in the development of personality disorders, 317–319
  traits relevant to personality disorders, 314–319
  *See also* Personality functioning; Trait models

Pessimistic anhedonia, 370t, 372t
PET studies. *See* Neuroimaging technologies
Pharmacotherapy
  anticonvulsants, 611–613
  antidepressants, 256, 277–278, 618–619, 622f
  atypical antipsychotics, 613–617
  borderline personality disorder and, 420, 605, 611–624, 619t, 622f
  cognitive analytic therapy (CAT) and, 499–500
  emotion regulation and, 277–278
  integrated modular treatment and, 657f
  neurotransmitter function and, 256, 261
  omega-3 fatty acids and, 617–618, 622f
  overview, 482–483, 611, 620–624, 622f
  psychoeducation and, 605
  research regarding, 619–620, 621
  resources for, 626–628
  trait assessment and, 369–370
  *See also* Treatment
Phenomenology, 35t, 107, 111
Phenotypic features, 230, 235–237, 237f, 238f. *See also* Genetic factors
Phobias, 159, 160
Physical abuse, 219, 305
Physical health, 221–222
Picture Arrangement Test, 284
PID-5 Brief Form (PID-5-BF), 353. *See also* Personality Inventory for DSM-5 (PID-5)
PID-5 Informant Rating Form (PID-5-IRF), 353–354. *See also* Personality Inventory for DSM-5 (PID-5)
Planning, 290, 294–295, 311–312
Porteus Maze Test, 290
Posttraumatic stress disorder (PTSD)
  borderline personality disorder and, 420
  dialectical behavior therapy (DBT) and, 530, 536, 539
  emotion regulation and, 277
  memory bias and, 294
  moral development and, 329
  neurotransmitter function and, 260
Practice-based evidence (PBE), 503–507, 504t
Predisposition/vulnerability model, 158, 158t. *See also* Bivariate models
Prevalence
  antisocial personality disorder and, 450
  childhood adversity and, 305
  early diagnosis and, 221
  obsessive–compulsive personality disorder and, 460–461
  overview, 169–170, 180–186, 181t, 183t, 185t, 186t, 192–193
  *See also* Epidemiology
Prevention, 221–223
Primary traits, 385–387, 386t
Problem solving
  borderline personality disorder and, 290, 294–295
  dialectical behavior therapy (DBT) and, 533–536
  memory bias and, 294
  systems training for emotion predictability and problem solving (STEPPS) and, 590
  violence reduction treatment and, 637

Procedural sequence object relations model (PSORM), 491
Prognosis, 170–171. *See also* Outcomes
Program implementation, 639–640
Progress monitoring, 387–388
Prosocial behavior, 373, 374–375
Proximity seeking, 126, 544–545
Psychiatric syndromes, 155–156, 160–164. *See also* Comorbidity
Psychiatry model, 7–8, 20
Psychic equivalence mode, 129. *See also* Mentalization
Psychoanalytic domain, 28–29, 30, 72, 102–103
Psychodynamic domain, 44, 111, 465–466, 636, 658f
Psychodynamic-interpersonal techniques (PI), 412
Psychoeducation
 dialectical behavior therapy (DBT) and, 533
 goals and contents of, 601–606, 602t
 integrated modular treatment and, 660–661, 667
 overview, 482, 600–601, 607
 peer psychoeducation, 606–607
 resources for, 607t–609t
 schema-focused therapy (SFT) and, 557–558, 563–564
 systems training for emotion predictability and problem solving (STEPPS) and, 587, 594
Psychological mechanisms, 18–19, 96, 319
*Psychopathic Personalities* (Schneider, 1923), 6
Psychopathic Personality Inventory (PPI)
 antisocial personality disorder and, 433–434, 435–436
 overview, 427, 429, 448–449, 448t
 triarchic model and, 430–431
Psychopathic Personality Inventory—Revised (PPI-R), 344–345
Psychopathy
 assessment and, 359, 447–450, 448t, 629
 biological factors and, 160–164
 callous–unemotional (CU) traits and, 324–325, 333
 childhood adversity and, 301–303
 clinical correlates and, 186–189
 cultural factors and, 90–91, 96
 early conceptualizations of personality disorder and, 5
 etiology and, 431–437
 factor hierarchy and, 78f
 historical overview of, 426–427
 inattention to in the medical model, 11
 integrated modular treatment and, 666
 mentalization and, 131, 542, 545–546
 overview, 101–105, 155–156, 417, 426–429, 629–630
 schema-focused therapy (SFT) and, 569
 subdimensions of, 427–429, 437–438
 traits relevant to personality disorders, 314
 transference-focused psychotherapy (TFP) and, 572, 573f
 treatment and, 453–454, 482, 629–641, 635f
 triarchic model, 429–431
 *See also* Antisocial personality disorder (ASPD); Comorbidity; Developmental psychopathology model

Psychopathy Checklist—Revised (PCL-R)
 antisocial personality disorder and, 433–434, 450–451, 453
 callous–unemotional (CU) traits and, 332–333
 overview, 344, 428, 429, 447–448, 448t, 449
 schema-focused therapy (SFT) and, 567
 triarchic model and, 431
 violence reduction treatment and, 633, 634, 641
Psychopathy Checklist—Youth Version (PCL-YV), 448t
Psychosis, 48–49, 246, 259
Psychosocial factors
 course of personality disorders and, 210–211
 historical overview of classification systems and, 51
 obsessive–compulsive personality disorder and, 463
 overview, 8–9, 229, 230–231, 651
 violence reduction treatment and, 637
Psychotherapy, 277–278, 483, 605, 616. *See also* Treatment
Psychoticism
 developmental factors and, 313, 314
 factor hierarchy and, 78f, 79
 neurotransmitter function and, 257
Punitive Parent mode, 561, 562t. *See also* Schema mode
Punitiveness, 535, 559t
Purpose to life, 384

Questionnaires, 342t–343t, 376, 557. *See also* Assessment

Rank-order stability, 206, 314, 320. *See also* Stability of personality disorders
Rapport, 387, 466
Reasoning and rehabilitation (R&R) therapy, 453
Recidivism
 antisocial personality disorder and, 452–454
 schema-focused therapy (SFT) and, 568
 treatment and, 453–454, 630–631, 640–641
Reciprocal role procedure (RRP), 491, 496, 499
Reciprocation, 495f, 536–537
Recognition, 501–502, 559t, 667
Reenactments, 490–491
Reflective mentalizing, 124–125. *See also* Mentalization
Reformulations, 499, 500–501
Regulatory processes
 callous–unemotional (CU) traits and, 330–331
 comorbidity and, 163
 integrated approach and, 381
 integrated modular treatment and, 657f, 659, 660–666
 overview, 648, 649
Reinforcement, 535, 588–589
Rejection, 331, 558, 559t, 603
Relationships
 borderline personality disorder and, 420, 422
 cognitive analytic therapy (CAT) and, 490–491

development of identity and, 117
dialectical behavior therapy (DBT) and, 528
mentalization and, 125–126, 133
multiple self-states model and, 496
obsessive–compulsive personality disorder and, 460, 469
schema-focused therapy (SFT) and, 564
systems training for emotion predictability and problem solving (STEPPS) and, 588, 591
Relaxation techniques, 591, 663
Reliability, 12, 397–398
Remorselessness, 370t, 429, 636
Repeatable Battery for the Assessment of Neuropsychological Status (RBANS), 286
Representations of other people, 143–144
Representations of the self, 103–104, 143–144
Representations of the world, 143–144
Reproducibility Project, 26
Research Domain Criteria (RDoC), 64–65, 155, 163–164, 355, 359
Resiliency, 41–42, 131–132, 302, 446
Response control, 294–295
Response inhibition, 290–291
Response styles, 145f, 148
Responsiveness, 316–317
Restricted emotional expression, 370t, 372t, 460, 672
Revised NEO Personality Inventory (NEO PI-R), 240. *See also* NEO Personality Inventory (NEO PI, NEO PI-R, and NEO-PI-3)
Revision, 501–502
Reward processing, 244, 310
Rigidity
 integrated modular treatment and, 655
 mentalization and, 132, 136, 545
 obsessive–compulsive personality disorder and, 460, 467, 470
 violence reduction treatment and, 636
Risk factors
 borderline personality disorder and, 231
 childhood adversity and, 301–302, 303, 305
 cultural factors and, 94–95
 early intervention and, 221–223
 gene–environment interactions and, 306
 overview, 218–220, 223, 233
 schema-focused therapy (SFT) and, 558
 suicidality and, 470
 violence reduction treatment and, 634–636, 635f
Risk taking, 394–395, 528
Risk–need–responsivity (RNR) framework, 630, 634–635, 640, 641
Robust mentalizing, 134–135. *See also* Mentalization
Role procedures, 116, 117, 493–494, 496
Rorschach test, 283
Ruff Figural Fluency Test, 287
Rule following, 311–312, 429, 467
Ryle, Tony, 489n

SAAB model, 408
SACB model, 408
Sadism, 370t, 372t
Sadistic personality disorder, 35, 54
Sadness, 560

# Subject Index

Safety
  antisocial personality disorder and, 429
  callous–unemotional (CU) traits and, 331
  integrated modular treatment and, 646, 659
  interpersonal reconstructive therapy (IRT) and, 398, 399
Sampling, 42, 203–205, 210
SASB Intrex, 405
Schedule for Affective Disorders and Schizophrenia—Lifetime Version (SADS-L), 175t, 178, 180
Schedule for Interviewing Borderlines (SIB), 178
Schedule for Nonadaptive and Adaptive Personality (SNAP), 75, 77t, 370
Schema mode
  cognitive-behavioral therapy for PDs (CBTpd) and, 514–515, 514f
  interventions and, 565–566
  overview, 104, 143, 567
  schema-focused therapy (SFT) and, 560–561, 562t–563t
  See also Schema-focused therapy (SFT); Schemas
Schema Mode Inventory, 557
Schema therapy. See Schema-focused therapy (SFT)
Schema therapy conceptual model, 566–567
Schema-focused therapy (SFT)
  cognitive-behavioral therapy and, 512, 514
  comparisons among the cognitive therapies and, 520, 521f
  diagnosis, assessment, and formulation and, 557–558
  integrated modular treatment and, 658f
  intervention strategies and methods of, 564–566
  overview, 143, 481–482, 483–484, 525, 555–557, 568–569
  research support for, 566–568
  systems training for emotion predictability and problem solving (STEPPS) and, 587
  theoretical orientations and, 558–564, 559t, 562t–563t
  treatment methods, 522–523
  See also Schemas
Schemas
  cognitive biases and, 144–148
  integrated modular treatment and, 658f, 666, 667–669
  origins and content of, 143–144
  overview, 141–142, 142f, 150, 558, 648, 650–651
  schema activation, 144
  schema avoidance, 560
  systems training for emotion predictability and problem solving (STEPPS) and, 589
  See also Schema mode; Schema-focused therapy (SFT); Self-schemas
Schizoid personality disorder (SPD)
  clinical correlates and, 186, 187, 188, 189
  demographic correlates, 189–191
  epidemiological studies, 178
  future editions of classification systems and, 63–64
  historical overview of classification systems and, 50t, 59–60
  mentalization and, 129
  neurotransmitter function and, 253–254
  overview, 34–35, 417
  parental psychopathology and, 303
  perinatal factors and, 218–219
  prevalence, 180–181, 181t, 182
  theoretical orientations and, 32–33
Schizophrenia
  clinical correlates and, 188
  comorbidity and, 158
  epidemiological studies, 179–180
  future editions of classification systems and, 63–64
  identity diffusion and, 113
  neurotransmitter function and, 258, 259
  obsessive–compulsive personality disorder and, 461
  overview, 104–105
Schizotypal personality disorder (STPD)
  clinical correlates and, 186, 188, 189
  comorbidity and, 158, 159
  epidemiological studies, 178, 179
  five-factor model (FFM) and, 75–76
  future editions of classification systems and, 63–64
  genetic factors and, 240, 246
  historical overview of classification systems and, 50t
  interpersonal reconstructive therapy (IRT) and, 394–395
  neuropsychological mechanisms and, 283
  neurotransmitter function and, 252, 257–259
  parental psychopathology and, 303
  perinatal factors and, 218–219
  prevalence, 181, 181t, 182
  in young people, 221
Schizotypy, 77t
Screening, 198, 499–500
Secure attachment, 127–128, 132–133
Secure base, 400–401
Security, 331, 380–381
Selective serotonin reuptake inhibitor (SSRI), 256, 277–278, 619, 622. See also Antidepressants; Pharmacotherapy
Self
  assessment and, 386t
  cognitive analytic therapy (CAT) and, 492–493
  integrated approach and, 381, 658f, 670–672
  mentalization and, 124, 125f, 129–132
  overview, 648–649
  schema-focused therapy (SFT) and, 559t
  transference-focused psychotherapy (TFP) and, 575
  See also Identity
Self pathology
  assessment and, 382, 383t, 384, 385
  clinical definition of PD and, 375
  diagnosis and assessment and, 338
Self-Aggrandizer mode, 563t
Self-awareness, 109, 661–662
Self-concept
  cultural factors and, 88
  identity diffusion and, 115
  lexical hypothesis and, 42
  mentalization and, 136
  overview, 109–110
  psychopathology and, 101–105
  See also Identity
Self-Concept and Identity Measure (SCIM), 115
Self-control, 316–317, 318–319, 559t
Self-criticism, 467, 561
Self-defeating personality disorder, 54
Self-defeating sadistic personality disorder, 50t
Self-destructive behaviors
  identity diffusion and, 114
  interventions and, 566
  psychoeducation and, 603
  schema mode and, 561
  schema-focused therapy (SFT) and, 564, 566
  transference-focused psychotherapy (TFP) and, 580
Self-directedness, 244, 373, 383t, 384, 394–395
Self-discipline, 559t
Self-disclosure, 536–537, 564
Self-efficacy, 384
Self-esteem
  assessment and, 380–381, 386t
  callous–unemotional (CU) traits and, 325
  cultural factors and, 94
  interpretational bias and, 147
  overview, 649, 651
Self-expression, 672–673
Self-harm
  assessment and, 373, 386t
  borderline personality disorder and, 420, 421–422, 423
  childhood adversity and, 305
  cultural factors and, 90
  dialectical behavior therapy (DBT) and, 528, 528–529
  mentalization and, 136
  neurotransmitter function and, 253, 256–257, 261
  overview, 372t
  pharmacotherapy and, 617
  schema mode and, 561
  schema-focused therapy (SFT) and, 567
  trait assessment and, 369–370, 370t
  See also Nonsuicidal self-injury (NSSI)
Self-identity, 18–19, 575
Self-injurious behavior (SIB), 276. See also Self-harm
Self-knowledge, 101–102, 375, 650, 655
Self-narrative, 110, 117, 649, 671. See also Narratives
Self-observation, 536
Self-orientation, 34–35
Self-perception, 376, 581
Self-referential knowledge, 101, 102, 670–671
Self-reflective thinking, 109–110, 373, 386t, 496, 654–655. See also Mentalization
Self-regulation
  childhood adversity and, 128
  clinical implications, 118–119
  developmental factors and, 217
  developmental psychopathology model and, 317
  identity and, 103, 113

Self-regulation *(cont.)*
  integrated modular treatment and, 646, 655, 657f, 659, 660–666
  overview, 103, 648
  transference-focused psychotherapy (TFP) and, 576, 577
Self-Report Psychopathy Scale-III (SRP-III), 448, 448t
Self-report questionnaires
  assessment and, 380
  identity diffusion and, 115
  overview, 351–353, 373, 376, 389
  psychopathy and, 428
  schema-focused therapy (SFT) and, 557
  stability and change and, 357–3598
  trait assessment and, 370
  *See also* Assessment
Self-representations
  assessment and, 379, 388
  childhood adversity and, 128
  identity diffusion and, 115
  integrated modular treatment and, 670–671
  mentalization and, 131
  transference-focused psychotherapy (TFP) and, 576–577
Self-schemas, 102, 386t, 667. *See also* Schemas
Self-soothing skills, 662–663
Self-states
  cognitive analytic therapy (CAT) and, 492–494, 500–501
  identity diffusion and, 114
  multiple self-states model and, 496
  overview, 104
Self-talk, 663–664
Semistructured interview, 575. *See also* Clinical interviews
Sensation seeking, 370t, 372t, 636
Sensitivity, 316–317, 397–398
Sequential diagrammatic reformulations (SDR)
  cognitive analytic therapy (CAT) and, 490, 492, 493–494, 501
  multiple self-states model and, 495–496, 497, 498f
Serotonin system
  arginine vasopressin (AVP) and, 262
  borderline personality disorder and, 275
  emotion regulation and, 277–278
  genetic factors and, 244, 245–246
  glutamate and, 260–261
  overview, 252–257
  *See also* Neurotransmitter systems
Serotonin-norepinephrine reuptake inhibitors (SNRIs), 619, 621–623, 622f. *See also* Pharmacotherapy
Severity
  assessment and, 382, 383t, 384
  dimensions of, 369
  transference-focused psychotherapy (TFP) and, 573f, 574, 576
  treatment and, 484–485
Severity Indices of Personality Problems (SIPP), 352
Sexual abuse, 116, 219, 304–305, 576
Sexual deviation personality disorder, 50t
Sexuality, 108–109, 112t, 370t, 371t
Shame, 518, 559t, 560
Shyness, 93, 316–317

Single-nucleotide peptide polymorphisms (SNPs), 243, 245–246
Skills training
  dialectical behavior therapy (DBT) and, 527, 529, 533–536
  integrated modular treatment and, 662–663
  systems training for emotion predictability and problem solving (STEPPS) and, 589–591, 593–595
  violence reduction treatment and, 636, 637–638
Sleep problems, 623
Social anxiety, 94–95, 319, 624
Social apprehensiveness, 370t, 372t
Social avoidance, 13–14, 20–21, 370t, 417, 666. *See also* Avoidance
Social factors
  callous–unemotional (CU) traits and, 325, 326–327
  disability and, 356
  genetic factors and, 246
  identity and, 107–108, 111, 113t
  integrated modular treatment and, 658f, 672–673
  isolation and, 559t
  learning and, 124, 135–136
  mentalization and, 131, 135–136
  moral development and, 328–329
  overview, 97, 135, 163, 305–306
  transference-focused psychotherapy (TFP) and, 581
  withdrawal and, 93, 417. *See also* Withdrawal
  *See also* Interpersonal factors
Social phobia, 94, 158, 216
Socialization, 316, 328–329, 330–331, 332
Sociopathic personality disturbance, 50t
Solution analysis, 533, 534
Specificity, 397–398
Spectrum model, 158, 158t. *See also* Bivariate models
Splitting, 114, 587–588, 634
Stability of personality disorders
  assessment and, 357–359
  borderline personality disorder and, 420–421
  cognitive analytic therapy (CAT) and, 494
  developmental psychopathology model and, 320
  longitudinal studies and, 205–208, 207f
  overview, 197, 208–211, 217–218
  traits relevant to personality disorders, 314–315, 316
  *See also* Course of personality disorders
Stages of change, 667. *See also* Change
STAIRWAYS program, 587, 594, 595, 595–596. *See also* Systems training for emotion predictability and problem solving (STEPPS)
Standardized Psychiatric Examination (SPE), 175t
Standards, unrelenting, 559t
State models, 125–126, 130–131
State–Trait Anger Expression Inventory (STAXI), 611–612
State–Trait Anxiety Inventory, 505
STEPPS. *See* Systems training for emotion predictability and problem solving (STEPPS)

Stopping rules, 38–42, 43
Stop-signal tasks, 290–291
Strange Situation, 127–128
Stress, 125f, 126, 244, 259–260, 302–303, 544–545
Stroop task, 276, 287, 290–291, 292
Structural analysis of social behavior (SASB) model
  case formulation and, 396, 397–398
  clinical applications of, 401–403, 402f
  comorbidity and, 408–409, 409t
  diagnosis and, 403, 405–408, 406t–407t
  diagnosis and assessment and, 339
  overview, 32–33, 394n, 399–400, 400f, 413, 414
  predictive principles, 401
  secure base and, 400–401
  structure of, 401
Structural Analysis of Social Behavior—Cyclic Maladaptive Pattern (SASB-CMP), 497
Structural interview, 378–380. *See also* Interviews, clinical
Structural model of psychopathology, 159
Structured clinical interview. *See* Clinical interviews
Structured Clinical Interview for DSM-III-R Personality Disorders (SCID-II), 178, 180
Structured Clinical Interview for DSM-III-R (SCID), 175t, 178
Structured Clinical Interview for DSM-IV Axis II (SCID-II)
  case formulation and, 397
  epidemiological studies, 176–177
  longitudinal studies and, 198
  overview, 354
  structural analysis of social behavior (SASB) model and, 405, 408
  transference-focused psychotherapy (TFP) and, 575
Structured Interview for DSM-III-R Personality Disorders (SIDP), 179, 192, 193, 198, 467
Structured Interview for DSM-III-R Personality Disorders-Revised (SIDP-R), 176
Structured Interview for DSM-IV Personality Disorders (SIDP-IV), 217, 241–242
Structured Interview for Personality Organization (STIPO), 379–380
Structured Interview for Personality Organization—Revised (STIPO-R), 379–380
Structured Interview for Schizotypy (SIS), 175t
Structured Interview of Personality Organization (STIPO), 115, 575
Structured interviews, 115. *See also* Assessment
Submissiveness, 59–60, 370t, 372t, 417, 469
Substance abuse
  antisocial personality disorder and, 433, 450–451
  borderline personality disorder and, 420
  cognitive analytic therapy (CAT) and, 494, 499
  cultural factors and, 90

## Subject Index

dialectical behavior therapy (DBT) and, 528, 538–539
early intervention and, 221–222
identity diffusion and, 114
obsessive–compulsive personality disorder and, 463
overview, 667
psychopathy and, 428
violence reduction treatment and, 636
Suicidality
antisocial personality disorder and, 450
assessment and, 386t
borderline personality disorder and, 274, 422, 423
cognitive-behavioral therapy for PDs (CBTpd) and, 525
cultural factors and, 90
dialectical behavior therapy (DBT) and, 527, 528–529, 538, 539
integrated modular treatment and, 663–664
memory bias and, 294
neurotransmitter function and, 252–254, 256–257, 261–262
obsessive–compulsive personality disorder and, 461–462, 469–470
psychopathy and, 428
schema mode and, 561
transference-focused psychotherapy (TFP) and, 581
Supervision, 529–530
Supportive dynamic therapy, 483–484
Suppression, 273, 665
Surrender, 142–143
Suspiciousness, 370t, 372t
Symptoms
antisocial personality disorder and, 445–446
assessment and, 386t
clinical correlates and, 186–189
cultural factors and, 96
developmental psychopathology model and, 320
disease model and, 4
early intervention and, 221–223
integrated approach and, 381, 657f
medical model and, 19–20
obsessive–compulsive personality disorder and, 459–460
overview, 649
precursor signs and symptoms, 218–220
psychoeducation and, 602t
traits relevant to personality disorders, 314–317
Synthesis, 646, 659, 670–673
Systematic Treatment Selection (STS), 377t, 378, 388
Systems approach, 587, 588–589
Systems training for emotion predictability and problem solving (STEPPS)
case example of, 595–596
components of, 589–591
format of, 591–595
overview, 481–482, 586–587, 597
research support for, 597
theoretical orientations and, 587–588

Taxonomy, 28, 31–35, 35f, 36f. See also Classification systems
Teleological mode, 129. See also Mentalization

Telephone consultation, 529
Temperament
antisocial personality disorder and, 432–433, 434–435
assessment and, 373
developmental factors and, 215–217
genetic factors and, 243–244
overview, 28–29, 30, 65, 311, 513
risk factors and, 219
Temperament and Character Inventory (TCI), 77t
Temporal instability, 72, 73, 112t
Termination, 502
Thematic Apperception Test (TAT), 146, 283
Theoretical integration, 647. See also Integrated treatment approach
Theoretical orientations
cognitive analytic therapy (CAT) and, 492–493
dialectical behavior therapy (DBT) and, 531–533
epistemic choices for structuring, 26–29
inductive-factor-trait models, 35–44, 36f
mentalization-based treatment (MBT) and, 543–544
multiple perspectives, 30–31, 33–35, 35t
overview, 29, 29f, 44–45
schema-focused therapy (SFT) and, 558–564, 559t, 562t–563t
single perspective, 29–30, 31–33
systems training for emotion predictability and problem solving (STEPPS) and, 587–588
taxonomically focused, 31–35, 35t
transference-focused psychotherapy (TFP) and, 575–577
Therapeutic alliance
assessment and, 387
integrated modular treatment and, 652–653, 656
mentalization and, 135, 136
motivation and, 656
obsessive–compulsive personality disorder and, 466
ruptures in, 653
violence reduction treatment and, 633
See also Therapeutic relationship
Therapeutic community (TC) approaches, 636
Therapeutic relationship
cognitive analytic therapy (CAT) and, 490–491, 495f, 502, 503
cognitive-behavioral therapy for PDs (CBTpd) and, 515–516, 520–522
dialectical behavior therapy (DBT) and, 530–531, 537–538
integrated modular treatment and, 652–653, 654, 656
mentalization-based treatment (MBT) and, 546, 549–550
motivation and, 656
schema-focused therapy (SFT) and, 564–565
transference-focused psychotherapy (TFP) and, 578–579
validation and, 654
See also Therapeutic alliance
Therapist ratings, 115. See also Assessment

Therapist stance, 543, 547–548, 578–579, 633–634. See also Clinician factors
Thoughts, 116, 466, 663–664
Threat perceptions, 145–146, 399
Threshold liability model, 236–237, 236f
Tolerance, 662
Tower of Hanoi task, 290
Tower of London task, 289, 290
Trail Making Test—Part B, 287
Trait constellations, 385–387, 386t
Trait models
antisocial personality disorder and, 446–447
assessment and, 337–338, 352–354, 355, 358
callous–unemotional (CU) traits and, 332
comorbidity and, 163
diagnosis and, 337–338
gene–environment interactions and, 306
integrated modular treatment and, 669–670
lexical hypothesis and, 42–43
longitudinal studies and, 198
measures for, 343t
mentalization and, 125–126
obsessive–compulsive personality disorder and, 468–471
overview, 35–44, 36f, 648, 650
See also Personality traits
Trait-dimensional model, 72, 74, 91–92, 369–370. See also Dimensional approaches to classification
Transactional models, 333
Transdiagnostic approach, 232, 539
Transference, 550. See also Transference-focused psychotherapy (TFP)
Transference-focused psychotherapy (TFP)
assessment and, 377t
diagnosis, assessment, and formulation and, 572–575, 573f, 574t
identity and identity diffusion and, 118–119
intervention strategies and methods of, 577–578, 578t
overview, 481–482, 483–484, 485, 571–572
process of, 579–580
research support for, 580–582
schema-focused therapy (SFT) and, 568
theoretical orientations and, 575–577
treatment relationship and, 578–579
Transtheoretical conceptualization, 104, 647
Trauma
callous–unemotional (CU) traits and, 325, 329–330, 331
childhood adversity associated with mental disorders and, 301–303
early experience of, 304–305
mentalization and, 126, 128–129
mentalization-based treatment (MBT) and, 544–545
neurotransmitter function and, 260, 263
overview, 232–233
schema-focused therapy (SFT) and, 558
Treatment
antisocial personality disorder and, 453–454
assessment and, 377–378, 377t, 386t, 387–388

Treatment *(cont.)*
  borderline personality disorder and, 422, 604–605, 621–624
  callous–unemotional (CU) traits and, 331–332
  childhood adversity and, 306
  clinical implications, 423
  cognitive theories and, 149–150
  comorbidity and, 163
  cultural factors and, 97
  diagnosis and, 21, 220–221, 337
  early intervention and, 221–223
  emotion regulation and, 277–278
  empirically based treatments, 481–485
  identity diffusion and, 116, 118–119
  integrated approach and, 381–387, 383*t*, 386*t*, 651
  interpersonal reconstructive therapy (IRT) and, 409–413, 411*f*
  mentalization and, 133–136
  neurotransmitter function and, 261
  obsessive–compulsive personality disorder and, 465–467, 471–472
  overview, 648
  psychoeducation and, 604–605
  psychopathy and, 453–454
  self-development and, 651
  violence and, 629–641, 635*f*
  *See also* Interventions; Pharmacotherapy; *individual treatment approaches*
Treatment planning, 367, 376, 381, 574
Treatment-resistant depression, 528, 539. *See also* Depression
Treatment-resistant PD, 339
Triarchic model, 429–431, 437, 438, 446–447, 451
Triarchic Psychopathy Measure (TriPM), 448*t*, 449, 452
Tridimensional model, 251–252
Tridimensional Personality Questionnaire (TPQ), 243–244

TriPM, 430–431, 433–434
Trust, 103–104, 327, 373, 545, 587
Twin studies
  antisocial personality disorder and, 436–437
  callous–unemotional (CU) traits and, 327
  childhood adversity and, 306
  identifying putative genes, 243
  obsessive–compulsive personality disorder and, 464
  overview, 238–243
  traits relevant to personality disorders, 315–316
  *See also* Family factors; Genetic factors

Uncertainty, 103–104

Validation, 533, 550–551, 558, 654
Values, 97, 108–109
Venturesomeness, 446
Verbal abuse, 219
Verbal episodic memory, 285–286. *See also* Memory processes
Violence
  antisocial personality disorder and, 452–453
  neurotransmitter function and, 253–254, 259–260
  overview, 629
  treatment and, 629–641, 635*f*
  *See also* Aggression; Antisocial behaviors; Violence reduction treatment
Violence Inhibition Mechanism (VIM), 329
Violence reduction treatment
  outcome evidence and, 640–641
  overview, 630–631, 641
  psychopathy and, 631–638, 635*f*
  treatment delivery, 638–640
  *See also* Treatment; Violence

Violence Risk Scale (VRS), 634–636, 635*f*, 640–641
Visual episodic memory, 286. *See also* Memory processes
Visual probe tasks, 292–293
Vocational aspirations, 108–109
VRS—Sexual Offender version (VRS-SO), 640–641
Vulnerabilities, 301–302, 559*t*, 566. *See also* Risk factors

Wakefulness, 259
Web-based treatment, 607
Wechsler Adult Intelligence Test—Revised (WAIS-R), 283–284, 285
Wechsler Memory Scale (WMS), 285–286
Weekly diary cards. *See* Diary cards
Wide Range Achievement Test, 285
Wideband Cross-Language Six (WCL6), 41–42, 44
Wisconsin Card Sorting Task (WCST), 259, 286–287
Wisconsin Personality Disorders Inventory (WISPI), 403, 405, 408, 413
Withdrawal, 79, 93, 417
WMS Logical Memory Test, 285–286
Working alliance. *See* Therapeutic alliance
Working memory, 259, 273. *See also* Memory processes

Young Parenting Inventory, 557
Young Schema Questionnaire, 515
Youth Psychopathic Traits Inventory (YPI), 240, 427, 430–431, 448*t*, 450
Youth Self-Report (YSR), 92

Zanarini Rating Scale for Borderline Personality Disorder (ZAN-BPD), 288
Zen, 531, 532
Zone of proximal development (ZPD), 494, 501–502